MEDICAL RADIOLOGY

Diagnostic Imaging and Radiation Oncology

Springer
Berlin
Heidelberg
New York
Barcelona
Hong Kong
London
Milan
Paris
Singapore
Tokyo

C. Bartolozzi · R. Lencioni (Eds.)

Liver Malignancies

Diagnostic and Interventional Radiology

With Contributions by

C. Bartolozzi · C. D. Becker · G. Bevilacqua · L. Bolondi · C. Bru · J. Bruix · F. Burresi
E. Buscarini · L. Buscarini · P. Busilacchi · M. A. Caligo · D. Campani · V. Cantisani
D. Caramella · R. Caudana · A. Cicorelli · D. Cioni · C. Colagrande · M. Coniglio · P. F. Conte
A. R. Cotroneo · L. Cova · L. Crocetti · A. M. De Gaetano · M. Dellanoce · G. Di Candio
A. Di Filippo · M. Di Giulio · F. Donati · I. Esposito · A. Falcone · C. Fava · F. S. Ferrari · R. Foroni
G. Galletti · F. Garbagnati · G. S. Gazelle · A. Giovagnoni · S. N. Goldberg · G. Granai
W. F. Grigioni · M. Grosso · R. Hammerstingl · N. Howarth · T. Ierace · R. Kayal · C. Lattes
R. Lencioni · D. A. Leung · E. Lezoche · T. Livraghi · G. Lucigrai · R. Manfredi · P. Marano
G. Maresca · B. Marincek · L. Masi · F. Maspes · Y. Menu · G. Morana · M. Moretti · F. Mosca
E. Neri · M. Oddone · A. Paganini · A. Paolicchi · T. Pfammatter · E. Pfanner · A. Pietrabissa
P. Pini · G. F. Pistolesi · G. Pizzi · M. Pocek · S. Pochon · G. Poggianti · G. L. Rapaccini
R. D. Redvanly · P. Ricci · A. Roche · S. Rossi · R. Roversi · G. Serafini · G. Simonetti · L. Solbiati
P. Stefani · E. Squillaci · F. Terrier · P. Tomà · M. Vaccari · G. Valeri · J. P. Vallée · A. Vecchioli
A. Veltri · T. J. Vogl

Series Editor's Foreword by

A. L. Baert

With 391 Figures in 977 Separate Illustrations, 66 in Color

Springer

C. Bartolozzi, MD, Professor and Chairman
R. Lencioni, MD
Division of Diagnostic and Interventional Radiology
Department of Oncology
University of Pisa
Via Roma 67
I-56125 Pisa
Italy

MEDICAL RADIOLOGY · Diagnostic Imaging and Radiation Oncology

Continuation of
Handbuch der medizinischen Radiologie
Encyclopedia of Medical Radiology

ISBN 3-540-64756-2 Springer-Verlag Berlin Heidelberg New York

Library of Congress Cataloging-in-Publication Data. Liver malignancies: diagnostic and interventional radiology / C. Bartolozzi ; R. Lencioni (eds.); with contributions by C. Bartolozzi ... [et al.] p. cm. -- (Medical radiology) Includes bibliographical references and index. ISBN 3-540-64756-2 (alk. paper) 1. Liver--Cancer--Imaging 2. Liver metastasies--Imaging. 3. Liver--Cancer--Interventional radiology. I. Bartolozzi, C. (Carlo), 1947- . II. Lencioni, R. (Riccardo), 1961- . III. Series [DNLM: 1. Liver Neoplasms--diagnosis. 2. Liver Neoplasms--therapy. 3. Diagnostic Imaging. 4. Radiology, Interventional--methods. WI 735 L784 1999] RC280.L5L5835.1999 616.99'436--dc21 DNLM/DLC for Library of Congress 99-23562 CIP

Printed in Germany

Typesetting: Verlagsservice Teichmann, Mauer

SPIN: 106 747 46 21/3135 – 5 4 3 2 1 0 – Printed on acid-free paper

Foreword

The detection and characterization of focal liver lesions remains a major challenge for every radiologist. It is of paramount importance to differentiate benign focal liver lesions – some of which, such as cysts and cavernous hemangioma, are quite common – from malignant tumors.

During the past decade enormous progress has been achieved in the differential diagnosis between benign and malignant liver tumors, mainly due to the improvements in Doppler and color ultrasonography, spiral CT and MRI. During the same period several non-surgical, percutaneous radiological techniques, such as transcatheter embolization, percutaneous ethanol ablation, percutaneous radiofrequency thermal ablation and interstitial laser photocoagulation and cryotherapy, have been developed. Relatively broad experience of the value of these methods for the treatment of primary and secondary liver malignancies has accumulated in several radiological centers, mainly in Europe and Japan. The Department of Radiology of the University of Pisa, under the chairmanship of Prof. C. Bartolozzi, has made important contributions in this field.

I am very grateful to Prof. Bartolozzi for accepting my invitation to edit this volume in our series Medical Radiology, together with his co-worker of many years, Dr. R. Lencioni. They have been able to ensure the collaboration of many outstanding specialists to this book, which provides up-to-date information on the radiological diagnosis and treatment of liver malignancies. I am convinced that radiologists, gastroenterologists and abdominal surgeons will find it a very useful source of information and that it will be well received by our colleagues. We would, however, welcome any constructive criticism.

Leuven — Albert L. Baert

Preface

In recent times, few fields in medicine have witnessed such impressive progress as the diagnosis and treatment of primary and secondary liver malignancies. The growing interest in this field is due on one hand to the increasing incidence of neoplastic diseases of the liver in many countries of the world and on the other to the development of new technologies, which have been successfully applied both to the diagnostic tools and to the therapeutic methods. Nowadays, in fact, it is possible to detect small neoplastic lesions of the liver at an early, preclinical stage and to reliably characterize them – both of which are prerequisites for planning an effective and radical therapeutic approach.

This book, written by leading experts worldwide, provides a comprehensive and up-to-date overview of the role of diagnostic and interventional radiology in respect of liver malignancies. Background chapters discuss anatomy, epidemiology, and clinicopathologic features of liver tumors: in this section, special attention is dedicated to new concepts in hepatocarcinogenesis and current nosological classification of diseases. Next, imaging features of primary and secondary tumors of the liver, including rare malignancies, are presented. Each of the diagnostic imaging techniques is carefully discussed and appraised, focusing on new developments in equipment and contrast agents. A large portion of the volume is dedicated to the interventional therapeutic approach to hepatic malignancies: full consideration, in particular, is given to newer sophisticated techniques of liver tumor ablation, which have rapidly become a viable alternative to surgery in many instances. The last part of the volume is dedicated to specific aspects of the general subject of liver malignancies, in order to provide a comprehensive perspective.

We hope that the book will fulfill the expectations of all our colleagues who are interested in this very important field.

Finally, we would like to express our deep appreciation to the Editor-in-Chief of the Medical Radiology series, Prof. Albert Baert, who gave us the opportunity to publish this volume in such a prestigious book series and provided us with continuous suggestions and support. We would also like to thank most sincerely all the authors for having spent so much time and effort in preparing truly outstanding contributions.

Pisa

C. Bartolozzi
R. Lencioni

Contents

Liver Metastases

Hepatocellular Carcinoma

Liver Metastases

I Introduction

1 Segmental Anatomy of the Liver

Y. Menu and R. Lencioni

CONTENTS

1.1 Introduction

The liver is the largest organ in the body. It occupies much of the right hypochondrial region of abdomen. Its left lobe extends across the epigastrium and projects a variable distance into the left hypochondrium. The liver has two major surfaces, a superior or diaphragmatic surface and an inferior or visceral surface. They are separated anteriorly and laterally by a sharply angled inferior margin. The diaphragmatic surface is highly convex, since it is molded by the inferior aspects of the diaphragm.

The liver can be subdivided in two different ways, an external lobation and segmentation (Friedman and Dachman 1994). The classical anatomic subdivision into four externally defined lobes is based on an approximately H-shaped or K-shaped series of indentations on the visceral surface of the liver. In contrast, the internal lobation and segmentation of the liver are based on the branching pattern of the portal vein, proper hepatic artery, and hepatic ducts, with the major hepatic veins occupying and helping to demarcate the planes between the lobes and segments.

Y. Menu, MD; Professor and Chairman, Department of Radiology, Hôpital Beaujon, 100 Bd. du Général Leclerc, F-92118 Clichy, France
R. Lencioni, MD; Division of Diagnostic and Interventional Radiology, Department of Oncology, University of Pisa, Via Roma 67, I-56125 Pisa, Italy

1.2 External Lobation

The H-shaped indentations on the visceral faces of the liver divide it into four externally defined lobes: the right, left, quadrate and caudate lobes. The right-hand limb of the H is formed by the fossa for gallbladder anteriorly and by a deep sulcus for the inferior vena cava posteriorly. The gallbladder fossa separates the anterior part of the externally defined right lobe from the quadrate lobe. The sulcus for the inferior vena cava separates the posterior portion of the right lobe from the caudate lobe. Between the gallbladder fossa and the sulcus for the inferior vena cava the right limb of the H is deficient where a caudate process connects the caudate lobe to the right lobe. On axial images the caudate process is insinuated between the portal vein and inferior vena cava. The left limb of the H is formed by two deep fissures that contain true ligaments in their depths. Anteriorly it is formed by the deep fissure for the ligamentum teres, which separates the anterior part of the externally defined left lobe from the quadrate lobe. Posteriorly it is formed by the fissure for the ligamentum venosum, which separates the posterior part of the left lobe (Friedman and Dachman 1994).

The ligamentum teres is the obliterated embryonic umbilical vein, while the ligamentum venosum is the obliterated embryonic ductus venosus. In the embryo these veins are continuous at their attachment to the left branch of the portal vein. The fissure for the ligamentum teres can be so deep that the left lobe of the liver often appears to be completely separate from the rest of the liver. Similarly, the depth of the fissure for the ligamentum venosum can cause the bulbous anteroinferior part of the caudate lobe (papillary process) to appear to be separate from the rest of the liver, so that it may be mistaken for an extrahepatic mass (Donosa et al. 1989). The porta of the liver forms the crossbar of the H and separates the quadrate from the caudate lobes.

An appreciation of the inferior slope of the liver from its posterior to its anterior aspect allows one to understand why in high-level axial sections the posteriorly situated caudate lobe separates the externally defined left lobe anteriorly and to the left from the externally defined right lobe posteriorly and to the right (Friedman and Dachman 1994). The caudate lobe is called caudate because of its appearance as a short, stubby tail, and not because of its caudal location, since it is one of the most cranially situated parts of the liver. In intermediate-level axial sections the porta and caudate process separate the right and left lobes.

1.3 Segmental Anatomy of the Liver

Segmental anatomy is crucial in order to precisely localize a focal lesion, to evaluate the possibility of a resection, find the adequate technique for resection, and finally to estimate the easiness or the difficulties of a biopsy or of any other percutaneous procedure. Segmental anatomy is the basis of modern hepatic surgery. Each segment, in fact, is supplied by a sheath containing branches of the hepatic artery and portal vein and a draining bile duct, which enters the middle of the segment. The venous drainage is by hepatic vein, which tends to run between segmental divisions (Couinaud 1957; Healy and Schroy 1953; Healy 1970; Michels 1996; Goldsmith and Woodburne 1957; Bismuth et al. 1988).

The hepatic veins are the main guides to liver segmental anatomy. The middle hepatic vein separates right and left liver, which is different from the left and right lobes. Two other anatomical landmarks also achieve separation between right and left liver: the left aspect of the inferior vena cava and the gallbladder (more precisely the gallbladder fossa). These three landmarks give the orientation of an oblique and slightly curved plane, which is very easy to delineate with real time ultrasound (US). This examination is probably the most accurate to precisely localize a focal lesion which would be located in the neighborhood of the separation between right and left liver (Fig. 1.1). Excepting the gallbladder fossa, there is no external landmark to localize the separation.

The right hepatic vein separates the anterior sector (between the middle and right hepatic veins) and the posterior sector (between the right hepatic vein and the posterior aspect of the right lobe). The left hepatic vein separates the left medial sector (between the left and the middle hepatic veins) and the left lateral sector (on the left of the left hepatic vein). The caudate lobe is limited by the portal trunk, the inferior vena cava (posteriorly), and the three hepatic veins (superiorly).

Right and left liver is not similar to right and left lobe. The separation between the right lobe and the left lobe is the transverse ligament, with a recognizable external fissure on the liver surface. It is clear that the right lobe is larger than the right liver, as it includes both the right liver and the left medial sector. The left lobe is smaller than the left liver as it does not include the left medial sector. Left lobe and left lateral sector are therefore two names for the same part of the liver.

1.3.1 Hepatic Segments

Sectorial anatomy, guided by the hepatic vein anatomy, is important, but it may be not sufficient to localize a lesion, and to understand localized liver resection. The basis of functional anatomy of the liver is the segment, which corresponds to the amount of liver parenchyma fed by a segmental portal vein.

1.3.1.1 Left Liver (Segments II, III, and IV)

The left portal vein divides into three branches: lateral posterior, lateral anterior and medial. The lateral posterior runs in the posterior part of the left lateral sector, and feeds half of it, also called segment II. The lateral anterior runs along the anterior part of the left lateral sector and feeds the other half, called segment III. The medial branch feeds the entire left medial sector, also called segment IV.

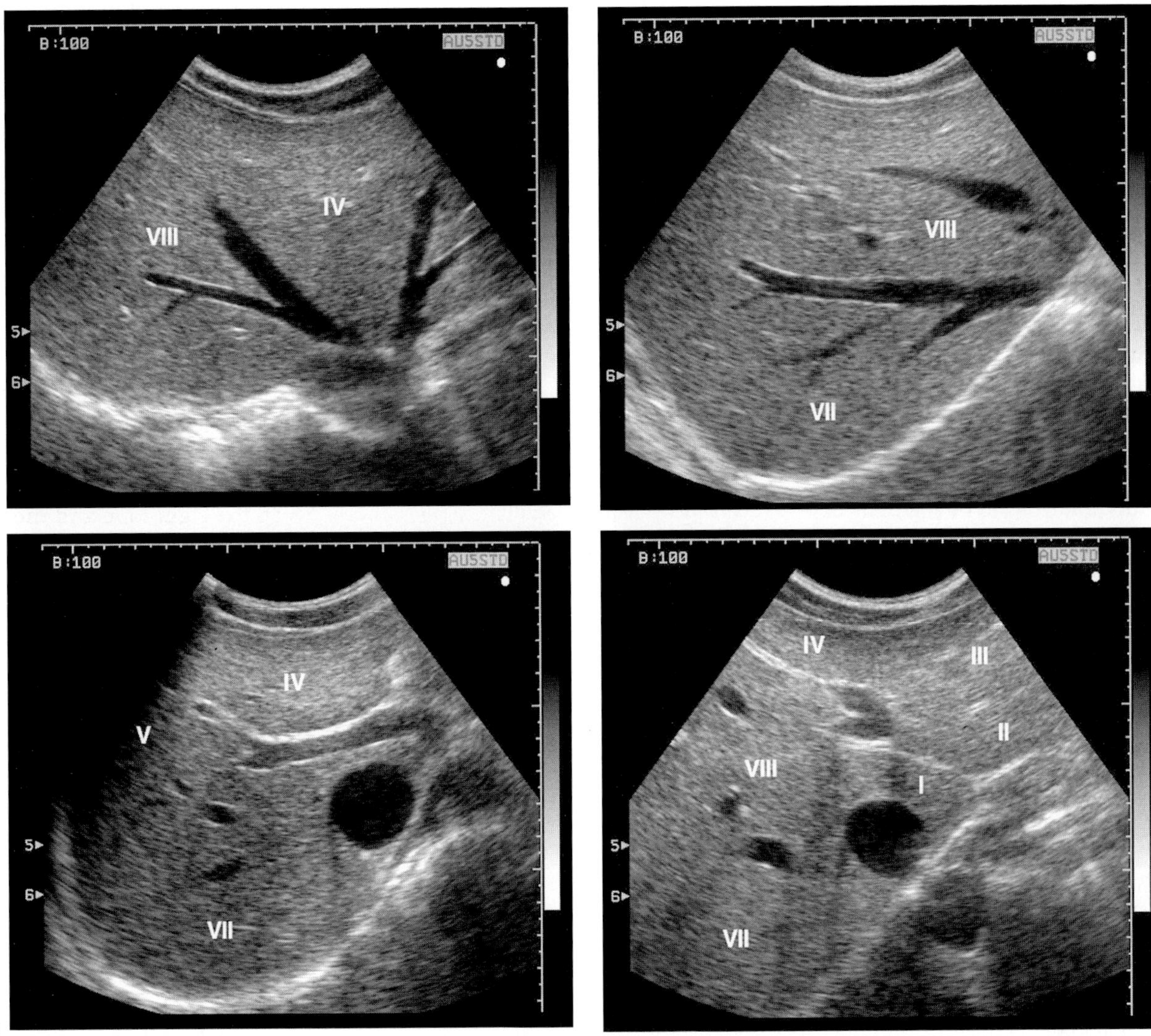

Fig. 1.1a–d. Segmental anatomy of the liver. US images showing **a** confluence of left and middle hepatic veins with identification of segments IV and VIII; **b** confluence of middle and right hepatic veins, with demonstration of segments VII and VIII; bifurcation of portal vein with segments IV, V, and VII; and inferior vena cava and left portal vein with evidence of segments I, II, III, IV, VII, and VIII

1.3.1.2
Right Liver (Segments V, VI, VII, and VIII)

The right portal vein divides into two branches, one anterior (for the right anterior sector) and one posterior (for the right posterior sector). The anterior branch divides into a superior branch, for the segment VIII, and inferior branch, for the segment V. Segment VIII is localized between the middle hepatic vein (left), the right hepatic vein (right), and the inferior vena cava (superior and posterior). It lies over the segment V. Segment V is localized between the middle hepatic vein and the gallbladder fossa (left), the right hepatic vein (right), and the surface of the liver (inferior and anterior). It lies under the segment VIII. Segment V does not reach the inferior vena cava. The posterior branch divides into a superior branch, for the segment VII, and inferior branch, for the segment VI. Segment VII is localized behind the right hepatic vein (right), and the inferior vena cava medial. It lies over the segment VI, and is hidden by the segment VIII when looking at the liver from the front. Segment VI is localized behind the right hepatic vein (right) and the surface of the liver (inferior and anterior). It lies under segment VII. Segment VI does not reach the inferior vena cava, but is usually located in front of the right kidney.

1.3.1.3 Segment I

Segment I is not fed by a single portal vein, and drains through multiple short hepatic veins to the inferior vena cava. Segment I is located between the portal trunk (anterior), the inferior vena cava (posterior), the liver surface (left), and is in complete continuity with segment VII on its right side.

1.3.1.4 Segment IX

Individualization of segment IX is a recent proposal from the major author of modern liver segmentation (COUINAUD 1998). This segment would be located in the right liver, in close relationship with the inferior vena cava. Segment IX is in close contact with the right aspect of the vena cava, rather symmetrical to segment I on the left side. Segment IX separates the segment VII from the vena cava, excepting the entrance of the right hepatic vein in the vena cava. Segment IX lies under the plane of the hepatic veins and extends from the posterior aspect of the liver posteriorly to segment I medially. No clear landmarks are available to delineate the anterior limits of segment IX and segments VII and VIII. Individualization of segment IX relies on the fact that many small portal branches arise from the portal arch. Branches arising from the left portal vein may feed some parts of segment IX. Also, as segment I, segment IX is drained by small hepatic veins entering either the caval axis directly, or the major hepatic veins. Segment IX and segment I together are the "dorsal sector," which is different from right and left liver. Individualization of dorsal sector may be important in understanding bleeding problems in resection or split liver transplantation.

1.3.2 Liver Resections

The terminology of different surgical procedures for resection of a focal process is as follows: left lobectomy is a resection of the left lateral sector (i.e., left lobe, or segments II and III); left hepatectomy is a resection of left lobe and segment I; right hepatectomy is the resection of segments V to VIII (and IX?); right lobectomy, also called trisegmentectomy, is the right hepatectomy associated with the resection of segment IV. Wedge resection and atypical resections try to make a resection with margins over 1 cm out of the tumor, but sparing liver parenchyma.

In a cirrhotic patient, only limited resections are possible, due to expected liver insufficiency. It is therefore crucial to define exactly the location of a neoplasm, for the most economic resection, or to decide an alternate treatment like percutaneous ablation.

1.4 Hepatic Vessels

1.4.1 Hepatic Artery

The origin and course of the hepatic artery can vary from person to person. Aberrant hepatic arteries are seen in up to 30–40% of individuals. Arteries within the liver travel with the portal vein radicles, which are normally larger. Within the porta hepatis, the hepatic artery may be seen anterior and slightly medial to the main portal vein, whereas the common hepatic duct is generally anterior and slightly lateral to the portal vein.

1.4.2 Portal Vein

As the portal vein approaches the liver, it is directed superiorly and to the right. The right portal vein appears to continue the course of the main portal vein but angles somewhat more to the right, forming a large obtuse angle with the main portal vein. The right portal vein varies from 0 to 3 cm in length before dividing into anterior and posterior segmental branches (PAGANI 1983). On axial sections the right portal vein is often directed somewhat posteriorly as well as to the right, because the right lobe is a relatively posteriorly situated lobe. The anterior segmental branch of the right portal vein courses to the right, superiorly and slightly anteriorly. The posterior segmental branch courses almost directly posteriorly. Hence, in anterior view or an anteroposterior (AP) portogram, it is seen end on (TAKAYASU et al. 1985). Both the anterior and posterior segmental veins give off a number of superiorly and inferiorly directed branches that supply their superior and inferior subsegments or areas (Fig. 1.2).

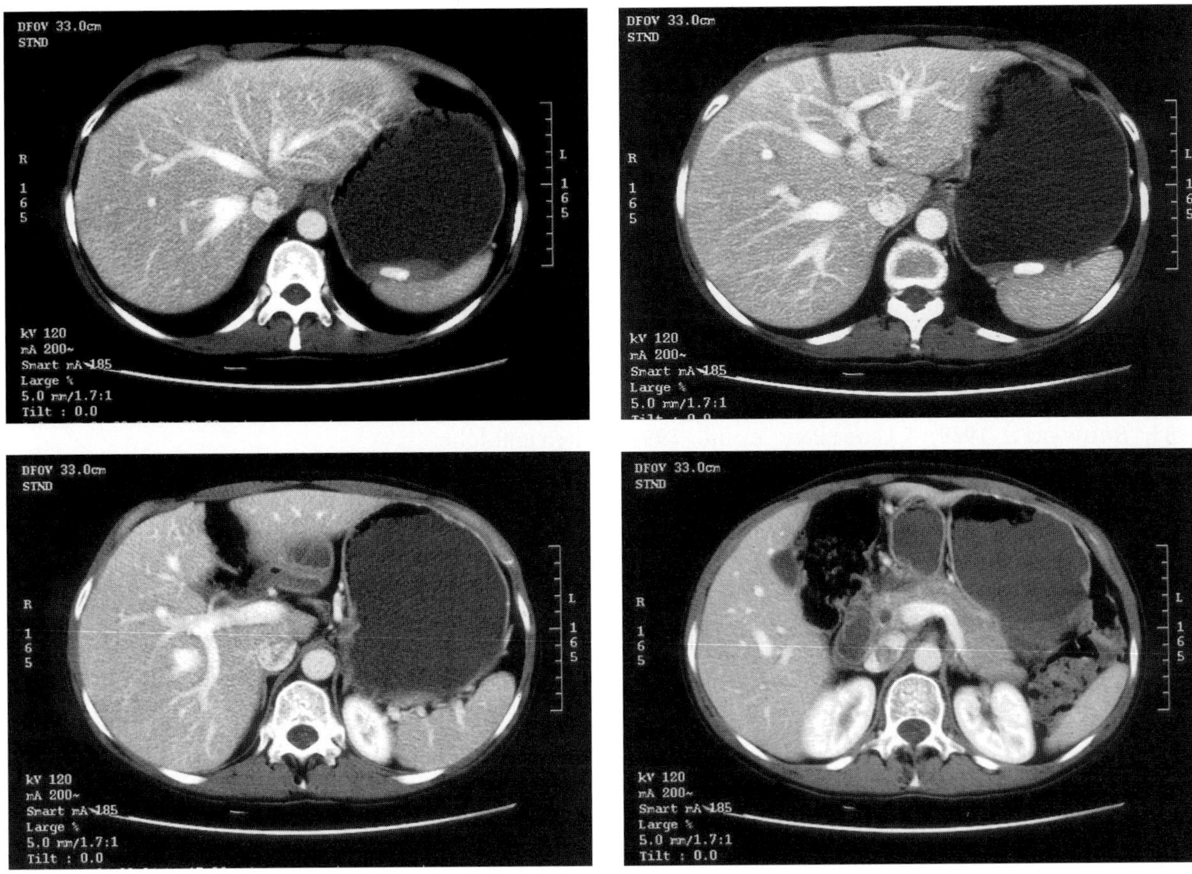

Fig. 1.2a–d. Cross-sectional imaging anatomy of the liver. Spiral CT images after intravenous injection of contrast material and hydric repletion of the digestive tract. Image through the superior aspect of the liver shows the right, middle, and left hepatic veins (**a**). Images caudal to **a** show left (**b**) and right (**c**) branches of the portal vein. Relationship with digestive tract is well depicted in **d**

The left portal vein arises from the main portal vein at a more acute angle than the right portal vein and courses to the left and forward for about 3–4 cm in what is called its transverse segment (Pagani 1983). It then turns directly forward in the depths of the fissure for the ligamentum venosum (umbilical fissure), in what is its umbilical segment. The umbilical segment ends blindly in the ligamentum teres. The umbilical segment of the left portal vein and the ligamentum teres are both surrounded by fat derived from the fat within the falciform ligament. Since in the average liver the umbilical segment of the left portal vein courses relatively directly forwards; it is seen end on in an anterior view or AP portogram.

The left portal vein gives off a number of what are typically called medial segmental branches into the quadrate lobe territory and a number of what are usually called lateral segmental branches into the area defined externally as the left lobe of the liver. Hence the medial segment of the internally defined left lobe includes the externally defined quadrate lobe and all of the liver volume directly above, where the quadrate lobe projects into the visceral. The lateral segment of left lobe of the liver is synonymous with the externally defined left lobe of the liver. However, the segmental terminology of the internally defined left lobe is somewhat confusing, since in the average-size liver the externally defined left lobe of the liver is typically in the midsagittal plane of the body while the quadrate lobe is to the right of the midsagittal plane. Therefore in most livers the internally named lateral segmental is actually medial to the more laterally located medial segment (Friedman and Dachman 1994). Both the medial and lateral segmental veins give off superiorly and inferiorly directed branches to supply superior and inferior subsegments or areas of these subsegments.

The caudate lobe of the liver is supplied by branches that arise from the proximal parts of both the right and left portal veins. Hence it is said to be split between right and left lobes of the liver.

1.4.3 Hepatic Veins

There are three major hepatic veins, which for part or all of their course run in the planes that separate each of the four major liver segments (Goldsmith and Woodburne 1957; Bismuth et al. 1988; Pagani 1983; Schwartz 1989; Lafortune et al. 1991; Nakamura and Tsuzuki 1981). In the proximal part of their course, near their termination in the inferior vena cava, the right, middle, and left hepatic veins have a relatively horizontal course (Fig. 1.2). Here they are visualized coursing relatively longitudinally in high-level axial sections and images. As they course distally, they gradually turn inferiorly to assume a more vertical course. Therefore in lower level axial sections and images the hepatic veins are cut more in cross section. In three dimensions, the hepatic veins are therefore oriented much like the staves of an open umbrella (Friedman and Dachman 1994).

In high-level axial images the left hepatic veins project almost directly forward relative to the inferior vena cava, and course temporarily in the intersegmental plane between the medial and lateral segments of the left lobe before entering the lateral segment, which they exclusively drain. They also usually receive a few tributaries from the upper portion of the medial segment. In high-level axial sections the middle hepatic vein courses to the right and anteriorly at an angle of 30–60° from the midsagittal or coronal planes. It enters the interlobar plane between the medial segment of the left lobe and the anterior segment of the right lobe. In this position it lies above and approximately parallel to the long axis of the gallbladder. The middle hepatic vein drains most of both the medial segment of the left lobe and the anterior segment of the left lobe. In about 85% of cases the middle hepatic vein joins the left hepatic vein just before the latter reaches the inferior vena cava (Nakamura and Tsuzuki 1981). In the other 15% of cases the middle hepatic vein empties independently into the inferior vena cava. In high-level axial sections and images the right hepatic vein typically courses to the right and slightly posteriorly to enter the intersegmental plane between the anterior and posterior segments of the right lobe. As it descends vertically, it runs in the interval between the bifurcation of the right portal vein into its anterior and posterior segmental branches. Therefore, in axial sections near the level of the liver porta, the transversely running right portal vein and its anterior and posterior segmental branches have a Y configuration, and the right hepatic vein is seen in cross section between the limbs of the Y.

A line constructed from the right hepatic vein to the point of bifurcation of the portal vein locates the intersegmental plane of the right lobe of the liver. The right hepatic vein drains the posterior segment and a small upper portion of the anterior segment of the right lobe.

In addition to receiving the main hepatic veins, the inferior vena cava also receives a highly variable number of smaller dorsal hepatic veins that typically enter the inferior vena cava at lower levels than the main hepatic veins. The number of significant dorsal hepatic veins can range from 3 to 14 (Nakamura and Tsuzuki 1981). These veins most commonly drain the posterior segment of the right lobe and the caudate lobe, which are the liver areas that are directly around the inferior vena cava.

1.4.4 Normal Variants

Major normal variants should be known as they may interfere with liver surgery. Liver resection and living related hepatic transplantation require an adequate evaluation of the precise anatomy of major vessels.

A large right inferior hepatic vein, draining segment VI is found in 15–20% of normal subjects. When a right inferior hepatic vein is present, the right hepatic vein is usually smaller, as it does not drain segment VI. In some cases, the right hepatic vein is absent, or limited to a very small vessel, when a large inferior right hepatic vein is associated with a predominant middle hepatic vein. There is a balance in territories drained by each hepatic vein. For surgical purposes, evaluation of the approximate territory drained by each hepatic vein is interesting, especially in order to prevent intraoperative bleeding.

Portal vein variants occur in 20% of cases. In most instances, the portal bifurcation is located higher than usual, and may be strictly intrahepatic, which may represent a surgical problem, when ligation of the right or left portal vein is required. The most usual abnormality is the left portal vein arising from the right portal vein or from the anterior branch or the right portal vein. Rarely, the right portal vein arises from the intrahepatic left portal vein; usually, the anterior branch of the right portal vein arises from the segment IV branch of the left portal vein.

1.5 Peritoneal Relationship of the Liver

The liver has some unique peritoneal and mesenteric relationships, which cause the upper portion of the greater peritoneal sac to be subdivided into four perihepatic recesses or spaces. The falciform ligament attaches anteriorly to the midline of the anterior abdominal wall above the umbilicus, and also to the diaphragm. From this point it extends upward and to the right, as a broad mesenteric sheet with a curved lower free border, to attach to the anterior portion of the superior or diaphragmatic surface of the liver. The falciform ligament is not a true ligament in the sense of being formed by dense, regularly arranged connective tissue. It is a mesentery made up of the two layers of visceral peritoneum separated by some loose connective tissue containing a variable amount of fat. However, within the lower, curved free margin of the falciform ligament there is a true ligament, the ligamentum teres, which as the obliterated embryonic umbilical vein begins below, at the umbilicus. At the inferior margin of the liver the ligamentum teres passes onto the visceral surface of the liver, where it occupies the deep fissure for the ligamentum teres and eventually becomes continuous with the left portal vein. The rest of the falciform ligament attaches to the diaphragmatic surface of the liver along a parasagittal plane situated to the right of the midline of the body. As the falciform ligament reaches the posterosuperior aspect of the liver, its right and left peritoneal leaves split apart like a T, to depart from the parasagittal plane and enter a nearly coronal plane where they form the right and left sides of the anterior or superior layer of the coronary ligament. Near the right and left borders of the liver, the anterior layer of the coronary ligament doubles acutely back on itself to form the respective right and left triangular ligaments, and then becomes the posterior or inferior layer of the coronary ligament. Between the anterior and posterior layers of the coronary ligament the liver is not peritonealized and therefore lies in direct contact with the diaphragm as the bare area of the liver.

The falciform and coronary ligaments delimit four important recesses or spaces of the greater peritoneal cavity around the liver. These are best visualized in sagittal sections. Between the liver and the diaphragm are two subphrenic or suprahepatic recesses that are separated from each other by the falciform ligament. The right subphrenic or suprahepatic recess or space is bounded superiorly and anteriorly by the diaphragm, inferiorly by the liver, posteriorly by the left side of the anterior layer of the coronary ligament, and on the right by the falciform ligament.

The coronary ligament helps to define two subhepatic recesses or spaces beneath the liver. The right subhepatic space is also known as the hepatorenal pouch of Morrison or Morrison's pouch. It is bounded superiorly by the posterior (inferior) layer of the coronary ligament, anteriosuperiorly by the right lobe of the liver, posteriorly by the diaphgram, and posteroinferiorly by the right kidney. When the patient is lying supine, as in the case for most imaging procedures, Morrison's pouch is the most gravitationally dependent area of the abdominal portion of the greater peritoneal sac. Hence it is the most frequent site of accumulation of ascitic or infectious fluids, which when the patient is supine tend to ascend the right lateral paracolic gutter to puddle in this recess.

The left subhepatic recess or space is also known as the hepatogastric space or pouch. It is bounded anterosuperiorly by the coronary ligament and the left lobe of the liver and posteroinferiorly by the stomach and lesser omentum. The two layers of the left side of the coronary ligament are in apposition at this point, so that there is no intervening bare area.

All of these perihepatic spaces assume a relatively gravitationally dependent position when the patient is in the supine position. Hence they can all puddle ascites or abscess fluid, with Morrison's pouch being most gravitationally dependent and also most likely to intercept fluid flowing superiorly in the right lateral paracolic gutter. The left subhepatic space is the least likely to puddle fluids, since it is relatively anteriorly located and has no right or left bounding structures unless there are adhesions. Hence, fluids accumulating in this recess tend to flow to the right, into Morrison's pouch, or to the left, into the more gravitationally dependent perisplenic spaces.

The caudate lobe of the liver has a relationship to the omental bursal (lesser peritoneal) sac. It is attached to the diaphragm above by the bare area of the liver. Inferiorly it protrudes into the superior part of the right side of the omental bursa. There is a superior recess of the right side of the omental bursa that extends upward behind and to the left of the caudate lobe. This superior recess is the most gravitationally dependent portion of the omental bursa when the patient is supine. Hence, small fluid collections within the omental bursa often tend to puddle posterior and to the left of the caudate lobe.

References

Bismuth H, Castaing D, Garden OJ (1988) Segmental surgery of the liver. Surg Ann 20:291–310

Couinaud C (1957) Le foie, etudes anatomiques et chirurgicales. Masson. Paris

Couinaud C (1998) The dorsal sector of the liver. Chirurgie 123:8–15

Donosa L, Martinez-Noguera A, Zidan A, Lora F (1989) Papillary process of the caudate lobe of the liver: sonographic appears. Radiology 173:631–633

Friedman AC, Dachman AH (1994) Radiology of the liver, biliary tract, and pancreas. Mosby, St. Louis.

Goldsmith NA, Woodburne RT (1957) The surgical anatomy pertaining to liver resection. Surg Gynecol Obstet 105:310–318

Healy JE (1970) Vascular anatomy of the liver. Ann NY Acad Sci 170:8–17

Healy JE, Schroy PC (1953) Anatomy of the biliary ducts within the human liver: analysis of prevaling pattern of branchings and major variations of the biliary ducts. Arch Surg 66:599–619

Lafortune M, Dauzat M, Pomier-Layrargues G, et al (1993) Hepatic artery: effect of a meal in healthy persons and transplant recipients. Radiology 187:391–394

Michels NA (1996) Newer anatomy of the liver and its variant blood supply and collateral circulation. Am J Surg 112:337–347

Nakamura S, Tsuzuki T (1981) Surgical anatomy of the hepatic veins and onferior vena cava. Surg Ginecol Obstet 152:43–50

Pagani JJ (1983) Intrahepatic vascular territories shown by computed tomography. Radiology 147:173–178

Schwartz SI (1989) Liver. In: Schwartz SI, Shires GP, Spencer FC (eds) Principle of surgery, vol II, McGraw Hill, New York

Takayasu K, Moryama M, Muramatsu Y, et al (1985) Intrahepatic portal vein branches studied by percutaneous transhepatic portography. Radiology 154:31–36

2 Clinico-pathological Classification of Liver Malignancies

G.L. RAPACCINI

CONTENTS

2.1 Introduction

Hepatic malignancies include primary and secondary (or metastatic) tumors. In children, primary tumors are the rule, and most are malignant. Primary liver malignancies are also more common in adult populations of sub-Saharan Africa, China, and other less industrialized areas of the world, but the majority of liver tumors diagnosed among adults in the developed areas are metastatic.

From a histological point of view, primary hepatic malignancies can be divided into three types according to their origins, i.e., those derived from the hepatocytes, those arising from the bile-duct epithelium, and those originating from the mesenchymal tissues of the liver. Some rare tumors (mixed type) include all three elements (Table 2.1).

Secondary liver tumors generally present the histotype of the primary neoplasm, and the clinical presentation will depend largely on the site of the primary tumor, as well as the size and number of hepatic metastases. For both primary and secondary tumors, the presence of underlying cirrhosis is highly significant since many of the initial symptoms of neoplastic involvement can be mistakenly attributed to this condition. In both cases, the clinical picture will also depend on the hormone-secreting characteristics of the neoplastic tissue, which are responsible for the so-called para-neoplastic syndrome.

G. L. RAPACCINI, MD; Professor, Department of Internal Medicine, A. Gemelli University Hospital, Largo A. Gemelli 8, I-00168 Rome, Italy

2.2 Hepatocyte

2.2.1 Hepatocellular Carcinoma

Hepatocellular carcinoma (HCC) is a common malignancy throughout the world with an estimated incidence of 300 000–1 000 000 new cases per year. It is the seventh most common cancer in men and the ninth in women. The highest incidence rates are found in sub-Saharan Africa and the Far East. Areas of low incidence include North America and north-

Table 2.1. Primary hepatic malignancies

Hepatocyte	Hepatocellular carcinoma Pre-neoplastic lesions Fibrolamellar carcinoma Hepatoblastoma
Bile duct epithelium	Cholangiocellular carcinoma Cystadenocarcinoma
Mesenchymal tissue	Angiosarcoma Epithelioid hemangio-endothelioma Sarcoma of the liver
Mixed	Hepato-cholangio-cellular carcinoma

ern Europe, while certain Mediterranean countries such as Spain, Italy, and Greece are in an intermediate position (Parkin et al. 1992; Bosch and Munoz 1991).

The geographic distribution of HCC is related to the etiology of the disease. In countries with low or intermediate incidence, most cases can be attributed to chronic hepatitis B (HBV) and / or C (HCV) that results in cirrhosis (Munoz and Bosch 1987; Colombo et al. 1989). In contrast, environmental and dietary factors are known to play major etiological roles in high-incidence areas. In Africa and Asia, for example, HCC seems to be related to the contamination of rice, grain and peanut stores by aflatoxin, a mycotoxin produced by the mold *Aspergillus flavius*, which is believed to have a direct carcinogenic effect in the liver (Enwonwu 1984; Collier et al. 1991). In these populations, HCC frequently develops in non-cirrhotic livers, but in some areas of Africa hepatitis B virus and aflatoxin may act as co-carcinogenic factors (Lutwick 1979). There is currently no experimental or clinical evidence that ethanol has direct carcinogenic effects in the liver. Nonetheless, it is thought to promote hepatic malignancy indirectly via: (a) its immunodepressant effects, which facilitate the development of HBV and HCV infections; (b) the induction of alcoholic cirrhosis; and (c) its well known oxidative effects, which deplete the anti-oxidative defense systems (Hardell et al. 1984). The suspicion that oral contraceptives might play a role in the genesis of liver cancer has yet to be confirmed in experimental or epidemiological studies.

On gross pathology, most HCCs fall into one of two categories. The nodular form, which is characterized by the presence of one or more encapsulated or non-encapsulated nodules, is seen predominantly in cirrhotic livers. The massive form, which consists in a large solitary tumor, is more frequent in developing countries, and, in most cases, there is no underlying cirrhosis. There is also a third so-called diffuse form, which is much less common than either of the former and is characterized by miliary infiltration of liver parenchyma (Anthony 1994).

Four different histological patterns can be distinguished: trabecular, pseudo-glandular, solid, and scirrhous (or sclerosing) (Gibson 1978). Depending on the cellular characteristics, these tumors are also described as well differentiated, moderately differentiated, poorly differentiated or undifferentiated (anaplastic) (Edmondson and Steiner 1954; Kondo et al. 1989; Nakashima et al. 1995). Occasionally, the malignant liver cells contain glycogen or fat stores that give them a clear, transparent appearance. The presence of bile stasis in the tumor cells is a marker of hepatocellular carcinoma, as are eosinophilic cytoplasmic inclusions representing deposits of alpha-fetoprotein, alpha1-antitrypsin, or ferritin (Kondo et al. 1989).

The clinical presentation of HCC depends largely on whether or not there is underlying cirrhosis. If so, the physical signs and symptoms of a small tumor will generally be indistinguishable from those of the chronic liver disease. When HCC develops in a normal liver, the clinical picture is usually that of advanced neoplastic disease.

In a patient with cirrhosis, the development of HCC is often heralded by an abrupt worsening of the clinical picture. In industrialized countries, where the typical HCC patient is an older individual (>50–60 years) with a long history of chronic, frequently viral, liver disease, the most common presenting symptoms are epigastric or right hypochondrial pain, weight loss or gain due to ascites (sometimes blood-stained), and jaundice (Kew and Popper 1984).

In the areas of highest incidence, where the tumor often develops in the absence of cirrhosis, the course of the disease is generally turbulent, and the diagnosis is always late (Kew and Geddes 1982). These patients are younger, generally about 40 years old, and they generally present with severe, often diffuse abdominal pain; weakness, weight loss, lack of appetite, and constipation may also be present. A few cases have been reported in which the sole presenting symptom was obstructive jaundice caused by biliary tree invasion (Chen et al. 1994). Rare cases have presented with an acute abdomen due to hemoperitoneum caused by tumor rupture into the abdominal cavity or a septic picture with fever and leukocytosis (Okuda et al. 1991).

Late extra-abdominal symptoms include cough and dyspnea caused by pulmonary metastases or right diaphragm involvement, and continuous back and/or chest wall pain due to osteolytic metastases in the ribs and vertebrae.

Finally, para-neoplastic manifestations, which are due to secretion of hormone-like substances by the tumor, can appear at any time during the course of HCC. One of the more frequent elements of the para-neoplastic syndrome is erythrocytosis, which occurs in about 10% of all HCC patients. It is thought to be caused by the synthesis of erythopoietin by the tumor tissue, though the latter has never actually been demonstrated (Kew and Dusheiko 1981). Hypoglycemia occurs in about 30% of all HCC patients, and in most cases it simply reflects high glucose consumption by a large, generally undifferentiated tumor. In the true para-neoplastic syndrome, however, the patient experiences severe hypoglycemic crises, often accompanied by neurological signs and even coma, which are caused by an insulin-like growth factor precursor (IGF-II) secreted by the tumor itself (Shapiro et al. 1990). In rare cases, patients with HCC present profound weakness, drowsiness, and lethargy caused by a hypercalcemic syndrome. The syndrome is unrelated to bone metastases and has been attributed to a parathyroid-like hormone produced by the tumor (Tamura et al. 1994). Occasional cases of HCC accompanied by hyperthyroidism (Helzberg et al. 1985) or pseudoporphyria (Pierach et al. 1984) have also been reported.

2.2.2 Preneoplastic Lesions

Liver cell dysplasia (LCD) and dysplastic (or adenomatous hyperplastic) nodules are not, strictly speaking, tumors of the liver, but as pre-neoplastic lesions they play major roles in the natural history of hepatocellular carcinoma. Liver cell dysplasia is a microscopic alteration that may be confined within a focal lesion; in some cases, however, there is diffuse involvement of the liver parenchyma affected by chronic disease. The features defined by Anthony et al. in 1973 include increases in the dimensions of both the cell and its nucleus (so that a normal nuclear/cytoplasmic ratio is maintained), accompanied by nuclear pleomorphism and hyperchromatism. Multinucleated cells may also be seen. This so-called large-cell dysplasia is to be distinguished from a less common form identified some 10 years later by Watanabe et al. (1983): this type of LCD (small cell dysplasia) is characterized by hepatocytes with a scarcity of cytoplasm and an increased nuclear/cytoplasmic ratio, which are sometimes crowded together in small foci.

Recent reports have confirmed the pre-neoplastic natures of LCD in a cirrhotic parenchyma (Borzio et al. 1991) and within the small discrete liver lesions discovered by ultrasound examination in cirrhotic patients (Caturelli et al. 1993).

These latter are the second type of pre-neoplastic lesion associated with cirrhosis. They are variously referred to as „macroregenerative nodules,“ „borderline lesions,“ „adenomatous hyperplastic nodules,“ and „dysplastic nodules“ (Wada et al. 1988; Arakawa et al. 1986). These lesions display high cellular proliferative activity (Anti et al. 1994; Orsatti et al. 1993), and their neoplastic potential has been well documented. In our experience, macro-regenerative nodules that are negative at the histological examination became hepatocellular carcinomas after a mean interval of 10 months (Rapaccini et al. 1990). The co-existence of dysplastic nodules and small hepatocellular carcinomas has been demonstrated in explanted cirrhotic livers (Ferrel et al. 1992), and HCC foci have also been found within these nodules (Fig. 2.1) (Arakawa et al. 1986; Pompili et al. 1991). All of the above findings support the theory that the development of HCC in cirrhotic liver begins with the simple regenerative nodule, which at some point in time evolves into an adenomatous hyperplastic nodule with dysplasia and, ultimately, with foci of HCC. Nevertheless, the possibility of de novo carcinogenesis without the preliminary steps cannot be excluded (Okuda et al. 1991).

2.2.3 Fibrolamellar Carcinoma

In 1980 Craig and co-workers described a variant of HCC characterized by large eosinophilic hepatocytes embedded in abundant fibrous tissue arranged in parallel bands (Fig. 2.2). Some of the histological features of this tumor are similar to those of focal nodular hyperplasia, but the hypothesis that fibrolamellar carcinoma arises from this benign lesion has been confirmed.

There are several differences between typical HCC and fibrolamellar carcinoma. The latter strikes a younger population (5–35 years of age), and both sexes are equally affected. Unlike HCC, fibrolamellar carcinoma generally develops in the absence of cirrhosis, does not appear to be related to previous HBV or HCV infection, and is not associated with elevated alpha-fetoprotein levels. Early reports hypothesized a relatively good prognosis for this neoplasm, the histological features of which are less malignant than those of HCC. However, this optimism has not been justified since most patients with fibrolamellar carcinomas present with advanced disease (manifested by abdominal pain and a palpable mass).

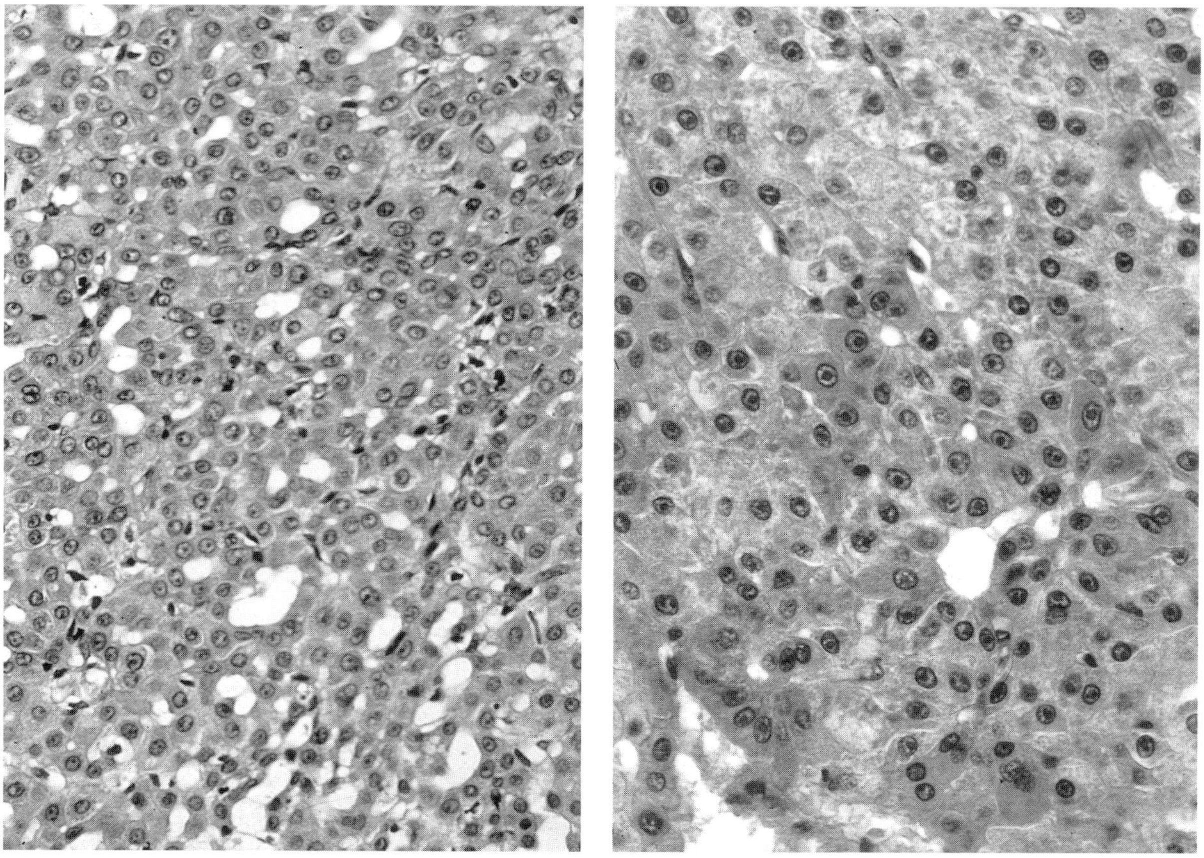

a b

Fig. 2.1a,b. Histologic samplings obtained in two different areas of the same same nodule: adenomatous hyperplasia with dysplasia (a); well-differentiated hepatocarcinoma (b). (Illustrations kindly provided by Prof. Fabio M. Vecchio, Department of Pathology, Catholic University of Rome)

2.2.4 Hepatoblastoma

Hepatoblastoma is the most common liver neoplasm during the first 4 years of life, but it is very rare in adults. It affects both sexes, but is more frequent in boys (Exelby et al. 1975). The tumor appears as a large mass (up to 25 cm in diameter), often encapsulated, with superficial vascular congestion; the core is composed of solid neoplastic tissue with areas of hemorrhage and sometimes calcification. In the mixed type (see below) fibrous septa may be present.

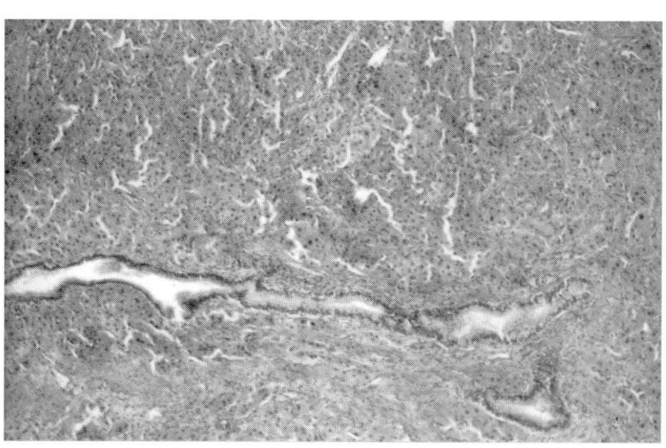

Fig. 2.2. Histologic features of fibrolamellar carcinoma: large, eosinophilic tumor cells are intermingled with bile ducts. (Illustration kindly provided by Prof. Fabio M. Vecchio, Department of Pathology, Catholic University of Rome)

From a histopathological point of view, hepatoblastomas are classified as epithelial or mixed (epithelial and mesenchymal) (Haas et al. 1989). The former is composed primarily of fetal hepatocytes and embryonic cells arranged in thin plates or pseudo-acinar structures (Fig. 2.3); sinusoids containing hematopoietic cells are sometimes found between the cellular plates. The mixed type contains mesenchymal tissue in various degrees of differentiation (mesenchyma, cartilage, striated muscle and even osteoid tissue) adjacent to the epithelial tissue; foci of squamous cells are sometimes present (Gururangan et al. 1992).

The clinical presentation of hepatoblastoma is that of a large mass that often distends the child's

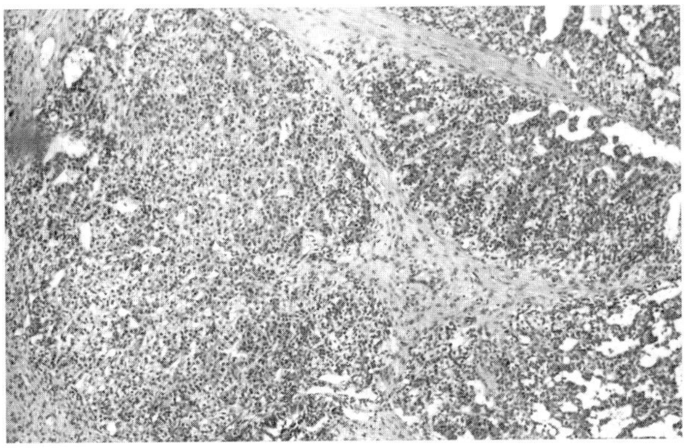

Fig. 2.3. Hepatoblastoma showing fetal epithelial pattern characterized by polygonal cells resembling hepatocytes arranged in cords with variable fat and glycogen. (Illustration kindly provided by Prof. Fabio M. Vecchio, Department of Pathology, Catholic University of Rome)

abdomen, accompanied by anorexia, vomiting, fever, and weight loss; jaundice is rare. Sexual precocity sometimes appears as a result of a pathological gonadotropin secretion by the tumor. Serum alpha-fetoprotein levels are usually high. Metastases can be found in the abdominal lymph nodes, the lungs, and, less commonly, the brain.

Genetic studies have documented an association between hepatoblastoma and abnormalities of a gene on chromosome 11 (Ding et al. 1994).

2.3 Bile Duct Epithelium

2.3.1 Cholangiocellular Carcinoma

Cholangiocarcinoma is usually classified on the basis of its site of origin: (1) the peripheral cholangiocarcinoma, which arises from intrahepatic bile ducts; (2) the hilar cholangiocarcinoma (Klatskin's tumor), which originates in the major bile ducts; and (3) the classical bile-duct carcinoma from the extrahepatic bile ducts (Ros et al. 1988).

Cholangiocarcinoma generally occurs during the sixth and seventh decades of life with a sex ratio of close to one. This tumor is rarer than hepatocellular carcinoma, but it is relatively frequent in some regions of the world such as the Far East. This geographical distribution may be related to the high prevalence of chronic biliary-tract infestations (*Clonorchis sinensis, Opisthorchis viverrini*) that characterizes these countries (Srivatanakul et al. 1991). In western countries the tumor generally complicates primary sclerosing cholangitis or congenital anomalies of the biliary tree (Kulkarni and Beatty 1977). Some cases have been correlated with previous administration of anabolic steroids or the radioactive contrast medium Thorotrast (Wogan 1976).

Peripheral cholangiocarcinoma presents as a large hepatic mass; sometimes the tumor is multifocal. Cholangiocellular carcinoma differs from HCC in that it is poorly vascularized, and invasion of the portal tree is an infrequent and late finding. Hilar and ductal cholangiocarcinomas grow into the walls of the bile ducts with invasion of the lumen, so obstructive jaundice is an early sign. There is dilatation of the biliary tree above the tumor, and in the rare longstanding cases that have been reported biliary cirrhosis was present (Sugihara and Kojiro 1987). Serum alpha-fetoprotein levels are always normal.

Histologically, cholangiocarcinoma resembles an adenocarcinoma with its tubular or acinar-glandular structures, and it may be difficult to differentiate this primary neoplasm from hepatic metastasis of an adenocarcinoma. The epithelial structures are frequently embedded in abundant fibrous tissue. The tumor may secrete mucus, but never bile, and the histochemical reaction for keratin is positive (Goodman et al. 1985). Metastases to the regional lymph nodes and lungs are common.

2.3.2 Cystadenocarcinoma

This rare neoplasm is seen predominantly in females. It arises from a cystoadenoma or a congenital biliary cyst and is, therefore, classified as a primary biliary tumor of the liver.

The patient reports a sensation of abdominal fullness, sometimes with pain. There may be significant weight loss. The physical examination reveals a large abdominal mass often in the right hypochondrium, which can be confirmed with various imaging techniques.

From a macroscopic point of view, cystadenocarcinoma is a large cystic mass containing bile-stained mucus and divided by internal septa. Microscopically the neoplastic tissue consists of epithelial cells arranged in papillary structures circumscribed by an abundant mesenchymal stroma (Wheeler and Edmondson 1985).

If surgical resection is possible, the prognosis is relatively good with survival up to 5 years.

2.4 Mesenchymal Tissue

2.4.1 Angiosarcoma

Angiosarcoma (also known as malignant hemangioendothelioma or Kupffer cell sarcoma) is a very rare neoplasm, but it is the most common hepatic tumor of mesenchymal origin. It displays a predilection for males and generally occurs during the sixth and seventh decades of life.

Angiosarcoma is a very interesting tumor because a number of etiologic factors have been identified in the last 50 years. The neoplasm was first described in German vintners who had been exposed to insecticides containing arsenic (Roth 1955). The literature also contains several cases of angiosarcoma attributed to past exposure (approximately 20 years before tumor diagnosis) to the contrast medium, thorium dioxide (Thorotrast), which is no longer used in radiology (Visfeldt and Poulsen 1972). Other iatrogenic cases have been caused by Fowler's solution, a potassium arsenite once used in the treatment of psoriasis (Regelson et al. 1968). There are also well documented cases that developed 10 years after exposure to vinyl chloride monomers, the metabolites of which exert a direct carcinogenic effect involving covalent binding of host DNA (Greech and Johnson 1974; Tamburro 1984). Rare cases have been described after prolonged use of anabolic steroids (Falk et al. 1979) or during the course of von Recklinghausen's disease (Lederman et al. 1987).

Angiosarcoma is a highly malignant tumor, and, therefore, symptoms and signs are those of a rapidly progressive and fatal disease. The patient complains of abdominal swelling and pain, weight loss, nausea and fever; jaundice may also be an early finding. The physical examination reveals hepatomegaly, and the liver is frequently tender with an irregular surface. Splenomegaly and ascites are sometimes present. An arterial bruit can sometimes be heard over the liver. In around 15% of all cases, acute hemoperitoneum occurs due to spontaneous tumor rupture.

Angiosarcomas are often multifocal tumors consisting of solid masses alternating with the characteristic blood-filled cysts; the masses are generally not encapsulated, and their borders are poorly defined. Microscopically the neoplastic tissue is characterized by elongated endothelial cells with clear cytoplasm and hyperchromatic nuclei that line dilated sinusoidal spaces. As the tumor grows, the dilated sinusoids become cavernous cavities with poorly defined borders. Infiltration of portal and hepatic venous radicles is early and massive (Ishak 1987). The neoplastic cells may be positive for factor VIII-related antigen.

The prognosis is usually quite poor because of the advanced stage at the time of the diagnosis. Radiation therapy is the only form of treatment that has proved palliative. Survival rarely exceeds 6 months, and death may be caused by fulminant disseminated intravascular coagulation.

2.4.2 Epithelioid Hemangioendothelioma

Epithelioid hemangioendothelioma, which is also quite rare, generally strikes young adult females. These tumors display a lower grade of malignancy than angiosarcoma, but the disease is somewhat progressive also with the appearance of distant metastasis. The first symptoms are abdominal pain, loss of weight and appetite, jaundice, and, occasionally, hemoperitoneum.

Macroscopically the liver presents multiple masses, which can complicate the differential diagnosis based on imaging techniques (Miller et al. 1992). The neoplastic tissue is composed of epithelioid cells that proliferate into the sinusoids and central hepatic veins (Fig. 2.4). Histochemical positivity

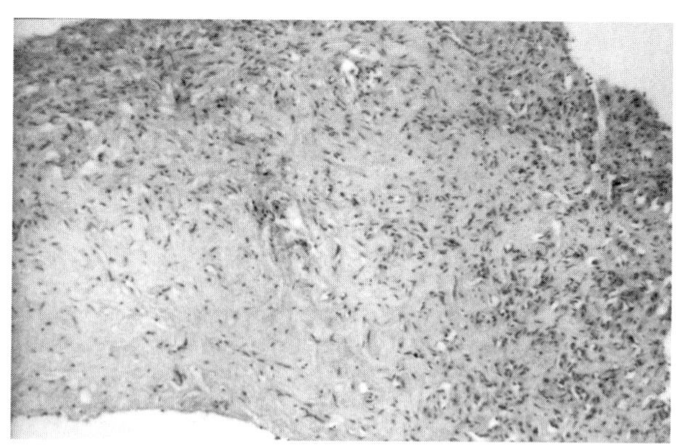

Fig. 2.4. Epithelioid hemangioendothelioma is characterized by dense fibrous stroma containing vacuolated spindle cells forming vascular lumina. (Illustration kindly provided by Prof. Fabio M. Vecchio, Department of Pathology, Catholic University of Rome)

for factor VIII antigen and lectins confirms the diagnosis.

For a young woman with epithelioid hemangioendothelioma, the treatment of choice is liver transplantation, which carries quite a good prognosis (Kelleher et al. 1989).

2.4.3 Sarcomas

Primary liver sarcomas are even less common than angiosarcoma and epithelioid hemangioendothelioma. They occur in both children and adults (Leuschner et al. 1990), are highly malignant, and survival rarely exceeds a few months. There is no effective treatment. The tumor presents as a large abdominal mass accompanied by fever and abdominal pain. It consists of a single solid-cystic mass with calcifications; invasion of the hepatic veins and the inferior vena cava are generally present at diagnosis. The histologic examination reveals the typical features of a sarcoma: a monotonous tissue composed of neoplastic fibrous elements that are positive for reticulin.

2.5 Mixed Tumors

2.5.1 Hepatocholangiocarcinoma

This tumor is also called mixed hepatocellular/cholangiocellular carcinoma since it presents typical cells of both carcinomas (Goodman et al. 1985). The elements of both tumors are variously combined within the same mass, so the neoplastic tissue may present stain positivity for both alpha-fetoprotein (HCC) and keratin (cholangiocarcinoma). These tumors may or may not be associated with underlying cirrhosis. The clinical presentation and course are generally similar to those of hepatocellular carcinoma.

References

Anti M, Marra G, Rapaccini GL, et al (1994) DNA ploidy pattern in human chronic liver diseases and hepatic nodular lesions flow cytometric analysis on echo-guided needle liver biopsies. Cancer 73:281–288

Anthony PP (1994) Tumors and tumor-like lesions of the liver and biliary tract. In: MacSween RNM, Antony PP, Scheuer PJ, et al (eds) Pathology of the liver. Churchill Livingstone, Edinburgh, p 635

Anthony PP, Vogel CL, Barker LF (1973) Liver cell dysplasia: a premalignant condition. J Clin Path 26:217–223

Arakawa M, Kage M, Matsumoto S, et al (1986) Frequency and significance of tumour thrombi in oesophageal varices in hepatocellular carcinoma associated with cirrhosis. Hepatology 6:419–422

Borzio M, Bruno S, Roncalli M, et al (1991) Liver cell dysplasia and risk of hepatocellular carcinoma in cirrhosis: a preliminary report. Br Med J 302:1312–1315

Bosch FX, Munoz N (1991) Hepatocellular carcinoma in the world: epidemiologic questions. In: Tabor E, Di Bisceglie AM, and Purcell RH (eds) Etiology, Pathology and Treatment of Hepatocellular Carcinoma in North America. Advances in Applied Technology Series, vol. 13. Gulf Publishing, Houston, p 35

Caturelli E, Fusilli S, Costarelli L, et al (1993) Focal ultrasound lesions in cirrhotic liver diagnosed as regenerative nodules by biopsy. A morphometric study. J Clin Gastroenterol 17:67–72

Chen MF, Jan YY, Jeng LB, et al (1994) Obstructive jaundice secondary to ruptured hepatocellular carcinoma into the common bile duct. Cancer 73:1335–1340

Collier JD, Carpenter M, Burt AD, et al (1991) Expression of mutant p53 protein in hepatocellular carcinoma. Gut 35:98–100

Colombo M, Kuo G, Choo QL, et al (1989) Prevalence of antibodies to hepatitis C virus in Italian patients with hepatocellular carcinoma. Lancet 2:1004–1006

Craig JR, Peters RL, Edmondson HA, et al (1980) Fibrolamellar carcinoma of the liver: a tumor of adolescents and young adults with distinctive clinico-pathologic features. Cancer 46:372–379

Ding SF, Michail NE, Habib NA (1994) Genetic changes in hepatoblastoma. J Hepatol 20:672–675

Edmondson HA, Steiner PE (1954) Primary carcinoma of the liver: a study of 100 cases among 48,900 necropsies. Cancer 7:462–503

Enwonwu CO (1984) The role of dietary aflatoxin in the genesis of hepatocellular cancer in the developing countries. Lancet 2:956–958

Exelby PR, Filler RM, Groshield JM (1975) Liver tumors in children with particular reference to hepatoblastoma and hepatocellular carcinoma. J Pediatr Surg 10:329–337

Falk H, Thomas LB, Popper H, et al (1979) Hepatic angiosarcoma associated with androgenic-anabolic steroids. Lancet 2:1120–1123

Ferrel L, Wright T, Lake J, et al (1992) Incidence and diagnostic features of macroregenerative nodules vs. small hepatocellular carcinoma in cirrhotic livers. Hepatology 16:1372–1381

Gibson JB (1978) International histological classification of the tumours. No.20. World Health Organization, Geneve, pp 20–22

Goodman ZD, Ishak KG, Langloss JM, et al (1985) Combined hepatocellular-cholangiocarcinoma: a histologic and immunohistochemical study. Cancer 55:124–135

Greech JL, Johnson MN (1974) Angiosarcoma of the liver in the manufacture of polyvinyl chloride. J Occup Med 16:150–151

Gururangan S, O'Meara A, MacMahon C, et al (1992) Primary hepatic tumours in children: a 26-year review. J Surg Oncol 50:30–36

Haas JE, Muczynski KA, Krailo M, et al (1989) Histopathology and prognosis in childhood hepatoblastoma and hepatocarcinoma. Cancer 64:1082–1095

Hardell L, Bengtsson NO, Jonsson U, et al (1984) Aetiological aspects of primary liver cancer with special regard to alcohol, organic solvents and acute intermittent porphyria – an epidemiological investigation. Br J Cancer 50:389–397

Helzberg JH, McPhee MS, Zarling EJ, et al (1985) Hepatocellular carcinoma: an unusual course with hyperthyroidism and inappropriate thyroid-stimulating hormone production. Gastroenterology 88:181–184

Ishak KG (1987) Malignant mesenchymal tumors of the liver. In: Okuda K, Ishak KG (eds) Neoplasms of the Liver. Springer-Verlag, Tokyo, pp 159–176

Kelleher MB, Iwatsuki S, Sheahan DG (1989) Epithelioid hemangioendothelioma of the liver. Clinicopathological correlation of 10 cases trated by orthotopic liver transplantation. Am J Surg Pathol 13:999–1008

Kew MC, Dusheiko GM (1981) Paraneoplastic manifestations of hepatocellular carcinoma. In: Chalmers TC, Berk PD (eds) Frontiers of Science in Liver Disease. Thieme-Stratton, New York, p 305

Kew MC, Geddes EW (1982) Hepatocellular carcinoma in rural southern African blacks. Medicine (Balt) 61:98– 108

Kew MC, Popper H (1984) The relationship between hepatocellular carcinoma and cirrhosis. Semin Liver Dis 4:136–146

Kondo F, Wada K, Nagato Y, et al (1989) Biopsy diagnosis of well-differentiated hepatocellular carcinoma based on new morphologic criteria. Hepatology 9:751–755

Kulkarni PB, Beatty EC (1977) Cholangiocarcinoma associated with biliary atresia. Am J Dis Child 131:442–444

Lederman SM, Martin EC, Laffey KT, et al (1987) Hepatic neurofibromatosis, malignant shwannoma and angiosarcoma in von Recklinghausen's disease. Gastroenterology 92:234–239

Leuschner I, Schmidt D, Harms D (1990) Undifferentiated sarcoma of the liver in childhood. Morphology, flow cytometry and literature review. Hum Pathol 21:68–73

Lutwick LI (1979) Relation between aflatoxins and hepatitis-B virus and hepatocellular carcinoma. Lancet 2:775–777

Miller WJ, Dood GD III, Federle MP, et al (1992) Epithelioid hemangioendothelioma of the liver: imaging findings with pathologic correlation. Am J Roentgenol 159:53–57

Munoz N, Bosch X (1987) Epidemiology of hepatocellular carcinoma. In: Okuda K, Ishak KG (eds) Neoplasms of the Liver. Springer-Verlag, Tokyo, pp 3–19

Nakashima O, Sugihara S, Kage M, et al (1995) Pathomorphologic characteristics of small hepatocellular carcinoma: A special reference to small hepatocellular carcinoma with indistict margins. Hepatology 22:101–105

Okuda K, Kondo Y, Nakano M, et al (1991) Hepatocellular carcinoma presenting with pyrexia and leukocytosis: report of five cases. Hepatology 13:695–700

Orsatti G, Theise ND, Thung SN, et al (1993) DNA image cytometric analysis of macroregenerative nodules (adenomatous hyperplasia) of the liver: evidence in support of their preneoplastic nature. Hepatology 17:621–627

Parkin DM, Muir CS, Whelan SL., et al (1992) Cancer Incidence in Five Continents, vol.5. IARC Publication, No.120. International Agency for Research on Cancer, Lyon

Pierach CA, Bossenmaier IC, Cardinal RA, et al (1984) Pseudoporphyria in a patient with hepatocellular carcinoma. Am J Med 76:545–548

Pompili M, Rapaccini GL, Gambassi G (1991) Review of adenomatous hyperplastic nodules in liver cirrhosis: pathologic features, imaging diagnosis and prognostic significance. Gastroenterology International 4:120–124

Rapaccini GL, Pompili M, Caturelli E, et al (1990) Focal ultrasound lesions in liver cirrhosis diagnosed as regenerating nodules by fine-needle biopsy. Follow-up of 12 cases. Dig Dis Sci 35:422–427

Regelson W, Kim U, Ospina J, et al (1968) Hemangio-endothelial sarcoma of the liver from chronic arsenic intoxication by Fowler's solution. Cancer 21:514– 522

Ros PR, Buck JL, Goodman ZD, et al (1988) Intrahepatic cholangiocarcinoma; radiologic-pathologic correlation. Radiology 167:689–693

Roth F (1955) Arsen-Leber-Tumoren (Hemangioendotheliom). Arch Pathol 60:493–499

Shapiro ET, Bell GI, Polonsky KS, et al (1990) Tumor hypoglycemia: relationship to high molecular weight insulin-like growth factor II. J Clin Invest 85:1672– 1679

Srivatanakul P, Parkin DM, Yiang Y-Z, et al (1991) The role of infection by Opisthorchis viverrini, hepatitis B virus, and aflatoxin exposure in liver cancer in Thailand. Cancer 68:2411–2417

Sugihara S, Kojiro M (1987) Pathology of cholangiocarcinoma. In: Okuda K, Ishak KG (eds) Neoplasms of the Liver. Springer-Verlag, Tokyo, pp 143–158

Tamburro CH (1984) Relationship of vinyl chloride and liver cancers: angiosarcoma and hepatocellular carcinoma. Semin Liver Dis 4:158–169

Tamura K, Kubota K, Take H, et al (1994) Parathyroid hormone-related peptide as a possible cause of hypercalcemia in a hepatocellular carcinoma patient. Am J Gastroenterol 89:644–645

Visfeldt J, Poulsen H (1972) On the histopathology of the liver and liver tumors in thorium dioxide patients. Acta Pathol Microbiol Scand 80 A:97–108

Wada K, Kondo F, Kondo Y (1988) Large regenerative nodules and dysplastic nodules in cirrhotic livers: a histopathologic study. Hepatology 12:592–597

Watanabe S, Okita K, Harada T, et al (1983) Morphologic studies of the liver cell dysplasia. Cancer 51:2197–2205

Wheeler DA, Edmondson HA (1985) Cystadenoma with mesenchymal stroma (CMS) in the liver and bile ducts: a clinicopathologic study of 17 cases, 4 with malignant change. Cancer 56:1434–1435

Wogan GN (1976)The induction of liver cancer by chemicals. In: Cameron HM, Linsell CA, Warwick GP (eds) Liver Cell Cancer. John Wiley, New York, pp 121–152

II Diagnostic Imaging

3 Carcinogenesis and Pathological Classification of Hepatocellular Carcinoma

M. Vaccari, C. Lattes, and W.F. Grigioni

CONTENTS

M. Vaccari, MD; Department of Pathology, Histology and Cytology, F. Addari Institute, S. Orsola Malpighi Hospital, Viale Ercolani 4/2, I-40138 Bologna, Italy
C. Lattes, MD; Department of Pathology, Histology and Cytology, F. Addari Institute, S. Orsola Malpighi Hospital, Viale Ercolani 4/2, I-40138 Bologna, Italy
W. F. Grigioni, MD; Professor, Department of Pathology, Histology and Cytology, F. Addari Institute, S. Orsola Malpighi Hospital, Viale Ercolani 4/2, I-40138 Bologna, Italy

3.1 Introduction

The fact that hepatocellular carcinoma (HCC) has different epidemiological distributions in different parts of the world has facilitated the identification of a series of associated risk factors (Johnson 1996). For instance, a clear association has been shown between HCC and hepatitis B virus (HBV) in areas of the world where HCC has a high incidence (China, Southeast Asia and northern Africa) (Johnson 1996). HCC is also now known to be associated with other risk factors such as hepatitis C virus (HCV), aflatoxins, sex hormones and some metabolic diseases (Johnson 1996; Graham and Alistar 1996). Moreover, there is no doubt that different combinations of risk factors account for the variations in incidence to be found in different geographical areas: for example, exposure to aflatoxin and carriage of hepatitis B surface antigen (HBsAg) are both significant risk factors, but the combination of the two exposes the individual to a much higher risk (Zeman et al. 1985). Furthermore, new diagnostic methods have been developed that allow direct assessment of risk factors. Thus, in recent years it has been possible to detect the HBV surface antigen (HBsAg) and HCC antibodies, and it is now also possible to reveal aflatoxin adducts of DNA in biological fluids as a measure of aflatoxin exposure (Ross et al. 1992).

The identification and quantification of risk factors and the development of cancer registries documenting the large geographical variations in the incidence of HCC allowed prevention strategies to be initiated, such as HBV immunization and ways of preventing exposure to aflatoxins. Moreover, in 70–90% of HCC there is association with hepatic cirrhosis, and all the factors linked to the development of HCC, including HBV, HCC and alcohol, also cause cirrhosis. Therefore, many screening programs are currently being implemented for secondary prevention of HCC in cirrhotic patients. Screening programs to identify early resectable lesions have been practised since the early 1970s, following the clinical observation that a substantial percentage of patients with HCC, particularly those with chronic HBV infection, have elevated serum levels of alpha-fetoprotein (AFP) (Munoz and Bosch 1987; Wanz and Blum 1991). Follow-up studies carried out in many countries on patients with cirrhosis with the application of sensitive and specific diagnostic methods such as real time ultrasonography and assays for serum AFP have made it possible to detect and treat HCCs at early stages (Okuda 1986; Colombo et al. 1991; Ebara et al. 1986). The identification of small liver lesions at early stages in the development of malignancy can greatly help to identify the morphological precursors of HCC, thereby adding to our knowledge of the morphological sequence of human liver carcinogenesis. At the moment, many lines of evidence suggest that the morphogenesis of HCC in cirrhotic patients is not identical to that occurring in non-cirrhotic subjects (Oka et al 1990; Shinigawa et al 1984; Sakamoto et al 1991; Tabarin et al 1987).

To understand the morphogenesis and prognosis of HCC, it is necessary to study the molecular mechanisms of liver cell transformation, and in the last few years the importance given to molecular markers has greatly increased. For example, dysfunction of genes involved in cell growth, differentiation and cell cycle control such as oncogenes, tumor suppressor genes and cyclins have been implicated during sequential carcinogenesis in the liver and other organs. These genes are involved in what are generally considered to be the three main stages of multistep carcinogenesis: that is to say, "initiation," "promotion" and "progression" (Mehta 1995).

3.2 Risk Factors and Pathogenesis

3.2.1 Hepatitis B Virus

The discovery of the HBsAg and the development of cancer registries in many countries allowed the association between HBV and HCC to be identified. The relative risk of patients with HBsAg of developing HCC varies from as much as 90% in high risk areas to 10% in low risk areas (Okuda et al. 1982). The association is known to be specifically confined to chronic HBV infection, as epidemiologic studies have found no increased risk among subjects who have cleared the virus after acute infection (Okuda et al. 1989).

The development of transgenic mice with HBV genes has led to new insights into HBV-induced liver carcinogenesis. Overexpression of the HBV large envelope protein leads to its cellular accumulation with consequent severe and prolonged cellular injury that triggers inflammation, regenerative hyperplasia, chromosomal aberrations and eventually HCC (Lau and Lai 1990). The increased expression of the specific cytochrome p450 may lead to increased production of carcinogenic metabolites (Beebe and Norman 1991). Ground-glass hepatocytes have been shown to be the direct precursors of foci of altered hepatocytes and their neoplastic descendants (Huang and Chisari 1995). High expression of the Hbx gene of HBV induces progressive morphological changes beginning with the development of foci of altered hepatocytes progressing into benign adenomatous hyperplasia (AH) and finally HCC (Kirby et al. 1994).

Viral integration into host DNA is found in 90% of HBsAg positive HCCs, as well as in liver tissue from chronic HBV hepatitis patients and healthy carriers (Toshkov et al. 1994). Integrated HBV DNA has also been found in some HCCs from HBsAg negative patients (Kim et al. 1991). Integrated HBV DNA is clonal (Shafritz et al. 1981), implying that viral integration precedes or accompanies malignant transformation. HBV integrates into DNA in a non-specific fashion, and leads to a variety of chromosomal abnormalities, including translocations, deletions and duplications (Paterlini et al. 1995). HBV integration could lead to HCC through the transactivation of cellular genes by the gene products of the integrated HBV DNA. The Hbx gene product is a novel serine-threonine protein kinase which acts as a non-specific transcriptional transactivator capable of altering cell growth and differentiation by catalyzing the phosphorylation of cellular factors (Shafritz and Kew 1981; Yaiginuma et al. 1987). In addition to the Hbx protein, the truncated pre-S2/S sequences have been found to have transcriptional transactivating activity (Spandau and Lee 1988; Twu and Schloemer 1987).

3.2.2 Hepatitis C Virus

The association of HCC with HCV infection is not as strong as with HBV. However, evidence is accumulating that HCV infection is an etiological factor in HCC development. Many cases of HCC are associated with the presence of HCV antibodies, although frequencies vary around the world (KEKULE et al. 1990; CASELMANN et al. 1990; BRUIX et al. 1989). In addition, HCV RNA can be identified in the serum of HCC patients (NISHIOKA et al. 1991; BAUR et al. 1992) and in HCC tissue (MANGIA et al.1994), where it is capable of active replications (BIUKH et al. 1993). HCV is the cause of most cases of post-transfusional non-A non-B (NANB) hepatitis (CHOU et al. 1991).

However, since HCV has no reverse trancriptase and is not a retrovirus it should in theory have no direct oncogenic potential. Many authors have attributed the association with HCC to the chronic liver disease which HCV can cause, while others, on the basis of prospective studies, suggest that HCV is an independent risk factor in patients with cirrhosis (OKUNO et al. 1994; SRIWATANAKUL et al. 1991; SIMONETTI et al. 1992; NAUMOV et al. 1994; CAPOROSO et al. 1991).

3.2.3 Aflatoxin

Aflatoxins are mycotoxins generated by the fungi *Aspergillus flavus* and *Aspergillus parasiticus*. Humans are exposed following ingestion of nuts and meal stored under the hot humid conditions in which these molds flourish. The carcinogenic action of the aflatoxins, especially aflatoxin B1 (AFB1), has been extensively studied in experimental models (IARC 1993; NEWBERNE and BUTLER 1969). It has been found that the presence of covalently bound albumin-AFB1 adducts in serum is associated with an increased risk of HCC (GOOPMAN et al. 1988). AFB1 is metabolized through an epoxidation pathway that produces an electrophilic DNA-binding metabolite which preferentially forms adducts with guanine. AFB1-induced HCC expresses single nucleotide mutations causing single amino acid substitutions. Gender-specific and genetic variations in phase I and II detoxification pathway enzymes may lead to differing levels of susceptibility to the effects of AFB1 (MCGLYNN et al. 1995). AFB1-induced HCC is thought to be independent of both direct DNA damage and the clonal selection of initiated hepatocytes during mitogenesis. While AFB1 alone is sufficient to induce HCC, AFB1 is often encountered in the presence of other liver carcinogens with which it may act synergistically (SLAGLE 1995).

3.2.4 Chronic Liver Disease

It is accepted that regardless of its etiology, cirrhosis is associated with the development of HCC, and that 70–90% of cases of HCC arise from cirrhotic liver. It is likely that carcinogenesis is associated with the large amount of regenerative changes occurring in the cirrhotic liver (SHEU et al. 1985; OKA et al. 1990; COLOMBO et al. 1991; CRAIG et al. 1991; KEW and POPPER 1984; FATTOVICH et al. 1995). In addition, several metabolic diseases show an association with HCC, including α1-antitrypsin deficiency (PROPST et al. 1994), tyrosinemia and porphyria cutanea tarda (SALATA et al. 1985). The incidence of HCC is also higher in the presence of hemochromatosis, but it is unclear if iron itself is pathogenic, or whether the increased cancer risk results solely from the cirrhotic process (DEUGNIER et al. 1993; STAL et al. 1995).

3.3 Morphogenesis

The main lesions involved in the morphogenesis of HCC in the cirrhotic liver are liver cell dysplasia, space occupying lesions, borderline lesions and minute HCCs in regenerative nodules of normal size. In non-cirrhotic liver, hepatocellular adenoma and hyperplastic tumor-like lesions are important.

3.3.1 Cirrhotic Liver

3.3.1.1 Liver Cell Dysplasia

The term liver cell dysplasia (LCD) was coined by ANTHONY et al. in 1973 to define a complex of morphological alterations in cirrhotic liver of a putatively premalignant nature. The term refers to the presence of cellular enlargement with normal nuclear-cytoplasmatic ratio, nuclear pleomorphism with hyperchromasia and multinucleation of liver cells. Enlargement is both nuclear and cytoplasmatic, and is generally two- to threefold. Intranuclear inclusions may be seen and nucleoli are prominent. These changes, when present, are multiple throughout the liver, and either occur in groups of liver cells or affect a whole cirrhotic nodule (Figs.

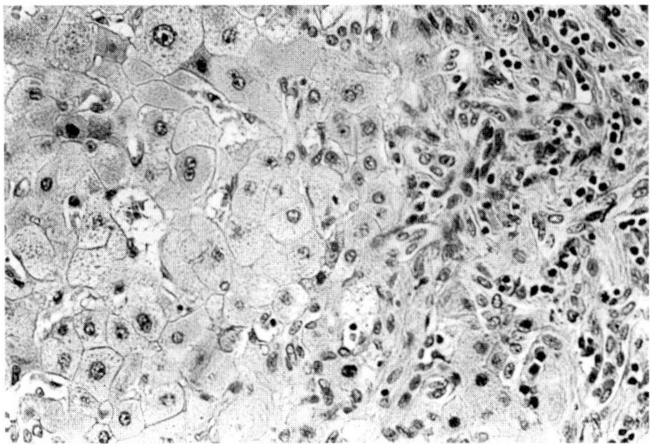

Fig. 3.1. Liver cell dysplasia in cirrhosis. Some hepatocytes show cellular enlargement and nuclear pleomorphism. ×40

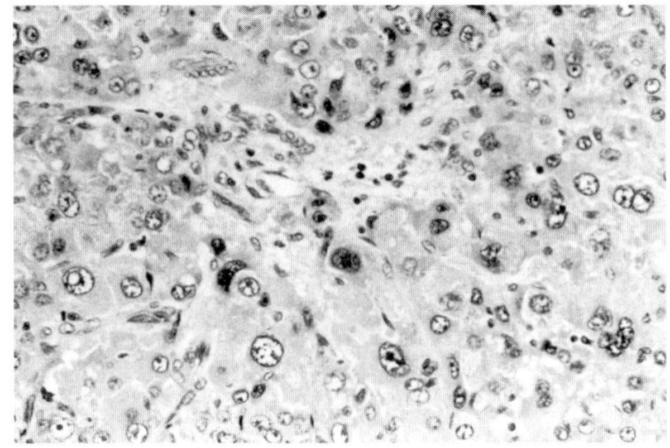

Fig. 3.2. Liver cell dysplasia in cirrhosis. The hepatocytes present large nuclei and cytoplasm. Several nuclei are pleomorphic with prominent nucleoli and occasionally multinucleations. ×40

3.1, 3.2). A close relation has been demonstrated between these cells and the presence of HBsAg (Akagi et al. 1984). Although the close relationship between dysplasia and HCC has subsequently been confirmed elsewhere (Omata et al. 1982; Ho et al. 1981), immunohistochemical studies on these cells led several groups of morphologists in Japan to reject the theory that the dysplastic cells are actually preneoplastic (Uchida et al. 1981; Okuda et al. 1980). AFP production was demonstrated by Okita et al. (1967) and by Popper (1979), but Roncalli et al. (1985) found no significant differences in production of AFP, carcinoembryonic antigen, and alpha-1-antitrypsin between cirrhotic, dysplastic and malignant cells. Uchida et al. (1981) failed to show a pattern of enzyme deviation seen in liver carcinoma cells, either in dysplastic liver cells or in liver cells bearing HBsAg. Studies in South Africa by Cohen and co-workers also addressed the premalignant nature of LCD (Choen et al. 1979; Choen and Berson 1986). Watanabe et al. (1983) later described a different type of liver dysplasia, which they named "small cell dysplasia" and suggested that this variety was more likely to be precancerous (Fig. 3.3). They classified dysplastic liver cells into two types - large and small both of which exhibited nuclear pleomorphism and multinucleation. However, whereas the large dysplastic cells had a normal nuclear-cytoplasmatic ratio and on electron microscopy exhibited the morphological features of regenerative cells, the small dysplastic ones were characterized by a decreased cytoplasm and an increased nuclear-cytoplasmatic ratio and had a tendency to produce small round foci or nodules. In the small dysplastic cells, the frequency of multinucleation was lower and the grade of pleomorphism smaller. Watanabe et al. (1983) suggested that these cells were more likely to be precancerous, owing to their greater similarity to cancer cells. Recently these data have been confirmed by several studies based on immunohistochemistry, morphometric analysis of nuclear size, DNA content and ploidy by cytofluorometry (Giannini et al. 1987; Roncalli et al. 1988, 1989; Henmi et al. 1985; Chen et al. 1984; Kagawa et al. 1984). Subsequently, the question as to whether LCD is a premalignant lesion has been discussed by several authors with contrasting findings (Nakashima et al. 1983; Suwangol and Jimarkorn 1980; Ho et al. 1981; Bartok et al. 1981; Paterson et al. 1989; Karhunen and Penttila 1987; Roncalli et al. 1985, 1986; Borzio et al. 1991). Some authors

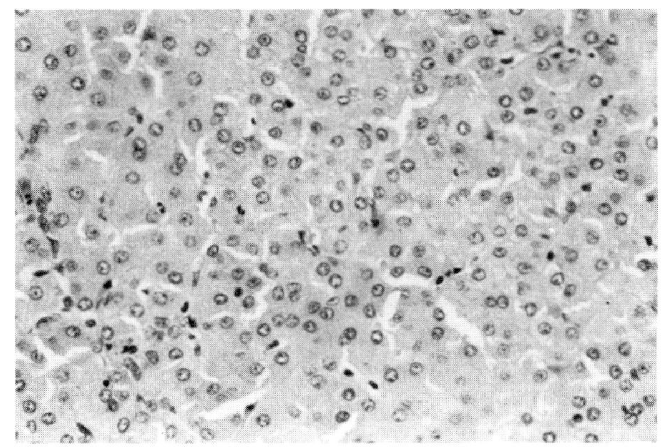

Fig. 3.3. Liver cell dysplasia (small cell type) in cirrhosis. The nodule is composed of small hepatocytes showing increased cellularity, nuclear crowding, and prominent nucleoli. The grade of pleomorphism is smaller than in large cell dysplasia. ×40

argue that evidence supporting the preneoplastic nature of LCD comes from some experimental liver carcinogenesis models in which preneoplastic lesions, such as hyperplastic nodules or areas, are known to regularly precede tumor development (PODDA et al. 1992; FABER and SARMA 1987; FABER 1976; SCHIRMACHER et al. 1991; EVARTZ et al. 1990; SELL and DUNSFORD 1989; SELL 1990). However, no direct evidence has yet been found in humans to document the development of HCC from these dysplastic cells. Indeed, in humans it is difficult to detect changes such as hyperplastic nodules, basophilic foci, clear cell change, oval cell proliferation and megalocytosis that can be seen during experimental liver carcinogenesis (ANTHONY 1987). ANTHONY affirms that megalocytosis may be the equivalent of LCD, but the other changes are never or hardly ever seen in man. Although it is still a matter of debate as to whether LCD is a premalignant change, patients in whom LCD is found on liver biopsy should be closely monitored for early detection of HCC by serial measurement of AFP and imaging techniques, especially in subjects who are cirrhotic or infected by HBV.

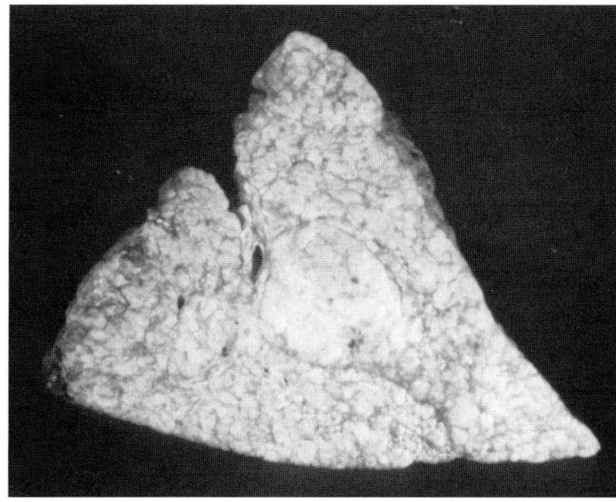

Fig. 3.4. Macroregenerative nodule. The cut surface of a cirrhotic liver shows a bulging macroregenerative nodule

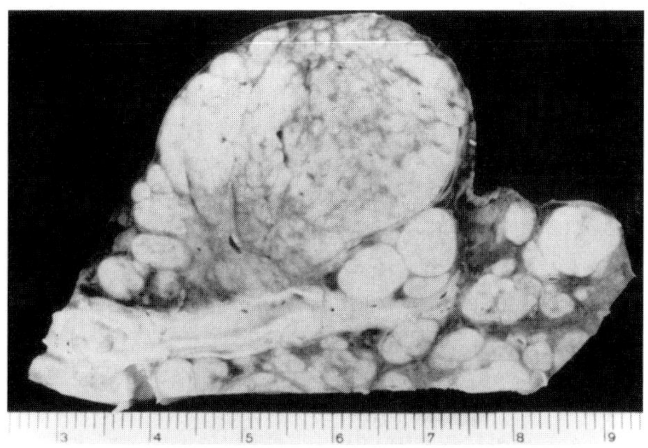

Fig. 3.5. Macroregenerative nodule. In this case of liver cirrhosis without hepatocellular carcinoma, there is present a sharply demarcated macroregenerative nodule of about 3 cm

3.3.1.2
Space Occupying Lesions

Space occupying lesions in cirrhotic livers have been variously defined as "adenomatous hyperplasia" (EDMONDSON 1976; TERADA et al. 1989b), "atypical adenomatous hyperplasia" (SAKAMOTO et al. 1991; TSUDA et al. 1988), "adenomatous hyperplastic nodules" (OHTA and NAKANUMA 1987; TERADA et al. 1990; ARAKAWA et al. 1986a), "small mass lesions in cirrhosis" (ARAKAWA et al. 1986b), "hepatocellular pseudotumor" (NAGASUE et al. 1984) and "macroregenerative nodules" (FURUYA et al. 1988, TERADA and NAKANUMA 1989a,b; TERADA et al. 1989b; WADA et al. 1988; GRIGIONI et al. 1989, 1991). Despite the varied nomenclature, these lesions are basically the same and show the main morphological features reported by EDMONDSON (1976) as adenomatous hyperplasia (AH). AH is usually detected in cirrhotic livers, sometimes with synchronous HCC, and ranges from 0.5 to 3 cm (or exceptionally even more) in diameter. These nodules can be distinguished from parenchyma by virtue of their expanding growth (Figs. 3.4, 3.5). Histologically, AH consists of hepatocytes that are occasionally larger than normal ones and are arranged in one-or-two-cell-thick plates, lacking a true capsule, and with a lobulated aspect. AH contains fibrous septa and frequently also portal tracts with portal veins, hepatic arteries and interlobular bile ducts. Although the majority of these nodules lack structural and cellular atypia, many cases of AH with internal foci of well differentiated HCC and/or foci with varying degrees of cellular and structural atypia – the so-called "atypical adenomatous hyperplasia" (AAH) – have been reported (Figs. 3.6, 3.7) (EDMONDSON 1976; TERADA et al. 1990; ARAKAWA et al. 1986a; GRIGIONI et al. 1989, 1991; TAKAYAMA et al. 1990; KONDO et al. 1990; OHNO et al. 1990; NAKANUMA et al. 1990). Thus, the imputed precancerous nature of AH seems to be justified.

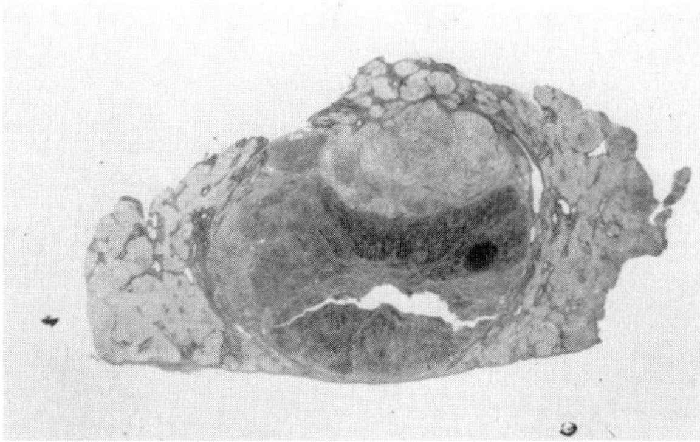

Fig. 3.6. Macroregenerative nodule. Low magnification view of a "nodule-in-nodule" lesion. A thin fibrous septum divides an adenomatous nodule (*left*) from an area with atypical aspects. ×10

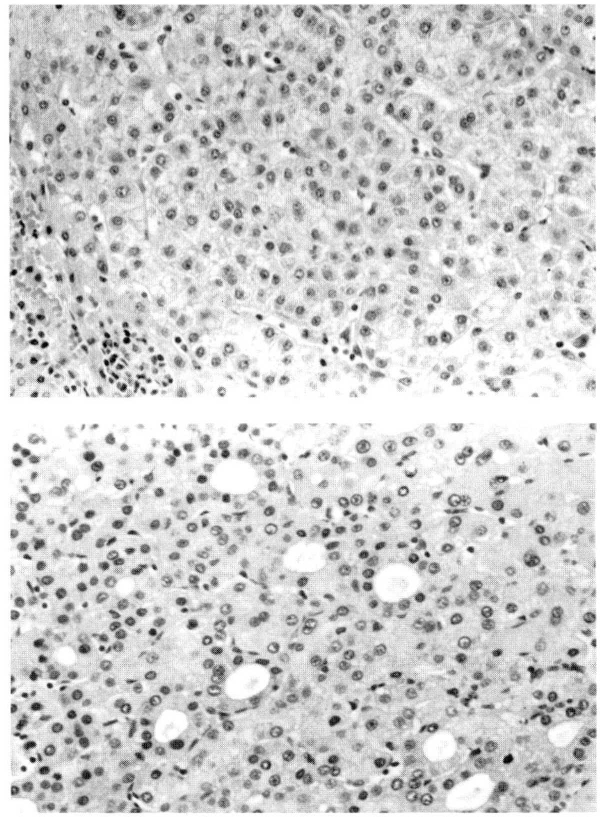

Fig. 3.7a,b. Macroregenerative nodule with HCC foci. **a** The cells of the nodule present mild distortion of cord structure as well as increased cellularity and N/C ratio. **b** The same nodule shows a focus of well-differentiated HCC with pseudoacinar formations. ×40

3.3.1.3 Borderline Lesions

In humans as well as in experimental models (Sell et al. 1991; Bannasch 1976), liver carcinogenesis seems to be a multistep process starting from hyperplastic nodules and reaching HCC via a continuous spectrum of lesions showing intermediate morphological features. In some lesions, the differential diagnosis between premalignant situations, expressed by cellular and/or structural atypia, and well-differentiated HCC (grade 1 on Edmondson's scale) is very difficult using routine histological procedures (Table 3.1). Acinar and trabecular arrangement, fibrosis, nuclear crowding, cytoplasm basophilia (Kondo et al. 1987,1989), Mallory bodies (Terada et al. 1989a; Nakanuma and Ohta 1985, 1986) and mitosis are the most common morphological criteria evaluated for early malignancy (Nonomura et al. 1990; Seki et al. 1990; Sano et al. 1989; Ganjey et al. 1988; Kuo et al. 1986; Govindarajan et al. 1990; Choen et al. 1986; Nagato et al. 1991; Kondo et al. 1988; Terasaki et al. 1991;Terada and Nakanuma 1991; Kenmochi et al. 1987). Nevertheless, a minimal combination of these aspects sufficient for a sure diagnosis of grade 1 HCC has yet to be established. Use of monoclonal antibodies such as Ki-67 (Grigioni et al. 1989), PCNA (Matsuno et al. 1990)

Table 3.1. Main pathological features of small nodular lesions involved in human hepatic carcinogenesis (cirrhotic patients)

Lesions	Common range of size (mm)	Nodule's tendency to enlarge	Small septa containing vessels and bile ducts	Foci of mild cellular or structural atypia	Foci of histologically proved HCC (grade II)	Fibrous stroma around the mass and compression of the sourrounding liver tissue	Fibrous capsule around the mass
CCN	1– 5	Absent	–	Absent	Infrequent	Fibrous stroma only	Absent
MRN type I	5–15	Absent	Present	Absent	Absent	Present	Absent
MRN type II	10–30	Present	Present	Present	Infrequent	Present	Absent
EL	10–20	Present	Absent	Present	Infrequent	Infrequent	Infrequent

CCN, common cirrhotic nodule; MRN, macroregenerative nodule; EL, equivocal lesion (possible HCC grade I); HCC, hepatocellular carcinoma; Grade, Edmondson's grade and bromodeoxiuridine (TARAO et al. 1989) seems to be promising in this respect. Cytochemistry of HCC tissue has yielded contrasting results, and in our experience its usefulness in evaluating the biology of borderline lesions is poor.

3.3.1.4
Minute Hepatocellular Carcinomas in Regenerative Nodules of Normal Size

Several Japanese authors (KONDO et al. 1983; KANAI et al. 1987; HIROOKA et al. 1990; NAKANUMA et al. 1986; FECHNER 1977) have reported minute HCCs (about 4 or 5 mm in diameter) without a background of AH, and also in our experience with Italian patients we have found very small HCCs lacking any apparent association with AH (GRIGIONI et al. 1989). These observations suggest the possibility of a direct transition from common cirrhotic nodules to HCC without an intermediate AH step. Both pathways (i.e. through the AH step and directly from a common cirrhotic nodule) are sometimes detected in the same liver, with the obvious diagnostic, therapeutic and prognostic implications. A comparison between the important frequency variations among different geographical areas regarding clinical morphological aspects and especially overall survival rates among HCC patients treated with the same procedures allows us to postulate that the different morphological pathways of HCC are related to different etiological and/or pathogenetic mechanisms involved in human liver carcinogenesis.

3.3.2
Non-Cirrhotic Liver

Precancerous conditions in non-cirrhotic liver are poorly defined. The main difficulties are the variable nomenclature referring to the same kinds of lesions investigated and the difficulty in distinguishing histologically hyperplastic benign liver lesions from hepatocellular adenoma, and the latter from well-differentiated carcinoma. In this way, some well-differentiated lesions can only be theoretically classified, and only after a long period of follow-up is it possible to verify the biological implications related to the original diagnosis.

3.3.2.1
Hepatocellular Adenoma

Hepatocellular adenoma (HCA) is a benign tumor of the liver that is often confused with focal nodular hyperplasia (FNH) or hamartoma (KERLING et al. 1983; GOLD et al.1978; ROOKS et al. 1979). It generally occurs in young women under the influence of oral contraceptives; a fact further corroborated by the detection of cytoplasmic progesterone receptors in the tumor cells and the occasional total regression of this tumor following discontinuation of the hormones (EDMONDSON 1976). These neoplasms have also been reported following anabolic androgen steroid therapy. Liver cell adenoma occurs in normal liver and usually ranges from a few cm to 15 cm or more in size (Fig. 3.8) (MARIANI et al. 1979; CHEN and BOCIAN 1983). Solitary HCAs normally do not display cytological atypias, while in HCAs some cellular and architectural abnormalities are frequently detected (Fig. 3.9) (LUI et al. 1980; SALISBURY and PORTMANN 1987). The magnitude of the risk for malignant transformation of both solitary and multiple HCAs has yet to be defined. Conflicting experiences have been reported and the percentage of malignancy ranges from 0% to 15%. A clear relationship between the number of HCA, their underlying etiologic factors and the risk of malignant transformation has been proposed.

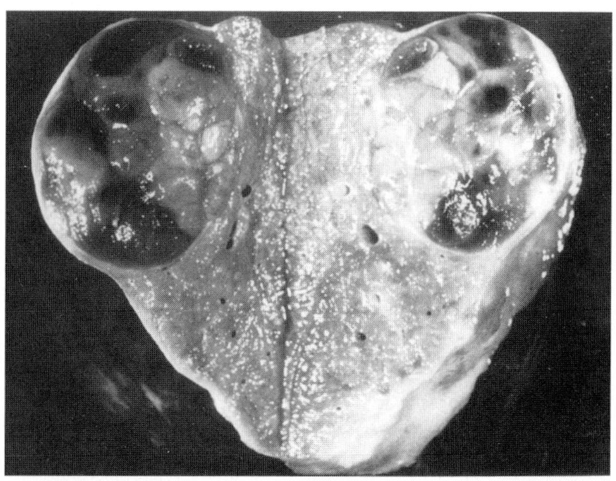

Fig. 3.8. Hepatocellular adenoma. A hepatocellular adenoma, resected in a 29-year-old woman, shows a widely hemorrhagic cut surface

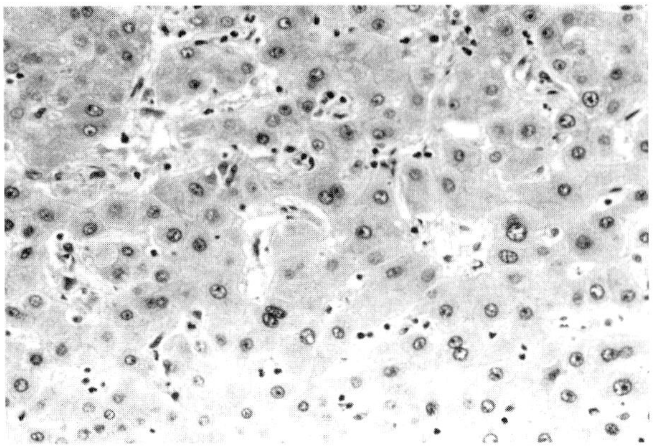

Fig. 3.9. Hepatocellular adenomatosis. Many multinucleate and pleomorphic hepatocytes are evident in this hepatocellular adenomatosis. Some cells show marked aspects of liver cell dysplasia. ×40

3.3.2.2 Hyperplastic Tumor-Like Lesions

FNH and nodular regenerative hyperplasia (NRH) are hyperplastic liver lesions with possible etiopathogenetic similarities. FNH is generally found in normal livers and appears as a single mass reaching less than 5 cm in size (Fig. 3.10). Histologically, FNH is composed of a mass of normal hepatocytes with a fibrous central stellate scar which divides the lesion into lobules (Gold et al. 1978; Stocker and Ishak 1981; Knowles and Wolff 1976; Vecchio et al. 1984). Cellular and/or structural atypia are highly exceptional, even though some authors have suggested that the fibrolamellar variant of hepatocellular carcinoma could represent the malignant counterpart of FNH (Strmeyer and Ishak 1981). NRH is a diffuse nodular lesion of the entire liver parenchyma (Fig. 3.11). Microscopically, the nodules are composed of normal hepatocytes arranged in liver plates two or three cells thick, compressing the peripheral parenchyma (Steiner 1959; Reynolds and Wanless 1984; Nakanuma et al. 1984; Sogaard 1981). Cytological and structural atypia and well-documented cases of HCC arising in NRH have been reported, suggesting that this lesion has a premalignant potential (Steiner 1959; Reynolds and Wanless 1984; Nakanuma et al. 1984; Sogaard 1981; Curry and Beattie 1996).

3.3.3 Conclusions

At present, it seems that the morphogenesis of human liver tumors can occur through different pathways. In non-cirrhotic liver, early development stages of HCC have been documented only in some hyperplastic tumor-like lesions, and the premalignant potentiality of various benign neoplastic lesions is not yet well defined. In cirrhotic liver, two morphological progressions in human carcinogenesis are well documented. Probably the most common progression pathway is via AH, which sometimes shows foci of cellular or structural atypia or clear-cut histologically proven HCC. A second possibility is a direct transition from common cirrhotic nodules to HCC without an intermediate step via AH. In some livers, both pathways are expressed.

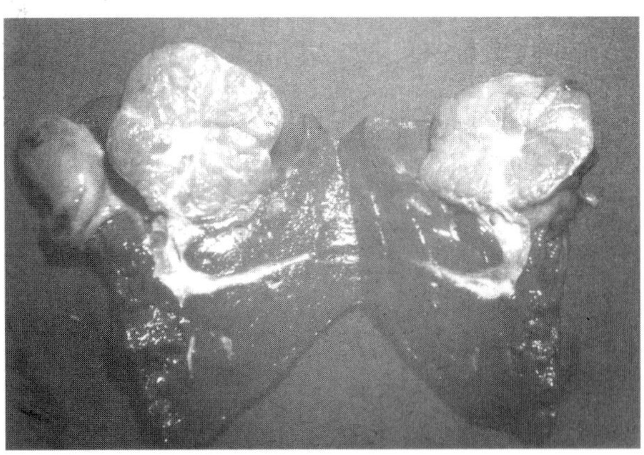

Fig. 3.10. Focal nodular hyperplasia. The cut surface of local nodular hyperplasia appears as a large, well-circumscribed mass with the typical central fibrous scar

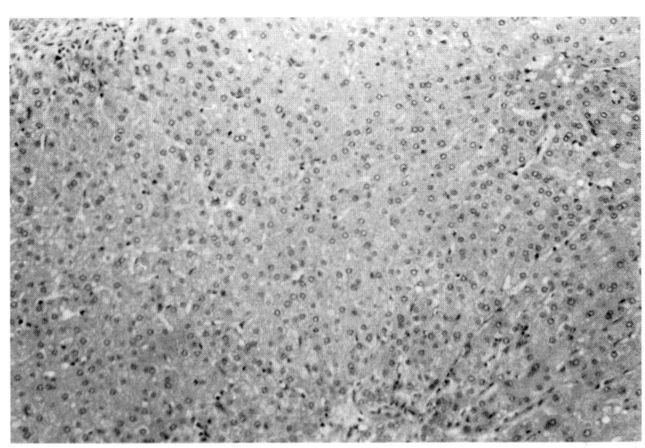

Fig. 3.11. Focal nodular hyperplasia. Microscopic aspect of focal nodular hyperplasia: *in the upper left corner*, thin fibrous septae with many small bile ductules are present. ×25

3.4 Molecular Markers

Epidemiologic and molecular studies suggest that at least three independent steps are required for the transformation of a normal hepatocyte into a neoplastic cell. It can be postulated that the genesis of HCC requires the activation of several oncogenes and the loss of two or more cancer suppressor genes (Buendia 1998). Liver carcinogenesis is therefore a multistep process involving DNA damage, fixation of mutation during cell proliferation, oncogene activation and loss of tumor suppressor genes function with malignant progression, regardless of the initiating cause (Hollstein et al. 1991).

The tumor suppressor gene p53 has been found to be abnormally expressed in a wide range of malignancies including HCC (Ozturk 1991). AFB1 is a well known mutagen and carcinogen which induces HCC. It has been found to be an important factor in inducing a high frequency of codon 249 mutation in the p53 gene. Experimentally, a high rate of p53 mutations was found in mice treated with AFB1, where a transversion mutation G→T is often observed on codon 247, as compared to codon 249 in humans (Lee et al. 1998). Independently of the 249 mutation, mutations and loss of heterozygosity in the p53 gene have been found in HBV-associated HCCs (Fujimoto et al. 1994; Ng et al. 1994). Overexpression of p53 has been described in some cirrhotic livers and in non-tumorous liver tissue from patients with HCC (Livni et al. 1995). This may indicate an abnormal or mutated p53 gene, which could precede development of HCC (Aguilar et al. 1994).

Mutational activation of the ras oncogene family occurs frequently in liver tumors in mice. Similar mutations have also been found in human HCCs (Ogata et al. 1991; Conte et al. 1994).

Other oncogenes such as c-myc and c-erb are also highly expressed during tumor development and progression. Although increased expression of proto-oncogenes is not necessary for cell proliferation, changes in oncogene expressions probably represent one of the multiple steps in HCC maintenance (Pascal et al. 1993; Ledda-Columbano et al. 1993).

Several growth factors have been implicated in liver carcinogenesis. Transforming growth factor β (TGF-β) levels are elevated in patients with HCC and increase tumor angiogenesis (Sun et al. 1955). Mesenchymal-epithelial interactions are also important in tumorigenesis. Kupffer cells play a central role in intrahepatic growth factor and cytokine production: the hepatic depletion of liver macrophages in cirrhosis may contribute to HCC development by altering the local production of growth factors and cytokines (Manifold et al. 1983; Kan et al. 1995).

In the last few years, molecular markers present in liver carcinogenesis have been characterized: although their functions have not yet become clear, their presence seems to indicate a higher risk of developing HCC. The markers most studied are silver staining nucleolar organizer regions (AgNORs) and the proliferating nuclear antigen (PCNA), an endogenous protein involved in the synthesis of the enzyme polymerase d, which is a marker for cellular proliferation (Metha 1995; Derenzini et al. 1993)

In summary, growing evidence supports a theory of liver carcinogenesis caused by multiple etiological agents via the dysregulation of biological signals and mechanisms controlling cell proliferation and death. To date, no molecular trigger has been identified, since most abnormalities seem only to aid tumor progression (Graham and Alistar 1996).

3.5 Primary Hepatic Tumors

Primary hepatic tumors are classified into three main groups: pseudo-tumoral lesions, benign lesions and malignant lesions. Neoplastic lesions are then distinguished into epithelial and mesenchymal ones on histogenetic grounds.

3.5.1 Benign Lesions

3.5.1.1 Pseudo-tumoral Lesions

3.5.1.1.1
Focal Nodular Hyperplasia

Focal nodular hyperplasia (FNH) is the most frequent benign hepatocellular lesion. Although it can occur in any age group, it is most often observed between the third and fifth decades of life (Berti et al. 1995). The male to female ratio is about 1:2.

Pathologic findings: FNH is a generally solitary, well circumscribed superficial lesion without a capsule, measuring 1–15 cm in diameter (on average around 5 cm). On cutting, a whitish depressed area of fibrosis can be seen in the center of the lesion with broad strands radiating to the periphery in a stellate configuration, dividing the lesion into nodules. Necrosis and hemorrhage are rare events.

Microscopically, all the components of the normal liver lobule are present, but there is not a true lobular structure: centrolobular veins may be completely obliterated and the nodular area can be supplied exclusively by peripheral enlarged sinusoids. Fibrous septa containing eccentrically thickened vessels and newly formed bile ducts converge on the central scar, which contains arteries with intimal hyperplasia, mural thickening and narrowing stenosis of the lumen in a dense connective tissue (Graig et al. 1989). Fat degeneration, PAS-diastase positive globules and Mallory bodies are sometimes seen. Mitosis and cellular atypia are rare events.

3.5.1.1.2
Biliary Hamartoma

This lesion, also known as von Meyenburg's or Moschowitz complex, is a fibrolipocystic disease of the liver and can be found in congenital hepatic fibrosis, Caroli's disease and polycystic autosomal dominant disease. Its detection is usually casual.

Pathologic findings: biliary hamartoma generally presents as multiple small whitish subcapsular nodules scattered throughout the liver. Microscopically, these nodules appear as a focal disorderly collection of bile ducts and ductules surrounded by abundant fibrous stroma: angles, ramifications and cystic dilatations are common. Isolated instances of malignant transformation have been reported (Lee 1994).

3.5.1.1.3
Macroregenerative Nodule

Macroregenerative nodules can arise on hepatic necrosis of any origin or on cirrhosis (in this case it is termed AH).

Pathologic findings: the lesion is composed of solitary or multiple nodules varying from 1 to 15 cm in size, which are found in the red-bluish necrotic liver stroma. It presents as an orange protruding nodule. Nodules arising in cirrhosis are usually green and their size is less than 3 cm.

Microscopically, the nodules look like the parenchymal nodules seen during cirrhosis: hepatocytes are arranged in two rows with connective septa containing bile ducts, vessels and various degrees of lymphocytic infiltration. Some nodules may present structural or cytological atypias and, in these cases, differential diagnosis with well-differentiated HCC is necessary. These latter lesions are also called type II macroregenerative nodules, atypical AH and borderline lesions, but it is still unclear whether they should be considered precancerous lesions (Okuda 1986; Grigioni et al. 1989).

3.5.1.1.4
Nodular Regenerative Hyperplasia

Nodular regenerative hyperplasia (NRH) indicates widespread hepatic nodules without fibrosis. NRH is a rare lesion detected by chance, and is associated with portal hypertension or other diseases such as Felty's syndrome.

Pathological findings: multiple whitish small nodules are present on the cut surface of the liver, which may be mistaken by the surgeon for metastatic carcinoma. Microscopically, they appear as nodules of hyperplastic hepatocytes arranged in multiple rows and surrounded by compressed atrophic parenchyma. Some authors have described rare cases with hepatocellular dysplasia and suggested this lesion may be precancerous (Wanless 1990).

3.5.1.1.5
Inflammatory Pseudotumor

Inflammatory pseudotumor is a benign lesion that can occur in either sex at any age.

Pathologic findings: the lesion is solitary, and varies in size from 2 to 25 cm in diameter. Microscopically, an inflammatory infiltration of spindle-shaped cells, foamy macrophages, lymphocytes and plasm cells presents around a central area composed of dense connective tissue (Horiuchi et al. 1990).

3.5.1.2 Benign Epithelial Lesions

3.5.1.2.1
Hepatocellular Adenoma

Hepatocellular adenoma (HCA) is a benign tumoral lesion that shows a predilection for females during the third to fifth decades of life.

Pathologic findings: HCA is usually a solitary subcapsular lesion measuring 5–15 cm in diameter. It displays a well-defined capsule and differs in its yellowish or hemorrhagic color from the surrounding liver (Fig. 3.12).

Microscopically, the hepatocytes appear normal or slightly enlarged, with pale or eosinophilic cytoplasm, and are organized in lamellae pervaded by sinusoids with compressed lumens. The lobular structure is not maintained and there are no portal fields or centrolobular veins. Vessels are thickened, and thrombi can sometimes cause hemorrhages, necrosis and scars. Mitoses and cellular atypias are infrequent (Kerlin et al. 1983). If there are more than four nodules the lesion is referred to as hepatic adenomatosis; in this case, structural and cytological

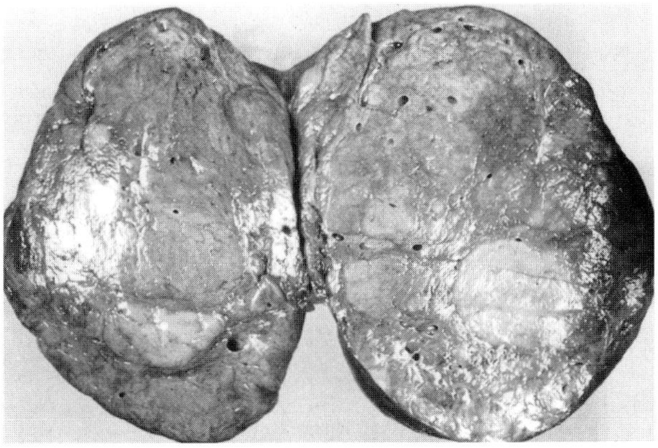

Fig. 3.12. Hepatocellular adenoma. A well circumscribed hepatocellular adenoma with bulging yellowish cut surface

abnormalities are often present (Lui et al. 1990; Salisbury and Portmann 1987). This latter lesion may have acinar structure, biliary pigments and slight atypia, and could be considered a precancerous lesion (Fig. 3.13) (Graig et al. 1989).

3.5.1.2.2
Bile Duct Adenoma
Bile duct adenoma is a rare benign tumor detected by chance which can be mistaken for metastatic carcinoma.

Pathologic findings: the lesion is generally solitary, subcapsular, less than 2 cm in diameter, well circumscribed and whitish with a dense central area. Microscopically, it is made up of small tubular structures with a virtual lumen, surrounded by cuboidal epithelium and fibrous stroma. In this lesion, inflammatory infiltration can be present.

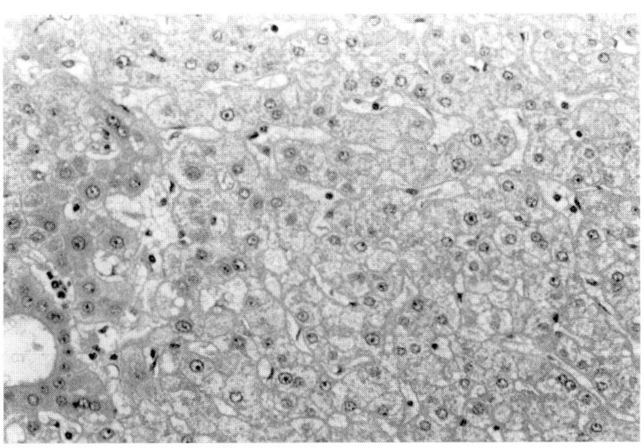

Fig. 3.13. Hepatocellular adenomatosis. Many multinucleated and pleomorphic hepatocytes are evident in this case of hepatocellular adenomatosis. Some cells show marked aspects of liver cell dysplasia. ×40

3.5.1.2.3
Biliary Cystadenoma
Biliary cystadenoma is a rare benign lesion which characteristically arises in women around 50 years old and is a cause of abdominal pain.

Pathologic findings: grossly, the lesions measure 2–25 cm, are multilocular and contain a mucinous or clear fluid. The tumors are lined by a single layer of cuboidal to tall columnar mucin-producing cells, which on occasion can be pseudostratified, polypoid, or papillary. The underlying layer of connective tissue is quite cellular and closely resembles ovarian stroma. This lesion may undergo malignant transformation, and if its excision is not complete, tends to recur.

3.5.1.2.4
Biliary Papillomatosis
Biliary papillomatosis is an extremely rare lesion characterized by a multicentric adenomatous proliferation of the biliary ducts. There are endoluminal brownish proliferations of the ducts which can be seen macroscopically. Microscopically, papillary biliary epithelium can be detected (Sternerg et al. 1994; Padfield et al. 1988).

3.5.1.3 Benign Mesenchymal Tumors

3.5.1.3.1
Hemangioma
Hemangioma is the most common benign tumor of the liver. It can arise at any age and in either sex. In most cases it is found incidentally.

Pathologic findings: the mass is usually solitary, smaller than 4 cm in diameter, and projects only slightly above the capsule. On cutting, a spongy appearance and dark red color are characteristic. Microscopically, it is constituted by widely dilated nonanastomotic vascular spaces lined by flat endothelial cells and supported by fibrous tissue. Thrombi in different stages of organization are often encountered. Hemangioma may become calcified, jalinized or ossified (Ishak 1988).

3.5.1.3.2
Rare Benign Mesenchymal Tumors
Altogether exceptional benign tumors include lipoma, fibroma, leiomyoma, lymphangiomatosis, chondroma, hemangioblastoma and mixoma.

3.5.2 Malignant Tumors

3.5.2.1 Malignant Epithelial Lesions

3.5.2.1.1
HEPATOCELLULAR CARCINOMA
Pathologic findings: HCC may present as a single large mass, as multiple nodules, or in the form of diffuse liver involvement. Some lesions are surrounded by a grossly distinct capsule. Tumors can measure from 1 to 30 cm in size (Fig. 3.14). Over the years, many macroscopic classifications have been proposed. The most widely used is Eggel's, which distinguishes three architectural patterns: massive, nodular and diffuse. More recent classifications are based on the growth pattern of the lesion and its connection with the surrounding parenchyma: whether it is expanding with sharp contours or infiltrating with undefined margins.

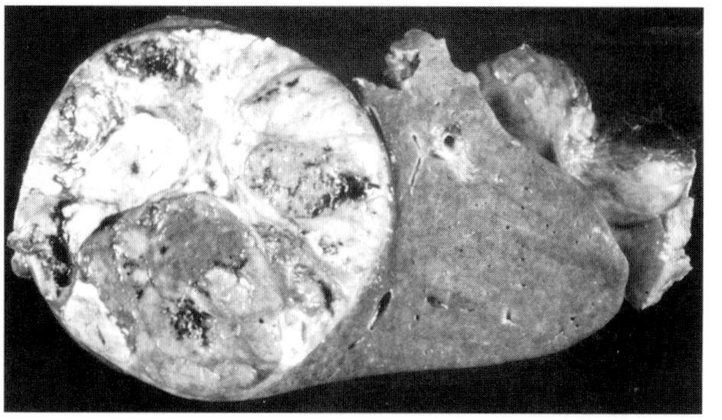

Fig. 3.14. Hepatocellular carcinoma. The pseudoadenomatous pattern of this hepatocellular carcinoma with extensive necrosis is a large mass and arose in a normal liver

Microscopically, HCC shows many variations, not only among different histologic types, but also within different fields of the same tumor. The principle architectural structure is trabecular, from which the other variants derive. The main variants are the pseudoglandular one, with enlargement of bile ducts or lysis at the center of the trabeculae, and the solid variety, in which the trabeculae are clustered together with compression of the sinusoids (Fig. 3.15). The transformed hepatocytes can be very similar to normal ones or quite undifferentiated. Cytologically, the cells can be classified as hepatocytic (the most frequent finding, with elements very similar to normal hepatocytes), clear cells, pleomorphic cells, giant cells, spindle cells or granular cells. Tumor differentiation is assessed in four grades according to Edmondson and Steiner's grading system. The tumor can be completely or partially capsulated, or may lack a capsule. Mallory's bodies, eosinophilic or PAS-positive intracytoplasmatic inclusions are frequent. The main histologic variants of HCC are: fibrolamellar, sclerosing, clear cell and sarcomatoid (GRAIG et al. 1989; MACSWEEN et al. 1987; COLOMBO 1992; CALLELA et al. 1992; OKUDA and ISHAK 1987).

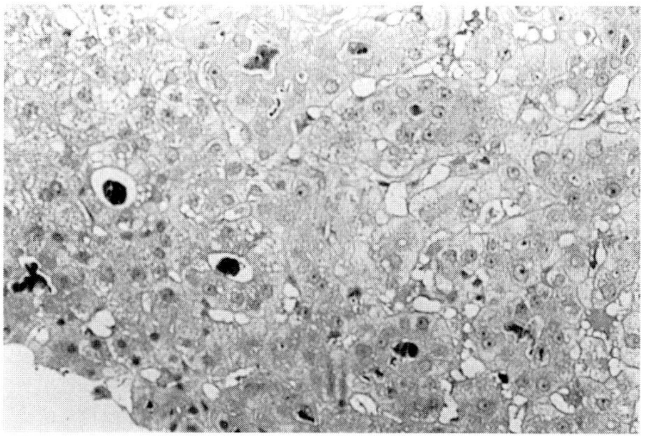

Fig. 3.15. Hepatocellular carcinoma. Microscopic aspect of trabecular hepatocellular carcinoma with nuclear atypia and bile production by tumor cells. +40

3.5.2.1.2
CHOLANGIOCELLULAR CARCINOMA
Cholangiocarcinoma is a malignant tumor arising from intra- or extrahepatic bile-duct epithelium or from hepatocytes. Intrahepatic cholangiocarcinomas are subdivided according to their location: of the hilus (Klatskin's tumor), of the central bile ducts, and peripheric.

Pathological findings: cholangiocarcinoma presents as a white-grayish solid mass from 2 to 15 cm in diameter, with undefined margins. Peripheric cholangiocarcinoma is seen as a single mass while the hilar and ductal varieties can be seen either as a single mass infiltrating the parenchyma, a mass surrounding a bile duct, or as a polyoid mass in the lumen of a bile duct. They usually arise in healthy livers, seldom in cirrhotic ones. The lesions have a scarlike appearance with a shiny central retraction.

Microscopically, the most common type is well-differentiated adenocarcinoma, showing glands with a small lumen; they are mucin producing (Klatskin's tumor) and are surrounded by abundant sclerotic tissue (Fig. 3.16). The possible variants of adenocarcinoma, all of which have been described, are: cystic, pleomorphic, papillary, signet-ring, and squamous

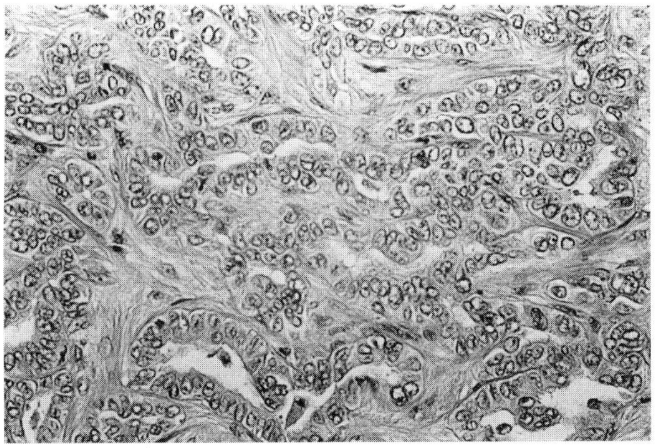

Fig. 3.16. Cholangiocarcinoma. Glandular structures grow in cellular nests, separated by fibrous stroma. ×40

differentiation. Cholangiocarcinoma disseminates both via the blood and lymphatically, infiltrating perineural, periductal and portal spaces (Nakajima et al. 1988; Ishak et al. 1984).

3.5.2.2
Malignant Mesenchymal Lesions

3.5.2.2.1
Angiosarcoma
This rare neoplasm is associated with exposure to radiation or some chemical agents. Most cases occur in elderly people, usually men. Prognosis is poor.

Pathologic findings: The entire liver is invaded by multiple spongy, white-grayish lumps of less than 5 cm, with well-defined margins. The tumor may occasionally present as a solitary lump. The non-neoplastic portion of the liver can be sclerotic or fibrotic.

Microscopically, malignant proliferating endothelial cells can be seen to line the walls of sinusoids or incompletely limited blood spaces. They proliferate into large clusters, sometimes forming pseudomasses, but without true cohesion. The cells are spindle-shaped with pale cytoplasm and pleomorphic or hyperchromatic nuclei. Frequent events are mitoses, thrombi and hemorrhages. The tumor also infiltrates the surrounding hepatic parenchyma, which can show hyperplasia, atrophy and fibrosis (Nakajima et al. 1988).

3.5.2.2.2
Epithelioid Hemangioendothelioma
This endothelial tumor mainly affects adult females. Its prognosis is favorable.

Pathologic findings: grossly the tumors are often multiple. The nodules are grayish, are smaller than 10 cm, and involve both hepatic lobes.

Microscopically, small groups of neoplastic endothelial cells infiltrate sinusoids and veins. The stroma, which is usually abundant, may have myxoid, sclerotic or calcifying features. The cells are plump, with an acidophilic cytoplasm that is often vacuolated. On the basis of the cytoplasm, hemangioendotheliomas can been classified as hepithelioid (with round cytoplasm) or dendritic (with starlike cytoplasm) (Lennert and Feller 1992).

3.5.2.2.3
Rare Malignant Mesenchymal Tumors
Primary sarcomas in the liver are exceptional and must be distinguished from metastatic tumors derived from sarcomas in other sites (particularly the retroperitoneum) and sarcomatoid liver cell carcinoma. Primary liver sarcomas arise in adults in the fifth or sixth decade of life, and have a poor prognosis (Ishak 1988; MacSween et al. 1987; Nakajima et al. 1988).

3.5.2.3
Malignant Lymphomas

The liver is a very infrequent primary site of malignant lymphoma (Lennert and Feller 1992). Most malignant lymphomas of the liver disseminate from other sites, frequently when the spleen is involved. Secondary involvement of the liver by non-Hodgkin's lymphomas or Hodgkin's disease is common in advanced stages.

References

Aguilar F, Harris CC, Sun T, Hollstein M, Cerutti P (1994) Geographic variation of p53 mutational profile in nonmalignant human liver. Science 264:1317–1319

Akagi G, Furuya K, Kanamura A, Chihara T, Otsuka H (1984) Liver cell dysplasia and hepatitis B surface antigen in liver cirrhosis and hepatocellular carcinoma. Cancer 54:315-320

Anthony PP (1987) Liver cell dysplasia: what is its significance? Hepatology 7:394-399

Anthony PP, Vogel CL Barker LF (1973) Liver cell dysplasia: premalignant condition. J Clin Pathol 26:217-220

Arakawa M, Kage M, Sugihara S, Nakashima T, Suenaga M, Okuda K. (1986a) Emergence of malignant lesions within an adenomatous hyperplastic nodule in a cirrhotic liver. Gastroenterology 91:198-202

Arakawa M, Kage M, Sugihara S, et al (1986) Small mass lesions in cirrhosis: transition from benign adenomatous hyperplasia to hepatocellular carcinoma. J Gastroenterol Hepatol 1:3-7

Bannasch P (1976) Cytology and cytogenesis of neoplastic (hyperplastic) hepatic nodules. Cancer Res 36:2555-2559

Bartok I, Remenar E, Toth J, Duschanek P, Kanyar B (1981) Clinicopathological studies of liver cirrhosis and hepatocellular carcinoma in a general hospital. Hum Pathol 12:794-798

Baur M, Hay U, Novaceck G, Dittrich C, Ferrenci P (1992) Prevalence of antibodies to hepatitis C virus in patients with hepatocellular carcinoma in Austria. Arch Virol 4(S):76-80

Beebe GW, Norman JE (1991) Study of the likelihood of hepatocellular carcinoma following the 1942 US Army epidemic of hepatitis B. In: Tabor E, Di Bisceglie AM, Purcell RH (eds) Etiology, Pathology and Treatment of Hepatocellular carcinoma in North America. Gulf Publishing Company, Houston, pp 3–15

Berti E, D'Errico A, Grigioni WF (1995) Classificazione delle neoplasie primitive epatiche nell'adulto. Il Fegato 1:5–10

Borzio M, Bruno S, Roncalli M,et al (1991) Liver cell dysplasia and risk of hepatocellular carcinoma in cirrhosis: a preliminary report. Br Med J 302:1312-1315

Bruix J, Barrera JM, Calvet X,et al (1989) Prevalence of antibodies to hepatitis C virus in Spanish patients with hepatocellular carcinoma and hepatic cirrhosis. Lancet 2: 1004–1006

Buendia MA. (1998) Hepatitis B viruses and cancerogenesis. Biomed and Pharmacother 52:34–43

Bukh J, Miller RH, Kew MC, Purcell RH (1993) Hepatitis C virus RNA in southern Africa blacks with hepatocellular carcinoma. Proc Natl Acad Sci USA 90:1848–1851

Callela F, Fabbretti G, Brisigotti M, et al (1992) Histological diagnosis of hepatocellular carcinoma. Ital J Gastroenterol 24:50–55

Caporoso N, Romano N, Marmo R (1991) Hepatitis C virus infection is an additive risk factor for development of hepatocellular carcinoma in patients with cirrhosis. J Hepatol 12:367–372

Caselmann WH, Meyer M, Kekule AS, Lauer U, Hofschneider PH, Koshy R (1990) A trans-activator function is generated by integration of hepatitis B virus preS/S sequences in human hepatocellular carcinoma DNA. Proc Natl Acad Sci USA 87:2970–2974

Chen KT and Bocian JJ (1983) Multiple hepatic adenomas. Arch Pathol Lab Med 107:274–276

Chen ML, Gerber MA, Thung SN (1984) Morphometric study of hepatocytes containing hepatitis B surface antigen. Am. J. Pathol. 114:217-222

Choen C, Berson SD (1986) Liver cell dysplasia in normal, cirrhotic, and hepatocellular carcinoma patients. Cancer 57:1535-1541

Choen C, Berson SD, Geddes EW (1979) Liver cell dysplasia. Association with hepatocellular carcinoma, cirrhosis and hepatitis B antigen carrier status. Cancer 44:1671-1679

Chou WH, Yoneyama T, Takeuchi K, Harada H, Saito J, Miyamura T (1991) Discrimination of hepatitis C virus in liver tissues from different patients with hepatocellular carcinomas by direct nucleotide sequencing of amplified cDNA of the viral genome. J Clin Microbiol 29:2860–2864

Cohen MB, Beckstead JH, Ferrel LD, Yen B.(1986) Enzyme histochemistry of hepatocellular neoplasms. Am J Surg Pathol 10:789-793

Colombo M, De Franchis R, Del Ninno E, et al (1991) Hepatocellular carcinoma in Italian patients with cirrohosis. N Engl J Med 325:675–680

Colombo M (1992) Hepatocellular carcinoma. J Hepatol 15:225–236

Colombo M, de Franchis R, Del Ninno E, Sangiovanni A, De Fazio C, Tommasini M, et al (1991) Hepatocellular carcinoma in Italian patients with cirrhosis. N Eng J Med 325:675–680

Conte D, Neri A, Fracchiolla NS, Croce LS, Lodi L, Fraquelli M, et al (1994) Analysis of p53 and *ras* gene mutations in hepatocellular carcinoma in Italy. Eur J Gastroenterol Hepatol 6:1005–1008

Craig, IR, Klatt, EC, Yu M (1991) Role of cirrhosis and the development of HCC: evidence from histologic studies and large population studies. In: Tabor E, Di Bisceglie AM, Purcell RH (eds) Etiology, Pathology, and Treatment of Hepatocellular carcinoma in North America. The Woodlands, New York, pp 103–109

Curry GW, Beattie AD (1996) Pathogenesis of primary hepatocellular carcinoma. Eur J Gastroenterology & Hepatology 8:850–855

Derenzini M, Trere' D, Olivieri F, et al (1993) Is high AgNOR quantity in hepatocytesassociated with increased risk of hepatocellular carcinoma in chronic liver disease? J Clin Pathol 36:727–729

Deugnier Y, Guyader D, Crantock L, Lopez J, Turlin B, Yaouanq J et al (1993) Primary liver cancer in genetic heamochromatosis: a clinical, pathological and pathogenetic study in 54 cases. Gastroenterology 104:228–234

Ebara M, Ohto M, Shinagawa T, et al (1986) Natural Histoty of minute hepatocellular carcinoma smaller than three centimeters complicating cirrhosis. A study in 22 patients. Gastroenterology 90:289-296

Edmondson HA (1976) Benign epithelial tumors and tumorlike lesions of the liver. In: Okuda K, Peters RL (eds) Hepatocellular carcinoma. Wiley, New York p 309-323

Evarts RP, Nakatsukasa H, Marsden ER, Hsia CC, Dunsford HA, Thorgeirsson SS (1990) Cellular and molecular changes in the early stages of chemical hepatocarcinogenesis in the rat. Cancer Res 50:3439-3445

Faber E, Sarma DSR (1987) Hepatocarcinogenesis: a dynamic cellular perspective. Lab Invest: 56:4-11

Faber E (1976) Hyperplastic areas, hyperplastic nodules and hyperbasophylic areas as putative precursor lesions. Cancer Res 36:2532-2541

Fattovich G, Giustina G, Schalm SW, Hadziyannis S, et al (1995) Occurrence of hepatocellular carcinoma and decompensation in Western European patients with cirrhosis type B. Hepatology 21:77–82

Fechner RE (1977) Benign hepatic lesions and orally administered contraceptives. Hum Pathol 8:255-261

Fujimoto Y, Hampton LL, Wirth PJ, Wang NJ, Xie JP, Thorgeirsson SS (1994) Alteration of tumor suppressor genes and allelic losses in human hepatocellular carcinomas in China. Cancer Res 54:281–285

Furuya K, Nakamura M, Yamamoto Y, Togei K, Otsuka H (1988) Macroregenerative nodule of the liver. A clinicopathologic study of 345 autopsy cases of chronic liver disease. Cancer 61:99-103

Ganjei SH, Nadji M, Albores-Saavedra J, Morales AR (1988) Histologic marker in primary and metastatic tumors of the liver. Cancer 62:1994-1997

Giannini A, Zampi G, Bartoloni F (1987) Morphogical precursors of hepatocellular carcinoma: a morphometrical analysis. Hepatogastroenterology 34:95-103

Gold JH, Guzman IJ, Rosai J (1978) Benign tumors of the liver. Pathologic examination of 45 cases. Am J Clin Pathol 70:6-14
Goopman JD, Cain LG, Kensler TW (1988) Aflatoxin exposure in human populations: measurements and relationship to cancer. CRC Crt Rev Toxicol 19: 113–145
Govindarajan S, Conrad A, Lim B, Valinluck B, Kim AM, Schmid P (1990) Study of preneoplastic changes of liver cells by immunohistochemical and molecular hybridization techniques. Arch Pathol Lab Med 114:1042-1047
Graham WC, Alistar DB (1996) Pathogenesis of primary hepatocellular carcinoma. Eur J Gastroenterol Hepatol 8:850–855
Graig JR, Peters RL, Edmondson HA (1989) Tumoers of the liver and intrahepatic bile ducts. AFIP 26
Grigioni WF, D'Errico A, Bacci F et al (1989) Small liver masses in cirrhotic patient. A pathological clue for the morphogenesis of human hepatocellular carcinoma. Acta Pathol Jpm 39:520–527
Grigioni WF, d'Errico A, Bacci F, Carella R, Mancini AM (1989) Small liver masses in cirrhotic patients. Acta Pathol Jpn 39:520-525
Grigioni WF, D'Errico A, Bacci F, Gaudio M, Mazziotti A, Mancini AM (1989) Primary liver neoplasm; evaluation of proliferative index using MoAb Ki 67. J Pathol 158:28-33
Grigioni WF, d'Errico A, Fortunato C, Cassisa A, Carella R, Mancini AM (1991) The morphogenenesis of human hepatocellular carcinoma. Ital J Gastroenterol 23:594-604
Henmi A, Uchida T, Shikata T (1985) Karyometric analysis of liver cell dysplasia and hepatocellular carcinoma. Evidence against precancerous nature of liver cell dysplasia. Cancer 55:2594-2599
Hirooka N, Nitta Y, Tsunoda T (1990) Microscopic incipient hepatocellular carcinoma found incidentally in a routine liver biopsy specimen. Hepatology 12:291–293
Ho JC, Wu PC, Mak TK (1981) Liver cell dysplasia in association with hepatocellular carcinoma, cirrhosis and hepatitis B surface antigen in Hong Kong: Int J Cancer 28:571-578
Hollstein M, Sidransky D, Vogelstein B, Harris CC (1991) p53 mutations in human cancers. Science 253:1708–1711
Horiuchi R, Uchida T, Koijima T, et al (1990) Inflammatory pseudotumor of the liver: clinicopathological study and rewiew of the literature. Cancer 65:1583–1590
Huang SN, Chisari FV, Strong (1995) Sustained hepatocellular proliferation precedes hepatocarcinogenesis in hepatitis B surface antigen transgenic mice. Hepatology 21:620–626
IARC Monogr Eval Carcinog Risks Hum (1993) Aflatoxins 56:245–395
Ishak KG, Sesterhenn IA, Goodman ZD et al (1984) Epitelioid hemangioendothelioma of the liver: a clinicopathological and follow-up study of 32 cases. Hum Pathol 15:839–852
Ishak KG (1988) Benign tumors and pseudotumoers of the liver. Appl Pathol 6:82–104
Johnson PJ (1996) The epidemiology of hepatocellular carcinoma. Eur J Gastroenterol Hepatol 8:845–849
Kagawa K, Deguchi T, Tomimasu H. (1984) Feulgen-DNA cytofluoremetry of the liver cell dysplasia (LCD) in the liver cirrhosis. Gastroenterology 81:82-87
Kan Z, Ivancev K, Lunderquist A, McCuskey PA, McCuskey RS, Wallace S (1995) *In vivo* microscopy of hepatic metastases: dynamic observation of tumor cell invasion and interaction with Kupffer cells. Hepatology 21:487–494
Kanai T, Hiroashi S, Upton MP, et al (1987) Pathology of small hepatocellular carcinoma. A proposal for a new gross classification. Cancer 60:810-819
Karhunen PJ, Penttila A (187) Preneoplastic lesions of human liver. Hepatogastroenterology 34:10-17
Kekule AS, Lauren U, Meyer M, Caselman VH, Hofschneider PH, Koshy R (1990) A trans-activator function is generated by integration of hepatitisB virus preS/S sequences in human hepatocelluar carcinoma DNA. Proc Nat Acad Sci USA 87: 2970–2974
Kenmochi K, Sugihara S, Koyiro M (1987) Relationship of histologic grade of hepatocellular carcinoma (HCC) to tumor size and demonstration of tumor cells of multiple different grades in single small HCC. Liver 7:18-23
Kerlin P, Davis GL, McGill DB, Weiland LH, Adson MA and Sheedy PF. (1983) Hepatic adenoma and focal nodular hyperplasia: clinicl, pathologic and radiologic features. Gastroenterology 84:994-1002
Kew MC, Popper H (1984) Relationship between hepatocellular carcinoma and cirrhosis. Semin Liver Dis 4: 136–145
Kim CM, Koike R, Saito I, Miyamura T, Jay G, (1991) HBx gene of hepatitis B virus induces liver cancer in transgenic mice. Nature 351:317–320
Kirby GM, Chemin I, Montesano R, Chisari FV, Lang, MA, Wild CP (1994) Induction of specific cytochrome p450 s involved in aflatoxin B1 metabolism in hepatitis B virus transgenic mice. Mol Carcinog 11:74–80
Knowles DM, Wolff M (1976) Focal nodular hyperplasia of the liver. A clinicopathologic study and review of the literature. Hum Pathol 7:533-539
Kondo F, Ebara M, Sugiura N (1990) Histological features and clinical course of large regenerative nodules: evaluation of their precancerous potentiality. Hepatology 12:592-602
Kondo F, Hirooka N, Wada K, Kondo Y (1987) Morphological clues for the diagnosis of small hepatocellular carcinomas. Virchows Arch A 411:15-22
Kondo F, Wada K, Kondo Y (1988) Morphometric analysis of hepatocellular carcinoma. Wirchows Archiv 413:425-431
Kondo F, Wada K, Nagato Y (1989) Biopsy diagnosis of well-differentiates hepatocellular carcinoma based on new morphologic criteria. Hepatology 9:751-758
Kondo Y, Niwa Y, Akikusa B, Takazawa K, Okabayashi A (1983) A histopathologic study of early hepatocellular carcinoma. Cancer 52:687-693
Kuo SH, Sheu JC, Chen DS, Sung JL, Lin CC, Hsu HC (1986) Cytophotometric measurements of nuclear DNA content in hepatocellular carcinomas. Hepatology 7:330-337
Lau JYN, Lai CL (1990) Hepatocarcinogenesis. Trop Gastroenterol. 11:9–24
Ledda-Columbano GM, Coni P, Simbula G, Zedda I, Columbano M (1993) Compensatory regeneration, mitogen-induced liver growth, and multistage chemical carcinogenesis. Environ Health Perspect 101:163–168
Lee CC, Liu JY, Lin JK, Chu JS, Shew JY (1998) p53 point mutation enhanced by hepatic regeneration in aflatoxin B1-induced rat liver tumors and preneoplastic lesions. Cancer Letters 125:1–7
Lee RG (1994) Diagnostic liver pathology. Mosby, St. Louis, pp 421–500
Lennert K, Feller AAC (1992) Histopathology of non-Hodgkin's lymphomas. Springer-Verlag, Berlin

Livni N, Eid A, Ilan Y, et al (1995) p53 expression in patients with cirrhosis with and without hepatocellular carcinoma. Cancer 75:2420–2426

Lui AF, Hiratzka LF, Hirose FM (1980) Multiple adenomas of the liver. Cancer 45:1001-1009

Mac Sween RNM, Anthony PP, Scheuer PJ (1987) Pathology of the liver. Churchill Livingstone, pp 574–645

Mangia A, Vallari D, Di Bisceglie A.M (1994) Use of confirmatory tests for hepatitis C viral infection in patients with hepatocellular carcinoma. J Med Virol 43:125–128

Manifold IH, Triger DR, Underwood JCE (1983) Kupffer-cell depletion in chronic liver disease: implications for hepatic carcinogenesis. Lancet 2:431–433

Mariani AF, Livingstone AS, Pereiras RV, Van Zuiden PE, Shiff ER (1979) Progressive enlargement of an hepatic cell adenoma. Gastroenterology 77:1319-1323

Matsuno Y, Hirohashi S, Furuya S, Sakamoto M, Mukai K, Shimosato Y (1990) Heterogeneity of proliferative activity in nodule-in-nodule lesions of small hepatocellular carcinoma. Jpn J Cancer Res 81:1137-1141

Mc Glynn KA, Rosvold EA, Lusthader ED,et al (1995) Susceptibility to hepatocellular carcinoma is associated with genetic variations in the enzymatic detoxification of aflatoxin B1. Proc Natl Acad Sci USA 14: 2384–2387

Mehta R (1995) The potential for the use of cell proliferation and oncogene expression as intermediate markers during liver carcinogenesis. Cancer Letters 93:85–102

Munoz N, Bosch X (1987) Epidemiology of hepatocellular carcinoma. In: Okuda K, Ishak KG (eds) Neoplasm of the liver, Vol I. Springer, Tokio, p 3

Nagasue N, Akamizu H, Yukaya H, Yuuki I (1984) Hepatocellular pseudotumor in the cirrhotic liver. Report of three cases. Cancer 54:2487-2491

Nagato Y, Kondo F, Kondo Y, Ebara M,Ohto M (1991) Histological and morphometrical indicators for a biopsy diagnosis of well-differentiated hepatocellular carcinoma. Hepatology 14:473-477

Nakajima T, Kondo T, Miyazaki M, et al (1988) A histopathological study of 102 cases of intrahepatic cholangiocarcinoma. Histologic classification and modes of spreading. Hum Pathol 19:1228–1234

Nakanuma Y, Ohta G (1985) Is Mallory body formation a preneoplastic change? A study of 181 cases of liver bearing hepatocellular carcinoma and 82 cases of cirrhosis. Cancer 55:2400-2405

Nakanuma Y and Ohta G (1986) Expression of Mallory bodies in hepatocellular carcinoma in man and its significance. Cancer 57:81-88

Nakanuma Y, Ohta G, Sasaki K (1984) Nodular regenerative hyperplasia of the liver associated with polyarteritis nodosa. Arch Pathol Lab Med 108:133-138

Nakanuma Y, Ohta G, Sugiura H, Watanabe K, Doishita K (1986) Incidental solitary hepatocellular carcinomas smaller than 1 cm in size found at autopsy: a morphologic study. Hepatology 6:631-637

Nakanuma Y, Terada T, Terasaki S, et al (1990) Atypical adenomatous hyperplasia in liver cirrhosis: low-grade hepatocellular carcinoma or bordeline lesions? Histopathology 17:27-32

Nakashima T, Okuda K, Kijoro M, Jimi A, Yamaguchi R, Sakamoto K (1983) Pathology of hepatocellular carcinoma in Japan: 232 consecutive cases autopsied in ten years. Cancer 51:863-867

Naumov NV, Chokshi S, Metivier E, Maerten G, Johnson PJ, Williams R (1994) HCV replication is an important factor for hepatocellular carcinoma development in patients with cirrhosis. Hepatology 20:285–289

Newberne PM, Butler WH (1969) Acute and chronic effects of aflatoxin on the liver of domestic and laboratory animals: a review. Cancer Res 29-236–250

Ng IO, Srivastava G, Chung LP, Tsang SW,Ng MM (1994) Overexpression and point mutations of p53 tumor suppressor gene in hepatocellular carcinomas in Hong Kong Chinese people. Cancer 74:30–37

Nishioka K, Watanabe J, Furuta S, et al (1991) A high prevalòence of antiboby to the hepatitis C virus in patients with hepatocellular carcinoma in Japan. Cancer 67:429–433

Nonomura A, Mizukami Y, Matsubara F, Nakanuma Y (1990) Identification of nucleolar organizer regions in non-neoplastic hepatocytes by the silver-staining technique. Liver 10:229-233

Ogata N, Kamimura T, Asakura H (1991) Point mutation, allelic loss and increased methylation of c-Ha-*ras* gene in human hepatocellular carcinoma. Hepatology 13:31–37

Ohno Y, Shiga J, Machinami R (1990) A histopathological analysis of five cases of adenomatous hyperplasia containing minute hepatocellular carcinoma. Acta Pathol Jpn 40:267-270

Ohta G, Nakanuma Y (1987)) Comparative study of the three nodular lesions in cirrhosis. Adenomatoid hyperplasia, adenomatoid hyperplasia with intermediate lesion, and small hepatocellular carcinoma. In: Okuda K, Ishak KG (eds) Neoplasm of the Liver. Springer-Verlag, Berlin, p 177

Oka H, Kurioka N, Kim K, et al (1990) Prospective study of early detection of hepatocellular carcinoma in patients with cirrhosis. Hepatology 12:680–687

Okita K, Kodama T, Haraka T (1977) Early lesions and development of primary hepatocellular carcinoma in man: association with hepatits B viral infection. Gastroenterol Jpn 12:51-55

Okuda K (1986) Early recognition of hepatocellular carcinoma. Hepatology 6:729-738

Okuda K, Ishak KG (1987) Neoplasms of the liver. Springer-Verlag, Berlin

Okuda K, Nakashima T, Obata T (1980) Hepatitis B virus and primary liver cell carcinoma In: Bianchi L, Gerok W, Sickinger K (eds) Virus and the liver. MTP Press, Lancaster, p 209

Okuda,K, Nakashima T, Sakamoto K (1982) Hepatocellular carcinoma arising in noncirrhotic and highly cirrhotic livers: a comparative study of histopathology and frequency of hepatitis B markers. Cancer 49:450-456

Okuda K, Nakashima T, Koijro M, Kondo Y, Wada K (1989) Hepatocellular carcinoma whithout cirrhosis in Japanese patients. Gastroenterology 97:140–145

Okuno H, Xie ZC, Lu BY, et al (1994) A low prevalence of anti-hepatitis C virus antibody in patients with hepatocellular carcinoma in Guangxi Province, Southern China. Cancer 73:58–62

Omata M, Mori J, Yokosuka O, Iwama S, Ito Y, Okuda K (1982) Hepatitis B virus antigens in liver tissue in hepatocellular carcinoma and advanced chronic liver disease. Relatioship to liver cell dysplasia. Liver 2:125-130

Ozturk M (1991) p53 mutation in hepatocellular carcinoma after aflatoxin exposure. Lancet 338:1356–1359

Padfield CJH, Ansell ID, Furness PN (1988) Mucinous biliary papillomatosis: a tumour in need of wider recognition. Histopathology 13:687–694

Pascale RM, Simile MM, Feo F (1993) Genomic abnormalities in hepatocarcinogenesis. Implications for a chemo-preventive strategy. Anticancer Research 13:1341–1356

Paterlini P, Poussin K, Kew M, Franco D, Brechot C (1995) Selective accumulation of the X trancript of hepatitis B virus in patients negatyive for hepatitis B surface antigen with hepatocellular carcinoma. Hepatology 21:313–321

Paterson AC, Kew MC, Duskeiko GM, Isaacson C (1989) Liver cell dysplasia accompanying hepatocellular carcinoma in southern Africa. Differences between urban and rural populations. J Hepatol 8:241-245

Podda M, Roncalli M, Battezzati PM, et al (1992) Liver cell dysplasia and hepatocellular carcinoma. Ital J Gastroenterol 24:39-43

Popper H (1979) Hepatocellular carcinoma: old and new problems. In: Davidson CS (ed) Problems in liver diseases. Georg Thieme, Stuttgart, chap. II

Propst T, Propst A, Dietze O, Judmayer G, Braunsteiner H, Vogel W (1994) Prevalence of hepatocellular carcinoma in alpha-1-antitrypsin deficiency. J Hepatol 21:1006–1011

Reynolds WJ, Wanless IR (1984) Nodular regenerative hyperplasia of the liver in a patient with rheumatoid vasculitis: a morphometric study suggesting a role for hepatic arteritis in the pathogenesis. J Rheumatol 11:838-843

Roncalli M, Borzio M, De Biagi G, et al (1985) Liver cell dysplasia and hepatocellular carcinoma: a histological and immunohistochemical study. Histopathology 9:209-213

Roncalli M, Borzio M, De Biagi G, et al (1986) Liver cell dysplasia in cirrhosis. A serologic and immunohistochemical study. Cancer 57:1515-1519

Roncalli M, Borzio M, Tombesi MV, Ferrari A, Servida E (1988) A morphometric study of liver cell dysplasia. Hum Pathol 19:471-476

Roncalli M, Borzio M, Brando B, Colloredo G, Servida E (1989) Abnormal DNA content in liver cell dysplasia: a flow cytometric study. Int J Cancer 44:204-210

Rooks JB, Org HW, Ishack KG (1979) Epidemiology of hepatocellular adenoma. The role of oral contraceptive use. JAMA 242:644-649

Ross RK, Yuan JM, Yu MC, et al (1992) Urinary aflatoxin biomarkers and risk of hepatocellular carcinoma. Lancet 339:943–946

Sakamoto M, Hirohashi S, Shimosato Y (1991) Early stages of multi-step hepatocarcinogenesis: adenomatous hiperplasia and early hepatocellular carcinoma: Hum. Pathol 22:172-176

Salata H, Cortes JM, de Salamanca RE, et al (1985) Porphiria cutanea tarda and hepatocellular carcinoma. J Hepatol 1:477–487

Salisbury JR, Portmann BC (1987) Oncocytic liver cell adenoma. Histopathology 11:533-537

Sano K, Fujioka Y, Nagashima K, et al (1989) Distributional variation of P-450 immunoreactive hepatocytes in human liver disorders. Hum Pathol 20:1015-1019

Schirmacher P, Held WA, Yang D, Biempica L, Rogler CE (1991) Selective amplification of periportal transitional cells precedes formation of hepatocellular carcinoma in SV40 large tag transgenic mice. Am J Pathol 139:231-237

Seki S, Sakaguchi H, Kawakita N, et al (1990) Identification a fine structure of proliferating hepatocytes in malignant and nonmalignant liver diseases by use of monoclonal antibody against DNA polymerase alpha. Hum Pathol 21:1020-1026

Sell S (1990) Is there a liver stem cell? Cancer Res 50:3811-3817

Sell S, Dunsford HA (1989) Evidence for the stem cell origin of hepatocellular carcinoma and cholangiocarcinoma. Am J Pathol 134:1347-1351

Sell S, Hunt JM, Dunsford HA, Chisari FV (1991) Synergy between hepatitis B virus expression and chemical hepatocarcinogens in transgenic mice. Cancer Res 51:1278-1282

Shafritz DA, Kew MC (1981) Identification of integrated hepatitis B virus DNA sequences in human hepatocellular carcinomas. Hepatology 1:1–3

Shafritz DA, Shouval D, Sherrnan HI, Hadziyannis SJ, Kew MC (1981) Integration of hepatitis B virus DNA into the genome of liver cells in chronic liver disease and hepatocellular carcinoma. Studies in percutaneous liver biopsies end post-mortem tissue specimen. N Enl J Med 305;1067–1073

Sheu JC, Shung JL, Chen DS, et al (1985) Early detection of hepatocellular carcinoma by real-time ultrasonograghy. A prospective study. Cancer 56:660–666

Shinagawa T, Ohto M, Kimura K, et al (1984) Diagnosis and clinical features of small hepatocellular carcinoma with emphasis on utility of real time ultrasonography. A study in 51 patients. Gastroenterology 86:495–499

Simonetti RG, Camma C, Fiorella F, et al (1992) Hepatitis C virus infection as a risk factor for hepatocellular carcinoma in patients with cirrhosis. Ann Intern Med 116:97–102

Slagle BL (1995) p53 mutations and hepatitis B virus: cofactors in hepatocellular carcinoma. Hepatology 21:597–599

Sogaard PE (1981) Nodular transfomation of the liver, alphafetoprotein and hepatocellular carcinoma. Hum Pathol 12:1052-1058

Spandau DF, Lee CH (1988) Trans-activation of viral enhancers by the hepatitis B virus X protein. J Virol 62: 427–434

Srivatanakul P, Parkin DM, Khlat M, et al (1991) Liver Cancer in Thailand: II. A case control study of hepatocellular carcinoma. Int J Cancer 48: 329–332

Stal P, Hulcrantz R, Moller L, Eriksson LC (1995) The effects of dietary iron on initiation and promotion in chemical hepatocarcinogenesis. Hepatology 21:521–528

Steiner PE (1959) Nodular regenerative hyperplasia of liver. Am J Pathol 35:943-946

Sternerg SS, Antonioli DA, Carter D, et al (1994) Diagnostic surgical pathology. Raven Press 2:1517–1580

Stoker JT, Ishak KG (1981) Focal nodular hyperplasia of the liver: a study of 21 pediatric cases. Cancer 48:336-339

Strmeyer FW, Ishak KG (1981) Nodular transformation (nodular "regenerative" hyperplasia) of the liver. A clinicopathologic study of 30 cases. Hum Pathol 12:60-63

Sun D, Kar S, Carr BI (1955) Differentially expressed genesis in TGF-beta1 sensitive and resistant human hepatoma cells. Cancer Letters 89:73–79

Suwangol P, Jimarkorn P (1980) Liver cell dysplasia in cirrhosis and liver cell carcinoma. J Med Assoc Thailand 63:382-386

Tabarin A, Boulac-Sage P, Boussarie L, Balabaud C, de Mascarel A,Grimaud J.A (1987) Hepatocellular carcinoma developed on non-cirrhotic livers. Sinusoids in hepatocellular carcinoma. Arch Pathol Lab Med 111:174-177

Takayama T, Makuuchi M, Hirohashi S, et al (1990) Malignant transformation of adenomatous hyperplasia to hepatocellular carcinoma. Lancet 336:1150-1157

Tarao K, Shimuzu A, Herada M (1989) Difference in the vitro uptake of bromodeoxiuridine between liver cirrhosis with and without hepatocellular carcinoma. Cancer 64:104-108

Terada T, Nakanuma Y (1989a) Iron-negative foci in siderotic macroregenerative nodules in human cirrhotic liver. A marker of incipient neoplastic lesions. Arch Pathol Lab Med 113:916-919

Terada T, Nakanuma Y (1989b) Survery of iron-accumulative macroregenerative nodules in cirrhotic livers. Hepatology 10:851-856

Terada T, Nakanuma Y (1991) Expression of ABH blood group antigens. Receptors of *Ulex Europaeus* agglutinin-1, and factor VIII-related antigen on sinusoidal endothelial cells in adenomatous hyperplasia in human cirrhotic livers. Hum Pathol 22:486-489

Terada T, Hoso M, Nakanuma Y (1989a) Mallory body clustering in adenomatous hyperplasia in human cirrhotic livers: report of four cass. Hum Pathol 20:886-889

Terada T, Nakanuma Y, Hoso M, Saito K, Sasaki M, Nonmura A. (1989b) Fatty macroregenerative nodule in non-steatotic liver cirrhosis. Virchows Arch. 415:131-134

Terada T, Kadoya M, Nakanuma Y, Matsui O (1990) Iron-accumulating adenomatous hyperplastic nodule with malignant foci in the cirrhotic liver. Histopathologic, quantitative iron, and magnetic resonance imaging in vitro studies. Cancer 65:1994-1999

Terasaki S, Terada T, Nakanuma Y, Nonomura A, Unoura M, Kobayashi K. (1991) Argyrophilic nucleolar organizer regions and alpha-fetoprotein in adenomatous hyperplasia in human cirrhotic livers. Am J Clin Pathol 95:850-854

Toshkov I, Chisari VF, Bannasch P (1994) Hepatic preneoplasia in hepatitis B virus transgenic mice. Hepatology 20:1162–1172

Tsuda H, Hirohashi S, Shimosato Y, Terada M, Hasegawa H (1988) Clonal origin of atypical adenomatous hyperplasia of the liver and clonal identity with hepatocellular carcinoma. Gastroenterology 95:1664-1667

Twu JS, Schloemer R.H (1987) Transcriptional trans-activating function of hepatitis B virus. J Virol 61:3448–3453

Uchida T, Miyata H, Shikata T (1981) Human hepatocellular carcinoma and putatyive precancerous disoders. Arch Pathol Lab Med 105:180-183

Vecchio FM, Fabiano A, Manna R, Massi G (1984) Fibrolamellar carcinoma of the liver: the malignant counterpart of focale nodular hyperplasia with oncocytic change. Am J Clin Pathol 81:521-524

Wada K, Kondo F, Kondo Y (1988) Large regenerative nodules and dysplastic nodules in cirrhotic livers: a histopathologic study. Hepatology 8:1684-1686

Wands JR, Blum HE (1991) Primary hepatocellular carcinoma. N Engl J Med 325:729-731

Wanless IR (1990) Micronodular transformation (nodular regenerative hyperplasia) of the liver: a report of 64 cases among 2500 autopsies and a new classification of hepatocellular nodules. Hepatology 11:787–797

Watanabe S, Okita K, Harada T, et al (1983) Morphologic studies of the liver cell dysplasia. Cancer 51:2197-2199

Yaiginuma H, Kobayashi H, Kobayashi M, et al (1987) Multiple integration site of hepatitis B virus DNA in hepatocellular carcinoma and chronic active hepatitis tissues from children. J Virol 61:1808–1813

Zeman SN, Melia WM, Johnson RD, Johnson PJ, Williams R (1985) Risk factors for the development of hepatocellular carcinoma in cirrhosis. A prospective study of 613 patients. Lancet 1:1357–1360

4 Epidemiology and Clinical Features of Hepatocellular Carcinoma

L. Bolondi, L. Masi, and P. Pini

CONTENTS

4.1 Epidemiology of Hepatocellular Carcinoma

4.1.1 Introduction

Hepatocellular carcinoma (HCC) is the most frequent malignant tumor of the liver. Worldwide, HCC is the seventh most common form of cancer in males and the ninth in females (Parkin et al. 1984): some 310000 to 1 million new cases occur each year (Parkin et al. 1992; Terry 1978).

There are variations in its frequency in different geographical areas; thus, it is the most common malignant tumor among males in western, middle and eastern Africa, the second most common in southern Africa and Southeast Asia, and the third most common among males in China. It is a relatively rare tumor in most parts of America, Europe, northern Africa and middle and eastern Asia (Parkin et al. 1984).

There are various risk factors that contribute to the development of HCC. These risk factors are different in different areas. During the last few decades a series of epidemiological and laboratory investigations have established an association between hepatitis B virus and HCC. There are laboratory and epidemiological studies indicating that aflatoxin plays an important role in the development of HCC in certain areas. Hepatitis C virus (HCV) infection is now recognized to be a major risk factor for HCC, evidenced by epidemiological and molecular studies.

4.1.2 Geographical Distribution

In many countries information on incidence is derived from a limited number of cancer registries, and only then is it possible to classify countries into broad risk categories. Despite these sources of inaccuracy, HCC has a peculiar geographic distribution. We can distinguish high risk areas (sub-Saharan Africa, Southeast Asia and China) with incidence rates of more than 20 per 100000 of the population per annum; intermediate risk areas (Japan and southern Europe) with incidence rates of 10–20 per 100000 of the population per annum and low risk areas (England, North and South America, Scandinavia, India and Australia) with incidence rates of less than 5 per 100 000 of the population per annum.

The incidence rate has increased substantially in Japan during the past three decades (Bosch and Munoz 1995), and slight increases have been recorded in a number of European countries, in some parts of North America and in Israel, India, and Puerto Rico (Parkin et al. 1992; Bosch and Munoz

L. Bolondi, MD; Professor and Chairman, Department of Internal Medicine, S. Orsola Malpighi Hospital, University of Bologna, Via Massarenti 9, I-40138 Bologna, Italy
L. Masi, MD; Department of Internal Medicine, S. Orsola Malpighi Hospital, University of Bologna, Via Massarenti 9, I-40138 Bologna, Italy
P. Pini, MD; Department of Internal Medicine, S. Orsola Malpighi Hospital, University of Bologna, Via Massarenti 9, I-40138 Bologna, Italy

1995). Some of these increases may be apparent rather than real, being attributable to changes over time in the composition of population or to increased efficiency of diagnosis.

Although mortality is a good indicator of incidence, considering the very poor survival in HCC, it also has serious limitations, particularly as a considerable proportion of cases are registered in national records as liver cancer of unspecified origin. Worldwide, mortality for HCC is actually 4% (WHO 1982).

4.1.3 Sex and Age Distribution

Men are generally more susceptible than women to HCC. The male/female ratio is 4/1. This higher proportion of males to females is especially evident among populations of high risk areas; moreover, this predominance is less marked in the low-risk populations of America and Europe. In patients in developed countries who have hepatocellular carcinoma but not cirrhosis, the sex distribution is approximately equal. The high occurrence of HCC in males could be explained by a higher susceptibility, genetic or acquired, or by a higher exposure to the environmental factors associated with HCC.

In all populations, independent of risk, the incidence rates increase progressively with age. In high risk populations, there is a shift toward the younger age group and the tumor is not infrequently seen in patients under 40 years of age. On the contrary, this phenomenon does not occur in populations with intermediate or low rates. Age at exposure to suspected risk factors might explain the higher differential in risk observed in the younger age-groups between high- and low-incidence populations. HCC is rare in children (Shorter et al. 1960).

4.1.4 Studies on Migrants

Persons who migrate from countries with a low incidence to those with a high incidence usually retain the low risk of their country of origin, even after several generations in their new environment (Parkin et al. 1992). The consequences for immigrants from countries with high incidence to countries where incidence is low differ, depending on the major risk factors for HCC in their country of origin and on whether hepatitis B virus infection, if this is the major risk factor, is acquired predominantly by the perinatal or the horizontal route (Parkin et al. 1992; Kew et al. 1986, 1987).

4.1.5 Risk Factors

Hepatocarcinogenesis is a complex incremental process that evolves over many years. Four major (and several minor) causal associations of the tumor have been identified, as shown in Table 4.1.

Table 4.1. Risk factors for HCC in humans

Major
Chronic HBV infection
Chronic HCV infection
Repeated exposure to aflatoxin b_1
Cirrhosis
Minor
Oral contraceptive steroids
Cigarette smokings
Hereditary hemochromatosis
Wilson's disease
α_1-Antitrypsin deficiency
Type I hereditary tyrosinemia
Glycogen storage disease (types 1 and 2)
Ataxia telangiectasia

4.1.5.1 Hepatitis B Virus

Several epidemiological studies and laboratory investigations have established that there is a strong and specific association between HBV and HCC. This association is restricted to the chronic HBV infection, characterized by the presence of HBsAg in the serum of patients.

Epidemiological Data. Chronic infection with HBV may cause as much as 80% HCC. Although an association between the virus and the tumor has been demonstrated in all populations, it is closest in ethnic Chinese and black Africans, as many as 80% of whom are still infected when they develop HCC (Beasley et al. 1982; Kew 1981).

Three types of epidemiological studies have been conducted:

- Correlation studies: These studies have demonstrated that there is a positive correlation between mortality from HCC and prevalence of

HBsAg (SZMUNESS 1978; MUNOZ and LINSELL 1982). Thus, those countries with a high prevalence of HBsAg (Southeast Asia and sub-Saharan Africa) also have the highest rates of HCC and populations with low rates of HCC (America and Europe) also have low prevalence rates of HBsAg carriers. An exception to this general pattern is represented by the Greenland Eskimo population, in which there is a high prevalence of HBsAg carriers and a low incidence rate of HCC.

- Case-control studies: These studies have shown that in the high-risk and in intermediate-risk populations the relative risk (RR) associated with the presence of HBsAg ranges from 10 to 20 (PRINCE et al. 1975; KEW et al. 1979; LAM et al. 1982; YEH et al. 1985; LINGAO et al. 1981; TRICHOPOPOULOS et al. 1987).
  On the contrary, the RR is higher in the low-risk populations, where the prevalence rates of HBsAg in the control population are very low.
- Cohort studies: These studies have compared the occurrence of HCC among HBsAg carriers with that of a noncarrier control population, demonstrating that the HBV infection precedes the development of HCC.

Indirect evidence that HBV infection precedes HCC is derived from the analysis of age-specific prevalence curves of HBsAg carriers in high-risk populations for HCC, showing a peak in the first decade of life (SZMUNESS et al. 1973). In this population, HBV perinatal infection could be one of the crucial factors in determining the risk of developing HCC. The high prevalence of HBsAg carriers in childhood among high-risk populations could explain the relatively common occurrence of HCC in younger age-groups in these populations.

In addition, sex distribution provides further epidemiological evidence of developing HCC on chronic HBV infection. The higher prevalence rates of HBsAg carriers among males fit quite well with the fact that males are more susceptible than females to developing HCC.

Laboratory Studies. The first studies were on the oncogenicity of the Hepadnaviridae virus family, to which HBV belongs. These studies demonstrated that Eastern woodchucks infected with these oncoviruses develop HCC within 2 years of infection. Similar outcomes have been obtained with Beechey ground squirrels infected with ground squirrel hepatitis virus (GERIN et al. 1991; MARION et al. 1987).

HBV DNA is integrated into cellular DNA in about 95% of patients with HBV-related tumors (ROBINSON 1992). The mechanism of viral involvement remains unclear. Evidence is accumulating, however, that both direct and indirect carcinogenic effects are operative.

Both the X gene (KIM et al. 1990) and the 3' truncated preS/S gene (KEKULE et al. 1990) have transactivating properties; the introduction of the preS/S gene into DNA of transgenic mice induces the development of HCC in the absence of chronic necroinflammatory hepatic disease. Integration also perturbs the function of cellular oncogenes and tumor suppressor genes, contributing to hepatocellular carcinogenesis (KEW 1996). Recently it has been demonstrated that pX (the product of the X gene) can interact with p53 protein, possibly interfering with its antitumor action (p53 is an important factor acting on regulation of apoptosis) (WANG et al. 1994; SHAFRITZ et al. 1981).

In addition, by increasing the cell turnover rate, chronic or recurring cycles of hepatocyte necrosis and regeneration induced by the virus may act as a promoter of hepatocarcinogenesis: the DNA of dividing cells is more susceptible to spontaneous mutation and to exogenous damage and there is insufficient time to repair damage DNA before the cell divides again, thus fixing the altered DNA in the progeny.

4.1.5.2 Hepatitis C Virus

Hepatitis C virus infection is now recognized to be a major risk factor for HCC, evidenced both by epidemiological and molecular studies (DI BISCEGLIE 1997).

HCV-related HCC appears to be most prevalent in areas with an intermediate risk for HCC, such as Europe and Japan, whereas in countries where HCC is most common, infection with the hepatitis B virus is the dominant cause of HCC.

Thus, in Japan, Italy and Spain, chronic HCV infection is the major risk factor for HCC, antibody to the virus or viral RNA being detected in the serum of as many as 83% of patients (KEW 1994). Not all countries in southern Europe are the same in this regard: in Greece, for instance, fewer than 20% of patients with HCC were found to be anti-HCV positive (HADZIYANNIS et al. 1995). A far smaller percentage of ethnic Chinese and black African patients have HCV-induced tumors, and in other countries HCV and HBV appear to account for a small but equivalent proportion of patients. It is not known if HBV and HCV interact in the hepatocarcinogenesis; patients with HCV-induced tumors are substantially older than those with HBV-induced tumors (KEW 1994).

The precise mechanism by which HCV infection results in HCC is not known. HCV acts as an indirect carcinogen by inducing chronic necroinflammatory hepatic disease, as confirmed by the fact that all reported HCV-related HCC have arisen in cirrhotic liver (KEW 1994).

HCV is an RNA virus and so its genome does not seem to become integrated in the host DNA. It has been noted recently that the HCV core protein has some potential direct carcinogenic effects in vitro (RAY et al. 1996a,b); several investigators have suggested that genotype 1b is associated with an increased risk of HCC compared with other genotypes (SILINI et al. 1996; TANAKA et al. 1996). This association between HCV genotypes 1b and HCC is not confirmed by a recent, longitudinal study conducted in Italy (BENVEGNU et al. 1997).

Because not all patients with HCV infection develop HCC, efforts have been aimed at determining which patients are at particular risk. Alcohol consumption appears to significantly worsen the course of chronic hepatitis C, perhaps accelerating the development of cirrhosis. In a study of patients with established cirrhosis (KEW et al. 1997), the 10-year rate of HCC was 19% in those with cirrhosis caused by alcohol alone, 57% in those with HCV-related cirrhosis, and 81% among those with HCV infection who consumed more than 120 g alcohol per day. Thus, it seems that alcohol consumption may both accelerate the development of cirrhosis and the appearance of HCC after cirrhosis is established.

4.1.5.3 Aflatoxins

Aflatoxins are mycotoxins elaborated by *Aspergillus flavus*, a ubiquitous fungus contaminating many staple foodstuffs in tropical and subtropical regions. There are four major members of this group (aflatoxins β_1, β_2, γ_1 and γ_2). Aflatoxin β_1 is a major risk factor for HCC in certain geographic regions (NEWBERNE 1984).

Epidemiologic correlations studies have shown a positive correlation between exposure to this mycotoxin and the incidence of HCC (NEWBERNE 1984; ROSS et al. 1992). Each of them indicates that incidence of HCC rises with the increase of aflatoxin in the diet.

In the Philippines, assessment of aflatoxin exposure was attempted using a dietary recall questionnaire and a table which provided measurements of aflatoxin in the local foodstuffs. In cases of HCC, there was exposure to a higher aflatoxin load per day than in matched controls (BULATAO-JAIME et al. 1982).

Epidemiological studies dealing with aflatoxin are often confounded by the simultaneous high rate of HBV infection in the same population.

During recent years evidence has emerged of a possible link between heavy exposure to aflatoxin and the presence of a specific inactivating point mutation in the p53 tumor-suppressor gene in HCC, suggesting one way in which this mycotoxin may contribute to hepatocellular carcinogenesis (HSU et al. 1991; BRESSAC et al. 1991).

4.1.5.4 Cirrhosis

Cirrhosis is a dynamic condition of varied etiology with different malignant potentials. The simple morphological classification of macronodular and micronodular is useful in explaining the association of cirrhosis with liver cancer. In ethnic Chinese and black Africans cirrhosis appears usually in the macronodular form, being the consequence of HBV infection, whereas in other populations it is commonly of the micronodular variety and is usually caused by chronic HCV infection, alcohol abuse or both.

Whether HCC is an inevitable consequence of cirrhosis per se is uncertain.

There is no agreement as to the oncogenic potential of the different types of cirrhosis. The essential point to determine is whether the etiological agents of the cirrhosis also cause HCC, the regenerative process associated with any cirrhosis leads by itself to HCC, or both mechanisms are involved. Probably, the role of cirrhosis is different in different incidence areas: in high risk areas, cirrhosis and HCC have the same etiology (viruses, alcohol or both); in low risk areas cirrhosis antedates the development of HCC and it is the cause of hepatocellular cancerogenesis.

4.1.5.5 Minor Risk Factors

Tobacco Smoking. Controversy exists over whether this is a minor risk factor for HCC, but the bulk of evidence suggests it is. However, these results are based on death certificates, which are known to be unreliable as diagnostic sources of primary liver cancer.

Sex Hormones. A statistically significant correlation has been demonstrated between the use of contraceptive steroids and the occurrence of HCC (TAVANI et al. 1993). The study has been conducted in countries with a low incidence of HCC. The risk is directly related to the duration of use. Moreover, the increased risk persists for approximately 10 years after the drugs are stopped.

Hereditary Hemochromatosis (HHC). This is a disease characterized by iron overload, genetically determined by an inappropriate increase in intestinal iron absorption. All patients with HHC have increased hepatic iron stores; abnormalities in serum aminotransferase levels are present in 30–50% of patients and the majority of patients develop cirrhosis (NIEDERAU et al. 1985; ADAMS et al. 1991; BACON and SADIQ 1995). As many as 45% of persons suffering from hereditary hemochromatosis develop HCC. HCC occurs only in patients with cirrhosis; a few patients, however, develop the tumor in the absence of cirrhosis, suggesting a direct carcinogenic role of iron in hepatocarcinogenesis (KEW 1990), perhaps by generating oxygen radicals (LOEB et al. 1988).

Wilson's Disease. This is an autosomal recessive disorder of copper overload, which can lead to cirrhosis. Patients with this disease rarely develop HCC, although in the presence of cirrhosis (POLIO et al. 1989). This has been attributed both to the cirrhosis and to oxidant stress secondary to accumulation of copper in the liver (TOKOL et al. 1994).

4.2 Clinical Features of Hepatocellular Carcinoma

4.2.1 Introduction

Patients with HCC are often unaware of its presence until the tumor has reached an advanced stage (KEW et al. 1971; BAGSHAVE and CAMERON 1976; KEW and GEDDS 1982).

Many patients with HCC have a past or current history of chronic liver disease, as shown in Table 4.2.

Table 4.2. Past history in patients with HCC (data from Liver Cancer Study Group 1982–1983)

History	No. of cases (yes/no)	Percentage
Acute hepatitis		
Confirmed	214/1378	15.5
Suspected	71/1378	5.2
Chronic hepatitis	678/1365	49.7
Liver cirrhosis	906/1485	61.0
Alcohol	510/1749	29.2
Drug-induced liver disease	8/1646	0.5
Prolonged use of medicines	102/1700	6.0

Before the late stage of HCC, the signs and the symptoms of patients are usually related to the condition underlying the tumor.

Clinical recognition of HCC is difficult. There are several reasons for this: none of the early clinical manifestations of HCC (if present) are pathognomonic; the liver is relatively inaccessible to the examining hand, and its large size allows the tumor to reach a large size before it can be felt or before invading adjacent structures.

In the low-incidence regions (but also in Japan, a country with intermediate incidence), HCC commonly develops as a complication of longstanding cirrhosis. The patient has few new symptoms, if any. One circumstance that should alert the clinician to the possible supervention of HCC in a cirrhotic liver is a sudden and unexplained change in the patient's condition: abdominal pain or weight loss can appear, ascites may become troublesome or blood-stained, and the liver can rapidly enlarge or hepatic failure may arise. In contrast, in populations at high risk of HCC, symptoms of coexisting cirrhosis are overshadowed by those of the tumor. In these populations the tumor has a large size and signs and symptoms are more florid; this aspect can help the diagnosis.

4.2.2 Symptoms

The most common – and frequently the first – complaint is right hypochondrial or epigastric pain (KEW et al. 1971; BAGSHAVE and CAMERON 1976; KEW and GEDDS 1982) (Table 4.3). Although sometimes severe, it is usually a dull continuous ache, which can become more intensive in the later stages

Table 4.3. Prevalence of clinical features of HCC

Symptoms	Prevalence (%)	Physical signs	Prevalence (%)
Abdominal pain	59–95	Hepatomegaly	54–98
Weight loss	34–71	Hepatic bruit	6–25
Weakness	22–53	Ascites	35–61
Abdominal swelling	28–43	Splenomegaly	27–42
Nonspecific gastrointestinal symptoms		Jaundice	4–35
	25–28	Wasting	25–41
Jaundice	5–26	Fever	11–54

of the disease. Two other symptoms often accompanying the pain are weakness and weight loss.

Other complaints are anorexia, dyspepsia, awareness of a mass in the upper abdomen, and constipation.

Jaundice is rarely present and is often obstructive (Kew and Paterson 1985).

Rarely, HCC presenting with acute abdomen when the tumor ruptures causes an hemoperitoneum; with bone pain due to skeletal metastases; with sudden paraplegia due to spinal metastases; or with cough or dyspnea as a result of multiple pulmonary metastases (Kew and Paterson 1985).

4.2.3 Physical Findings

As symptoms, physical findings are different according to the stage of the illness (Table 4.3). When the tumor is advanced, the liver is almost always enlarged, particularly in black African and ethnic Chinese patients; hepatic tenderness is common and may be severe. The surface of the enlarged and tender liver is smooth, irregular or frankly nodular. An arterial bruit can be heard over the tumor (Kew et al. 1971; Kew and Gedds 1982; Clain et al. 1976; Okuda and Nakashima 1984). It is rough in character, systolic in timing and not affected by the position of the patient.

Ascites can be present (Kew et al. 1971; Bagshave and Cameron 1976; Kew and Gedds 1982). Ascites, in the bulk, is the result of portal hypertension due to cirrhosis, but there are cases in which ascites is caused by vascular invasion or by involvement of peritoneum by the primary tumor or by metastases.

Splenomegaly can be present and it reflects cirrhosis and portal hypertension (Kew et al. 1971; Bagshave and Cameron 1976; Kew and Gedds 1982).

Progressive muscle wasting is the rule in the latter stages of the illness. A low-moderate and intermittent or remittent fever can be present (Kew et al. 1971; Bagshave and Cameron 1976; Kew and Gedds 1982).

4.2.4 Paraneoplastic Manifestations

Like other tumors, HCC may synthesize and secrete substances that are biologically active and in this way it can cause deleterious effects. Clinically recognizable effects are most often caused by secretion of hormones or hormone-like substances. Some paraneoplastic effects can precede the local effects of the tumor; thus, they may attract attention. In addition, some, such as hypoglycemia or hypercalcemia, have therapeutic indications (Table 4.4).

Polycythemia occurs in fewer than 10% of patients. If a patient with cirrhosis develops polycythemia, it can be that HCC has supervened. The pathogenesis of this phenomenon is not clear; recently, it has been demonstrated that erythrocytosis results from the secretion of erythropoietin by the tumor (Kew and Dusheiko 1981).

Another important paraneoplastic syndrome is hypoglycemia. It can be severe and manifests relatively early in the course of the illness; it can be the reason for which the patient is brought to medical attention. The hypoglycemia is believed to result from production by the tumor of a high-molecular weight form of the precursor of insulin-like growth factor II (pro-IGF II). This factor is bound less avidly as serum by IGF-binding protein than IGF II; consequently, it is far more readily accessible to peripheral tissues, where it can enhance glucose uptake to pathological levels (Daughaday et al. 1990).

Some patients can present hypercalcemia in the absence of skeletal metastases (Tamura et al. 1994).

Table 4.4. Paraneoplastic syndrome associated with HCC

Hypoglycemia
Polycythemia
Hypercalcemia
Sexual changes: isosexual precocity, gynecomastia, feminization
Systemic arterial hypertension
Water diarrhea syndrome
Porphyria
Carcinoid syndrome
Osteoporosis
Hypertrophic osteoarthropathy
Thyreotoxicosis
Thrombophlebitis migrans
Polymyositis
Neuropathy
Cutaneous markers: pityriasis rotunda, dermatomyositis, pemphigus foliaceus

This phenomenon has been attributed to production by the tumor of parathyroid hormone-related protein (Tamura et al. 1994). Hypercalcemia can be severe and the patient can be drowsy and lethargic.

Rarely, HCC can give cutaneous manifestations. In black Africans, a marker of the presence of HCC is pityriasis rotunda, consisting of single or multiple, round or oval, hyperpigmented, scaly lesions on the trunk that range in size from 0.5 to 25 cm (Berkowitz et al. 1989).

References

Adams PC, Kertesz AE, Valberg LS (1991) Clinical presentation of hemochromatosis: a changing scene. Am J Med 90:445–449

Bacon BR, Sadiq SA (1995) Hereditary hemochromatosis: diagnosis in the 1990's. Hepatology 22:372–379

Bagshave A, Cameron HM (1976) The clinical problem of liver cell cancer in a high incidence area. In: Cameron HM, Linsell DA, Warwick GP (eds) Liver Cell Cancer. Elsevier, Amsterdam, p 45

Beasley RP, Blumberg B, Popper H, et al (1982) Hepatitis B virus and hepatocellular carcinoma. In: Okuda KL, Mackay I (eds) Hepatocallular carcinoma. U.I.C.C., Geneva, p 60

Benvegnu L, Pontisso P, Cavalletto D, et al (1997) Lack of correlation between hepatitis C virus genotypes and clinical course of hepatitis C virus-related cirrhosis. Hepatology, 25:211–215

Berkowitz I, Hodkinson HJ, Kew MC, et al (1989) Pityriasis rotunda as a cutaneous marker in hepatocellular carcinoma. A comparison of its prevalence in other disease. Br J Dermatol 120:545–551

Bosch FX, Munoz N (1995) Hepatocellular carcinoma in the world: epidemiologic question. In: Tabor E, Di Bisceglie AM, Purcell RH (eds) Etiology, pathology and treatment of hepatocellular carcinoma in North America. Advances in uppled technology series, vol 13. Gulf Pubblishing, Houston, pag 35

Bressac B, Kew MC, Wands JR, et al (1991) Selective G to T mutations of p53 gene in hepatocellular carcinoma from southern Africa. Nature 350:429–436

Bulatao-Jaime J, Almero EM, Castro CA, et al (1982) A case-control dietary study of primary liver cancer risk from aflatoxin exposure. Int J Epidemiol 11:112–119

Clain D, Wartnaby K, Sherlock S (1966) Abdominal arterial murmurs in liver disease. Lancet 2:516–519

Daughaday WH, Wu JC, Lee SD, et al (1990) Abnormal processing of abnormal pro-IGF II in patients with hepatoma and in some HBV-positive asymptomatic individuals J Lab Clin Med 115:555–559

Di Bisceglie AM (1997) Hepatitis C and hepatocellular carcinoma. Hepatology 26:34S-38 S

Gerin JL, Cote PJ, Korba BE, et al (1991) Hepatitis B virus and liver cancer: the woodchuck as an experimental model of hepadnavirus-induced liver cancer. In: Hollinger FB, Lemon SM and Magrolis HS (eds) Viral hepatitis and liver disease. Williams & Wilkins, Baltimore, p 556

Hadziyannis S, Tabor E, Kaklamani E, et al (1995) A case-control study of hepatitis B and C virus infections in the etiology of hepatocellular carcinoma. Int J Cancer 60:627–631

Hsu IC, Metcalf RA, Sun T, et al (1991) Mutational hotspot in the p53 gene in human hepatocellular carcinomas. Nature 350:427–431

Kekule A, Lauer U, Meyer M, et al (1990) The pre-S2/S region of the integrated hepatitis B virus DNA encodes a transcriptional activator. Nature 353:457–462

Kew MC (1981) The hepatitis B virus and hepatocellular carcinoma. Semin Liver Dis 1:59–63

Kew MC (1990) Pathogenesis of hepatocellular carcinoma in hereditary hemochromatosis: occurence in non-cirrhotic patients. Hepatology 11:1806–1813

Kew MC (1994) Hepatitis C virus and hepatocellular carcinoma. FEMS Microbiol Rev 14:211–219

Kew MC. (1996) Hepatitis B virus-induced hepatocellular carcinoma. GI Cancer 1: 143–148

Kew MC, Dusheiko GM (1981) Paraneoplastic manifestations of hepatocellular cárcinoma. In:Chalmers TC, Berk PD (eds) Frontiers of science in liver disease. Stratton-Thieme, New york, p. 305

Kew MC, Gedds EW (1982) Hepatocellular carcinoma in rural sothern African blacks. Medicine (Balt) 61:98–103

Kew MC, Paterson AC (1985) Unusual clinical presentation of hepatocellular carcinoma. J Trop Gastroenterol 84:1092–1096

Kew MC, Dos Santos HA, Sherlock S (1971) Diagnosis of primary cancer of the liver. Br Med J 4:408–415

Kew MC, Desmyter J, Bradburne AF, et al (1979) Hepatitis B virus infection in southern African blacks with hepatocellular cancer. J Natl Cancer Inst 62:517–520

Kew MC, Kassianides C, Hodkinson J, et al (1986) Hepatocellular carcinoma in urban-born blacks: frequency and relation to hepatitis B virus. Br Med J 293:1339–1342

Kew MC, Kassianides C, Berger EL, et al (1987) Prevalence of chronic hepatitis B virus infection in pregnant balck women living in Soweto. J Med. Virol 22:263–269

Kew MC, Yu MC, Kedda M, et al (1997) The relative roles of hepatitis B and C viruses in the ethiology of hepatocellular carcinoma in southern Africans blacks. Gastroenterol 112:184–187

Kim CM, Koike K, Saito A, et al (1990) HBx gene of hepatitis B virus induces liver cancer in transgenic mice. Nature, 351:317–324

Lam KC, Yu MC, Leung JWC, et al (1982) Hepatitis B virus and cigarette smoking: risk factors for hepatocellular carcinoma in Hong Kong. Cancer Res 42:5246–5248

Lingao AL, Domingo EO, Nishioka K (1981) Hepatitis B virus profile of hepatocellular carcinoma in the Philippines. Cancer 48:1590–1595

Loeb LA, James EA, Waltersdorph AM, et al (1988) Mutagenesis by the auto-oxidation of iron with isolated DNA. Proc Natl Acad Sci USA 85:3918–3922

Marion PL, Oshiro LS, Popper H, et al (1987) Groundsquirrel hepatitis and hepatocellular carcinoma. In Robinson WS, Koike K, Will H (eds) Hepadnaviruses. Alan R Liss, New York, p 337

Munoz N, Linsell A (1982) Epidemiology of primery liver carncer. In: Correa P, Haeszel W (eds) Epidemiology of cancer of the digestive tract. The Hague, Nijhoff, pp161–195

Newberne PN (1984) Chemical carcinogenesis: mycotoxins and other chemicals to which humans are exposed. Semin Liver Dis. 4:122–127

Niederau C, Fischer R, Sonnenberg A, et al (1985) Survival and causes of death in cirrhotic and non cirrhotic patients with primary hemochromatosis. N Engl J Med 313:1265–1269

Okuda K, Nakashima T (1984) Primary carcinoma of the liver. In: Berk JE, et al (eds) Bockus-Gastroenterology 4th edn, vol.5. Saunders, Philadelphia, pp 3315–3376

Parkin DM, Stjernswärd J, Muir CS (1984) Estimates of the worldwide frequency of twelve major cancers. Bull Wld Hlth Org 62:163–182

Parkin DM, Muir CS, Whelan SL, et al (1992) Cancer incidence in five continents vol 5. IARC Pubblication, No 120. Lyon, International Agency for Research on cancer.

Polio J, Enriquez RE, Chow A, et al (1989) Hepatocellular carcinoma in Wilson's disease; case report and review of the literature. J Clin Gastroenterol 11:220–226

Prince AM, Szmuness W, Michon J, et al (1975) A case-control study of the association between primary liver cancer and hepatitis B infection in Senegal. Int J Cancer 16:376–383

Ray RB, Lagging LM, Meyer K, et al (1996a) Hepatitis C virus core protein cooperates with ras and trasforms primary rat embryo fibroblasts to tumorigenic phenotype. J Virol 70:4438–4443

Ray RB, Meyer K, Ray R (1996b) Suppression of apoptotic cell death by hepatitis C virus core proteine. Virology 226:176–182

Robinson WS (1992) The role of hepatitis B virus in the developement of hepatocellular carcinoma. J Gastroenterol Hepatol 7:622–629

Ross RK, Yuan JM, Yu MC, et al (1992) Urinary aflatoxin biomarkers and risk of hepatocellular carcinoma. Lancet 339: 943–947

Shafritz DA, Shouval D, Sherman HI, et al (1981) Integration of hepatitis B virus DNA into the genome of liver cells in chronic liver disease and hepatocellular carcinoma. N Engl J Med 305:1067–1073

Shorter RG, Baggenstoss AH, Logan GB, et al (1960) Primary carcinoma of the liver in infancy and childhood. Pediatrics 25:191–197

Silini E, Bottelli R, Asti M, et al (1996) Hepatitis C virus genotypes and risk of hepatocellular carcinoma in cirrhosis: a case-control study. Gastrenterol 11:199–205

Szmuness W (1978) Hepatocellular carcinoma and the hepatitis B virus: evidence for a causal association. Prog Med Virol 24:40–69

Szmuness W, Prince AM, Diebolt G, et al (1973) The epidemiology of hepatitis B infection in Africa: results of a pilot survey in the Republic of Senegal. Am J Epidemiol 98:104–110

Tamura K, Kubota K, Take H, et al (1994) Parathyroid hormone-related peptide as a possible cause of hypercalcemia in a hepatocellular carcinoma patient. Am J Gastroenterol 89:644–649

Tanaka K, Hiroaka T, Ikematsu H, et al (1996) Hepatitis C virus infection and risk of hepatocellular carcinoma among Japanese: possible role of type 1 b (II) infection. J Natl Cancer Inst 88:742–746

Tavani A, Negri E, Parazzini F, et al (1993) Female hormone utilization and risk of hepatocellular carcinoma. Br J Cancer 67: 635–639

Terry WD (1978) Primary cancer of the liver. In: Kaplan HS, Tsuchitani PJ (eds) Cancer in China. Alan R Liss, New York, p 101

Tokol RJ, Twedt T, McKim J, et al (1994) Oxidant injury to hepatic mithocondria in patients with liver disease and Bedlington terriers with copper toxicosis. Gastroenterol 107:1788–1792

Trichopopoulos D, Day N, Kaklamani E, et al (1987) Tobacco smoking, hepatitis B virus and ethanol consumption in the etiology of hepatocellular carcinoma. Int J Cancer

Wang WX, Forrester K, Yeh H, et al (1994) Hepatitis B virus protein inhibit p53 sequence specific DNA binding, transcriptional activity and association with transcription factor ERCC3. Proc Natl Acad Sci USA, 91:2230–2234

World Health Organization (1982) World health statistics, annual 1978–1982. Vital statistics and causes of death. WHO, Geneva

Yeh FS, Mo CC, Luo S, et al (1985) A serological case-control study of primary hepatocellular carcinoma in Guangxi, China. Cancer Res 45:872–873

5 Ultrasound and Doppler Ultrasound of Hepatocellular Carcinoma

R. LENCIONI and Y. MENU

CONTENTS

R. LENCIONI, MD; Division of Diagnostic and Interventional Radiology, Department of Oncology, University of Pisa, Via Roma 67, I-56125 Pisa, Italy
Y. MENU, MD; Professor and Chairman, Department of Radiology, Hôpital Beaujon, 100 Bd. du Général Leclerc, I-92118 Clichy, France

5.1 Introduction

Despite the advancements of CT and MR imaging, ultrasonography (US) has continued to improve and to develop as well as to have enormous applications, implications, and importance in diagnostic imaging of the liver. While gray-scale imaging has improved significantly, so that the definition of subtle lesions only a few millimeters in size is now possible, recent years have seen the most exciting advances in Doppler US technology. The development of power Doppler imaging has substantially improved perception of tumor vascularity. The introduction of US contrast media in combination with harmonic imaging has even further enlarged the potential uses of this technique. This article explores the most recent advances in gray-scale and Doppler US of the liver, with emphasis on their clinical applications for the study of hepatocellular carcinoma (HCC). US currently plays a fundamental role in the diagnostic and therapeutic management of patients with HCC.

5.2 Gray-Scale Ultrasound

5.2.1 Technique

In western Europe and North America, US represents the largest sales among imaging machines. Among the radiological community, the market share of high quality machines is tending to increase, representing 50% of sales of the top ten machines in 1997 in the United States. This is a consequence of the obvious improvement of the method during the last few years, and significant advances in image quality and color Doppler imaging. Although routine surveys of patients for the detection of liver masses can still be performed with machines of average quality, special examinations like Doppler evaluation of liver tumors, with or without contrast media, require higher quality. The main advances in US rely on probe technology and computerization of the signal. Whatever the type of US scanner used, attention should be paid to probe frequency and image focusing. When purchasing a machine, general ergonomy is of major interest, as well as objective (and subjective) image quality.

5.2.1.1
Ergonomy

Ergonomy of the machine itself is an important topic. It should be stressed that not all machines would be convenient for mobile bedside US. Although very recent machines tend to benefit from the miniaturization of the computer components, and are high performance machines with acceptable size, many devices are not adapted for bedside examination. This has to be considered because emergency and post-surgical bedside machines are being developed, especially in the case of liver transplantation. Although smaller machines are necessary, the quality of color Doppler images has to be stressed, because the evaluation of vessels, and especially the hepatic artery, is the main interest with such patients.

For upper abdominal imaging, sector scanning, either with mechanical probes or curved arrays, is best adapted to patient morphology, because an intercostal approach is always necessary to examine the entire liver. It is observed that almost all probes are now curved arrays. These probes have many advantages: the absence of mechanics improves reliability; increasing the number of elements allows better focalization of gray-scale image, a higher rate of image acquisition, and a higher signal to noise ratio in Doppler signal sampling. It is now possible to acquire high-resolution images with a color Doppler signal, and multiple focal zones without having the penalty of a slowed rate of image refreshment. Mechanical probes still have two advantages: a better focalization in the perpendicular axis to the slice, and a smaller contact area with the skin allowing better examination through small windows. The former advantage will not last for more than a few years as electronic sector probes with perpendicular focalization develop. Concerning the size of the probe, phased-array sector probes – such as those dedicated to cardiac imaging – provide the same advantage, and the image quality increases. It could be anticipated that most examinations of the abdomen would be made with electronic sector probes in the near future.

Another advantage of ultrasonography is the guidance of intervention, for instance biopsy or percutaneous thermal ablation. A special needle guide could help guidance by itself, with a fixed route appearing on the image. Most operators, especially experienced ones, prefer the hand-held method. When purchasing a device, attention should be paid to the compatibility of the probes with the sterilization technique, which should be attested by the vendor.

Machines which allow several transducers to be connected at the same time have a clear advantage, as the time required to shift from one probe to another is minimized. Three probes could be currently connected to many modern machines, but many still allow only two simultaneous connections. Whether switching of the probe is easy or not is another interesting point to consider when purchasing the machine, accessibility being very poor in some machines. Although liver imaging does not require more than two probes, and usually no more than one, in most cases, it should be anticipated that future developments would include a specialized transducer, necessitating more frequent probe switching. As an example, 3D imaging may require dedicated probes.

5.2.1.2
Frequency

Modern US devices are real-time, high-resolution machines. Many modern transducers allow a large bandwidth emission/reception. Image properties can be chosen in order to fit the patient's morphologic appearance. Preference can be given to higher frequency signals (5–7 MHz) in thin patients, and whether low frequency signals give better signals (2–4 MHz) in large patients. Spatial resolution increases when using higher frequency, but, conversely, signal attenuation increases too. Depending on the device, selection of the main frequency is automatic or manual. In some machines, the operator chooses the main frequency, whereas in other devices the best frequency is chosen while selecting "optimization" programs.

In less sophisticated machines, the frequency cannot be changed, either due to fixed excitation of the probe, or more likely in relation to a simplified signal analysis, focussing on the nominal probe frequency. Even if large bandwidth analysis provides an optimized image, an excellent diagnostic examination can still be done with a simpler machine. As a compromise, 3.5 MHz is the average frequency for all-purpose examinations. A 5-MHz probe is useful in thin adults and children.

5.2.1.3 Focusing

Focusing is crucial as the spatial resolution of the image depends on the width of the US beam. In order to differentiate two spots, the beam width should be inferior to the distance between these two spots. Focusing is the method for narrowing the beam in the area of interest. Different methods can be used, depending on the transducer technology. With electronic probes, focusing is obtained with a calculated delay of excitation of the different crystals, and arrangements in signal reception. Different groups of crystals are dedicated to a focal area. When multiplying the focal areas, time for signal acquisition and signal treatment increases, leading to a slower rate of images. New probes with more than 128 crystals and improved computing capabilities allow extensive focusing with no penalty for high-quality machines, but are not always available with low- or mid-segment machines.

When examining the liver, the focus should be set from 5 to 12 cm in depth. With single focal area machines, it is recommended to set the focal area to two-thirds of the distance between the skin and the diaphragm, as the resolution deteriorates more rapidly distally than proximally to the selected area. No equipment can provide optimal focusing of the whole image. It is then mandatory to focus on different zones in order to obtain an optimal examination of liver depth and surface.

5.2.1.4 Gain Curve

It is commonplace to stress the fact that attenuation of the US beam is different from one patient and examination to another, due to patient morphology, depth of the region of interest, and other patient characteristics. As a consequence, settings of the beam will not be convenient for every patient. It is recommended to start the examination with a test image of the liver through the intercostal approach, where fat planes are the smallest. On this image a general and localized gain should be set in order to make the liver appear homogeneous from the surface to depth, with a clear differentiation of liver surface from the superficial planes, echo-free vessels and gallbladder, the liver appearing as mid-gray. Only minimal modification of the settings should be necessary for the rest of the examination.

5.2.1.5 Other Parameters

Screen controls should not be modified, as they should be set to optimal for all examinations. Settings concerning pre- and post-processing are essentially subjective and the image appearance can be set in order to sharpen or smooth the image, depending on personal preference.

5.2.2 Ultrasound Screening of Hepatocellular Carcinoma

The liver is an excellent organ for evaluation by means of US, especially for the detection of focal lesions. US is the preferred routine hepatobiliary imaging method worldwide: it is easy to perform, largely accessible, and has a low cost. Moreover, acceptance by the patient is good to excellent, which is mandatory for a technique dedicated to routine survey. Furthermore, even if high level equipment is required to perform cutting-edge techniques like harmonic imaging or quantification of enhancement after contrast media injection, adequate diagnostic examinations can be performed with low- or mid-priced devices.

Since the mid-1970s, the recognition of the close association of HCC with cirrhosis has stimulated the development of clinical programs for the early detection of HCC in cirrhotic patients (Kabayashi et al. 1985; Okuda 1986). Extensive screening for HCC was made possible by the application of sensitive and specific diagnostic methods, such as assays for serum alpha-fetoprotein (AFP) and real-time US. US has been the imaging method of choice for screening high-risk patient populations, such as cirrhotic patients and patients infected with hepatitis B and C viruses (Bruix et al. 1989; Beasley et al. 1981; Takano et al. 1995). This resulted in great success in detecting small HCCs less than 2–3 cm in diameter and early-stage well differentiated HCCs. Based on this screening protocol, approximately 20–30% of the HCC nodules currently detected are less than 2 cm in diameter, and 50–60% are less than 5 cm in diameter. In only 15–20% of the small HCC cases (less than 2 cm) is the AFP level increased to more than 20 ng/ml (Colombo et al. 1991).

Thus, regular screening of high-risk patients by US is undoubtedly important in the early detection of small HCC in the clinical setting, especially in countries where HCC is prevalent (Tanaka et al. 1986, 1990a; Pateron et al. 1994). The most commonly used screening protocol includes regular follow-up of high-risk patients with US examination and serum AFP measurement every 3–6 months (Bartolozzi et al. 1995; Choi et al. 1989a; Ricca Rosellini et al. 1992).

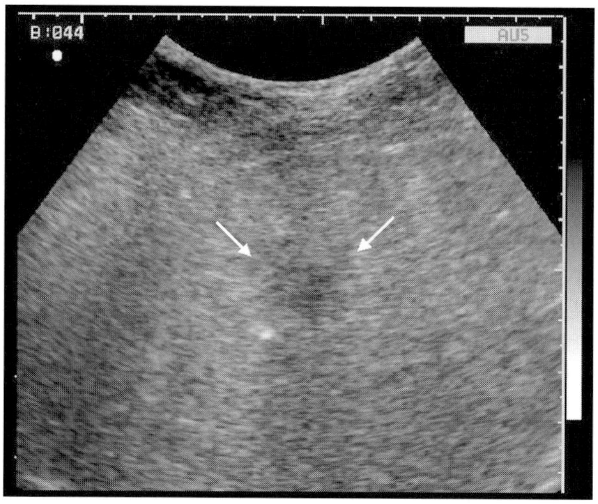

Fig. 5.1. Small hepatocellular carcinoma of the poorly demarcated nodular type (*arrow*). The lesion shows an irregular and blurred margin on the US image

5.2.3 Ultrasound Features of Hepatocellular Carcinoma

5.2.3.1 Small Hepatocellular Carcinoma

Morphologically, small HCC tumors less than 3 cm in greatest dimension usually show a nodular configuration and may be divided into four types: single nodular type, single nodular type with extranodular growth, contiguous multinodular type, and poorly demarcated nodular type (Buscarini et al. 1991, 1996; Ikeda et al. 1994; Takayasu et al. 1990).

Small, classical, nodular type HCC is a sharply demarcated lesion, which may or may not be encapsulated. Pathologically, the tumor capsule is seen in about 50–60% of small HCC lesions. On US, the shape of the tumor appears round or oval, and its boundary is sharp and smooth. The US detection rate of the capsule is low in small tumors because the capsule is thin and poorly developed. The fibrous capsule is seen as a peripheral hypoechoic halo. However, depiction of peripheral halo may also be due to compressed liver tissue at the periphery of the tumor (so called "pseudocapsule"). The presence of the fibrous capsule is commonly said to produce a typical US feature of HCC, represented by lateral shadows. More probably this phenomenon is not unique to HCC and depends on the incidence of the US beam on the lateral profile of a round mass acting as a refracting lens (Ros et al. 1990). The single nodular type with extranodular growth, the contiguous multinodular type, and the poorly demarcated nodular type show a nodular configuration with an irregular or blurred margin on US images (Fig. 5.1) (Choi et al. 1989b; Honda et al. 1992; Okuda et al. 1977; Shinagawa et al. 1984).

There are three types of internal echogenicity in HCC: hypoechoic, isoechoic, and hyperechoic (Kanno et al. 1989). When the nodule is small, the internal echo pattern tends to be hypoechoic (Fig. 5.2).

Sometimes small HCCs may exhibit a hyperechoic pattern, which is indicative of fatty metamorphosis, clear cell change, pseudoglandular arrangement of the cancer cells, peliotic changes of the vascular space in the tumor, or sclerotic changes in the tumor (Fig. 5.3).

More than half of small HCC nodules present with a hypoechoic pattern, about one-third present with a hyperechoic pattern, whereas a minority of lesions present with an isoechoic pattern, frequently with a peripheral hypoechoic halo (Fig. 5.4).

Many HCC are homogeneous, but some are found to be heterogeneous and consist of a mosaic. Internal mosaic architecture is a typical feature of large HCC and is characterized by components separated by thin septa. The different components may show various echogenicities on US images, particularly if areas of different degrees of differentiation or different degrees of fatty metamorphosis are present (Fig. 5.5).

Another characteristic US feature of HCC is posterior echo enhancement, which is produced by the softness of the tumor compared with the surrounding cirrhotic tissue. This feature may serve to detect isoechoic lesions (Fig. 5.6) (Boultbee 1979; Wernecke et al. 1992; Tanaka et al. 1983; Sakaguchi et al. 1992).

5.2.3.2 Advanced Hepatocellular Carcinoma

Advanced HCC lesions are classified into three major types: expansive nodular type, infiltrative type, and diffuse type (Buscarini et al. 1991, 1996).

The typical expansive type of HCC is a sharply demarcated lesion, which may be unifocal or multifocal. Most expansive HCC lesions have a well-developed fibrous capsule. The capsule may be depicted by US in up to 60–70% of large, encapsulated lesions on macroscopic pathologic examination (Figs. 5.7, 5.8) (Ros et al.1990). Internal architecture is typically characterized by mosaic pattern, with components of different echogenicity separated by thin septa (Fig. 5.9). In large lesions, mosaic architecture should not be confused with uneven US appearance caused by degeneration, necrosis, or bleeding.

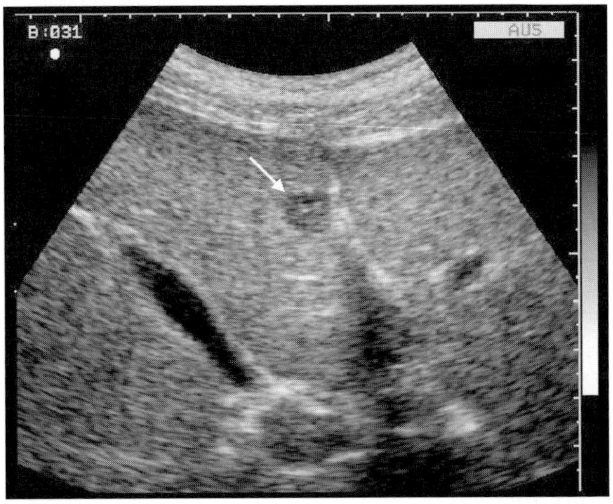

Fig. 5.2. Small hepatocellular carcinoma. The tiny lesion (*arrow*) appears hypoechoic with respect to surrounding liver parenchyma

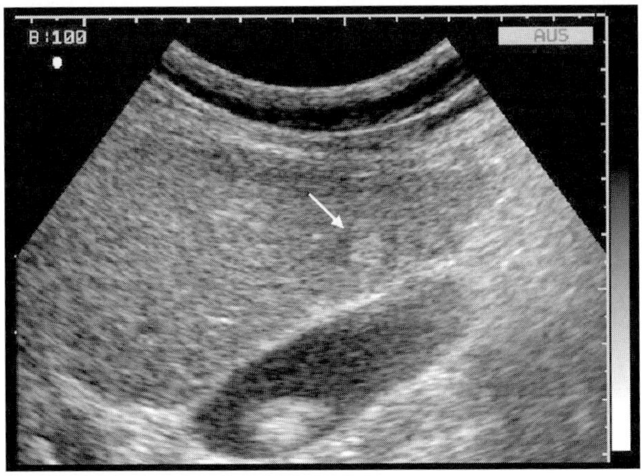

Fig. 5.3. Small hepatocellular carcinoma with hyperechoic pattern (*arrow*). Biopsy showed a well-differentiated tumor of Edmondson grade 1

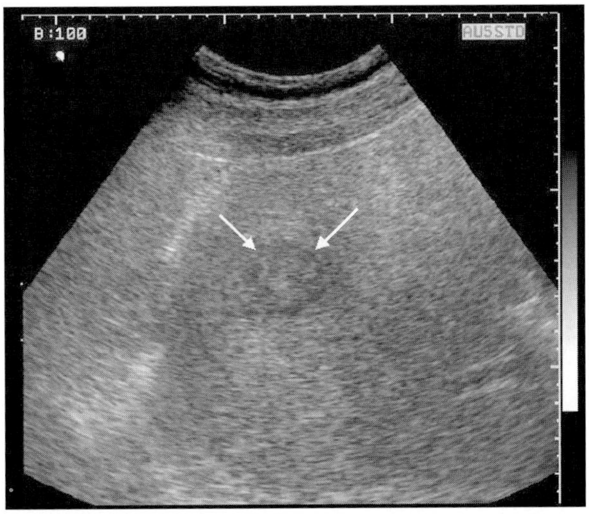

Fig. 5.4. Small hepatocellular carcinoma (*arrows*). The lesion appears isoechoic to liver parenchyma with a peripheral hypoechoic halo

The infiltrative type HCC is characterized by an irregular and indistinct tumor-nontumor boundary. This type is demonstrated as a mainly uneven area with unclear margins (Fig. 5.10). The tumor forms strands into surrounding tissue, which frequently invade vascular structures, particularly portal vein branches.

HCC, in fact, has a great propensity for invading and growing into the portal vein, eliciting tumor thrombi (Fig. 5.11). Infiltrative HCC may create a massive involvement of the liver, replacing large parts of the parenchyma. The diffuse type is by far the most unusual presentation of HCC. This type is characterized by numerous nodules of small size scattered throughout the liver. The nodules do not fuse with each other and are visualized as diffusely distributed hypoechoic lesions (Okuda et al. 1977; Honda et al. 1992).

In addition to these morphological features, HCC has the typical tendency to give small or minute satellite nodules, called "daughter" lesions. These nod-

a

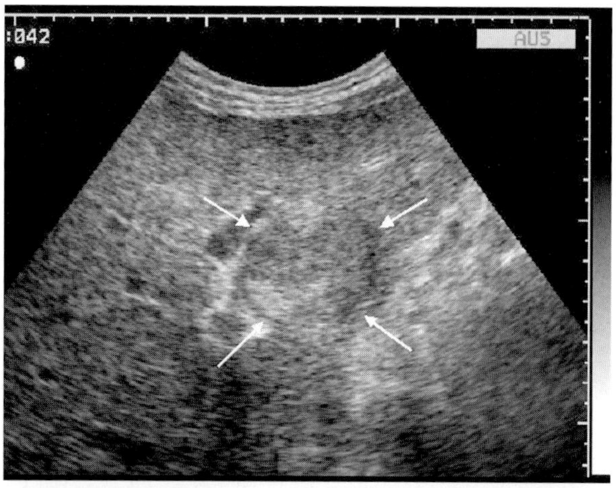

b

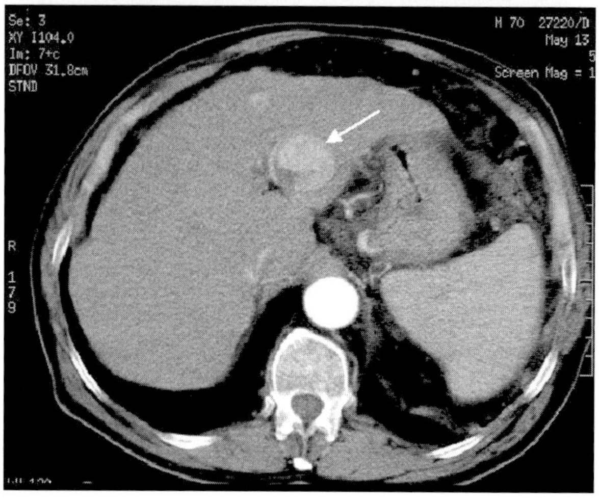

Fig. 5.5a,b. Small hepatocellular carcinoma with internal mosaic architecture. The lesion (*arrows*) shows hypoechoic and hyperechoic portions on the US image (**a**). On spiral CT, hypoechoic and hyperechoic areas showing different degrees of attenuation are depicted within the tumor (*arrow*). A daughter lesion is also depicted in the spiral CT image

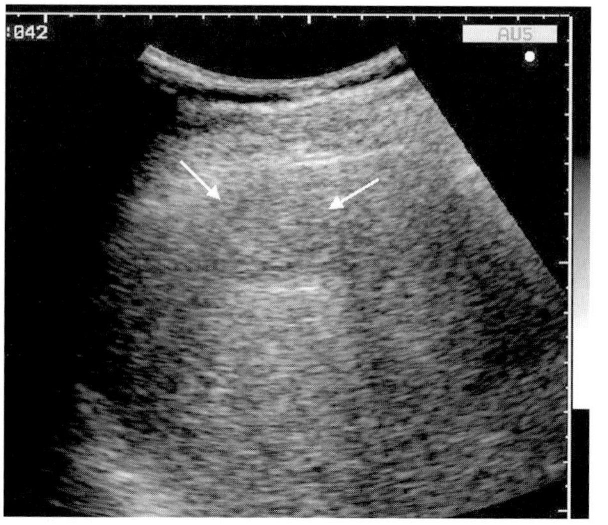

Fig. 5.6. Hepatocellular carcinoma with hypoechoic pattern and posterior echo enhancement (*arrows*)

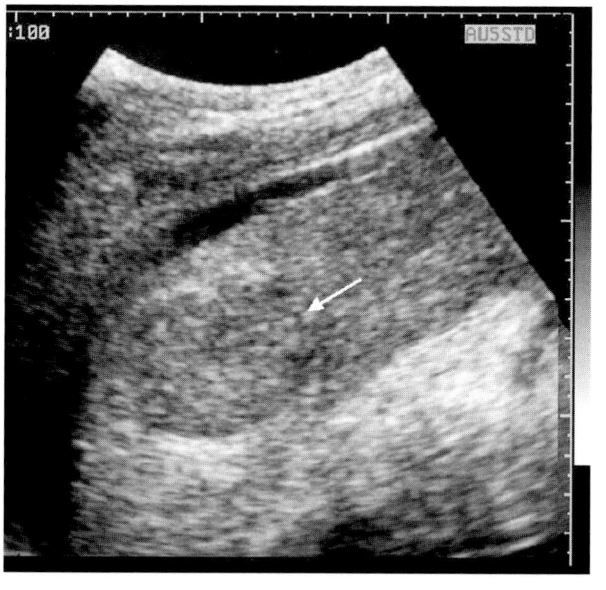

Fig. 5.7. Expansive type hepatocellular carcinoma. The lesion (*arrow*) appears well demarcated with respect to surrounding liver parenchyma, although the capsule is not depicted

ules represent intrahepatic metastases developed via the portal vein branches and are frequently located in the vicinity of the main tumor. Identification of these satellite lesions is of the utmost importance for therapeutic planning, and represents one of the most challenging issues in HCC patients. Satellite lesions should be distinguished from multiple small HCC tumors caused by multicentric development. Such a distinction is important since the presence of intrahepatic metastases indicates a more advanced stage and is associated with a worse prognosis (Hayashi et al. 1987; Okuda et al. 1985) (Fig. 5.12).

Unusual histopathologic characteristics of HCC may modify the typical US appearance of this tumor (Yoshikawa et al. 1988). These unusual histopathologic characteristics include marked fatty change, massive necrosis, abundant fibrous stroma (sclerosing type HCC), sarcomatous change, and calcifications. When fatty metamorphosis is severe, US shows hyperechoic areas within the tumor. When the degree of fatty deposition differs among internal por-

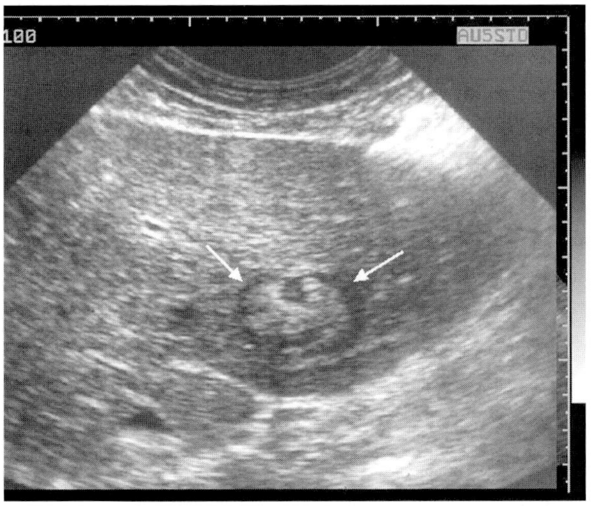

Fig. 5.8. Expansive type hepatocellular carcinoma. The lesion (*arrows*) shows an inhomogeneous internal pattern with a thick peripheral halo corresponding to the capsule

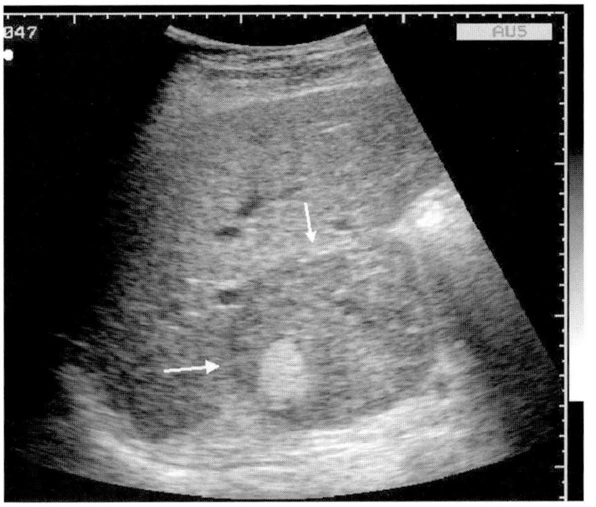

Fig. 5.10. Infiltrative-type hepatocellular carcinoma. The lesion (*arrows*), which shows internal mosaic architecture, is demonstrated as an uneven area with unclear margins, which strands into surrounding tissue

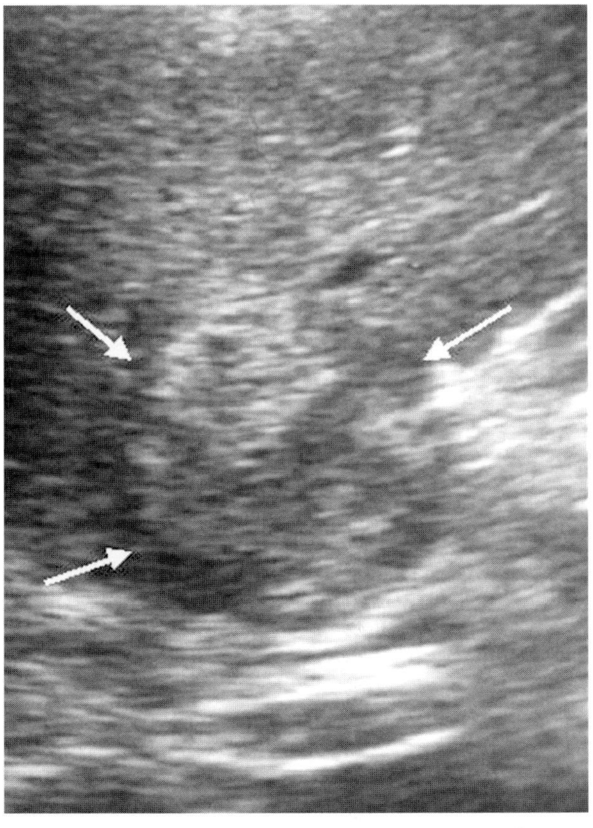

Fig. 5.9. Large hepatocellular carcinoma (*arrows*) with internal inhomogeneity due to hypoechoic and hyperechoic areas

tions of the tumor, the typical mosaic architecture can be visualized. However, in the case of diffuse fatty metamorphosis of the lesion, differential diagnosis from lipomatous tumors may not be achieved by US. Spontaneous massive necrosis within HCC is shown as an internal hypo-anechoic area, similar to other necrotic tumors. HCC with abundant fibrous stroma (sclerosing type HCC) and HCC with sarcomatous change (which is a very rare histotype) demonstrates internal inhomogeneity, frequently with hyperechoic pattern, but their appearance is nonspecific. The presence of calcifications is uncommon in HCC, being detected in about 0.2–1% of tumors. Calcifications, however, are not rare in fibrolamellar carcinoma and in mixed cholangiocellular-hepatocellular carcinoma (Tanaka et al. 1983; Sakaguchi et al. 1992; Boultbee 1979).

5.2.4 Differential Diagnosis by Gray-Scale Ultrasound

The differential diagnosis of a suspected HCC raises different issues in the setting of a nodular lesion detected in a patient with liver cirrhosis or in the case of a tumor developed in an otherwise normal liver (Trevisani et al. 1995).

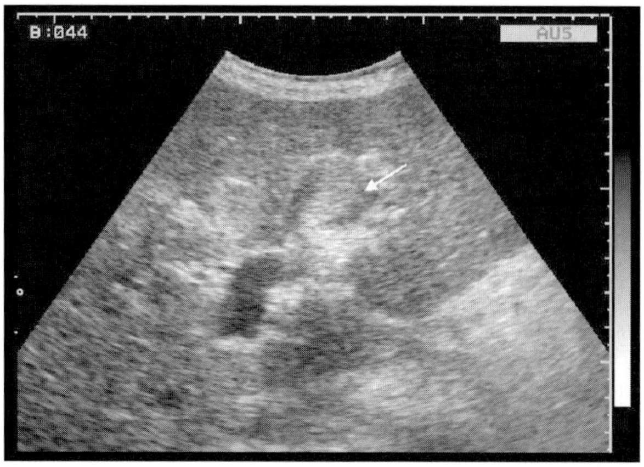

Fig. 5.11. Infiltrative-type hepatocellular carcinoma. US image shows diffuse tumor involvement of the liver parenchyma, without clear-cut evidence of a mass. Neoplastic thrombosis (*arrow*) is depicted in the portal vein

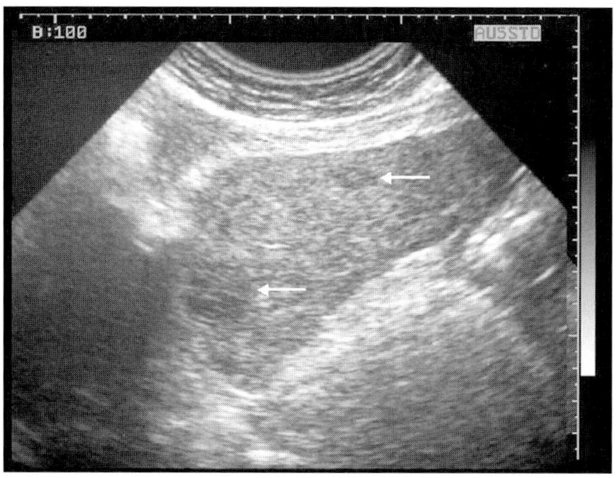

Fig. 5.12. Hepatocellular carcinoma with satellite lesions. The main tumor and the tiny satellite nodule (*arrows*) show similar hypoechoic appearance

5.2.4.1 Differential Diagnosis of Lesions in Cirrhotic Liver

Currently, efforts are directed toward making the diagnosis of HCC developed in cirrhotic livers at an early preclinical stage (Sheu et al. 1985a; Oka et al. 1990; Cottone et al. 1983). With this aim, particular attention is directed to characterizing even very small nodules detected by US screening. Along with progress in early diagnosis, various new information on the pathomorphologic characteristics and developmental process of early-stage HCC has been obtained through the histologic examination of resected lesions, explanted livers, and autopsy specimens (Lencioni et al. 1994).

HCC is currently thought to develop through two main pathways: a de novo carcinogenesis and a multistep progression. Multistep development is considered to be the most frequent model of hepatocarcinogenesis in cirrhotic livers. This model includes the transition from large regenerative nodules (or macroregenerative nodules) to dysplastic nodules (or borderline lesions), to early HCC (very well differentiated tumor of Edmondson grade 1), and, finally, to overt HCC (advanced tumor of Edmondson grade 2 or greater). HCC (Edmondson and Steiner 1954) usually develops as a focus of well-differentiated cancer within a dysplastic lesion (Arakawa et al. 1986). When the tumor grows to 1–1.5 cm in diameter, de-differentiation of well differentiated cancer cells occurs: cancer tissue at lower histologic grades proliferates within the well-differentiated cancerous nodule (early-advanced HCC), replaces the well-differentiated tissue that has weak proliferative activity, and then starts to grow expansively developing into advanced HCC (Calvet et al. 1990; Cottone et al. 1989; Ebara et al. 1986) (Fig. 5.13).

Therefore, when examining the echo texture of cirrhotic livers, we have to face a wide spectrum of hepatocellular nodular lesions, ranging from frankly benign nodules, to equivocal or borderline lesions, to clear-cut malignancies (Fig. 5.14). The distinction between these different histologic entities appears to be essential because of course it substantially affects patient prognosis and treatment planning. Unfortunately, there is enough variability and overlap in the US appearance of hepatocellular nodular lesions developed on a cirrhotic background to make a definite distinction problematic. In addition, the possibility of a nonhepatocellular nodular lesion incidentally found in a cirrhotic liver, like an hemangioma or a metastasis, should not be completely disregarded. The US appearance of HCC may be indistinguishable from either a hemangioma or a metastasis (Fig. 5.15). In view of the close association of HCC and cirrhosis, every solid focal liver lesion emerged in a cirrhotic liver should be regarded as an HCC unless a different diagnosis has been proved (Choi et al. 1993; Freeman et al. 1986).

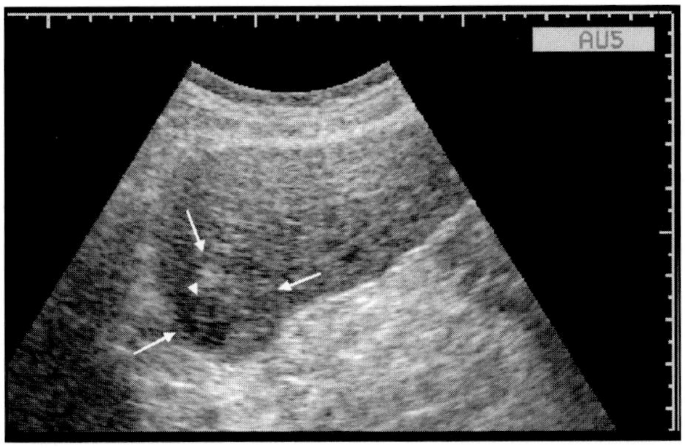

Fig. 5.13. Hepatocellular carcinoma developed within a dysplastic nodule. The dysplastic lesion is isoechoic with respect to surrounding liver parenchyma (*arrows*). Within the larger nodule, a hypoechoic area is depicted (*arrowhead*), reflecting malignant change

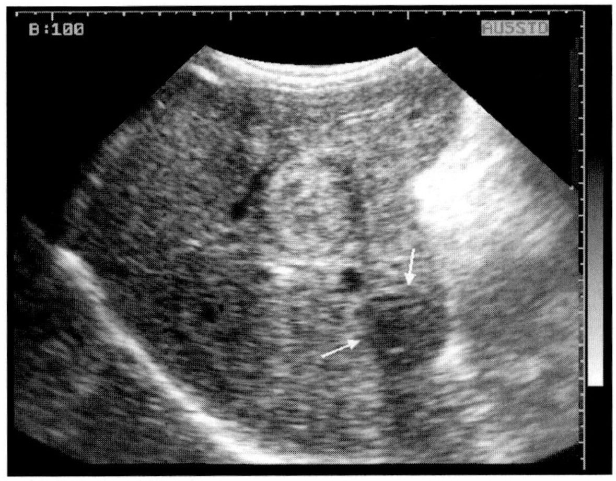

Fig. 5.14. Dysplastic nodule in the vicinity of a small hepatocellular carcinoma. The neoplastic lesion, which was proved to represent well-differentiated hepatocellular carcinoma with fatty degeneration on pathologic examination following liver transplantation, appears hyperechoic. The dysplastic lesion, which did not contain tumor foci, is homogeneously hypoechoic (*arrows*)

5.2.4.2
Differential Diagnosis of Lesions in Otherwise Normal Liver

The diagnosis of HCC developed in a noncirrhotic liver is usually made at an advanced stage, as no US survey has been performed (Sheu et al. 1985b). Differential diagnosis is usually more difficult, as a number of different entities must be taken into account (Choi et al. 1993).

If the tumor has an expansive growth, typical features suggesting HCC, such as tumor capsule and internal mosaic architecture, should be accurately searched for (Kamin et al. 1979). Expansive HCC lesions should be distinguished in the first place from metastatic nodules and benign tumors. Liver metastases have a variety of presentations (Yoshida et al. 1987), which are described in detail in the relevant chapter. Benign liver tumors include, among others, hemangioma, focal nodular hyperplasia, and hepatocellular adenoma (Melato et al. 1989; Kawasaki et al. 1978).

Hemangioma is the most common benign tumor of the liver. The incidence has been evaluated as being from 2% to 7% in autopsy series. The shape of an hemangioma is round or oval, and its boundary is lobulated and finely irregular. The hyperechoic pattern is by far the most frequent. However, about 20% of hemangiomas may appear hypoechoic or isoechoic with a peripheral hyperechoic rim. The most typical location is in apposition to either an hepatic vein or the hepatic capsule. Posterior echoes are even or enhanced, and lateral shadows are absent. US usually allows a confident diagnosis of he-

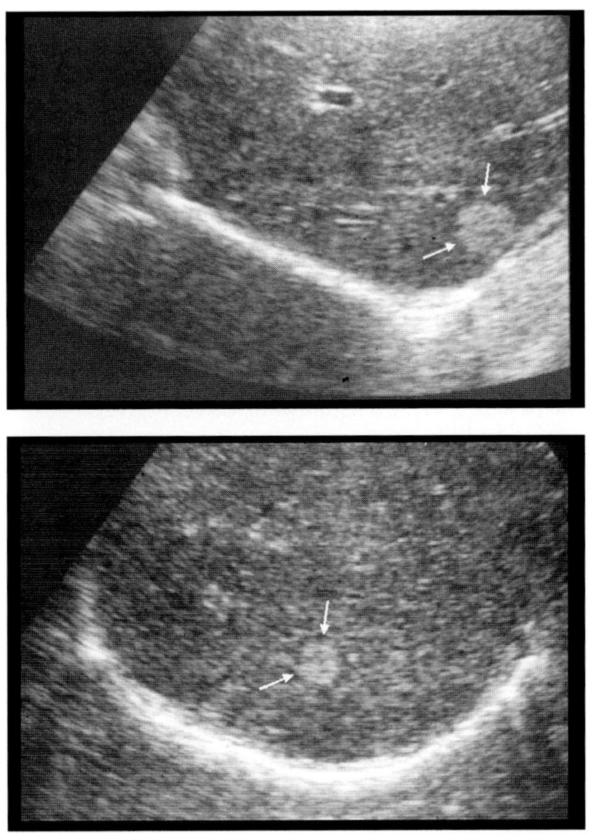

a

b

Fig. 5.15. Hepatic hemangioma (**a**) and small hyperechoic hepatocellular carcinoma (**b**) (*arrows in* **a** and **b**). The two lesions cannot be reliably distinguished based on US findings mangiomas with typical hyperechoic appearance, provided that the lesion is detected in a patient with neither history of malignancy nor chronic liver disease.

Focal nodular hyperplasia (FNH) is a nodule composed of benign-appearing hepatocytes occurring in a liver that is otherwise histologically normal or nearly normal. The lesion is supplied by large arteries accompanied by fibrous stroma containing ductules. The stroma is usually prominent, forming a stellate "scar." FNH is a congenital or acquired anomaly of the arterial supply leading to focal hyperperfusion of the parenchyma. It is usually asymptomatic and detected as an incidental finding. All ages may be affected, with marked female predominance. This lesion usually pursues a benign course, with no risk of rupture, hemorrhage or malignant change. The US features of FNH are nonspecific: the lesion appears as a rounded or oval mass usually ranging from 2 to 10 cm. It can be isoechoic or slightly hyperechoic and can lead to a mass effect. In very few cases, a stellate hyperechoic structure corresponding to the central scar may be detected.

Hepatocellular adenoma is a benign neoplasm composed of hepatocytes occurring in a liver that is otherwise histologically normal or nearly normal. Portal tracts, ducts, and ductular differentiation are usually not seen. Sinusoidal dilatation or peliosis may be present. There is usually no fibrous capsule. Adenoma usually arises in the setting of hepatocellular stimulation (oral contraceptive, anabolic steroids, or abnormal carbohydrate metabolism). Adenoma is often asymptomatic and detected as an incidental finding. It may regress after withdrawal of the stimulus. Adenoma may undergo possible rupture, hemorrhage, or malignant change (rare). As in the case of FNH, US usually allows recognition of the tumor, but has no histological specificity. The mass may appear round or oval, and its US structure may be variable. The center of the mass may appear heterogeneous because of the frequency of necrosis or bleeding causing a hypoechoic area.

In infiltrating lesions, invasion of portal vein branches suggests HCC. Other kinds of malignancy which may resemble infiltrative HCC include, beside rare primary tumors, intrahepatic cholangiocellular carcinoma and fibrolamellar carcinoma.

Intrahepatic cholangiocellular carcinoma, originating in small intrahepatic ducts, represents 10% of all cholangiocarcinomas. It is the second most common primary malignancy and is usually seen in the seventh decade. There is no association between cholangiocarcinoma and liver cirrhosis. Characteristically, an abundant fibroblastic stroma is present in this tumor, which is histologically a sclerosing adenocarcinoma. The US appearance is usually that of a potato- or cauliflower-like mass and the boundary is coarsely irregular. There is frequently a thick marginal hypoechoic zone and its internal side is blurred. The internal echoes have a target-like distribution, and a hypoechoic central area may be observed. Dilated bile ducts are one of the characteristic signs of biliary obstruction by the cholangiocarcinoma. A partially dilated bile duct with irregular walls and partial occlusion are important findings of this kind of malignancy.

Fibrolamellar carcinoma represents only 2% of hepatocellular malignancies. Typically, this neoplasm occurs in young people and is not associated with underlying cirrhosis. Most often, fibrolamellar carcinoma appears as a solitary, large, firm circumscribed mass with lobulated borders. More than two-thirds of reported cases have involved the left lobe. A prominent central fibrous scar with a radiating fibrous septa may be present (Wernecke et al. 1992).

5.2.5 Ultrasound Staging of Hepatocellular Carcinoma

Accurate staging is necessary to determine the best treatment method for HCC. US findings may provide useful information regarding the extent of the tumor, although US alone is usually insufficient to define accurately the degree of intrahepatic and extrahepatic spread of the tumor (Garbagnati et al. 1991).

Staging of HCC includes the assessment of: (a) number, size, location, and characteristics of the tumor nodules; (b) vascular invasion by the tumor; and (c) extrahepatic metastases. All these factors should be accurately evaluated, as they affect therapeutic options as well as the patient's prognosis (Buscarini et al. 1991, 1996).

Gray-scale US may provide an accurate assessment of the number and size of HCC lesions (Fig. 5.16). However, US examination of the entire liver is sometimes impossible because of the patient's habitus, intervening bones, or colonic interposition, especially in small cirrhotic livers. In addition, the US detection rate of small intrahepatic metastatic nodules is low.

US location of the segment in which the tumor exists is done in relation to hepatic and intrahepatic portal veins. However, when a small lesion is located at the boundary of the segments, it is not easy to determine the segmental anatomy. The characteristics of the lesion, particularly with regard to the type of tumor growth (expanding or infiltrating), are usually well defined by US. US identification of the tumor capsule is accurate in large tumors, but is less reliable in small lesions, which usually have a thin and poorly developed fibrous capsule (Dodd et al. 1992).

Vascular invasion by the tumor is a crucial staging factor (Subramanyam et al. 1984; Mathieu et al. 1988) (Fig. 5.17). A tendency to grow into the portal veins, eliciting tumor thrombi, is a peculiar feature of HCC. US allows accurate identification of tumor thrombi in the main portal veins. Tumor thrombi are shown as solid masses in the blood vessels often in contiguity with the main tumor. Identification of tumor invasion in peripheral (segmental or subsegmental) portal vein branches is unreliable by US (Jackson et al. 1983; Dodd et al. 1995). Lymphatic metastases in HCC are not common. They may be seen in about 10–15% of autopsy cases, especially in the hepatic hilar lymph nodes. Extrahepatic hematogenous metastases are usually associated with advanced-stage tumors. The lung is the commonest site of metastases, followed by the bone and the adrenal gland. US is valuable for the diagnosis of adenopathies and adrenal metastatic disease (Boultbee 1979; Honda et al. 1992; Sakaguchi et al. 1992; Tanaka et al. 1983; Yuki et al. 1990).

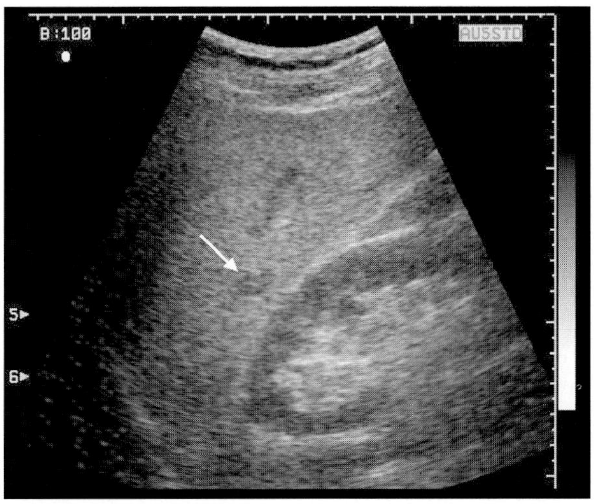

Fig. 5.16. Tiny intrahepatic metastatic nodule of hepatocellular carcinoma (*arrow*). US demonstration of the small lesion changed the therapeutic approach for the main tumor, which was located in a different hepatic segment (not shown)

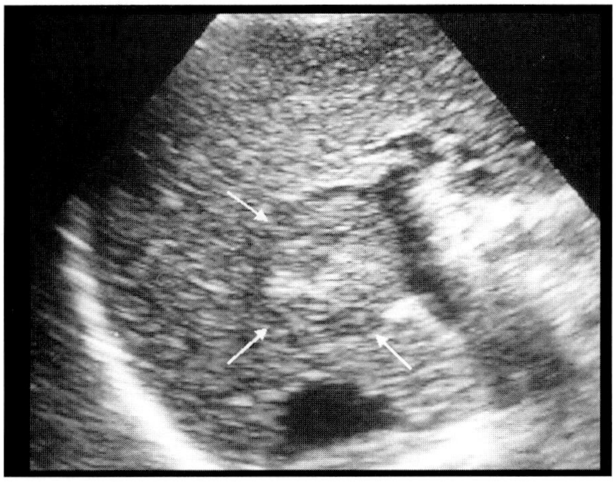

Fig. 5.17. Hepatocellular carcinoma. The large lesion displaces the portal vein and causes initial invasion of the vessel. Tumor thrombosis has not yet developed

5.3 Doppler Ultrasound

Doppler imaging is a part of liver examination. Every single US examination, particularly in a cirrhotic patient, should include at least an evaluation of the portal vein flow. Continuous wave Doppler is an excellent method for the detection and analysis of flow, but the lack of spatial selection lessens its use for abdominal purposes, as multiple vessels are commonly seen, and recorded all together, within a single beam. Pulsed Doppler, color-coded, and power Doppler have the capability to record the signal from an area that is chosen on gray-scale imaging.

5.3.1 Technique

5.3.1.1 Pulsed Doppler

Pulsed Doppler remains the reference method for quantitative evaluation of the flow. Spectral analysis allows measurements of flow velocity and indices, unobtainable by color or power Doppler. No significant advances in pulsed Doppler have been encountered in recent years. In most cases, pulsed Doppler recording of a flow in the vessel follows localization by color image. This is mandatory for small vessels that are very difficult to see in B-mode images, like intrahepatic arteries or vessels in a tumor. One should be cautious as to the delay in spectrum acquisition. In some machines, it may take a few seconds to shift from color Doppler to pulsed Doppler recording. As we are looking at small vessels, in a very mobile area, due to breathing, any delay is deleterious to the quality of the examination. The very first quality of a machine dedicated to liver imaging is to be able to perform a pulsed Doppler "on-the-fly," with no delay at all, preferably with a single button which is easy to switch without looking at the keyboard. Even with high-resolution machines such a delay may be encountered.

Duplex scanning is the possibility of recording simultaneously a B-mode image and a pulsed signal. There is a slight degradation of Doppler signal, but it still may be sufficient for the identification of the type of flow – i.e., is it a vein or an artery – or for a general survey of the liver. Triplex scanning is the association of B-mode image in real time, pulsed Doppler and color or power Doppler.

Pulsed Doppler gain can be set in every machine. The optimal setting is as follows: during a spectrum record, gain is increased until noise signal appears in the background above and under the spectrum. The gain is then lowered, until the noise disappears.

Frequency of emission depends on the transducer. On most probes, the frequency used for the image and for Doppler measurements is the same. Generally, the Doppler signal is better with a lower frequency. On a large bandwidth transducer, the B-mode signal could be preferentially acquired with higher components of the spectrum, while the Doppler signal may benefit from lower frequencies. The main frequency may be manually switched on some devices. It is advisable to choose a lower frequency when Doppler is the main interest of the examination, and higher when Doppler is ancillary.

The *angle of the ultrasonic beam* with the vessel should be reduced as much as possible. Measurements of velocity are accurate only when the angle is inferior to 60°. This is the consequence of the basic equation of the Doppler effect. This is never a problem within the liver, due to the orientation of most vessels, and the possibility of recording flow with a subcostal or an intercostal approach. Recording of the inferior vena cava or the portal trunk may be difficult, especially in the lower part of the porta hepatis, as the beam is generally perpendicular to the vessel. Patient position should be changed, for instance from supine to lateral decubitus, to provide a more favorable approach. Other vessels are sometimes difficult to record for the same reasons, like the left gastric vein and the common hepatic artery. Another problem is the evaluation of the beam angle with small tortuous vessels. When a very small vessel is recorded in a tumor, it is generally impossible to see it. This may be true with branches or hepatic artery. Exact calculation of the velocity is very hazardous.

Pulse repetition frequency (PRF) is a major setting in pulsed Doppler. According to Shannon's law, a Doppler frequency could be correctly identified by samples only if sampling frequency is at least twice as high as observed frequency. This means that an artery with a Doppler frequency of 3 kHz needs a sampling frequency (PRF) of 6 kHz at least. PRF should be set manually in a few machines. In most instances the optimal PRF is calculated depending on the depth of the sampling area and characteristics of the transducer, especially nominal frequency. Usually, a manual setting of the PRF remains available. As a rule, the higher available PRF should be used in order to avoid aliasing. A „high PRF" capability is implemented on most machines, allowing better differentiation of flow, but a high PRF also introduces a spatial aliasing represented on the images by multiple gates. One should be cautious, using high PRF, with the exact location of the vessel in order to identify precisely the examined vessel. When performing a Doppler examination of tumor vascularity, low PRF values may be necessary to investigate tiny vessels with a low-velocity blood flow.

Setting of the sampling gate is also important. For the examination of small vessels, the gate width could be as large or even slightly larger than the vessels, in order to be able to record the flow even if there is a faint movement. In larger vessels, the gate should be smaller than the vessel in an artery, to minimize the artifacts linked to wall motion. Conversely, if measurement of flow and mean velocity is required, sample volume should be set to cover exactly the diameter of the vessel.

Different filters may be applied to the image, in order to minimize the noise and signal arising from the vessel walls, from the heart, and from body motion. Most of these signals have a low frequency and are controlled by a "wall-filter." One pitfall is that these filters, when switched on, may hide a venous signal, which is a low frequency. On most machines, there are preset settings called "slow flow", "high velocity" and "average" with predefined settings corresponding to expected flow velocity.

5.3.1.2 Color Doppler Ultrasound

Color Doppler has been one of the most significant advances in US. One of the major problems of color Doppler has been the considerable number of measurements and calculations required for the reconstruction of a single image. Each should be acquired several times, one for gray-scale recording, and two or more for evaluation of the Doppler signal. In order to maintain Doppler signal quality and image refreshment rate, analysis of only a small part of the image is recommended. This is still true with midsized machines, but high quality machines now have enhanced color Doppler function, due to probes with multiple channels and increased computing power. On these machines, an excellent color Doppler signal can be recorded in a large area, with no marked slowing of refreshment rate.

It should be remembered that color Doppler, despite recent advances, remains a qualitative examination, even if the color scale may give an idea of the flow. As color Doppler sensitivity is lower than that of pulsed Doppler, it may happen that despite negative color imaging, pulsed Doppler is able to record a flow. Although this situation is becoming less and less frequent, it can still happen in the case of slow flow in the portal vein in a cirrhotic patient. As a rule, diagnosis of vein obstruction cannot rely on color Doppler examination only. Most settings are similar to those of pulsed Doppler.

Gain is set as in pulsed Doppler: while acquiring a single slice the gain is increased until color signal clearly appears outside the vessels, in the liver parenchyma. Gain is lowered until the extravascular color signal disappears. During this acquisition, the patient is not breathing at all, and the slice is preferably made on the right lobe via the intercostal approach rather than on the left lobe, to avoid cardiac artifacts.

Concerning *the angle of the ultrasonic beam*, it is crucial to remember that color Doppler will not detect all the vessels included in the image, as some of them might be seen with a large angle. The same slice, with only a slight reorientation of the transducer, will show different vessels and/or a different appearance of the same vessels.

When fishing for vessels, without any idea of the possible orientation, size and type of flow, it is preferable to start the examination with a higher sampling frequency and the lowest filters. When the vessels are detected, the correct sampling and filters are applied.

5.3.1.3 Power Doppler Ultrasound

Power Doppler US is a relatively new Doppler technique which was developed in an attempt to overcome some of the drawbacks of conventional color Doppler imaging. Conventional color Doppler US, in fact, is based on the mean Doppler frequency shift and is therefore subject to several limitations. In the mean frequency mode, in fact, noise can look like flow in any direction. Hence, if the color gain is too high or the Doppler display threshold too low, noise will dominate the image and make the identification of true flow impossible. Turning down the color gain will eliminate artifacts, but will also greatly reduce sensitivity. Moreover, color Doppler imaging is angle dependent, and therefore it loses sensitivity to flows that are perpendicular to the sound field. Finally, as it is a frequency detection technique, color Doppler US has the potential to alias.

The principle of power Doppler US is simple: color Doppler cannot include low frequency signals because the signal is so small that it is impossible to know if the blood is flowing forward or backward. Color Doppler also makes an attempt to identify the level of flow, although this remains semi-quantitative. With power Doppler, no attempt is made to detect the flow direction or to give an evaluation of blood velocity. Only the quantity of signal is considered, and coded on B-mode image with a single color. Information is binary (flow or no flow), but this is very complementary to pulsed Doppler, which is able to provide flow direction and velocity identification. A crucial point is that in the power Doppler mode, noise – which has a uniformly low power – assumes a homogeneous appearance (corresponding to a background that can be cancelled from the screen) even when the gain is increased greatly over the level at which noise obscures the conventional color Doppler image. A color gain increase of 10–15 dB can therefore be attained, resulting in increased sensitivity to depict blood flow. Other advantages power Doppler has over color Doppler US are that it is essentially angle independent and is not subject to aliasing, so it elicits more precise, angiogram-like pictures without the salt-and-pepper appearance of conventional color Doppler imaging. The major pitfall of power Doppler is its sensitivity to the motion artifacts.

5.3.1.4 Ultrasound Contrast Agents

Although contrast media for US were developed a long time ago, few molecules are available on the market today. Nevertheless, it is an emerging topic in liver US, as new molecules are able to pass through the pulmonary filter, and then enhance the sonographic signal in the arterial compartment.

Some products are only intravascular media, with an uneven distribution after injection. These agents are mainly microbubbles coated with a stabilized envelope. Echo enhancement is in part due to the reflectivity of the microbubbles. These particles have a very different impedance from flowing blood and are strong reflectors. Reflectivity is proportional to the fourth power of the bubble diameter, and to the bubbles' concentration. Additional action is the so-called "stimulated acoustic emission" or "sonoscintigraphy": when a microbubble is hit by a strong sound wave, it may explode, producing a short and very strong noise which is read by the transducer as a Doppler signal, producing a color spot where the bubble exploded. Although preliminary, this may give rise to additional work on appropriate settings to especially enhance this mechanism, and to record the phenomenon.

The first commercially available contrast media in Europe was Levovist, a galactose-based microbubble agent: trials show a marked increase in diagnostic confidence in liver imaging, and a reduced percentage of nondiagnostic examinations (Bolondi et al. 1998). Liver enhancement lasts for a few minutes (Catalano et al. 1998), and Doppler signal in the vessels is constantly increased (+15 dB). There is a twofold enhancement of the detection of intratumoral vessels in a series of hepatocellular carcinomas (Tanaka et al. 1998). Other molecules are expected to be available soon as many pharmaceutical groups are developing research on US contrast media. A preliminary list would include Albunex from Molecular Biosystems Inc., Quantison from Andaris, Echogen from Sonus Pharmaceutical Abbott, Optison from Molecular Biosystems Inc., Sonovue from Bracco, Imagent from Alliance Pharmaceutical Co., and NC 100–100 from Nycomed Amersham, but other companies are still in the competition. This illustrates the fact that contrast media in US are now a major concern for companies, as even if only a small percentage of US examinations need contrast media, this would nevertheless represent a large number of patients worldwide. Expected improvements are a longer lasting action. More recently, molecules which are intended to be more specific have been presented, accumulating in target tissues like the reticulo-endothelial system, which would be of major interest for liver US (Forsberg et al. 1998). Finally, it is not clear if settings of US scanners will be convenient for contrast imaging with any pharmaceutical, or if an adjustment of settings will be necessary for each agent. US may then be different from other imaging modalities, like CT, where interaction of iodine with X-rays is similar from one agent to another.

One track for research is the application of harmonic imaging to contrast enhanced US. The principle of harmonic imaging is described in the next topic. The advantage of harmonic imaging with contrast media is that it eliminates backscattered echo and allows differentiation of backscatter from microbubbles (Schwarz et al. 1997). Harmonic imaging with contrast media has proved to allow the detection of very small vessels (down to 40 μm), and very slow flow (Calliada et al. 1998). Contrast media may be interesting for the examination of the portal system in patients with a very slow flow, in order to differentiate slow flow and thrombosis. Identification of abnormal vessels (collateral veins, tumor vessels) could also be an interesting area.

5.3.1.5 Harmonic Imaging

Despite the fact that harmonic imaging was first dedicated to contrast media, it appears that it enhances gray-scale images too. The basic idea of harmonic imaging is the following: any tissue receiving a sound wave may absorb it and then release a reflected beam at different frequencies. In contrast harmonic imaging, the harmonic frequency energy is produced by the reflection on the microbubble itself. In tissue harmonic imaging, the harmonic wave is generated gradually while the ultrasonic beam progresses through the tissue (Thomas and Rubin 1998). Building the image with a second harmonic echo allows the image to be cleaned from the noise, especially in the superficial areas, because proximal echoes are less likely to produce harmonic wave. Second harmonic imaging may not be the only way to record the signal. It has been suggested, and experimentally proved, that recording the subharmonics of the main frequency may be helpful (Shankar et al. 1998). Although the technology has not stabilized (narrow bandwidth vs large bandwidth), it appears that harmonic imaging is an interesting advance in liver examination. It is currently available in most high-end scanners, but it will probably be implemented within a few years on the mid-tier machines. One can anticipate that tissue harmonic imaging will be a standard method for the assessment of the liver in the near future.

5.3.1.6 Time-Intensity Curves

Time-intensity wash-in–wash-out curves represent a recent development in the US technology applied to contrast-enhanced Doppler imaging. The objective of this analysis is to evaluate time/intensity data of Doppler signals within the organ or the lesion under examination after intravenous bolus injection of an US contrast agent. High speed technology is needed to calculate the data analysis in different areas of interest and to provide automatic data elaboration and curve visualization, allowing quick comparison among curves obtained in healthy and pathologic tissues. Double-image display (color or power Doppler contrast-enhanced image plus wash-in/wash-out curves is currently possible, as well as visualization of multi-graphic displays. Selectable automatic measures (curve velocity, velocity ratio, curve area, point-to-point time calculation) may be performed on graphs, and row graph data may be saved in digital format. Box re-sizing and moving elaboration also enable the accurate calculation of enhancement curves even in small targets, such as in the case of hepatic lesions.

Time-intensity wash-in–wash-out curves allow the contrast enhancement pattern of the lesion to be investigated and objectified. The Doppler US examination is performed by injecting a bolus of a microbubble contrast agent and by performing continuous imaging of the lesion, in the harmonic power Doppler mode, for 2–3 min. The enhancement curve of the lesion showing the variation of the average pixel power inside the color box over time is then immediately provided by a dedicated software program implemented on the US system (Lencioni et al. 1998).

5.3.1.7 Three-Dimensional Imaging

Three-dimensional imaging was developed a long time ago, but has not yet gained wide acceptance for liver imaging. The principle is not different from 3D imaging in CT or MR. Acquisition of contiguous slices allows the calculation of the data in a volume. These data may then be displayed in 2D images on different planes. This is especially useful for the reconstruction in a coronal plane, which could not be directly acquired during sonographic examination. The best application has been found in obstetrics ultrasonography, in order to show anatomical details like lips, or to obtain the exact plane for a specified measurement. Data can be represented in 3D images if a single element is extracted from acquisition volume. Again, this has been helpful for the evaluation of the external morphology of a fetus. Liver volume in the fetus can be estimated (Laudy et al. 1998). In liver imaging, 3D images can be useful for the representation of vessels, after a color Doppler acquisition. Contrast media may help in enhancing the signal from the examined vessel, especially using second-harmonic imaging in order to eliminate the artifacts (Campani et al. 1998). Three-dimensional imaging may be performed on the ultrasound scanner or reconstructed after data transfer on another workstation. Three-dimensional imaging is a reality from a technical point of view, but application to the adult liver has not yet been studied.

5.3.2 Doppler Ultrasound Features of Hepatocellular Carcinoma

On color Doppler US, HCC is usually displayed as a vascular-rich region containing intratumoral signals with a pulsatile arterial Doppler spectrum, corresponding to the characteristic findings of hypervascularity on angiography. A basket pattern, which is a fine blood-flow network surrounding the tumor nodule, and tumor vessels flowing into the tumor and branching within it, are the characteristic findings of HCC (Choi et al. 1996; Lencioni et al. 1996b).

These findings are almost always depicted in large HCC lesions, and are frequently associated with very high Doppler shifts (Numata et al. 1993, 1997; Oka et al. 1990; Shimamoto et al. 1987, 1992). It has been reported that, when employing Doppler shifts of 4.5 kHz or more as a positive finding for HCC, the specificity may be as high as 95%, and the sensitivity is also rather high at 70%. In small HCC lesions, however, the sensitivity of such findings is substantially lower. Indeed, the current technology of color Doppler imaging is still inferior to angiography (Reinhold et al. 1995; Lencioni et al. 1996b). According to our experience, color signals may be detected in no more than 70% of HCC lesions 3 cm or less in greatest dimension. The observed features were those of vessels running toward the center of the tumor or along its periphery. On Doppler spectral analysis, a pulsatile flow with a typical arterial waveform was demonstrated in less than 50% of lesions: the peak systolic frequency shift ranged from 0.44 to 3.85 kHz (mean, 1.21 kHz) and the resistive index ranged from 0.31 to 0.64 (mean, 0.49). The lack of arterial flow in some small HCC lesions may suggest that their neovasculature has not yet fully developed, due to their small size; however, in several other instances, hypervascularity was already present (as confirmed by angiography or other imaging studies), but color Doppler US was not sufficiently sensitive to demonstrate it.

In our series (Lencioni et al. 1996b), some small HCC lesions in which no arterial flow was detected on color Doppler US showed the presence of a draining venous vessel with constant-flow at the periphery of the tumor. This feature was first reported by Tanaka et al. (1992), who demonstrated that the detection of a constant-flow efferent tumor vessel continuing to a portal branch was a characteristic finding of HCC, probably reflecting an overflow into the portal system caused by tumor blockade of the normal outflow route from the sinusoid space to the hepatic venous system.

Power Doppler US proved to be significantly more accurate than color Doppler US in assessing vascularity of HCC (Rubin et al. 1994; Bude and Rubin 1996). In our study, among 75 HCC lesions which showed an arterial hypervascular supply on angiography, intratumoral pulsatile flow was detected in 92% of cases by power Doppler US and in only 73% of cases by conventional color Doppler imaging. Correlation of Doppler studies with angiographic findings also showed that power Doppler US, like conventional color Doppler US, had no false positives in diagnosing tumor hypervascularity. All lesions in which arterial signals were seen on power Doppler US, in fact, were confirmed to be truly hypervascular tumors on angiography (Lencioni et al. 1996b).

Of interest, the detectability rate of power Doppler signals in angiographically hypervascular tumors was not affected by the size of the lesion or by its location within the liver parenchyma. In contrast, with conventional color Doppler imaging, the detectability rate of pulsatile arterial flow was significantly lower in lesions smaller than 2 cm or located 9 cm or more from the skin surface (Lencioni et al. 1996b). This proves that power Doppler US is more sensitive than color Doppler US in depiction of weak signals coming from tiny or remotely located nodules (Bude and Rubin 1996; Rubin et al. 1994). Indeed, the mean peak systolic frequency shift calculated on power Doppler spectra in our series was significantly lower than that obtained with conventional color Doppler imaging, which suggests that also low and fine blood flows – not detected by using the mean-frequency mode – were measured (Lencioni et al. 1996b).

The use of US contrast agents may add further information to the color and power Doppler studies (Tano et al. 1997; Fujimoto et al. 1994; Albrecht et al. 1998). After administration of a US contrast agent, hypervascular HCCs show strong, rapid intratumoral enhancement in the arterial phase (i.e., within 45 s after the start of the injection). The observable features included the evidence of several well-defined intratumoral vessels running toward the center of the tumor and along its periphery or multiple internal vascular pedicles (Fujimoto et al. 1994; Kim et al. 1998). In our experience (Bartolozzi et al. 1998), contrast-enhanced Doppler imaging studies significantly outperformed unenhanced Doppler US, and provided information similar to that obtained with more complex imaging modalities, such as dual-phase spiral CT, dynamic MR imaging, or angiography (Fig. 5.18).

In our series, on unenhanced color Doppler US performed before PEI, intratumoral blood flow signals were depicted in 35 (65%) of 54 lesions. Twenty-four to 35 s after injection of the US contrast agent (mean±standard deviation, 27±4 s), 47 (87%) of the 54 lesions (in 40 of the 42 patients) showed strong intratumoral enhancement, including 12 lesions with no signs of internal vascularity at the precontrast examinations. The augmentation of the color Doppler signal persisted for 204–362 s (mean±standard deviation, 261±41 s).

Color Doppler US studies are very useful in evaluating portal vein thrombosis. As patients with cirrhosis are at high risk of developing portal vein thrombosis, this phenomenon cannot be immediately related to the presence of HCC, despite the well-known propensity of this tumor of invading the portal vein branches. Moreover, in rare situations, portal vein thrombosis is the unique detectable feature of the tumor. With color Doppler US, the peculiar aspect seen in cases of malignant thrombosis is the presence of pulsatile arterial flow within the thrombus. This finding is the expression of hypervascular neoplastic tissue growing into the portal vein and corresponds to the arteriographic „thread and streaks“ sign first described in 1975 by Okuda et al. (1975). In our experience, this sign always indicated

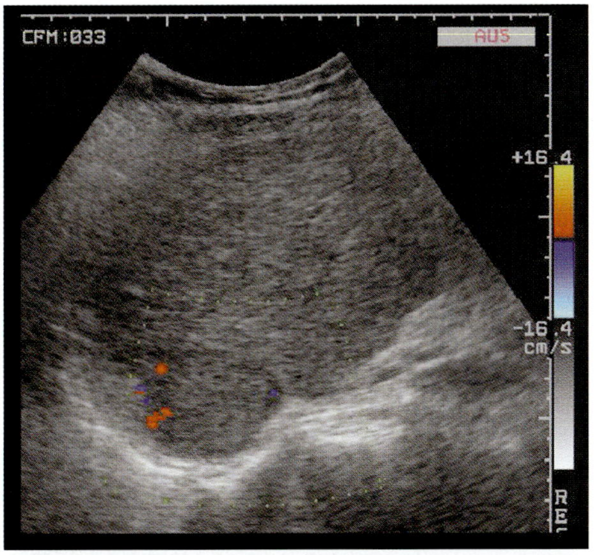

a

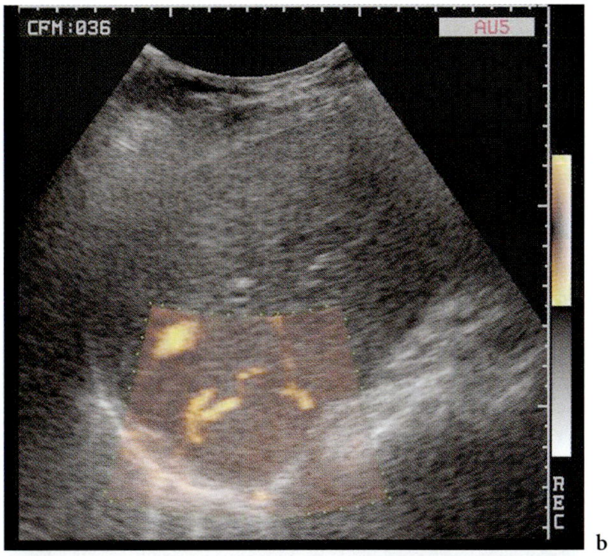

b

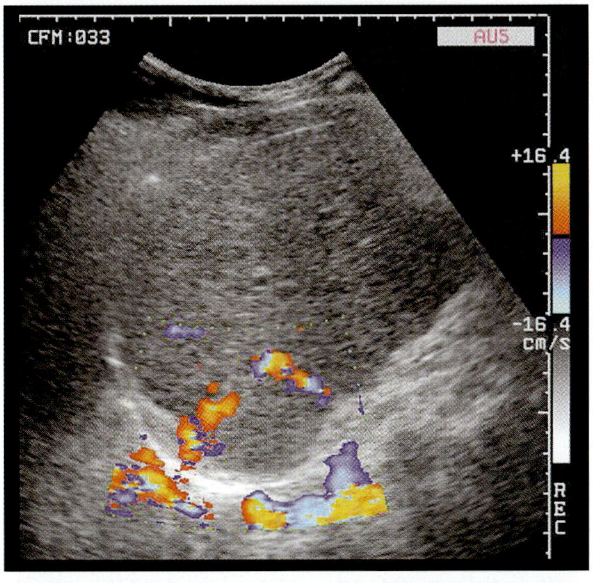

c

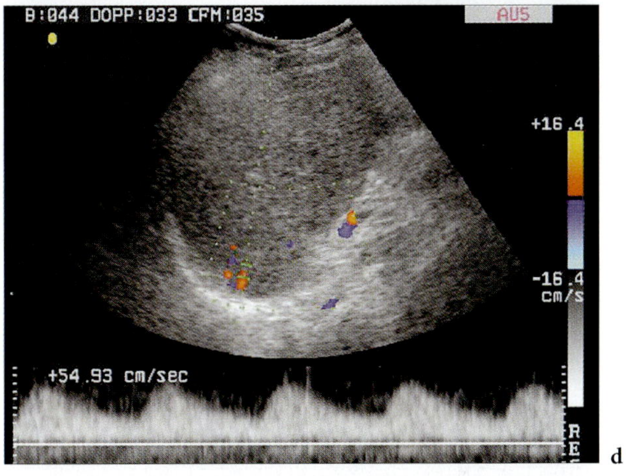

d

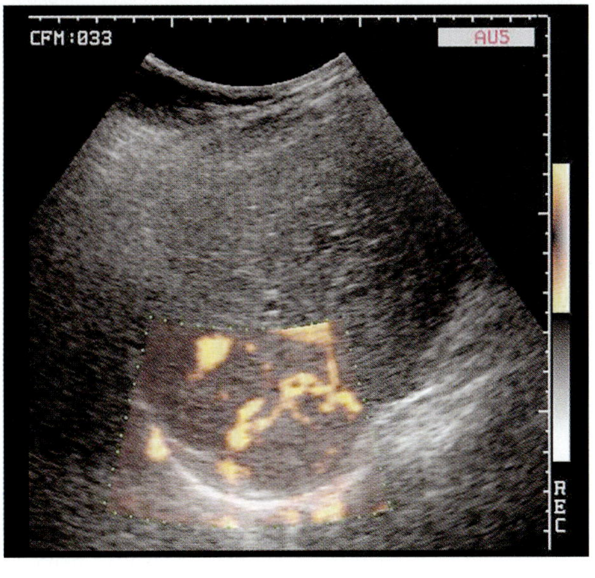

e

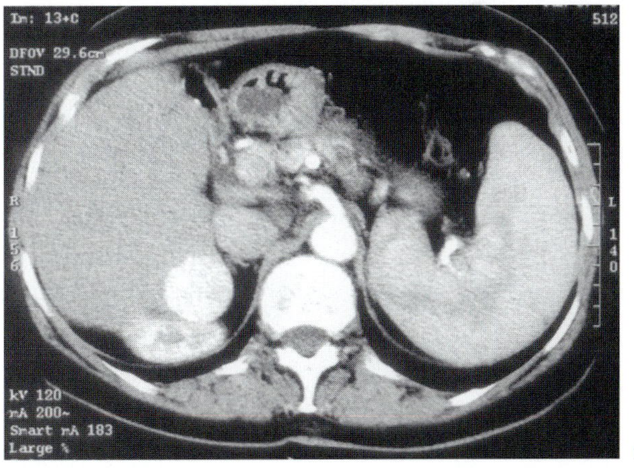

f

Fig. 5.18a–f. Doppler US study of hepatocellular carcinoma. Conventional color Doppler US shows small color dots within the tumor (**a**). On power Doppler US, intratumoral vessels are clearly depicted (**b**). Following the administration of a microbubble contrast agent, the tumor shows early enhancement in the arterial phase on color Doppler US (**c**). Spectral analysis confirms the presence of arterial vessels with a pulsatile Doppler waveform (**d**). Contrast-enhanced power Doppler US provides an accurate depiction of the vascular network of the lesion (**e**). Spiral CT in the arterial phase confirms a hypervascular tumor (**f**) tumor extension into the portal vein and was never observed in benign thromboses (LENCIONI et al. 1995). The sensitivity of color Doppler US in detecting pulsatile flow within tumor thrombi may be increased by using the power mode in combination with microbubble contrast agents: enhancement of the thrombus in the arterial phase will indicate malignant thrombosis (Fig. 5.19).

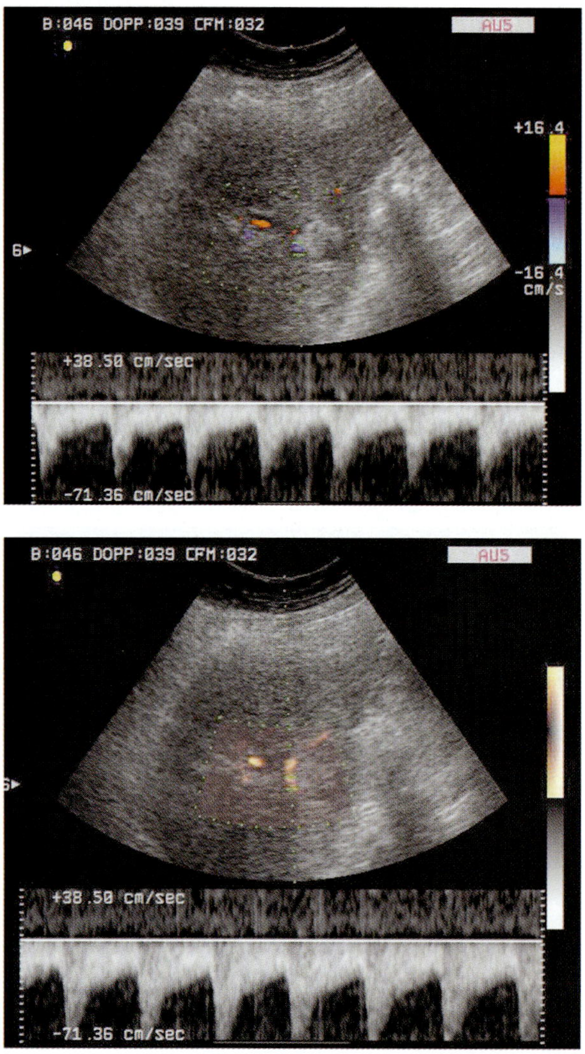

Fig. 5.19. Contrast-enhanced Doppler US of portal vein thrombosis in the color (**a**) and the power (**b**) mode. Enhancement within the thrombus is seen in the early phase following contrast injection, and pulsatile arterial flow is recorded. These findings indicate malignant thrombosis due to vascular invasion by hepatocellular carcinoma

5.3.3 Differential Diagnosis by Doppler Ultrasound

The use of Doppler US aims to aid differential diagnosis of tumors by its ability to demonstrate tumor vessels. In the case of focal hepatic lesions, color Doppler US attempts to identify the vascularity of a lesion and provide a diagnosis on the basis of morphologic and quantitative assessment of blood flow.

5.3.3.1 Differential Diagnosis of Lesions in Cirrhotic Liver

In patients with liver cirrhosis and a nodular lesion detected by US screening, color Doppler US may help differentiate HCC from nonneoplastic hepatocellular lesions, such as macroregenerative or dysplastic nodules. Along with progression from regeneration to cancer, in fact, hepatocellular nodular lesions show a change in the blood supply: the intranodular portal blood supply tends to decrease and, in contrast, the intranodular arterial supply tends to increase in the path from benign to malignancy (TANAKA et al. 1990b; YASHURA et al. 1988; TAYLOR et al. 1987; OHNISHI and NOMURA 1989).

Macroregenerative and dysplastic nodules, as well as early HCC, have a predominantly portal blood supply, while overt HCC lesions are supplied almost exclusively by hepatic arterial branches. The neoangiogenesis of nontriadal arteries, which is the pathologic substratum of tumor hypervascularity, relates especially to the presence of HCC tissue of Edmondson grade 2 or greater.

The different blood supply to the lesion is therefore an important feature that may help differentiate among small hepatocellular lesions emerging in a cirrhotic liver. In fact, while small, overt HCC tumors show a typical hypervascular pattern, with clear-cut intratumoral pulsatile flow on color or power Doppler US and early, arterial-phase enhancement after administered microbubble US contrast agents, early-stage HCC and regenerative or dysplastic lesions fail to exhibit this hypervascular feature (Figs. 5.20, 5.21) (TANAKA et al. 1992; MATSUI et al. 1991; LENCIONI et al. 1996a).

The different blood supply of overt HCC tumors and dysplastic or early-stage HCC lesions is even better depicted by analysis of time-intensity enhancement curves with harmonic power Doppler US. In a pilot clinical study, overt HCC lesions (tumors confirmed as hypervascular lesions by spiral CT or dynamic MR imaging) showed a rapid peak of

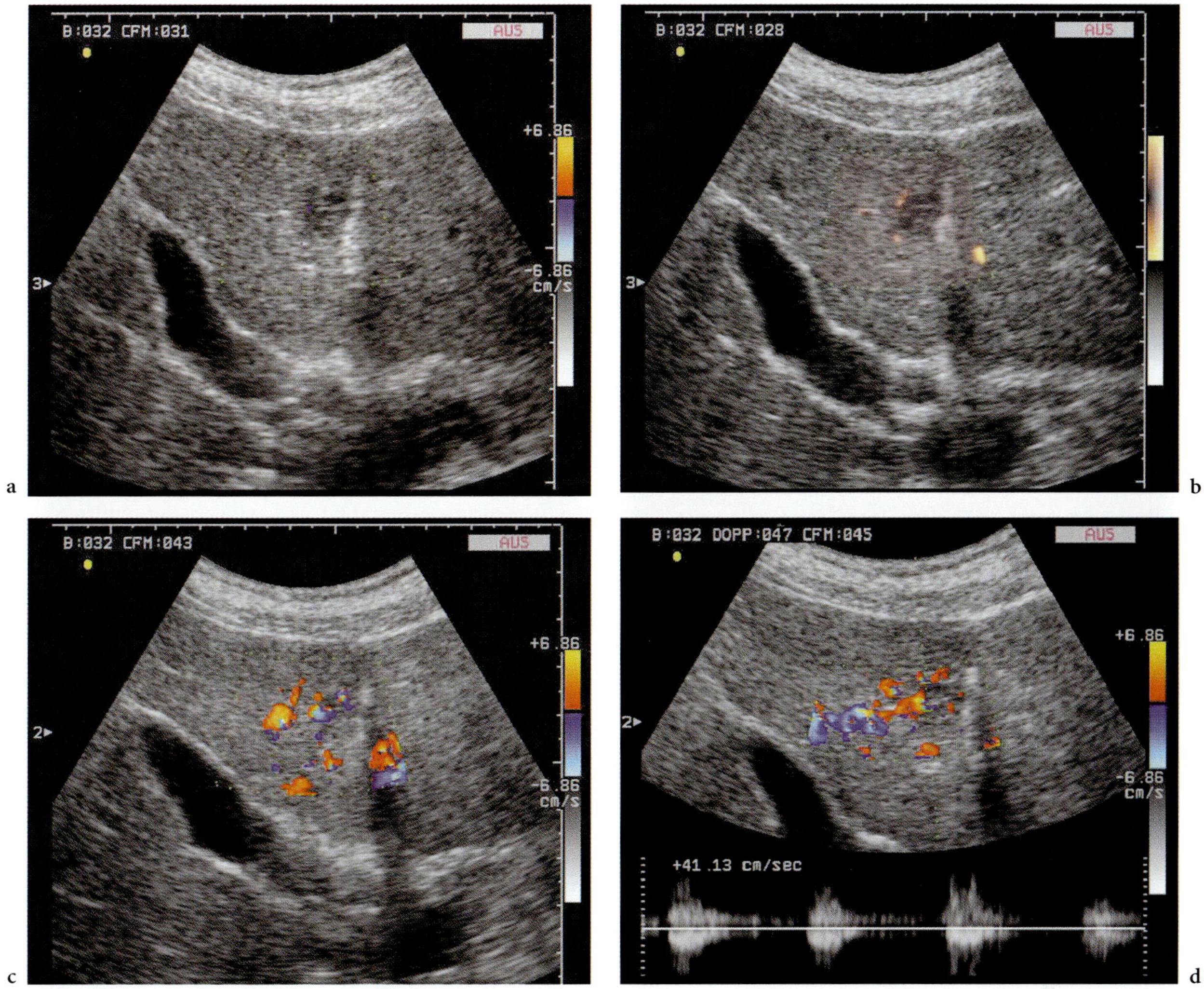

Fig. 5.20a–d. Doppler US study of a small nodular lesion which has emerged in a cirrhotic liver (same case as in Fig. 5.2). Unenhanced color (**a**) and power (**b**) Doppler US fail to show intratumoral blood flow. After contrast injection, rapid enhancement is seen with harmonic color Doppler US within the small lesion, reflecting an arterial hypervascular supply (**c**). Spectral analysis of harmonic signals confirms pulsatile arterial flow (**d**)

enhancement in the early arterial phase (25–48 s after the start of injection; mean±SD, 34±6 s), followed by a rapid decrease during the delayed phase (type 1 curve) (Fig. 5.22). In contrast, early-stage, well-differentiated HCC tumors of Edmondson grade 1 (which were seen as hypovascular tumors on spiral CT or dynamic MR imaging) showed a type 2 curve, characterized by slight, progressive enhancement but no peak in the early phase and a slow decrease in the delayed phase (Fig. 5.23).

In our series, macroregenerative or dysplastic lesions showed either a type 2 curve (similar to that of early-stage HCC) or a complete absence of enhancement throughout the harmonic power Doppler imaging study (type 3 curve).

We therefore found a strong agreement between enhancement pattern on harmonic power Doppler US and tumor vascularity as assessed by spiral CT or dynamic MR imaging. Hence, we believe that evaluation of the enhancement pattern in harmonic power Doppler imaging is a valuable noninvasive means for investigating tumor vascularity in hepatocellular lesions and that, despite considerable overlap between early-stage tumors and macroregenerative or dysplastic nodules, this technique might have the potential to help characterize nodular lesions which have emerged in a cirrhotic liver (Lencioni et al. 1999).

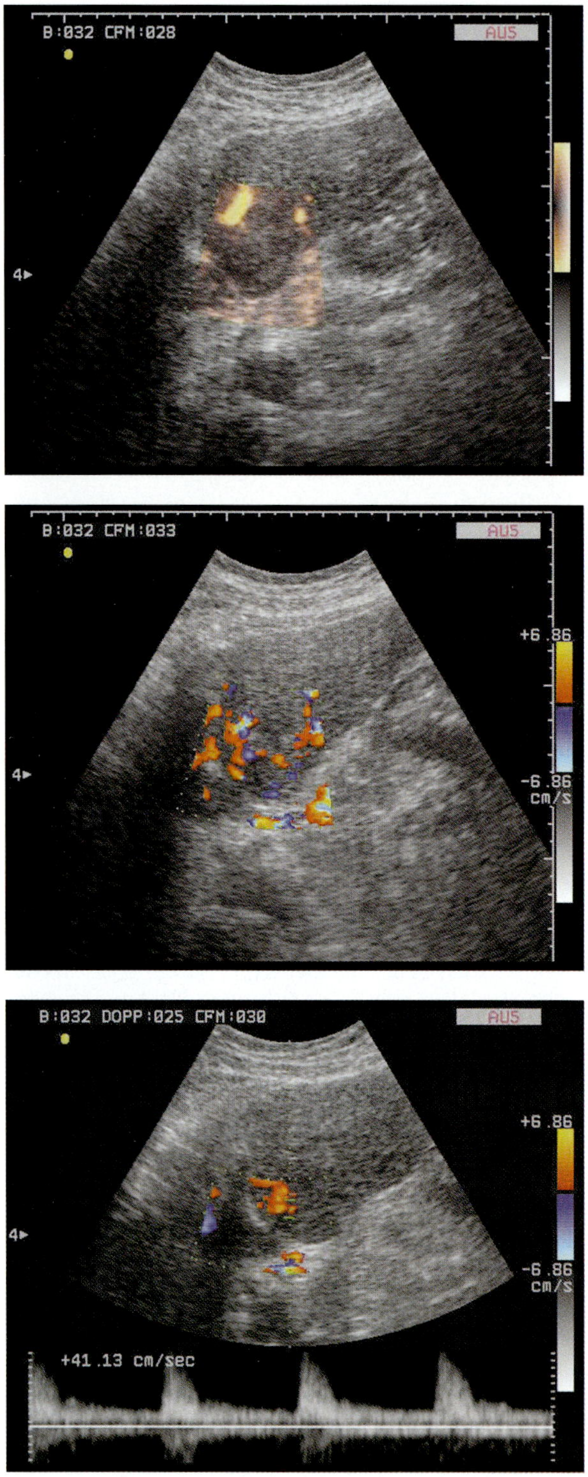

a

b

c

Fig. 5.21a–c. Doppler US study of a small hepatocellular carcinoma which has emerged in a dysplastic lesion (same case as in Fig. 5.13). Unenhanced power Doppler US does not show intratumoral flow (**a**). Contrast-enhanced color Doppler US image shows tumor vessels located around the neoplastic focus (**b**). On spectral analysis, arterial blood supply is observed (**c**)

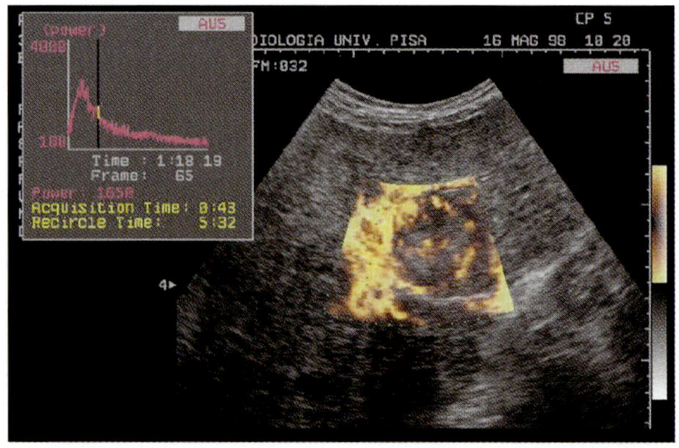

Fig. 5.22. Time-intensity curve of hepatocellular carcinoma (same case as in Fig. 5.5). The lesion demonstrates a clear-cut hypervascular pattern, with a rapid peak of enhancement in the early arterial phase followed by a rapid decrease during the delayed phase. Spiral CT and angiography confirmed a hypervascular tumor

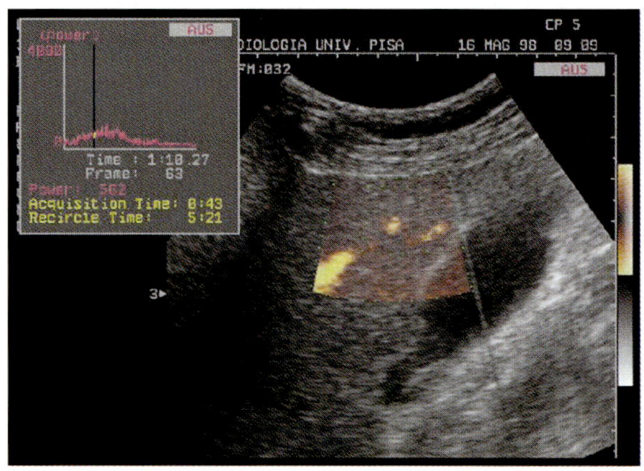

Fig. 5.23. Time-intensity curve of well-differentiated (Edmondson grade 1) hepatocellular carcinoma (same case as in Fig. 5.3). The lesion shows slight, progressive enhancement with no peak in the early phase and a slow decrease in the delayed phase. Spiral CT and angiography confirmed a hypovascular tumor

5.3.3.2
Differential Diagnosis of Lesions in Otherwise Normal Liver

As previously discussed, the diagnosis of HCC developed in a noncirrhotic liver is far more difficult, as a number of different entities must be taken into account. It is important to state that the color Doppler features described above for HCC may help make the diagnosis in the context of a cirrhotic patient, but are less helpful in the clinical setting of a patient with a focal lesion and an otherwise normal liver

(Yashura et al. 1988; Taylor et al. 1987; Tanaka et al. 1990b; Ohnishi and Nomura 1989; Nino-Murcia et al. 1992; Bartolozzi et al. 1997).

The detection of a pulsatile arterial blood flow within the lesion is not specific for HCC. Some other benign and malignant tumors are typically hypervascular. Morphologic analysis of tumor vascularity is also nonspecific: the typical color Doppler features of HCC, namely the "basket pattern" and the "vessel within the tumor," may be depicted also in other kinds of lesions. Hepatocellular adenoma, for instance, typically shows a basket pattern with peritumoral arteries, frequently associated with intratumoral vessels with a venous Doppler spectrum. Intratumoral arteries, however, are not a typical finding in hepatocellular adenoma, but are characteristically found in FNH. In FNH, vessels with a pulsatile Doppler spectrum typically radiate from the center to the periphery of the lesion, and may be associated with either pulsatile or continuous peripheral flow (Bartolozzi et al. 1997; Yashura et al. 1988; Taylor et al. 1987; Tanaka et al. 1990b; Ohnishi and Nomura 1989; Nino-Murcia et al. 1992).

5.4 Conclusions

US is the initial examination performed in most patients clinically suspected of having an hepatic malignancy, as it enables a rapid, accurate, and noninvasive assessment of liver parenchyma. US is an ideal technique for screening patients with chronic liver disease for early detection of HCC, and has been a fundamental tool for understanding the natural history of this tumor. In many cases, US findings enable a confident characterization of the tumor, especially when the HCC develops on a cirrhotic background. US examination can also provide useful information regarding the stage of the tumor, although it is easy to underestimate the presence of tiny satellite nodules or tumor invasion into segmental or subsegmental portal vein branches (Tanaka et al. 1986).

With recent advances in instrumentation and the introduction of US contrast media, color Doppler US currently provides an accurate depiction of tumor vascularity in HCC (Tanaka et al. 1989). Doppler US studies may help differentiate HCC from nonneoplastic hepatocellular lesions arising in cirrhotic livers, such as macroregenerative or dysplastic lesions. Moreover, information on tumor vascularity may help select the most appropriate nonsurgical treatment for small HCC lesions. Tumors showing an arterial hypervascular supply at Doppler US, in fact, might well be suitable for treatment by transcatheter arterial chemoembolization, as the response of HCC to therapeutic arterial embolization is closely related to the degree of neovascularization of the lesion. In contrast, tumors without signs of hypervascularity on power Doppler imaging might be best treated with percutaneous ethanol injection, whose efficacy is not impaired by the lack of arterial blood supply to the tumor. Finally, Doppler US is a tool for monitoring the therapeutic response of the tumor to interventional treatments.

References

Albrecht T, Urbank A, Mahler M, et al (1998) Prolungation and optimization of Doppler enhancement with a microbubbles US contrast agent by using continuous infusion: preliminary experience. Radiology 207:339–347

Arakawa M, Kage M, Sugihara S, Nakashima T, Suenaga M, Okuda K (1986) Emergence of malignant lesions within an adenomatous hyperplastic nodule in a cirrhotic liver. Observations in five cases. Gastroenterology 91:198–208

Bartolozzi C, Lencioni R, Caramella D, Palla A, Bassi AM, Di Candio G (1995) Small hepatocellular carcinoma: detection with US, CT, MR imaging, DSA and Lipiodol-CT. Acta Radiol 37:69–74

Bartolozzi C, Lencioni R, Paolicchi A, Moretti M, Armillotta N, Pinto F (1997) Differentation of hepatocellular adenoma and focal nodular hyperplasia of the liver: comparison of power Doppler imaging and conventional color Doppler sonography. Eur Radiol 7:1410–1415

Bartolozzi C, Lencioni R, Ricci P, et al (1998) Hepatocellular carcinoma treatment with percutaneous ethanol injection: evaluation with contrast-enhaced color Doppler US. Radiology 209:387–393

Beasley RP, Hwang LY, Lin CC, Chien CS (1981) Hepatocellular carcinoma and hepatitis B virus. Lancet 2:1129–1133

Bolondi L, Gaiani S, Gebel M (1998) Portohepatic vascular pathology and liver disease: diagnosis and monitoring. Eur J Ultrasound 7:41–52

Boultbee J (1979) Gray scale ultrasound in hepatocellular carcinoma. Clin Radiol 30:547–552

Bruix J, Calvet X, Costa J, et al (1989) Prevalence of antibodies to hepatitis C virus in Spanish patients with hepatocellular carcinoma and hepatic cirrhosis. Lancet 2:1004–1006

Bude RO, Rubin JM (1996) Power Doppler sonography. Radiology 200: 21–23

Buscarini L, Fornari F, Canaletti R, et al (1991) Diagnostic aspects and follow up of 174 cases od hepatocellular carcinoma: second report. Oncology 48:26–30

Buscarini L, Di Stasi M, Buscarini E, et al (1996) Clinical presentation, diagnostic work-up and therapeutic choices in two consecutive series of patient with hepatocellular carcinoma. Oncology 53:204–209

Calliada F, Campani R, Bottinelli O, Bozzini A, Sommaruga MG (1998) Ultrasound contrast agents: basic principles. Eur J Radiol 27(S):157–160

Calvet X, Bruix J, Bru C, et al (1990) Natural history of hepatocellular carcinoma in Spain. Five year's experience in 249 cases. J Hepatol 10:311–317

Campani R, Bottinelli O, Calliada F, Coscia D (1998) The latest in ultrasound: three-dimensional imaging. Eur J Radiol 27(S):183–187

Catalano O, Cusati B, Esposito M, Trivellini V, Lobianco R, Siani A (1998) The correlation between Doppler echography with a contrast medium and CT in the study of a hepatocarcinoma submitted to chemoembolization. Radiol Med (Torino) 95:608–613

Choi BI, Park JH, Kim BH, Kim SH, Han MC, Kim CW (1989a) Small hepatocellular carcinoma: detection with sonography, computed tomography (CT), angiography and Lipiodol-CT. Br J Radiol 62:897–903

Choi BI, Kim CW, Ham MC, et al (1989b) Sonographic characteristics of small hepatocellular carcinoma. Gastrointest Radiol 14:255–261

Choi BI, Takayasu K, Han MC (1993) Small hepatocellular carcinomas and associated nodular lesion of the liver. Paythology, pathogenesis, and imaging findings. AJR 160:1177–1187

Choi BI, Kim TK, Han JK, et al (1996) Power versus conventional color Doppler sonography: comparison in the depiction of vasculature in liver tumors. Radiology 200:55–58

Colombo M, De Franchis R, Del Ninno E, et al (1991) Hepatocellular carcinoma in Italian patient with cirrhosis. N Engl J Med 325:675–680

Cottone M, Maceno MP, Maringhini A, et al (1983) Ultrasound in the diagnosis of hepatocellular carcinoma associated with cirrhosis. Radiology 147:517–519

Cottone M, Vordone R, Fusco G, et al (1989) Asymptomatic hepatocellular carcinoma in Child's A cirrhosis. A comparison of natural history and surgical treatment. Gastroenterology 96:1566–1571

Dodd GD, Miller WJ, Baron RL, Skoinick ML, Campbell WL (1992) Detection of malignant tumors in end-stage cirrhotic livers: efficacy of sonography as a screening technique. AJR 159:727–733

Dodd GD, Memel BS, Baron RL, Eichner L, Santiguida LA (1995) Portal vein thrombosis in patient with cirrhosis: does sonographic detection of intrathrombus flow alllow differentiation of benign and malignant thrombus? AJR 165:573–577

Ebara M, Ohto M, Shinagawa T, et al (1986) Natural history of minute hepatocellular carcinoma smaller than three centimeters complicating cirrhosis. A study in 22 patients. Gastroenterology 90:289–298

Edmondson HA, Steiner PA (1954) Primary carcinoma of the liver. Cancer 7:462–471

Forsberg F, Merton DA, Liu JB, Needleman L, Goldberg BB (1998) Clinical applications of ultrasound contrast agents. Ultrasonics 36:695–701

Freeman MP, Vick CW, Taylor KJW, Carithers RL, Brewer WH (1986) Regenerating nodules in cirrhosis: appearance with anatomic correlation. AJR 146:533–536

Fujimoto M, Moriyasu F, Nishikawa K, et al (1994) Color Doppler sonography of hepatic tumors with a galactose-based contrast agent. Correlation with angiographic findings. AJR 163:1099–1104

Garbagnati F, Spreafico D, Marchianò A, Salvetti M, Segura C, Piragine G (1991) Staging of hepatocellular carcinoma by ultrasonography, computed tomography, and angiography: the role of CT combined with arterial portography. Gastrointest Radiol 16:225–228

Hayashi N, Yamamoto K, Tamaki N, et al (1987) Metastatic nodules of hepatocellular carcinoma: detection with angiography, CT, and US. Radiology 165:61–63

Honda H, Onitsuka H, Murakami J, et al (1992) Characteristic findings of hepatocellular carcinoma: an evaluation with compatative study of US, CT, and MRI. Gastrointest Radiol 17:245–249

Ikeda K, Saitoh S, Koida I, et al (1994) Imaging diagnosis of small hepatocellular carcinoma. Hepatology 20:82–87

Jackson VP, Martin-Simmerman P, Becker GJ, Holden RW (1983) Real-time ultrasonographic demonstration of vascular invasion by hepatocellular carcinoma. J Ultrasound Med 2:277–280

Kabayashi K, Sugimoto T, Makino H, et al (1985) Screening methods for early detection of hepatocellular carcinoma. Hepatology 5:1100–1105

Kamin PD, Bernardino ME, Green B (1979) Ultrasound manifestations of hepatocellular carcinoma. Radiology 131:459–461

Kanno T, Kurioka N, Kim S, et al (1989) Implications of hypoechoic lesions in small hepatocellular carcinoma. Gastroenterol Jpn 24:528–534

Kawasaki H, Sakaguchi S, Irisa T, Hirayama C (1978) Value of B-scan ultrasonography in the diagnosis of liver cancer. Am J Gastroenter 69:436–442

Kim AY, Choi BI, Han JK et al (1998) Hepatocellular carcinoma: power Doppler US with a contrast-agent-preliminary results. Radiology 209:135–140

Laudy JA, Janssen MM, Struyk PC, Stijnen T, Wallenburg HC, Wladimiroff JW (1998) Fetal liver volume measurement by three-dimensional ultrasonography: a preliminary study. Ultrasound Obstet Gynecol 12:93–96

Lencioni R, Caramella D, Bartolozzi C, Di Coscio G (1994) Long term follow-up study of adenomatous hyperplasia in liver cirrhosis. Ital J Gastroenterol 26:163–168

Lencioni R, Caramella D, Sanguinetti F, Battolla L, Falaschi F, Bartolozzi C (1995) Portal vein thrombosis after percutaneous ethanol injection for hepatocellular carcinoma: value of color Doppler sonography in distinguishing chemical and tumor thrombi. AJR 164:1125–1130

Lencioni R, Mascalchi M, Caramella D, Bartolozzi C (1996a) Small hepatocellular carcinoma: differentiation from adenomatous hyperplasia with color doppler US and dynamic Gd-DTPA-enhanced MR imaging. Abdom Imaging 21: 41–48

Lencioni R, Pinto F, Armillotta N, Bartolozzi C (1996b) Assessment of tumor vascularity in hepatocellular carcinoma: comparison of power Doppler US and color Doppler US. Radiology 201:353–358

Lencioni R, Cioni D, Donati F, Bartolozzi C (1999) Contrast-enhancement pattern in harmonic power Doppler imaging: value in characterization of hepatic tumors. Radiographics (in press)

Mathieu D, Guinet C, Bouklia-Hassane A, Vasile N (1988) Hepatic vein involvement in hepatocellular carcinoma. Gastrointest Radiol 13:55–60

Matsui O, Kadoya M, Kameyana T, et al (1991) Benign and malignant nodules in cirrhotic livers. Distinction based on blood supply. Radiology 178:493–497

Melato M, Laurino L, Mucli E, Valente M, Okuda K (1989) Relationship between cirrhosis, liver cancer, and hepatic metastases. An autopsy study. Cancer 64:455–459

Nino-Murcia M, ralls PW, Jeffrey RB, et al (1992) Color flow Doppler characterization of focal hepatic lesions. AJR 159:1195–1197

Numata K, Tanaka K, Mitsui K, Morimoto M, Inoue S, Yonezawa H (1993) Flow characteristics of hepatic tumors at color Doppler sonography: correlation with arteriographic findings. AJR 160:515–521

Numata K, Tanaka K, Kiba T, et al (1997) Use of hepatic tumor index on color Doppler sonography for differentiating large hepatic tumors. AJR 168:991–995

Ohnishi K, Nomura F(1989) Ultrasonic Doppler studies of hepatocellular carcinoma and comparison with other hepatic focal lesions. Gastroenterology 97:1489–1497

Oka H, Kurioka M, Kim K, et al (1990) Prospective study of early detection of hepatocellular carcinoma in patients with cirrhosis. Hepatology 12:680–687

Okuda K (1986) Early recognition of hepatocellular carcinoma. Hepatology 6:729–738

Okuda K, Musha H, Yoshida T, et al (1975) Demonstration of growing casts of hepatocellular carcinoma in the portal vein by celiac angiography: the tread and streaks sign. Radiology 117:303–309

Okuda K, Musha H, Nakajima J, et al (1977) Clinicopathologic features of encapsulated hepatocellular carcinoma: a study of 26 cases. Cancer 40:1240–1245

Okuda K, Ohtsuki T, Obata H, et al (1985) Natural history of hepatocellular carcinoma and prognosis in relation to treatment: study of 850 patients. Cancer 56:918–928

Pateron D, Gonne N, Trinchet J, et al (1994) Prospective study of screening of hepatocellular carcinoma in caucasian patients with cirrhosis. J Hepatol 20:65–71

Reinhold C, Hammers L, Taylor CR, Quedes-Case CL, Holland CK,Taylor KJW (1995) Characterization of focal hepatic lesions with duplex sonography: findings in 198 patients. AJR 164:1131–1135

Ricca Rosellini S, Arienti V, Nanni O, et al (1992) Hepatocellular carcinoma. Prognostic factors and survival analysis in 135 italian patients. J Hepatol 16:66–72

Ros PR, Murphy BJ, Buck JL, Olmedilla G, Goodman Z (1990) Encapsulated hepatocellular carcinoma: radiologic findings and pathologic correlation. Gastrointest Radiol 15:233–237

Rubin JM, Bude RO, Carson PL, Bree RL, Adler RS (1994) Power Doppler US: A potentiallly useful alternative to mean frequency-based color Doppler US. Radiology 190:853–856

Sakaguchi S, Tohara K, Oka Y (1992) Ultrasonographic diagnosis of hepatocellular carcinoma. In: Tobe T, Kameda H, Okudaira M, et al (eds) Primary liver cancer in Japan. Springer-Verlag, Tokyo, p 115

Schwarz K, Chen X, Steinmetz S, Phillips D (1997) Harmonic imaging with Levovist. J Am Soc Echocardiogr 10:1–10

Shankar P, Dala Krishna P, Newhouse VL (1998) Advantages of subharmonic over second harmonic backscatter for contrast-to-tissue echo enhancement. Ultrasound Med Biol 24:395–399

Sheu JC, Chen DS, Sung JL, et al (1985a) Hepatocellular carcinoma: US evolution in the early stage. Radiology 155:463–467

Sheu JC, Sung JL, Chen DS, et al (1985b) Growth rate of asymptomatic hepatocellular carcinoma and its clinical implications. Gastroenterology 89:259–266

Shimamoto K, Sakuma S, Ishigaki T, Makino M (1987) Intratumoral blood flow: evaluation with color Doppler echography. Radiology 165:683–685

Shimamoto K, Sakuma S, Ishigaki T, et al (1992) Hepatocellular carcinoma: evaluation with color Doppler US and MR imaging. Radiology 182:149–153

Shinagawa T, Ohto M, Kimura K, et al (1984) Diagnosis and clinical features of small hepatocellular carcinoma with emphasis on the utility of realtime ultrasonography. A study of 51 patients. Gastroenterology 86:495–502

Subramanyam BR, Balthazar EJ, Hilton S, Lefleur RS, Horii SC, Raghavendra BN (1984) Hepatocellular carcinoma with venous invasion. Sonographic-angiographic correlation. Radiology 150:793–796

Takano S, Yokosuka O, Imazeki F, et al (1995) Incidence of hepatocellular carcinoma in chronic hepatitis B and C. A prospective study of 251 patients. Hepatology 21:650–655

Takayasu K, Moriyama N, Muramatsu Y, et al (1990) The diagnosis of small hepatocellular carcinomas: efficacy of various imaging procedures in 100 patients. AJR 155:49–54

Tanaka S, Kitamura T, Imaoka S, Sasaki Y, Taniguchi H, Ishiguro S (1983) Hepatocellular carcinoma: sonographic and histologic correlation. AJR 140:701–707

Tanaka S, Kitamura T, Ahshima A, et al (1986) Diagnostic accuracy of ultrasonography for hepatocellular carcinoma. Cancer 58:344–347

Tanaka S, Kitamura T, Nakanishi K, Okuda S, Kojima J, Fujimoto I (1989) Recent advances in ultrasonographic diagnosis of hepatocellular carcinoma. Cancer 63:1313–1317

Tanaka S, Kitamura T, Nakanishi K, et al (1990a) Effectiveness of periodic checkup by ultrasonography for the early diagnosis of hepatocellular carcinoma. Cancer 66:2210–2214

Tanaka S, Kitamura T, Fujita M, et al (1990b) Color Doppler flow imaging of liver tumors. AJR 143:509–514

Tanaka S, Kitamura T, Fujita M, et al (1992) Small hepatocellular carcinoma. Differentation from adenomatous hyperplastic nodule with color Doppler flow imaging. Radiology 182:161–165

Tanaka S, Kitamura T, Fujita M, Yoshioka F (1998) Value of contrast-enhanced color Doppler sonography in diagnosing hepatocellular carcinoma with special attention to the „color-filled pattern". J Clin Ultrasound 26:207–212

Tano S, Ueno N, Toliyama T, et al (1997) Possibility of differentiating small hyperechoic liver tumors using contrast-enhanced color Doppler ultrasonography: a preliminary study. Clin Radiol 52:41–45

Taylor KJW, Ramos I, Morse SS, et al (1987) Focal liver masses. Differential diagnosis with pulsed Doppler US. Radiology 164:643–647

Thomas J, Rubin DN (1998) Tissue harmonic imaging: why does it work? J Am Soc Echocardiogr 11:803–808

Trevisani F, D'Intino PE, Caraceni P, et al (1995) Etiologic factors and clinical presentation of hepatocellular carcinoma. Differences between cirrhotic and noncirrhotic Italian patient. Cancer 75:2220–2232

Wernecke K, Henke L, Vassallo P, et al (1992) Pathologic explanation for hypoechoic halo seen on sonograms of malignant liver tumors: an in vitro correlative study. AJR 159:1011–1016

Yashura K, Kimuram K, Ohto M, et al (1988) Pulsed Doppler in the diagnosis of small liver tumors. Br J Radiology 61:898–902

Yoshida T, Matsue H, Okazaki MD, Yoshino M (1987) Ultrasonographic differentiation of hepatocellular carcinoma from metastatic liver cancer. J Clin Ultrasound 15:431–437

Yoshikawa J, Matsui O, Takashima T, et al (1988) Fatty metamorphosis in hepatocellular carcinoma: radiologic features in 10 cases. AJR 151:717–720

Yuki K, Hirohashi S, Sakamoto M, Kanai T, Shimosato Y (1990) Growth and spread of hepatocellular carcinoma. A review of 240 consecutive autopsy cases. Cancer 66:2174–2179

6 Computed Tomography of Hepatocellular Carcinoma

C. BARTOLOZZI, F. DONATI, D. CIONI, L. CROCETTI, and R. LENCIONI

CONTENTS

C. BARTOLOZZI, MD; Professor and Chairman, Division of Diagnostic and Interventional Radiology, Department of Oncology, University of Pisa, Via Roma 67, I-56125 Pisa, Italy
F. DONATI, MD; Division of Diagnostic and Interventional Radiology, Department of Oncology, University of Pisa, Via Roma 67, I-56125 Pisa, Italy
D. CIONI, MD; Division of Diagnostic and Interventional Radiology, Department of Oncology, University of Pisa, Via Roma 67, I-56125 Pisa, Italy
L. CROCETTI, MD; Division of Diagnostic and Interventional Radiology, Department of Oncology, University of Pisa, Via Roma 67, I-56125 Pisa, Italy
R. LENCIONI, MD; Division of Diagnostic and Interventional Radiology, Department of Oncology, University of Pisa, Via Roma 67, I-56125 Pisa, Italy

6.1 Introduction

Computed tomography (CT) currently plays a fundamental role in the screening, differential diagnosis, staging, and evaluation of response to treatment of hepatocellular carcinoma (HCC) (OLIVER et al. 1996). HCC is a hypervascular tumor which is best depicted by CT images obtained during the predominantly arterial phase of contrast enhancement. Hence, the use of a spiral scanner is mandatory when studying this kind of malignancy to perform an accurate examination of the entire liver parenchyma (RUMMENY and MARCHAL 1997). This article will focus on spiral CT features of HCC lesions and on the role of CT for screening, differential diagnosis, and staging of HCC. The usefulness of spiral CT for the assessment of tumor response will be discussed in the relevant chapter.

6.2 Technique

6.2.1 Dual-Phase Spiral CT

Evaluation of patients with suspected HCC requires a carefully standardized examination protocol (MITSUKAKI et al. 1996; OLIVER et al. 1996; TUBLIN et al. 1999). Obtaining unenhanced scans is mandatory. In fact, since patients with HCC usually also have liver cirrhosis, macroregenerative or dysplastic nodules containing iron deposits may be occasionally found. These lesions are well depicted on unenhanced CT images, as they have a higher attenuation than liver parenchyma owing to the intranodular content of iron (Fig. 6.1).

Unenhanced and dual-phase contrast-enhanced spiral CT examination is performed by obtaining a volume acquisition covering the entire liver parenchyma during a single suspended respiration. A 7-mm collimation and a 1:1 pitch in a cranial-cau-

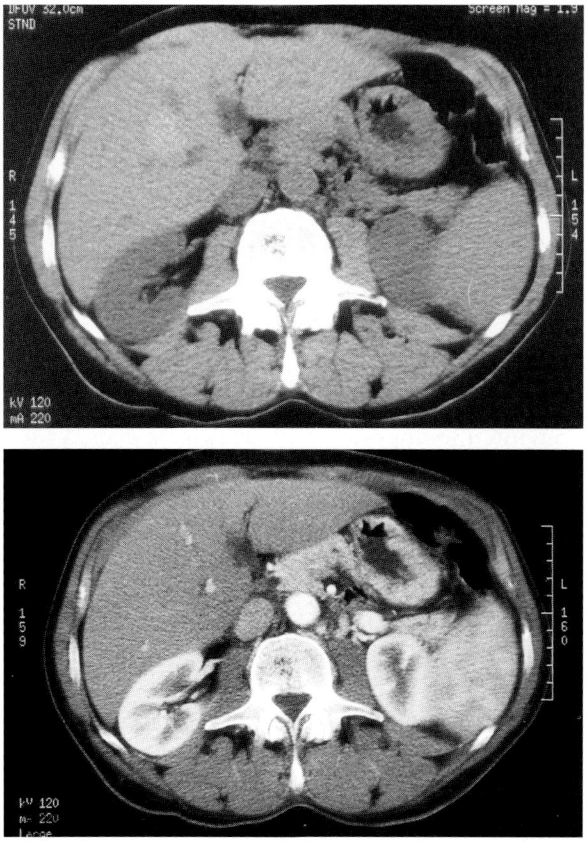

a

b

Fig. 6.1a,b. Macroregenerative nodule containing iron deposits. The lesion appears hyperdense in the baseline scan (**a**), and fails to enhance in the arterial phase image, becoming undetectable (**b**)

dal direction beginning at the top of the liver are used. For the dual-phase contrast-enhanced study, patients receive 130–150 ml nonionic contrast material at a rate of 3–5 ml/s. CT is initiated 20 s (if using an infusion rate of 5 ml/s) or 25 s (if using an infusion rate of 3 ml/s) after the start of contrast injection to obtain arterial-phase images. The liver is imaged in 20–30 s (Bonaldi et al. 1995). Portal venous phase images are then obtained beginning at 65–70 s (if using an infusion rate of 5 ml/s) or 70–75 s (if using an infusion rate of 3 ml/s) after the start of contrast injection (Choi et al. 1996; Mitsukaki et al. 1996). Delayed phase images may also be useful in selected cases, particularly to evaluate tumor characteristics such as the presence of a capsule (Fig. 6.2).

6.2.2
Angiographically Assisted CT Techniques

The combination of CT and angiography allows the performance of accurate CT studies for the detection and characterization of HCC (Kanematsu et al. 1999). There are three combinations of CT and angiography: CT during the injection of contrast material into the hepatic artery (CT arteriography), CT during arterial portography (CTAP), and CT performed after the intra-arterial injection of iodized oil (Lipiodol CT). These are accurate but invasive procedures that are mainly used to overcome the limitations of conventional CT in the detection and evaluation of small HCC lesions (Merine et al. 1990). Following the introduction of spiral scanners, the indications for angiographically assisted CT techniques have been restricted to selected cases (Nelson et al. 1990; Small et al. 1993; Tourel et al. 1995).

6.2.2.1
CT Arteriography

In CT arteriography (CTA), contrast material is injected directly into the proper or common hepatic artery or, if not possible, into the celiac artery. With conventional nonspiral CT scanners, 10–15 ml of contrast material are injected at a rate of 1–3 ml/s during the scanning of each slice of the liver. After the introduction of spiral machines, it has become possible to obtain high-quality CTA images of the entire liver during a single breathhold. Contrast material is injected at a rate of 3–5 ml/s during the scanning of the entire liver. Scanning is initiated 5 s after the start of contrast injection (Rubin et al. 1993).

6.2.2.2
CT during Arterial Portography

Before spiral CTAP, limited visceral angiography must be performed to place the tip of a 5F catheter in the proximal superior mesenteric artery. With conventional nonspiral machines, 70–100 ml of contrast material are injected at a rate of 0.5–1.5 ml/s during sequential scanning of the liver with incremental changes in the position of the table. The scanning is started around 20 s after the initiation of the infusion. With spiral systems, it is possible to increase the rate of injection up to 3 ml/s, examining the whole liver parenchyma during a single suspended respiration. Scanning is started 30 s after beginning of contrast administration (Bluemke et al. 1995; Hori et al. 1998; Kanematsu et al. 1997, 1998; Merine et al. 1990).

6.2.2.3
Lipiodol CT

To perform Lipiodol CT, a complete angiographic study of the arterial supply to the liver must per-

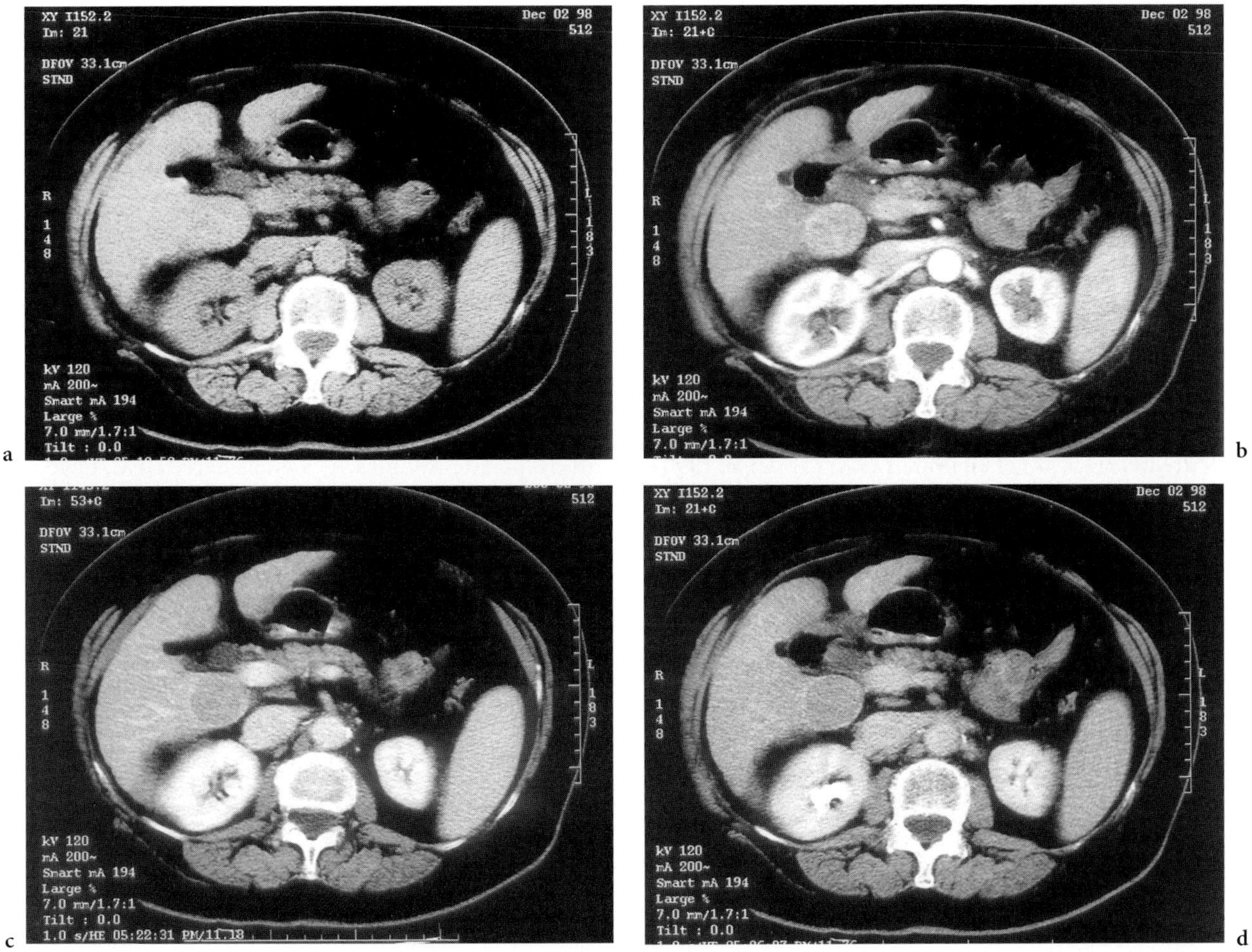

Fig. 6.2a–d. Small hepatocellular carcinoma. The lesion is isoattenuating with respect to liver parenchyma in the baseline scan (**a**), and stands out in the arterial phase image (**b**). The tumor is nearly isodense to liver in the portal venous phase (**c**) and in the delayed phase (**d**). The tumor capsule is not depicted in the baseline scan (**a**), in the arterial phase image (**b**), and in the portal venous phase image (**c**), but may be appreciated in the delayed phase image as a peripheral rim of enhancement (**d**)

formed as a preliminary step. Then, 10–20 ml of iodized oil (Lipiodol UltraFluid, Laboratories Guerbet, France) mixed with 50–100 mg of epirubicin hydrochloride are injected. The anticancer-in-oil emulsion must be injected with the catheter tip advanced into either the proper hepatic artery, after the emergence of the gastroduodenal and cystic arteries, or in both the right and left hepatic arteries. When accessory or replaced hepatic arteries are found, repeated catheterizations and injections must be performed so that the emulsion could reach the whole liver parenchyma to identify any possible lesion. The final step of the procedure is the injection of absorbable gelatin sponge particles.

Three to 4 weeks after the procedure, unenhanced CT of the liver is performed to evaluate areas of retained Lipiodol (Lencioni et al. 1997). If the washout of the iodized oil from the liver parenchyma is still incomplete on CT scans obtained 3–4 weeks after Lipiodol injection, CT may be repeated 1–2 weeks later (Bisollon et al. 1998; Choi et al. 1997; Merine et al. 1990).

6.3 CT Features of Hepatocellular Carcinoma

6.3.1 Dual-Phase Spiral CT

6.3.1.1 Small Hepatocellular Carcinoma

Along with progress in early diagnosis, various new information on the pathomorphologic characteristics and developmental process of early-stage HCC has been obtained through the histologic examination of resected lesions, explanted livers, and autopsy specimens (Choi et al. 1993).

Currently, HCC is thought to develop through two main pathways: a de novo carcinogenesis and a multistep progression. Multistep development is considered to be the most frequent model of hepatocarcinogenesis in cirrhotic livers. This model includes the transition from frankly benign nodules (large regenerative nodules or macroregenerative nodules) to equivocal lesions (dysplastic nodules or borderline lesions), to early HCC (very well differentiated tumor of Edmondson grade 1), and, finally, to overt HCC (advanced tumor of Edmondson grade 2 or greater) (Kanai et al. 1987; Takayama et al. 1990). HCC usually develops as a focus of well-differentiated cancer within a dysplastic lesion. When the tumor grows to 1–1.5 cm in diameter, de-differentiation of well-differentiated cancer cells occurs: cancer tissue at lower histologic grades proliferates within the well-differentiated cancerous nodule (early-advanced HCC), replaces the well-differentiated tissue that has weak proliferative activity, and then starts to grow expansively, developing into advanced HCC (Kim SR et al. 1998).

Along with progression from regeneration to cancer, hepatocellular nodular lesions shows a change in the blood supply. In fact, the intranodular portal blood supply tends to decrease and, in contrast, the intranodular arterial supply tends to increase in the path from benign to malignancy. Macroregenerative and dysplastic nodules, as well as early HCC, have a predominantly portal blood supply, while overt HCC lesions are supplied almost exclusively by hepatic ar-

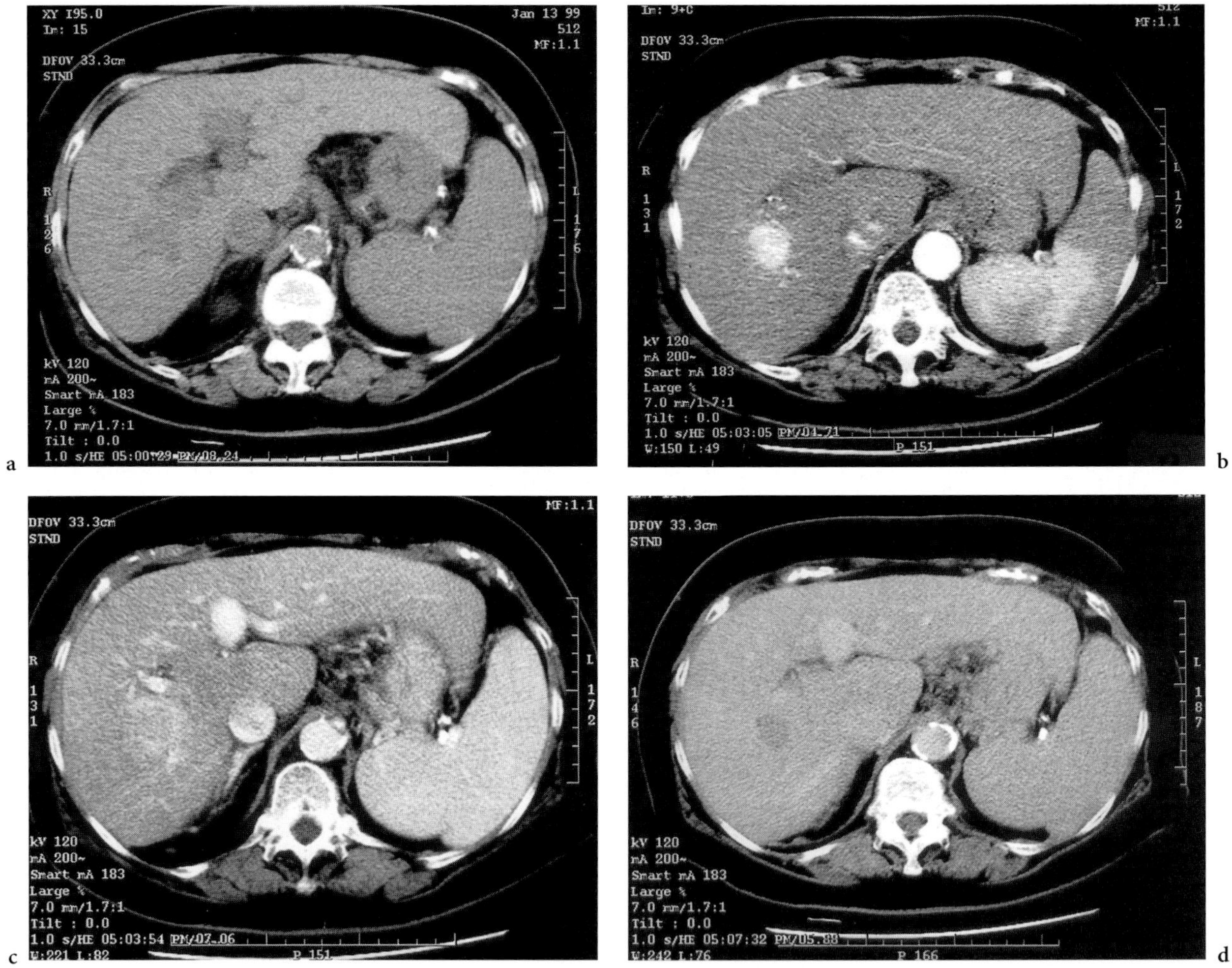

Fig. 6.3a–d. Small, overt, hepatocellular carcinoma. The tumor is slightly hypoattenuating in the baseline scan (**a**). The lesion shows a clear-cut hypervascular pattern and stands out in the arterial phase spiral CT image (**b**) against the faintly enhanced liver parenchyma. Rapid wash-out of contrast material is observed in the portal venous phase image (**c**), in which the lesion is not detectable. The tumor is hypoattenuating in the delayed phase (**d**)

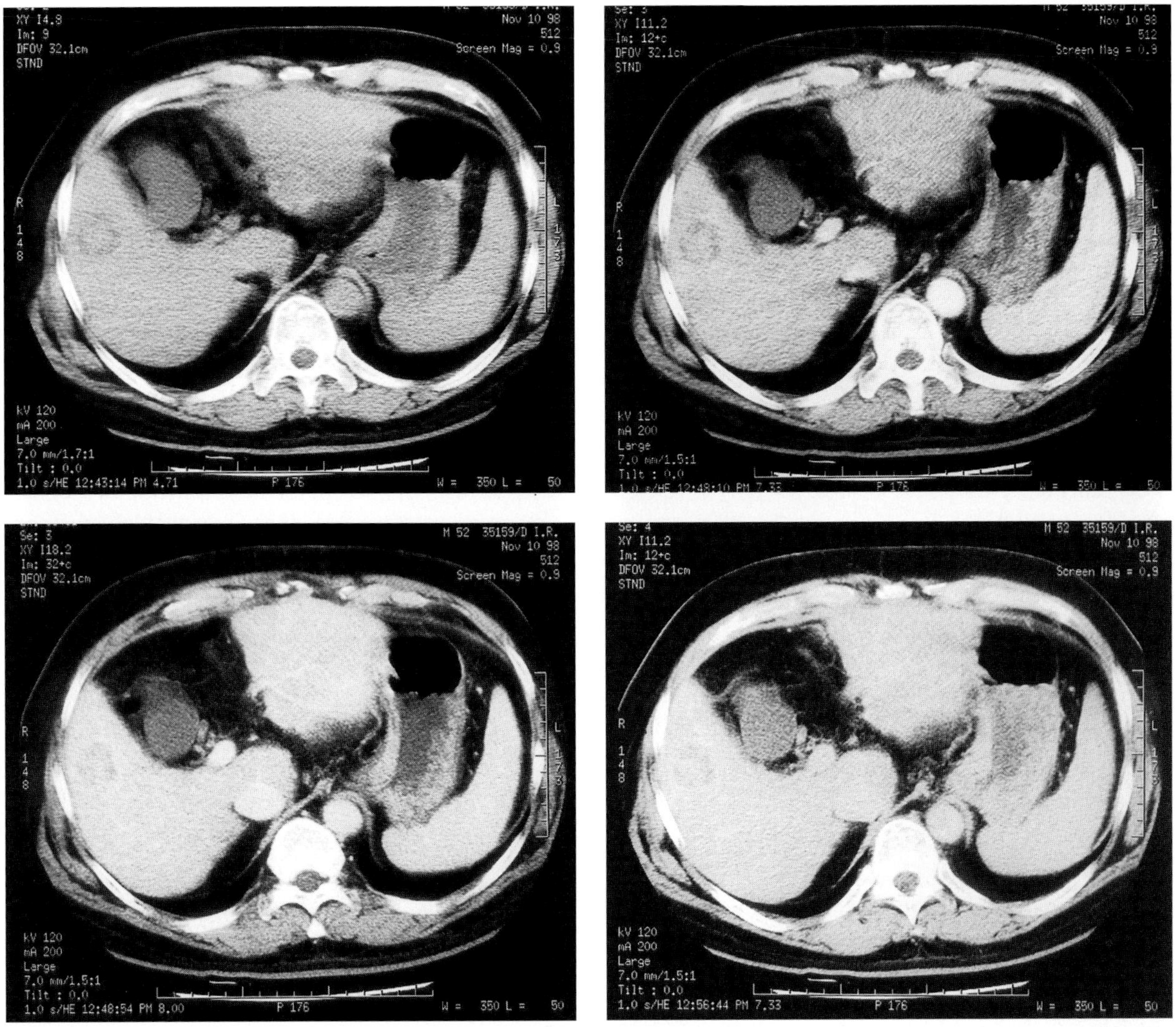

Fig. 6.4a–d. Early-stage, hypovascular hepatocellular carcinoma. The lesion is depicted as a slightly low-attenuating nodule in the precontrast spiral CT image (**a**). The lesion fails to enhance in the arterial phase image (**b**), and appears hypoattenuating with respect to surrounding liver parenchyma in the portal venous phase (**c**) and in the delayed phase (**d**)

terial branches (Nakakuma et al. 1993). The neoangiogenesis of nontriadal arteries, that is the pathologic substratum of tumor hypervascularity, relates to the presence of HCC tissue of Edmondson grade 2 or greater (Lencioni et al. 1996).

The different blood supply to the lesion is the single most important CT feature that may help differentiate among small hepatocellular lesions which have emerged in a cirrhotic liver (Lee et al. 1997). In fact, while small, overt HCC tumors show a typical hypervascular pattern, with clear-cut enhancement in the predominantly arterial phase and rapid washout in the portal venous phase (Fig. 6.3), early-stage HCC and regenerative or dysplastic lesions fail to exhibit this feature and appear isoattenuating or hypoattenuating with respect to surrounding liver parenchyma on dual-phase spiral CT images (Fig. 6.4) (Bonaldi et al. 1995; Choi et al. 1996; Rofflett et al. 1995). These early-stage lesions usually appear hyperintense on T1-weighted MR images and almost isointense to liver on T2-weighted MR images. The lack of arterial blood supply is also well depicted by dynamic contrast-enhanced MR images (Fig. 6.5).

Morphologically, small HCC tumors less than 3 cm in greatest dimension usually show a nodular configuration and may be divided into four types: single nodular type, single nodular type with extranodular growth, contiguous multinodular type, and poorly demarcated nodular type (Hollett et al. 1995).

Small, classical, nodular type HCC is a sharply demarcated lesion, which may or may not be encapsulated (Figs. 6.6, 6.7). Pathologically, the tumor capsule is seen in about 50–60% of small HCC lesions. The CT detection rate of the capsule by is low in small tumors because the capsule is thin and poorly developed. The capsule is seen as a peripheral rim that is hypoattenuating on unenhanced and arterial-phase contrast-enhanced images and hyperattenuating on delayed contrast-enhanced images (Fig. 6.7) (Ros et al. 1990).

The single nodular type with extranodular growth, the contiguous multinodular type, and the poorly demarcated nodular type show a nodular configuration with an irregular or unclear margin on CT images (Figs. 6.8, 6.9) (Oliver et al. 1996).

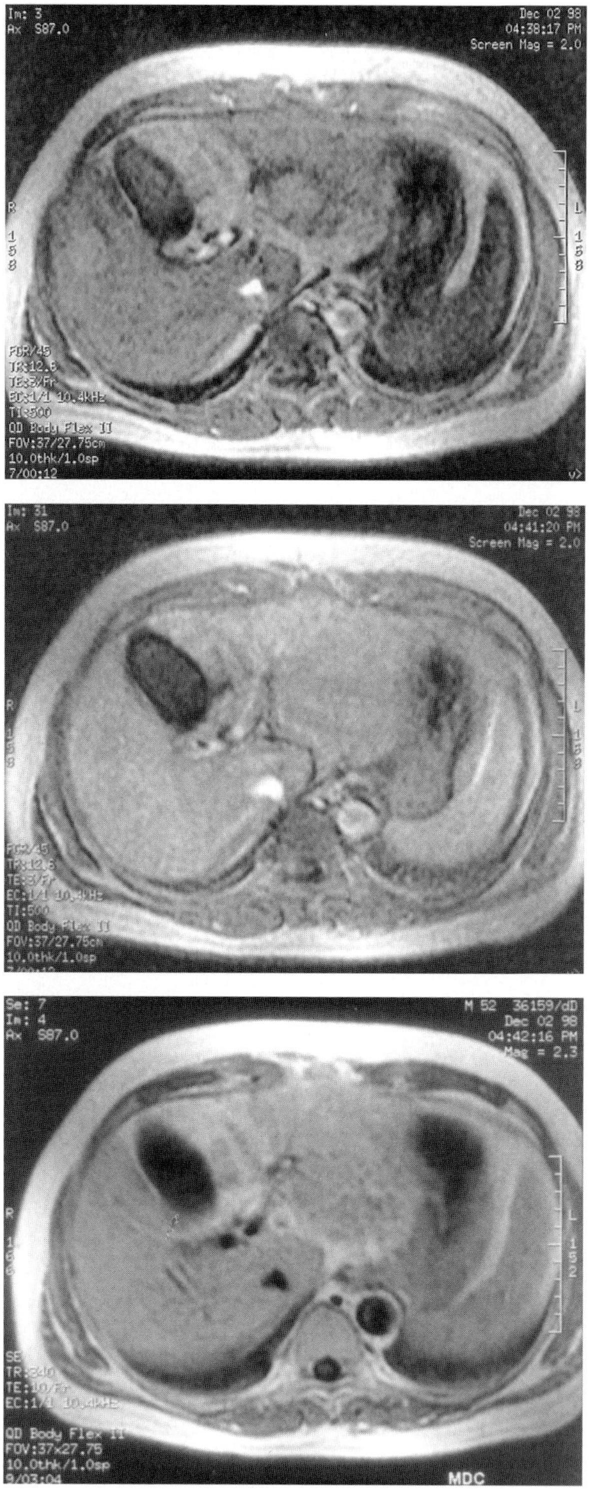

Fig. 6.5a–c. Early-stage, hypovascular hepatocellular carcinoma (same case as in Fig. 6.4). The lesion is depicted as a hyperintense nodule in the unenhanced gradient-echo T1-weighted MR image (**a**). The lesion fails to enhance in the arterial phase gradient-echo image (**b**), and appears isointense with respect to surrounding liver parenchyma in the delayed contrast-enhanced spin-echo image (**c**)

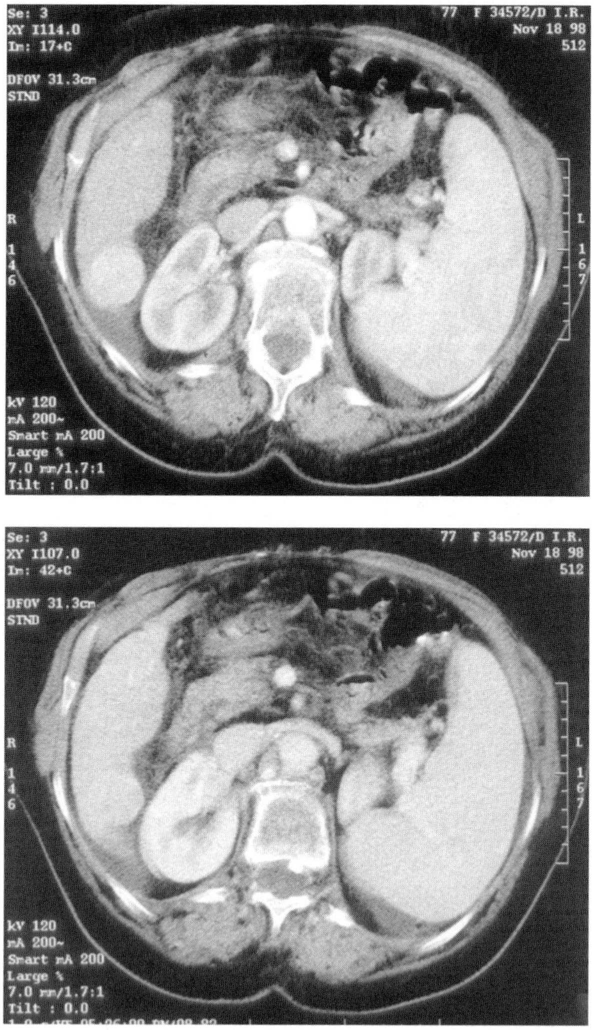

Fig. 6.6a,b. Small, nodular type hepatocellular carcinoma. The lesion is well depicted in the arterial phase spiral CT image (**a**). In the portal venous phase, the tumor becomes isoattenuating to liver (**b**). The tumor capsule is not depicted

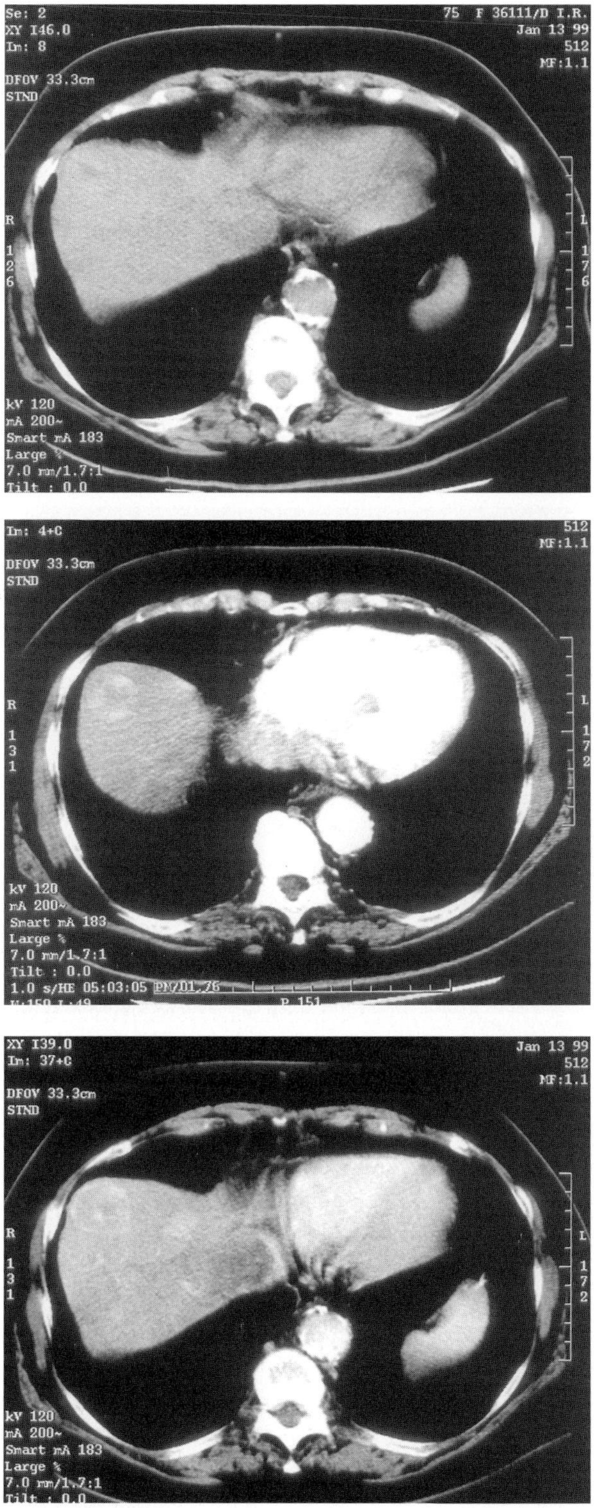

a

b

c

Fig. 6.7a–c. Small, nodular type, encapsulated hepatocellular carcinoma. The thin capsule is seen as a peripheral rim that is hypoattenuating on unenhanced (**a**) and arterial-phase contrast-enhanced images (**b**) and hyperattenuating on delayed contrast-enhanced images (**c**)

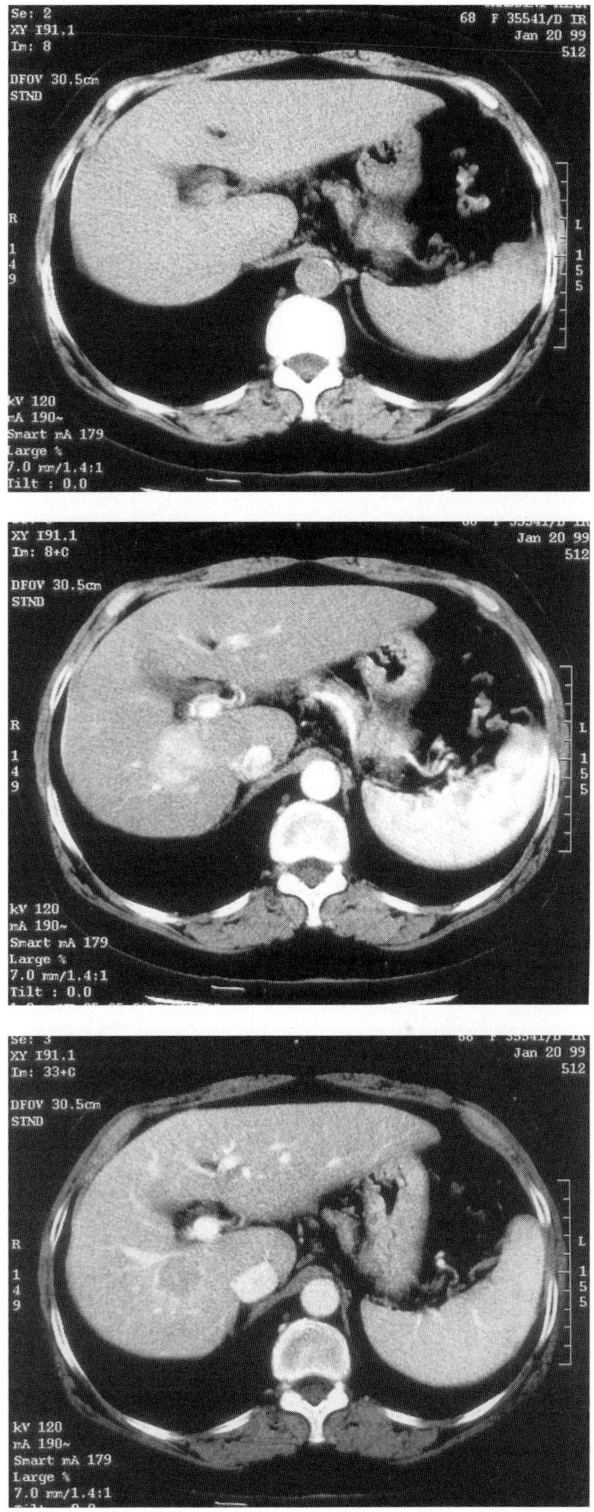

a

b

c

Fig. 6.8a–c. Small, nodular type hepatocellular carcinoma with extranodular growth. The tumor appears isodense in the baseline scan (**a**), hyperdense in the arterial phase (**b**) and hypodense in the portal venous phase (**c**). The lesion shows nodular configuration with irregular margins and incomplete encapsulation

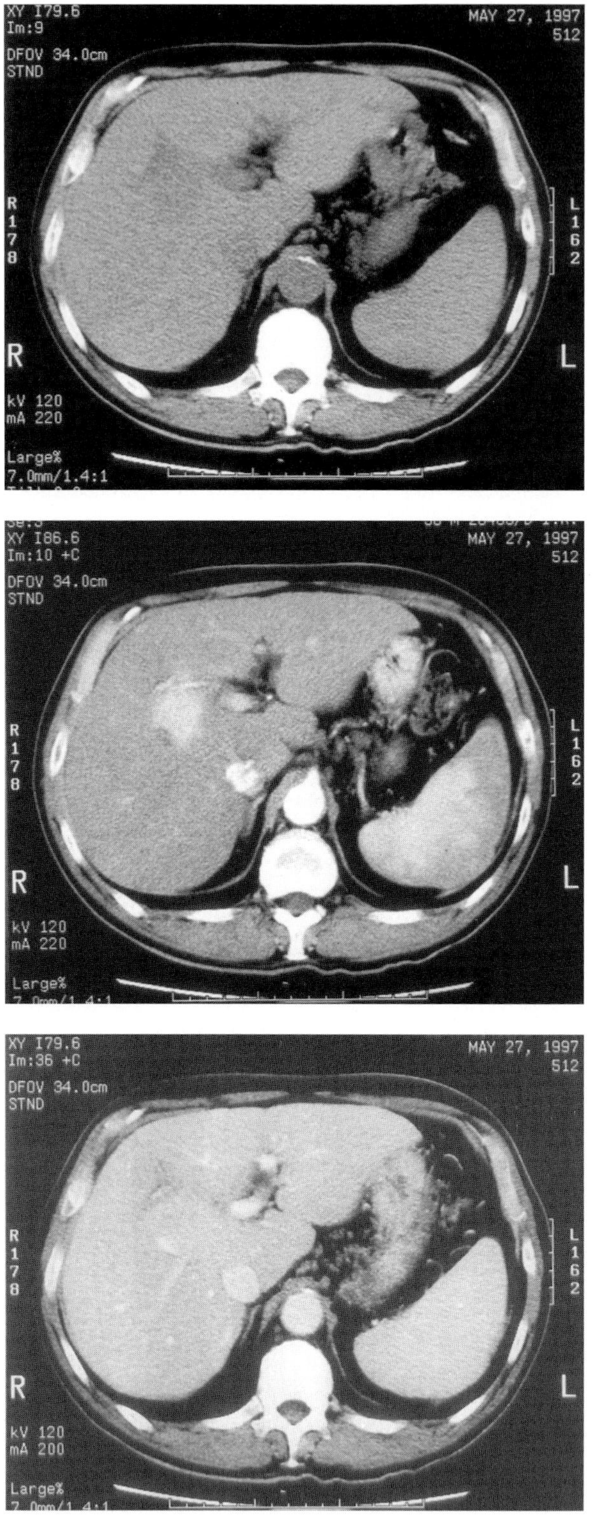

Fig. 6.9a–c. Small, poorly demarcated, nodular type hepatocellular carcinoma. The tumor appears hypodense in the baseline scan (**a**), slightly hyperdense in the arterial phase (**b**) and isodense in the portal venous phase (**c**) of the spiral CT study. The lesion shows nodular configuration with irregular and unclear margin

6.3.1.2 *Advanced Hepatocellular Carcinoma*

Advanced HCC lesions are classified into three major types: expansive nodular type, infiltrative type, and diffuse type.

The typical expansive type of HCC is a sharply demarcated lesion, which may be unifocal or multifocal. Typical features of expansive type HCC include tumor capsule and internal mosaic architecture. Most expansive HCC lesions have a well-developed fibrous capsule. The capsule may be depicted by CT in up to 70–80% of large, encapsulated lesions on macroscopic pathologic examination. The fibrous capsule is demonstrated by CT as a hypoattenuating

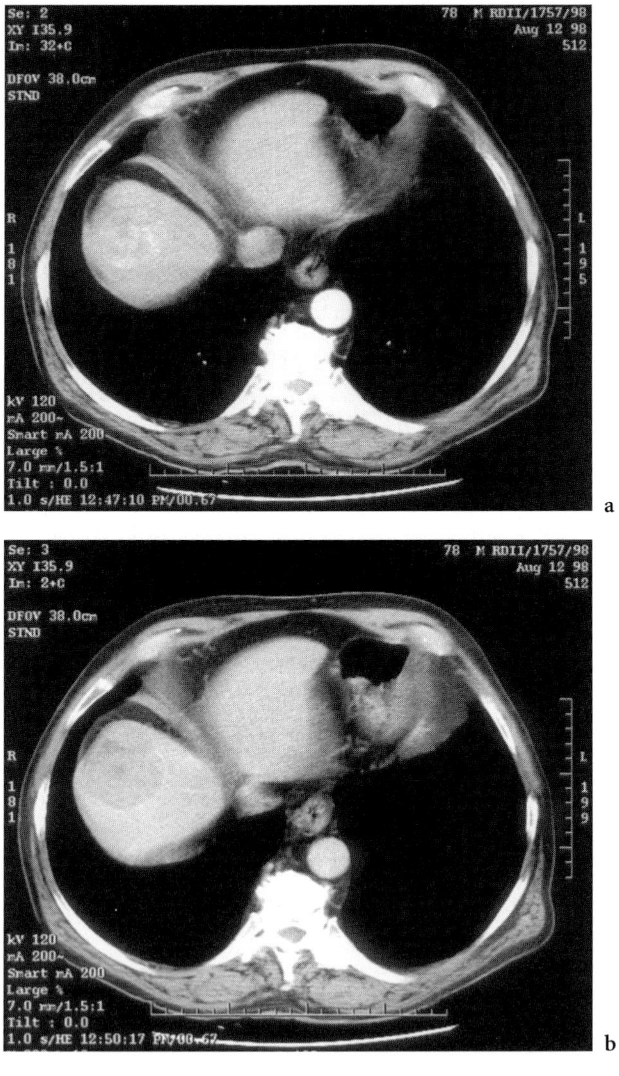

Fig. 6.10a,b. Large, encapsulated hepatocellular carcinoma. Spiral CT images obtained in the arterial (**a**) and the portal venous phase (**b**). The capsule is depicted as a thin enhancing rim in the portal venous phase image

rim which enhances in the delayed phase (Fig. 6.10). Internal mosaic architecture is characterized by components separated by thin septa (Fig. 6.11). The different components may show various attenuation indexes on precontrast CT images, particularly if areas of well-differentiated tumor with different degrees of fatty metamorphosis are present (Ros et al. 1990).

The infiltrative type HCC is characterized by an irregular and indistinct tumor-nontumor boundary. This type is demonstrated as a mainly uneven area with unclear margins (Fig. 6.12). The tumor strands into surrounding tissue, and frequently invades vascular structures, particularly portal vein branches

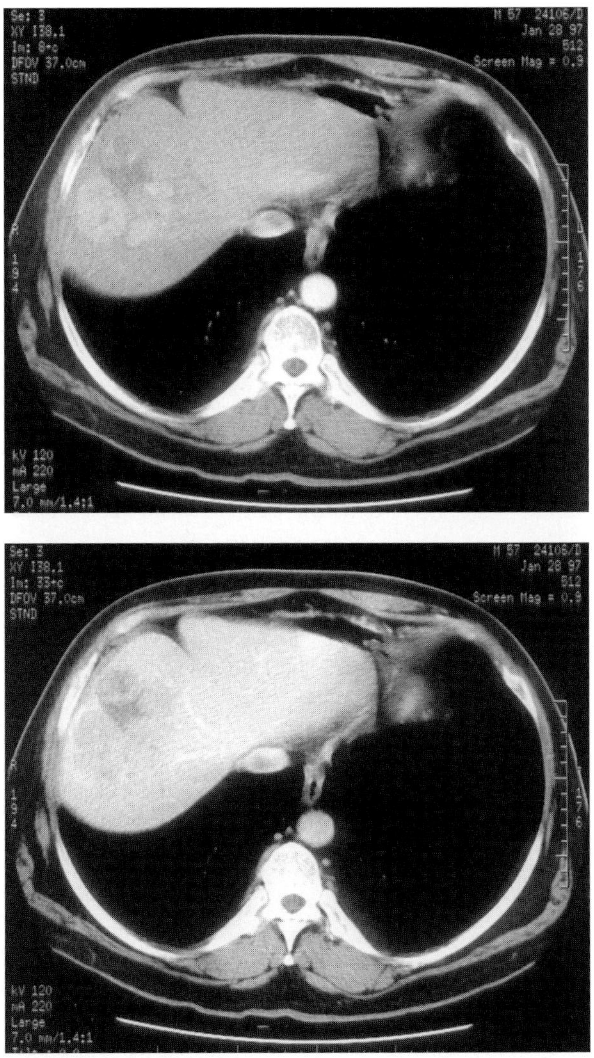

Fig. 6.11a,b. Hepatocellular carcinoma with internal mosaic architecture and intratumoral septa. Spiral CT images obtained in the arterial (**a**) and the portal venous phase (**b**). Different components of the tumor show various attenuation

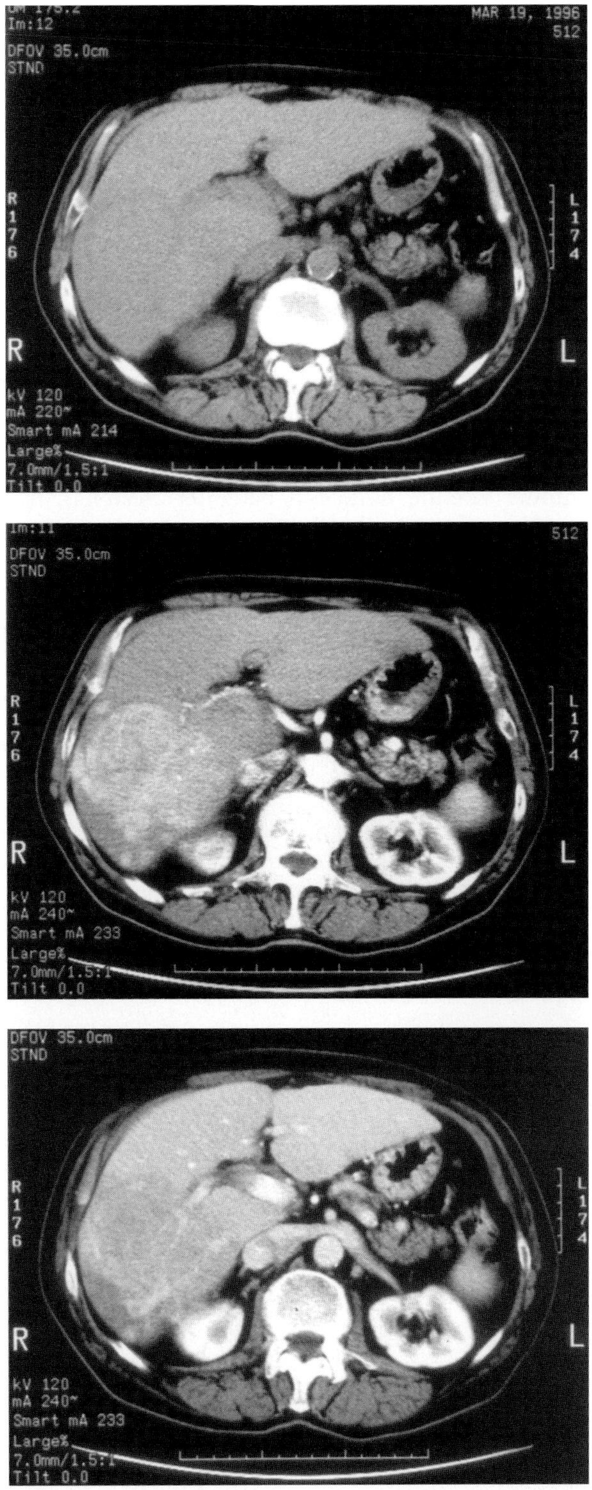

Fig. 6.12a–c. Infiltrative type hepatocellular carcinoma. The tumor is hardly detectable in the baseline scan (**a**) and is depicted by arterial phase (**b**) and portal venous phase (**c**) spiral CT images as an uneven area with irregular borders and inhomogeneous enhancement which strands into surrounding tissue. Tiny satellite nodules are also detected in the vicinity of the main tumor

(Choi 1995). HCC, in fact, has a great propensity for invading and growing into the portal vein, eliciting tumor thrombi (Fig. 6.13). Identification of neoplastic thrombosis of the portal vein is a crucial staging and prognostic factor (Novick and Fishman 1998). Infiltrative HCC may create a massive involvement of the liver, replacing large parts of the parenchyma. The diffuse type is by far the most unusual presentation of HCC. This type is characterized by numerous nodules of small size scattered throughout the liver. The nodules do not fuse with each other and are visualized as diffusely distributed hypodense lesions (Oliver et al. 1996).

In addition to these morphological features, HCC has the typical tendency of giving out small or minute satellite nodules ("daughter" lesions), frequently located in the vicinity of the main tumor. These nodules represent intrahepatic metastases that are usually developed via the portal vein branches. Identification of these satellite lesions is of the utmost importance for therapeutic planning, and represents one of the most challenging issues in HCC patients (Fig. 6.14) (Oi et al. 1996). Satellite lesions should be distinguished from multiple small HCC tumors caused by multicentric development. Such a distinction is important since the presence of intrahepatic metastases indicates a more advanced stage and is associated with a worse prognosis. In the case of multicentric development, multiple small tumors may exhibit a different enhancement pattern on spiral CT, reflecting a different degree of tumor differentiation (Choi et al. 1997; Lencioni et al. 1997).

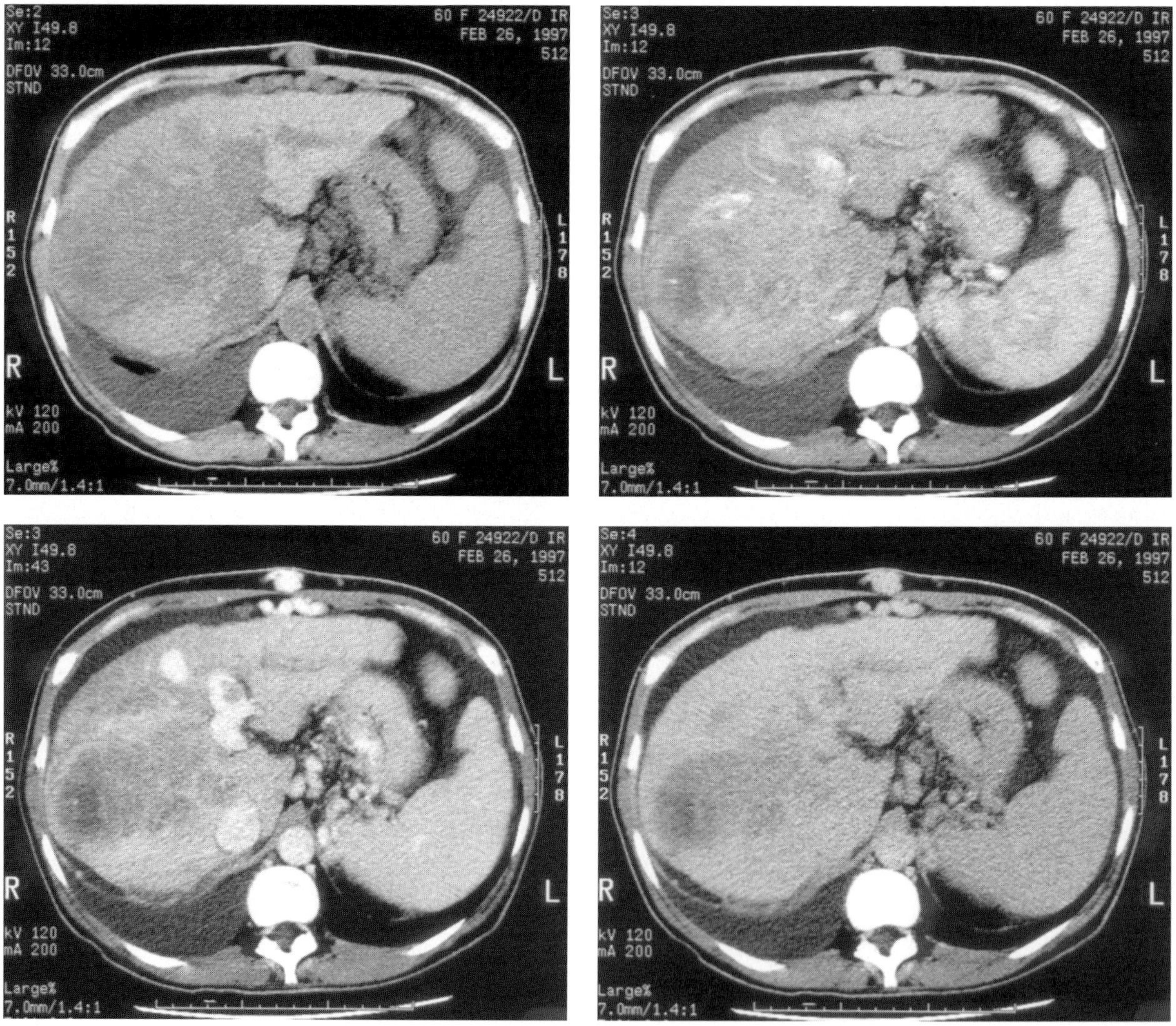

Fig. 6.13a–d. Infiltrative type hepatocellular carcinoma with tumor thrombus in the portal vein. Spiral CT images obtained in baseline (**a**), arterial (**b**), portal (**c**), and delayed phase (**d**) show a huge tumor mass replacing a large part of the liver parenchyma, invading the portal vein branches and eliciting neoplastic thrombosis

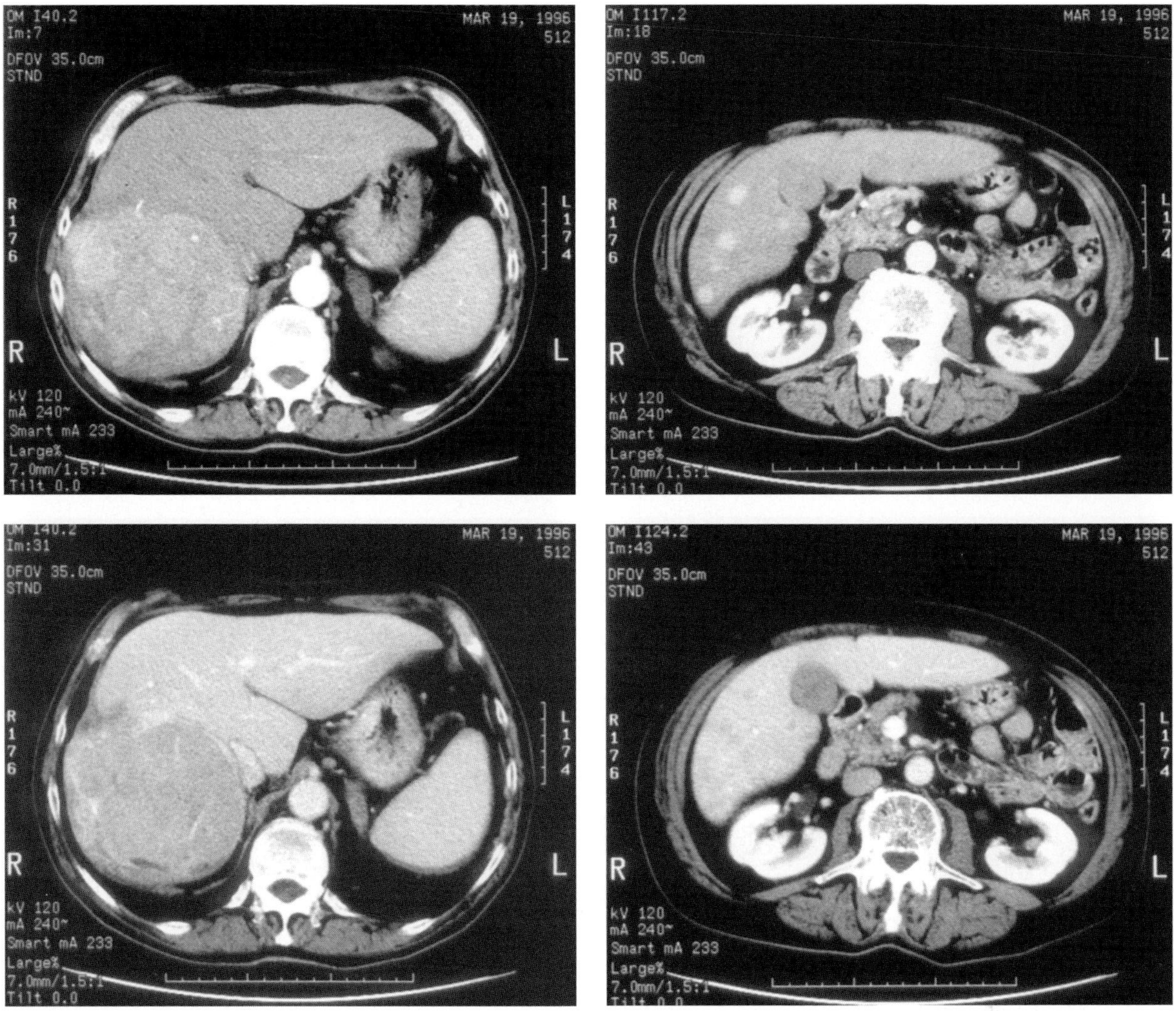

a b c d

Fig. 6.14a–d. Hepatocellular carcinoma with multiple satellite lesions. The main tumor and the daughter nodules are well depicted in the arterial phase spiral CT images due to their clear-cut enhancement (**a,b**). In the portal venous phase images (**c,d**), the main tumor and the satellite lesions appear hypoattenuating with respect to surrounding liver parenchyma

6.3.1.3
Unusual CT Features of Hepatocellular Carcinoma

Unusual histopathologic characteristics of HCC may modify the typical CT appearance of this tumor. These unusual histopathologic characteristics include marked fatty change, massive necrosis, abundant fibrous stroma (sclerosing type HCC), sarcomatous change, copper accumulation, and calcifications (Freeny et al. 1992).

When fatty metamorphosis is severe, CT usually shows areas of negative attenuation value within the tumor, allowing the diagnosis of the fat component (Fig. 6.15). When the degree of fatty deposition differs among internal portions of the tumor, the mosaic architecture can be visualized and the diagnosis of HCC made. However, in the case of diffuse fatty metamorphosis of the lesion, differential diagnosis from lipomatous tumors may not be achieved by CT (Yoshikawa et al. 1988).

Spontaneous massive necrosis within HCC is shown as a non-enhanced area, similar to other necrotic tumors (Fig. 6.16). HCC with abundant fibrous stroma (sclerosing type HCC) demonstrates hypovascularity on arterial-phase CT images and shows delayed enhancement (Yamashita et al. 1993; Yoshikawa et al. 1992). The same enhancement pattern may be seen in HCC with sarcomatous change, which is a very rare histotype. These CT features are commonly seen in lesions with a rich fibrous component, such as confluent hepatic fibrosis in cirrhotic

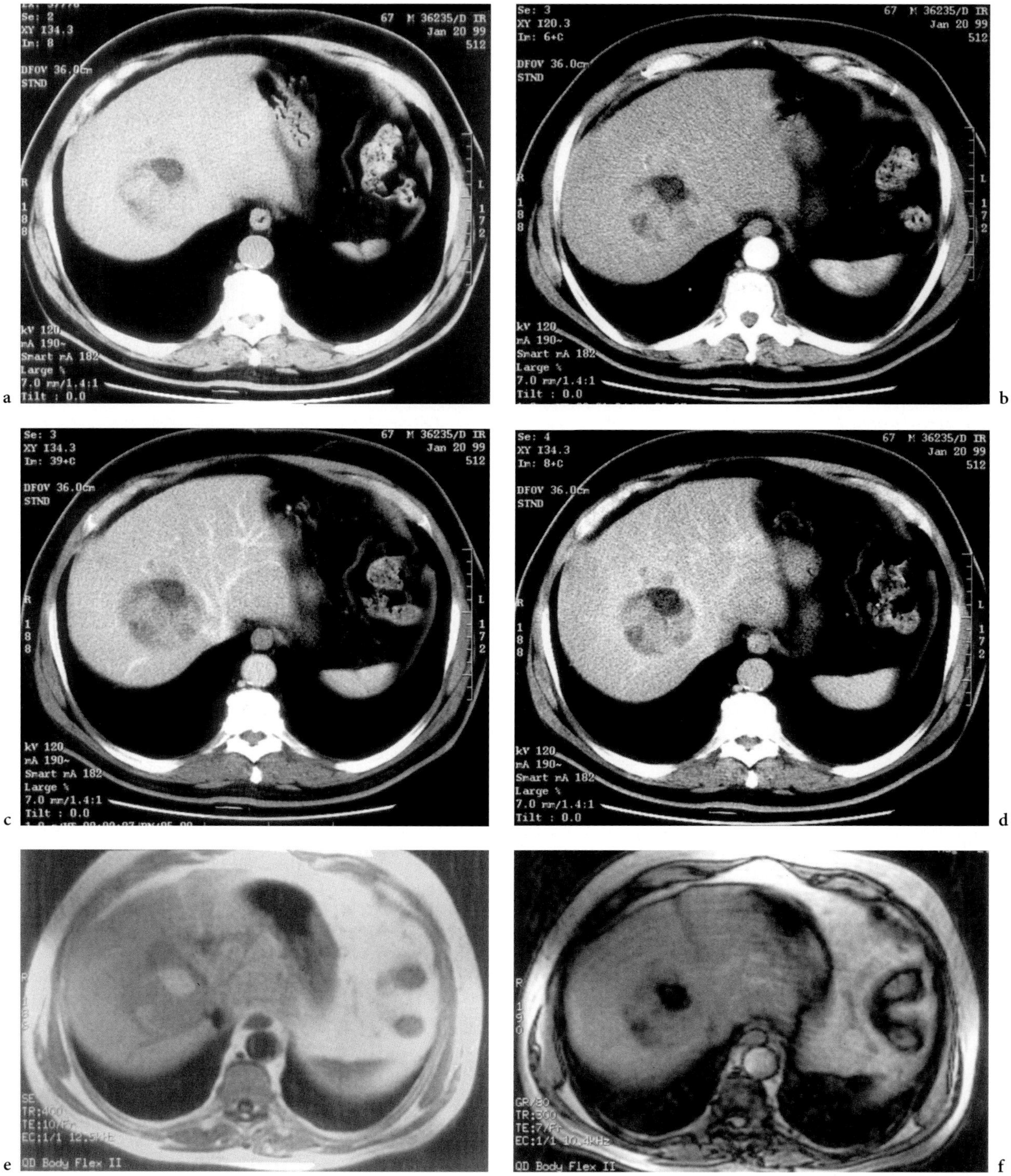

Fig. 6.15a–f. Hepatocellular carcinoma with fatty metamorphosis. Spiral CT images obtained in the precontrast phase (**a**), arterial phase (**b**), portal venous phase (**c**), and delayed phase (**d**). The lesion shows internal areas that are markedly hypoattenuating due intratumoral fatty accumulation. MR imaging confirms the presence of areas of fatty change, which appear hyperintense in the spin echo T1-weighed image (**e**) and hypointense in the gradient-echo out-of-phase T1-weighted image (**f**)

liver and cholangiocellular carcinoma (OHTOMO et al. 1993).

Deposition of copper and copper-binding protein in some HCC lesions has been recognized, resulting in increased attenuation on precontrast CT images (KITAGAUA et al. 1991). The presence of calcifications is uncommon in HCC, being detected in about 0.2–1% of tumors. Calcifications, however, are not rare in fibrolamellar carcinoma and in mixed cholangiocellular-hepatocellular carcinoma.

6.3.2 Angiographically Assisted CT Techniques

6.3.2.1 *CT Arteriography*

CTA is based on the fact that all but very few HCC tumors are fed from the hepatic artery. On CTA images, HCC lesions show high-attenuation blushes compared with the surrounding normal liver and stand out against the faintly enhanced normal parenchyma. Therefore, even small but overt HCC tumors may be well depicted. With CTA, however, early-stage, well-differentiated HCC tumors with immature neovascularity fail to enhance and are not distinguished from liver parenchyma (TAKAYASU et al. 1995b).

Variations in vascular anatomy, flow-related artifacts, and altered hemodynamics due to the associated chronic liver disease may significantly change the patterns of enhancement and produce both false-negative and false-positive results. Familiarity with the hemodynamics and the disease processes, and correlation of the CT findings with those seen on hepatic angiograms, will help avoid these pitfalls (RUBIN et al. 1993; UEDA et al. 1998).

6.3.2.2 *CT during Arterial Portography*

CTAP is based on the reverse pathologic substratum with respect to CTA, that is, on the fact that almost no HCC tumors are fed by the portal vein. This procedure produces dense enhancement of portal venous blood, so that the arterially supplied overt HCC lesions are highlighted as negative defects (Fig. 6.17). The liver is markedly increased in attenuation, and even small tumor deposits may be depicted as definitely hypodense areas. Well-differentiated, early-stage HCC tumors, however, maintain a portal blood supply (although usually decreased with re-

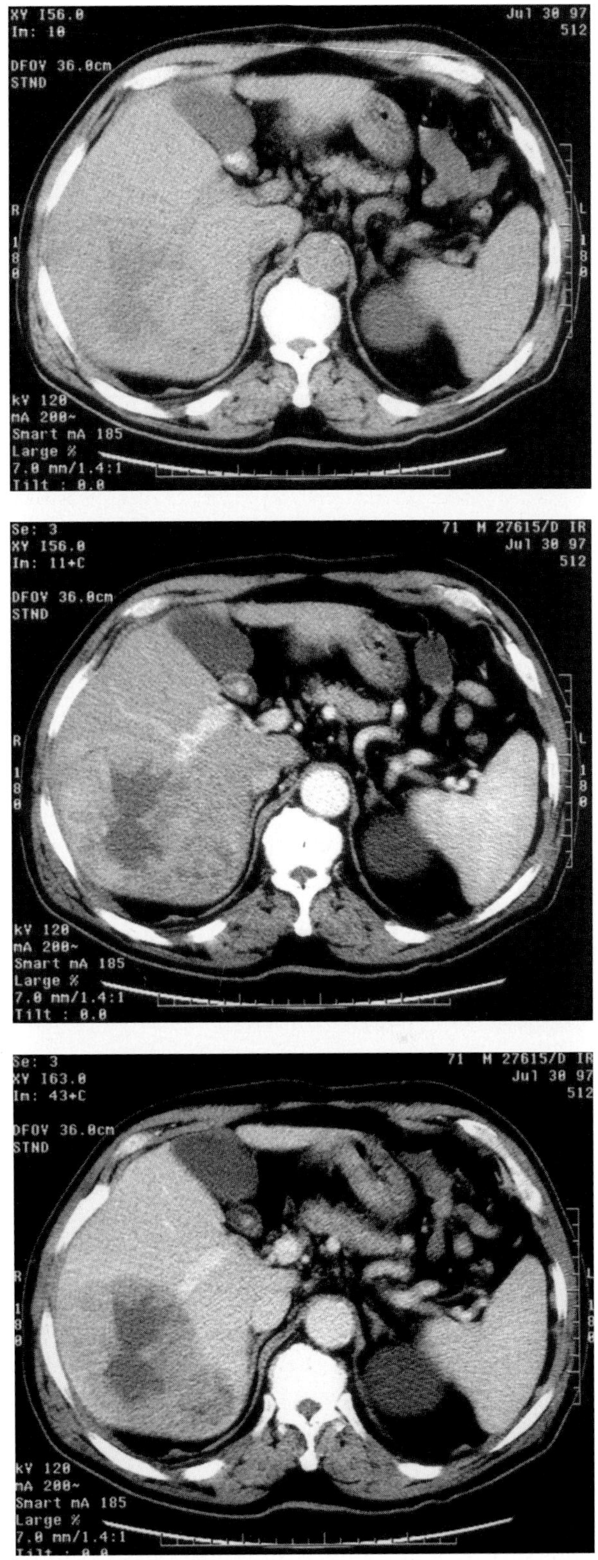

a b c

Fig. 6.16a–c. Large hepatocellular carcinoma with internal necrosis. The necrotic portion is depicted as a low attenuating area in the precontrast spiral CT image (**a**), which fails to enhance in the arterial (**b**) and the portal (**c**) phases

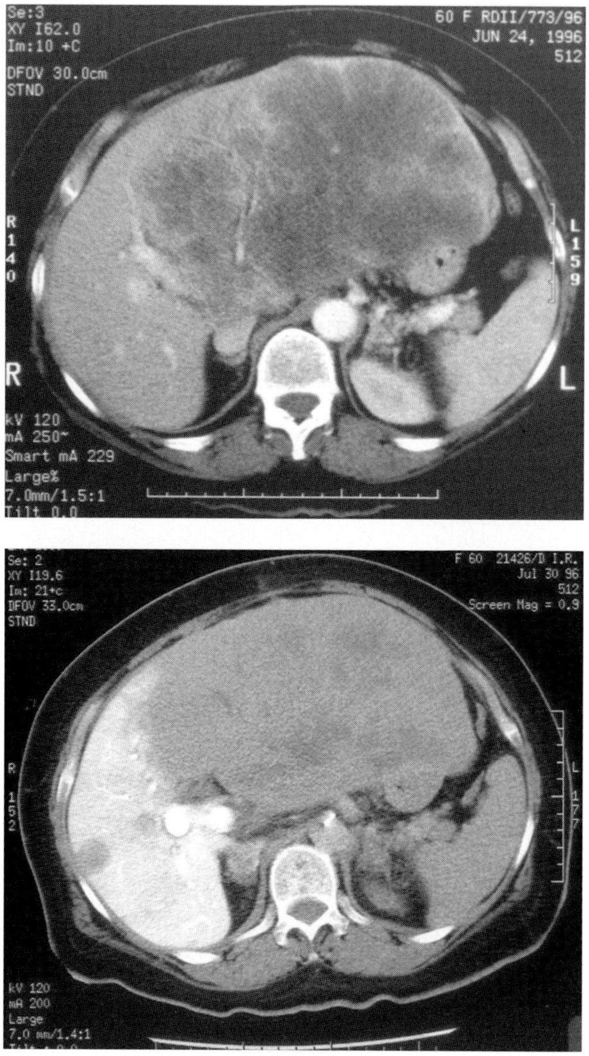

a
b

Fig. 6.17a,b. Spiral CT during arterial portography. Large tumor mass is detected in the left lobe by conventional spiral CT image (**a**). Further evaluation with spiral CT during arterial portography reveals a 1-cm neoplastic nodule in the right lobe undetected by previous studies (**b**)

spect to that of normal liver or regenerative nodules) and may exhibit a faint hypodensity with respect to liver parenchyma, being hardly detectable (Bluemke et al. 1995; Takayasu et al. 1995b).

Many reports have shown that this technique has a very high detectability rate for small, overt HCC tumors. However, CTAP lacks specificity, as almost every focal lesion in the liver, including benign lesions such as hemangiomas and small cysts, assumes the same hypoattenuating appearance and therefore may simulate tumor (Matsui et al. 1994). Moreover, this technique has the drawback that nontumorous portal vein perfusion defects, unrelated to tumor deposits, can occur due to altered hemodynamics, particularly in the presence of liver cirrhosis. False-positive rates as high as 20–30% for patient analysis, in fact, have been reported, making CTAP unreliable for the correct prediction of positive tumor involvement (Hori et al. 1998; Kanematsu et al. 1997, 1998; Merine et al. 1990).

6.3.2.3 Lipiodol CT

Lipiodol is the iodinated ethyl ester of the fatty acid of poppy seed oil and contains 37–38% iodine by weight. When Lipiodol is injected into the hepatic artery, most of the iodized oil droplets flow into HCC lesions by virtue of the increased blood supply to the tumor. Once deposited in the tumor, the Lipiodol droplets disappear at a far slower rate compared with those deposited in the normal liver tissue. In fact, while iodized oil undergoes rapid washout from the noncancerous liver parenchyma, usually leaving an unappreciable amount 3-4 weeks after the intra-arterial injection, it remains for months or years within HCC nodules.

The reason for the selective and prolonged retention of Lipiodol in HCC lesions has yet to be fully clarified. Some authors suggested that trapping of the oil in the irregular, tortuous, and poorly contractile vessels of the tumor, as well as the abnormally increased permeability of these vessels, may be involved. Moreover, it has been hypothesized that the slow disappearance of Lipiodol from HCC lesions may be explained with the absence of lymphatic vessels and Kupffer cells in the tumorous tissue.

On CT scans acquired 3–4 weeks after intra-arterial injection of Lipiodol, HCC lesions appear as highly hyperattenuating areas compared with nontumorous liver tissue (Fig. 6.18). Many published reports have shown that Lipiodol-CT has a high detectability rate for tiny HCC nodules (Bartolozzi et al. 1996; Merine et al. 1990; Lencioni et al. 1997). Findings on Lipiodol CT are quite specific for the diagnosis of HCC, provided that correct diagnostic criteria are used. Small, rounded, circumscribed areas of dense Lipiodol retention on CT scans obtained 3–4 weeks after the intra-arterial injection of the iodized oil have a 90% positive predictive value for being true satellite neoplastic foci in the clinical setting of a cirrhotic patient with HCC (Bisollon et al. 1998; Choi et al. 1997; Lencioni et al. 1997; Tourel et al. 1995).

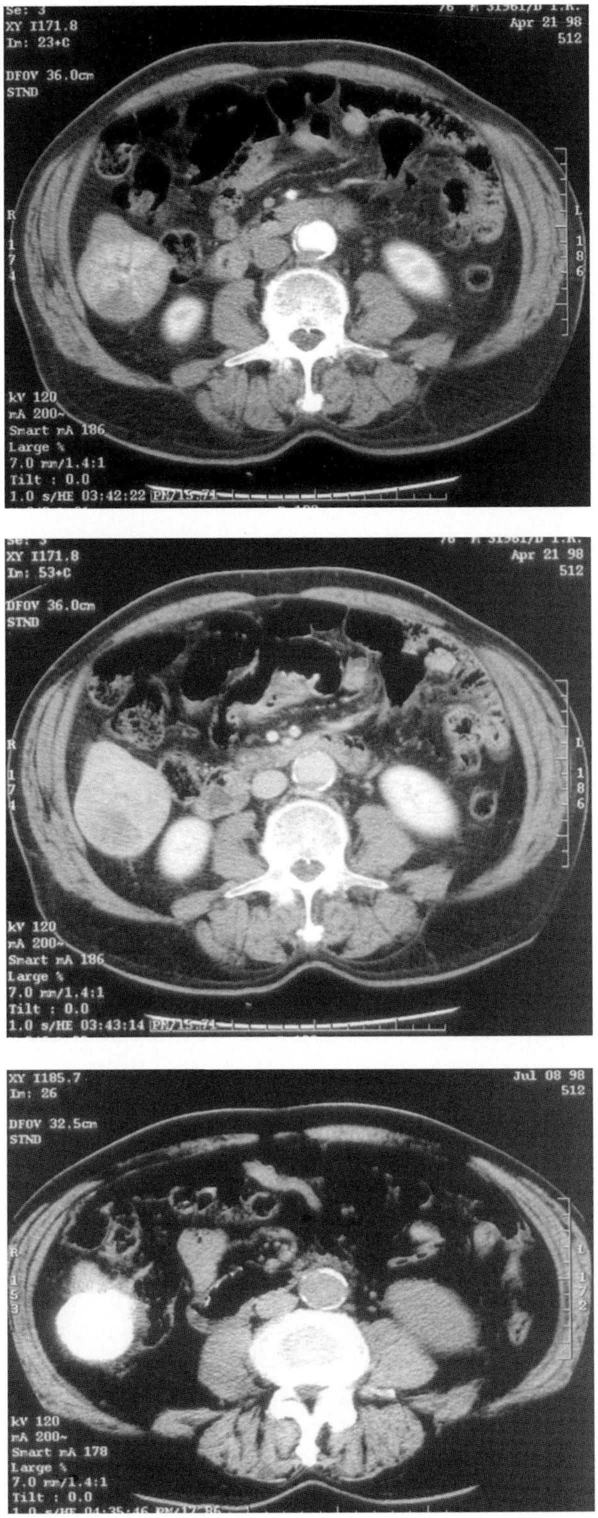

a b c

Fig. 6.18a–c. Lipiodol CT. Hepatocellular carcinoma is depicted by conventional spiral CT images acquired in the arterial (**a**) and the portal (**b**) phases. On unenhanced CT scan obtained 4 weeks after intra-arterial injection of iodized oil, the lesion appears homogeneously hyperattenuating due to massive retention of Lipiodol (**c**)

6.4 Role of CT in Screening

In Western countries, as well as in Japan, HCC emerge in cirrhotic livers in more than 90% of cases. Patients with liver cirrhosis, in fact, have long been identified as being a high-risk group for the development of HCC. Since the mid-1970s, the recognition of the close association of HCC with cirrhosis has stimulated the development of clinical programs for the early detection of HCC in cirrhotic patients (Nakakuma et al. 1993).

Extensive screening for HCC was made possible by the application of widely available diagnostic methods, such as assay for serum alpha-fetoprotein (AFP) and real-time ultrasonography (US). As a result of widespread screening programs, an increasing number of tumors have been identified at a treatable stage (Takayasu et al. 1990). The use of US as the imaging modality of choice for screening has been widely accepted, although US examination of the entire liver is sometimes impossible because of the patient's habitus, intervening bones, or colonic interposition, especially in small cirrhotic livers (Dodd et al 1992).

Conventional CT, performed by using nonspiral scanners, did not provide any substantial advantage over US for early detection of HCC. The sensitivity of conventional CT in the detection of small HCC lesions, in fact, was inferior to that of US in most published series.

Currently, the increasing availability of spiral scanners opens new prospects for HCC screening (Oliver et al. 1996). Despite the low sensitivity in the detection of early-stage, hypovascular HCC nodules (well-differentiated tumors of Edmondson grade 1, which usually have weak proliferative activity), spiral CT has a very high detection rate for small, overt, hypervascular HCC lesions (tumors that are small in size but have already undergone the de-differentiation process, starting their progression toward advanced HCC) (Hollett et al. 1995). Spiral CT can therefore guarantee an objective and comprehensive survey of the liver parenchyma, detecting small tumors which necessitate timely therapeutic intervention (Fig. 6.19) (Choi et al. 1996; Lee et al. 1997; Ueda et al. 1995). The use of spiral CT could be recommended in high-risk patients, such as those with abnormal (above 200 ng/ml) or increasing AFP levels, and negative US findings (Fig. 6.20) (Takayasu et al. 1995a).

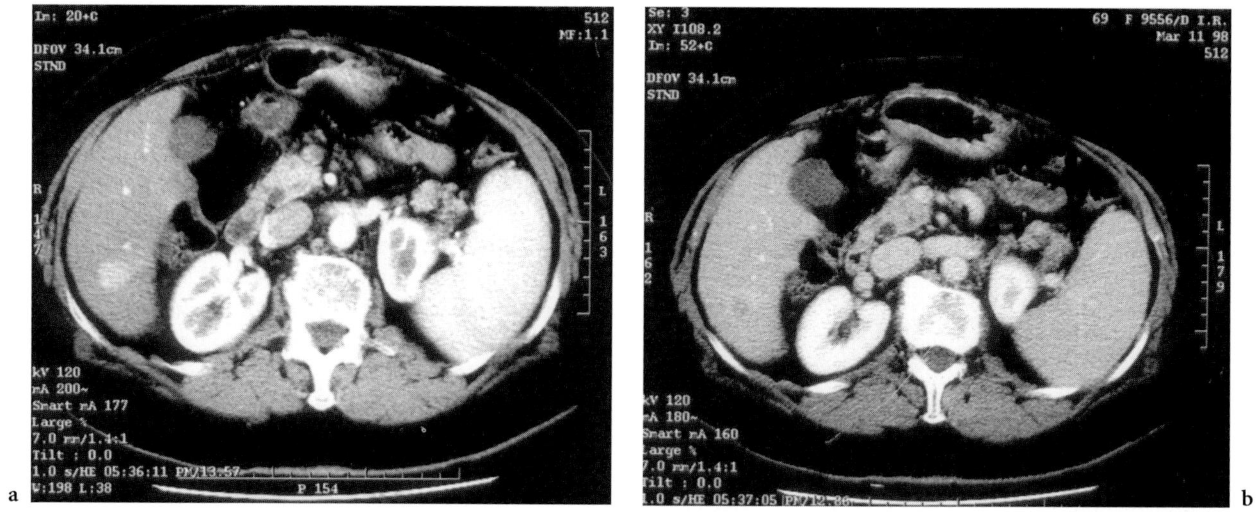

Fig. 6.19a,b. Small hepatocellular carcinoma detected by spiral CT. The lesion shows typical features in the arterial (**a**) and in the portal (**b**) phase images despite the small size

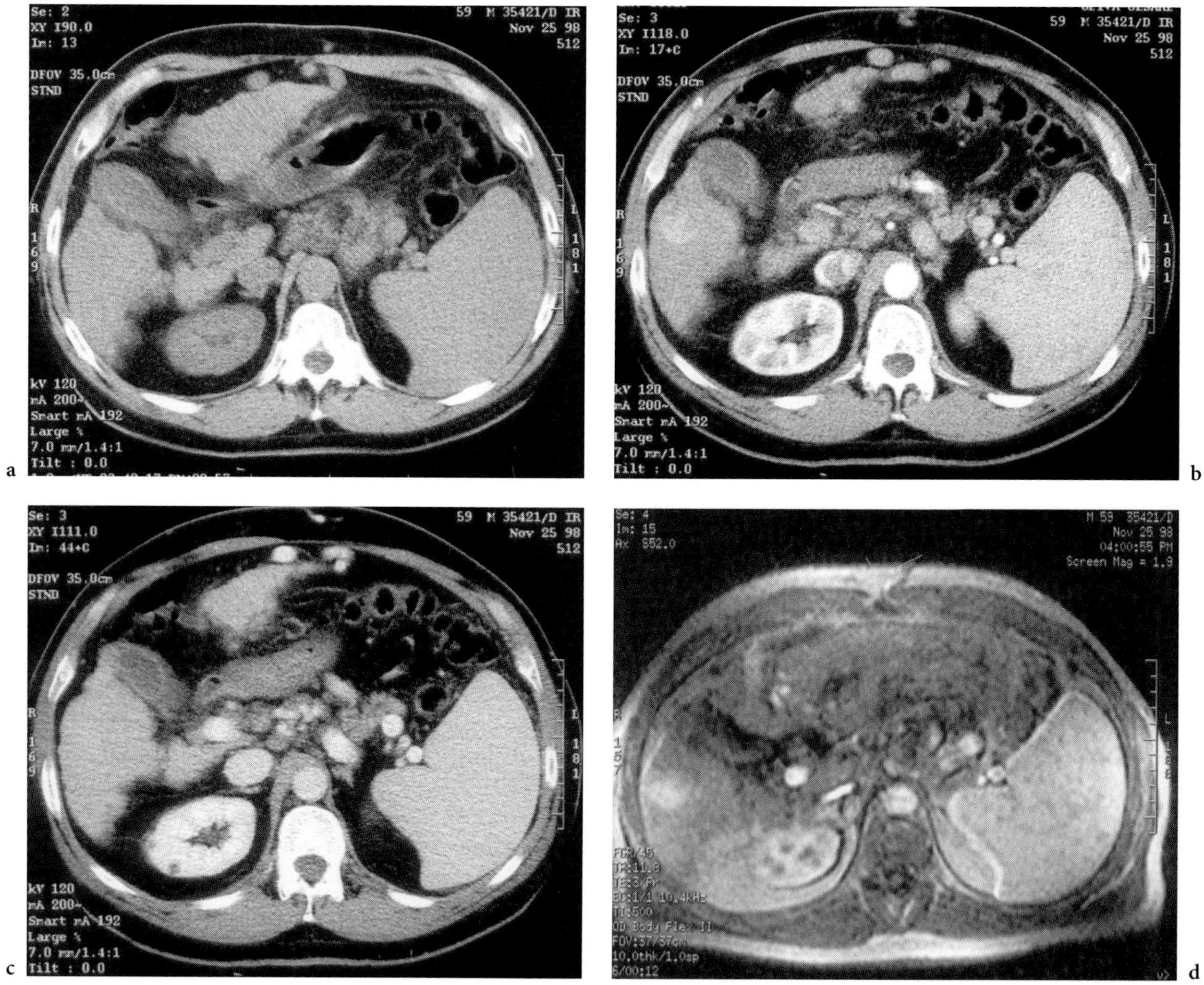

Fig. 6.20a–d. Tiny hepatocellular carcinoma detected by spiral CT in patients with abnormal AFP level and negative US examination. The small lesion is undetectable in the baseline scan (**a**), appears slightly hyperattenuating in the arterial phase (**b**), and is again undetectable in the delayed phase (**c**). Contrast-enhanced gradient-echo T1-weighted MR image in the arterial phase confirms the presence of the small neoplastic nodule (**d**)

6.5 CT Differential Diagnosis of Hepatocellular Carcinoma

The differential diagnosis of a suspected HCC raises different issues in the setting of a nodular lesion detected in a patient with liver cirrhosis or in the case of a tumor developed in an otherwise normal liver.

6.5.1 Differential Diagnosis of Lesions in Cirrhotic Liver

Currently, efforts are being directed toward making the diagnosis of HCC developed in cirrhotic livers at an early preclinical stage. With this aim, patients with chronic liver disease are carefully followed with AFP level measurement and US examination performed at regular intervals. Hence, particular attention is directed to characterizing even very small nodules detected by US screening (Nakakuma et al. 1993; Oliver et al. 1996). Every solid focal liver lesion which has emerged in a cirrhotic liver should be regarded as an HCC unless a different diagnosis has been proved (Lencioni et al. 1996).

6.5.1.1 Differential Diagnosis of Hypervascular Lesions

If the lesion shows a typical hypervascular pattern, with clear-cut enhancement in the predominantly arterial phase and rapid wash-out in the portal venous phase, the diagnosis of HCC is very likely. If the additional features of a peripheral rim of delayed enhancement (corresponding to the capsule) or internal mosaic architecture are seen, the diagnosis of HCC can be confidently assumed (Fig. 6.21) (Bonaldi et al. 1995; Choi et al. 1996; Lee et al. 1997; Ros et al. 1990). Biopsy confirmation may not be required in such instances. Mosaic architecture should not be confused with uneven CT densities in tumors caused by degeneration, necrosis, or bleeding.

If these typical morphological features of HCC are not depicted, HCC must be differentiated from other hypervascular lesions which may be occasionally found in cirrhotic livers. These include, among others, small hemangiomas and hypervascular metastases (Kim TK et al. 1998; Matsui et al. 1991; van Hoe et al. 1997).

Hemangiomas usually appear as low-attenuating lesions on precontrast CT images, and show peripheral nodular or globular enhancement in arterial-phase images with progressive centripetal fill-in. Prolonged enhancement is typically seen in the delayed phase. On the other hand, classical HCC nodules are usually opacified throughout the entire tumor on arterial-phase images, and become hypodense in the delayed phase. Tiny hemangiomas, however, may sometimes exhibit the same homogeneously hypervascular pattern as small HCC (Hanafusa et al. 1997; Jang et al. 1998). In these cases, CT differential diagnosis may be not be possible and further investigation with MRI is recommended (Fig. 6.22).

Hepatic metastases are uncommon in the clinical setting of a cirrhotic patient, and hypervascular metastases resembling HCC are uncommon among hepatic metastases. Nevertheless, this diagnostic dilemma may occur if the patient has a clinical history of extrahepatic malignancy or there is any clinical or laboratory suspicion of an extrahepatic tumor. In this case, imaging findings alone may not allow a differential diagnosis, and biopsy may be recommended (Fig. 6.23) (Oliver et al. 1997).

6.5.1.2 Differential Diagnosis of Hypovascular Lesions

The detection of a small hypovascular lesion in a cirrhotic patient may be due to either a dysplastic/well-differentiated hepatocellular nodule or, less frequently, to a non-cirrhotic-related lesion, such as an hepatic metastasis (Nakakuma et al. 1993; Matsui et al. 1991; van Hoe et al. 1997).

Differentiation among the histologically varied grades of dysplastic and well-differentiated neoplastic hepatocellular lesions is not achievable by CT. It has to be considered, however, that a reliable clear cut differentiation between dysplastic lesions and early-stage well-differentiated cancer is not possible either with imaging modalities or biopsy, as dysplastic nodules may contain microscopic foci of HCC. Following new information of hepatocarcinogenesis, dysplastic nodules are now considered as lesions with high malignant potential (Krinsky et al. 1998). Therefore, these borderline lesions are currently considered eligible for interventional procedures such as percutaneous ethanol injection or radiofrequency thermal ablation, like small HCC nodules.

Hypovascular metastases may exhibit peculiar features such as a necrotic center and vascular rim. Enhanced rims of neovascularity, or peripheral high-density rims resulting from congested, dilated

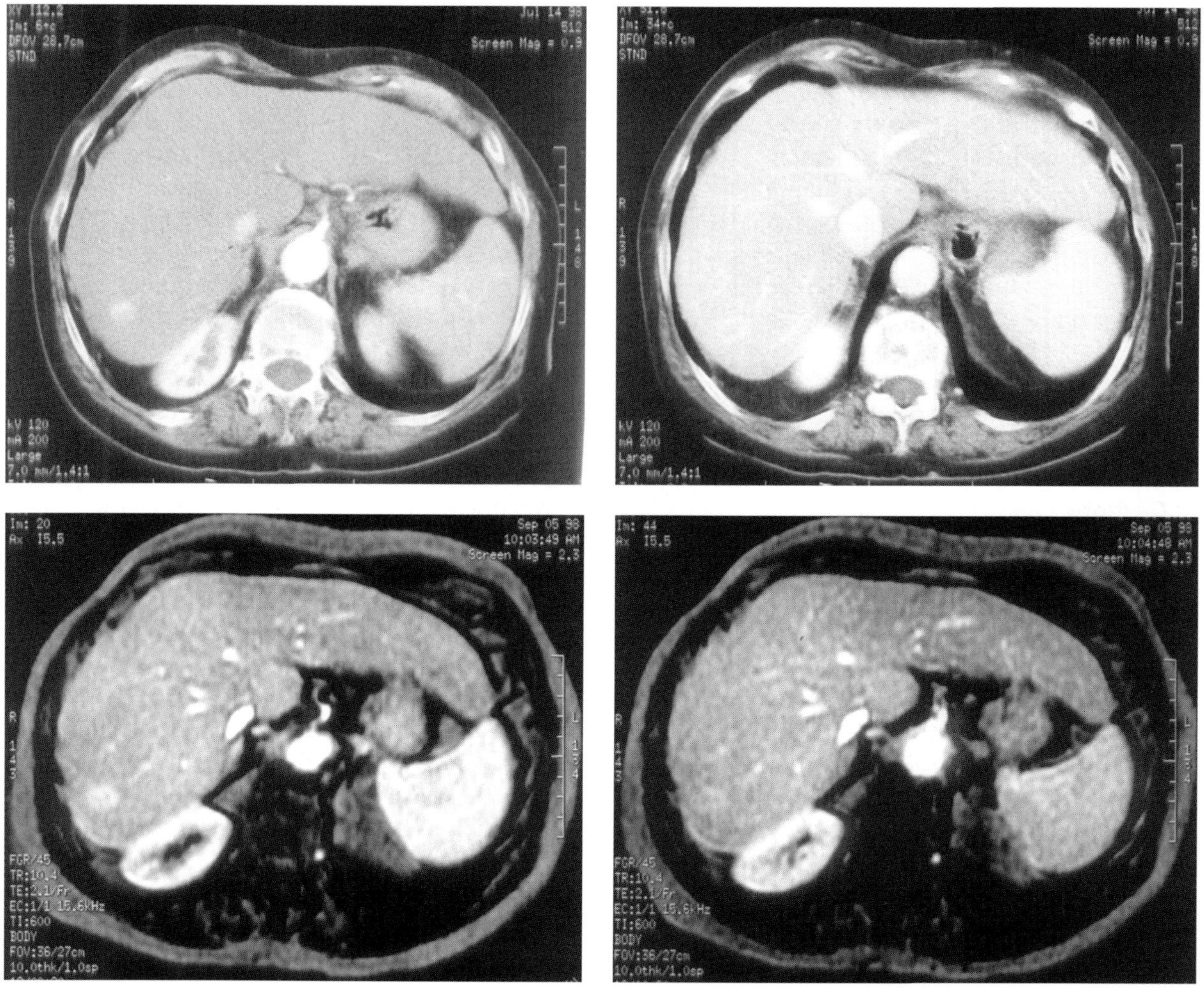

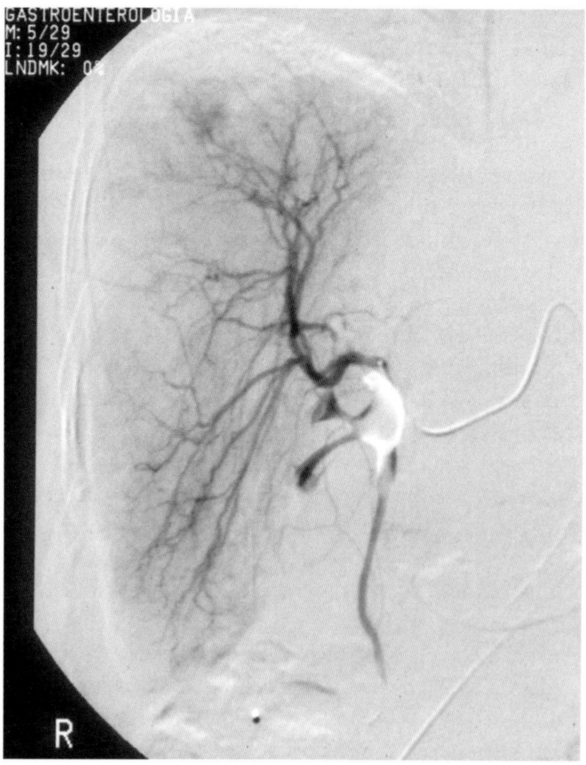

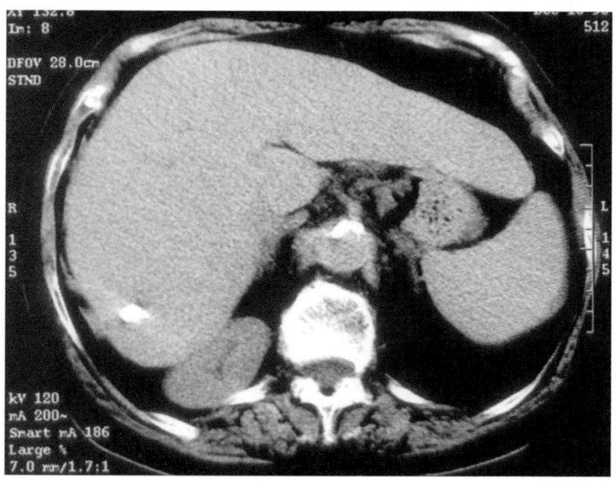

Fig. 6.21a–f. Small hepatocellular carcinoma characterized by spiral CT in patient with liver cirrhosis. The small lesion is hyperattenuating in the arterial phase (**a**), and isoattenuating in the portal phase (**b**). A thin peripheral rim of enhancement corresponding to the tumor capsule is depicted in the portal phase image (**b**). Contrast-enhanced gradient-echo T1-weighted MR images acquired in the arterial (**c**) and the portal venous phase (**d**) confirm CT findings. Digital subtraction angiography shows a small hypervascular tumor (**e**). On CT scan obtained 4 weeks after Lipiodol transcatheter arterial chemoembolization (**f**), dense and homogeneous retention of iodized oil is seen

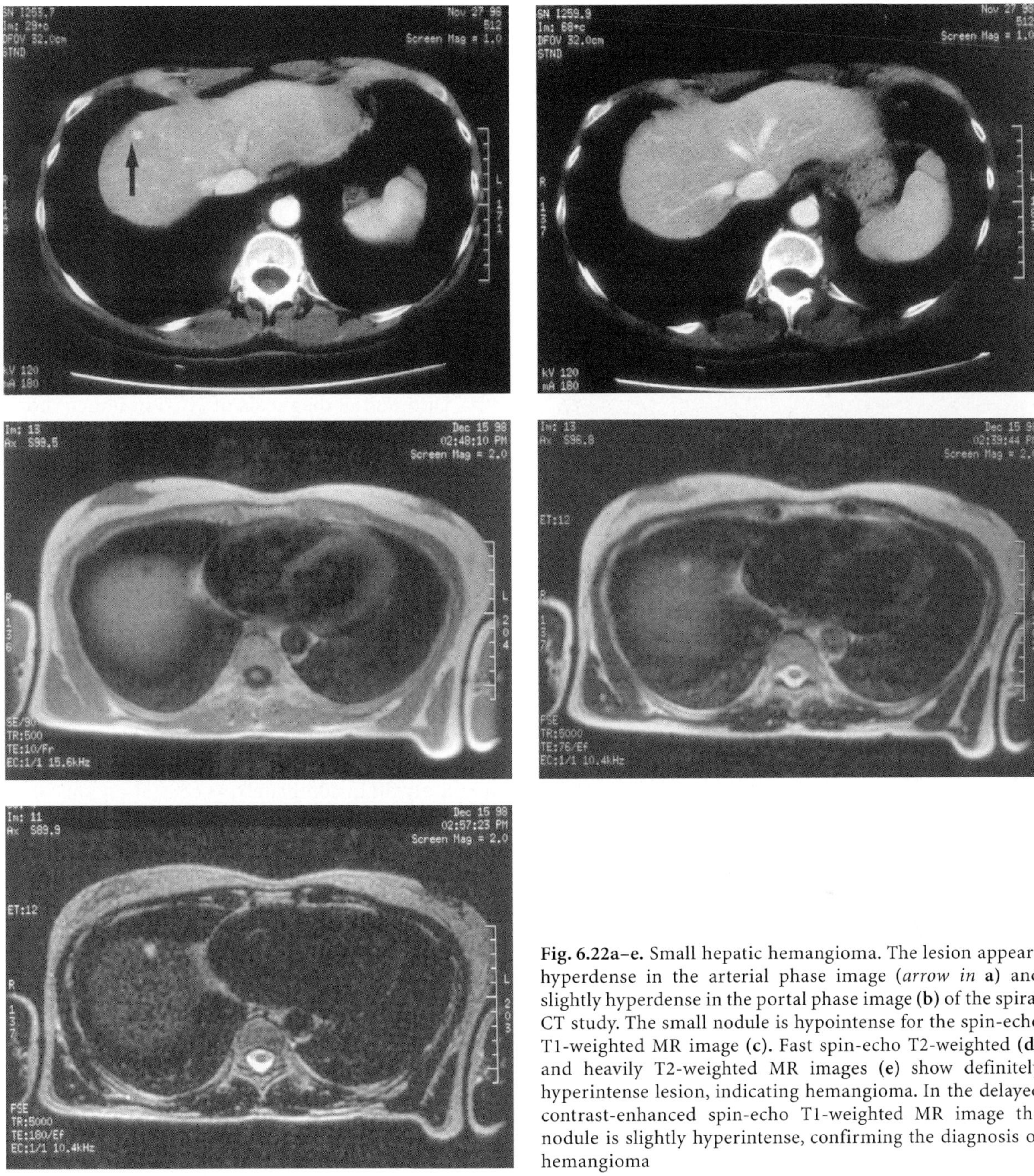

Fig. 6.22a–e. Small hepatic hemangioma. The lesion appears hyperdense in the arterial phase image (*arrow in* **a**) and slightly hyperdense in the portal phase image (**b**) of the spiral CT study. The small nodule is hypointense for the spin-echo T1-weighted MR image (**c**). Fast spin-echo T2-weighted (**d**) and heavily T2-weighted MR images (**e**) show definitely hyperintense lesion, indicating hemangioma. In the delayed contrast-enhanced spin-echo T1-weighted MR image the nodule is slightly hyperintense, confirming the diagnosis of hemangioma

sinusoids outside a hypovascular tumor, may be best depicted in arterial phase images. Prolonged enhancement is sometimes seen in the center of metastases in delayed scans. The combination of delayed and prolonged central enhancement producing high-central density and relatively low-peripheral density mass strongly suggests metastatic carcinoma.

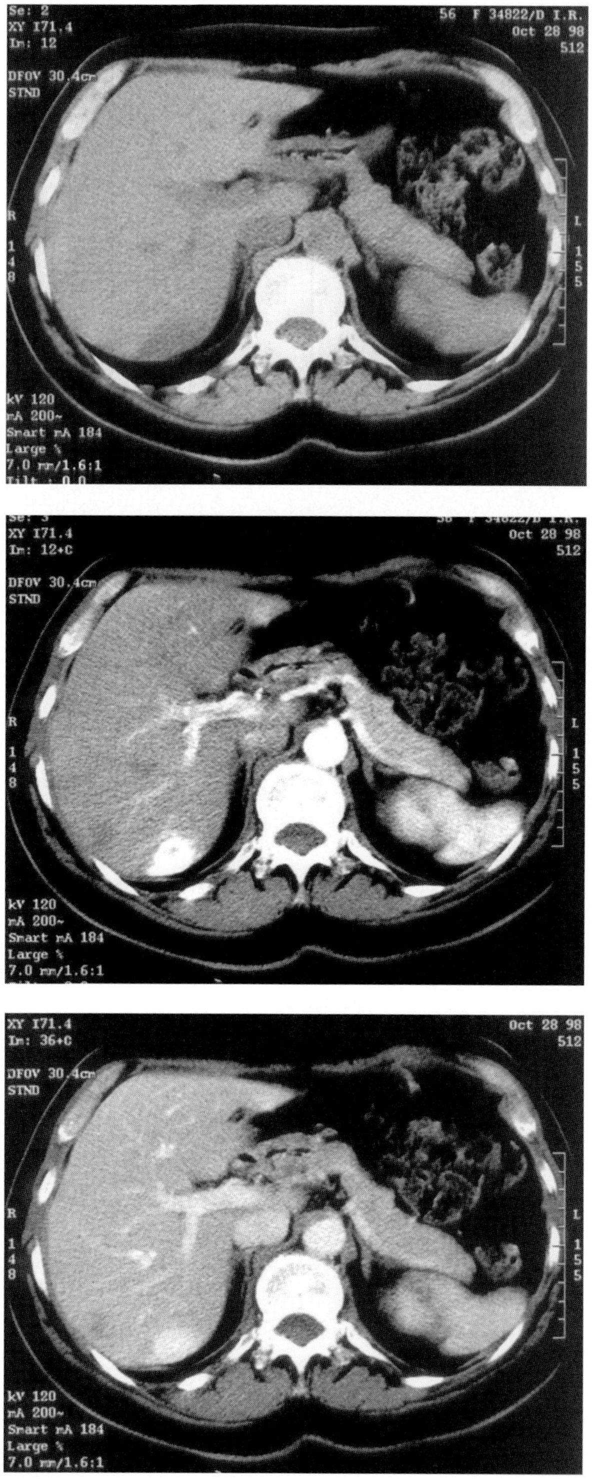

a
b
c

Fig. 6.23a–c. Hypervascular hepatic metastasis. The lesion is hypoattenuating in the baseline scan (**a**), and shows clear cut enhancement in the arterial phase (**b**). Persistent enhancement is seen in the delayed phase (**c**)

6.5.2
Differential Diagnosis of Lesions in Non-Cirrhotic Liver

The diagnosis of HCC developed in a non-cirrhotic liver is usually made at an advanced stage, as no US survey has been performed. Differential diagnosis is usually more difficult, as a number of different entities must be taken into account.

If the tumor has an expansive growth, typical features suggesting HCC, such as tumor capsule and internal mosaic architecture (including areas of fatty degeneration), may be observed. In infiltrating lesions, invasion of portal vein branches may suggest HCC. Differential diagnosis of HCC in noncirrhotic livers includes a variety of benign and malignant entities (Grossholz et al. 1998; van Hoe et al. 1997).

Expansive HCC lesions without signs of vascular invasion should be distinguished in the first place from benign tumors. These include, among others, hemangioma, focal nodular hyperplasia, and hepatocellular adenoma.

Hemangiomas are well-demarcated masses that are hypodense with respect to normal liver and typically show peripheral nodular or globular enhancement in arterial-phase images with progressive centripetal fill-in. Prolonged enhancement is typically seen in the delayed phase. Large hemangiomas, however, rarely fill in completely, as central regions of fibrosis or thrombosis remain hypodense (Hanafusa et al. 1997; Jang et al. 1998).

Focal nodular hyperplasia and hepatocellular adenoma typically occur in young patients and predominantly in females. Focal nodular hyperplasia usually has a typical biphasic enhancement on spiral CT: in the arterial phase, the peripheral portion of the lesion shows clear cut enhancement, becoming definitely hyperdense with respect to adjacent hepatic parenchyma, while the central portion, which corresponds to the stellate scar, does not enhance. In the delayed phase images, the peripheral portion of the lesion appears isodense with respect to the surrounding normal liver, while the central scar demonstrates late enhancement. Hepatocellular adenoma is depicted as a nonspecific well-defined mass; areas of increased density may be observed on unenhanced scans, corresponding to recent intratumoral hemorrhage.

HCC which has emerged in noncirrhotic liver should also be distinguished from other kinds of malignancy (Fernandez and Redvanly 1998). These include, beside metastases and rare primary tumors, intrahepatic cholangiocellular carcinoma and fibrolamellar carcinoma.

Intrahepatic cholangiocellular carcinoma, originating in small intrahepatic ducts, represents 10% of all cholangiocarcinomas. It is the second most common primary malignancy and is usually seen in the seventh decade. There is no association between cholangiocarcinoma and liver cirrhosis. Characteristically, an abundant fibroblastic stroma is present in this tumor, which is histologically a sclerosing adenocarcinoma. Two CT configurations predominate in cholangiocarcinoma. The first is a well-defined hypodense mass with a slightly denser internal component on unenhanced scans. Injection of contrast medium produces prominent enhancement of the large internal component. The second appearance is that of a hypodense mass of variable homogeneity (sometimes with low-attenuating internal regions), and variable shape and sharpness of contour showing peripheral enhancement. Septated or streaked internal enhancement may be seen. Delayed scans may show accumulation of contrast medium within the tumor after washout from the normal liver, which seems to be correlated with the fibrous component. Proximal biliary dilatation is often present in either of the two configurations of the disease, while it is relatively uncommon in HCC (Ros et al. 1988; Tillich et al. 1998).

Fibrolamellar carcinoma represents only 2% of hepatocellular malignancies. Typically, this neoplasm occurs in young people and is not associated with underlying cirrhosis. Most often, fibrolamellar carcinoma appears as a solitary, large, firm circumscribed mass with lobulated borders. More than two-thirds of reported cases have involved the left lobe. A prominent central fibrous scar with radiating fibrous septa may be present. The scar usually does not enhance after contrast administration, although accumulation of contrast in delayed scans, resembling the behavior of the central stellate scar commonly seen in focal nodular hyperplasia, has been reported. The major CT clue to the diagnosis of fibrolamellar carcinoma is the presence of central stellate or trabecular calcifications, which are seen in 30–70% of cases. In HCC, calcifications may occur in the sclerosing type, which is characterized by intense fibrosis: this kind of malignancy, however, typically arises at an older age.

6.6 CT Staging of Hepatocellular Carcinoma

Accurate staging is necessary to determine the best treatment method for HCC. Spiral CT is an ideal technique for staging, as it provides reliable detection of both intrahepatic and extrahepatic spread of the tumor. Staging of HCC includes the assessment of: (a) number, size, location, and characteristics of the tumor nodules; (b) vascular invasion by the tumor; and (c) extrahepatic metastases. All these factors should be accurately evaluated, as they affect therapeutic options as well as patient's prognosis.

Dual-phase spiral CT provides accurate assessment of the number and size of HCC lesions, enabling identification of even small intrahepatic metastatic nodules (Oi et al. 1996). These tiny tumor deposits, in fact, are usually hypervascular, like the main tumor, and therefore well depicted in the arterial phase images (Fig. 6.24). The availability of spiral scanners has substantially restricted the indication of more complex and invasive angiographically assisted CT techniques, such as CTAP or Lipiodol CT, for detection of satellite lesions (Kanematsu et al. 1997; Choi et al. 1997; Lencioni et al. 1997). However, if a surgical therapeutic approach is being considered, more precise preoperative staging by Lipiodol CT is still recommended (Bisollon et al. 1998; Nelson et al. 1990; Small et al. 1993; Tourel et al. 1995).

CT location of the segment in which the tumor exists is done in relation to hepatic and intrahepatic portal veins. Segmental location is usually made on portal venous phase spiral CT images, in which intrahepatic veins are well opacified. However, when a small lesion is located at the boundary of the segments, it is not easy to determine segmental anatomy (Fasel et al. 1996, 1998). CTAP is the best CT technique for this purpose, as it provides accurate delineation of the intrahepatic vein branches (Kanematsu et al. 1997; Soyer et al. 1994).

The characteristics of the lesion, particularly with regard to the type of tumor growth (expanding or infiltrating) are usually well defined by spiral CT. CT identification of the tumor capsule is accurate in large tumors, but is less reliable in small lesions, which usually have a thin and poorly developed fibrous capsule (Ros et al. 1990).

Vascular invasion by the tumor is a crucial staging factor (Choi 1995). Tendency to grow into the portal veins, eliciting tumor thrombi, is a peculiar feature of HCC. Spiral CT allows accurate identification of tumor thrombi in the main portal veins. Tumor

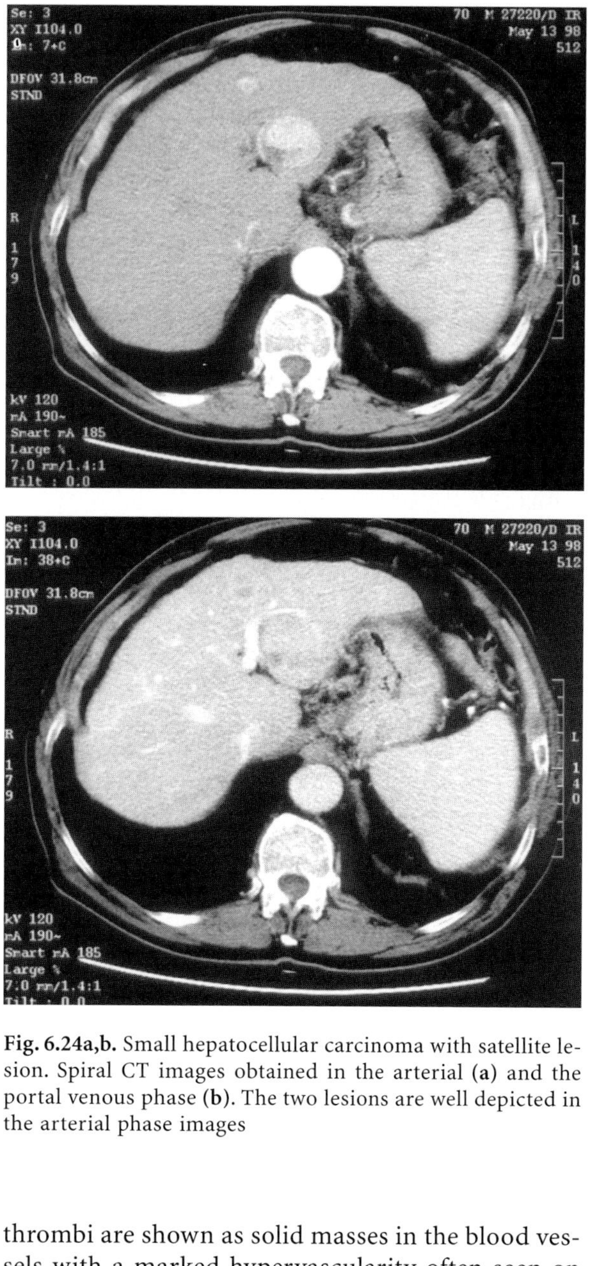

a

b

Fig. 6.24a,b. Small hepatocellular carcinoma with satellite lesion. Spiral CT images obtained in the arterial (**a**) and the portal venous phase (**b**). The two lesions are well depicted in the arterial phase images

thrombi are shown as solid masses in the blood vessels with a marked hypervascularity often seen on arterial-phase spiral CT images. Arteriovenous shunting may be present within thrombi. The hepatic segment in which the feeding portal vein is obstructed demonstrates hyperperfusion abnormality on arterial-phase CT images, as a result of arterial compensation and lack of dilution of the enhanced arterial blood with the unenhanced portal blood. Identification of tumor invasion in peripheral (segmental or subsegmental) portal vein branches is unreliable by spiral CT and requires the use of CTAP. CTAP visualizes portal vein perfusion defects caused by thrombi as wedge-shaped hypodense areas including the tumor (Novick and Fishman 1998).

Lymphatic metastases in HCC are not common. They may be seen in about 10–15% of autopsy cases, especially in the hepatic hilar lymph nodes. Extrahepatic hematogenous metastases are usually associated with advanced-stage tumors. The lung is the most common site of metastases, followed by the bone and the adrenal gland. CT is valuable for the diagnosis of adenopathies and distant metastatic disease, except for bone metastases.

References

Bartolozzi C, Lencioni R, Caramella D, Palla A, Bassi AM, Di Candio G (1996) Small hepatocellular carcinoma. Detection with US, CT, MR imaging, DSA, and Lipiodol-CT. Acta Radiol 37:69–74

BisollonT, Rode A, Baricel B, et al (1998) Diagnostic value and tolerance of Lipiodol computed tomography for the detection of small hepatocellular carcinoma: correlation with pathologic examination of explanted livers. J Hepatol 28:491–496

Bluemke DA, Soyer P, Chan B, et al (1995) Spiral CT during arterial portography: techniques and application. Radiographics 15:633–637

Bonaldi VM, Bret PM, Reinhold C, Atri M (1995) Helical CT of the liver: value of an early hepatic arterial phase. Radiology 197:357–363

Choi BI (1995) Vascular invasion by hepatocellular carcinoma. Abdom Imaging 20:277–278

Choi BI, Takayasu K, Han MC, et al (1993) Small hepatocellular carcinomas and associated nodular lesions of the liver: pathology, pathogenesis and imaging findings. AJR 160:1177–1187

Choi BI, Cho GM, Han JK, et al (1996) Spiral CT for the detection of hepatocellular carcinoma: relative value of arterial and late phase scanning. Abdom Imaging 21:440–444

Choi BI, Lee HJ, Han JK, Choi DS, Seo JB, Han MC (1997) Detection of hypervascular nodular hepatocellular carcinomas: value of triphasic helical CT compared with iodized-oil CT. AJR 168:219–224

Dodd GD, Miller WJ, Baron RL, et al (1992) Detection of nalignant tumors in end-stage cirrhotic livers: efficacy of sonography as a screening technique. AJR 159:727–733

Fasel JH, Gailloud P, Terrier F, Mentha G, Sprumont P (1996) Segmental anatomy of the liver: a review and a proposal for an international working nomenclature. Eur Radiol 6:834–837

Fasel JH, Selle D, Evertsz CJ, Terrier F, Peitgen HO, Gailloud P (1998) Segmental anatomy of the liver: poor correlation with CT. Radiology 206:151–156

Fernandez MP, Redvanly RD (1998) Primary hepatic malignant neoplasms. Radiol Clin North Am 36:333–348

Freeny PC, Baron RL, Teefey SA (1992) Hepatocellular carcinoma: reduced frequency of typical findings with dynamic contrast enhanced CT in a non Asian population. Radiology 185:143–148

Grossholz M, Terrier F, Rubbia L, et al (1998) Focal sparing in the fatty liver as a sign of an adjacent space-occupying lesion. AJR 171:1391–1395

Hanafusa K, Ohashi I, Gomi N, Himeno Y, Wakita T, Shibuya H (1997) Differential diagnosis of early homogeneously enhancing hepatocellular carcinoma and hemangioma by two-phase CT. J Comput Assist Tomogr 21:361–368

Hollett MD, Jeffry RB Jr, Nino-Murcia M, et al (1995) Dual-phase helical CT of the liver: value of arterial phase scans in the detection of small (<1.5 cm) malignant hepatic neoplasms. AJR 164:879–884

Hori M, Murakami T, Kim T, et al (1998) Sensitivity of double-phase helical CT during arterial portography for detection of hypervascular hepatocellular carcinoma. J Comput Assist Tomogr 22:861–867

Jang HJ, Choi BI, Kim TK, et al (1998) Atypical small hemangiomas of the liver: "bright dot" sign at two-phase spiral CT. Radiology 208:543–548

Kanai T, Hirohashi S, Upton M, et al (1987) Pathology of small hepatocellular carcinoma: a proposal for a new gross classification. Cancer 60:810–819

Kanematsu M, Oliver JH III, Carr B, Baron RL (1997) Hepatocellular carcinoma: the role of helical biphasic contrast-enhanced CT versus CT during arterial portography. Radiology 205:75–80

Kanematsu M, Kondo H, Enya M, Yokoyama R, Hoshi H (1998) Nondiseased portal perfusion defects adjacent to the right ribs shown on helical CT during arterial portography. AJR 171:445–448

Kanematsu M, Hoshi H, Yamawaki Y, et al (1999) Angiographically assisted helical CT of the liver. AJR 172:97–105

Kim SR, Hayashi Y, Matsuoka T, et al (1998) A case of well-differentiated minute hepatocellular carcinoma with extrahepatic metastasis. J Gastroenterol Hepatol 13:892–896

Kim TK, Choi BI, Han JK, Chung JW, Park JH, Han MC (1998) Nontumorous arterioportal shunt mimicking hypervascular tumor in cirrhotic liver: two-phase spiral CT findings. Radiology 208:597–603

Kitagaua K, Matsui O, Kadoya M, et al (1991) Hepatocellular carcinomas with excessive copper accumulation: CT and MR findings. Radiology 180:623–628

Krinsky GA, Theise ND, Rofsky NM, Mizrachi H, Tepperman LW, Weinreb JC (1998) Dysplastic nodules in cirrhotic liver: arterial phase enhancement at CT and MR imaging – a case report. Radiology 209:461–464

Lee HM, Lu DS, Krasny RM, Busuttil R, Kadell B, Lucas J (1997) Hepatic lesion characterization in cirrhosis: significance of arterial hypervascularity on dual-phase helical CT. AJR 169:125–30

Lencioni R, Mascalchi M, Caramella D, Bartolozzi C (1996) Small hepatocellular carcinoma: differentiation from adenomatous hyperplasia with color Doppler US and dynamic Gd-DTPA-enhanced MR imaging. Abdom Imaging 21:41–48

Lencioni R, Pinto F, Armillotta N, et al (1997) Intrahepatic metastatic nodules of hepatocellular carcinoma detected at Lipiodol-CT: imaging-pathologic correlation. Abdom Imaging 22:253–258

Matsui O, Kadoya M, Kameyama T, et al (1991) Benign and malignant nodules in cirrothic livers: distinction based on blood supply. Radiology 178:493–497

Matsui O, Takahshi S, Kadoya M, et al (1994) Pseudolesion in segment IV of the liver at CT during arterial portography: correlation with aberrant gastric venous drainage. Radiology 193:31–35

Merine D, Takayasu K, Wakao F (1990) Detection of hepatocellular carcinoma: comparison of CT during arterial portography with CT after intraarterial injection of iodized oil. Radiology 175:707–710

Mitsukaki K, Yamashita Y, Ogata I, et al (1996) Multiple phase helical-CT of the liver for detecting small hepatomas in patients with liver cirrhosis: contrast-injection protocol and optimal timing. AJR 167:753–757

Nakakuma Y, Terada T, Ueda K, et al (1993) Adenomatous hyperplasia of the liver as a precancerous lesion. Liver 13:1–9

Nelson RC, Chezmar JL, Sugarbaker TH, et al (1990) Preoperative localization of focal liver lesions to specific liver segments: utility of CT during arterial portography. Radiology 176:89–94

Novick SL, Fishman EK (1998) Portal vein thrombosis: spectrum of helical CT and CT angiographic findings. Abdom Imaging 23:505–510

Ohtomo K, Baron RJ, Dodd GD, et al (1993) Confluent hepatic fibrosis in advanced cirrhosis: appearance at CT. Radiology 188:31–35

Oi H, Murakami T, Kim T, et al (1996) Dynamic MR imaging and early-phase helical CT for detecting small intrahepatic metastases of hepatocellular carcinoma. AJR 166:369–374

Oliver JH III, Baron RL (1996) Helical biphasic contrast-enhanced CT of the liver: technique, indications, interpretation and pitfalls. Radiology 201:1–14

Oliver JH III, Baron RL, Federle MP, et al (1996) Detecting hepatocellular carcinoma: value of unenhanced or arterial phase CT imaging or both, used in conjunction with conventional portal venous phase contrast-enhanced CT imaging. AJR 167:71–77

Oliver JH III, Baron RL, Federle MP, Jones BC, Sheng R (1997) Hypervascular liver metastases: do unenhanced and hepatic arterial phase CT images affect tumor detection? Radiology 205:709–715

Rofflett MD, Jeffrey RB, Nino Murcia M, et al (1995) Dual phase helical CT of the liver: value of arterial phase scans in the detection of small (< 1.5 cm) malignant hepatic neoplasms. AJR 164:879–884

Ros PR, Buck JL, Goodman ID, et al (1988) Intrahepatic cholangiocarcinoma: radiologic-pathologic correlation. Radiology 167:689–693

Ros PR, Murphy BJ, Back JL, et al (1990) Encapsulated hepatocellular carcinoma: radiologic findings and pathological correlation. Gastrointest Radiol 15:233–237

Rubin GD, Dake MD, Napel SA, et al (1993) Three dimensional spiral CT angiography of the abdomen: initial clinical experience. Radiology 186:147–152

Rummeny EJ, Marchal G (1997) Liver imaging. Clinical applications and future perspectives. Acta Radiol 38:626–630

Small WC, Mehard WB, Langmo LS, et al (1993) Preoperative determination of the resectability of hepatic tumors; efficacy of CT during arterial portography. AJR 161:319–322

Soyer P, Bluemke DA, Bliss DF, et al (1994) Surgical segmental anatomy of the liver: demonstration with spiral CT during arterial portography and multiplanar reconstruction. AJR 163:99–103

Takayama T, Makuuchi M, Hirahashi S, et al (1990) Malignant transformation of adenomatous hyperplasia to hepatocellular carcinoma. Lancet 336:1150–1153

Takayasu K, Moriyama N, Muramatsu Y, et al (1990) The diagnosis of small hepatocellular carcinomas: efficacy of various imaging procedures in 100 patients. AJR 155:49–54

Takayasu K, Furukawa H, Wakao F, et al (1995a) CT diagnosis of early hepatocellular carcinoma: sensitivity, findings, and CT pathologic correlation. AJR 164:885–890

Takayasu K, Muramatsu Y, Furukawa H, et al (1995b) Early hepatocellular carcinoma: appearance at CT during arterial portography and CT arteriography with pathologic correlation. Radiology 194:101–105

Tillich M, Mischinger HJ, Preisegger KH, Rabl H, Szolar DH (1998) Multiphasic helical CT in diagnosis and staging of hilar cholangiocarcinoma. AJR 171:651–658

Tourel PG, Pageaux GP, Coste V, et al (1995) Small hepatocellular carcinoma in patients undergoing liver transplantation: detection with CT after injection of iodized oil. Radiology 197:377–380

Tublin ME, Tessler FN, Cheng SL, Peters TL, McGovern PC (1999) Effect of injection rate of contrast medium on pancreatic and hepatic helical CT. Radiology 210:97–101

Ueda K, Kitigawa K, Kadoya M, et al (1995) Detection of hypervascular hepatocellular carcinoma by using spiral volumetric CT: comparison of US and MR imaging. Abdom Imaging 20:547–554

Ueda K, Matsui O, Kawamori Y, et al (1998) Differentiation of hypervascular hepatic pseudolesions from hepatocellular carcinoma: value of single-level dynamic CT during hepatic arteriography. J Comput Assist Tomogr 22:703–708

van Hoe L, Baert AL, Gryspeerdt S, et al (1997) Dual-phase helical-CT of the liver: value of an early phase acquisition in the differential diagnosis of non-cystic focal lesions. AJR 169:1185–1192

Yamashita Y, Fan ZM, Yamamoto H, et al (1993) Sclerosing hepatocellular carcinoma: radiologic findings. Abdom Imaging 18:347–351

Yoshikawa J, Matsui O, Takashima T, et al (1988) Fatty methamorphosis in hepatocellular carcinoma: radiologic features in 10 cases. AJR 151:717–720

Yoshikawa J, Matsui O, Kadoya M, et al (1992) Delayed enhancement of fibrotic areas in hepatic masses: CT-patholgic correlation. J Comput Assist Tomogr 16:206–211

7 Magnetic Resonance Imaging of Hepatocellular Carcinoma

T.J. Vogl and R. Hammerstingl

CONTENTS

T. J. Vogl, MD, Professor; Department of Radiology, Johann Wolfgang Goethe University, Frankfurt am Main, Theodor Stern Kai 7, D-60590 Frankfurt am Main, Germany
R. Hammerstingl, MD; Department of Radiology, Johann Wolfgang Goethe University, Frankfurt am Main, Theodor Stern Kai 7, D-60590 Frankfurt am Main, Germany

7.1 Introduction

Hepatocellular carcinoma (HCC) is extremely common in sub-Saharan Africa and the Far East. In high incidence areas it presents in young to middle-aged adults with an 8:1 male predominance, a relatively acute onset of symptoms, and a rapid clinical course. In contrast in the United States and Europe it is relatively uncommon and occurs predominantly in elderly individuals (2.5:1 male predominance). HCC frequently develops on the basis of alcohol- or hepatitis-related cirrhosis, which presents with an insidious onset of symptoms and a more protracted clinical course. In the following, imaging features concerning the morphology of HCC in unenhanced and contrast-enhanced MRI are presented. Special emphasis is placed on the differential diagnostic criteria versus other hepatic tumors.

7.2 Imaging Modalities

For the diagnosis of focal liver lesions ultrasound and spiral computed tomography (CT) are recommended as screening modalities. These are defined to represent noninvasive fast imaging techniques with a high sensitivity in the detection of lesions and an efficient diagnostic accuracy in the differential diagnosis of liver tumors. In the pretherapeutic staging of hepatic lesions, double phase spiral CT, CT during arterial portography (CTAP) and magnetic resonance imaging (MRI) provide detailed information concerning segmental anatomy with excellent delineation of the topographical relationship of vascular, biliary and abdominal structures (De Santis et al. 1992; Itai et al. 1986; Itoh et al. 1987; Kanematsu et al. 1987; Ueda et al. 1995).

Unenhanced MRI helps the diagnosis of focal liver lesions because of the qualitative information on morphology provided by T2- and T1-weighted sequences. Advanced MRI protocols, like gradient-echo, fast spin-echo and fat suppression, are becoming the noninvasive imaging techniques of choice for investigating the liver nowadays (Rummeny et al. 1989a,c). Nevertheless plain imaging techniques have to deal with some limitations in the diagnosis of focal liver disease due to a lack of contrast between the lesion and normal liver parenchyma and an overlap in the morphologic findings of benign and malignant tumors provided by different pulse sequences (Blakeborough et al. 1997).

As shown in clinical studies, the use of liver contrast agents is one way of obtaining higher contrast between normal liver tissue and tumorous tissue, together with greater sensitivity. A variety of contrast media, extracellular, hepatobiliary and tissue-specific MR contrast agents, have been investigated in clinical studies to improve the differential diagnostic potential of the modality.

7.3 MR Imaging

7.3.1 MR Protocols and Technical Factors

Key factors that influence the diagnostic quality of MR imaging are: relative T1 and T2 relaxation times of lesion and liver, pulse sequences utilized and presence of artifacts. The first two factors can be influenced via sequence selection and the use of special contrast agents. The third factor depends on the technical equipment of the MR scanner as well as the degree of field strength and the available software options. Moreover, the breathhold technique reduces artifacts and motion to a high degree and is becoming available with newer equipment (Ohtomo et al. 1997).

The *sequence protocol* for imaging of the liver includes unenhanced proton density, T2-weighted and T1-weighted spin echo (SE) sequences as well as T1-weighted gradient echo (GRE) sequences in axial orientation. Alternatively fat-suppressed T2- and T1-weighted sequences can be obtained. Newer scanner modalities offer the advantage of fast imaging techniques such as turbo spin echo, half-Fourier single-shot fast spin-echo (HASTE) sequences, and faster T1-weighted GRE imaging (Blakeborough et al. 1997; Ichikawa et al. 1998).

Dynamic studies can be performed with a T1-weighted GRE sequence during administration of an extracellular or hepatobiliary contrast medium over a period of 5 min. Contrast-enhanced scans include T1-weighted SE conventional and fat-suppressed as well as T1-weighted GRE sequences.

Iron oxide-enhanced studies should be performed using T2- as well as T1-weighted sequences. Unenhanced and contrast-enhanced studies are compared. Dynamic studies during fast injection of iron oxides can be obtained using either T2- or T1-weighted GRE-imaging protocols (Stark et al. 1988).

7.3.2 MR Imaging Criteria

A variety of quantitative and qualitative criteria are used for contrast-enhanced liver imaging to improve diagnosis of focal liver lesions (Itai et al. 1986; Itoh et al. 1987; Ohtomo et al. 1997).

Qualitative criteria: images can be interpreted and assessed for homogeneity and form of the lesions, the presence or absence of morphologic features such as necrosis, central scar, surrounding capsule, and contrast enhancement (Bartolozzi et al. 1994).

Quantitative criteria are the number and size of the lesions, as well as involved hepatic segments, S/N (signal to noise), C/N (contrast to noise), percentage enhancement and percentage signal intensity loss. Signal intensity is read directly from the monitor for lesion and normal liver parenchyma using operator-defined regions of interest (ROI). For lesions with cystic components, care should be taken to measure signal intensity only in solid portions of the tumor (outside the regions of capsule or scar). Major hepatic and portal vessels should be avoided when measuring the signal intensity of normal liver parenchyma. ROIs are placed identically on unenhanced and contrast-enhanced sequences.

The percentage signal intensity loss (PSIL) of lesions and of normal liver parenchyma (region of interest technique) is calculated using unenhanced and superparamagnetic iron oxide (SPIO)-enhanced images as follows:

$$PSIL = \frac{SI_{postcontrast} - SI_{precontrast}}{SI_{precontrast}} \cdot (-100)$$

where $SI_{precontrast}$=signal intensity of tissue using unenhanced scans and $SI_{postcontrast}$=signal intensity using contrast-enhanced scans.
The degree of contrast enhancement is described using static and dynamic imaging after administra-

tion of gadolium-chelates/hepatobiliary agents as follows:

$$\textit{Percentage enhancement: } PE = \frac{SI_{postcontrast} - SI_{precontrast}}{SI_{precontrast}} \cdot 100$$

Depending on the clinical situation, a number of distinct objectives need to be achieved:

- Identification or presence of liver disease (focal or diffuse)
- Improvement in lesion detection
- Characterization of liver lesions
- Lesion localization: liver segments/anatomical situation concerning resectability
- Vascular situation: invasion of vessels
- Documentation of extrahepatic disease

MR imaging helps in providing excellent diagnostic information as a general screening examination of focused protocol of liver disease.

7.3.3 Contrast Agents

7.3.3.1 *Classes of Contrast Agents*

Concerning MR imaging of the liver there are two major classes of contrast agents: these substances, infact, act indirectly by their effects on T1- and T2-weighted imaging (relaxation time). There are positive enhancing paramagnetic agents that increase tissue signal intensity. On the other hand, susceptibility agents produce a negative enhancement by decreasing signal intensity depending on the used MRI sequence protocol. Positive agents reduce T1 relaxivity to a greater extent than T2 relaxivity. At a higher concentration T2 could also be reduced. Negative agents usually reduce T2 relaxivity but to some extent also demonstrate a T1 effect (Brasch 1992).

7.3.3.2 *Extracellular Contrast Media*

Extracellular contrast agents are nonspecific paramagnetic substances, enhancing the extracellular fluid spaces. Among other indications these contrast media are frequently applied in the diagnosis of tumorous lesions, inflammation, vascular pathologies, and MR angiography. After intravenous administration these substances are rapidly cleared from the intravascular space to the interstitial space (Peterson et al. 1996). The biodistribution is nonspecific, and they are rapidly excreted by the kidneys (Mahfoutz et al. 1993a,b; Weinmann et al. 1984).

The usual clinical dose of these gadolinium chelates is 0.1 mmol/kg body wt. This substance group includes several different products. Gadopentetate dimeglumine – Gd-DTPA – Magnevist (Schering, Germany) was the first MR imaging contrast agent approved for clinical use (Rocklage et al. 1991; Vogl et al. 1992, 1997c). It exemplifies paramagnetic metal ion complexes, producing positive enhancement. Other gadolinium complexes include Dotarem (Guerbet, France), Omiscan (Nycomed, USA), ProHance (Bracco, Italy), and Gadovist (Schering, Germany). Additionally nonionic contrast agents are available with a lower osmolality than Magnevist potentially offering greater safety for high-dose studies and rapid bolus injection (Tweedle 1997).

7.3.3.3 *Hepatobiliary Contrast Media*

Liver specific contrast agents require lower doses, as they accumulate in the liver, and functional information about the liver parenchyma may be obtained if contrast uptake is related to liver function. *Hepatobiliary contrast agents* are substances rapidly eliminated from the blood with excretion through the biliary and renal systems. They appear with high T1 relaxivity in liver parenchyma. Liver-specific contrast agents can be used in a similar way to nonspecific contrast agents for lesion characterization in the early vascular phase using dynamic imaging with rapid bolus injection.

Gd-EOB-DTPA – Eovist (Schering, Germany) – is a lipophilic modification of the chelate Gd-DTPA with hepatobiliary distribution (Reimer et al. 1996).

Gd-BOPTA – MultiHance (Bracco, Italy) – is a novel lipophilic chelate with hepatobiliary distribution. It is intravenously administered in a dose of 0.1 mmol/kg body wt. (0.5 mol/l).

Mn-DPDP – Teslascan (Nycomed, USA) – is a hepatobiliary contrast agent that enhances liver parenchyma, facilitating depiction of hypointense liver tumors (Bernardino et al. 1992; Elizondo et al. 1991; Liou et al. 1994).

Liver-specific contrast agents can be used in a similar way to nonspecific contrast agents for lesion characterization in the early vascular phase using dynamic imaging with rapid bolus injection.

Gd-EOB-DTPA and Gd-BOPTA show an uptake by the hepatocytes through an organic anion transporter; Mn-DPDP demonstrates an uptake due to the ability of the hepatocytes to excrete metal ions.

7.3.3.4
Tissue-Specific Contrast Media

Superparamagnetic iron oxides (SPIO) are small particles of iron oxide with crystals of small size surrounded by stabilizing agents such as mannitol, citrate and dextran. They produce a significant signal loss on T2-weighted images due to shortening of T2 relaxation time. A T1 effect is observed as well. The specific uptake of intravenously administered AMI-25 particles by the reticuloendothelial system enables visualization of phagocyte activity throughout the liver and spleen (Hamm et al. 1994; Stark et al. 1988; Weissleder 1994).

The iron oxide *AMI-25 – Endorem* (Guerbet, Paris) – is available for clinical use. It is administered in a dosage of 10/15 μmol/kg body wt. The contrast medium is diluted in 100 ml of 5% glucose solution and infused over 30 min using a biphasic infusion protocol. Postcontrast MR images should be obtained between 30 min and 3 h after commencing infusion.

Another *SPIO SHU 555A – Resovist* – is in clinical phase III trials. It contents of 0.5 mol Fe/l, 40 mg/ml mannitol and 2 mg/ml lactic acid. The microparticles have a mean diameter of 61 nm. The drug is administered via bolus injection and therefore delivers dynamic imaging (Brasch 1992; Shamsi et al. 1998).

7.4
Precontrast MR Imaging of Hepatocellular Carcinoma

The MR appearance of HCC can be divided into three basic categories: a solitary mass, multiple masses (multinodular) or diffuse parenchymal involvement. Furthermore the degree of fibrosis, the amount of fatty tissue within the tumorous mass, as well as the possibility of tumor necrosis and hemorrhage will vary the appearance of the lesion (Bartolozzi et al. 1994; Itai et al. 1986; Martin et al. 1995).

In addition to the imaging sequences employed, the magnetic field strength, the technical design of the MR scanner and the accompanying proprietary technology of the scanner's manufacturer enable a variety of imaging patterns (Choi et al. 1990).

7.4.1
Solitary Hepatocellular Carcinoma

On unenhanced T1-weighted scans the solitary mass is often well defined and distinct from normal liver parenchyma documenting a moderately hypointense (Figs. 7.1, 7.2) signal intensity (fibrotic lesions) relative to the liver (Hirai et al. 1991; Kelekis et al. 1998; Yamashita et al. 1993). Patterns of isointense

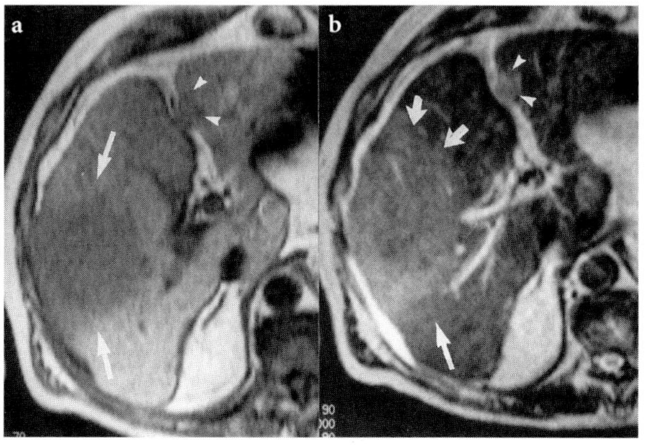

Fig. 7.1a,b. Multinodular hepatocellular carcinoma. **a** A lesion in the right liver lobe (*arrow*) with inhomogeneities in the margin is documented in an unenhanced T1-weighted GRE sequence (TR/TE/FA=154/6/70°). Probable documentation of a satellite in the left liver lobe (*arrowheads*). **b** Using a T2-weighted sequence a moderate hyperintense lesion is depicted (*arrows*). The inhomogeneities in the margin of the lesion appear as infiltrations of the huge tumor mass (*small arrows*). There is a second lesion in the left liver lobe (*arrowheads*)

Fig. 7.2a–g. Large HCC tumor. **a** Using a moderate T2-weighted sequence (TR/TE=2000/45), a hyperintense HCC nodule was visualized in the left liver lobe segment 3. **b** T2-weighted imaging (TR/TE=2000/90) also documented a hyperintense tumorous lesion. **c** Using a T1-weighted sequence (TR/TE=550/15), hypointense signal intensity of the HCC lesion was observed in the left liver lobe segment 3. Singular hyperintense foci were delineated. **d** T1-weighted gadolinium-enhanced imaging documented a moderate enhancement of the tumorous lesion demarcating the inhomogeneous inner structure to a high degree. Delineation of a possibly capsular structure. **e,f** Dynamic T1-weighted GRE sequence (TR/TE/FA=154/6/70°). **e** Using an unenhanced scan a hypointense signal lesion was visualized with a hypointense pseudocapsule. **f** Fifteen seconds postinjection of gadolinium the HCC showed a hypervascular appearance with almost isointensity to liver parenchyma. Documentation of a nonenhancing capsule. **g** Five minutes postinjection of gadolinium a more hypointense enhancement of the tumorous lesion was depicted with the beginning of enhancement of parts of the capsule ▷

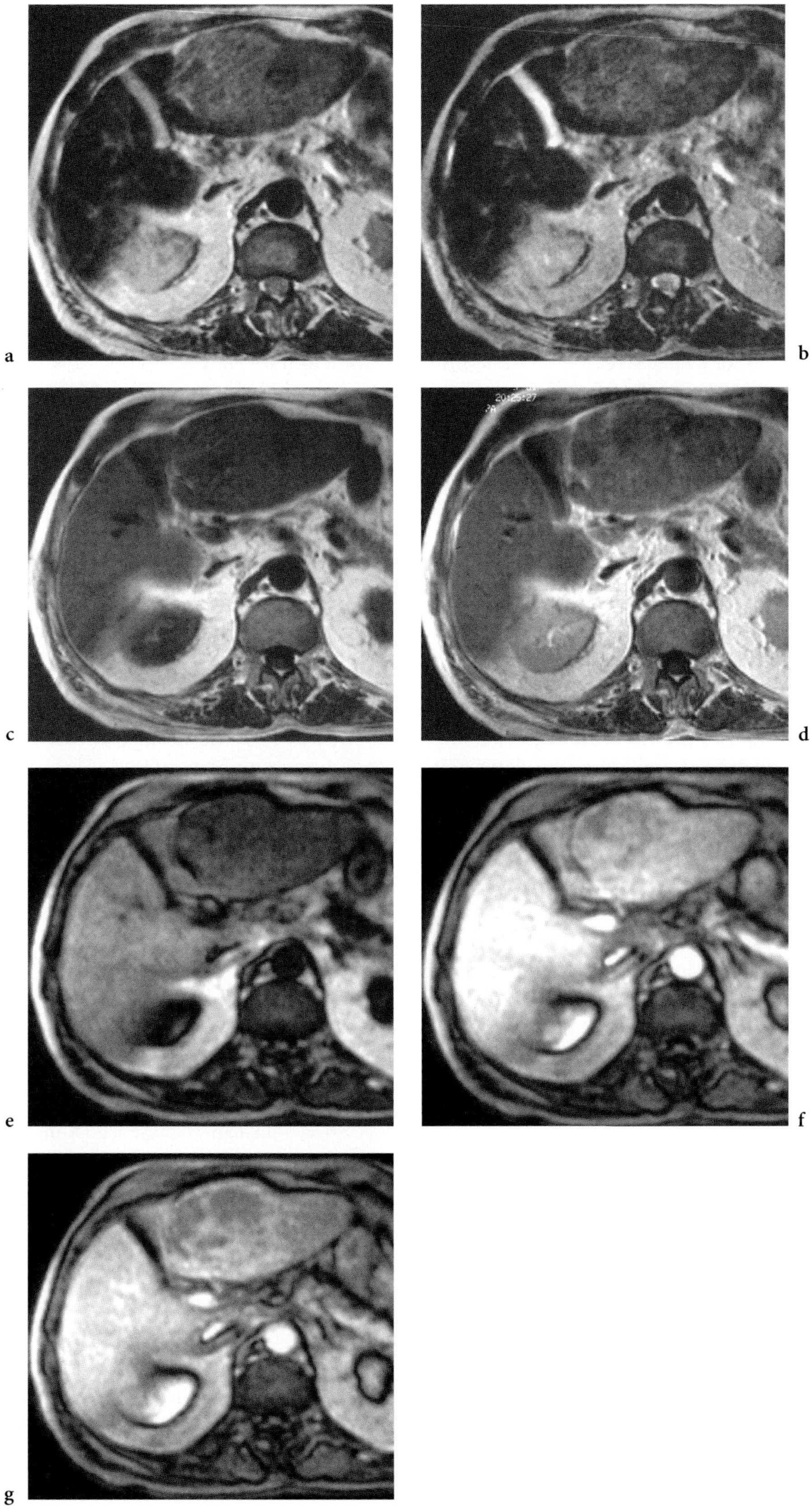

signal intensity are often seen in well-differentiated (Figs. 7.3) and early HCC. High signal intensity on T1 may be due to steatosis, hemorrhagic necrosis, intracellular glycogen, or copper deposition (EBARA et al. 1991; KITAGAWA et al. 1991; MATSUZAKI et al. 1997; HONDA et al. 1997; MITCHELL et al. 1991). High signal intensity on T1-weighted imaging is helpful due to the fact that only a few other lesions have this finding (benign conditions with fat). Fat and glycogen are more common in small, well-differentiated HCC nodules, probably reflecting a defective release of these components by partially functioning hepatocytes (MARTIN et al. 1995). Because of the abnormal low signal of iron overloaded liver, variable grade of lesion hyperintensity relative to surrounding parenchyma is a common finding of HCC superimposed on hemochromatosis on all sequences (HONDA et al. 1997). Mixed signal intensity is also depicted. The border of the lesion is smooth, irregular, or lobulated (BARTOLOZZI et al. 1994).

The lesion is usually moderate hyperintense using T2-weighted imaging (Figs. 7.1, 7.2) (KELEKIS et al. 1998). Only in a few cases is an isointense pattern depicted, generally when well differentiated. It is therefore indistinguishable from metastatic disease and other tumors of the liver (7.4). The high intensity on T2-weighted imaging correlates with the grade of malignancy in nodular lesions of cirrhotic liver according to histopathologic studies (BARTOLOZZI et al. 1984; INOUE et al. 1993; KANEMATSU et al. 1997). No significant difference can be observed comparing signal intensities of trabecular and pseudoglandular forms of tumors. Moreover, hyperintense foci on T2-weighted scans (Fig. 7.3) are found in large tumors with peliotic changes of intratumoral sinusoids. Spontaneous coagulation necrosis may lead to hypointense signal intensity on T2 in a few HCC nodules (DE SANTIS et al. 1992; HIRAI et al. 1991).

7.4.1.1 Inner Structure

A mosaic pattern is a common MRI finding in HCC. Intratumoral, linear-like hypointense areas are detected on T1-weighted scans and a nonuniform signal on T2-weighted imaging. Histopathologic correlation reveals intratumoral septa and a variety of histopathological findings within the tumorous tissue (BARTOLOZZI et al. 1994; INOUE et al. 1993).

The great majority of HCC lesions appear with inhomogeneous signal intensity. Internal heterogeneity is a common feature especially on T2-weighted imaging. Large lesions are often more inhomogeneous compared to smaller ones.

Central necrosis presents itself usually with hypointensity on T1- as well T2-weighted imaging. In the case of liquefaction a change in hyperintensity may be documented. Hyperintense foci inside the nodules on T2-weighed scans are likely to be intratumoral sinusoidal dilation due to peliotic change (Fig. 7.3).

Due to the frequent intrahepatic portal vein occlusion by the lesions, perfusion defects are seen with a difference of signal intensities in normal liver parenchyma. These areas are delineated with hyperintensity using T2-weighted imaging and hypointensity using T1-weighted scans.

Calcification is mostly documented in fibrolamellar HCC with hypointensity on T1- as well as T2-weighted imaging (CASEIRO-ALVES et al. 1996; TITELBAUM et al. 1988).

Fat-suppressed imaging techniques are useful for the diagnostic differentiation of present steatosis versus blood correlating with hyperintense signal intensity on T1-weighted imaging. The presence of fatty tissue is more likely combined with HCC than with metastatic disease, although the overall frequency of fatty tissue in the Western population is documented to be very low.

The differential diagnosis of fat containing liver tumors includes various lesions such as lipoma, adenoma, angiomyolipoma, and focal fatty infiltration (MARTIN et al. 1995).

Fig. 7.3a–g. Solitary HCC nodule in distinct liver cirrhosis. **a** Using a moderate T2-weighted sequence (PD-weighted; TR/TE=2000/45), a moderate hyperintense lesion is documented in liver segment 4 with a hypointense capsule and hyperintense foci inside and a heterogeneous inner structure. **b** T2-weighted imaging (TR/TE=2000/90) demonstrated the lesion with hyperintense signal intensity compared to distinct cirrhotic liver parenchyma. **c** A T1-weighted spin echo sequence (TR/TE=550/15) delineated the HCC as almost isointense to moderately hypointense with a hypointense capsule compared to the surrounding liver parenchyma. **d** The lesion was depicted with moderate enhancement using delayed gadolinium-enhanced static T1-weighted imaging with a moderate enhancement of the capsule. **e** Using a T1-weighted GRE sequence (TR/TE/FA=154/6/70°) delineated the HCC as almost isointense with an inhomogeneous inner structure and a hypointense pseudocapsule. **f** Gadolinium-enhanced delayed breathhold imaging revealed the tumorous lesion with a hypointense signal intensity compared to the surrounding liver parenchyma. Inhomogeneous central structures were visualized much better compared to unenhanced imaging. Documentation of a hyperintense enhancement of the pseudocapsule. **g** Dynamic imaging using a ▷

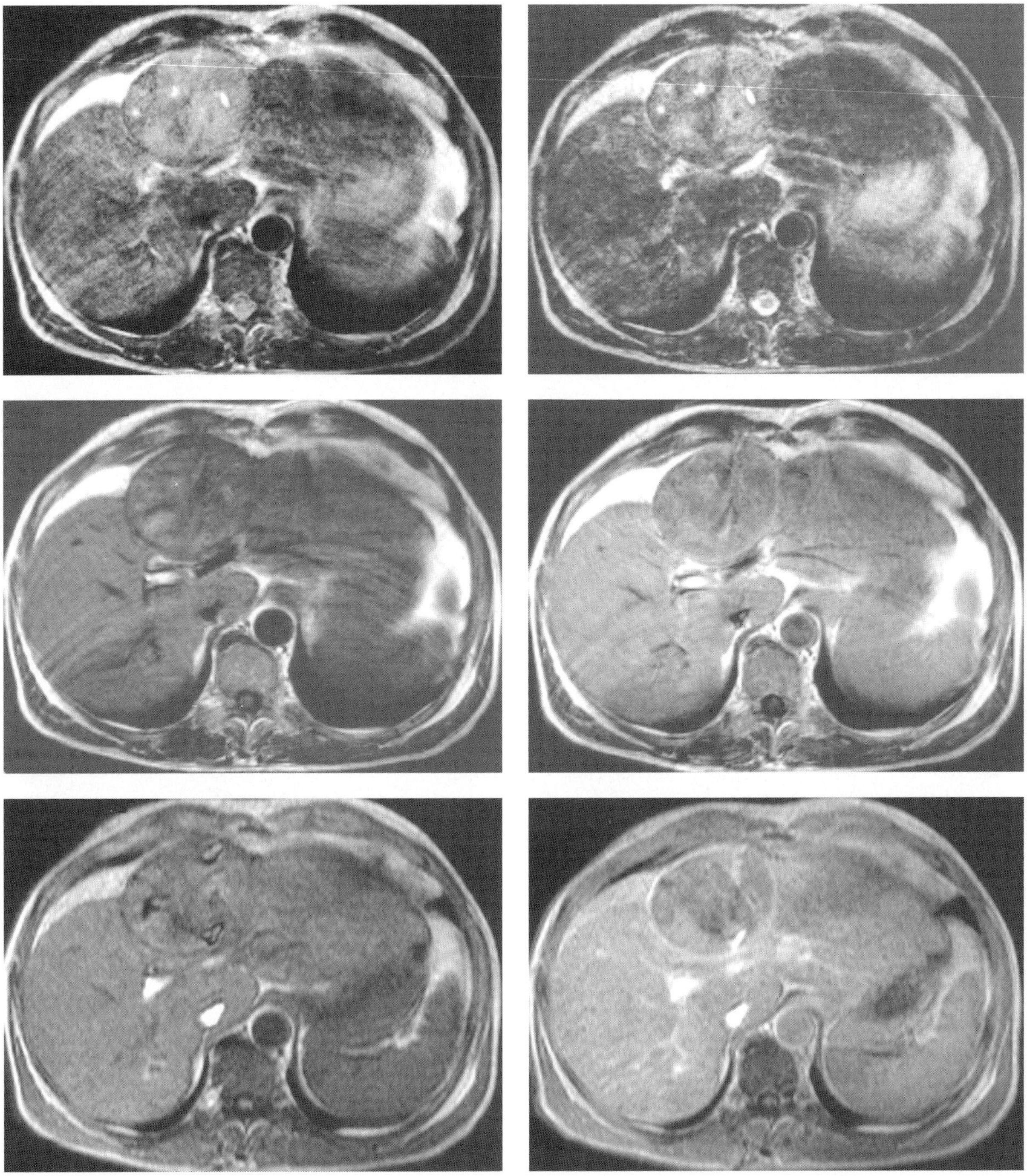

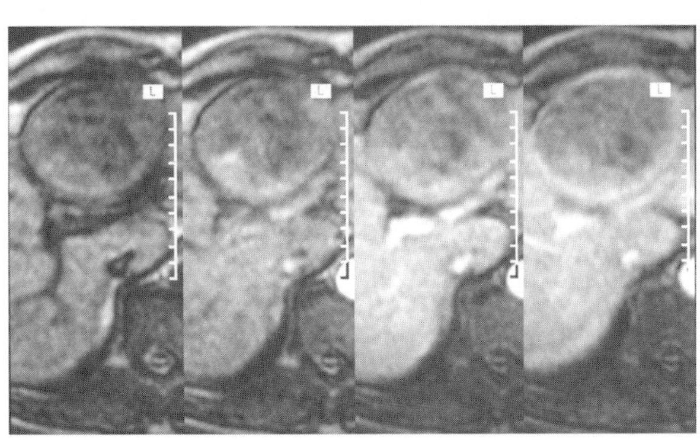

T1-weighted GRE sequence (TR/TE/TI/FA a=7/3/350/8°) in a single slice technique imaging every 5 s over a time period of 5 min. Unenhanced imaging **(ga)** presented a hypointense inhomogeneous lesion with a hypointense capsule. Imaging 15 s postinjection of gadolinium **(gb)** documented an early uptake of contrast material in the lesion. No enhancement of capsule. In the medium dynamic phase (2 min p.i.) **(gc)** signal intensity of the lesion changed to isointensity compared to liver parenchyma. Again a nonenhancing capsular structure was visualized. In the late dynamic study (5 min p.i.) **(gd)**, a hyperintense enhancement of the pseudocapsule was detected. Documentation of a more hypointense signal of the tumor compared to the liver

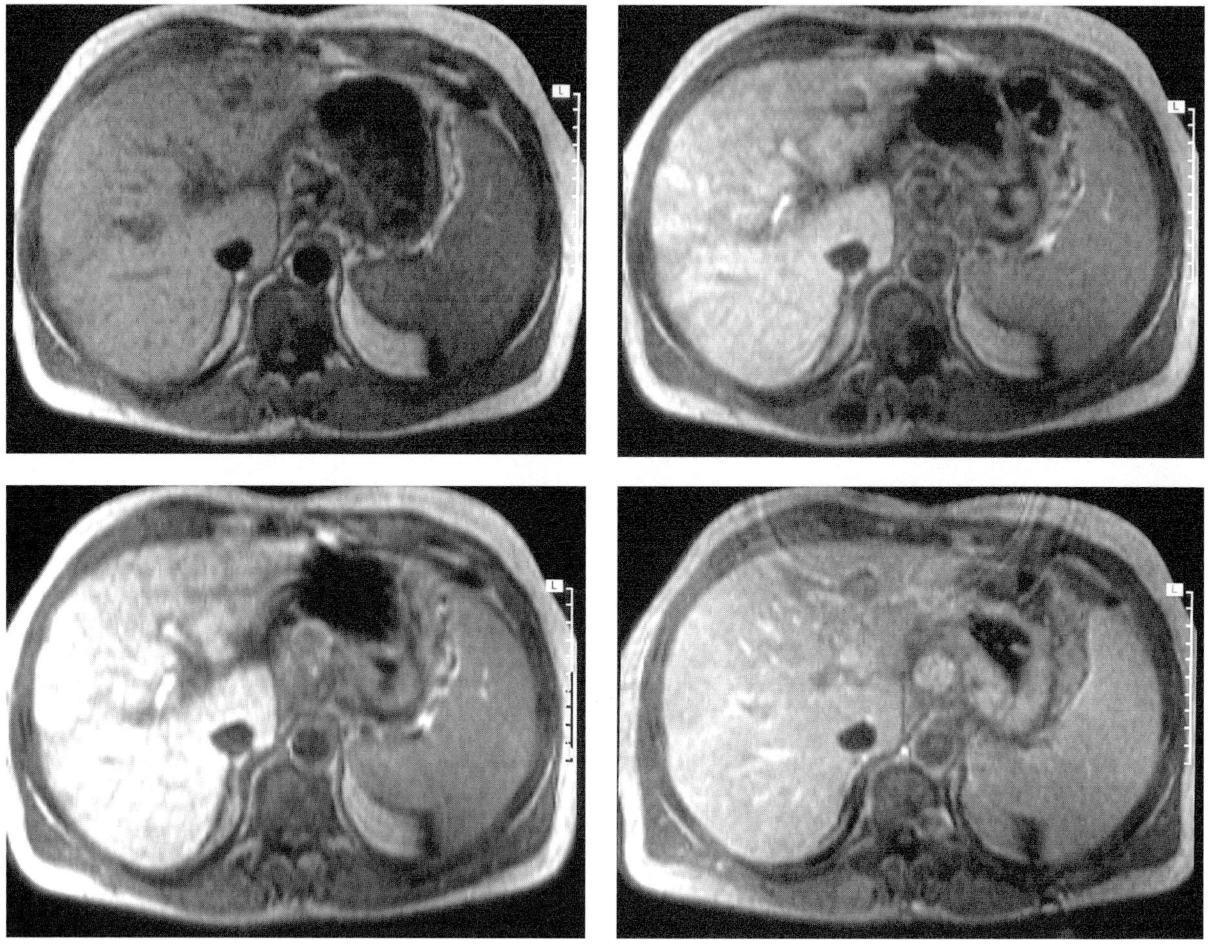

Fig. 7.4a–d. Diffuse hepatocellular carcinoma. **a** Using an unenhanced T1-weighted GRE sequence, no lesion could be clearly detected. **b** Gd-EOB-DTPA-enhanced imaging revealed a diffuse enhancement in the right liver lobe 20 min postinjection using a dose of 25 μmol/kg body wt. A demarcation of the lesion in diagnostic quality was not achieved. **c** Excellent delineation of a diffuse HCC in the right liver lobe 45 min postinjection of Gd-EOB-DTPA. **d** Using Gd-DTPA in a standard dose the diffuse infiltration could not be visualized. Isointense demarcation of the HCC

Fig. 7.5a–h. Nodular HCC in hepatic steatosis hepatis. **a** Delineation of isointense HCC lesions in the right liver lobe using an unenhanced T1-weighted GRE sequence (TR/TE/FA=154/6/70°). **b** Twenty minutes postinjection of Gd-EOB-DTPA (dose of 12.5 μmol) better demarcation of the HCC nodules compared to liver parenchyma. Documentation of a hyperintense rim enhancement. **c** Improvement in contrast and delineation of lesions versus liver parenchyma 45 min postinjection of Gd-EOB-DTPA. Better visualization of rim enhancement. **d** Gd-DTPA revealed an isointensity of lesion with a reduced delineation compared to Gd-EOB-DTPA-enhanced imaging. **e,f** Dynamic imaging using Gd-EOB-DTPA-enhanced T1-weighted GRE sequence (TR/TE/FA=100/5/70°). Unenhanced imaging (**e**) presented a hypointense tumorous lesion. Improvement of lesion-to-liver contrast using Gd-EOB-DTPA-enhanced scans (**f** 45 s p.i.; **g** 20 min p.i.). Forty-five minutes (**h**) postinjection a hyperintense rim enhancement was documented ▷

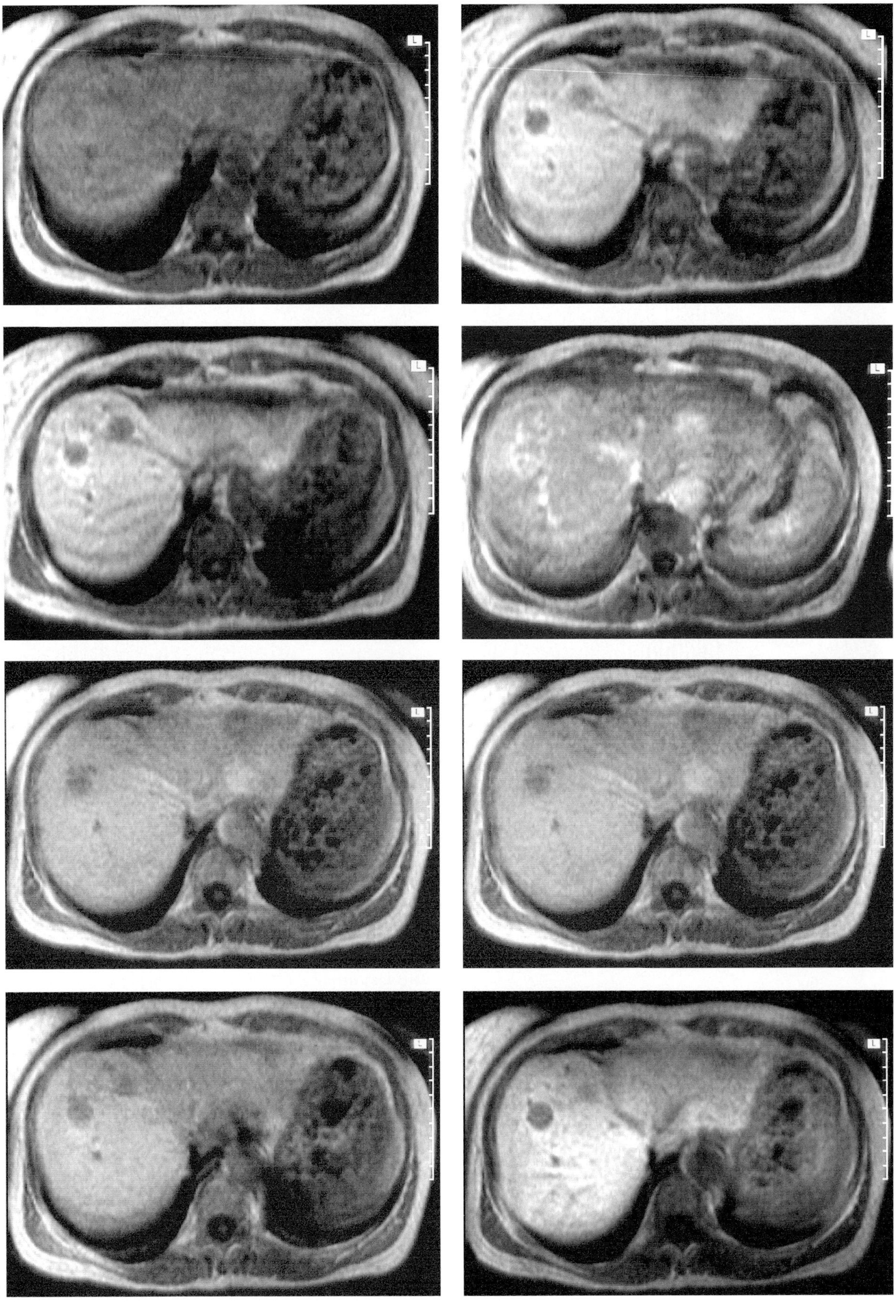

a b c d e f g h

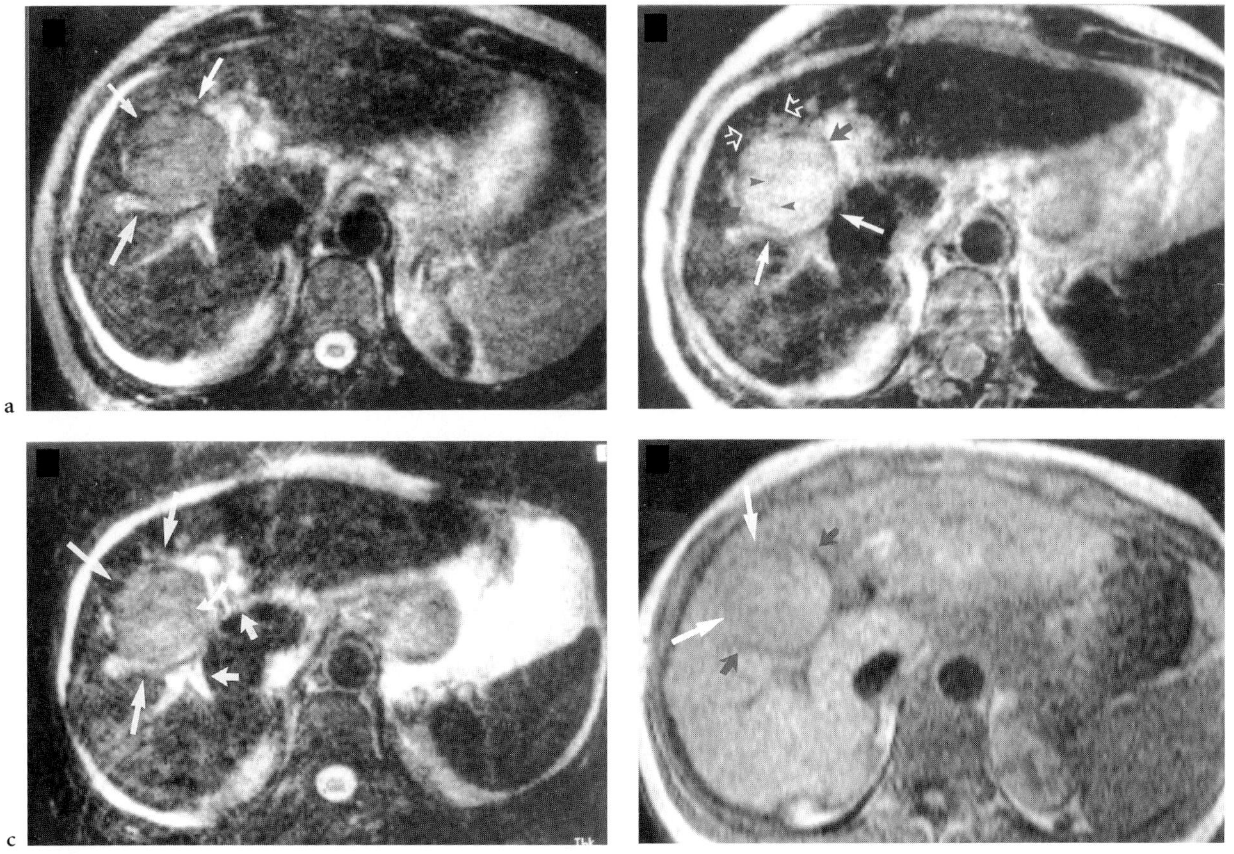

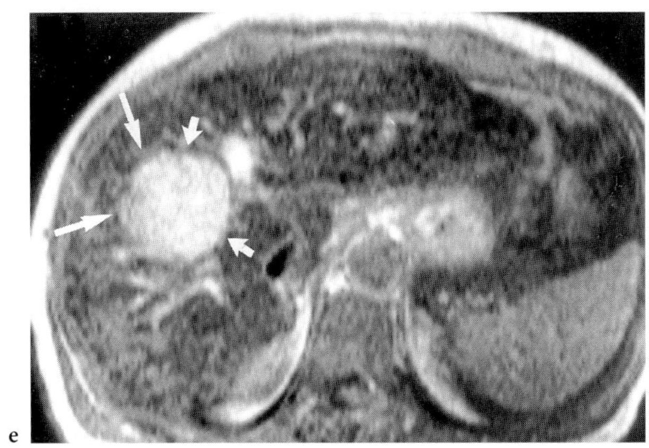

Fig. 7.6a–e. Well differentiated hepatocellular carcinoma. **a** In an unenhanced PDw sequence (TR/TE=2000/45) a 5+6-cm hyperintense lesion is seen in the right liver lobe segment 8 with inhomogeneities in the margin. Possible visualization of a capsule. **b** Using SPIO-enhanced imaging the lesion demonstrates no significant signal loss (*arrow*). In the margin inhomogeneities show an uptake of SPIO anterior to the hyperintense lesion (*open arrows*). A capsule (*black arrow*) is clearly delineated using SPIO-enhanced imaging. **c** Spots with some enhancement are documented (*curved arrow*) using T2-weighted fat-suppressed techniques. Infiltrations of vessels (*small arrows*) are delineated using SPIO-enhanced imaging. **d** T1-weighted GRE (TR/TE/FA=154/6/70°) imaging reveals a hypointense lesion (*arrows*) with a hypointense capsule (*black arrows*). **e** A hyperintense hypervascularized lesion (*arrows*) is depicted with a hypointense capsule (*small arrows*) using SPIO-enhanced T1-weighted GRE imaging

7.4.1.2 Capsule

Encapsulated lesions are rare in series from western countries compared to series from Asia. A thin rim with a hypointense signal intensity is documented on T1-weighted imaging due to its fibrotic composition (Figs. 7.3, 7,5, 7,6, 7.7). T2-weighted scans delineate a single ring with hypointense signal intensity (Figs. 7.3, 7.6a) or a double ring with inner hypointensity and outer hyperintensity. Capsules are more likely seen on T1-weighed scans. Histopathology reveals two-layered capsules with a thin fibrous inner zone and an outer zone consisting of compressed small vessels and bile ducts (Choi et al. 1990; Imaeda et al. 1994).

7.4.1.3 *Central Scarring*

Inflammatory central scars have been reported in some cases with hypointense signal intensity on T1-weighted images and hyperintensity on T2-weighted scans. Moreover, collagenous central scars are delineated within some HCC nodules with hypointensity on T1- as well as on T2-weighted imaging (RUMMENY et al. 1989b).

7.4.1.4 *Edema*

Edema is a diagnostic feature generally associated with malignant liver lesions. It is also observed in HCC nodules. Signal intensity of edema is hyperintense using T2-weighted images surrounding the lesion. It might reflect the anatomic distribution of venous or lymphatic infiltration as a wedge-shape sign.

7.4.1.5 *Vascularity*

HCC nodules are generally hypervascular tumors, predominantly supplied by the hepatic arterial system. Hypovascular necrotic areas may be seen especially in large tumors according to the heterogeneous internal architecture.

7.4.2 Multinodular Hepatocellular Carcinoma

Encapsulation is demonstrated in fewer multinodular HCC lesions compared to solitary mass. On T1-weighted unenhanced images, less contrast is documented between lesion and normal liver parenchyma. Using T2-weighted scans the nodules are most evident (Fig. 7.8, 7.9).

7.4.3 Diffuse Hepatocellular Carcinoma

The diffuse form of HCC is poorly marginated and no capsule is seen (Fig. 7.10, 7.11) T2-weighted unenhanced images demonstrate an improved lesion to liver contrast compared to T1-weighted scans.

7.4.4 Early Hepatocellular Carcinoma

Adenomatous hyperplasia with malignant foci presents a variable MRI appearance. Typically these lesions have a lower diameter. They show isointense signal intensity on T1-weighted imaging, in some cases hyperintense signal (Fig. 7.12). On T2-weighted scans hyperintense signal is visualized. Nevertheless mixed patterns of signal intensity are observed (Fig. 7.12). A nodule-in-nodule appearance suggests early HCC in cirrhotic liver parenchyma (SABEK et al. 1995). The nodule demonstrates a hypointense periphery resulting from iron deposition with an isointense iron poor center (HONDA et al. 1997). This pattern correlates with early carcinoma or dysplasia within a regenerative nodule (MURAMATSU et al. 1991).

7.4.5 Fibrolamellar Hepatocellular Carcinoma

Fibrolamellar HCC (FLHCC) is an uncommon, rare neoplasm of the liver. It usually occurs in a younger population, lacks specific association with cirrhosis or parenchymal liver disease, and has no definite sex predilection. Presently FLHCC is of unknown cause. It is frequently resectable and potentially curable (TITELBAUM et al. 1988).

Most often FLHCC is a solitary large lobulated mass. MRI reveals the tumor with a partial or complete capsule. Large thin-walled veins are verified within the capsule and fibrous septa.

A depressed central fibrous scar with bulging margins and fibrous septa is documented. Classically the scar is of low signal intensity on both T1- and T2-weighted images in contrast to the central scar of FNH. In this tumor it appears hyperintense on T2-weighted images. In some cases, however, hyperintense scars have been reported in FLHCC. Therefore the findings of FLHCC are in some circumstances confused with focal nodular hyperplasia (CASEIRO-ALVES et al. 1996).

Large areas of necrosis are missing in most cases. Calcification is present in these tumors and more unusually in HCC. In general, tumors have been iso- or hypointense to the liver on T1-weighted images and iso- to hyperintense on T2-weighted sequences (CASEIRO-ALVES et al. 1996).

7.4.6 Secondary Signs

Using unenhanced MR imaging generalized hepatomegaly or a localized bulge in the liver contour caused by HCC may be seen. Secondary signs of HCC, including ascites and hepatomegaly, are well documented using T2- as well as T1-weighted imaging.

The disease has a propensity to invade the portal vein, hepatic veins, or both with frequently visualized intratumoral vessels. Extension into the inferior vena cava is depicted in some cases. Tumor thrombus might be identified within the inferior vena cava and the portal vein.

7.4.7 Differential Diagnosis

Regenerative nodules are a common feature of liver cirrhosis. Using MR imaging these lesions appear as small hypointense nodular lesions on both T1- and T2-weighted imaging (Fig. 7.13). HCC are depicted usually with high signal intensity on T2-weighted images. Histopathological findings have shown hemosiderin deposits in many of these nodules. Usually these nodules are more homogeneous than HCC lesions.

Adenomatous hyperplasia is defined as regenerative nodules with dysplastic histology. These lesions are iso-hyperintense using T1-weighted imaging like well-differentiated HCC nodules. Unlike malignant lesions adenomatous hyperplasia provides a smooth margin. There is no evidence of capsule.

Early advanced HCC may have a dominant early component with a small HCC nodule leading to a nodule-within-nodule appearance. It has been considered as a transitional tumor between early HCC and advanced HCC associated with chronic liver disease. Central hypointensity surrounded by hyperintensity on T1-weighted images is depicted. Using T2-weighted scans central hyperintensity is documented (Fig. 7.14) (Sabek et al. 1995; Winter et al. 1994).

The differentiation of *adenoma* versus well-differentiated HCC remains a diagnostic challenge due to the similarity of morphologic features (Fig. 7.15). A mixed pattern is also documented for adenomas such as internal heterogeneity due to central necrosis, hemorrhage, a hypointense capsule, and central scarring. Clinical data may help the diagnosis.

FNH shows typically moderate hypointense to isointense signal intensity using T1-weighted imaging. On T2-weighted scans this lesion is isointense to slightly hyperintense (Figs. 7.16, 7.17). No capsule is evident, whereas a central scar is depicted in most cases with hypointensity on T1-weighted (Fig. 7.17) and hyperintensity on T2-weighted imaging (Fig. 7.16).

7.5 Extracellular-Agent-Enhanced MR Imaging of Hepatocellular Carcinoma

7.5.1 Dynamic Imaging

Dynamic MRI scanning is provided by fast imaging techniques following bolus administration of gadolinium chelates. Dynamic enhanced T1-weighted imaging is based on the comprehensive analysis of the arterial and venous phase enhanced sequences (Tweedle 1997; Vogl et al. 1992, 1997c; Yamashita et al. 1994).

The degree of enhancement on dynamic gadolinium-enhanced images corresponds to the degree of vascularity of lesion (Kelekis et al. 1998). Accordingly the enhancement of HCC nodules in the early arterial phase is delineated with a mixed pattern: peripheral, central, mixed, complete or nonexistent. In most cases enhancement is present due to hypervascularity of lesions. HCC nodules enhance more than the surrounding liver parenchyma (Fig. 7.2). HCC lesions show variable degrees of hyperintensity in relation to the normal liver parenchyma in the first minute after injection of gadolinium. The maximum lesion-to liver contrast is depicted in the very early arterial phase (Fig. 7.3). The peak of enhancement of the HCC nodules is reached about 45 s postinjection. A nodule-within-nodule appearance is observed in about 30% of the lesions in the early arterial phase imaging. Usually the enhancement is heterogeneous. Tumor enhancement decreases in the middle phase leading to isointensity in comparison to surrounding liver parenchyma (Fig. 7.3) (Peterson et al. 1996).

Necrotic areas document no enhancement in the central zone (Lencioni et al. 1996; Marchal et al. 1993).

Mahfouz et al. (1993b) reported the peripheral washout as a specific sign of malignancy in dynamic gadolinium-enhanced MRI. HCC lesions were depicted on dynamic imaging most frequently with inhomogeneity of enhancement (heterogeneous enhancement), intralesional nonenhancing areas, and typical late enhancement of a pseudocapsule (Figs. 7.2, 7.3) (Choi et al. 1990; Hammerstingl et al. 1997; Imaeda et al. 1994; Kim et al. 1995; Mafhouz et al. 1994).

Muramatsu et al. (1997) stated the so-called wedge sign on T1-weighted contrast-enhanced images associated with liver tumors, indicating intraductal tumor extension in intrahepatic bile ducts.

7.5.2 Delayed Imaging

On delayed postcontrast scans a mixed or peripheral enhancement is seen in HCC lesions. Enhancement is heterogeneous (Figs. 7.2, 7.3) (Peterson et al. 1996). The pseudocapsule shows delayed enhancement (Fig. 7.3). This is due to the large extracellular spaces of the capsular region, which include vascular lakes within the compressed liver parenchyma. In some cases a peripheral hyperintense halo is documented on early delayed postcontrast scans corresponding to a fibrous capsule with no enhancement in the early phase of dynamic imaging (Choi et al. 1990; Imaeda et al. 1994; Mahfouz et al. 1994).

7.5.3 Differential Diagnosis

Regenerating nodules are observed as hypovascular-hypointense nodules in the early phase of gadolinium-enhanced images. They reveal a lower positive enhancement with postextracellular contrast agents with a better demarcation in contrast to surrounding liver parenchyma using delayed imaging (Fig. 7.13).

Adenomatous hyperplasia shows enhancing features similar to the surrounding liver parenchyma, due to a prevalent portal vein vascular supply (Lencioni et al. 1996).

Early HCC reveals similar enhancement criteria as adenomatous hyperplasia.

Early advanced HCC usually shows hypervascularity using dynamic studies.

Adenomas show early enhancement on dynamic MR studies. They present as homogeneous lesions with isointensity in some cases using contrast-enhanced imaging. In general adenomas present a mixed pattern in correlation with internal heterogeneity due to necrosis/hemorrhage/capsule/scar.

In contrast to HCC a homogeneous enhancement of *FNH nodules* presents a rapid isointensity in the early to medium phase of gadolinium-enhanced dynamic studies (Fig. 7.17). In comparison with HCC nodules a slightly stronger and earlier enhancement is reported (Fig. 7.17). In contrast enhancement of FNH is homogeneous. In the early arterial phase the central scar is depicted with a nonenhancing hypointense signal (Fig. 7.17) changing to hyperintensity (enhancement) (Fig. 7.17) in the late phase (Caseiro-Alvez et al. 1996; Mahfouz et al. 1993a).

For *metastatic infiltrations* a peripheral enhancement is delineated in the majority of cases. Also there is an overlap in the enhancement pattern between hypervascular malignant HCC and FNH, the combination of unenhanced, dynamic and static enhanced images enabling a differential diagnosis with a high degree of certainty (Hammerstingl et al. 1998).

On dynamic gadolinium-enhanced evaluation of *fibrolamellar* HCC, a diffuse heterogeneous enhancement is noted early with a prompt return to homogeneous, isointense signal intensity. This is nonspecific and overlaps with the enhancement pattern of other primary tumors (Corrigan and Semelka 1995).

7.6 Hepatobiliary-Agent-Enhanced MR Imaging of Hepatocellular Carcinoma

7.6.1 Gd-EOB-DTPA-Enhanced MR Imaging

Gd-EOB-DTPA is a safe hepatobiliary contrast agent, which provides a strong and persistent enhancement of normal hepatic parenchyma based on its uptake by hepatocytes (Hamm et al. 1995). This contrast agent can be administered as a bolus injection allowing additional dynamic imaging. The potential of adding diagnostic information can be achieved on the differences in vascularity and the extent of extracellular space of the focal hepatic lesions comparable to extracellular contrast agents. Therefore both the characterization and the detection of liver lesions are improved in a single examination. Moreover it allows good delineation of the biliary passages. This helps the diagnosis of early infiltration of the bile ducts.

Our data showed a biphasic contrast effect in normal liver parenchyma using dynamic T1-GRE images. The maximum percentage enhancement was 45 min p.i. for Gd-EOB-DTPA (50 μmol/kg body wt.). Lower signal intensities were documented for patients suffering from liver cirrhosis (Reimer et al. 1996).

HCC nodules are surrounded by a rim of high signal intensity in the early phase of dynamic imaging (starting 15 s up to 5 min p.i.) (50 μmol of Gd-EOB-DTPA). The peripheral enhancement of metastases is usually less than for HCC nodules (Bellin et al. 1994; van Beers et al. 1994). In patients with FNH the dynamic Gd-EOB-DTPA-enhanced (higher doses) images revealed a contrast enhancement similar to Gd-DTPA.

Our protocol documents a statistically significant difference of percentage enhancement of malignant liver lesions (HCC, metastases) compared to benign liver tumors (FNH, hemangiomas) for all five doses of Gd-EOB-DTPA tested in this study (20 min after injection of contrast medium) ($P<0.05$) (Reimer et al. 1997; Harisinghani et al. 1997).

Improved detection of hepatic lesions is enabled using Gd-EOB-DTPA-enhanced imaging in comparison with Gd-DTPA-enhanced MRI. Differential diagnostic information comparable to Gd-DTPA-enhanced imaging is provided using Gd-EOB-DTPA in higher doses (Hamm et al. 1995; Marchal et al. 1993; Reimer et al. 1996; van Beers et al. 1994; Vogl et al. 1996b).

7.6.2 Gd-BOPTA-Enhanced MR Imaging

Gd-BOPTA results in significant enhancement of normal liver tissue compared to unenhanced imaging (Caudana et al. 1996). A reproducibly increased enhancement of liver parenchyma is documented after intravenous administration of 0.1 mmol/kg body wt. due to the uptake of the contrast agent by the hepatocytes. Qualitative and quantitative analysis reveal a biphasic pattern of contrast enhancement using intravenous Gd-BOPTA. The maximum liver enhancement is yielded in the perfusion phase with a peak of signal intensities 10 min postinjection. A plateaulike constant signal intensity is documented over approximately 1 h. A statistically significant enhancement of normal liver tissue is seen up to 8 h postinjection. A high degree of enhancement and contrast of the gallbladder as well as the biliary tract compared to surrounding liver tissue is recorded.

Improved lesion detection is documented using dynamic study protocols. Differential diagnostic information is increased using dynamic T1-weighted imaging as well as static postcontrast delayed scans.

Our group was able to document an improved characterization of HCC lesions using dynamic imaging using Gd-BOPTA. A rapid increase in signal intensity during the early, arterial phase in well-differentiated HCC lesions was depicted followed by a progressive decrease in signal intensity. This is due to the fact that well-differentiated HCC retain some hepatocellular function, with uptake of hepatospecific contrast agents. The enhancement was mainly seen in the periphery of the lesion. Dynamic sequences showed a substantial relationship between the rapid and high increase in signal intensity of HCCs in the perfusion phase and their morphologic features. Undifferentiated or poorly differentiated HCC lesions showed no rapid increase in signal intensity (Inoue et al. 1993).

Well-differentiated HCCs presented themselves with a hypointense rim before injection and both hypo- and hyperintense rims immediately after injection compared to normal liver parenchyma. A double-ring sign in larger well-differentiated nodular HCC lesions was delineated (Imaeda et al. 1994).

In the middle phase a single-rim enhancement was detected in most HCCs. Enhancement during the venous perfusion phase is generally an indication of venous vascularity, and possibly increased cellular uptake in peritumoral vital tissue. The nonenhancing peripheral rim was defined as a capsule of lesions (Caudana et al. 1996).

7.6.3 Mn-DPDP-Enhanced MR Imaging

After intravenous administration of Mn-DPDP, normal liver parenchyma enhances significantly with a persisting longlasting enhancement (hours). A wide imaging window is provided.

Mn-DPDP is nonenhancing in undifferentiated HCC, metastases, intrahepatic cholangiocarcinomas, and lymphomas. Consequently, contrast-to-noise ratio and demarcation of malignant liver tumors improve compared to unenhanced imaging. Detection rate is increased versus nonenhancing techniques (Fretz et al 1990; Seneterre et al. 1996).

Mn-DPDP accumulates in well differentiated hepatocellular carcinoma. Other liver specific contrast agents are usually nonenhancing in this malignancy (Rofsky et al. 1993). According to the composition of the hepatocytes liver tumors demonstrate an uptake of the contrast agent. Benign lesions such as FNH and regenerative nodules demonstrate an uptake of this liver-specific contrast agent and result in different enhancement compared with metastatic infiltration and undifferentiated HCC. Its role in the characterization of focal hepatic lesions is restricted to the rough differentiation of hepatocellular from nonhepatocellular (or hepatocyte versus nonhepatocyte lesion) tumors (Bernardino et al. 1991; Vogl et al. 1993; Liou et al. 1994; Marchal et al. 1993).

Murakami et al. (1996) stated that the degree of tumor enhancement of HCC correlated with the histologic differentiation. Significantly greater enhancement of Mn-DPDP was seen in well-differentiated lesions than in poorly differentiated ones. Imaging in cirrhotic liver demonstrated a decreased enhancement of Mn-DPDP in patients with confluent/diffuse fibrosis and siderotic regenerating nodules. An increased enhancement was delineated in benign regenerating nodules (Elizondo et al. 1991; Inoue et al. 1993; Ni et al. 1993).

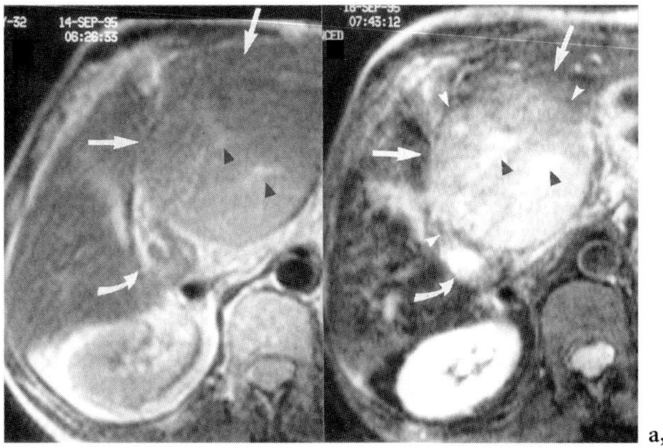

a,b

Fig. 7.7a,b. Solitary huge hepatocellular carcinoma. **a** Documentation of a nearly isointense huge HCC (*arrows*) in the left liver lobe segment 3 using a moderate T2-weighted sequence (PD-weighted sequence: TR/TE=2000/45). **b** Using SPIO-enhanced T2-weighted sequences no signal loss of the lesion (*arrows*) is documented with hyperintense foci in the center due to fatty infiltration (*black arrowheads*). A hypointense capsule is observed (*arrowheads*). Documentation of a compressed vena cava inferior (*curved arrow*)

7.7 SPIO-Enhanced MR Imaging of Hepatocellular Carcinoma

7.7.1 Imaging Criteria

Using SPIO-enhanced imaging normal liver parenchyma demonstrates an uptake of the contrast agent owing to its endothelial and Kupffer cells. A negative enhancement or loss of signal intensity of normal liver parenchyma is seen using moderate and heavily T2-weighted images because of the more effective T2 shortening with these sequences (Hamm et al. 1994; Stark et al. 1988; Vogl et al. 1997a).

Malignant liver lesions such as HCC usually demonstrate no change in signal intensity comparing unenhanced and SPIO-enhanced T2-weighted images (Figs. 7.6, 7.7). This leads to an improvement of the contrast-to-noise ratio but also of the signal-to-noise ratio of lesions with a decreased signal intensity of liver parenchyma and a high signal intensity of malignant tumors. Thus lesion demarcation as well as visualization and delineation is improved and the detection rate of focal liver lesions is increased comparing unenhanced and SPIO-enhanced MRI (Fig. 7.9b) (Denys et al. 1994; Vogl et al. 1996c).

Nevertheless in some cases well differentiated HCC (Asian population, Japan) demonstrate an uptake of the contrast medium due to the presence of Kupffer cells.

Low SPIO concentrations also increase the signal intensity on T1-weighted imaging because of their T1 effect (Fig. 7.6). HCC nodules demonstrate a moderate hyperintense to hyperintense signal intensity according to their vascularity using T1-weighted sequences (Figs. 7.6, 7.8) (Oudkerk et al. 1997). Therefore SPIO agents are available as positive enhancers for a short period after intravenous administration with the possibility of vascular information (Hahn et al. 1990; Scharf et al. 1998).

7.7.2 Dynamic Imaging

Minimal amounts of Resovist induce a high reduction of signal intensity by shortening the T2 relaxation time. Data from clinical studies proved that bolus injection of Resovist was well tolerated (Reimer et al. 1995). The quantitative evaluation al-

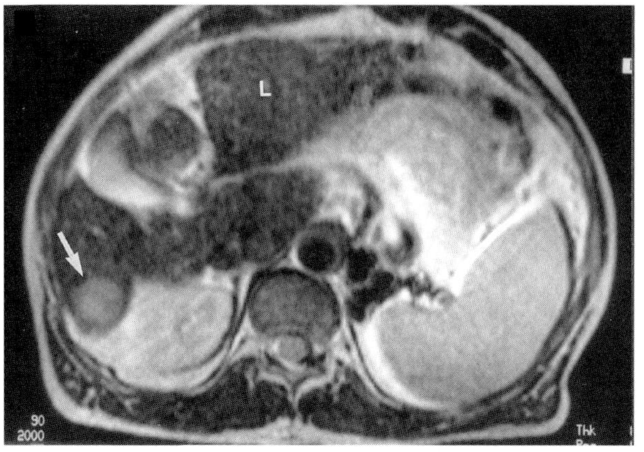

a

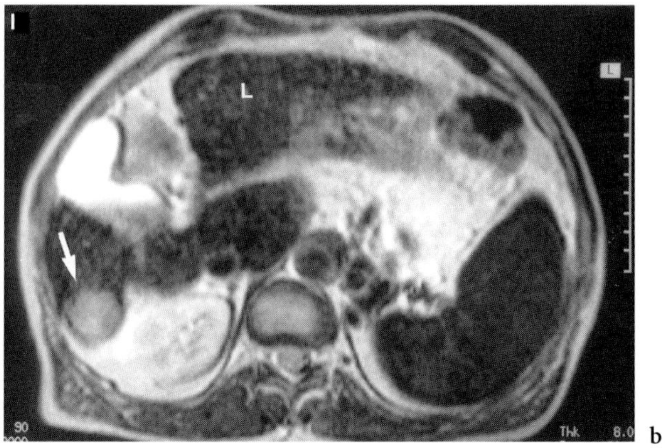

b

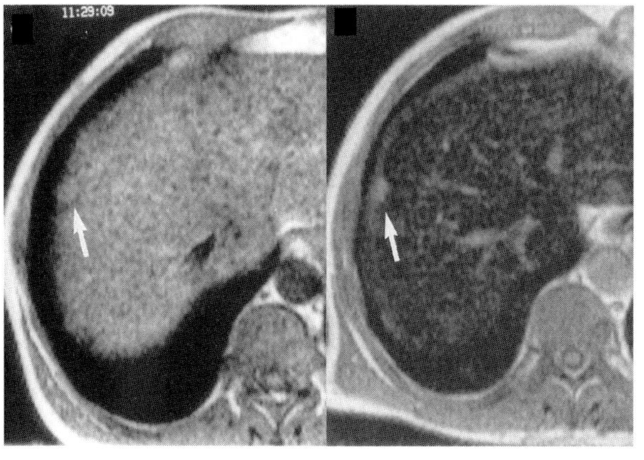

c,d

Fig. 7.8a–d. Poorly differentiated hepatocellular carcinoma. **a** Documentation of a 2+2-cm large hyperintense lesion in the right liver lobe segment 6 (*arrow*) using an unenhanced T2-weighted sequence (TR/TE=2000/45). **b** On SPIO-enhanced scans a significant signal loss of normal liver parenchyma (*L*) is seen in contrast to no decrease of signal intensity of the hepatocellular carcinoma (*arrow*). **c** On unenhanced T1-weighted GRE images a nearly isointense lesion with a hypointense capsule is detected (*arrows*). **d** Using the SPIO-enhanced sequence a nonenhancing hyperintense HCC nodule (*arrow*) is delineated compared with the decrease in signal intensity of liver cirrhotic parenchyma. Liver transplantation verified this lesion

lows more detailed information on the characteristics of liver tumors using early dynamic and late static enhancement. Clinical studies proved the capability of dynamic SPIO-enhanced T_2-weighted and T_1-weighted imaging protocols for the evaluation of the perfusion phase (Hamm et al. 1994; Kim et al. 1995; Vogl et al. 1997b).

Using T2-weighted dynamic imaging hypervascular lesions like FNH, an earlier signal loss appeared than with normal liver parenchyma. To some extent the same phenomenon could be observed in hypervascular HCC. Using a dynamic T2-weighted protocol, a reproducible sudden drop-out phenomenon was observed in hypervascular HCC nodules. This phenomenon resulted in a rapid signal loss in the perfusion phase followed by a short increase in signal (Hahn et al. 1990).

No significant signal loss of the HCC could be documented using Resovist-enhanced static sequences. Due to a high signal loss of the surrounding liver parenchyma the contrast between HCC nodules and the liver parenchyma was improved, also allowing a better delineation of the lesion (Denys et al. 1994).

Regenerating nodules presented a relatively low percentage signal intensity loss in comparison to normal liver parenchyma (Kawamori et al. 1992; Yamamoto et al. 1995).

Resovist-enhanced proton density-weighted and T_2-weighted sequences greatly improve the depiction and delineation of liver tumors by modifying the liver-to-tumor contrast. Metastases lacking RES could be visualized with a better contrast to the normal liver parenchyma (Bellin et al. 1994; Fretz et al. 1990; Hammerstingl et al. 1998; Marchal et al. 1989; Seneterre et al. 1996). This refers to the lesion's rim and especially to the lesion's center, where isointense or slightly hyperintense liver parenchyma using unenhanced scans turns to hypointense tissue using Resovist-enhanced images. The results of our study using Resovist enhanced MRI prove an increased detection rate and an improved depiction quality in patients with liver metastases.

Regardless of histopathology of the lesion, we observed better results using proton density-weighted and T_2-weighted Resovist enhanced images than FLASH-2D scans concerning the quality of delineation and contrast.

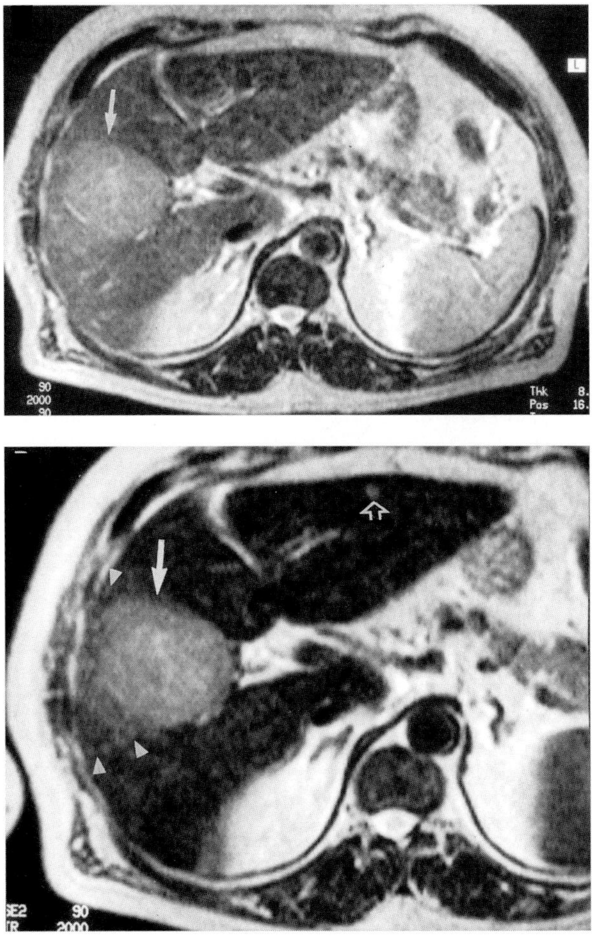

Fig. 7.9a,b. Multinodular hepatocellular carcinoma. **a** On a T2-weighted unenhanced sequence (TR/TE=2000/90) a large hyperintense lesion is documented in the right liver lobe (*arrow*). **b** Using a T2-weighted SPIO-enhanced sequence (TR/TE=2000/90), improved delineation of the large hyperintense lesion in the right liver lobe (*arrow*) is seen with infiltration in the surrounding liver parenchyma (*small arrows*). A satellite lesion is depicted in the left liver lobe (*open arrow*)

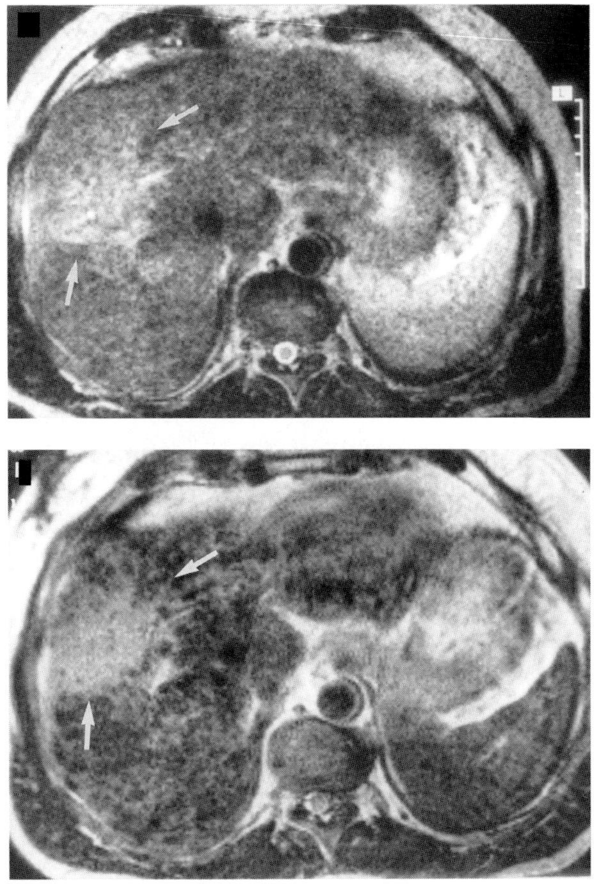

Fig. 7.10a,b. Undifferentiated hepatocellular carcinoma in liver cirrhosis. **a** Using an unenhanced PDw image (TR/TE=2000/45), a 7×6-cm hyperintense lesion (*arrows*) is delineated in the right liver lobe with central inhomogeneities and unsharp margins. **b** The PDw image (TR/TE=2000/45) after intravenous administration of SPIO allows an accurate delineation of the involved segments of the right liver lobe (*arrows*) due to marked signal loss of the normal liver parenchyma, which is presented with an inhomogeneous texture due to liver cirrhosis

Further studies using the new SPIO formulation Resovist should be directed towards to a more detailed analysis of the dynamic protocol for its use in the characterization of hypervascular tumors like hepatocellular carcinoma and adenoma (Hahn et al. 1990). Resovist enhanced MR imaging is going to become a diagnostic means with excellent capabilities for both the detection and differentiation of hepatic tumors with the advantage of a bolus intravenous injection (Kopp et al. 1997; Shamsi et al. 1998; Vogl et al. 1996a,c).

7.7.3 Differential Diagnosis

Hyperplastic or *regenerative nodules* show a change in signal intensity postcontrast with a decrease (loss of signal) comparing sequences of unenhanced and SPIO-enhanced imaging (Fig. 7.12) (Kawamori et al. 1992).

Adenoma shows hyper-isointense lesions on T2-weighted SPIO-enhanced images (Fig. 7.15). Using T1-weighted scans, lesions appear moderately hyperintense when SPIO-enhanced (Fig. 7.15).

FNH nodules are moderately hyperintense on T2-weighted images when unenhanced, revealing a de-

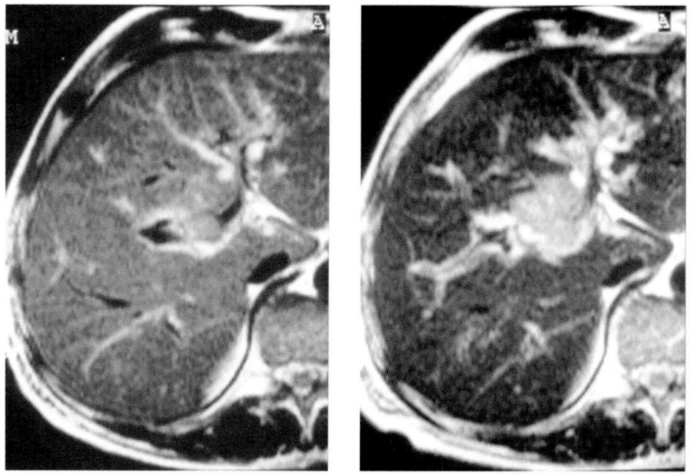

a b

Fig. 7.11a,b. HCC in liver cirrhosis (patient suffering from hepatitis C). **a** In a male patient pre liver transplantation a hyperintense lesion in segment 8 of the liver is delineated using T2-weighted turbo spin echo sequence (TR/TE=2000/90). **b** Using T2w TSE sequence postcontrast almost no change in signal intensity of the lesion is documented. Significant signal loss of liver parenchyma

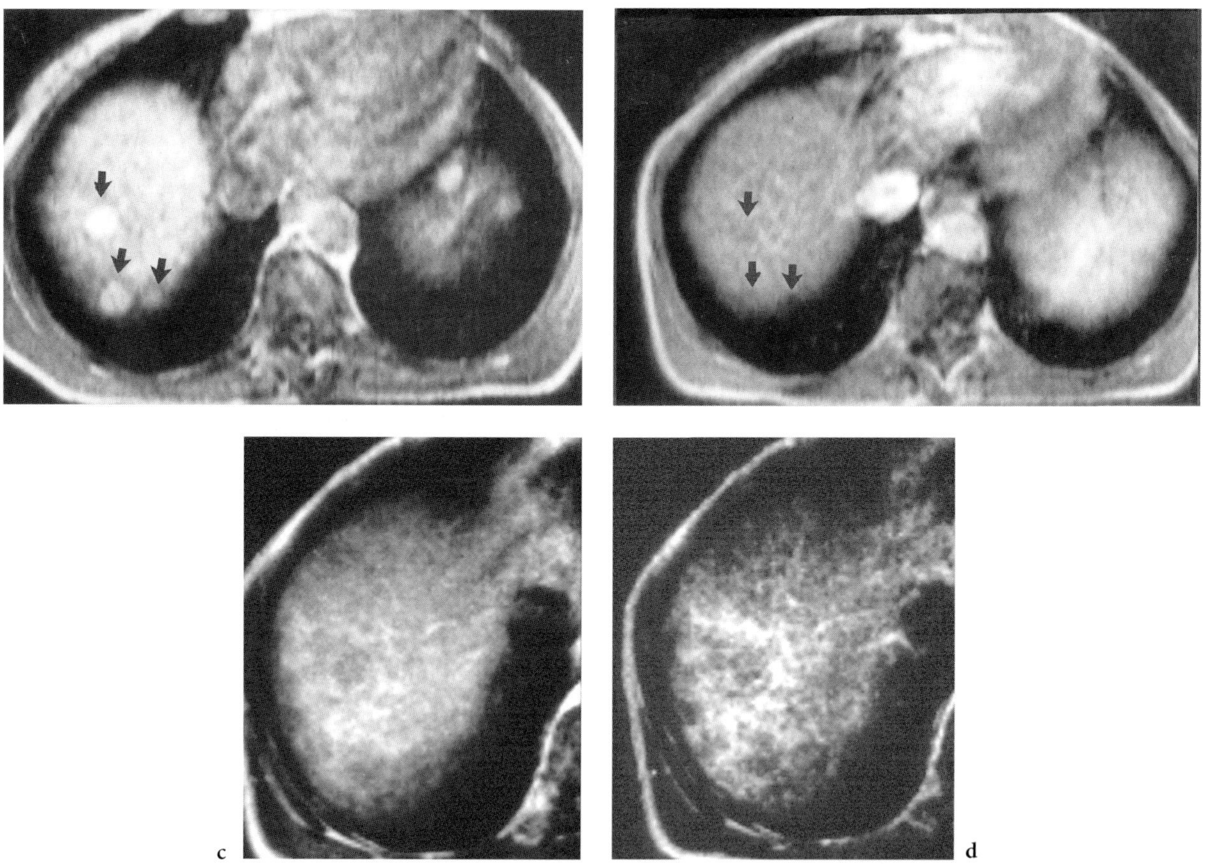

a b c d

Fig. 7.12a–d. Hyperplastic regenerating nodules. **a** Using a T1w GRE sequence (TR/TE/FA=154/6/70°) unenhanced hyperintense lesions are delineated in the right liver lobe (*arrows*) in a female patient suffering from hepatitis and scheduled for liver transplantation. **b** On SPIO-enhanced T1-weighted GRE scans a signal loss of the lesions is documented with hypo- to isointensity in contrast to liver parenchyma (*arrows*). The diagnosis of regenerating nodules was revealed by histopathology after liver transplantation. **c** In a moderate T2-weighted spin echo sequence (PD-weighted; TR/TE=2000/45), hypointense nodules were delineated. **d** Using a moderate SPIO-enhanced T2-weighted sequence, a significant signal loss of cirrhotic liver parenchyma and of the nodules is documented

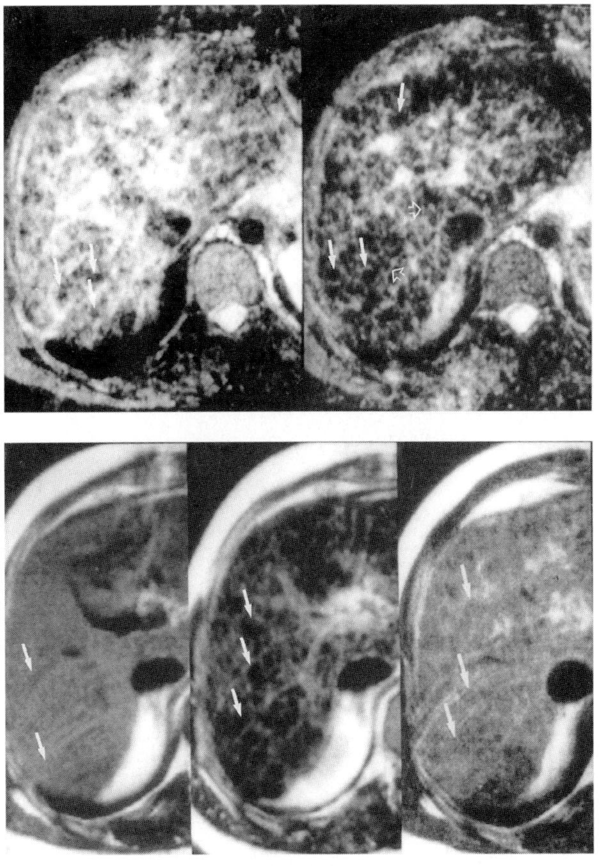

a,b

c,d,e

Fig. 7.13a–e. Acute stadium of Wilson's disease. **a** Proton-density weighted sequence (TR/TE=2000/45). Using unenhanced scans hypointense nodules (*arrows*) and high intensity septa (*open arrows*) are seen. **b** SPIO-enhanced MRI reveals hypointense nodules with loss of signal intensity (*arrows*). Detection rate has improved. **c** T1-weighted sequence (TR/TE=550/15). Documentation of hypointense nodules versus normal liver parenchyma (*arrows*) using unenhanced scans. **d** SPIO-enhanced images depict hypointense nodules (*arrows*). **e** Using Gd-DTPA enhanced MRI a positive enhancement of nodules (*arrows*) versus liver parenchyma is seen

crease in SPIO-enhanced signal (Figs. 7.16, 7.17). Lesions change from isointense to moderately hyperintense using T1-weighted images (Caseiro-Alvez et al. 1996; Oudkerk et al. 1997).

Hemangiomas are lesions with a markedly hyperintense signal intensity using unenhanced and SPIO-enhanced T2-weighted sequences. A hypointense intensity is documented for lesions on T1-weighted images with a change to hyperintensity post SPIO due to a T1 effect (Harisinghani et al. 1997).

Metastastic infiltrations document no significant loss of signal intensity on T2-weighted SPIO-en-

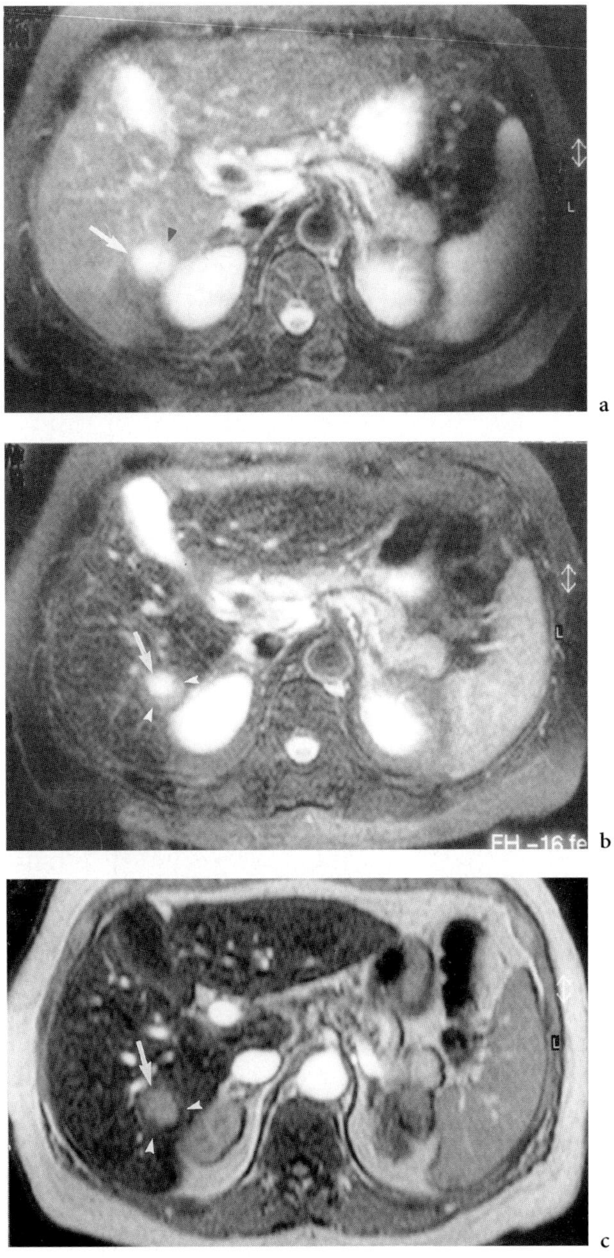

a

b

c

Fig. 7.14a–c. HCC in adenoma (nodule-in-nodule appearance). **a** A T2-weighted unenhanced fat suppressed turbospin echo sequence (TR/TE=2000/90) revealed a better demarcation of the hyperintense lesion compared to conventional scans (*arrow*). Delineation of an isointense signal intensity in the periphery (*black arrowhead*). **b** Using SPIO-enhanced T2-weighted fat suppressed turbospin echo sequence (TR/TE=2000/90), the lesion is seen with hyperintensities in the center (*arrow*) and isointense signal in the peripheral zone (*arrowhead*). A significant percentage signal intensity loss can be documented in the periphery. **c** T1-weighted gradient echo sequence (TR/TE/FA=30/5/30°), unenhanced. Documentation of a change of signal intensity postcontrast in the center to hyperintensity (*arrow*). The peripheral zone provides an uptake of contrast material with near isointensity compared to cirrhotic liver parenchyma (*arrowheads*)

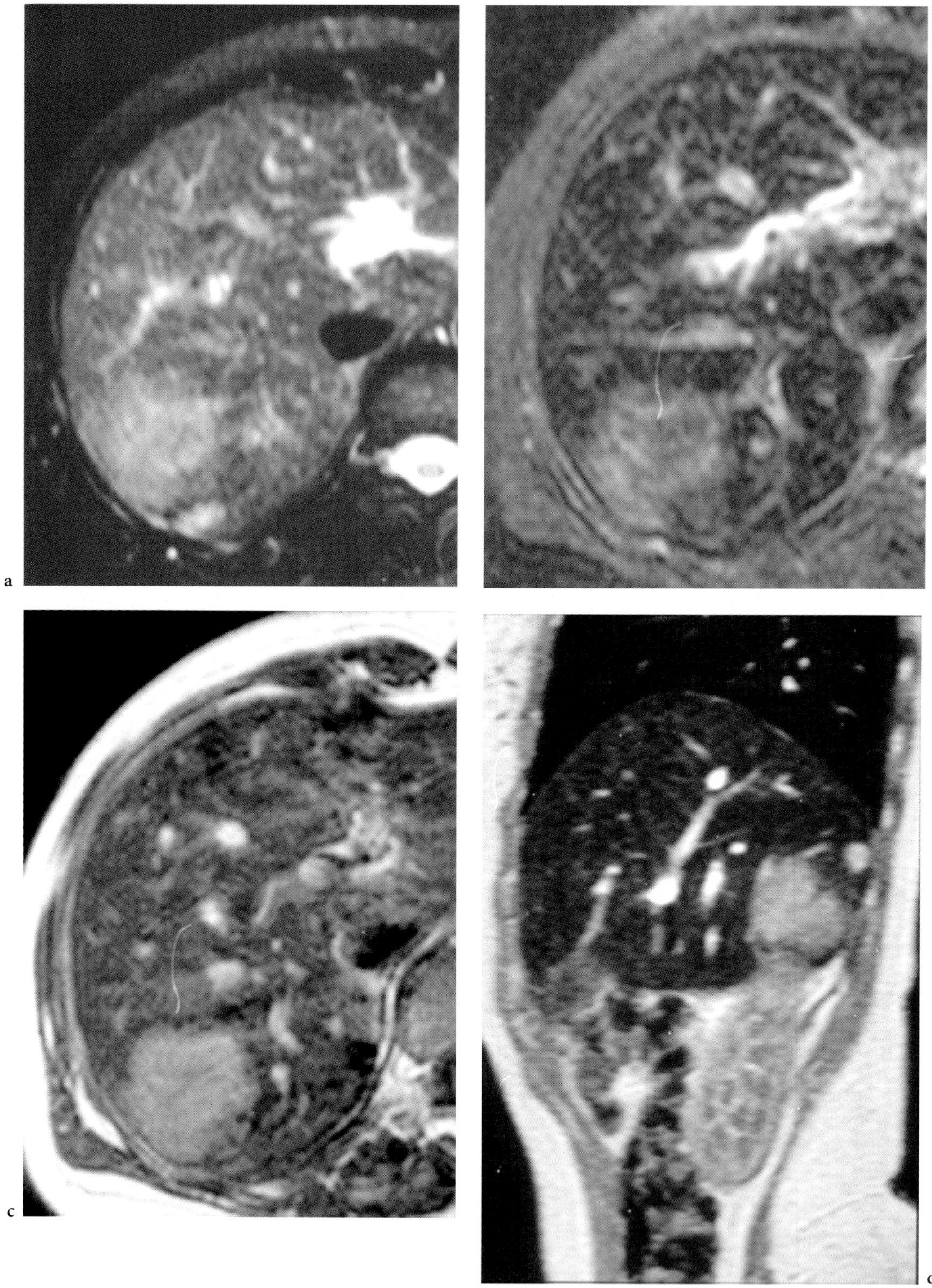

Fig. 7.15a–d. Multinodular adenoma. **a** In a female patient pre liver transplantation a hyperintense lesion in segment 7 of the liver is delineated using a T2-weighted fat saturated turbospin echo sequence. **b** Using a SPIO-enhanced T2w TSE-FS sequence, a moderate decrease of signal intensity of the lesion is documented. Significant signal loss of liver parenchyma. **c** In a T1w SE sequence a SPIO-enhanced hyperintense signal of the lesion is visualized due to a T1 effect. **d** Using a SPIO-enhanced T1w GRE sequence in a sagittal slice orientation a second lesion is depicted

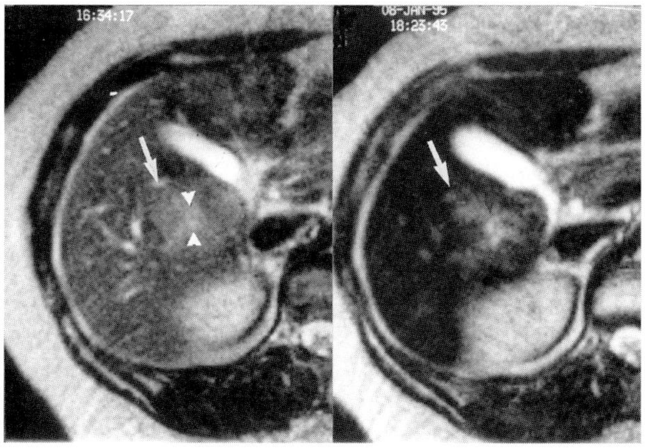

a,b

Fig. 7.16a,b. FNH. **a** In an unenhanced PDw sequence (TR/TE=2000/45), a hyperintense lesion (*arrow*) is visualized in the right liver lobe segment with an inhomogeneous margin to the surrounding liver parenchyma. Compression of the gallbladder with postprandial clinical symptoms. No delineation of capsule. Probable existence of central scar tissue (*arrowheads*). **b** After administration of SPIO a significant signal loss of the FNH nodule (*arrow*) and also of normal liver parenchyma is delineated. Documentation of a hyperintense unenhancing central scar (*arrowheads*). No additional nodules

hanced images (Bellin et al; 1994; Fretz et al. 1990; Hammerstingl et al. 1998; Marchal et al. 1989; Seneterre et al. 1996).

7.7.3.1 Discussion

The reticuloendothelial system with its Kupffer cells comprises only 2% of the liver volume, but its properties make it interesting for use as a vehicle for superparamagnetic coated iron oxide particles such as AMI-25 for contrast-enhanced MR imaging (Stark et al. 1988). Superparamagnetic iron oxides have been thoroughly investigated and produce a significant signal loss on T2-weighted images due to shortening of T2 relaxation time. The potential of these small crystalline ferrite particles as a tissue-specific contrast agent for liver and spleen and therefore in the diagnosis of liver tumors has been reported (Bellin et al. 1994; Vogl et al. 1997a). The specific uptake of intravenously administered SPIO particles by the reticuloendothelial system enables visualization of phagocyte activity throughout the liver and spleen. This is due to the significant signal loss in proton density-weighted and T2-weighted sequences. The quantitative evaluation of this phagocyte activity is not yet possible (Hamm et al. 1994).

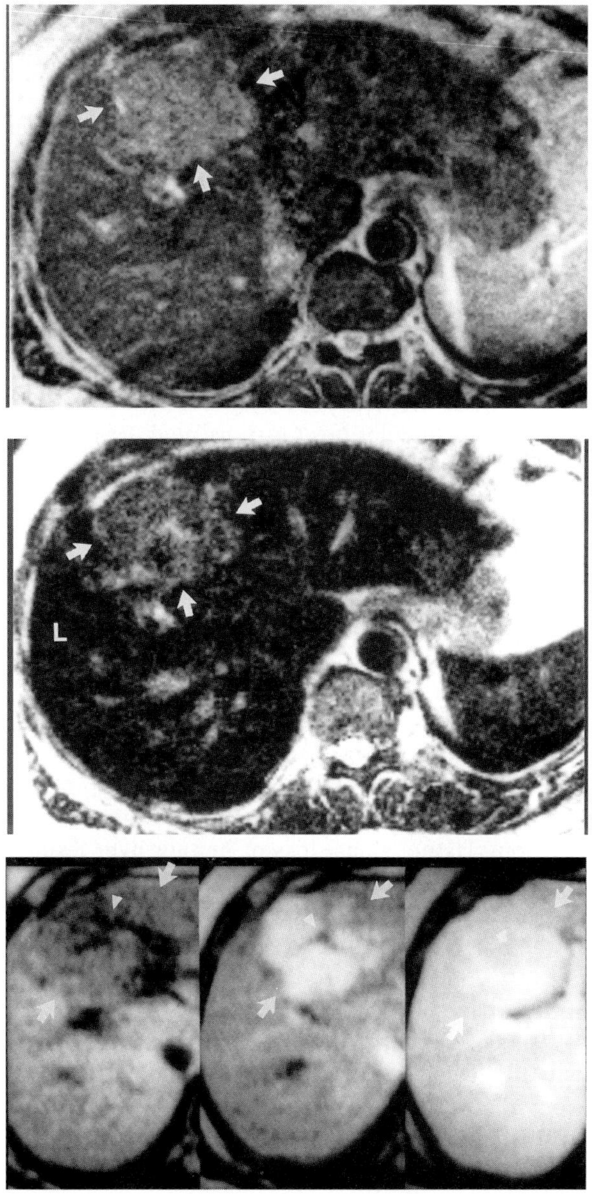

a b c

Fig. 7.17a–c. FNH. **a** T2-weighted sequence (TR/TE=2000/45), unenhanced. Demarcation of a hyperintense lesion in the right liver lobe segment 4 (*arrows*) versus normal liver parenchyma. No visualization of scar tissue or capsule, unenhanced. **b** SPIO-enhanced T2-weighted imaging shows a decrease in signal intensity of the lesion with moderate hyperintensity versus liver parenchyma (*arrows*). Documentation of a central scar (*arrowheads*).**c** T1-weighted GRE dynamic imaging (TR/TE/FA/TI=6.5/3/15°/350), unenhanced and during intravenous administration of gadolinium. **ca** Delineation of a hypointense (*arrows*) and central scar tissue (*arrowhead*) using unenhanced imaging. **cb** Hyperintense enhancement 15 s postintravenous injection of gadolinium (*arrows*). Documentation of hypointense scar tissue (*arrowhead*). **cc** Nearly isointense signal intensity of the lesion in the right liver lobe 5 min postintravenous injection of gadolinium (*arrows*). Enhancement of the central scar tissue (*arrowheads*)

SPIO-enhanced MR imaging has proven to be an effective imaging tool for the detection and differentiation of focal liver lesions (Denys et al. 1994; Fretz et al. 1990; Hammerstingl et al. 1997). Optimal imaging qualities can be achieved using a proton density and T2-weighted sequence in conventional and fat suppressed techniques. Significant signal loss of primary benign liver lesions (FNH, adenoma, hemangioma, and regenerating nodules) can be documented in these sequences (Kawamori et al. 1992). Additionally T1-weighted sequences have to be performed in order to detect and define lesion specific enhancement especially for the differential diagnosis of benign liver lesions (Scharf et al. 1998).

HCC usually cannot absorb these agents because Kupffer cells are lacking, but this is variable and depends on the grading of these tumors and on the presence of normal liver parenchyma within the tumor. Clinical studies demonstrated a significant but variable signal loss of well differentiated HCC. In undifferentiated HCC no contrast enhancement was delineated and the signal loss was similar to the pattern seen for the secondary metastatic process. Metastases also show a lack of reticuloendothelial cells and therefore no appreciable signal loss (Bellin et al. 1994; Fretz et al. 1990; Seneterre et al. 1996).

A long lasting signal loss of benign liver lesions after administration of SPIO was first described for hemangiomas by Hahn et al (1990), more recently for hemangioma and FNH by Denys et al (1994). This phenomenon is probably based on the uptake of iron oxide particles by macrophages or endothelial cells of the hemangioma. Hepatic lesions which contain phagocytes, such as FNH, adenoma, regenerating nodules, and some well-differentiated hepatocellular carcinomas, demonstrate signal loss, which is comparable in intensity to that of normal liver parenchyma.

Summing up, detection rate of focal liver lesions is increased using SPIO-enhanced sequences in comparison to unenhanced protocols (Hammerstingl et al. 1997). The detection of smallest lesions using iron oxide particle MR imaging might be limited in some cases. T2-weighted SE sequences demonstrated some limitations in the differentiation of small secondary lesions from intrahepatic vessel structures. Using fat-saturated sequences and fast T2-weighted GRE sequences may help to solve this problem. MR imaging during the early period of contrast agent administration could be a better option because of intrahepatic and intravascular signal loss due to circulating superparamagnetic particles (Hahn et al. 1990). Moreover, the use of T1-weighted SE sequences provides another alternative to solve the problem of the low signal of liver lesions.

7.7.4 USPIO-Enhanced MR Imaging of Hepatocellular Carcinoma

Ultrasmall superparamagnetic iron oxides (USPIO) are tissue-specific MR contrast agents with an increased T1 effect compared to SPIO. These dextran-coated particles have been used as blood-pool contrast agents due to their long half-life in blood. This relatively long half-life provides a wide imaging window during the intravascular phase. They are not immediately phagocytized by the reticuloendothelial system due to their small size. Perfusion phase and enhancement phase show an increased delay between both phases.

Intravascular contrast agents lead to improved lesion detection due to the larger blood volume of liver parenchyma and a comparatively smaller blood volume of solid tumors.

Imaging during the intravascular phase allows differentiation of vascularized lesions and other liver tumors/lesions due to their extent of vascularity. These agents can improve the lesion-to-liver contrast on T1-weighted imaging as positive enhancers. On T2-weighted imaging they act as negative enhancers. One such substance (AMI-227, Sinerem, Guerbet, France, Adv. M.) is in clinical phase III trials.

Mergo et al. (1996) stated a ring enhancement as a characteristic sign for malignancy using AMI-227 intravenously in patients with focal liver lesions. This attests to the significant blood-pool effects of USPIO particles. Harisinghani et al. (1977) documented a significantly lower degree of enhancement on T1-weighted images and of signal intensity drop on T2-weighted images in malignant liver masses compared to hemangiomas.

7.8 Summary

Various studies so far have documented the superiority of MRI for the diagnosis and differential diagnosis of the various patterns of hepatocellular carcinomas. Contrast enhanced studies could further improve the diagnosis of this oncologic disease. Nowadays MRI is considered to be superior to ultrasound, CT and even CTAP for the majority of clinical questions in liver cirrhosis and associated malignant liver disease (LENCIONI et al. 1996; UEDA et al. 1995; KANEMATSU et al. 1997). Our data and the experience of various groups favor the routine use of contrast agents to further improve the sensitivity and specificity of MRI. The diagnosis of focal hepatic lesion on MR imaging is improved concerning focal lesion detection and focal lesion characterization (DE SANTIS et al. 1992).

We strictly favor the use of negative contrast agents in all patients with underlying liver cirrhosis, fibrosis or postinterventional therapeutic strategies. Moreover, detection rate is increased using SPIO-enhanced MRI. It should therefore be used for the preoperative evaluation of patients with primary or secondary hepatic neoplasms.

In patients without known underlying liver disease, extracellular agents might be equal to hepatocellular agents with an improved characterization of lesions (various differential criteria for diagnostic imaging).

Further research is being currently directed towards the use of dynamic protocols and a more precise differential diagnosis of HCC nodules versus regenerating liver disease.

References

Bartolozzi C, Lencioni R, Caramella D, Paolicchi A, Russo R, Romani R (1994) The magnetic resonance and histological correlations in hepatocellular carcinoma. Radiol Med 87:90–95

Bellin M, Zaim S, Auberton E, et al (1994) Liver metastases: safety and efficacy of detection with superparamagnetic iron oxide in MR imaging. Radiology 193:657–663

Bernardino ME, Young SW, Lee JKT, et al (1992) Hepatic MR imaging with Mn-DPDP: safety, image quality, and sensitivity. Radiology 183:53–58

Blakeborough A, Ward J, Wilson D, et al (1997) Hepatic lesion detection at MR imaging: a comparative study with four sequences. Radiology 203:759–765

Brasch RC (1992) New directions in the development of MR imaging contrast media. Radiology 183:1–11

Caseiro Alves F, Zins M, Mahfouz AE, et al (1996) Calcification in focal nodular hyperplasia: a new problem for differentiation from fibrolamellar hepatocellular carcinoma. Radiology 198:889–892

Caudana R, Morasna G, Pirovano GP (1996) Focal malignant hepatic lesions: MR imaging enahnced with gadolinium benzyloxy-propionictetra-acetate (BOPTA) – preliminary results of phase II clinical application. Radiology 199:513–520

Choi BI, Lee GK, Kim ST, Han MC (1990) Mosaic pattern of encapsulated hepatocellular carcinoma: correlation of magnetic resonance imaging and pathology. Gastrointest Radiol 15:238–240

Corrigan K, Semelka RC (1995) Dynamic contrast-enhanced MR imaging of fibrolamellar hepatocellular carcinoma. Abdom Imaging 20:122–125

De Santis M, Romagnoli R, Cristani A, et al (1992) MRI of small hepatocellular carcinoma: comparison with US, CT, DSA, and Lipiodol-CT. J Comput Assist Tomogr 16:189–197

Denys A, Arrive L, Servois V, et al (1994) Hepatic tumors: detection and characterization at 1-T MR imaging enhanced with AMI-25. Radiology 193:665–669

Ebara M, Watanabe S, Kita K, et al (1991) MR imaging of small hepatocellular carcinoma: effect of intratumoral copper content on signal intensity. Radiology 180:617–621

Elizondo G, Fretz C, Stark DD, et al (1991) Preclinical evaluation of Mn-DPDP: new paramagnetic hepatobiliary contrast agent for MR imaging. Radiology 178:73–78

Fretz CJ, Stark DD, Metz CE, et al (1990) Detection of hepatic metastases: comparison of contrast-enhanced CT, unenhanced MR imaging, and iron oxide-enhanced MR imaging. AJR 155: 763-770

Hahn PF, Stark DD, Weissleder R, Elizondo G, Saini S, Ferrucci JT (1990) Clinical application of superparamagnetic iron oxide to MR imaging of tissue perfusion in vascular liver tumors. Radiology 174:361–366

Hamm B, Staks T, Taupitz M, et al (1994) Contrast-enhanced MR imaging of liver and spleen: first experience in humans with a new superparamagnetic iron oxide. JMRI 4: 659–668

Hamm B, Staks T, Muhler A (1995) Phase I clinical evaluation of Gd-EOB-DTPA as a hepatobiliary contrast agent: safety, pharmacokinetics, and MR imaging. Radiology 195:785–792

Hammerstingl R, Vogl ThJ, Schwarz W (1997) Detection and differential diagnosis of focal liver lesions: comparison of iron oxide-enhanced and gadolinium-enhanced MRI in the same patient. Results of a ROC analysis. Radiology 205(P):318-322

Hammerstingl R, Vogl ThJ, Schwarz W (1998) Contrast-enhanced MRI of focal liver lesions: differentiation and detection of primary and secondary liver lesions using Resovist-enhanced versus gadolinium-enhanced MRI in the same patient. Acta Radiol 5:75–79

Harisinghani M, Saini S, Weissleder R, et al (1997) Differentiation of liver hemangiomas from metastases and hepatocellular carcinomas at MR imaging enhanced with blood-pool contrast agent code-7227. Radiology 202:687–691

Hirai K, Aoki Y, Majima Y, et al (1991) Magnetic resonance imaging of small hepatocellular carcinoma. Am J Gastroenterol 86:205-210

Honda H, Kaneko K, Kanazawa Y, et al (1997) MR imaging of hepatocellular carcinomas: effect of Cu and Fe contents on signal intensity. Abdom Imaging 22:60–66

Ichikawa T, Haradome H, Hachiya J, Nitatori T, Araki T (1998) Diffusion-weighted MR imaging with a single-shot echoplanar sequence: detection and characterization of focal hepatic lesions. AJR 170:397–402

Imaeda T, Kanematsu M, Mochizuki R, Goto H, Saji S, Shimokawa K (1994) Extracapsular invasion of small hepatocellular carcinoma: MR and CT findings. J Comput Assist Tomogr 18:755–760

Inoue E, Kuroda C, Fujita M, et al (1993) MR features of various histological grades of small hepatocellular carcinoma. J Comput Assist Tomogr 17:75–79

Itai Y, Ohtomo K, Furui S, Minami M, Yoshikawa K, Yashiro N (1986) MR imaging of hepatocellular carcinoma. J Comput Assist Tomogr 10:963–968

Itoh K, Nishimura K, Togashi K, et al (1987) Hepatocellular carcinoma: MR imaging. Radiology 164:21–25

Kanematsu M, Hoshi H, Murakami T, et al (1997) Detection of hepatocellular carcinoma in patients with cirrhosis: MR imaging versus angiographically assisted helical CT. AJR 169:1507–1515

Kawamori Y, Matsui O, Kadoya M, Yoshikawa J, Demachi H, Takashima T (1992) Differentiation of hepatocellular carcinomas from hyperplastic nodules induced in rat liver with ferrite-enhanced MR imaging. Radiology 183:65–72

Kelekis NL, Semelka RC, Worawattanakul S, et al (1998) Hepatocellular carcinoma in North America: a multiinstitutional study of appearance on T1-weighted, T2-weighted, and serial gadolinium-enhanced gradient-echo images. AJR 170:1005–1009

Kim T, Murakami T, Oi H, et al (1995) Detection of hypervascular hepatocellular carcinoma by dynamic MRI and dynamic spiral CT. J Comput Assist Tomogr 19:948–954

Kitagawa K, Matsui O, Kadoya M, et al (1991) Hepatocellular carcinomas with excessive copper accumulation: CT and MR findings. Radiology 180:623–628

Kopp AF, Laniado M, Dammann F, et al (1997) MR imaging of the liver with Resovist: safety, efficacy, and pharmocaodynamic properties. Radiology 204:749–756

Lencioni R, Mascalchi M, Caramella D, Bartolozzi C (1996) Small hepatocellular carcinoma: differentiation from adenomatous hyperplasia with color Doppler US and dynamic Gd-DTPA-enhanced MR imaging. Abdom Imaging 21:41–48

Liou J, Lee JK, Borrello JA, Brown JJ (1994) Differentiation of hepatomas from nonhepatomatous masses: use of MnDPDP-enhanced MR images. Magn Reson Imaging 12:71–79

Mahfouz AE, Hamm B, Taupitz M (1993a) Hypervascular liver lesions: differentiation of focal nodular hyperplasia from malignant tumors with dynamic gadolinium-enhanced MR imaging. Radiology 186:133–138

Mahfouz AE, Hamm B, Wolf KJ (1993b) Dynamic gadopenteteate dimeglumine-enhanced MR imaging of hepatocellular carcinoma. Eur Radiol 3:453–458

Mahfouz AE, Hamm B, Wolf KJ (1994) Peripheral washout: a sign of malignancy on dynamic gadolinium-enhanced MR images of focal liver lesions. Radiology 190:49–52

Marchal G, Van HP, Demaerel P, et al (1989) Detection of liver metastases with superparamagnetic iron oxide in 15 patients: results of MR imaging at 1.5 T. AJR 152:771–775.

Marchal G, Zhang X, Ni Y, Hecke PVan, Yu J, Baert AL (1993) Comparison between Gd-DTPA, Gd-EOB-DTPA, and Mn-DPDP in induced HCC in rats: a correlation study of MR imaging, microangiography, and histology. Magn Reson Imaging 11:665–674

Martin J, Sentis M, Zidan A, et al (1995) Fatty metamorphosis of hepatocellular carcinoma: detection with chemical shift gradient-echo MR imaging. Radiology 195:125–130

Matsuzaki K, Sano N, Hashiguchi N, Yoshida S, Nishitani H (1997) Influence of copper on MRI of hepatocellular carcinoma. JMRI 7(3):478–481

Mergo P, Helmberger T, Nicolas A, et al (1996) Ring enhanement in ultrasmall superparamagnetic iron oxide MR imaging: a potential new sign for characterization of liver lesions. AJR 166:379–384

Mitchell DG, Palazzo J, Hann HW, Rifkin MD, Burk DL, Rubin R (1991) Hepatocellular tumors with high signal on T1-weighted MR images: chemical shift MR imaging and histologic correlation. J Comput Assist Tomogr 15:762–769

Murakami T, Baron RL, Peterson MS (1996) Hepatocellular carcinoma: MR imaging with Mangafodipir Trisodium (Mn-DPDP). Radiology 200:69–77

Muramatsu Y, Nawano S, Takayasu K, et al (1991) Early hepatocellular carcinoma: MR imaging. Radiology 181:209–213

Muramatsu M, Takayasu K, Furukawa Y, et al (1997) Hepatic tumor invasion of bile ducts: Wedge-shaped sign on MR images. Radiology 205:81–85

Ni Y, Marchal G, Yu J, et al (1993) Experimental liver cancers: Mn-DPDP-enhanced rims in MR-microangiographic-histologic correlation study. Radiology 188:45–51

Ohtomo K, Matsuoka Y, Abe O, et al (1997) High-resolution MR imaging evaluation of hepatocellular carcinoma. Abdom Imaging 22:182–186

Oudkerk M, Heuvel AG, Wielopolski P, et al (1997) Hepatic lesions: detection with ferumoxide-enhanced T1-weighted MR imaging. Radiology 203:449–456

Peterson MS, Baron RL, Murakami T (1996) Hepatic malignancies: usefulness of acquisition of multiple arterial and portal venous phase images at dynamic gadolinium-enhanced MR imaging. Radiology 201:337–345

Reimer P, Rummeny EJ, Daldrup HE, et al (1995) Clinical results with Resovist: a phase 2 clinical trial. Radiology 195:489–496

Reimer P, Rummeny EJ, Shamsi K, et al (1996) Clinical results with Gd-EOB-DTPA: dose finding, safety aspects, and pulse sequences evaluation within a hase II trial. Radiology 199:177–183

Reimer P, Rummeny EJ, Daldrup HE, et al (1997) Enhancement characteristic of liver metastases, hepatocellular carcinomas, and hemangiomas with Gd-EOB-DTPA: preliminary results with dynamic MR imaging. Eur Radiol 7:275–280

Rocklage SM, Worah D, Kim SH (1991) Metal ion release from paramagnetic chelates: what is tolerable? Magn Reson Med 11:509–519

Rofsky NM, Weinreb JC, Bernardino ME, et al (1993) Hepatocellular Tumors: characterization with Mn-DPDP-enhanced MR imaging. Radiology 188:53–59

Rummeny E, Saini S, Wittenberg J, et al. (1989a) MR imaging of liver neoplasms. AJR 152:493–499

Rummeny E, Weissleder R, Sironi S, Stark DD, et al (1989b) Central scars in primary liver tumors: MR features, specificity, and pathologic correlation. Radiology 171:323–326

Rummeny E, Weissleder R, Stark DD, Saini S, et al (1989c) Primary liver tumors: diagnosis by MR imaging. AJR 152:63–72

Sadek AG, Mitchell DG, Siegelman ES, Outwater EK, Matteucci T, Hann HW (1995) Early hepatocellular carcinoma that develops within macroregenerative nodules: growth rate depicted at serial MR imaging. Radiology 195:753–756

Scharf J, Hoffmann V, Lehnert T, et al (1998) Pseudolesions at T1-weighted gradient-echo imaging after administration of superparamagnetic iron oxide: comparison with portal perfusion abnormalities at CT during arterial portography. Radiology 207:67–72

Seneterre E, Taourel, Bouvier Y, et al (1996) Detection of hepatic metastases: ferrumoxides-enhanced MR imaging versus unenhanced MR imaging and CT during arterial portography. Radiology 200:785–792

Shamsi K, Balzer T, Saini S, et al (1998): Superparamagnetic iron oxide particles (SHU 555 A): evaluation of efficacy in three doses for hepatic MR imaging. Radiology 206:365–371

Stark DD, Weissleder R, Elizondo G, et al (1988) Superparamagnetic iron oxide: clinical applicaation as a contrast agent for MR imaging of the liver. Radiology 168:297–301

Titelbaum DS, Burke DR, Meranze SG, Saul SH (1988) Fibrolamellar hepatocellular carcinoma: pitfalls in nonoperative diagnosis. Radiology 167:25–30

Tweedle MF (1997) The ProHance story: the making of a novel MRI contrast agent. Eur Radiol 7:225–230

Ueda K, Kitagawa K, Kadoya M, Matsui O, Takashima T, Yamahana T (1995) Detection of hypervascular hepatocellular carcinoma by using spiral volumetric CT: comparison of US and MR imaging. Abdom Imaging 20:547–553

van Beers BE, Grandin C, Pauwels S, et al (1994) Gd-EOB-DTPA enhancement pattern of hepatocellular carcinomas in rats: comparison with Tc-99m-IDA uptake. JMRI 4:351–354

Vogl ThJ, Pegios W, McMahon C, et al (1992) Gadobenate dimeglumine – a new contrast agent for MR imaging: preliminary evaluation in healthy volunteers. AJR 158:887

Vogl ThJ, Hamm B, Schnell B, et al (1993) Mn-DPDP enhancement patterns of hepatocellular lesions on MR images. JMRI 3:51-56

Vogl ThJ, Hammerstingl R, Schwarz W (1996a) Magnetic resonance iamging of focal liver lesions. Comparison of the superparamagnetic iron oxide Resovist versus Gadolinium-DTPA in the same patient. Investigative Radiology 31:696–708

Vogl ThJ, Kümmel S, Hammerstingl R, et al (1996b) Liver tumors: comparison of MR imaging with Gd-EOB-DTPA and Gd-DTPA. Radiology 200:59-63

Vogl TJ, Hammerstingl R, Schwarz W (1996c) Superparamagnetic iron oxide-enhanced versus gadolinium-enhanced MR imaging for differential diagnosis of focal liver lesions. Radiology 198:881–887

Vogl ThJ, Hammerstingl R, Schwarz W (1997a) Iron oxide-enhanced MR imaging of focal liver lesions: clinical single center outcome study in 700 patients. Radiology 205(P):457-452

Vogl ThJ, Schwarz W, Hammerstingl R (1997b) Dynamic and static SPIO-enhanced MR imaging in focal liver lesions. Radiology 205(P):456-461

Vogl ThJ, Stupavsky A, Pegios W, Hammerstingl R (1997c) Hepatocellular carcinoma: Evaluation with dynamic and static gadobenate dimeglumine-enhanced MR imaging and histopathologic correlation. Radiology 205:721–728

Weinmann MJ, Brasch RC, Press WR, et al (1984) Characteristics of gadolinium-DTPA complex: a potential NMR contrast agent. AJR 142:619–624

Weissleder R (1994) Liver MR imaging with iron oxides: toward consensus and clinical practice. Radiology 193:593–595

Winter TCr, Takayasu K, Muramatsu Y, et al (1994) Early advanced hepatocellular carcinoma: evaluation of CT and MR appearance with pathologic correlation. Radiology 192:379–387

Yamamoto H, Yamashita Y, Yoshimatsu S, et al (1995) Hepatocellular carcinoma in cirrhotic livers: detection with unenhanced and iron oxide-enhanced MR imaging. Radiology 195:106–112

Yamashita Y, Fan ZM, Yamamoto H, et al (1993) Sclerosing hepatocellular carcinoma: radiologic findings. Abdom Imaging 18:347–351

Yamashita Y, Fan ZM, Yamamoto H, et al (1994) Spin-echo and dynamic gadolinium-enhanced FLASH MR imaging of hepatocellular carcinoma: correlation with histopathologic findings. JMRI 4:83–90

Yamashita Y, Mitsuzaki K, Yi T, et al (1996) Small hepatocellular carcinoma in patients with chronic liver damage: prospective comparison of detection with dynamic MR imaging and helical CT of the whole liver. Radiology 200:79–84

8 Angiography and Angiographically Assisted Techniques

C. FAVA, M. GROSSO, and A. VELTRI

CONTENTS

8.1 Introduction

The past few years have witnessed a spectacular increase in the options for studying the hepatic and portal vessels, in part because of the introduction of new techniques and in part due to advances in techniques already in use. This chapter will illustrate the invasive methods for studying the hepatic vessels based on the equipment used for registering the image, such as the angiography unit (conventional angiography), sonography (sonographic angiography), and computed tomography (CT) (CT during arterial portography and Lipiodol CT). In this context, the role of traditional angiography has changed, losing its previous diagnostic leadership to some of the newer techniques (and their various associations).

C. FAVA, MD; Professor, Department of Radiological Sciences, University of Turin, Via Genova 3, I-10126 Turin, Italy
M. GROSSO, MD; Department of Radiological Sciences, University of Turin, Via Genova 3, I-10126 Turin, Italy
A. VELTRI, MD; Department of Radiological Sciences, University of Turin, Via Genova 3, I-10126 Turin, Italy

However, since percutaneous arterial catheterism is the basis for all these techniques, the execution of various examinations in association with each other during a single diagnostic imaging session has become the rule in centers where hepatocellular carcinoma (HCC) is studied and treated.

Whereas the techniques based on segmentation using CT or US do not require a particularly selective catheterization, arteriographic studies using hydrosoluble contrast agents require greater skill on the part of the operator, with execution of superselective catheterizations (sometimes with coaxial techniques) or else simultaneous arterial and venous accesses. This type of approach is currently associated with (or preceding) a therapeutic procedure performed through the catheter. Although the procedures described are usually performed in association (and frequently, it should be remembered, in a single session), the techniques and their results will be first addressed individually and, subsequently, the value of their various associations in reference to the defined goals (both diagnostic and/or therapeutic) will be examined.

8.2 Angiography

The role angiography plays in the diagnosis of HCC has undergone considerable changes related, on one hand, to the evolution of the technique itself and angiographic materials, and, on the other hand, to the development of competing methods. Since the second half of the 1970s, in fact, the introduction and progressive growth of sonography and CT has gradually reduced the diagnostic role of angiography, and further competition has occurred with the subsequent growth of magnetic resonance imaging (MRI). Further competition has subsequently been developed in techniques based on arterial catheterism and injection of contrast media, but employing contrast agents other than iodated ones and different methods of image extraction (US, CT).

However, the terrain which angiography has lost in its diagnostic role has been amply compensated by what has been gained in its therapeutic role due to the transcatheter treatment techniques developed since the 1980s, so that today the diagnostic angiographic study constitutes the preliminary phase of a therapeutic plan aimed, more or less directly, at treating the neoplasm.

This different goal has, in any case, emphasized the importance of the technical aspect of arterial catheterization, which, in turn, has become less important in the angiographic-type methods competing on the diagnostic level (sonographic angiography using CO_2 microbubbles, CT arterial portography, Lipiodol CT).

8.2.1 Equipment and Technique

Technical advancements in the equipment have greatly influenced the evolution of angiographic techniques. Currently, angiographic examinations are exclusively performed using digital equipment, characterized by rather modest spatial resolution (particularly when the images are photographed on radiographic film) but high contrast resolution. These characteristics allow for a high sensitivity in demonstrating the capillary phase opacification and, in more general terms, the overall parenchymal opacification of the entire organ. The ideal equipment has a large format (14") intensifier and a 512×512 matrix (or, even better, 1024×1024) with a generator power of 100 kW. This qualitative standard is available in most angiographic suites. The employment of digital equipment permits use of modest flow rates for the contrast agent and, therefore, the possibility of using fine caliber catheters (4–5F) and, sometimes, coaxial systems.

A complete vascular study of the liver requires catheterization of the celiac axis and its branches as well as the superior mesenteric artery due to the frequent presence (20% of cases) of an accessory branch to the right hepatic lobe originating from the superior mesenteric artery, requiring its systematic opacification. On the other hand, the direct origin from the aorta of a branch of the hepatic artery is exceptional (Lamarque 1974).

The arterial study is naturally completed with the opacification of the venous vessels of the portal circulation, which occurs during the late phase after injection of the superior mesenteric artery, the celiac axis, or the splenic artery. To obtain good quality images, it is important during digital subtraction angiography (DSA) to maintain a good mask for the entire period of image acquisition. It is therefore indispensable that the patient maintains a good apnea and receives adequate instructions to this end (as well as be informed on the importance of his collaboration). Some authors recommend administration of oxygen to the patient (Ikeda et al. 1994). In this way, even patients in a precarious condition are able to maintain the 20 s of apnea necessary to acquire good images of the spleno-portal (or mesentero-portal) axis. In our experience, even a simple hyperventilation (60–120 s) immediately performed before the injection can significantly influence the possibility of maintaining the apnea.

With injection of the contrast agent into the superior mesenteric artery, the venous return can be enhanced by employing a vasodilator (Venitrin or similar nitrates). Many authors also recommend the use of drugs with an antispastic action (Buscopan) in order to eliminate or reduce the effects of peristalsis on image subtraction.

A complete angiographic study of the liver should, therefore, be articulated by means of the following selective studies:

- Superior mesenteric artery (injection of 20–25 ml of contrast at 4–5 ml/s): in order to evaluate the presence of the above mentioned anatomic variant and to obtain visualization of the mesenteric venous bed and, therefore, the portal vein with its intrahepatic portal branches.
- Celiac axis (25–30 ml of contrast agent at 5–6 ml/s): in order to demonstrate the distribution of the hepatic vessels as well as anatomic variations in their origin; in particular, this study permits documentation of the eventual presence of branches supplying the left lobe segment (predominantly segments II and III) originating from the left gastric artery (Lamarque 1974); during the venous return phase, the splenic vein is visible as well as the portal vein and its intraparenchymal branches, in normal conditions; in pathologic situations, frequently found in the population of patients made up of cirrhotic patients with portal hypertension, the anatomical and flow-related alterations are evident.
- Splenic artery (25–30 ml of contrast agent at 5–6 ml/s): selective catheterization of this vessel is performed when the venous return after injection of the celiac axis does not determine an adequate opacification of the spleno-portal axis or whenever it is desirable to evaluate the portal circula-

tion exclusively, with opacification only of the portal circulation without an arterial hepatic parenchymal phase (in alternative to mesenteric venous return).

- Common or proper hepatic artery (8–12 ml of contrast agent at 2–3 ml/s; many authors recommend greater quantity of contrast media, up to 20 ml), with the goal of demonstrating the arterial alterations of the hepatic parenchyma with greater enhancement and in the absence of superimposition of the venous return; in order to achieve this, it is advisable to maintain low injection rates (<3 ml/s) even if it is necessary to inject a greater total quantity of contrast agent.

The selective study of the common or proper hepatic artery is frequently followed by superselective studies particularly if a transcatheter treatment is planned. Injections using progressively lesser amounts of contrast media at a low flow rate (<1 ml/s) are performed, even manually. Selective catheterization is a very variable technique, depending on both the operator's experience and the patient's anatomical configuration.

Our group has developed a simple method, which allows a complete arterial evaluation in 90% of patients: a flexible 5F Shepherd hook type catheter (Boston Scientific, Watertown, MA) is advanced into the abdominal aorta and selective injections of the celiac axis and superior mesenteric artery are then performed; next, superselective studies of the celiac axis are performed by catheterizing both the splenic and hepatic arteries using a 0.35- or 0.38-caliber hydrophilic guidewire (Terumo, Japan), whose curved tip allows for easier guidability; once the guidewire has been advanced deep inside the vessel, the catheter is advanced over it; the minimal friction of the guidewire along with the good degree of rigidity allows for considerable selective advancement of the catheter along the vessel to be examined.

The same procedure can be utilized for superselective study of the superior mesenteric artery (particularly important when a hepatic branch originates from it). It is therefore possible to greatly reduce the examination time by using a single catheter for a complete angiographic study of the hepato-spleno-mesenteric arterial area.

In certain anatomical conditions (in particular, in longilineal subjects whose mesenteric artery and celiac axis originate at an acute angle), it may necessary to employ some of the other catheters, such as Simmonds II and III. With an acute angle it may not always be possible to advance the guidewire into the vessel's secondary branches or even to pass the catheter into the vessel.

In relatively recent times, variations in technique have been proposed (above all by Japanese authors) designed to improve the sensitivity of angiography in detecting or in revealing afferent and efferent vessels. Takahashi et al. (1990) prefers two successive injections in the celiac axis, separated by 25 s, acquiring the images only during the second injection. In this fashion, the mask comprises a portal parenchymal phase (due to the first injection) with the aim of increasing the sensitivity. With this technique, called hepatoportal subtraction angiography, the sensitivity increases to 92% (in comparison to 71% for conventional DSA, 42% for US, 39% for conventional CT, and 90% for Lipiodol CT in the same patients).

Kanazawa et al. (1995) subsequently proposed occlusion of the hepatic veins draining the portion of the hepatic parenchyma containing the nodule by using a catheter for venous occlusion. With this procedure, the number of venous collecting vessels opacified is increased as well as the intensity of capillary blush within the lesion. Rather than increasing the amount of diagnostic information available, the authors use this method in order the improve the therapeutic results during transcatheter treatment.

8.2.2 Radiologic Findings

The images obtained by the angiographic examination are directly dependent on the pathological characteristics of the lesion undergoing study. The most significant angiographic characteristic of HCC is the hypervascularization of the lesion, which can be identified with greatest clarity in the capillary phase, during which a more intense accumulation of contrast medium inside the lesion differentiates it from the surrounding parenchyma (tumor stain). This accumulation is not constant, being more apparent in approximately 80% of the nodular forms (Kido et al. 1971; Sumida et al. 1986). The size of the node can influence the angiographic findings in that in small HCC, as Ikeda points out, an evident capillary hypervascularization is present in 73.7% of nodes measuring from 16 mm to 20 mm and in 59.2% of nodules measuring <15 mm (Ikeda et al. 1994).

The two forms usually considered, the nodular type (single or multiple nodules, encapsulated) and the infiltrative type, are translated into characteristic and distinct angiographic patterns (Sumida et al. 1986).

The nodular lesion (Figs. 8.1–8.3) is characterized, in the arterial phase of the angiographic study, by a very rich tumor vascularization with a tree-branch pattern or, in contrast, by an artery of increased caliber supplying it (KIDO et al. 1971). The presence of neovasculature is very characteristic in the nodular forms and is found in 95% of cases (ROVERSI 1989) being found also in lesions which do not have a significant tumor stain. The dilatation of the artery supplying the neovasculature is also a constant finding, and demonstrable even in eventual satellite nodules.

During the arteriolo-capillary and capillary phase (generally 15–20 s after the start of injection) the above cited tumor stain becomes apparent. This finding can be angiographically demonstrated with DSA in, at the most, 80% of cases and with

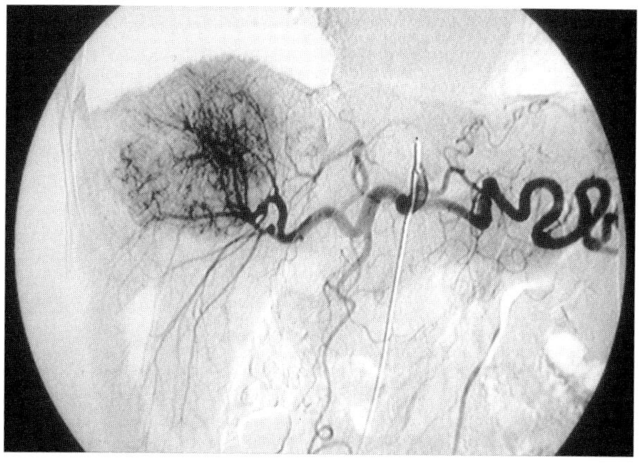

a

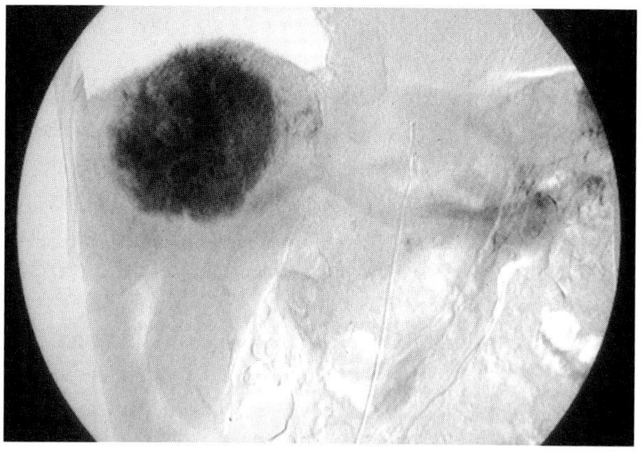

b

Fig. 8.1a,b. Angiographic study of the nodular form of HCC. **a** Arterial and arteriolar phases: characteristic tree-branching pattern of the nodule's afferent arterioles, with dilatation of the tributary arterial branch. **b** Tumor stain, intense even if not very homogeneous (as typically found in voluminous nodules, subject to necrosis). The nodule (accompanied by a small satellite lesion) is clearly delimitated, as usually seen in encapsulated tumors

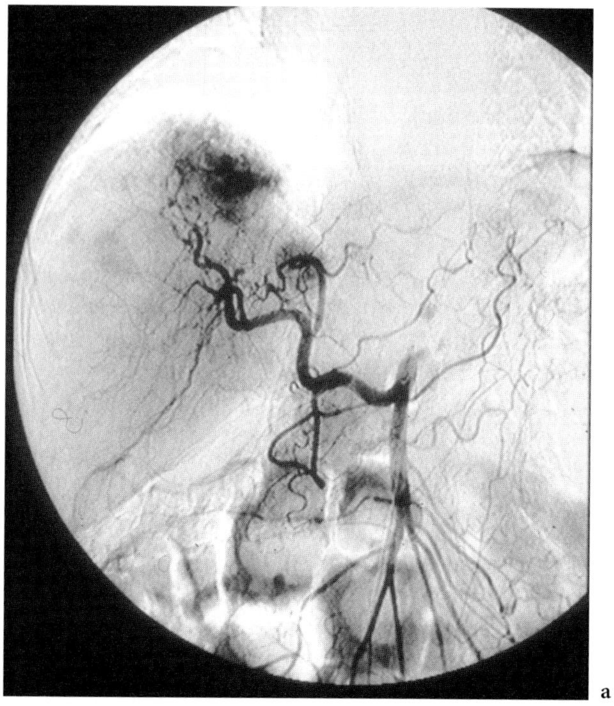

a

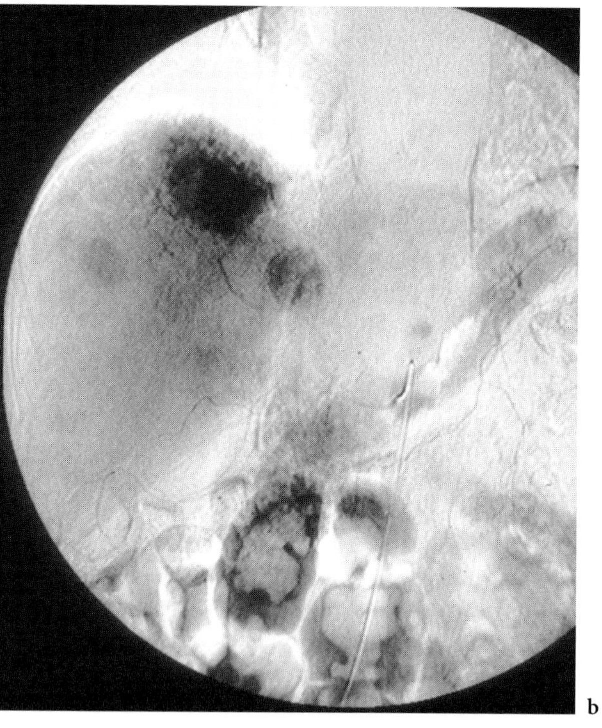

b

Fig. 8.2a,b. Extensive multifocal HCC in both hepatic lobes. a Arterial phase: ectasia of the tributary vessels supplying the large sized nodules. Anatomical variations of vascularization are frequently found: the origin of an hepatic vessel from the superior mesenteric artery (in this case, not frequent, all the liver is supplied by the mesenteric artery, from which the gastroduodenal artery also originates). **b** A tumor stain of discrete intensity is seen in all the nodules, which appear well delimitated greater difficulty in small sized nodules (IKEDA et al. 1994).

Prognostically, the absence of an angiographically demonstrable tumor stain is considered a negative factor. Probably, the absence of tumor stain is due, in most cases, other than its lightness, to the difficulty in differentiating the focal hyperaccumulation from the background inhomogeneity frequently found in cirrhotic livers. This seems confirmed by the observation that some nodules (IKEDA et al. 1994) not demonstrated angiographically can be detected with other imaging methods (carbon dioxide enhanced ultrasonography) also based on demonstration of the vessels (71.2% vs 59.2% of sensitivity in demonstrating nodules <2 cm).

Further confirmation can be found in the results reported by TAKAHASHI et al. regarding the technique proposed by his group, called hepatoportal subtraction angiography, which presumes elimination of the inhomogeneity of the parenchymal hepatogram. With this procedure, even though a less selective catheterization was used in comparison to traditional hepatic DSA (celiac axis, common or proper hepatic artery), in a series of 84 hepatomas the sensitivity increased from 71% to 92% ($P<0.002$). Furthermore, as pointed out above, the tumor stain can be enhanced by altering the hemodynamic conditions employing sectorial occlusion of the drainage system (KANAZAWA et al. 1995), a rather complex procedure which is justified only by the utility of the subsequent phase of therapy via the catheter.

In the diffuse form (Fig. 8.4), the degree of hypervascularization is usually minor. Dilatation of the afferent vessels is generally not present and the tumor stain can be demonstrated with less frequency and intensity (SUMIDA et al. 1986). In contrast to the nodular form, the delimitation of the mass appears indistinct and, usually, the capillary phase of enhancement is fleeting.

With both forms (nodular and diffuse), additional angiographic signs can be found in a high percentage of cases:

- The presence of a shunt between the neoplastic arterial bed and the venous system
- The presence of neoplastic thrombi in the portal system

The arterio-venous shunts (usually arterio-portal) are present in a percentage of cases, which is very variable in the reported literature. The presence of small shunts with the peritumoral venules should be considered distinct from important hemodynamic findings of reflux portal filling (Fig. 8.4). This last finding has been reported by ROVERSI (1989) to be

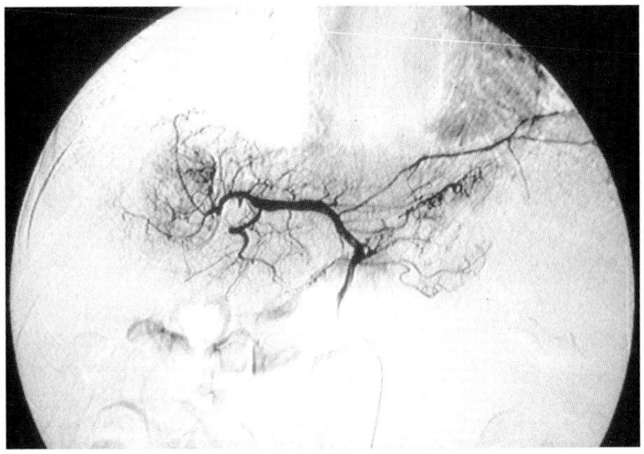

Fig. 8.3. Voluminous HCC in the IV hepatic segment. Another frequent anatomic variant is seen: the origin of the hepatic vessels supplying the left lobe from the left gastric artery. In the case shown, the entire left lobe is supplied by this artery

present in about 10% of cases of HCC, while the small perilesional fistulas, probably present in all cases, are angiographically demonstrable in two-thirds of cases (OKUDA et al. 1977). The arterio-venous fistulas, believed by some to be pathognomonic of HCC, are actually present in other pathologies: cavernous hemangiomas, regenerative nodules, sequels of intervention on the parenchyma, and cirrhosis (ROVERSI 1989). Angiography still represents today the most sensitive method for demonstrating arterio-venous fistulas.

Neoplastic thrombi are present in various case studies in percentages as high as 33% (SUBRAMANYAN et al. 1984). The alteration is due to the progressive colonization of the portal vein by a mass of neoplastic tissue which finds, in the vessel wall, a kind of capsule. The mass has an arterial type vascularization, and the vessels which supply it are often visible during contrast injection of the proper hepatic artery, giving the finding of a typical appearance (thread and streak sign). According to some authors, this finding (portal thrombosis associated with thread and streak sign) is pathognomonic of HCC, without any demonstrated false positives (OKUDA et al. 1977). It occurs both in the nodular form and in the diffuse form (even if it is more frequent in the former).

8.2.3 Current Role of Angiography

In studies conducted with pathological correlation, angiography has a modest sensitivity in revealing

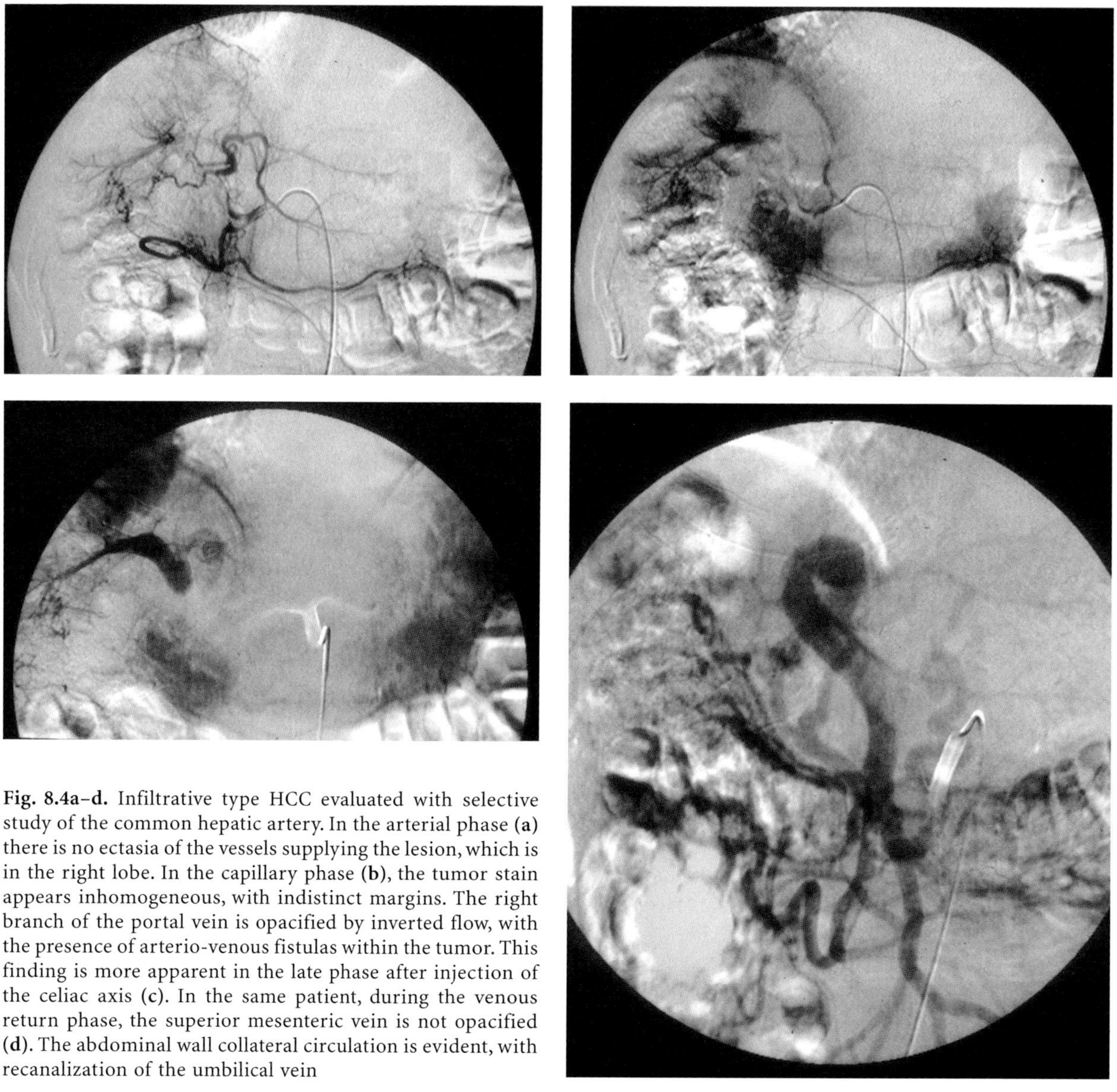

a b c d

Fig. 8.4a–d. Infiltrative type HCC evaluated with selective study of the common hepatic artery. In the arterial phase (**a**) there is no ectasia of the vessels supplying the lesion, which is in the right lobe. In the capillary phase (**b**), the tumor stain appears inhomogeneous, with indistinct margins. The right branch of the portal vein is opacified by inverted flow, with the presence of arterio-venous fistulas within the tumor. This finding is more apparent in the late phase after injection of the celiac axis (**c**). In the same patient, during the venous return phase, the superior mesenteric vein is not opacified (**d**). The abdominal wall collateral circulation is evident, with recanalization of the umbilical vein

HCC nodules, which does not reach 60% in detecting lesions less than 2 cm in diameter (Ikeda et al. 1994), attributable to the frequent absence of hypervascularization (which is the only concrete positive sign for this method). Even in typification, the value of angiography is limited. The focal lesions to take into consideration in the differential diagnosis are cavernous hemangioma, regenerative nodule, focal nodular hyperplasia, adenoma (all benign lesions), as well as cholangiocarcinoma and metastases.

In comparison to other non-invasive techniques (US, CT, and MRI), angiography does not offer superior elements regarding lesion typification, even if it frequently provides some particular types of information (characteristic disposition of the vessels in hemangioma; stellate aspect of the nodule in focal nodular hyperplasia; intense and early blush, without any dishomogeneities, in adenoma) tied to the type of image extraction furnished by the method.

With the exception of regenerative nodule in cirrhosis, for which the ability of angiography to formulate a diagnosis is modest, the diagnostic accuracy of the method reflects the values of noninvasive imaging techniques.

The method offers some advantages in differentiating cavernous hemangioma, where the diagnostic accuracy is close to 100% (Roversi 1989). In cases which are still equivocal after non-invasive studies have been performed, angiography is justified, above all in cirrhotic patients.

Therefore, more than for the detection of lesions and their differential diagnosis, the utility of angiography should be looked for in its other capabilities:

- Furnishing information on the vascular (and pathological) anatomy
- Providing the background information for a possible transcatheter treatment

Regarding the anatomical information, the method is still the most precise instrument for providing a vascular map of the liver, both arterial and venous. On the arterial side, the examination is useful for demonstrating the presence of possible anatomical variants, whose knowledge is essential in planned transcatheter treatment. The angiographic study is also very effective in showing the morphology of the portal circulation and the rheological alteration of the venous bed, due to arterio-venous fistulas, neoplastic thrombosis or possible cirrhosis. If present, collateral circulation can also be clearly depicted.

In demonstrating fistulas or other flow anomalies, angiography is currently the most sensitive instrument available to the clinician, with the only inconvenience being its invasiveness.

The performance of a diagnostically oriented catheterization is a required first step when the eventual goal is therapy by means of transcatheter chemoembolization in that it provides the anatomic, pathologic, and functional information necessary to carry out an effective treatment. And it is in this phase of treatment, which usually follows the diagnostic phase in the same session, that the technical component of catheterization finds its role, in order to place the embolization materials, both selectively and superselectively, in the most appropriate sites.

8.3 Sonographic Angiography with Intra-arterial Injection of CO_2 Microbubbles

Among the experimental techniques for the study of hepatic tumors, sonographic angiography performed with intra-arterial injection of CO_2 microbubbles has recently been introduced, first reported by MATSUDA and YABUUCHI in 1986 and then tested on more than 100 small HCC nodules by KUDO et al. (1992a,b). The technique utilizes the transcatheter injection of carbon dioxide, which allows for real-time visualization of the intralesional distribution of blood flow and provides sonographic angiography patterns correlated with the various tumor types; furthermore, the CO_2 increases the sonographic contrast, facilitating the detection of small intraparenchymal lesions. On the basis of data reported up to now, it is possible to recognize a typical pattern for HCC (even if it is not pathognomonic) and to further increase the sensitivity of sonography in the detection of additional satellite nodules surrounding a primary focus.

8.3.1 Methods and Results

The technique consists of superselective catheterization of the hepatic artery followed by injection, at a velocity of 1–2 ml/s, of a mixture of 10 ml of CO_2, 10 ml of heparinized saline solution and 5 ml of the patient's blood. The patient must hold a constant apnea for at least 15 s, during which the sonographic scanning plane which best shows the lesion and surrounding parenchyma is maintained. A conventional sonographic scanner equipped with a variable frequency (3.5–5 MHz) convex transducer is used to observe the arrival and distribution of the gaseous contrast agent. The examination is videotaped in order to review it at the end of the procedure; the arterial phase, during which the CO_2 reaches the nodule and the surrounding parenchyma, lasts only a few seconds, and at the end of this phase the liver parenchyma becomes so hyperechoic as to be no longer explorable with sonography. Overall, the time added to the angiographic examination (always performed preliminarily in the reported studies to date), necessary in preparing the carbon dioxide microbubbles and injecting them under sonographic visualization, is less than 10 min.

KUDO et al. (1992a,b) have divided the examination into three phases, with a variable duration depending on the case. He has distinguished: an "early" phase which lasts 5–10 s and ends with the complete enhancement of the parenchyma surrounding the lesion; an "intermediate" phase which can last up to 60 s after the injection of the contrast medium and during which the enhancement is immodified; and a "late" phase, lasting 2 min, during which the CO_2 is progressively washed out of the liver. Based on this subdivision of the examination time, KUDO et al. (1992a,b) have described different possible sonographic angiography patterns. Above all, they distinguished hypervascular, isovascular, and hypovascular lesions based on the comparison of the tumor's vascularity with that of the surrounding parenchyma. The hypervascular lesions are, in turn, divided into four types: (1) nodules with peripheral centripetal arterial flow, giving rise to a homogeneous enhancement or to a "mosaic" pattern enhancement; (2) nodules with "spotty" hyperechoic enhancement; (3) nodules which are hypervascular only in their peripheral portions; and (4) nodules with central arterial inflow and dense, marked centrifugal enhancement. The results obtained by Kudo et al. (1992a,b) regarding HCC demonstrate a hypervascular pattern in 90% of cases, an isovascular pattern in 6% of cases, and a hypovascular pattern in the remaining 4%. In particular, the pattern of centripetal arterial flow with homogeneous or mosaic enhancement has, according to the Japanese authors, a sensitivity of 90% and a specificity of 89%, as well as a positive predictive value and a negative predictive value of, respectively, 93% and 84%.

Regarding the detection of small-sized (diameter less than 3 cm) hypervascular HCC nodules, Kudo et al. (1992a,b) give sonographic angiography a sensitivity of 86%, significantly greater than that of traditional angiography (63%) or digital subtraction angiography (70%), and comparable only to that of Lipiodol CT (82%).

The technique was modified in a trial conducted on 48 patients (21 with multifocal or unifocal HCC) at the Institute of Radiology of the University of Turin (Italy). In particular, the subdivision of the phases was modified and standardized. Considering the greater importance of the early and late patterns of the lesions, the videotaping was interrupted after 15 s (corresponding to the early phase according to Kudo et al. 1992a,b). Observation is then recommended after 10 min, outside of the angiography suite and after catheter removal, if necessary (Veltri et al. 1994). If hemangioma is suspected, a check after 30–60 min should be performed because this type of lesion has longer-lasting enhancement. In the experience of the Italian researchers, HCC also is a hypervascular lesion (18/21 cases or 85.7%), with rapid, centripetal, complete enhancement persisting into the late scans (Fig. 8.5). There are, however, two variants which are worth mentioning: the possibility of nodules enhancing mainly in their peripheral portion, found in two discrete-sized nodules (Fig. 8.6); and the finding, in one case, of intense intralesional spotty enhancement in the late phase (considered typical for hemangioma by Kudo et al.). Both patterns were compared to the histological results and seem to correlate with areas of necrosis.

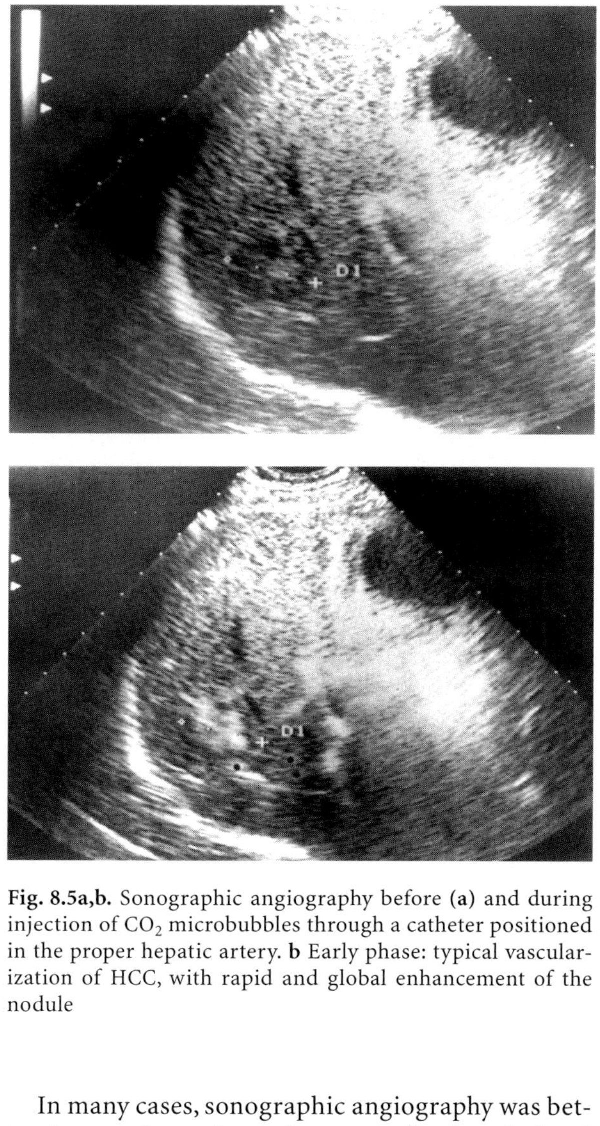

a

b

Fig. 8.5a,b. Sonographic angiography before (**a**) and during injection of CO_2 microbubbles through a catheter positioned in the proper hepatic artery. **b** Early phase: typical vascularization of HCC, with rapid and global enhancement of the nodule

In many cases, sonographic angiography was better than angiography at demonstrating intralesional vascularization, allowing for detection of some scarcely vascularized HCCs. Persistence of the contrast medium, which is washed out of healthy parenchyma earlier than degenerative nodules, into the late phase permits detection of additional small nodules not seen on preliminary US scanning due to the increased contrast resolution (Kudo et al. 1992; Veltri et al. 1994) (Fig. 8.7).

Overall, the method seems simple, sensitive, cost effective and without side effects or complications, except for the onset of transient epigastralgia after CO_2 injection.

a

b

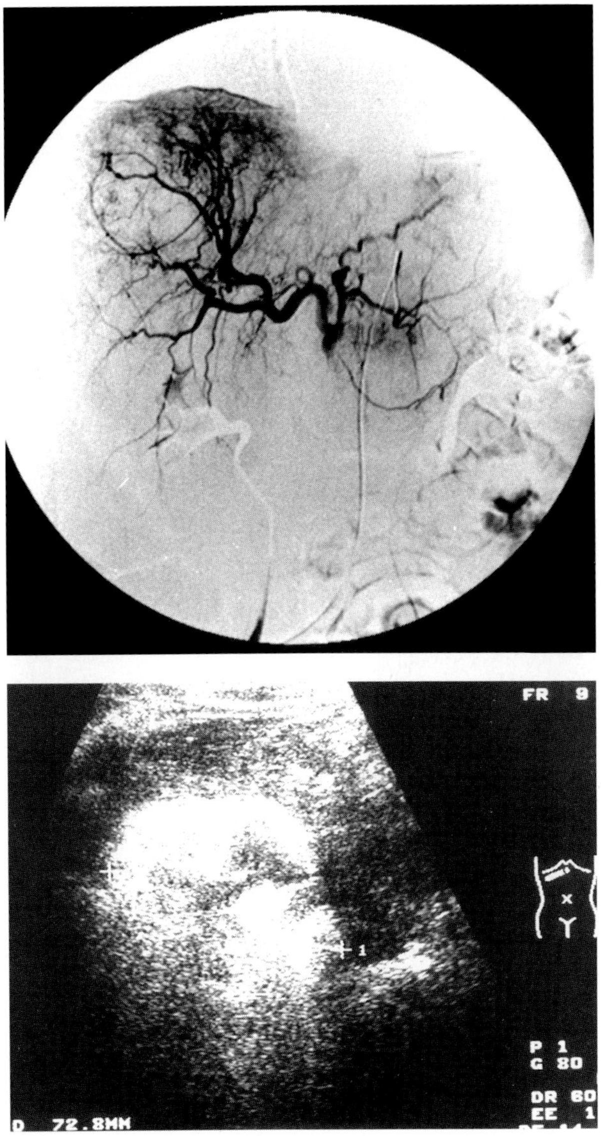

Fig. 8.6. a,b. a Angiography: large "hypovascular" HCC, vascularized only in its periphery, due to central necrosis. **b** Sonographic angiography, late phase: "atypical" pattern, with inhomogeneous, mostly peripheral enhancement

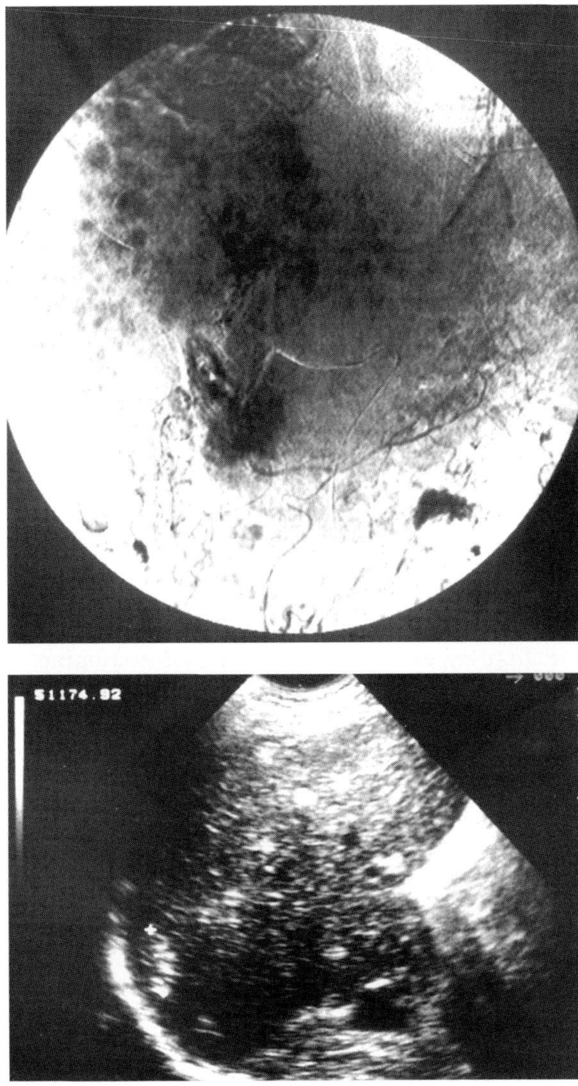

a

b

Fig. 8.7a,b. Diffuse small HCC nodules. **a** Digital angiography. **b** Sonographic angiography, late phase: multiple hyperechoic lesions not visible on preliminary US scan

8.3.2 Conclusion

The early diagnosis of HCC is justified by the improvement of surgical and non-surgical therapeutic choices which have significantly modified the prognosis of this pathology. This has brought about the improvement of the techniques already in common use (US, CT, etc.) and the development of new techniques (color-Doppler US, MRI, etc.) (Taylor et al. 1987; Heiken et al. 1989); moreover, good results have been obtained by combined imaging, such as Lipiodol-CT (Puech et al. 1987; Merine et al. 1990), CT during arterial portography (Heiken et al. 1989; Merine et al. 1990) and CT arteriography (Freeny and Marks 1983), all having high diagnostic accuracy in typifying and staging the disease. Sonographic angiography also is a useful integration of two imaging methods: angiography has the advantage of highlighting the vasculature whereas sonography allows for real time intralesional observation (Matsuda and Yabuuchi 1986); it is therefore possible to study the vascularization of a hepatic nodule optimally and dynamically. On the other hand, the contrast medium renders even small nodules visible, increasing the sensitivity of sonography in determining the tumor extension. Sonography during the late phase can be essential in cases which are equivocal during sonography or angiography.

In conclusion, sonographic angiography utilizing CO_2 microbubbles can provide additional diagnostic information in the characterization and staging of HCC. Considering the minimal added cost and operator's work, sonographic angiography should be performed at the end of the angiographic examination; this integrated technique could be a new "arm" in the diagnosis of hepatic tumors.

8.4 CT during Arterial Portography

The first experience with computed tomography during arterial portography (CTAP) for detection of hepatic neoplasm was reported by Hise et al. (1980). This technique is based on portal enhancement of the liver by infusion of contrast material through the superior mesenteric or the splenic artery.

The portal vein is responsible for 70% of the liver's vascularization and the hepatic artery supplies the other 30% while hepatic tumors, especially HCC, are almost entirely supplied by the hepatic artery.

During CTAP the enhancement of the normal liver parenchyma is very intense; hepatic tumors are detected as areas of poorly enhancing focal lesions and the contrast difference between the lesion and the normal liver is greater during CTAP than during CT after intravenous contrast material injection (Fig. 8.8).

CT during hepatic arteriography (CTA) had been described by Prado et al. in 1979 but this technique has been used less frequently than CTAP; the reason is due to the high prevalence of perfusion abnormalities caused by the anomalous origin of the hepatic artery, present in about 40% of cases, and by the arterial hemodynamic changes due to hepatic tumor and to cirrhosis.

CTA has recently been proposed in combination with CTAP utilizing helical CT with promising results not only in detecting hepatic tumors but also in characterizing the lesions (Kanematsu et al 1997a,b; Murakami et al 1997).

The techniques of CTAP and of CTA are standardized and will be described below.

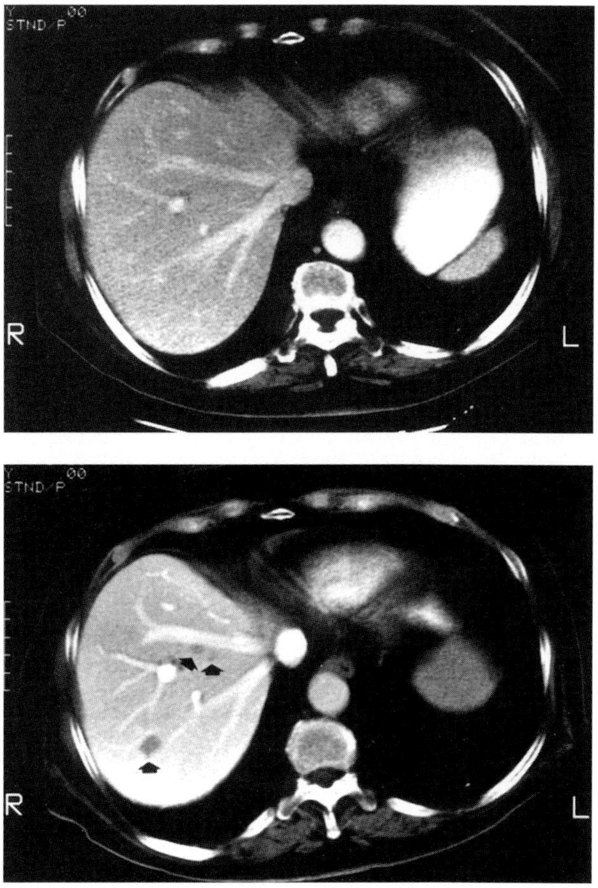

a

b

Fig. 8.8. **a** CT during intravenous injection of contrast agent does not demonstrate any hepatic focal nodules. **b** CT during arterial portography detects three focal lesions of variable size (5–12 mm) in the right hepatic lobe, probably secondary lesions

8.4.1 Technique

Transfemoral angiography is performed with selective studies of celiac axis and mesenteric artery using a 5F visceral catheter (Shepered Hook or Mikaelson catheter).

Digital subtraction angiography is performed to evaluate the hepatic vascular anatomy and the patency of the portal vein; the amount of iodated contrast material should be minimized (dose <50 ml).

Some authors recommend not performing a preliminary angiographic study to reduce the contrast material injection before CTAP to 5/10 ml (Leone et al. 1996); contrast medium retained inside the tumors reduces the difference in attenuation values between normal liver and hepatic tumors during CTAP.

The catheter for CTAP is most commonly placed in the superior mesenteric artery; in cases in which a replaced or accessory right hepatic artery arises from the superior mesenteric artery, the tip of the catheter is advanced sufficiently far into the artery to avoid reflux of the contrast agent into the hepatic artery.

Some authors have suggested that CTAP performed with catheterization of the splenic artery presents some advantages, such as greater hepatic enhancement, fewer non-tumoral perfusion defects and less discomfort for the patient, but these findings were not confirmed by McDermott et al. (1996) (Little et al. 1994). Splenomegaly can increase splenic venous blood flow by tenfold and is a limitation in utilizing the splenic approach, especially in patients with cirrhosis.

Injection of vasodilating agent into the mesenteric artery (40 mg of papaverine hydrochloride or 10 mg of tolazoline) before infusion of contrast material has been suggested in order to improve hepatic enhancement (Soyer et al 1993; Graf et al 1994).

There are some differences in the technical procedure when CTAP is performed using either helical CT or non-spiral CT (Soyer et al 1994; Baron 1994).

Using non-spiral CT, 150 ml of nonionic contrast agent (iodine concentration 300 mg/ml) is injected with a power injector at a rate of 2.0 ml/s; scanning is initiated after 20 s from start of injection.

Using spiral CT, 150 ml of nonionic contrast agent (iodine concentration 200–220 mg/ml) is injected at a rate of 3 ml/s; the scan delay is 30 s. A volumetric acquisition during a single breath-hold (acquisition time 24/30 s, slice thickness 8 mm with 4 mm overlap) eliminates motion artifact and improves tumor detection.

Different techniques are described for CTA combined with CTAP (Kanematsu et al. 1997a,b; Murakami et al. 1997; Toshiyuki et al. 1995). Kanematsu et al. (1997a,b) propose using two 5F angiographic catheters placed in the superior mesenteric artery and hepatic artery by the Seldinger technique bilaterally or unilaterally through the femoral artery; in the case of a unilateral approach, two catheters are placed in one femoral artery and the second access is performed 1 cm caudal to the first access site. Murakami et al. (1997) employ a single cobra triple-lumen balloon catheter.

CTAP is performed by injecting contrast agent either into the splenic artery through a side-hole in the catheter proximal to the balloon inflated into the common hepatic artery or into the superior mesenteric artery through an end-hole in the catheter; CTA is performed by injecting contrast material either into the common hepatic artery from the end-hole or into the accessory right hepatic artery through a side-hole proximal to the inflated balloon in the mesenteric artery. CTA is performed by injecting 70 ml of nonionic contrast material (iodine concentration 150–200 mg/ml) at a rate of 1.7 ml/s; scan acquisition begins 3 s after the initiation of the injection. CTAP is performed 10 min after CTA by Kanematsu et al. (1997b), while Murakami et al. (1997) first perform CTAP and then CTA.

8.4.2 Radiologic Findings

With CTAP, hepatic tumors are visualized as rounded, low-attenuation, solid lesions, well delineated from the normal liver parenchyma enhanced by portography, provided that one completes the scanning rapidly before recirculation brings contrast agent into the hepatic artery (Soyer et al 1994; Baron 1994) (Figs. 8.8, 8.9). The tumors must be differentiated from non-tumoral perfusion defects or pseudo-lesions (Ohashi et al. 1995).

The perfusion defects are categorized as flat, peripheral wedge, lobar or segmental hypoperfusion and gravity defects. The flat perfusion defect, or pseudolesion, is an elongated lesion anterior to the porta hepatis, in segment 4A or 4B, present in 14% of CTAP and is due to anomalous drainage of the gastric vein (Fig. 8.10). The peripheral wedge defect is a small subcapsular area of low attenuation considered to be a physiological variation in portal perfusion. Pseudolesions may also be recognized adjacent to the gallbladder and to the falciform ligament; these lesions have typical aspects and seldom cause false-positive results.

The presence of cirrhosis and portal hypertension may produce hemodynamic alterations causing problems in CTAP interpretation; the presence of arterial-portal venous shunt is also a possible cause of pseudolesion.

HCC often involves the portal vein branch so the hypoattenuating areas are larger than the tumors and satellites nodules are not detected (Figs. 8.9, 8.11). Also the central tumors may compress the portal hilum and be responsible for a diffuse non-diagnostic hypoperfusion of liver parenchyma (Kanematsu et al. 1997).

Despite the high sensitivity of CTAP for lesion detection, its specificity for lesion characterization is low; combining CTAP with CTA can significantly

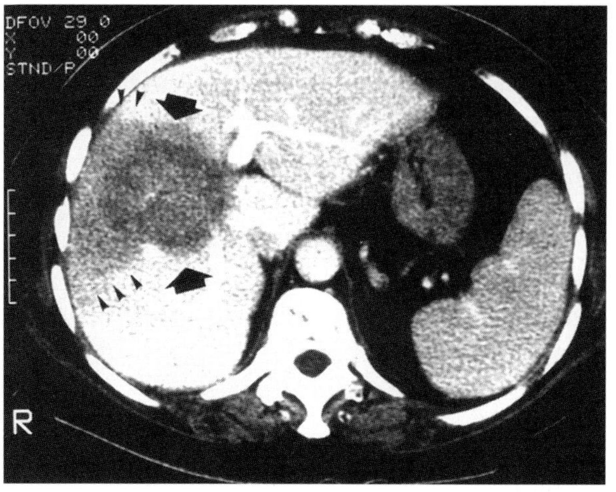

Fig. 8.9. The neoplastic lesion (*large arrows*) appears hypodense in comparison to the healthy hepatic parenchyma surrounding it. *The small arrows* indicate normal parenchyma with lesser density posterior to the lesion. This artifact is due to compression of the portal system by the space occupying lesion

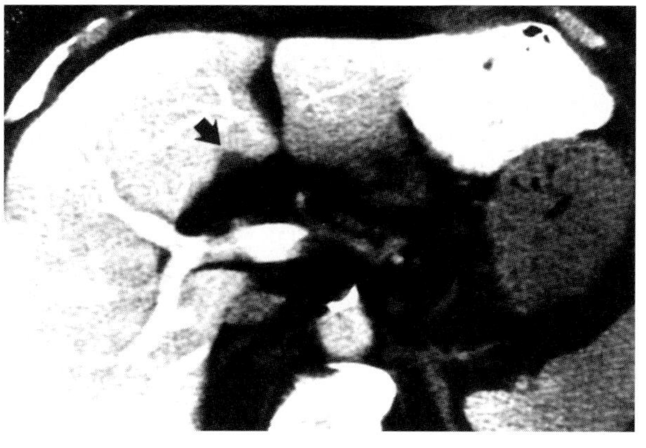

Fig. 8.10. Typical triangular shaped perfusion defect of the IV hepatic segment, just anterior to the portal vein, due to anomalous perfusion in this region

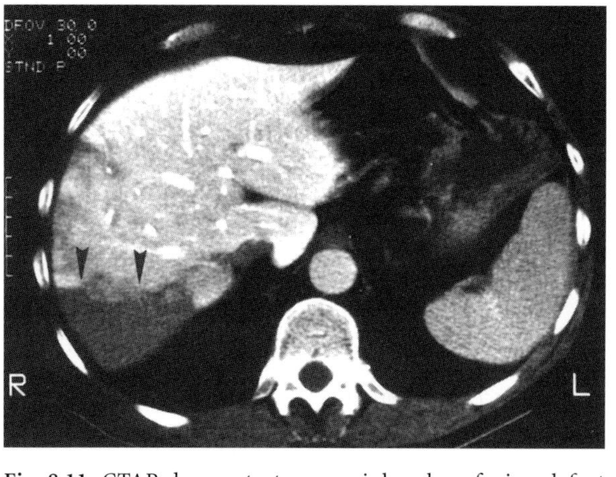

Fig. 8.11. CTAP demonstrates a peripheral perfusion defect (*straight line sign*) in the right hepatic lobe caused by compression of a portal vein branch

improve the characterization and specificity of hepatic lesions that are detected compared with those obtained with CTAP alone.

The enhanced characteristics on CTA may help to characterize portal perfusion defects seen during CTAP: HCC shows homogeneous to heterogeneous enhancement patterns, metastases show ring enhancement and non-tumoral perfusion abnormalities show homogeneous enhancement or do not show any focal enhancement on CTA.

8.4.3 Results

Sensitivity of CTAP for tumor detection is very high and reported to be 84–93% and this technique provides a tumor nodule detection rate exceeding conventional TC by 30–40% (Soyer et al 1994; Baron 1994). In contrast with its high sensitivity, the specificity of CTAP is low; many lesions during CTAP appear as an area of hypodensity including cysts, hemangiomas and other benign lesions; even though most of these lesions may be considered benign based on prior imaging studies (US, MR). The frequency of false-positive lesions with CTAP has been reported to be approximately 15%, but may be lower when CTA is associated with CTAP (Soyer et al. 1994).

For HCC nodules less than 1 cm, the sensitivity of CTAP is 60% (Utsunomiya et al. 1992); this low detection rate seems to be related to the hemodynamic alterations secondary to portal hypertension with hepatofugal collaterals and to the presence of regenerative nodules and periportal fibrosis.

In conclusion, CTAP has a very high sensitivity in detection of hepatic tumors but presents false positives and some limitations in patients with cirrhosis. Its findings must be integrated with sonography and MR imaging to obtain the best results.

8.5 Lipiodol CT

In the last 20 years, the introduction of new therapeutic (both surgical and radiological) approaches for HCC has contributed to the significant increase of survival at 5 and 10 years (Bruix 1997). Staging of this neoplasm is a fundamental part of the diagnostic work-up, since it will condition the therapeutic choices, particularly regarding the possibility of liver transplantation (OLT). It has, in fact, been demonstrated that the post-OLT survival of patients affected with HCC in early stages (I and II according to UICC classification) is similar to that of transplanted patients without HCC (68–85%) (Lohmann et al. 1995), while it drops below 50% when the tumor is in an advanced stage, even down to 0–15% in stage IVa (Pichmayr et al. 1995).

In order to correctly stage the neoplasm, numerous diagnostic imaging techniques have been proposed, including US, CT, MR, angiography, and Lipiodol CT, but no clear diagnostic protocol has yet emerged (Bartolozzi et al. 1996; Dalla Palma et al. 1995). In particular, the use of Lipiodol-CT is still controversial due to the differing values of diagnostic accuracy and predictive values reported in the literature (Pozzi Mucelli et al. 1995).

8.5.1 Method and Results

Lipiodol ultra fluid (Guerbet, Aulnay-sous-Bois, France) is an oil-based contrast medium composed of folic acid ethylic esters (extracts of poppyseed oil) conjugated with iodine. Ethyl esterification, instead of glyceryl esterification, was preferred in order to obtain a more fluid preparation. The iodine is in a 48% concentration, which is greater than the concentration used in hydrophilic contrast agents.

The contrast medium selectively accumulates inside the HCC nodule (Fig. 8.12), but the mechanism of accumulation is only partially known. HCC is a highly vascularized nodule, with the arterial supply prevailing over the portal supply, which undergoes a progressive involution as the nodule increases in size; this creates a "siphon effect", which causes accumulation of Lipiodol inside the lesion. Furthermore, tumor neoangiogenesis favors the passage of contrast medium into the intercellular space: arterial vessels are tortuous and irregular, with their caliber moderately increased and with segment lacking the tunica muscularis. Finally, the wash-out of Lipiodol from the lesion seems slow for at least two reasons: the insufficient portal vascularization (the main mechanism responsible for non-neoplastic wash-out) and the absence of reticuloendothelial cells; some authors also believe that the lack of lymphatic vessels in HCC delays wash-out of the contrast medium. Lastly, during the neoplastic transformation of hepatocytes, the plasma membrane may undergo a biochemical modification, rendering it more lipophilic; this would favor adhesion of Lipiodol to the membrane and its subsequent endocytosis into the neoplastic cell (Pozzi Mucelli et al. 1995).

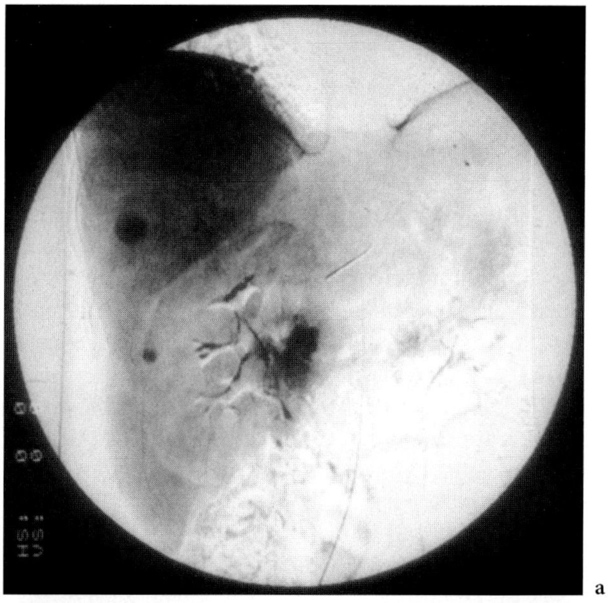

a

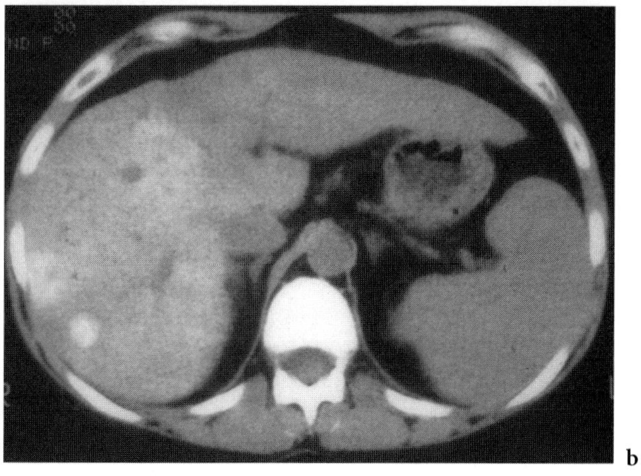

b

Fig. 8.12. a Angiography shows two hypervascular HCC nodules in the right liver lobe. **b** Lipiodol-CT: the iodized oil selectively accumulates inside the lesions, with homogeneous enhancement of the nodules (type I according to Bruneton's classification)

The ability of Lipiodol to concentrate selectively in HCC cells was recognized in the 1970s and was employed in anatomical-radiological studies (Nakakuma et al. 1985). In the 1980s, this property was applied to both therapeutic purposes, being used as a vehicle for chemotherapy agents in chemoembolization (Konno et al. 1984), as well as for diagnostic purposes, to detect on subsequent CT scan the nodules of HCC (Maki et al. 1985).

The method consists of slowly injecting into the proper hepatic artery (beyond the origins of the gastroduodenal and cystic arteries) 10 ml of Lipiodol, which is a sufficient quantity for eventual uptake into the neoplastic nodules. Follow-up CT scanning is then performed on the whole liver (contiguous scans of 1 cm thickness) at 3 weeks after administration of Lipiodol, which is the time necessary for the non-neoplastic parenchyma to eliminate the contrast medium. The method is, therefore, discretely invasive since it is necessary to selectively catheterize the proper hepatic artery via transfemoral arterial access (Pozzi Mucelli et al. 1995).

The patterns of Lipiodol CT have been covered in the literature. Among the most complete studies are those of Bruneton et al. (1988) and the Liver Cancer Study Group of Japan in 1989.

The Liver Cancer Study Group of Japan (1989) has recognized two types of HCC based on its characteristics on Lipiodol CT: (1) massive form, with diffuse enhancement with Lipiodol of ample areas of the liver; (2) nodular form, which can present in various forms: as a single lesion, a single lesion with small satellite nodule(s), multiple separate lesions, and multiple confluent lesions.

Bruneton et al. (1988), on the other hand, have emphasized the anatomical-radiological correlation, describing four types of enhancement corresponding to four types of vascularization: type I: a hypervascular nodule with diffuse and homogeneous enhancement; type II: a hypovascular nodule with no uptake of Lipiodol; type III: centrally hypovascular nodule, with peripheral enhancement; type IV: predominantly hypovascular nodule with areas of irregular uptake of contrast agent. According to these researchers, and according to most case studies, the most frequent finding is that of a hypervascular nodule, with intense and homogeneous uptake of Lipiodol (type I) (Fig. 8.12).

Absence of lesion enhancement may possibly be explained by the lesion's scarce vascularization (more frequent in case of small-sized nodules) or by the insufficient quantity of Lipiodol employed. The presence of "spots" of Lipiodol within a solitary lesion is due to the presence of necrotic areas within the tumor. The diagnostic accuracy and the predictive values of Lipiodol CT are still being discussed in the literature.

Numerous studies have reported the sensitivity (in respect to lesion identification and not patient detection) with variable values (ranging from 53% to 100%) (Arakawa et al. 1996; Bartolozzi et al. 1994; Lencioni et al. 1997; Ngan 1990; Roversi et al. 1989; Takayasu et al. 1990; Taourel et al. 1995; Valls et al. 1994, 1995; Veltri et al. 1996), but most frequently with high values (greater than 90%); in

Table 8.1. Sensitivity of Lipiodol CT (literature data)

Author	Year	Sensitivity
Roversi	1989	100%
Ngan	1990	97%
Takayasu	1990	93%
Bartolozzi	1994	95%
Valls	1994	70%
Valls	1995	74%
Taourel	1995	53%
Arakawa	1996	77%
Veltri	1996	78%
Lencioni	1997	70%

our experience, comparing the results of Lipiodol CT with the histological study of the explanted liver, the sensitivity of the method is inferior (around 75%) (Veltri et al. 1998) (Table 8.1). Many of the above mentioned studies, however, are inadequate in their reference standard, consisting in some cases of other radiological studies (Pozzi Mucelli et al. 1995; Bartolozzi et al. 1994; Dalla Palma et al. 1997), and in other cases of biopsies or histological examination of resected portions (Bartolozzi et al. 1996; Lencioni et al. 1997); infrequently the histological study of the entire organ was performed. When the "gold standard" was the histological examination of all the hepatic parenchyma explanted during OLT, the results regarding the diagnostic accuracy of Lipiodol CT have been redimensioned; such studies are relatively rare in the literature: we cite the studies by Valls et al. (1994, 1995) and Taourel et al. (1995), who report a sensitivity of 74% and 53%, respectively, with a high number of false negatives. In this regard, other authors have demonstrated that the number of false negatives increases when nodules less than 2 cm in diameter are considered: Yoshimatsu et al. (1989), who have obtained a sensitivity of 64%, attribute the increase in false negatives to the greater degree of differentiation and to the lesser degree of vascularization of small lesions; lastly, also in detecting small lesions the sensitivity of Lipiodol CT was lower when the control selected was the pathologic examination (Lencioni et al. 1997) instead of other radiological methods (Bartolozzi et al. 1994).

Overall, our study, like other detailed studies recently reported in the literature, demonstrates that Lipiodol CT does not have a significantly greater sensitivity in comparison to other imaging methods.

Studies on the specificity of Lipiodol CT are less numerous and many authors have emphasized the need to investigate this aspect (Lencioni et al. 1997;

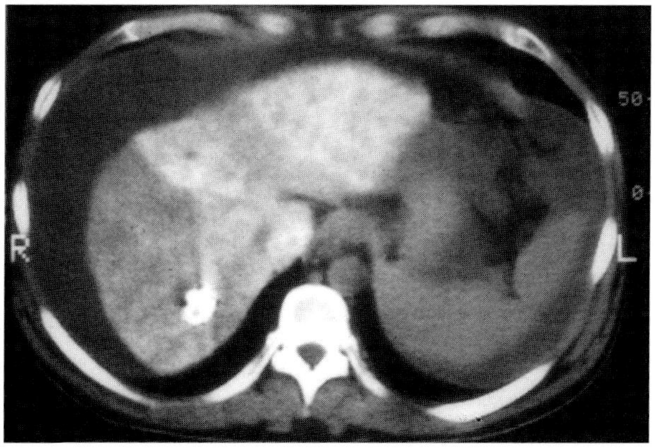

Fig. 8.13. False positive: at the pathological examination, the intense focal uptake of Lipiodol corresponded to a hemangioma

Itai 1997). The number of false positives weighs heavily on the specificity and the positive predictive value, which are particularly low in our experience (specificity 63.8%, positive predictive value for single lesion 70.5%, positive predictive value for patient detection 72.9%) (Veltri et al. 1998). Even Taourel, in the above cited work, reports a positive predictive value (75%) similar to ours (Taourel et al. 1995). In these studies, the focal lesions responsible for false positives were hemangiomas (Veltri et al. 1998) (Fig. 8.13), regenerative nodules and aspecific uptake areas (Taourel et al. 1995).

For this reason, when Lipiodol is employed to take advantage of its sensitivity, a confirmation of the detected nodule must be obtained; in fact, Ferris et al. (1995), who have evaluated candidates for OLT, attribute to Lipiodol CT the capacity of detecting nodules not seen with other imaging methods, but emphasize the need for histological confirmation due to the possibility of false positives.

8.5.2 Conclusion

Lipiodol CT is one of the methods employed in staging HCC. After the initial enthusiasm, its role is being reviewed because of a more critical evaluation of its sensitivity and specificity and since more accurate methods have emerged (helical CT) or are promising (MR imaging with hepatospecific contrast agents). Lipiodol CT, however, still remains an important prognostic indicator when performed after chemoembolization, in order to evaluate its result. In this case it evaluates the accumulation of Lipiodol within the lesion, which is proportional to the efficacy of therapy and considered indicative for the necessity of other complementary treatments, such as alcoholization.

8.6 Summary

Angiographic studies and imaging techniques based on arterial catheterization, when considered individually, have a sensitivity and/or specificity which are generally modest. Regarding the sensitivity, the poorest results are those of DSA, especially for small sized nodules (<60% in nodules whose diameter is less than 2 cm). The other techniques which have the advantage of presenting the information as a "tomographic" image, and are therefore, by definition, more analytic, habitually give better results: sensitivity of 86% for sonographic angiography, 82% for Lipiodol CT in detecting nodules down to 3 cm in diameter, in comparison with the 70% sensitivity for DSA; sensitivity of 90% for CT during arterial portography. If the sensitivity for these techniques is satisfactory or even high, as in CT during arterial portography, the specificity remains modest for all of the methods. Even the technique which elicited, in our opinion, the greatest enthusiasm, Lipiodol CT, revealed itself to be plagued with a high rate of false negatives and false positives. The diagnostic accuracy of the method is estimated to be modest in controlled studies comparing findings to surgical transplantation specimens, with a positive predictive value of 70–75%. The association of several techniques improves the diagnostic yield, in respect to both sensitivity and specificity. The association of techniques with an angiographic approach is feasible, with execution of several studies possible (for example, DSA+sonographic angiography+CT arterial portography; DSA+Lipiodol CT). In the literature, the advantages of association with non-angiographic techniques has been emphasized. However, in daily practice, a significant port of the lesion-type diagnoses is still performed using fine needle aspiration (usually US-guided). In fact, the examinations performed with angiographic techniques, even in association, have a specificity such that, not infrequently, it is necessary to perform other diagnostic tests.

In conclusion, angiography, whose catheterization phase forms the basis of all the other types of examinations, is currently considered, from many viewpoints, to be an insufficiently reliable technique. But it is angiography's particular role in establishing access to the vascular bed by means of a more or less selective catheterization that is the qualifying element of this procedure, which constitutes the preliminary and essential phase of all forms of loco-regional treatment of HCC via the catheter.

References

Arakawa A, Nishiharu T, Matsukawa T, et al (1996) Detection of hepatocellular carcinoma by intrarterially enhanced ultrasonography with CO_2 microbubbles. Comparison with DSA, dynamic CT, and Lipiodol CT. Acta Radiol 37:250–254

Baron R (1994) Detection of liver neoplasm: techniques and outcomes. Abdom Imaging 19:320–324

Bartolozzi C, Lencioni R, Caramella D, et al (1994) Stadiazione del carcinoma epatocellulare. Confronto tra ecografia, Tomografia Computerizzata, Risonanza Magnetica, angiografia digitale e Tomografia Computerizzata con Lipiodol. Radiol Med 88:429–436

Bartolozzi C, Lencioni R, Caramella D, et al (1996) Small hepatocellular carcinoma. Detection with US, CT, MR imaging, DSA, and Lipiodol CT. Acta Radiol 37:69–74

Bruix J (1997) Treatment of hepatocellular carcinoma. Hepatology 25:259–262

Bruneton JN, Kerboul P, Grimaldi, et al (1988) Hepatic intrarterial Lipiodol: technique, semeiologic patterns and value for hepatic tumors. Gastrointest Radiol 13:45–51

Dalla Palma L, Pozzi Mucelli R, Sponza M, et al (1995) Valutazione comparativa dell'ecografia, della Tomografia Computerizzata, dell'angiografia, della Lipiodol-TC nel bilancio di estensione dell'epatocarcinoma. Studio multicentrico. Radiol Med 89:270–277

Dalla Palma L, Pozzi Mucelli R, Sponza M, et al (1997) La diagnostica mediante immagini e la terapia interventistica dell'epatocarcinoma. Studio multicentrico su 290 casi. Radiol Med 94:30–36

Ferris IV, Marsh JW, Little AF, et al (1995) Presurgical evaluation of the liver transplant candidate. Radiol Clin North Am 33:497–520

Freeny PC, Marks WM (1983) Computed tomographic arteriography of the liver. Radiology 148:193–197

Graf O, Dock WI, Lammer J, et al (1994) Determination of optimal time window for liver scanning with CT during arterial portography. Radiology 190:43–47

Heiken JP, Weyman PJ, Lee JKT, et al (1989) Detection of focal hepatic masses: prospective evaluation with CT, delayed CT, CT during arterial portography, and MR imaging. Radiology 171:47–51

Hise N, Hiramatsu K, Narimatsu Y, et al (1980) Detection of hepatic neoplasms by computed tomography in portal hepatogram phase. Jpn J Clin Radiol 25:529–534

Ikeda K, Saitoh S, Koida I, et al (1994) Imaging diagnosis of small hepatocellular carcinoma. Hepatology 20:82–87

Itai Y (1997) Lipiodol CT for hepatocellular. Abdom Imaging 22:259–260

Kanazawa S, Yasui K, Doke T, et al (1995) Hepatic arteriography in patients with hepatocellular carcinoma: change in findings caused by balloon occlusion of tumor-draining hepatic veins. AJR 165:1415–1419

Kanematsu M, Hoshi H, Imaeda T, et al (1997) Detection and characterization of hepatic tumors: value of combined helical CT hepatic arteriography and CT during arterial portography. AJR 168:1193–1198

Kanematsu M, Hoshi H, Yamada T, et al (1997) Overestimating the size of hepatic malignancy on helical CT during arterial portography: equilibrium phase CT and pathology. J Comput Assist Tomogr 21:713–719

Kido C, Sasaki T, Kaneko M (1971) Angiography of primary liver cancer. AJR 113:70–75

Konno T, Maeda U, Iwai K, et al (1984) Selective targeting anti-cancer drug and simultaneous image enhancement in solid tumors by arterially administred lipid contrast medium. Cancer 54:2367–2374

Kudo M, Tomita S, Tochio H, et al (1992a) Small hepatocellular carcinoma: diagnosis with US angiography with intraarterial CO2 microbubbles. Radiology 182:155–160

Kudo M, Tomita S, Tochio H, et al (1992b) Sonography with intraarterial infusion of carbon dioxide microbubbles (sonographic angiography): value in differential diagnosis of hepatic tumors. AJR 158:65–74

Lamarque JL (1974) Artériographie hépatique. Masson et Cie, Paris

Lencioni R, Pinto F, Armillotta N, et al (1997) Intrahepatic metastatic nodules of hepatocellular carcinoma detected at Lipiodol CT: imaging-pathologic correlation. Abdom Imaging 22:253–258

Leone A, Violino P, Ghirardo D (1996) Il ruolo della portografia con tomografia computerizzata nella diagnosi di metastasi epatiche da neoplasie del colon-retto. Radiol Med 91:86–90

Little A, Baron R, Peterson M (1994) Optimizing CT portography: a prospective comparison of injection into the splenic versus superior mesenteric artery. Radiology 193:651–655

Liver Cancer Study Group of Japan (1989) The general rules for the clinical and pathological study of primay liver cancer. Jpn J Surg 19:98–129

Lohmann R, Bechstein WO, Langrehr JM, et al (1995) Analysis of risk factors for recurrence of hepatocellular carcinoma after ortothopic liver transplantation. Transplant Proc 27:1245–1246

Maki S, Konno T, Maeda H (1985) Image enhancement in Computerized Tomography for sensitive diagnosis of liver cancer and semiquantitation of tumor selective drug targeting with oily contrast medium. Cancer 56:751–757

Matsuda Y, Yabuuchi I (1986) Hepatic tumors: US contrast enhancement with CO2 microbubbles. Radiology 161:701–705

McDermott V, Lawrance J, Paulson E, et al (1996) CT during arterial portography: comparison of injection into the splenic versus superior mesenteric artery. Radiology 199:627–631

Merine D, Takayasu K, Wakao F (1990) Detection of hepatocellular carcinoma: comparison of CT during arterial portography with CT after intraarterial injection of iodized oil. Radiology 175:707–710

Murakami T, Oi H, Hori M, et al (1997) CT arterial portography and CT arteriography with a triple-lumen balloon catheter. Acta Radiol 38:553–557

Nakakuma K, Tashiro S, Hiraoka T, et al (1985) Hepatocellular carcinoma and metastatic cancer detected by iodised oil. Radiology 154:15–17

Ngan H (1990) Lipiodol Computerized Tomography: how sensitive and specific is the technique in the diagnosis of hepatocellular carcinoma? Br J Radiol 63:771–775

Ohashi I, Ina H, Gomi N, et al (1995) Hepatic pseudolesion in the left lobe around the falciform ligament at helical CT. Radiology 196:245–249

Okuda K, Musha H, Yamasaki T, et al (1977) Angiographic demonstration of intrahepatic arterio-portal anastomoses in hepatocellular carcinoma. Radiology 122:53–58

Pichmayr R, Weimann A, Oldhafer KJ, et al (1995) Role of liver transplantation in the treatment of unresectable liver cancer. World J Surg 19:807–813

Pozzi Mucelli RS, Cova M, Pagnan L, et al (1995) Lipiodol TC. In: Dalla Palma L (ed) L'epatocarcinoma. Diagnostica per immagini e terapia interventistica. Edizioni Lint, Trieste, pp 89–98

Prado A, Wallance, Benardio ME, Lindeller MMS (1979) Computed tomography arteriography of the liver. Radiology 130:697–701

Puech JL, Rousseau H, Portalez D, et al (1987) Lipiodolisation artérielle hépatique et diagnostic scanographique des tumeurs malignes du foie. Ann Radiol 30:193–201

Roversi R (1989) Angiografia digitale dell'epatocarcinoma. Tecnica, diagnostica e terapia transcatetere. Aulo Gaggi, Bologna

Roversi R, Ricci S, Rossi C, et al (1989) Il Lipiodol ultrafluid nella diagnostica per immagini dell'epatocarcinoma su cirrosi. Radiol Med 78:44–52

Soyer P, Lachekeb, Levesque M (1993) CT arterial portography of the abdomen: effect of injecting papaverine into the mesenteric artery on hepatic contrast enhancement. AJR 169:1213–1215

Soyer P, Bluemke D, Fishman E (1994) CT during arterial portography for the preoperative evaluation of hepatic tumors: how, when, and why. AJR 163:1325–1331

Subramanyan BR, Balthazar EJ, Hilton S, et al (1984) Hepatocellular carcinoma with venous invasion. Radiology 150:793–797

Sumida M, Ohto M, Ebara M, et al (1986) Accuracy of angiography in the diagnosis of small hepatocellular carcinoma. AJR 147:531–536

Takahashi K, Saito K, Tamura K, et al (1990) Hepatic neoplasms: detection with hepatoportal subtraction angiography – a new technique of DSA. Radiology 177:243–248

Takayasu K, Moriyama N, Murutsu Y, et al (1990) The diagnosis of small hepatocellular carcinoma: efficacy of various imaging procedures in 100 patients. AJR 155: 49–54

Taourel PG, Pageaux GP, Coste V, et al (1995) Small hepatocellular carcinoma in patients undergoing liver transplantation: detection with CT after injection of iodised oil. Radiology 197:377–380

Taylor KJW, Ramos I, Morse SS, et al (1987) Focal liver masses: differential diagnosis with pulsed Doppler US. Radiology 164:643–647

Toshiyuki I, Koij T, Yoichi W, et al (1995) CT evaluation of hepatic tumors: comparison of CT with infusion hepatic arteriography, and simultaneous use of both techniques. AJR 164:1407–1412

Utsunomiya T, Matsumata T, Adachi E, et al (1992) Limitations of current preoperative liver imaging techniques for intrahepatic metastatic nodules of hepatocellular carcinoma. Hepatology 16:694–701

Valls C, Pamies JJ, Sancho C, et al (1994) Computed Tomography after Lipiodol chemoembolization in hepatocellular carcinoma. Eur Radiol 4:238–242

Valls C, Figueras J, Pamies JJ, et al (1995) Preoperative TNM staging of hepatocellular carcinoma in hepatic transplantation: value of Lipiodol Computed Tomography. Transpl

9 Cholangiocellular Carcinoma

R. MANFREDI, G. MARESCA, A. VECCHIOLI, C. COLAGRANDE, G. GALLETTI, and P. MARANO

CONTENTS

9.1 Epidemiology

Cholangiocarcinoma is a primary malignancy arising from the bile duct epithelium (CRAIG et al. 1989). The relative incidence of cholangiocarcinoma among primary liver cancer reported in autopsy series ranges from 5% to 30% (HOYNE and KERNOHAN 1947; EDMONDSON and STEINER 1954; MACDONALD 1956; MORI 1967; SAN JOSE et al. 1965; CRUICKSHANK 1961; PATTON and HORN 1964). Risk factors for cholangiocarcinoma are primary sclerosing cholangitis, choledocal cyst, familial polyposis, congenital hepatic fibrosis, infection with *Clonorchis siniensis* (Chinese liver fluke), and history of exposure to thorium dioxide (Thorotrast).

Cholangiocarcinoma is a disease of older individuals; the average age at diagnosis is 65 years; but most patients with risk factors often develop this neoplasm at a much younger age. The cancer occurs slightly more frequently in males than females.

According to the site of origin, cholangiocarcinomas can be classified into two types: intrahepatic and extrahepatic (ROS et al. 1988; OKUDA et al. 1977; KLATSKIN 1965). The term cholangiocarcinoma should be used for intrahepatic lesions whereas bile duct carcinoma should be preferred for extrahepatic neoplasms (SAUL 1994).

The intrahepatic or peripheral cholangiocarcinoma represents 10% of all cholangiocarcinomas, arises in small intrahepatic ducts, and, although rare, is the second most common primary malignant liver tumor after hepatocellular carcinoma. It is an adenocarcinoma arising from the internal wall of the small bile ducts, peripheral to the right or left hepatic ducts and grows exophytically into the liver as a focal mass (ROS et al. 1988).

Bile duct carcinomas include tumors occurring at the common hepatic duct and its bifurcation, also referred to as Klatskin's tumors (70%), and tumors arising in the distalmost common bile duct (CBD) (10–20%). In this latter location, sometimes tumors can be hardly differentiated from those originating from the ampulla, head of the pancreas, or duodenal wall; therefore malignancies of this area are usually lumped together under the term periampullary tumors, and will not be discussed in this chapter.

9.2 Clinical Findings

The symptoms of peripheral cholangiocarcinoma are non-specific: anorexia, weight loss, vague gastrointestinal symptoms, ill defined upper abdominal discomfort, and elevated serum alkaline

R. MANFREDI, MD; Department of Radiology, A. Gemelli University Hospital, Largo A. Gemelli 8, I-00168 Rome, Italy
G. MARESCA, MD; Professor, Department of Radiology, A. Gemelli University Hospital, Largo A. Gemelli 8, I-00168 Rome, Italy
A. VECCHIOLI, MD; Department of Radiology, A. Gemelli University Hospital, Largo A. Gemelli 8, I-00168 Rome, Italy
C. COLAGRANDE, MD; Professor, Department of Radiology, A. Gemelli University Hospital, Largo A. Gemelli 8, I-00168 Rome, Italy
G. GALLETTI, MD; Department of Radiology, A. Gemelli University Hospital, Largo A. Gemelli 8, I-00168 Rome, Italy
P. MARANO, MD; Professor and Chairman, Department of Radiology, A. Gemelli University Hospital, Largo A. Gemelli 8, I-00168 Rome, Italy

phosphatase and bilirubin levels. All these symptoms appear after the tumor has been enlarged. Therefore, early diagnosis is more unusual. On the contrary, the main signs and symptoms of hilar cholangiocarcinoma are similar to those of extrahepatic bile duct carcinomas. Jaundice is usually the first sign and, if not, it begins shortly after the onset of pain in the right upper quadrant. If cholangiocarcinoma exists at the junction of the right and left hepatic ducts within the liver, the onset of jaundice is early and in such cases even a small tumor may cause jaundice. Cholangitis is unusual as a presenting symptom (Klatskin 1965).

9.3 Pathology

Cholangiocarcinoma has traditionally been divided into three separate types, based on the appearance and location of the lesion. Cholangiocarcinomas developing in the peripheral duct system, referred to as intrahepatic or peripheral neoplasms, are clinically silent, allowing unchecked growth of the mass. According to the tumor growth, it has been termed bulky exophytic because of its mass-like qualities, or diffuse sclerosing because of its smooth stricture effect on the intrahepatic biliary tree.

Grossly, the liver involved with cholangiocarcinoma is usually enlarged partly due to the tumor itself and partly due to hydrohepatosis or to associated cholangitis with or without abscess formation. However, in some instances, especially in hilar cholangiocarcinomas, there may be no increase in the weight of the liver. The gross appearance of cholangiocarcinoma is that of a grayish white, firm, solid and fibrous mass. Cut surfaces are usually sclerotic gray white or pale white, with dense fibrous stranding. Characteristically this malignancy has a large central core of fibrotic tissue relatively devoid of malignant cells. Most of the cancer cells are located in the tumor's periphery.

Sometimes daughter nodules are irregularly distributed throughout the liver. This form of tumor is not highly vascularized; hemorrhage, necrosis and cystic degeneration are uncommon. Portal thrombosis, when it does appear, is usually a result of secondary cholangitis and not of tumor thrombosis. The surrounding liver parenchyma is smooth and usually non-cirrhotic, but may be deeply stained with bile, a feature that contrasts with the tumor itself, which is not pigmented.

The majority of cholangiocarcinomas (up to 70%) occur at the common hepatic duct (CHD) and its bifurcation, also referred to as Klatskin's tumor. At this location the tumor produces a localized stricture, giving rise to its descriptive terms: focal stenosis or infiltrating stenosis. The frequent mode of spread is local extension from the biliary tree invading the liver. This appearance has implications for radiologic diagnosis and prognosis given the uncertainty of obtaining a surgical cure after transductal spread.

Bile duct carcinomas developing in the common bile duct appear as a rounded intraluminal mass, usually within the mid-extrahepatic biliary tree at the distal common hepatic duct or at the common bile duct. This polypoid of the papillary variety should bring the patient to medical attention relatively early, thus improving the prognosis.

Microscopically, cholangiocarcinoma represent an adenocarcinoma with a glandular appearance arising from the epithelium of the bile ducts. Mucus secretion and calcification are sometimes found, but there is no bile production. Occasionally cholangiocarcinomas of larger hepatic duct branches are papillary. The neoplastic cells provoke a variable desmoplastic reaction; therefore the tumor mass most often lies in a connective tissue stroma, but the degree of desmoplastic reaction among the cholangiocarcinomas varies considerably.

Most cholangiocarcinomas are well-differentiated adenocarcinomas but undifferentiated forms may occur. It is often impossible to histologically distinguish cholangiocarcinomas from carcinoma of the extrahepatic bile ducts and other adenocarcinomas that have metastasized to the liver.

The liver bearing a hilar cholangiocarcinoma (Klatskin's tumor) microscopically shows a typical appearance of biliary obstruction, the predominant features being moderate to marked bile stasis, portal fibrosis, ductal proliferation, and periportal inflammatory reaction.

9.4 Imaging Findings

The imaging findings of cholangiocarcinomas depend on the tumor location: intrahepatic and peripheral to the hilus, hilar, or in the distal common hepatic duct or common bile duct. Other features determining imaging findings are morphology of the tumor and its type of growth: (1) exophytic, to the ductal

Table 9.1. Pathologic-radiologic correlation

Pathologic feature	Imaging findings
Calcification	US: hyperechoic with shadowing CT: hyperdensity
Fibrosis	US: hypoechoic area CT: hypodense area MRI: hypointensity
Mucin	CT: hypodensity MRI: hyperintensity
Hypovascularity	Doppler US: scanty signals CT: hypodensity during the arterial phase MRI: hypointensity during the arterial phase Angiography: early phase: peripheral enhancement; capillary phase: central zone of hypovascularity

wall, with intrahepatic growth; (2) scirrhous infiltrating neoplasm causing stricture; and (3) polypoid neoplasm bulging into the bile duct lumen (Table 9.1).

9.4.1 Intrahepatic Cholangiocarcinoma

About 20–30% of cholangiocarcinomas are exophytic, intrahepatic masses (Thorsen et al. 1984; Nesbit et al. 1988). Intrahepatic cholangiocarcinomas may also be polypoid or focally stenotic. Excluding the exophytic intrahepatic type, about three-fourths of cholangiocarcinomas manifest as a focal stricture, and one-fourth are polypoid or diffusely stenotic. Most polypoid cholangiocarcinomas are intrahepatic, whereas some affect the extrahepatic bile ducts (Kokubo et al. 1988).

9.4.1.1 Ultrasound

The nodular pattern is more frequently seen (94.4%) compared to the infiltrative pattern (5.6%). In the nodular pattern, a single mass is frequently observed, predominantly located in the posterior segments of the liver parenchyma. Small nodules (<3 cm) most frequently appear hypo- or isoechoic, whereas the nodules larger than 3 cm are predominantly hyperechoic (Fig. 9.1). When multiple lesions are present, the larger mass shows higher echogenicity compared to the daughter nodules. An hypoechoic halo is observed in one-third of cases.

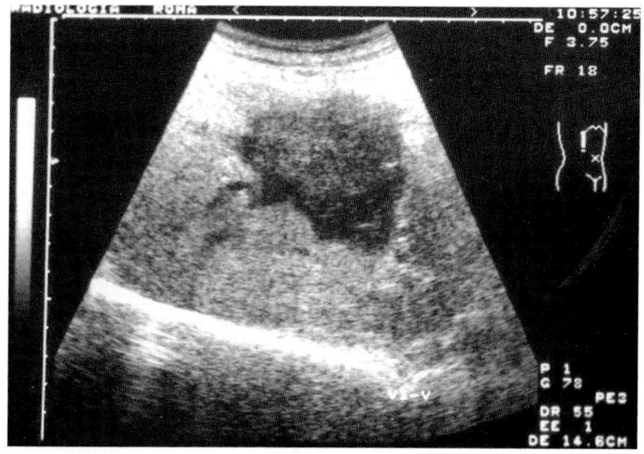

Fig. 9.1. Intrahepatic cholangiocarcinoma: ultrasound. Sonography shows a cholangiocarcinoma, in the VI–V hepatic segments, that appears hypoechoic compared to adjacent liver parenchyma

Because of the peripheral location of the mass, bile duct obstruction is not often seen and, when present, it is a helpful sign for the differential diagnosis with hepatocellular carcinoma (Table 9.2). Sometimes, the central portion of the tumor may appear hypoechoic, due to the presence of necrosis, or hyperechoic with acoustic shadowing, due to the presence of calcification. The infiltrative pattern of growth of cholangiocarcinoma appears as diffuse architectural changes of an hepatic lobe. Because of its hypovascular feature, cholangiocarcinoma shows scanty color signals on color Doppler ultrasound; this is a helpful sign for the differential diagnosis with hepatocellular carcinoma that is typically hypervascular.

9.4.1.2 Computed Tomography

Unenhanced CT scan shows a hypodense mass, either solitary or with multiple satellite nodules

Table 9.2. Criteria for differential diagnosis between cholangiocarcinoma and hepatocellular carcinoma

Feature	Cholangio-carcinoma	HCC
Biliary duct dilatation	Yes	No
Calcification, fibrosis, mucin secretion	Yes	No
Retraction of the liver capsule	Yes	No
Portal vein infiltration	Rare	Frequent
Extrahepatic extension	Frequent	Rare

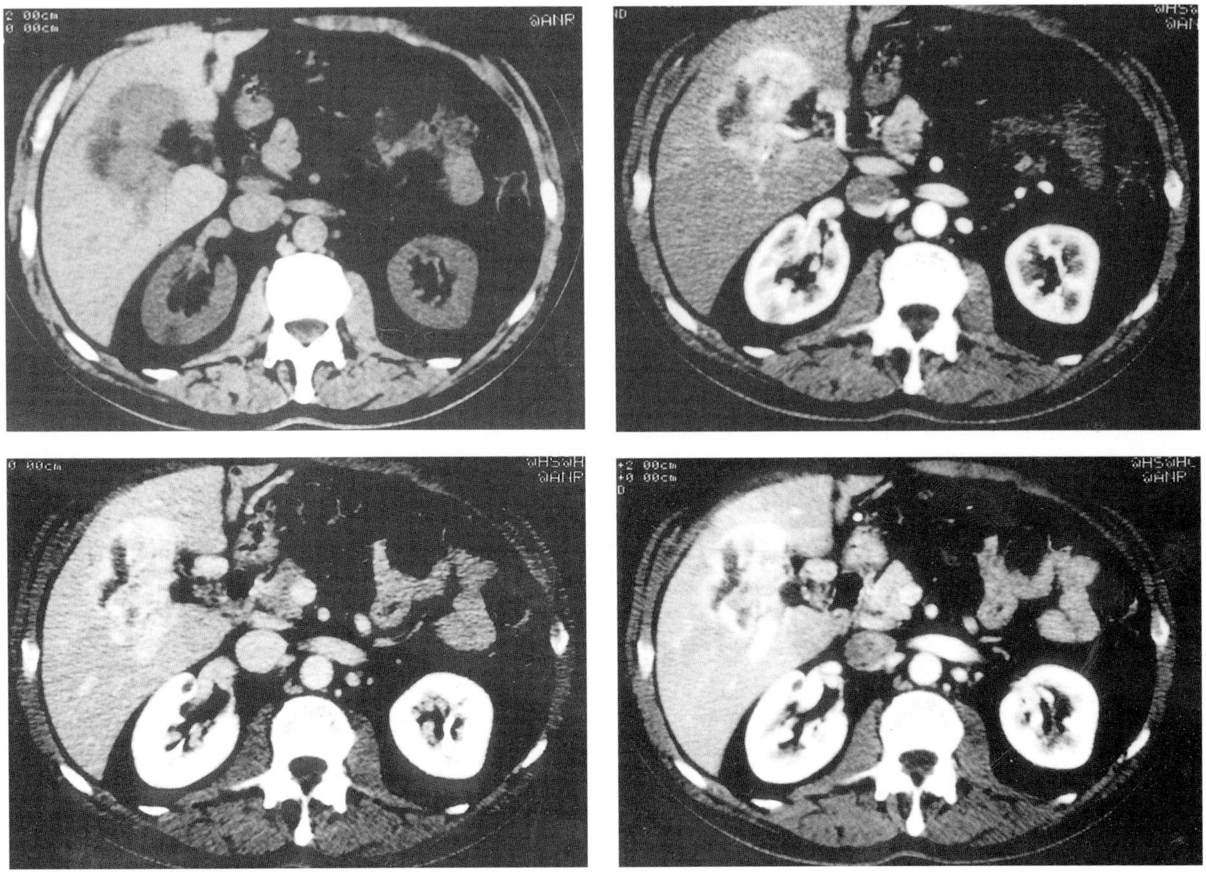

a b c d

Fig. 9.2a–d. Intrahepatic cholangiocarcinoma: CT. Unenhanced CT (**a**) shows an hypodense focal liver mass in the V–VI segment. A peripheral hypodense area is observed adjacent to the gallbladder (**b**). Because of its hypovascular nature, cholangiocarcinoma shows a peripheral incomplete rim-like contrast enhancement, during the arterial phase with progressive filling in with contrast medium during the portal venous (**c**) and equilibrium phase (**d**)

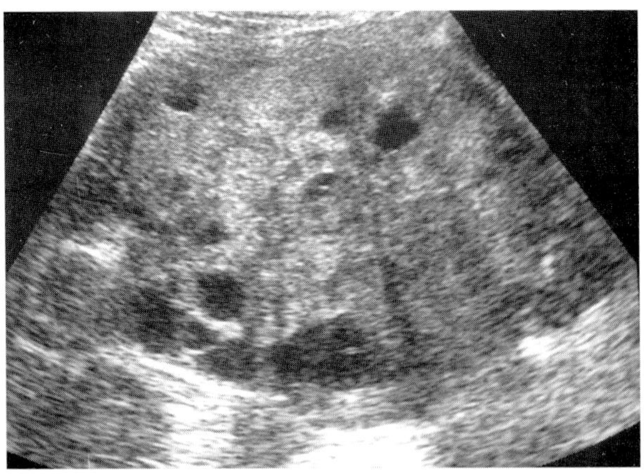

Fig. 9.3. Intrahepatic cholangiocarcinoma with microcystic changes: ultrasound. Sonography shows a large cholangiocarcinoma that appears hyperechoic, with hypoechoic central areas due to necrosis

(Fig. 9.2). Calcification may be seen, in the central portion of the lesions, on unenhanced CT scan, in mucin-secreting cholangiocarcinomas. The most common pattern of contrast enhancement in peripheral cholangiocarcinoma is that of a peripheral area of thin, mild, incomplete, rimlike contrast enhancement on CT scans obtained at both the hepatic arterial and portal venous phase (Fig. 9.2) (Kim et al. 1997).

The distinctive intratumoral appearance of peripheral cholangiocarcinoma on two-phase spiral CT scans is that of markedly low attenuation mixed with amorphous areas of slightly high attenuation during both the arterial and portal venous phase (Fig. 9.2) (Kim et al. 1997). The areas of marked low attenuation in peripheral cholangiocarcinoma corresponded to diffuse, microcystic changes of necrosis of the comedo type (Fig. 9.3).

The areas of slightly high attenuation in the masses probably correspond to mucinous sub-

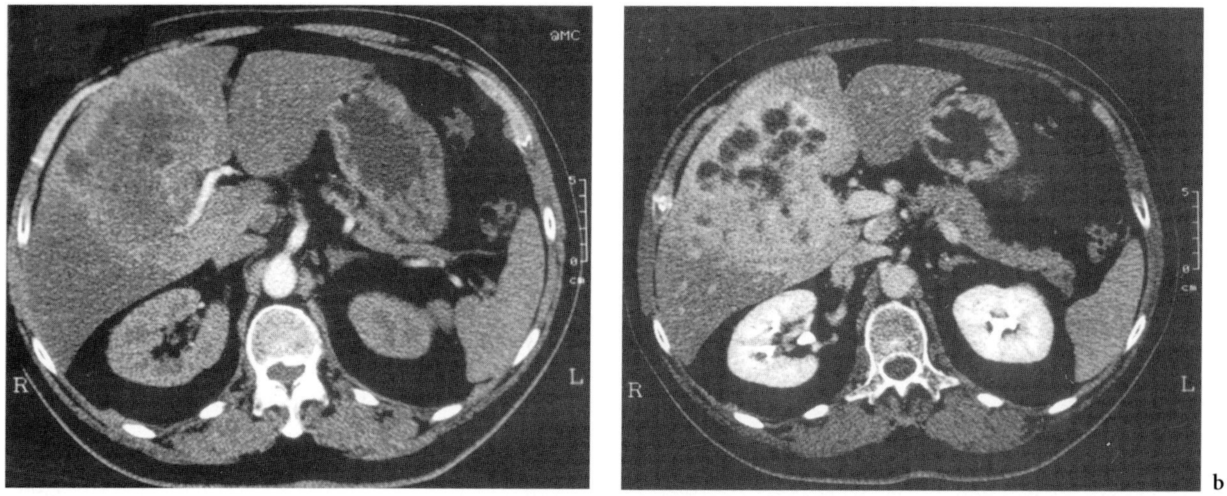

Fig. 9.4a,b. Intrahepatic cholangiocarcinoma with microcystic changes: CT (same patient as in Fig. 9.3). **a** Dynamic CT scan during the arterial phase show a mild peripheral rim-like contrast enhancement. **b** CT scan during the equilibrium phase shows central low density areas due to microcystic changes of necrosis

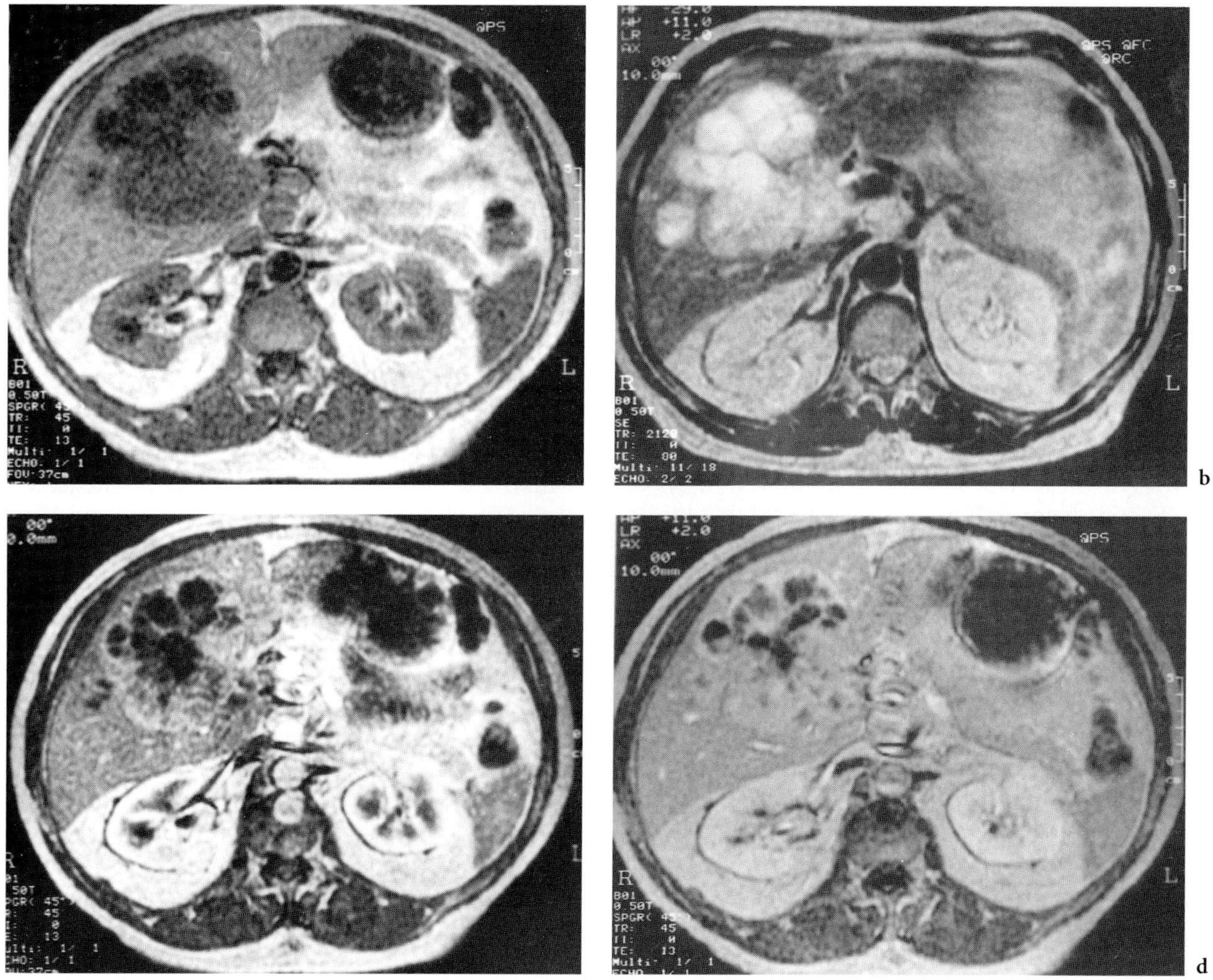

Fig. 9.5a–d. MR imaging of intrahepatic mucin producing cholangiocarcinoma (same patient as in Figs. 9.3 and 9.4). **a** Axial T1-weighted images show a hypointense lesion in the right hepatic lobe. On T2-weighted images (**b**) the lesion appears hyperintense, with cystic hyperintense areas due to mucin production. These areas do not show any enhancement following contrast medium injection (**c,d**)

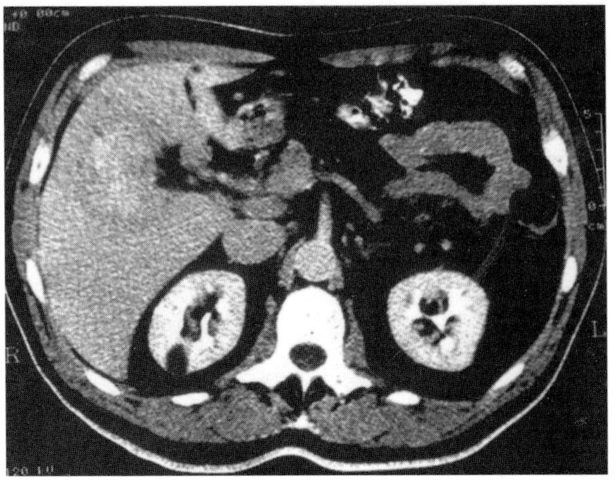

Fig. 9.6. Intrahepatic cholangiocarcinoma: delayed CT scan. Cholangiocarcinoma appears slightly hyperdense compared to adjacent liver parenchyma

stances within those masses, which may be nicely depicted by either CT (Fig. 9.4) or MR imaging (Fig. 9.5) (Kim et al. 1997).

Intrahepatic cholangiocarcinomas show an enhancement greater than that of normal liver parenchyma, on post-equilibrium-phase contrast enhanced images (Fig. 9.6). This occurs in 74% of the patients undergoing delayed imaging (Lacomis et al. 1997). Delayed imaging is therefore useful in detecting intrahepatic cholangiocarcinoma nodules, differentiating them from dilated bile ducts or fatty infiltration of the liver, and better defining tumor margins.

In addition, although not necessary for diagnosis, delayed enhancement can be helpful as a target for CT-guided biopsy. It has been suggested that the delayed enhancement characteristics of cholangiocarcinoma may be due to contrast material retention within the fibrous stroma inherent within these tumors (Takayasu et al. 1990; Honda et al. 1993).

Besides fibrosis, other factors affect the delayed enhancement: distribution of fibrosis (Lacomis et al. 1997), tumor grading, and better differentiated tumors are more likely to show delayed contrast material retention than poorly differentiated ones (Lacomis et al. 1997).

The contrast enhancement pattern of cholangiocarcinoma differs from that of hepatocellular carcinoma or other hypervascular tumors, which most commonly have predominantly high attenuation during the hepatic arterial phase and isoattenuation or low attenuation during the portal venous phase (Oliver et al. 1996). Furthermore, most cholangiocarcinomas occur in non-cirrhotic livers, frequently cause bile duct dilatation, do not have a pseudocapsule, may have intratumoral calcification, and rarely show vessel invasion. Extension through the hepatic capsule and invasion of organs adjacent to the liver is common in intrahepatic cholangiocarcinoma, but rare in hepatocellular carcinoma. The invasion of vascular structures around the liver is rare in cholangiocarcinoma. All these criteria are helpful for the differential diagnosis between cholangiocarcinoma and hepatocellular carcinoma, which represent the two most common primary liver neoplasms (Table 9.2).

Hypovascular metastases, especially from adenocarcinoma of the gastrointestinal tract, may have a pattern similar to that of peripheral cholangiocarcinoma and the differential diagnosis can be very difficult (Choi et al. 1995). Clues for the differential diagnosis between metastases and intrahepatic cholangiocarcinoma are unknown primary tumor, a relatively large tumor size, and other ancillary findings such as segmentary or subsegmentary bile duct dilatation, and retraction of liver capsule (Kim et al. 1997).

Sometimes, a papillary intrahepatic cholangiocarcinoma produces abundant mucin that may calcify, resulting in a well-marginated cystic mass that resembles biliary cystoadenocarcinoma. The mucin may also obstruct the duct lumen distal to the carcinoma (Itai et al. 1983).

9.4.1.3 MR Imaging

The MR imaging appearance of cholangiocarcinoma is that of a non-capsulated tumor, hypointense on T1-weighted images and hyperintense on T2-weighted images (Fig. 9.7). The signal intensity of the tumor is variable according to the amount of fibrosis, necrosis, and mucinous material within the tumor. Central hypointensity may be seen on T2-weighted images, corresponding to fibrosis (central scar). Importantly, a central scar can be a reliable feature for differentiating primary liver neoplasm from metastases on MR imaging evaluation (Ishak et al. 1984; Rummeny et al. 1989). Mucinous cholangiocarcinoma is one of the subtypes of cholangiocarcinomas, according to predominant features, and can be extremely hypointense on T1-weighted images and hyperintense on T2-weighted images, due to large mucinous lakes within the tumor.

On dynamic MR imaging studies the size of the tumor influences the enhancement pattern. Small tumors (2–4 cm) may enhance homogeneously and

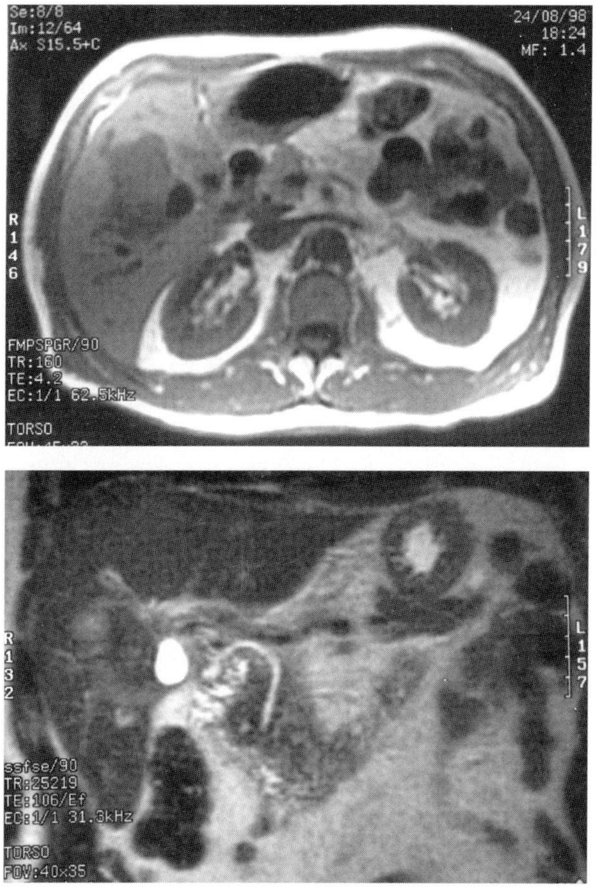

a

b

Fig. 9.7a,b. Intrahepatic cholangiocarcinoma: MR imaging (same patient as in Fig. 9.6). Cholangiocarcinoma appears hypointense on axial T1-weighted MR images (**a**) and hyperintense with a central hypointense area on coronal T2-weighted images. A peripheral hyperintense cyst can also be observed

simulate an hepatocellular carcinoma (ADJEI et al. 1995); in larger tumors, minimal to moderate peripheral enhancement is evident followed by progressive and concentric filling in the tumor with contrast material (Fig. 9.8) (SOYER et al. 1995). Pooling of contrast within the tumor on delayed MR images can be a finding suggestive of the diagnosis of peripheral cholangiocarcinoma; however, incomplete central filling is also noted on delayed images. This characteristic enhancement pattern may reflect the a large amount of fibrous tissue and neovascularity at the periphery of the lesion.

The central scar may enhance with gadolinium on delayed images, but becomes isointense with the tumor rather than hyperintense as is seen in focal nodular hyperplasia (SOYER et al. 1995).

Although some authors have stressed that the portal and hepatic veins are not commonly invaded

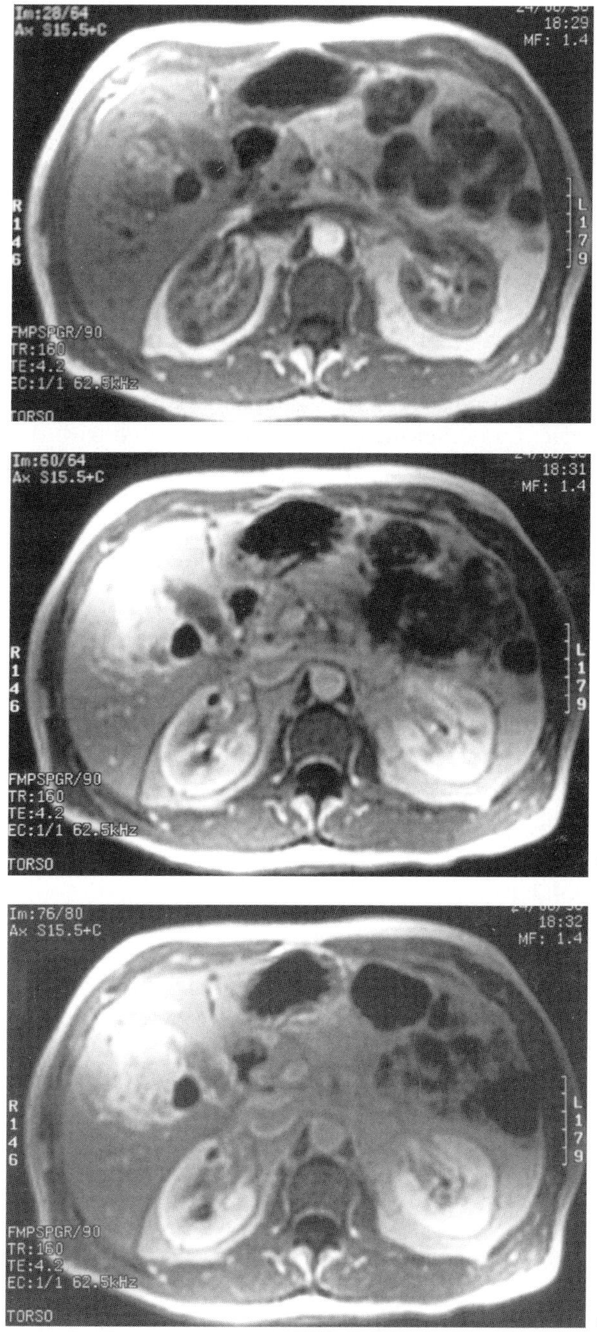

a

b

c

Fig. 9.8a–c. Dynamic MR imaging (same patient as in Figs. 9.6 and 9.7). The cholangiocarcinoma appears hypovascular compared to adjacent liver parenchyma, with a moderate peripheral enhancement during the arterial phase (**a**); with progressive and concentric filling of contrast material during the portal venous (**b**) and equilibrium (**c**) phase

and make this a differentiating point from hepatocellular carcinoma (ROS 1988), most authors believe the portal vein is commonly involved with tumor and emphasize the role of MR imaging in this field

(Soyer et al. 1995; Sugihara and Kojiro 1987; Tani et al. 1991). Dilatation of the peripheral portion of the intrahepatic biliary ducts is occasionally seen in peripheral cholangiocarcinomas, especially in patients associated with clonorchiasis (Choi et al. 1998).

9.4.1.4 Angiography

Angiographically, intrahepatic cholangiocarcinoma is predominantly hypovascular, thin vessels corresponding to the fibrous nature of its tumor (Fig. 9.9) (Kaude and Rian 1971). Encasement of hepatic arteries and other major vessels is associated with the degree of sclerosis resulting from the tumor.

9.4.2 Hilar Cholangiocarcinoma

Cholangiocarcinoma most often occurs at the confluence of the right and left bile duct and the proximal common hepatic duct (Fig. 9.10) (Bismuth and Malt 1979). These so-called Klatskin's tumors are usually scirrhous and cause almost invariably biliary dilatation (Klatskin 1965).

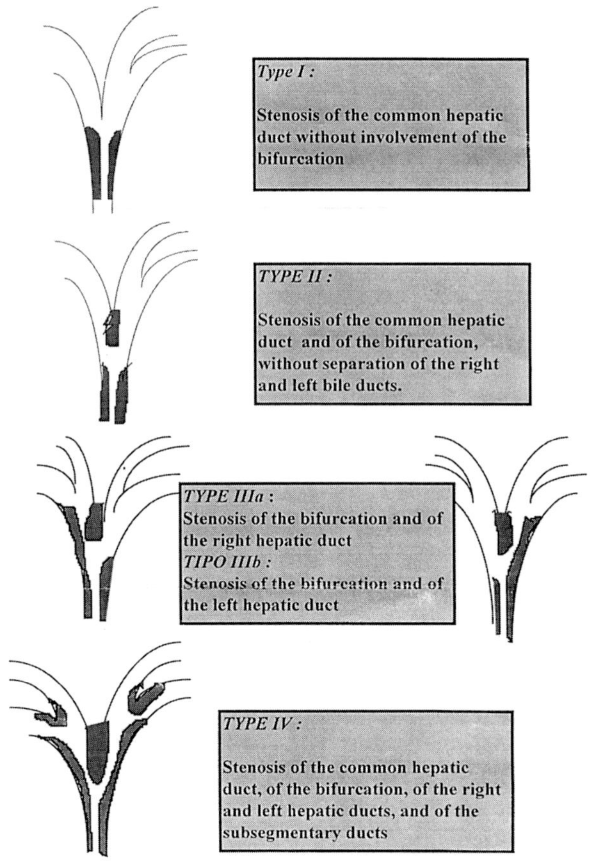

Fig. 9.10. Scheme representing the location of hilar cholangiocarcinoma

9.4.2.1 Ultrasound

Klatskin's tumor has a variable morphology that can be categorized as nodular, infiltrative or polypoid, according to the pathologic classification (Adam and Benjamin 1992). Nodular mural thickening is the most frequent finding (56%) evident as discrete, usually smooth masses with associated mural thickening. Infiltrative lesions are second in frequency (26%): they locally spread in the periductal tissue and cause the ducts to become irregular in caliber. The focal irregularity of the involved ducts can be used to establish the sonographic diagnosis of infiltrative Klatskin's tumor (Fig. 9.11) (Hann et al. 1997). The polypoid variety (18%) is most easily recognized because of its intraluminal growth that causes expansion of the ducts (Hann et al. 1997).

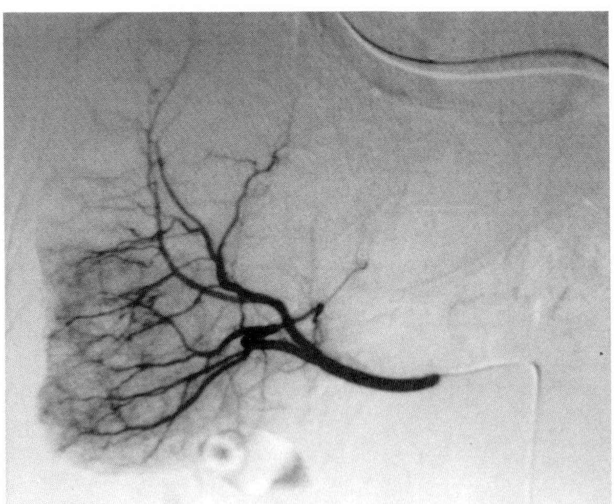

Fig. 9.9. Intrahepatic cholangiocarcinoma: selective digital subtraction angiography of the hepatic artery. Angiography of the VI hepatic segment, with neoformed circulation, without arterio-venous shunts, and with initial tumor stain

The sonographic appearance of Klatskin's tumor includes duct dilatation, isolation of the right and left bile duct segments, mass or bile duct wall thickening at the hilus, and lobar atrophy with crowded, dilated ducts (Fig. 9.11). Biliary duct dilatation is almost invariably present in Klatskin's tumor, and can be a useful sign in the differential diagnosis with other hepatic tumors.

Ultrasound is accurate for revealing the level of bile duct obstruction but it shows a mass only in 21–

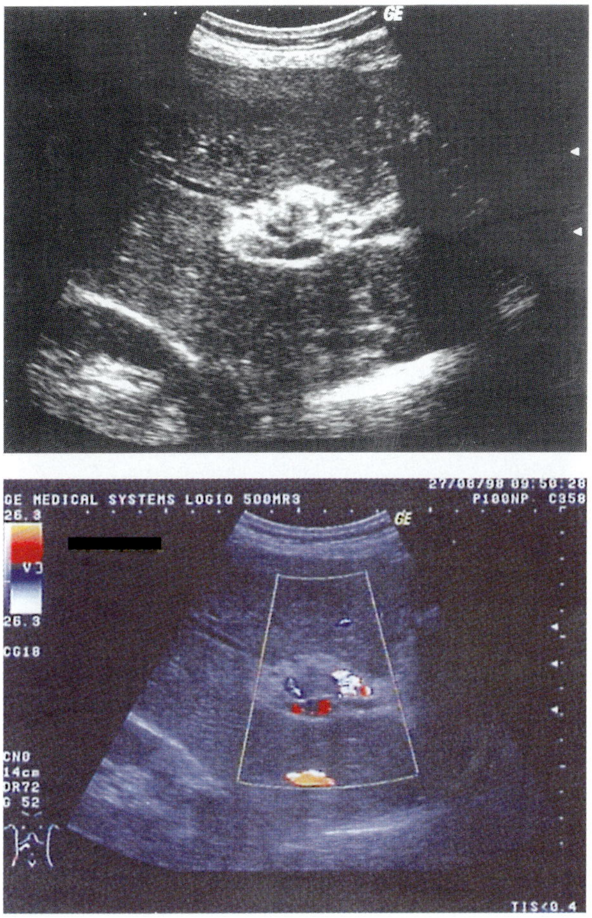

Fig. 9.11a,b. Hilar cholangiocarcinoma (Klatskin's tumor): ultrasound. **a** Sonography shows an isoechoic mass at confluence of the right and left hepatic ducts, with bile duct dilatation. **b** Doppler ultrasound shows patency of the portal bifurcation

74% of patients (Nesbit et al. 1988; Kokubo et al. 1988; Itai et al. 1983; Nichols et al. 1983; Choi et al. 1989; Garber et al. 1983). When a mass is seen, it is most often small, poorly defined and isoechoic to hepatic parenchyma in 50–65% of cases, and the bile duct wall underlying the mass is poorly defined (Fig. 9.11) (Looser et al. 1992; Hann et al. 1997). These features are a reflection of the submucosal growth of the neoplasm.

Sonography is, however, unable to evaluate the real extension of the neoplasm in the underlying hepatic parenchyma, because of the ill-defined margins of the tumor, resulting most often in an underestimation of the hepatic parenchyma infiltration by Klatskin's tumor (Fig. 9.12).

Because the location at the hilus is critical, these tumors may produce biliary obstruction while the

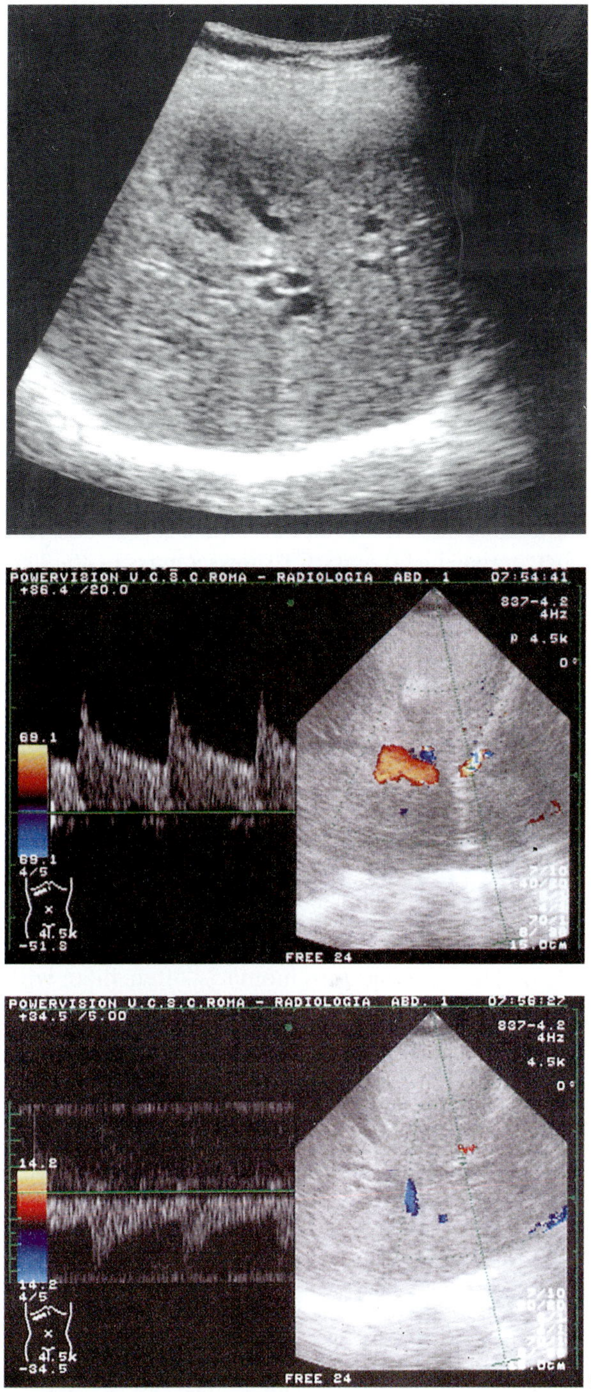

Fig. 9.12a–c. Hilar cholangiocarcinoma (Klatskin's tumor): ultrasound. **a** Infiltrative Klastkin's tumor; the mass is not directly visualized but there is the dilatation of the intrahepatic bile ducts with separation of the right and left hepatic ducts. Color Doppler ultrasound shows patency of the right portal vein (**b**) and thrombosis of the left portal vein with hypertrophy of the left hepatic artery (**c**)

tumor is still small. However, tumors confined to one lobe may present at a later stage because unilateral obstruction may not lead to clinical jaundice. When the lobar atrophy is seen, sonograms show crowded and dilated ducts within the atrophic lobe.

Portal vein involvement is present in 41–63% of cases (Hann et al. 1997; Looser et al. 1992). The high frequency of portal vein involvement reflects the locally infiltrative pattern of spread that is seen in Klatskin's tumors. Color Doppler ultrasound is able to define portal vein involvement, whereas it is not helpful in characterizing tumor mass.

9.4.2.2 Computed Tomography

CT is more sensitive than ultrasound in detecting an obstructive ductal mass. CT shows a mass in 40–90% of hilar cholangiocarcinomas. The mass is usually small and hypodense to the surrounding normal liver parenchyma on unenhanced scans (Fahim et al. 1962; Bloustein 1977; Nesbit et al. 1988; Choi et al. 1988). Some tumors become hyperdense during dynamic scanning (Fig. 9.13); others show tumor enhancement 8–15 min after the contrast medium injection (Takayasu et al. 1990).

Lobar hepatic atrophy with marked dilatation and crowding of bile ducts is seen on CT scans in approximately one-fourth of patients with hilar cholangiocarcinoma (Nesbit et al. 1988; Carr et al. 1985). The cholangiocarcinoma is often hilar with dominant involvement of the duct supplying the atrophied segment. Lobar atrophy with biliary dilatation strongly suggests the diagnosis of cholangiocarcinoma, although long-standing biliary obstruction from surgical trauma or focal biliary obstruction can cause similar findings (Vazquez et al. 1985; Walter et al. 1976).

The liver parenchyma and hepato-duodenal ligament are commonly invaded in Klatskin's tumor, appearing as dense masses in the hypodense tissue of the ligament.

Lymphatic metastases most commonly involve the porta-caval, superior and posterior pancreaticoduodenal lymph nodes. Retroperitoneal lymphadenopathy, peritoneal spread, and proximal intestinal obstruction occur in advanced stages of hilar cholangiocarcinoma. Both CT and ultrasound tend to understage hilar cholangiocarcinoma, as local tumor extension, peritoneal spread, and metastases in normal sized lymph nodes may not be appreciated.

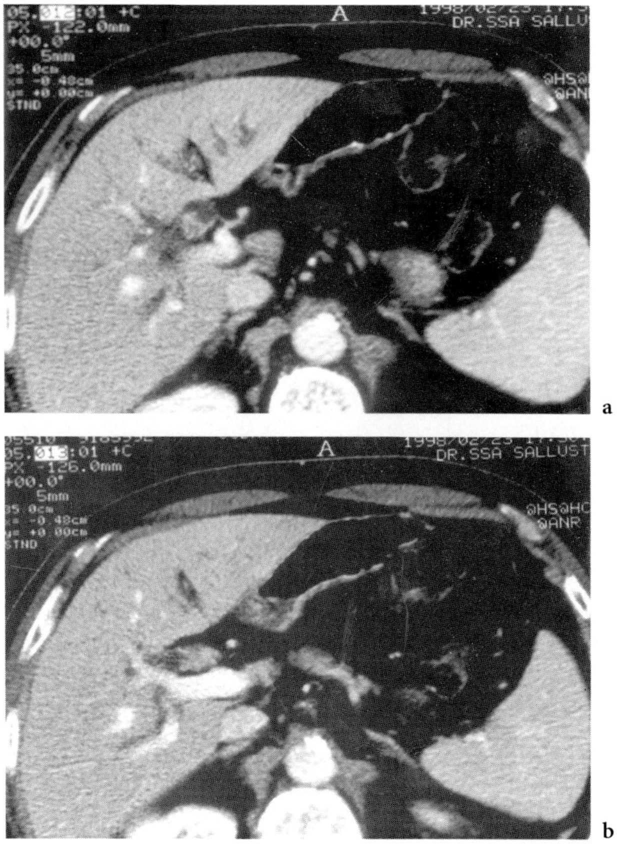

Fig. 9.13a,b. Hilar cholangiocarcinoma: CT. **a** CT scan during the portal venous phase shows a dilatation of the common hepatic duct, with thickening of the posterior wall of the duct. **b** In the CT scan caudad to **a** there is a complete filling of the ductal lumen by the mass

9.4.2.3 MR imaging

On MR images, Klatskin's tumors are often small in size (<5 cm) at presentation with prominent ductal dilatation. The lesion appears hypointense to the liver on T1-weighted images and with high signal intensity on T2-weighted images (Fig. 9.14).

Hilar cholangiocarcinomas are typically hypovascular tumors and show an enhancement pattern that differs from that of intrahepatic cholangiocarcinoma. The peripheral enhancement with progressive concentric filling, typical of peripheral cholangiocarcinoma, is rarely seen in hilar cholangiocarcinoma.

The enhancement pattern of hilar cholangiocarcinoma is varied: some tumors show immediate diffuse enhancement with retention of contrast material on delayed images (Fig. 9.14); others show periductal enhancement. There is a small percentage

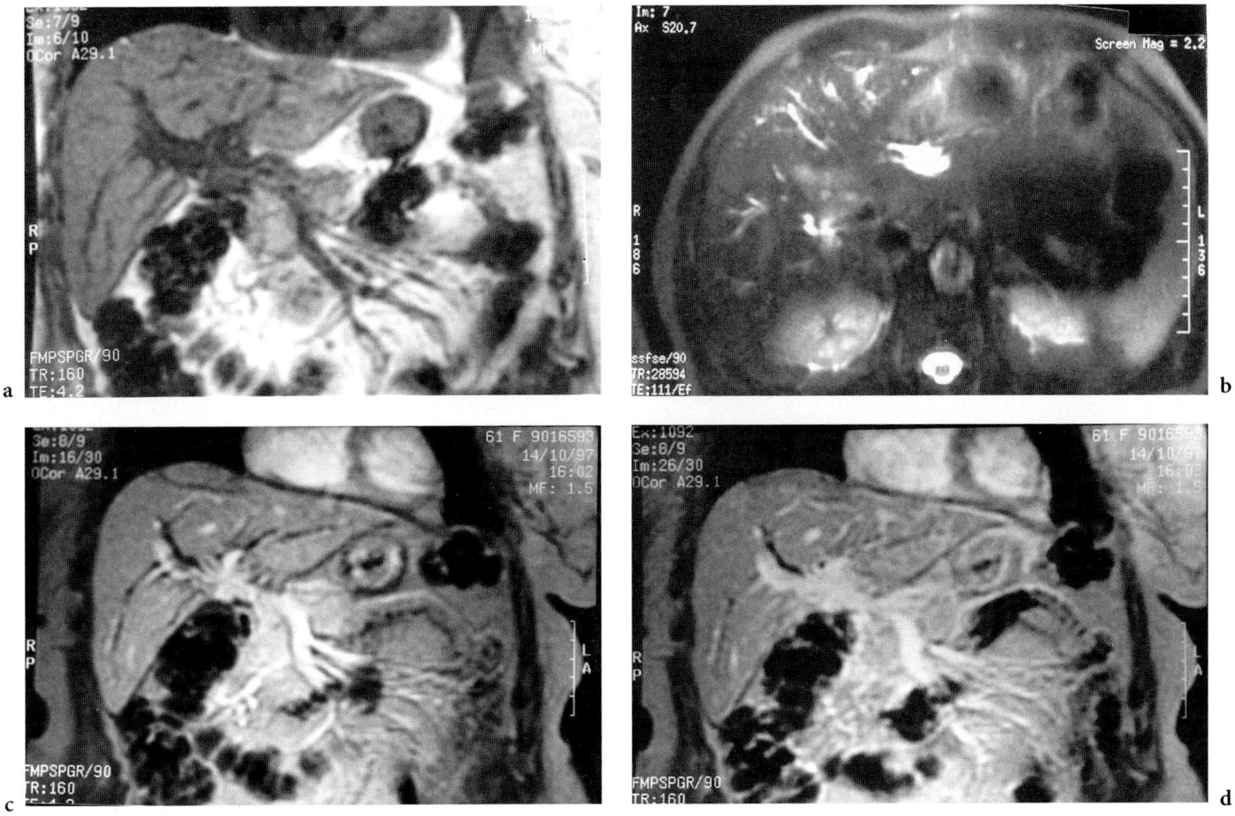

Fig. 9.14a–d. Hilar cholangiocarcinoma: MR imaging. **a** Coronal oblique T1-weighted image shows a hypointense mass at the hepatic hilum. **b** Axial T2-weighted image shows a hyperintense mass at the hepatic hilum. **c** On the coronal oblique plane, during the portal venous phase of the dynamic study, the mass enhances, and dilated intrahepatic biliary are easily differentiated from intrahepatic vessels. **d** Hilar cholangiocarcinoma retains contrast material on the delayed scan

of hypervascular hilar cholangiocarcinomas; however, the immediate diffuse enhancement seen with other hypervascular liver lesions is rarely seen (Guthrie et al. 1996).

Increased signal intensity in hepatic parenchyma in areas of ductal dilatation on unenhanced T1-weighted images is reported, but the etiology of this signal intensity change remains unclear (Choi et al. 1998).

The central scar is an unusual feature of the hilar cholangiocarcinoma, differently to what happens in the peripheral type.

Satellite nodules are less commonly seen in hilar cholangiocarcinoma, compared to intrahepatic cholangiocarcinoma, which is in keeping with the much earlier manifestation of lesion situated at the hilum (Whithey et al. 1993; Ros 1988).

Intraluminal projection associated with a mass lesion can be seen in patients with hilar cholangiocarcinoma and these intraluminal filling defects are usually larger than 1 cm (McCarthy et al. 1985). Dynamic imaging in the coronal oblique plane is particularly useful for distinguishing vessels from bile ducts and for demonstrating intraluminal extension of a tumor.

Recently MR cholangiography (MRCP), used in conjunction with MR imaging, has been introduced to evaluate the extent of the tumor in the bile ducts. MRCP with half Fourier techniques can produce excellent cholangiographic imaging. With this technique, hilar obstruction and subsequent dilatation of separated bile ducts can be easily diagnosed (Fig. 9.15). MRCP has advantages over direct cholangiographies, including non-invasiveness, and possible visualization of isolated bile ducts. However, the spatial resolution of MRCP seems to be still inferior to endoscopic retrograde cholangiography. Therefore MRCP has become recognized as an accurate and noninvasive alternative to endoscopic retrograde cholangiography in the evaluation of suspected hilar cholangiocarcinoma (Fulcher and Turner 1997).

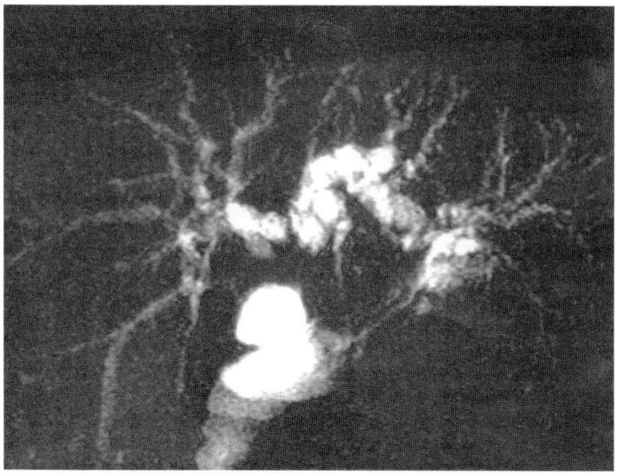

Fig. 9.15. Hilar cholangiocarcinoma: MR cholangiography (MRCP) acquired in the coronal oblique plane shows a filling defect in the proximal common hepatic duct, involving the confluence of the right and left hepatic ducts, and dilatation of the intrahepatic bile ducts

MRCP permits visualization of the ductal irregularity and narrowing characteristics of hilar cholangiocarcinoma and more accurately allows determination of the extent of proximal disease, in association with cross-sectional imaging that evaluates parenchymal invasion, leading to a greater accuracy to preoperative staging.

Preoperative assessment of resectability in cholangiocarcinoma typically requires the use of angiography to determine vessel involvement. Dynamic contrast enhanced MR imaging is comparable to angiography in the assessment of the portal vasculature in patients with cholangiocarcinoma (Guthrie et al. 1996). The coronal oblique plane is especially useful for showing the relationship of the lesion to the portal veins, because the whole of the portal veins are typically seen on one or two sections, hilar lesions are more easily localized, and the coronal anatomy is similar to that seen on surgery.

9.4.2.4 Direct Cholangiographic Techniques

Cholangiography defines the presence and in part the extent of hilar cholangiocarcinoma. The cholangiographic appearance of cholangiocarcinoma reflects its name: focal stenotic or infiltrating stenotic; although its appearance is variable. Klatskin's tumor appears as a ductal stenosis of the right and left and common hepatic ducts, with smooth shoulders or irregular tapering ducts. It is usually 1–3 cm in length but may be longer, as it encompasses most of the extrahepatic duct or invades the liver. The contour may be smooth or moderately irregular. These neoplastic strictures tend to branch and may extend into the secondary order biliary radicles. Isolation of segments of bile ducts is common. Cholangiography often underestimates the extent of submucosal spread of cholangiocarcinoma.

The peripheral cholangiocarcinoma gives the intrahepatic ducts an encased or scalloped appearance. The smooth, variable length stricture affects adjacent ducts within the same hepatic territory. This appearance is usually not mistaken for the peripherally invading Klatskin tumor, but care is required not to interpret these findings as sclerosing cholangitis.

Although the description of the three types of cholangiocarcinoma appears straightforward, at times the cholangiographic differentiation may be difficult – especially between focal stenosis and papillary lesions. Polypoid cholangiocarcinoma, when small, is visualized as a sessile papillary excrescence protruding into the duct lumen. However, when the polypoid lesion grows, at the expense of the bile duct lumen, there is slow progress toward the near-total obstruction of the lumen. In this case the contrast medium is able to define only the rounded surface interface, causing a cap or meniscus. making the exact origin of the mass difficult to define.

Furthermore, hilar cholangiocarcinoma should be differentiated cholangiographically from extrinsic strictures (lymphadenopathy) and benign intrinsic strictures. Lymphadenopathy compresses and displaces rather than invades the extrahepatic ducts. Benign strictures almost invariably occur after cholecystectomy or distal gastric surgery, are short, and cause symmetric narrowing of the common hepatic bile duct. Rarely are lymphoma or sarcoidosis of the bile ducts indistinguishable from cholangiocarcinoma (Tartar and Balfe 1990).

Direct cholangiographies are able to combine diagnostic capabilities with therapeutic ones; therefore they should be performed in the work-up of patients with suspected cholangiocarcinoma, either to evaluate the extension of neoplasm before surgical intervention, or to perform palliative treatment.

References

Adam A, Benjamin IS (1992) The staging of cholangiocarcinoma. Clin Radiol 46:299–303

Adjei ON, Tamura S, Sugimara H, et al (1995) Contrast enhanced MR imaging of intrahepatic cholangiocarcinoma. Clin Radiol 50:6–10

Bismuth H, Malt RA (1979) Current concepts in cancer: carcinoma of the biliary tract. New Engl J Med 301:704–706

Bloustein PA (1977) Association of carcinoma with congenital cystic conditions of the liver and bile ducts. Am J Gastroenterol 67:40–46

Boring CC, Squires TS, Tong T (1993) Cancer statistics, 1993. Cancer 43:7–23

Carr DH, Hadjis NS, Banks LM, et al (1985) Computed tomography of hilar cholangiocarcinoma: a new sign. AJR 145:53–56

Choi BI, Park JH, Furui S, Yashiro N, Ohtomo K, Ilio M (1988) Computed tomography of primary intrahepatic biliary malignancy. Radiology 169:149–153

Choi Bl, Lee JH, Han MC, et al (1989) Hilar cholangiocarcinoma: comparative study with sonography and CT. Radiology 172:689–692

Choi BI, Han JK, Cho JM et al (1995) Characterization of focal hepatic tumors: value of two-phase scanning with spiral computed tomography. Cancer 76:2434–2442

Choi BI, Kim TK, Han JK (1998) MRI imaging of clonorchiasis and cholangiocarcinoma. JMRI 8:359–366

Craig JR, Peters RL, Edmondson HA (1989) Tumors of the liver and intrahepatic bile ducts. Fascicle 26, 2nd series. Washington DC, Armed Forces Institute of Pathology, pp 123–222

Cruickshank AH (1961) The pathology of 111 cases of primary hepatic malignancy collected in the Liverpool region. J Clin Pathol 14:120–131

Edmondson HA, Steiner PE (1954) Primary carcinoma of the liver: a study of 100 cases among 48,900 necropsies. Cancer 7:462–503

Fahim RB, McDonald JR, Richards JC (1962) Carcinoma of the gallbladder: a study of its modes of spread. Ann Surg 156:114–124

Fulcher AS, Turner MA (1997) HASTE MR cholangiography in the evaluation of hilar cholangiocarcinoma. AJR 169:1501–1505

Garber SJ, Donald JJ, Lees WR (1983) Cholangiocarcinoma: ultrasound features and correlation with survival. Abdom Imaging 18:66–69

Guthrie JA, Ward J, Robinson PJ (1996) Hilar cholangiocarcinoma: T2-weighted spin-echo and gadolinium enhanced FLASH MR imaging. Radiology 201:347–351

Hann LE, Greatrex KV, Bach AM, Fong Y, Blumgart LH (1997) Cholangiocarcinoma at the hepatic hilus: sonographic findings. AJR 168:985–989

Honda H, Onitsuka H, Yasumori K, et al (1993) Intrahepatic peripheral cholangiocarcinoma: two-phased dynamic incremental CT and pathologic correlation. J Comput Assist Tomogr 17:397–402

Hoyne RM, Kernohan JW (1947) Primary carcinoma of the liver: a study of 31 cases. Arch Intern Med 79:532–554

Ishak KG, Sesterhenn IA, Goodman ZD, et al (1984) Epithelioid hemangioendothelioma of the liver: A clinicopathologic and follow-up study of 32 cases. Hum Pathol 15:839–852

Itai Y, Araki T, Furui S, et al (1983) Computed tomography of primary intrahepatic biliary malignancy. Radiology 147:485–490

Kaude J, Rian R (1971) Cholangiocarcinoma. Radiology 100:573–580

Kim TK, Choi BI, Han JK, et al (1997) Peripheral cholangiocarcinoma of the liver: two-phase spiral CT findings. Radiology 204:539–543

Klatskin G (1965) Adenocarcinoma of the hepatic duct at its bifurcation within the porta hepatis: an unusual tumor with distinctive clinical and pathological features. Am J Med 38:241–256

Kokubo T, Itai Y, Ohtomo K, et al (1988) Mucin-hypersecreting intrahepatic biliary neoplasms. Radiology 168:609–614

Lacomis JM, Baron RL, Oliver JH, Nalesnik MA, Federle MP (1997) Cholangiocarcinoma: delayed CT contrast enhancement patterns. Radiology 203:98–104

Looser C, Stain SL, Baer HU, Triller J, Blumgart LH (1992) Staging of hilar cholangiocarcinoima by ultrasound and duplex sonography: a comparison with angiography and operative findings. Br J Radiol 65:871–877

MacDonald RA (1956) Cirrhosis and primary carcinoma of the liver: changes in their occurrence at the Boston City Hospital 1897–1954. New Engl J Med 255:1179–1183

McCarthy RL, LaRusso NF, May GR, et al (1985) Cholangiocarcinoma complicating primary sclerosing cholangitis: cholangiographic appearances. Radiology 156:43–46

Mori W (1967) Cirrhosis and primary cancer of the liver-comparative study in Tokyo and Cincinnati. Cancer 20:627–631

Nesbit GM, Johnson CD, James EM, et al (1988) Cholangiocarcinoma: diagnosis and evaluation of resectability by CT and sonography as procedures complementary to cholangiography. AJR 151:933–938

Nichols DA, MacCarty RL, Gaffey TA (1983) Cholangiographic evaluation of bile duct carcinoma. AJR 141:1291–1294

Okuda K, Kubo Y. Okazaki N, et al (1977) Clinical aspects of intrahepatic bile duct carcinoma including hilar carcinoma: a study of 57 autopsy-proven cases. Cancer 39:232–246

Oliver JH, Baron RL, Federle MP, Rockette HP (1996) Detecting hepatocellular carcinoma: the relative added value of using noncontrast and/or arterial phase imaging in conjunction with conventional portal venous phase contrast CT. AJR 167:71–77

Patton RB, Horn RC Jr (1964) Primary liver carcinoma. Autopsy study of 60 cases. Cancer 17:757–768

Ros PR, Buck JL, Comdr LT, Goodman ZD, et al (1988) Intrahepatic cholangiocarcinoma: radiology-Pathologic Correlation. Radiology 167:689–693

Rummeny E, Weissleder R, Stark DD, et al (1989) Primary liver tumors: diagnosis by MR imaging. AJR 152:63–72

San Jose D, Cady A, West M, et al (1965) Primary carcinoma of the liver, analysis of clinical and biochemical features of 80 cases. Am J Dig Dis 10:657–673

Saul SH (1994) Masses of the liver. In: Stemberg SS (ed) Diagnostic Surgical Pathology, 2nd edn. Raven Press, New York, pp 1543–1545

Soyer PA, Bluemke DA, Sibert A, et al (1995) MR imaging of intrahepatic cholangiocarcinoma. Abdom Imaging 20:126–130

Sugihara S, Kojiro M (1987) Pathology of cholangiocarcinoma. In: Nakashima T, Kojiro M (eds) Hepatocellular Carcinoma: an atlas of its pathology. Springer Verlag, Tokyo, pp 191–211

Takayasu K, lkeya S, Mukai K, et al (1990) CT of hilar

cholangiocarcinoma: late contrast enhancement in six patients. AJR 154:1203–1206
Tani K, Kubota Y, Yamaguchi T, et al (1991) MR imaging of peripheral cholangiocarcinoma. J Comput Assist Tomogr 15:975–978
Tartar VM, Balfe DM (1990) Lymphoma in the wall of the bile ducts: radiologic imaging. Gastrointest Radiol 15:53–57
Thorsen MK, Quiroz F, Lawson TL, et al (1984) Primary biliary carcinoma: CT evaluation. Radiology 152:479–483
Vazquez JL, Thorsen MK, Dodds WJ, et al (1985) Atrophy of the left hepatic lobe caused by a cholangiocarcinoma. AJR 144:547–548
Walter JF, Bookstein JJ, Bouffard EV (1976) Newer angiographic observations in cholangiocarcinoma. Radiology 118:19–23
Whithey WS, Herfkens RJ, Brooke JR et al (1993) Dynamic breathhold multiplanar spoiled gradient-recalled MR imaging with gadolinium enhancement for differentiating hepatic hemangiomas from malignancy at 1.5 T. Radiology 189:863–870

10 Rare Primary Malignancies of the Liver

R. Manfredi, G. Maresca, A.R. Cotroneo, A.M. De Gaetano, and P. Marano

CONTENTS

10.1 Introduction

Primary malignant neoplasms of the liver are classified by the cell of origin (Table 10.1). In this chapter, primary malignant liver tumors are discussed: hepatoblastoma, arising from hepatocytes; cystoadenoma and cystoadenocarcinoma, arising from biliary cells; epithelioid hemangioendothelioma, angiosarcoma and other mesenchymal sarcomas, arising from mesenchymal tissue; and finally primary lymphoma, arising from lymphomatous tissue.

Table 10.1. Malignant liver tumors

Hepatocellular origin
Hepatocellular carcinoma
Fibrolamellar carcinoma
Hepatoblastoma
Cholangiocellular origin
Cholangiocarcinoma
Cystoadenocarcinoma
Mesenchymal origin
Angiosarcoma
Epithelioid hemangioendothelioma
Leiomyosarcoma
Fibrosarcoma
Malignant fibrous histiocytoma
Primary lymphoma

R. Manfredi, MD; Department of Radiology, A. Gemelli University Hospital, Largo A. Gemelli 8, I-00168 Rome, Italy
G. Maresca, MD; Professor, Department of Radiology, A. Gemelli University Hospital, Largo A. Gemelli 8, I-00168 Rome, Italy
A.R. Cotroneo, MD; Professor, Department of Radiology, A. Gemelli University Hospital, Largo A. Gemelli 8, I-00168 Rome, Italy
A.M. De Gaetano, MD; Department of Radiology, A. Gemelli University Hospital, Largo A. Gemelli 8, I-00168 Rome, Italy
P. Marano, MD; Professor and Chairman, Department of Radiology, A. Gemelli University Hospital, Largo A. Gemelli 8, I-00168 Rome, Italy

10.2 Hepatoblastoma

10.2.1 Incidence and Clinical Presentation

Hepatoblastoma is the most frequent primary hepatic neoplasm in the pediatric age group (Nelson et al. 1996), constituting 43% of all tumors (Davey and Cohen 1996). The tumor is often detected before 3 years of age (Boechat et al. 1988; Geoffray et al. 1987), with a median survival of 1 year (Friedburg et al. 1989). Hepatoblastoma is more frequent in males than in females, with a ratio of 3:2 (Davey and Cohen 1996). It is not associated with underlying cirrhosis but is more common in patients with hemihypertrophy, Beckwith-Weideman syndrome, Wilm's tumor, glycogen storage disease, diaphragmatic and umbilical hernias, and Meckel's diverticulum (Davey and Cohen 1996; Nelson et al. 1996; Rosai 1996). Rare occurrence in siblings has been observed (Horowitz et al. 1987).

Presentation is most often due to enlargement of an abdominal mass with a few cases manifesting fever, pain, weight loss, and vomiting (Nelson et al. 1996); jaundice is rarely observed. The serum alphafetoprotein is elevated in 66% (Haaga et al. 1994) to 90% (Davey and Cohen 1996) of cases.

10.2.2 Pathologic Findings

Hepatoblastoma is a malignant tumor of hepatocyte origin, which often contains mesenchymal components (Ishak and Glunz 1967). On macroscopic inspection, hepatoblastoma is a solid, well-defined, sometimes lobulated mass, surrounded by a pseudocapsule (Boechat et al. 1988; Rosai 1996). Although it is usually solitary, multiple lesions can be observed in less than 20% of cases (Davey and Cohen 1996; Rosai 1996). Areas of necrosis and calcification are frequently present (Boechat et al. 1988).

Microscopically, it can be classified as an epithelial or mixed (epithelial-mesenchymal) neoplasm. Epithelial hepatoblastoma is composed of fetal or embryonal malignant hepatocytes or a combination of these (Boechat et al. 1988; Marti-Bonmati et al. 1993). These cells are associated with extramedullary hematopoiesis pseudocapsule (Boechat et al. 1988; Rosai 1996). Mixed hepatoblastoma has both an epithelial (hepatocyte) component and a mesenchymal component, consisting of primitive mesenchymal tissue and osteoid material and/or cartilage, which is responsible for the calcification seen on imaging studies.

The histologic classification has prognostic implications: the epithelial type, particularly if it has fetal hepatocytes, has a better prognosis. Embryonal epithelial cells are more primitive than fetal epithelial and mesenchymal cells, and tumors with this histologic type have a worse prognosis.

10.2.3 Imaging Findings

10.2.3.1 Ultrasound

Sonographically, hepatoblastoma appears as an echogenic mass that may have shadowing and echogenic foci corresponding to intratumoral calcification. Hyperechoic and/or cystic areas, corresponding to hemorrhage within the tumor, and/or necrotic areas may be present as well (Kaude et al. 1981). Hepatoblastoma is associated with high Doppler frequency shifts that correlate with the neovascularity typical of this tumor (Bates et al. 1990).

10.2.3.2 Compted Tomography

On unenhanced scans, hepatoblastoma appears as a solid hypodense mass, which may occupy large portions of the liver. Fifty percent of hepatoblastomas show calcifications, which are particularly extensive

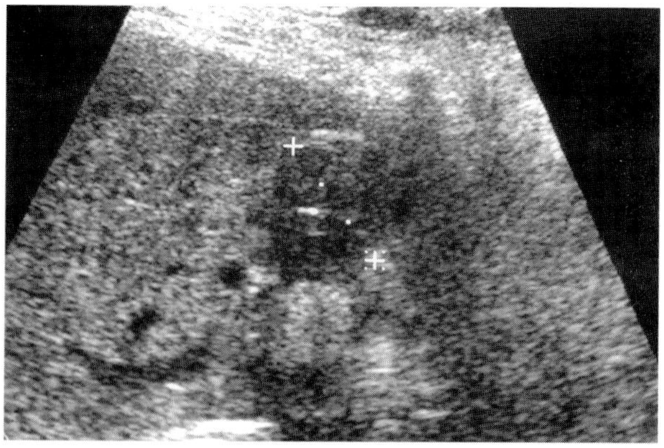

Fig. 10.1. Cystoadenocarcinoma: ultrasound. On sonographic scan, cystoadenocarcinoma appears hypoechoic, with intralesional hyperechoic septa

in mixed hepatoblastoma. Frequently a lobulated pattern caused by bands of fibrosis can be seen (DACHMAN et al. 1987). After contrast medium administration, the tumor appears hyperdense, because of its hypervascular nature. Occasionally invasion of the perihepatic vessels or other structures can be demonstrated (DACHMAN et al. 1987).

10.2.3.3 MR Imaging

Hepatoblastoma has a lower signal intensity on T1-weighted images than adjacent normal liver parenchyma, with eventual areas of higher signal intensity representing hemorrhage (DAVEY and COHEN 1996; SILVERMAN and KUH 1993; STARK and BRADLEY 1992). The tumor shows a heterogeneous increased signal intensity on T2-weighted images. Epithelial type hepatoblastoma may have a more homogeneous pattern than mixed type (POWERS et al. 1994).

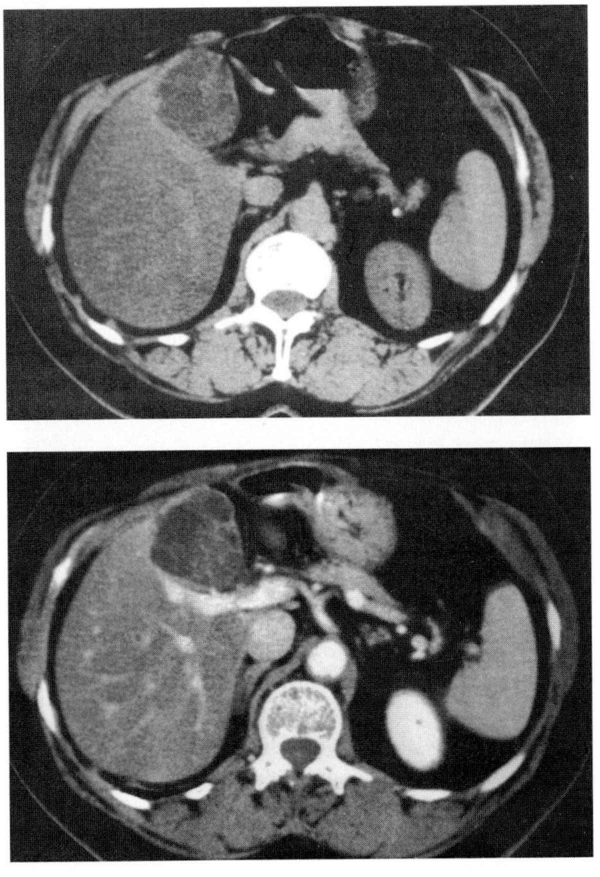

a

b

Fig. 10.2a,b. Cystoadenocarcinoma: CT. **a** Unenhanced CT scan shows a hypodense mass, with central hyperdense areas, in the IV segment of the liver. **b** CT scan during the portal venous phase shows a hypodense mass with internal enhancing septations

MR imaging is extremely helpful in surgical planning owing to its multiplanar capabilities and exquisite depiction of vascular anatomy. Specifically, MR imaging more reliably demonstrates the inferior vena cava and hepatic veins invasion than does CT. There is a variable enhancement pattern after i.v. gadolinium contrast material injection.

10.2.3.4 Angiography

Angiographically, hepatoblastoma is hypervascular and occasionally has a „spoke wheel“ pattern, similar to that of focal nodular hyperplasia, which is due to the presence of multiple fibrous septa and bands. Arterio-venous shunting is uncommon and invasion of the vessels is rare (SMITH et al. 1983). Hypovascular or avascular zone resulting from hemorrhage can occur within the tumor.

10.3 Biliary Cystoadenoma and Cystoadenocarcinoma

10.3.1 Incidence and Clinical Presentation

Cystoadenomas and cytoadenocarcinomas are rare and represent less than 5% of all intrahepatic cysts of biliary origin (ISHAK et al. 1977). They are probably congenital in origin because of the presence of aberrant bile ducts. Approximately 90% of these neoplasms occur in women who are usually in middle age (median of diagnosis 38 years of age) (BUETOW et al. 1995). When present, the symptoms are those of a growing abdominal mass. Right upper quadrant abdominal pain, occasionally irradiating to the scapula, is the chief finding in 60% of patients at presentation (EDMONSON 1976).

10.3.2 Pathologic Findings

Biliary cystoadenoma and cystoadenocarcinoma are currently considered forms of the same disease, with cystoadenoma being a benign neoplasm with malignant potential and cystoadenocarcinoma being an overt malignant neoplasm. Transformation of cystoadenoma to cystoadenocarcinoma is a recognized complication (ISHAK et al. 1977; WHEELER and

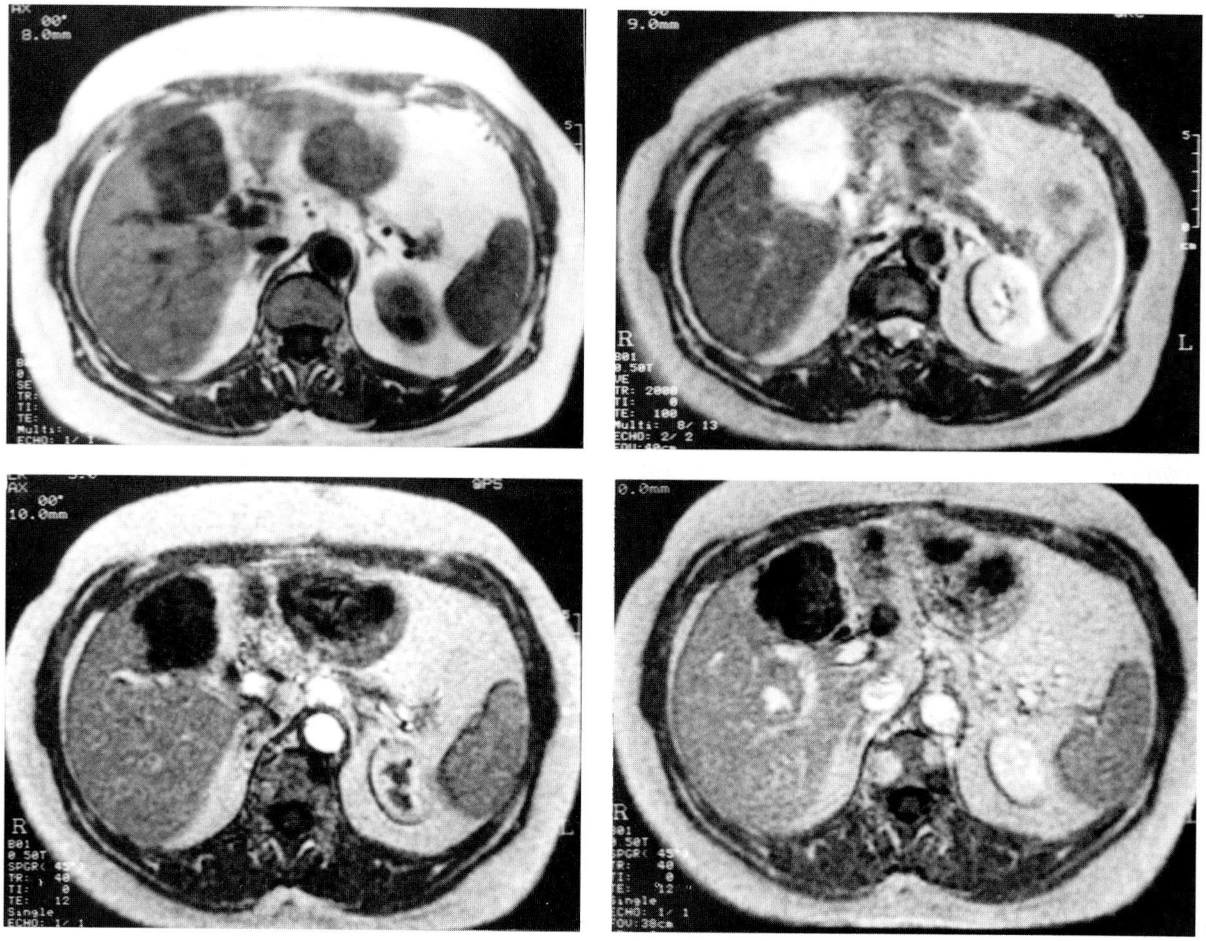

a b c d

Fig. 10.3a–d. Cystoadenocarcinoma: MR imaging. **a** Axial T1-weighted image shows a hypointense focal liver lesion in the IV segment. **b** On T2-weighted image the lesion shows a fluid-like signal intensity. **c** The lesion is hypovascular compared to the surrounding liver parenchyma, on the dynamic scanning after the IV injection of contrast medium, with enhancing internal

Edmondson 1985). They originate from the mucinous-secreting epithelium of the biliary ducts.

Most of the lesions are intrahepatic; less than 10% are extrahepatic, arising in the extrahepatic biliary ducts. Connections to the biliary tree may be seen, but are uncommon.

Macroscopically, these tumors vary from a few centimeters to large multicystic structures, 15–18 cm in greatest diameter. Most of the tumors are solitary, with a smooth or bosselated surface. On cut section, the neoplasm is composed of multiple communicating cysts, of variable size, with a variable amount of internal septations, papillary excrescences or mural nodules seen on the tumor wall (Buetow et al. 1995; Ishak et al. 1977). Occasionally there is one large cyst with many small locules around the periphery (Edmonson 1976).

Histologically they show similar features to those of mucinous cystic tumors that arise in the pancreas and in the ovary. They are commonly mucinous, but a serous variety is also present. The cysts are multilocular and contain mucoid material; the cystic walls are lined by columnar, cuboidal or even flattened epithelium. Just beneath this biliary-like epithelium there is a compact mesenchymal stroma, containing closely bound spindle cells, which bears some resemblance to ovarian stroma; this is found only in women. A minority of lesions do not contain ovarian stroma and these may be found in both men and women.

10.3.3
Imaging Findings

10.3.3.1
Ultrasound

The pathologic features of the lesion have been shown to correlate with the imaging features on ultrasound (US), CT, and MR imaging. However, there are no consistent morphologic or imaging features that would consistently distinguish neoplasms with ovarian-like stroma from those without it (BUETOW et al. 1995). Features such as nodularity and thickened septation are associated with biliary cystoadenocarcinoma; the lack of nodularity is associated with cystoadenoma. Ultrasound demonstrates a cystic-like lesion, multiloculated, and hypoechoic with intralesional septa and mural nodules on the cystic walls (Fig. 10.1).

10.3.3.2
Computed Tomography

On CT scans, these tumors are large, low attenuating intrahepatic masses with thick irregular walls, that enhance following the i.v. administration of iodinated contrast media (Fig. 10.2) (MURPHY et al. 1989; AGILDERE et al. 1991; KOROBKIN et al. 1989).

10.3.3.3
MR Imaging

On MR imaging, findings include a multiloculated septated mass, with variable signal intensity, within the solid and cystic component on T1- and T2-weighted images (Fig. 10.3), depending on the composition of the cystic fluid, which may be serous, mucinous, bilious, hemorrhagic, or a combination of these fluids (BUETOW et al. 1995). Furthermore, low signal intensity within the wall on T2-weighted images may represent hemorrhage. The internal septation, mural nodules and papillary projections enhance following the i.v. administration of gadolinium compounds (Fig. 10.3). Radiographically, it is impossible to distinguish cystoadenomas from cystoadenocarcinomas, except for the presence of distant metastases, adenopathy or other signs of widespread malignancy, in the case of cystoadenocarcinoma. Although cystoadenocarcinomas tend to have more solid components and be more irregular than cystoadenomas, these are not reliable signs.

10.3.3.4
Angiography

Angiographically cystoadenoma and cystoadenocarcinoma are avascular tumors that may demonstrate peripheral neovascularity if there is a large solid component.

10.4
Epithelioid Hemangioendothelioma

10.4.1
Incidence and Clinical Presentation

Epithelioid hemangioendothelioma (EHE) is a rare malignant hepatic neoplasm of vascular origin that develops in adults. It should not be confused with infantile hemangioendothelioma, which occurs predominantly in young children. Only recently has EHE been recognized as a distinct entity. It is a solid tumor primarily composed of epithelioid-appearing endothelial cells. The tumor has a variable clinical course between that of benign endothelial tumors (hemangiomas) and malignant angiosarcomas. Most patients survive 5–10 years after diagnosis. Unlike most primary malignant hepatic tumors, two-thirds of patients affected are women, in the third or fourth decade of life (DEAN et al. 1985). The clinical signs and symptoms of patients with EHE are non-specific: EHE is usually discovered incidentally, although jaundice and liver failure may be present. Rare manifestations include hemoperitoneum (CHOI et al. 1989) and Budd-Chiari syndrome (FUKAYAMA et al. 1984). No risk factors of specific causes of hepatic EHE are known.

10.4.2
Pathologic Findings

Macroscopically, multifocal nodules varying in size from a few millimeters to several centimeters are seen. These nodules tend to coalesce, as they grow, to form large confluent masses, usually in the periphery of the liver, owing to the extension of the tumor through the tributaries of the portal and hepatic veins (DEAN et al. 1985; FURUI et al. 1989). Because EHE replaces hepatic parenchyma slowly over several years, compensatory enlargement of uninvolved portions of the liver can be seen (RADIN et al. 1988; CLEMENTS et al. 1986; ECKSTEIN and RAVICH 1986).

These solid tumors characteristically have a dense fibrotic hypovascular central core and a peripheral hyperemic rim. At the outer edge of these tumors is often a narrow avascular zone where hepatic sinusoids and small vessels are infiltrated by advancing tumor (Miller et al. 1992).

The hepatic capsule overlying an EHE is frequently retracted inward, which is thought to be due to fibrosis induced by the tumor. This capsular retraction is an unusual feature in malignant lesions of the liver, and is suggestive of EHE (Oliver 1996).

Microscopically, the tumors are composed of dendritic spindle-cells and epithelioid round cells within abundant matrix of myxoid and fibrous stroma. Neoplastic cells invade and eventually obliterate sinusoids, terminal hepatic veins, and portal veins. About 30% of patients may demonstrate progressive sclerosis and eventual calcification.

10.4.3 Imaging Findings

The radiologic findings seen in patients with hepatic EHE correlate well with the pathologic composition of the tumors.

10.4.3.1 Ultrasound

Sonographically, EHEs appear as multiple nodules that grow and coalesce forming large confluent masses. The echo pattern of EHEs tends to be nonspecific. EHE lesions tend to be solid and predominantly hypoechoic, relative to surrounding normal liver parenchyma. Occasionally lesions are isoechoic or hyperechoic to surrounding hepatic parenchyma with central hypoechoic rims (Miller et al. 1992).

10.4.3.2 Computer Tomography

Unenhanced CT images often provide better tumor conspicuity and more accurate evaluation of tumor extent than do enhanced CT images (Miller et al. 1992; Radin et al. 1988; Furui et al. 1989). On unenhanced CT images EHE lesions are of uniformly low attenuation relative to surrounding liver parenchyma. Calcification may be seen. Following the administration of i.v. contrast material, most lesions remain relatively hypodense centrally, while the hypervascular peripheral portion of the tumor enhances appreciably. If present, the outer avascular zone remains relatively unenhanced, giving the characteristic target appearance to the lesion (Miller et al. 1992). If no avascular zone is present, the hyperemic outer margin of the tumor will often be isodense to adjacent enhancing hepatic parenchyma, which can result in significant underestimation of lesion size on unenhanced CT images (Oliver 1996).

10.4.3.3 MR Imaging

Similar features of EHE may also be seen on MR images. Concentric alteration in signal intensity, corresponding to the regions of different histology, can be seen both on short TR/TE images and long TR/TE images. MR images demonstrate subcapsular nodules of increased signal intensity on T2-weighted images similar to that of most malignancies, but not as intense as the characteristic high signal intensity of hepatic hemangiomas. Faint peripheral enhancement can be seen after the administration of gadolinium (Ohtomo et al. 1992).

10.5 Angiosarcoma

10.5.1 Incidence and Clinical Presentation

Angiosarcomas are malignant neoplasms derived from endothelial cells that occur primarily in adults with exposure to a variety of chemical agents (inorganic arsenic, vinyl chloride) (Locker et al. 1979; White et al. 1993; Corrigan and Semelka 1995) and radiation [radium, thorium oxide (Thorotrast)] (Kojiro et al. 1985; Ito et al. 1988). Although primary angiosarcoma accounts for less than 2% of all primary liver neoplasm (Corrigan and Semelka 1995), it is regarded as the most common sarcoma of the liver, occurring more frequently than fibrosarcoma malignant fibrous histiocytoma and leiomyosarcoma (Buetow et al. 1994).

Primary hepatic angiosarcomas are highly aggressive and have an extremely poor prognosis. The median survival after diagnosis is 6 months. This tumor metastasizes early, with 60% of patients having metastases at presentation (Locker et al. 1979). The most common sites for metastases are lung and spleen (Locker et al. 1979; Buetow et al. 1994).

Association with hemochromatosis, von Recklinghausen's disease, and alcoholic cirrhosis has also been noted (Locker et al. 1979; MacMahon et al. 1947; Tavares et al. 1979). It occurs four times more frequently in males; it is 30 times less common than hepatocellular carcinoma (Ishak 1976).

10.5.2 Pathologic Findings

Macroscopically, there are two patterns of growth: multifocal nodules (seen approximately in 71% of cases) and large solitary mass (Buetow and Midkiff 1997). The tumor nodules varies in size from pinpoint foci to large nodules measuring several centimeters in diameter. The nodules may have a dark, red-brown appearance due to the presence of areas of internal hemorrhage (Kojiro et al. 1985).

When angiosarcoma appears a solitary, large mass it does not have a capsule and frequently contains large cystic areas filled with blood debris (Ishak 1976).

Microscopically, hepatic angiosarcomas are composed of malignant vascular cells that may form poorly organized vessels, variable in size from cavernous to capillary, trying to form sinusoids. These vessels are lined with malignant endothelial cells. Tumor cells tend to growth along preformed vascular channels, particularly the sinusoid, and may form solid nodules or cavitary spaces.

Thorotrast particles can be found within the malignant endothelial cells in cases of Thorotrast-induced angiosarcoma.

10.5.3 Imaging Findings

10.5.3.1 Ultrasound

On ultrasound scan, angiosarcomas appear as either single or multiple hyperechoic masses (Fig. 10.4). The echo architecture is heterogeneous because of hemorrhage of various ages. Multiple color signals are detected on color Doppler ultrasound (Fig. 10.4).

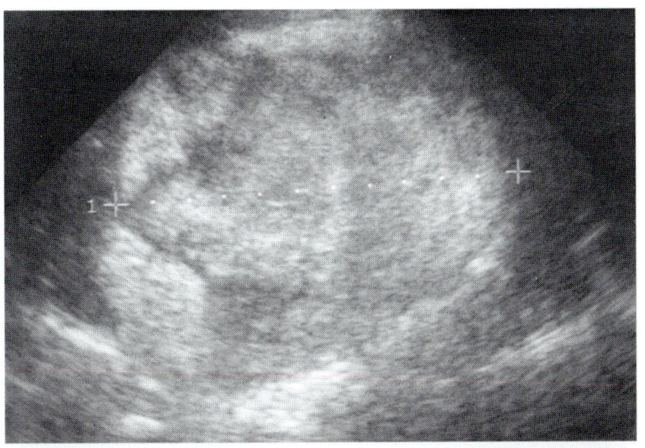
a

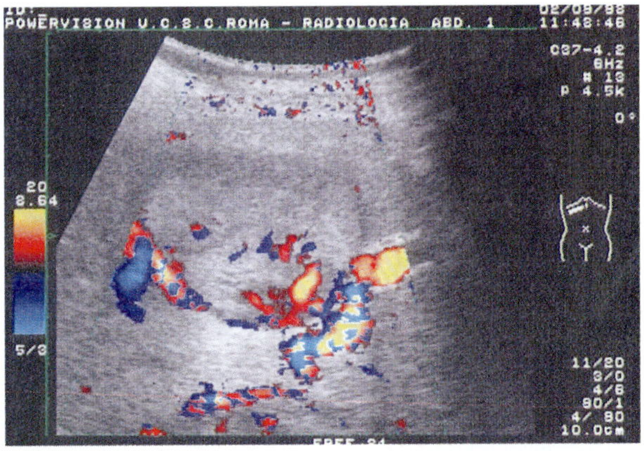

b

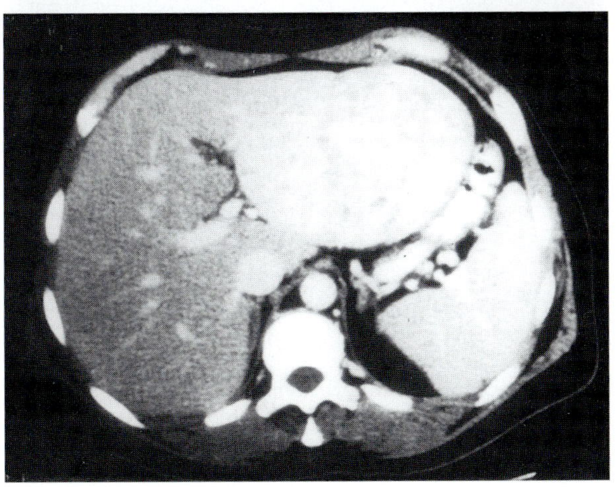
c

Fig. 10.4a–c. Angiosarcoma: ultrasound and CT. **a** On ultrasound scan, angiosarcoma appears hyperechoic compared to adjacent liver parenchyma, with peripheral hypoechoic halo. **b** Color Doppler ultrasound shows multiple color signals predominantly at the periphery of the lesion. **c** Contrast enhanced CT of the same patient shows intense and heterogeneous contrast enhancement

10.5.3.2
Computed Tomography

Most hepatic angiosarcomas are of low attenuation of unenhanced CT images (Fig. 10.5). High attenuation areas can be seen in tumors with fresh hemorrhage. The elevated attenuation values are best seen on unenhanced images. Areas of near water density may be seen in tumors with old hemorrhage.

In cases of prior Thorotrast exposure, high density nodules can be seen in the liver, spleen and lymph nodes on unenhanced CT images. Dynamic enhanced CT images of angiosarcoma can show enhancement patterns similar to those seen in cavernous hemangiomas, which should not be surprising given the cavernous vascular changes that occur in angiosarcoma (Fig. 10.5) (Itai and Teraoka 1989; Mahoney et al. 1982). Even angiosarcomas with central hemorrhage or necrosis have substantial and prolonged peripheral enhancement that can mimic large hemangiomas, which commonly do not fill in completely with contrast material (Buetow et al. 1994).

10.5.3.3
MR Imaging

With MR imaging, the signal intensity features of angiosarcoma are similar to those that may be seen in hemangioma. Both tumors contain abundant blood-filled vascular spaces, which may exhibit high signal intensity on T2-weighted MR images (Fig. 10.6) (Itai and Terako 1989; Ohtomo et al. 1992). Peripheral enhancement after gadolinium administration may be seen but it is not of the dense, discontinuous and globular pattern that is typically seen in cases of hemangioma (Fig. 10.6c,d) (Buetow et al. 1995). Usually the tumor exhibits a heterogeneous signal intensity on T2-weighted images that is far less intense than that of fluid such as cerebrospinal fluid (due to the presence of proteinacious material) (Fig. 10.6).

10.5.3.4
Angiography

Angiographically, angiosarcomas have been reported to show a peripheral stain late in the arterial phase with puddling of contrast material from the

a
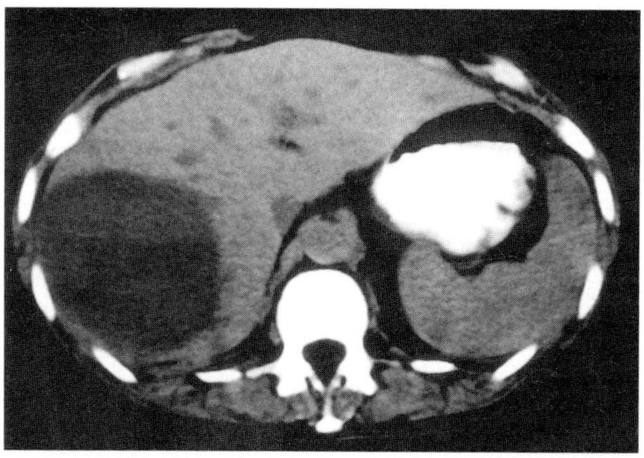

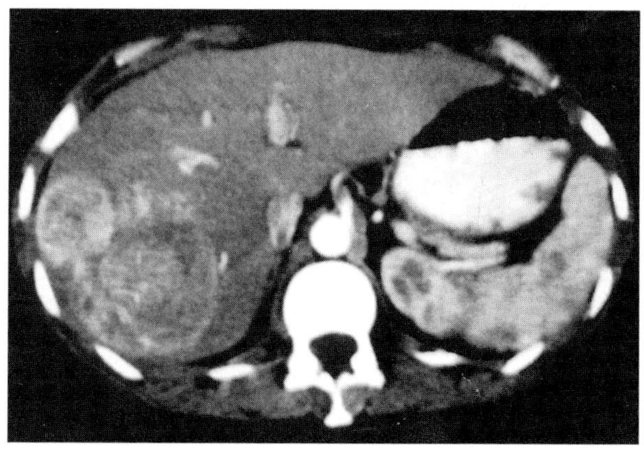
b

c
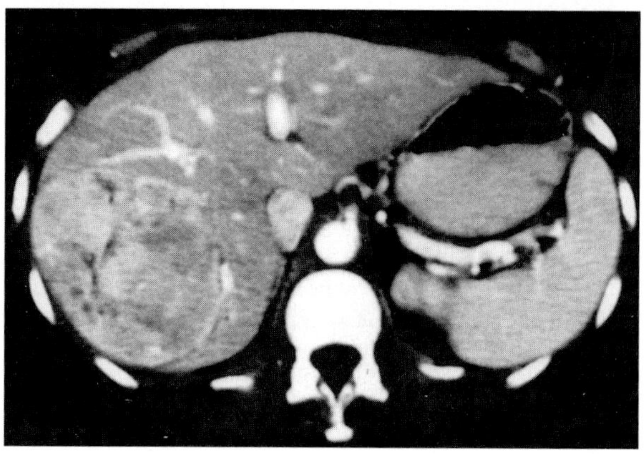

Fig. 10.5a–c. Angiosarcoma: CT. **a** Unenhanced CT scan shows a well-marginated, hypodense focal liver lesion in the right lobe. The lesion is hypervascular compared to adjacent liver parenchyma, with hyperdense areas predominately located at the periphery of the lesion (**b**) with progressive filling of the lesion with contrast medium, during the portal venous phase (**c**)

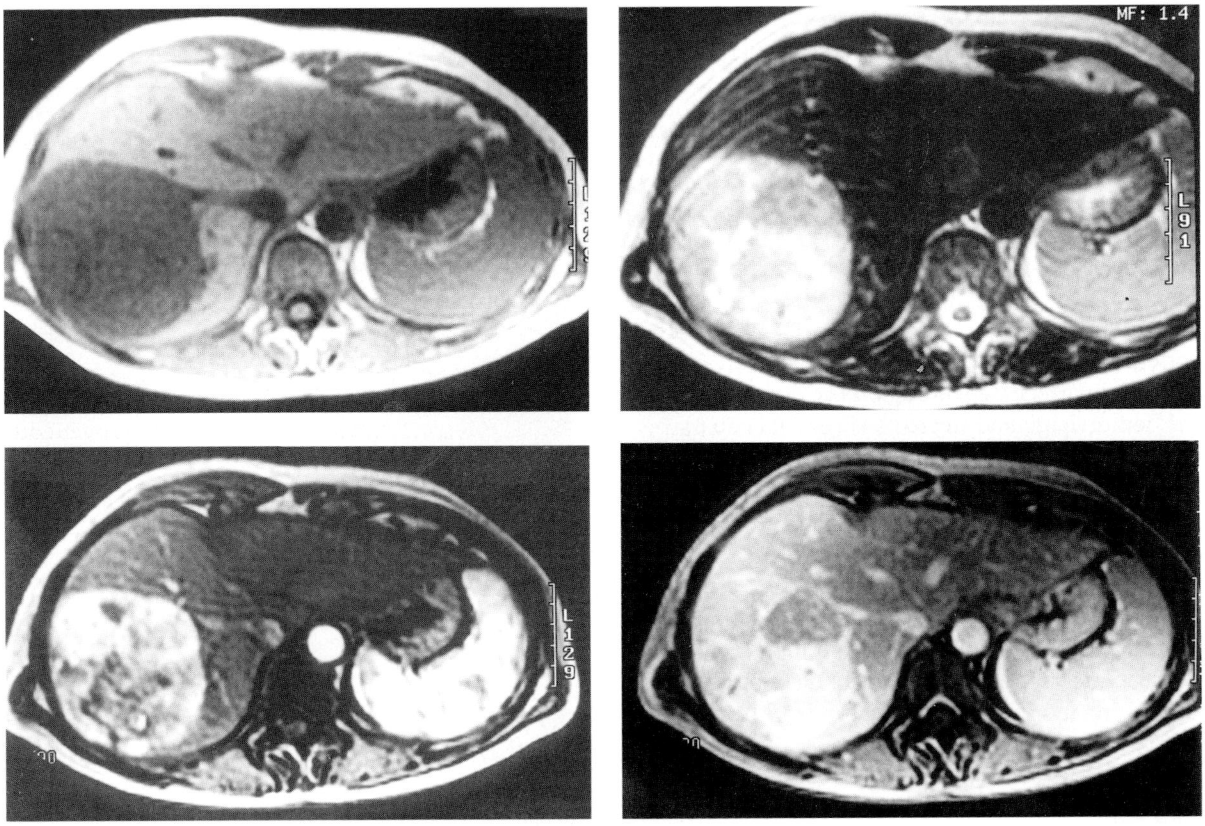

Fig. 10.6a–d. Angiosarcoma: MR imaging. **a** Axial T1-weighted image shows a well-marginated, hypointense mass in the right hepatic lobe. The lesion appears heterogeneously hyperintense on T2-weighted image (**b**). On dynamic scanning the lesion is hypervascular, with predominately peripheral enhancement, without, however, the discontinuous and globular pattern typically seen in hemangiomas (**c**) and delayed retention of contrast medium (**d**)

midarterial phase to the late venous phase (Stephens and Johnson 1994; Whelan et al. 1976). This stain is supposed to distinguish hepatic angiosarcomas from hemangiomas (Whelan et al.1976). However, many authors feel that distinguishing hepatic angiosarcomas from other hypervascular tumors of the liver can be extremely difficult (Stephens and Johnson 1994; Buetow et al. 1994).

10.6 Other Sarcomas

10.6.1 Incidence and Clinical Presentation

Other sarcomas of the liver include leiomyosarcoma, malignant fibrous histiocytoma, and fibrosarcoma. These are all rare tumors, leiomyosarcoma being the most common (Ishak 1987). Malignant fibrous histiocytoma has become increasingly common since the 1960s and 1970s, when it was introduced as a separate pathologic entity and subsequently popularized.

These lesions demonstrate no significant sex predilection and usually occur in patients between 40 and 60 years of age (Ishak 1987). In a recent review of the literature there were 54 cases of primary hepatic leiomyosarcoma. The male-to-female ratio was 25:26 and the mean age at diagnosis was 54 years (Gates et al. 1995).

10.6.2 Pathologic Findings

These tumors consist of malignant sarcomatous cells corresponding to the respective criteria used for each entity (Enzinger and Weiss 1983). Grossly, these lesions present large solitary masses on the background of a normal non-cirrhotic liver. There are variable amounts of internal hemorrhage and necrosis.

10.6.3 Imaging Findings

10.6.3.1 Ultrasound

Sonography demonstrates a large mass, with a variable echo pattern depending on the degrees of internal hemorrhage and necrosis (Figs. 10.7, 10.8).

10.6.3.2 Computed Tomography

Similarly on CT scan, both leiomyosarcomas and malignant fibrous histiocytoma have a similar appearance: a large noncalcified, hypodense, homogeneous mass that exhibits heterogeneous peripheral enhancement after contrast medium administration (Fig. 10.9).

10.6.3.3 MR Imaging

MR imaging demonstrates a signal intensity that is variable on T1- and T2-weighted images; more frequently they appear as hypointense masses both on T1- and T2-weighted images (Fig. 10.10). Enhancement of the viable portions of the tumor are usually seen peripherally.

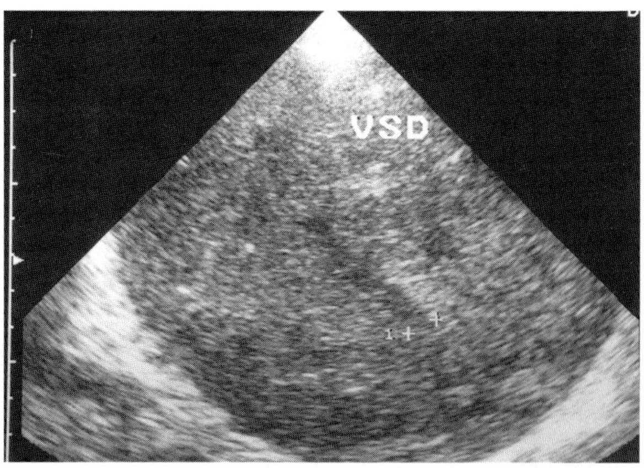

Fig. 10.7. Leiomyosarcoma sonography. Leiomyosarcoma appears as an ill-defined isoechoic mass compared to adjacent liver parenchyma, encasing intrahepatic vessels (right hepatic vein)

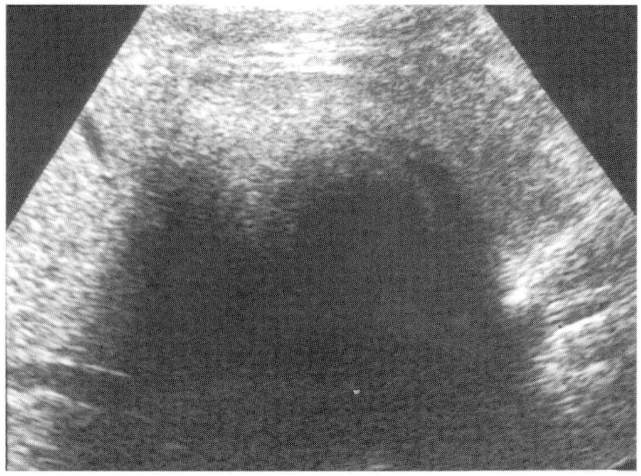

Fig. 10.8. Malignant fibrous histiocytoma: ultrasound. Sonographic scan shows a hypoechoic lesion, with posterior shadowing

10.7 Lymphoma

10.7.1 Incidence and Clinical Presentation

Primary hepatic lymphoma is a rare disease (Weissieder et al. 1988; Sanders et al. 1989; Ryan et al. 1988; Gazelle et al. 1994). Lymphoma is considered to be a primary neoplasm of the liver when the tumor is limited to hepatic parenchyma. Hepatic lymphoma is usually seen in association with systemic disease, both non-Hodgkin's (Sanders et al. 1989) and Hodgkin's lymphoma, and recently has been seen with increased association in patients immunocompromised by AIDS (Bacchi et al. 1996; Siskin et al. 1995) or pharmacologic immunosuppression (Nyberg et al. 1986; Ziegier et al. 1984; Penn et al. 1969; Harris et al. 1987). The lymphomatous process in these patients includes a spectrum of lymphoproliferation from benign B-cell hyperplasia to malignant monoclonal non-Hodgkin's lymphoma (List et al. 1987; Nalesnik et al. 1988a,b). Post-transplant lymphoproliferative disease (PTLD) is mainly of B-cell origin, although up to 11% may arise from T-cell lymphocytes (Penn 1990). A strong association has been identified between PTLD and Epstein-Barr virus (Oliver 1996). Up to 80% of patients with PTLD are infected with this virus at the time of lymphoma diagnosis (List et al. 1987; Nalesnik et al. 1988a,b).

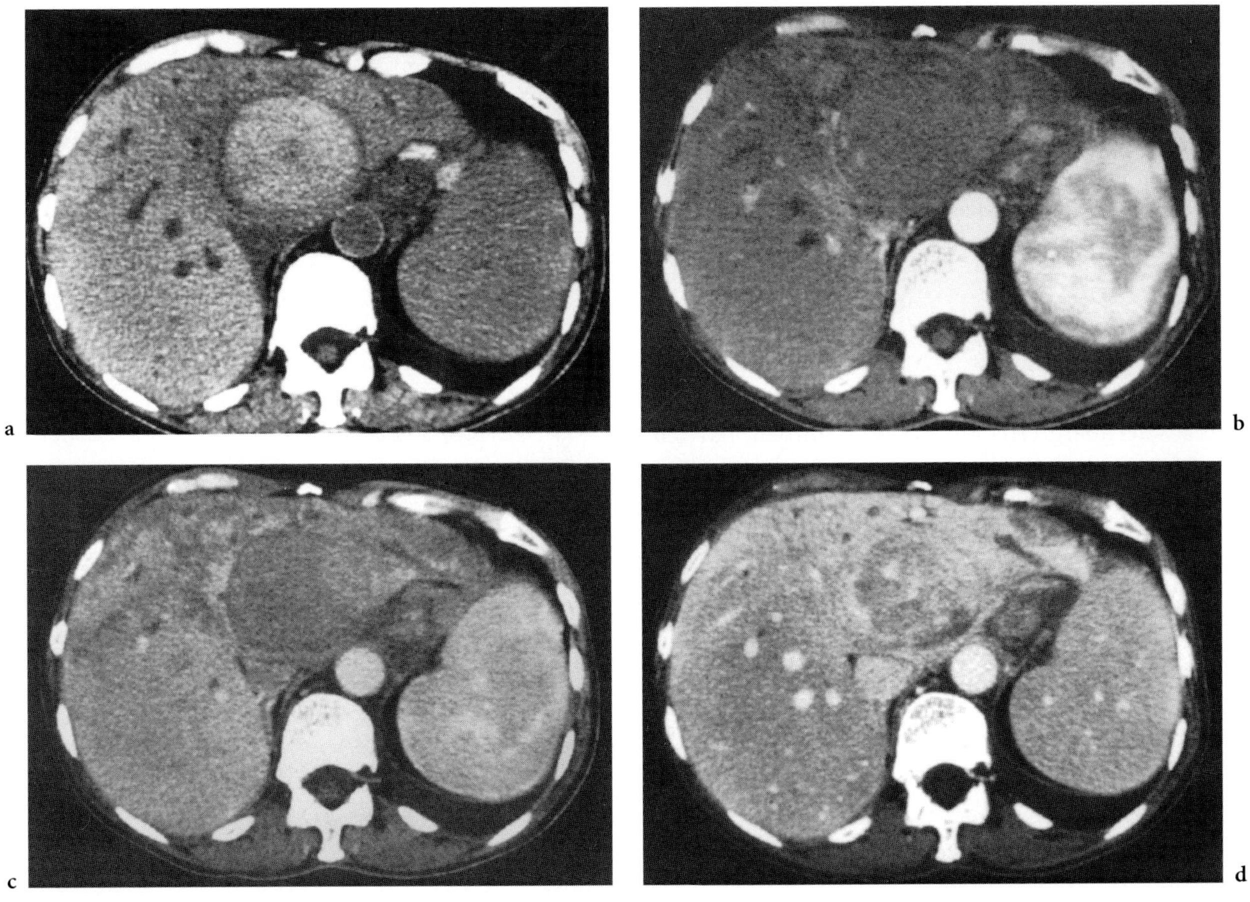

Fig 10.9a–d. Malignant fibrous histiocytoma: CT. **a** On unenhanced CT scan, malignant fibrous histiocytoma appears hyperdense compared to adjacent liver parenchyma, non-calcified, with a peripheral hypodense rim. The lesion is hypodense during the arterial phase (**b**), indicating its hypovascularity, showing mild, inhomogeneous peripheral enhancement during the portal venous (**c**) and delayed phase (**d**)

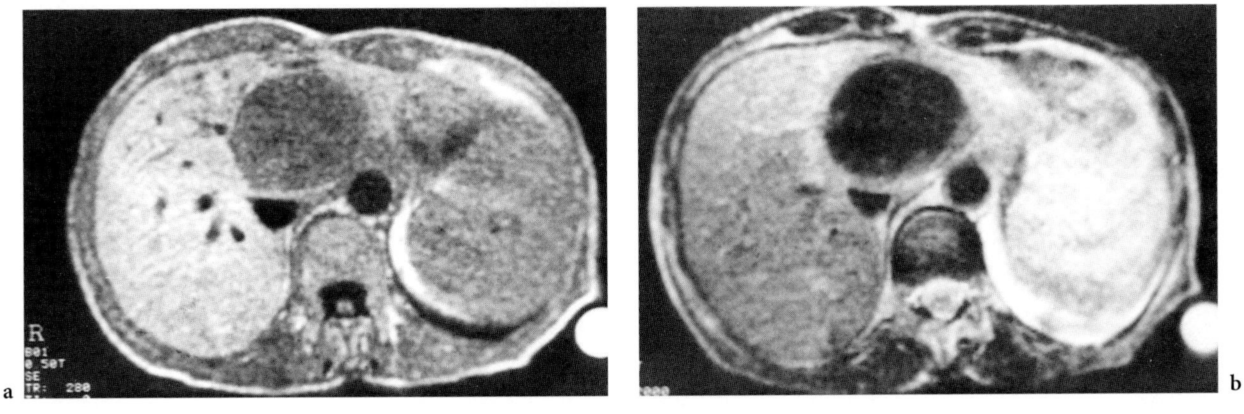

Fig. 10.10a,b. Malignant fibrous histiocytoma: MR imaging. MR imaging shows a hypointense lesion both on T1- (**a**) and T2-weighted images (**b**) in the left liver lobe

10.7.2 Pathologic Findings

Grossly, nodular and diffuse forms of hepatic lymphoma are seen. Hodgkin's disease occurs more often as miliary lesions than masses (Ros 1994). Early in the disease liver parenchyma involvement is microscopic, but with time small nodules from a few millimeters to several centimeters in size develop (Sherlock and Dooley 1993).

Microscopically, in patients with Hodgkin's disease, a Reed-Sternberg variant type of cell is accepted as evidence for liver involvement. Typical Reed-Sternberg cells are rarely identified, particularly in biopsy specimens. In non-Hodgkin's lymphoma, the lymphocytic form tends to be miliary, whereas the large cells or histiocytic varieties are nodular or tumoral (Jaffe 1987).

In both Hodgkin's and non-Hodgkin's lymphoma, initial involvement is seen in the portal areas, because this is where the majority of the lymphatic tissue of the liver is found (Ros 1994).

10.7.3 Imaging Findings

10.7.3.1 Ultrasound

On ultrasound studies, hepatic lymphoma appears as a hypoechoic mass or masses in the nodular form of the disease, sometimes with a cystic-like appearance (Fig. 10.11) (Ginaldi et al. 1980). In the diffuse form, the echogenicity of the hepatic parenchyma may be normal or the overall architecture of the liver may be altered (Shirkhoda et al. 1990).

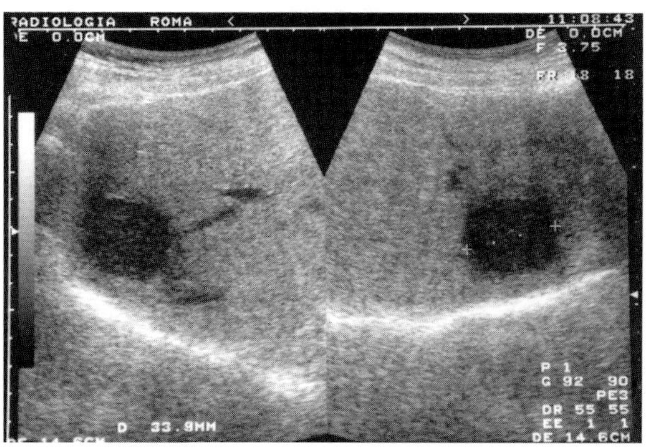

Fig. 10.11. Lymphoma: ultrasound. On ultrasound scan, the tumoral form of lymphoma appears as a homogeneous, hypoechoic mass

10.7.3.2 Computed Tomography

CT is currently the preferred imaging modality for evaluating hepatic lymphoma, with a specificity of almost 90% and a sensitivity of almost 60% (Castellino et al. 1984). On CT these tumors appear as large discrete masses with decreased attenuation relative to surrounding liver parenchyma on both unenhanced and portal venous phase enhanced images (Fig. 10.12) (Sanders et al. 1989). The degree of necrosis and presence of calcification may vary.

10.7.3.3 MR Imaging

On MR images these tumors are hypointense on T1-weighted images and isointense to the spleen on T2-weighted images (Fig. 10.13) (Gazelle et al. 1994). Although the appearance of primary lymphoma on any single imaging study is not specific for lymphoma, the integration of these findings on several different imaging studies may suggest the diagnosis.

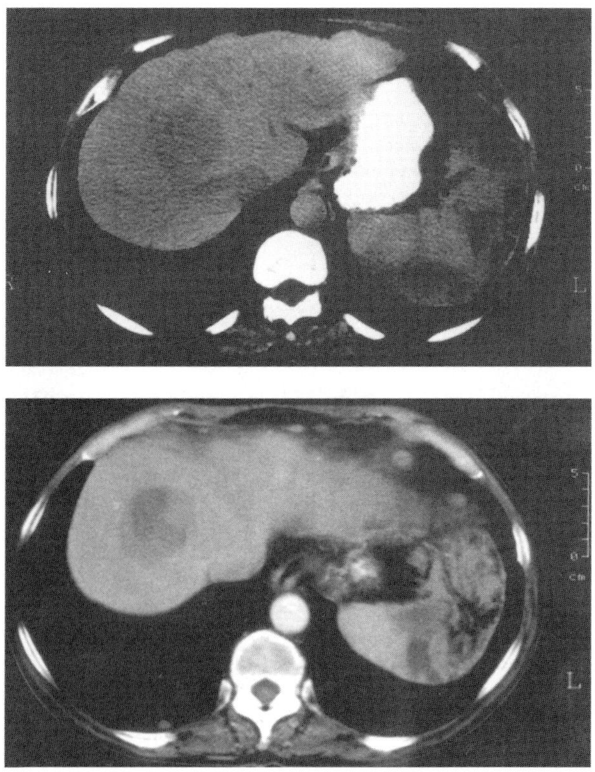

a

b

Fig. 10.12a,b. Lymphoma: CT. **a** On unenhanced scan lymphoma appears as a homogeneous hypodense lesion. **b** On contrast enhanced CT scan, lymphoma appears as a large, well-defined hypodense mass

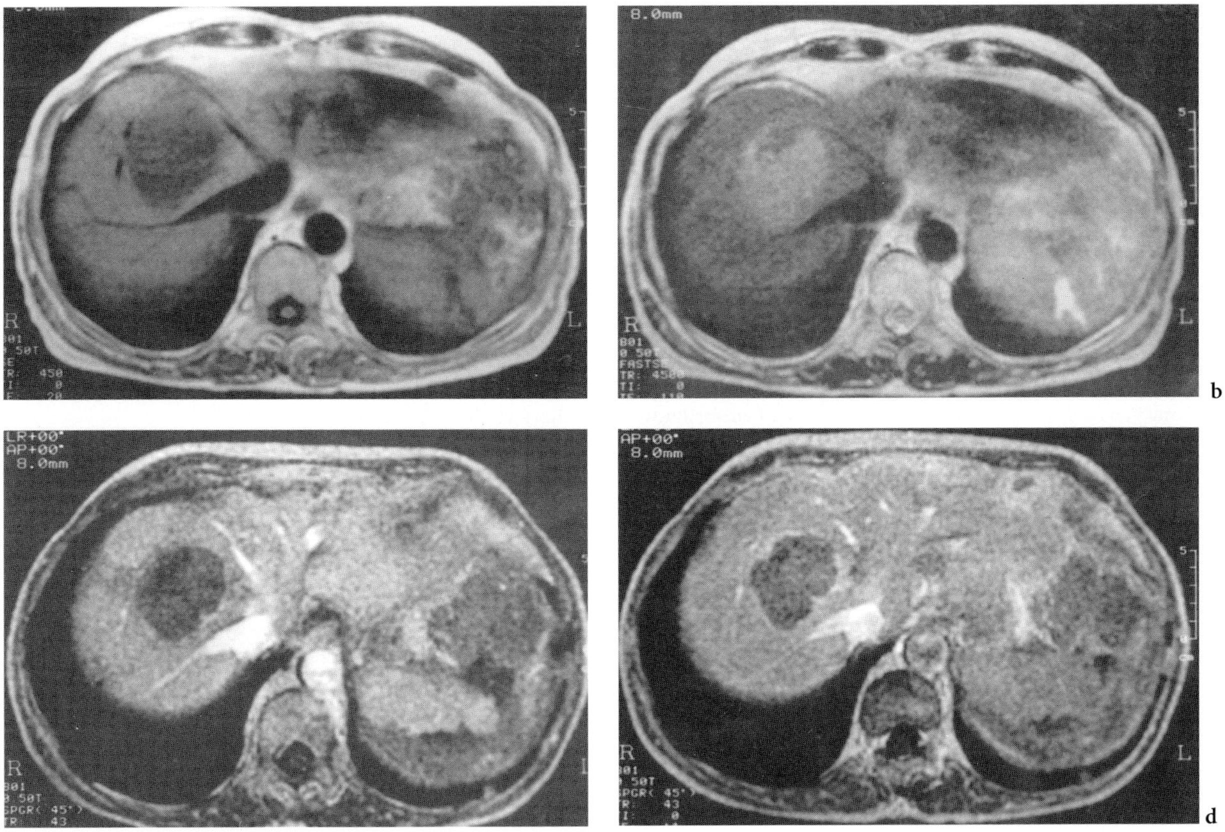

Fig. 10.13a–d. Lymphoma: MR imaging. **a** Axial T1-weighted image shows a well-defined hypointense lesion in the VIII hepatic segment. **b** The lesion appears homogeneously hyperintense on T2-weighted images. **c** On dynamic MR images, focal lymphoma is hypovascular, with a mild peripheral rim on delayed image (**d**)

References

Agildere AM, Haliloglu M, Akhan O (1991) Biliary cystadenoma and cystadenocarcinoma. AJR 156:1113

Bacchi MM, Rabenhorst SH, Soares FA, et al (1996) AIDS-related lymphoma in Brazil. Histopathology, immunophenotype, and association with Epstein-Barr virus. Am J Clin Pathol 105:230–237

Bates SM, Keller MS, Ramos IM, et al (1990) Hepatoblastoma: detection of tumor vascularity with duplex Doppler US. Radiology 176:505–507

Boechat MI, Kanganlow H, Ortega J, et al (1988) Primary liver tumors in children: Comparison of CT and MR imaging. Radiology 169:727–732

Buetow PC, Midkiff RB (1997). Primary malignant neoplasms in the adult. MRI Clin North Am 5:289–318

Buetow PC, Buck JL, Ros PR, et al (1994) Malignant vascular tumors of the liver: radiologic-pathologic correlation. RadioGraphics 14:153-166

Buetow PC, Buck JL, Pantongrag-Brown L, et al (1995) Biliary cystadenoma and cystadenocarcinoma: Clinical-imaging-pathologic correlation with emphasis on the importance of ovarian stroma. Radiology 196:805–810

Castellino RA, Hoppe RT, Blank N, et al (1984) Computed tomography, lymphography and staging laparotomy in colon correlations in staging of Hodgkin disease. AIR 143:37–41

Choi BL, Lim JH, Han MC, et al (1989) Biliary cystadenoma and cystadenocarcinoma: CT and sonographic findings. Radiology 171:57–61

Clements D, Hubscher S, West R, et al (1986) Epithelioid hemangioendothelioma of the liver: a case report. J Hepatol 2:441–449

Corrigan K, Semelka RC (1995) Dynamic contrast-enhanced MR imaging of fibrolamellar hepatocellular carcinoma. Abdom Imaging 20:122–125

Craig JR, Peters RL, Edmondson HA (1989) Tumors of the liver and intrahepatic bile ducts. In: Atlas of tumor pathology, Second Series, Fascicle 26. Armed Forces Institute of Pathology, Washington DC

Dachman AH, Parker RL, Ros PR, et al (1987) Hepatoblastoma: a radiologic-pathologic correlation in 50 cases. Radiology 164:15–19

Davey MS, Cohen MD (1996) Imaging of gastrointestinal malignancy in childhood. Radiol Clin North Am 34:717–742

Dean PJ, Haggitt RC, O'Hara CJ (1985) Malignant epithelioid hemangioendothelioma of the liver in young women: Relationship to oral contraceptive use. Am J Surg Pathol 9:695–704

Eckstein RP, Ravich RMB (1986) Epithelioid hemangioendotheiioma of the liver: report of two cases histologically mimicking venoocciusive disease. Pathology 18:459–462

Edmonson HA (1976) Benign epithelial tumors and tumorlike lesions of the liver. In: Okuda K, Peters RL (eds) Hepatocellular carcinoma. Wiley, New York, pp 309–330

Enzinger FM, Weiss SW (1983) Soft-Tissue Tumors. Mosby Year-Book, St. Louis

Freeney PC, Baron RL, Teefey SA (1992) Hepatocellular carcinoma: Reduced frequency of typical findings with dynamic contrast-enhanced CT in a non-Asian population. Radiology 182:143–148

Friedburg H, Kauffmann GW, Bohm N, et al (1989) Sonographic and computed tomographic features of embryonal rhabdomyosarcoma of the biliary tract. Pediatr Radiol 14:436–438

Fukayama M, Nihei Z, Takizawa T, et al (1984) Malignant epithelioid hemangioendothelioma of the liver spreading throughout the hepatic veins. Virchows Arch A 404:275–287

Furui S, Itai Y, Ohtomo K, et al (1989) Hepatic epithelioid hemangioendothelioma: Report of five cases. Radiology 171:63–68

Gates LK Jr, Cameron AJ, Nagorney DM, et al (1995) Primary leiomyosarcoma of the liver mimicking liver abscess. Am J Gastroenterol 90:649–652

Gazelle GS, Lee MJ, Hahn PF, et al (1994) US, CT and MRI of primary and secondary liver lymphoma. J Comput Assist Tomogr 18:412–415

Geoffray A, Couanet D, Montagne JP, et al (1987) Ultrasonography and computed tomography for diagnosis and follow-up of biliary duct rhabdomyosarcomas in children. Pediatr Radiol 17:127–131

Ginaldi S, Bernadino M, Jing B, et al (1980) Ultrasonographic patterns of hepatic lymphoma. Radiology 136:427–431

Haaga JR, Lanzieri CF, Sartoris DJ, et al (1994) Computed Tomography and Magnetic Resonance Imaging of the Whole Body, 3rd edn. Mosby-Year Book, St. Louis, pp 909–919

Harris KM, Schwartz ML, Slasky BS, et al (1987) Post-transplantation cyclosporine-induced lymphoproliferative disorders: clinical and radiologic manifestations. Radiology 162:697–700

Horowitz ME, Etcubanas E, Webber BL, et al (1987) Hepatic undifferentiated (embryonal) sarcoma and rhabdomyosarcoma in children. Results of therapy. Cancer 59:396–402

Ishak KG (1976) Mesenchymal tumors of the liver. In: Okuda K, Peter RL (eds) Hepatocellular Carcinoma. John Wiley & Sons, New York, pp 228–587

Ishak KG (1987) Malignant mesenchymal tumors of the liver. In: Okuda K, Ishak KG (eds) Neoplasms of the Liver. Springer Verlag, New York, pp 121–156

Ishak KG, Glunz PR (1967) Hepatoblastoma and hepatocarcinoma in infancy and childhood. Report of 47 cases. Cancer 20:396–422

Ishak KG, Willis GW, Cummins SD, et al (1977) Biliary cystadenoma and cystadenocarcinoma. Report of 14 cases and review of the literature. Cancer 39:322–338

Itai Y, Teraoka T (1989) Angiosarcoma of the liver mimicking cavernous hemangioma on dynamic CT. J Comput Assist Tomogr 13:910–912

Ito Y, Kojiro M, Nakashima T, et al (1988) Pathomorphologic characteristics of 102 cases of Thorotrast-related hepatocellular carcinoma, cholangiocarcinoma, and hepatic angiosarcoma. Cancer 62:1153–1162

Jaffe ES (1987) Malignant lymphoma: pathology of hepatic involvement. Semin Liver Dis 7:257–268

Kaude JV, Felman AU, Hawkins IF Jr (1980) Ultrasonography in primary hepatic tumors in early childhood. Pediatr Radiol 9:77–83

Kojiro M, Nakashima T, Ito Y, et al (1985) Thorium dioxide-related angiosarcoma of the liver. Pathomorphic study of 29 autopsy cases. Arch Pathol Lab Med 109:853–857

Korobkin MT, Stephens DH, Lee JKT, et al (1989) Biliary cystadenoma and cystadenocarcinoma: CT and sonographic findings. AJR 153:507–511

List AF, Greco FA, Vogier LB (1987) Lymphoproliterative diseases in immunocompromised hosts: the role of Epstein-Barr virus. J Clin Oncol 5:1678–1689

Locker GY, Doroshow JH, Swelling LA, et al (1979) The clinical features of hepatic angiosarcoma: a report of four cases and a review of the English literature. Medicine 58:48–63

MacMahon HE, Murphy AS, Bates MI (1947) Endothelial-cell sarcoma of the liver following thorotrast injections. Am J Pathol 23:585–611

Mahoney B, Jeffrey RB, Federle MP (1982) Spontaneous rupture of hepatic and splenic angiosarcoma demonstrated by CT. AJR 183:965–966

Marti-Bonmati L, Ferrer D, Menor F, et al (1993) Hepatic mesenchymal sarcoma: MRI findings. Abdom lmaging 18:176–179

Miller JH (1981) The ultrasonographic appearance of cystic hyperplastoma. Radiology 138:141–143

Miller WJ, Dodd GD, Federle MP, Baron RL (1992) Epithelioid hemangioendothelioma of the liver: imaging findings with pathologic correlation. AJR 159:53–57

Murphy BJ, Casillas J, Ros PR, et al (1989) The CT appearance of cystic masses of the liver. RadioGraphics 9:307–322

Nalesnik MA, Jatfe R, Starzl TE, et al (1988a) The pathology of posttransplant lymphoproliferative disorders occurring in the setting of cyclosporine A-prednisone immunosuppression. Am J Pathol 133:173–192

Nalesnik MA, Makowka L, Starzl TE (1988b) The diagnosis and treatment of posttransplant lymphoproliferative disorders. Curr Probl Surg 25:367–472

Nelson WE, Behrman RE, Kliegman RM, et al (1996) Nelson Textbook of Pediatrics, 15th edn. WB Saunders Company, Philadelphia, pp 1472–1473

Nyberg DA, Jetfrey RB, Federle MP, et al (1986) Lymphomas: evaluation by abdominal CT. Radiology 159:59–63

Ohtomo K, Tsutomu A, Itai Y, et al (1992) MR imaging of malignant mesenchymal tumors of the liver. Gastrointest Radiol 17:58–62

Oliver JH (1996) Malignant hepatic neoplasms, excluding hepatocellular carcinoma and cholangiocarcinoma. In: Freeney (ed) Radiology of the liver, biliary tract, and pancreas. American Roentgen Ray Society, U.S.A.

Penn I, Hammond W, Brettschneider L, et al (1969) Malignant lymphomas in transplantation patients. Transplant Proc 1:106–112

Penn I (1990) Cancers complicating organ transplantation (editorial) N Engl J Med 323:1767–1768

Powers C, Ros PR, Stoupis C, et al (1994) Primary liver neoplasms: MR imaging with pathologic correlation. Radiographics 14:459–482

Radin DR, Craig JR, Colletti PM, et al (1988) Hepatic epithelioid hemangioendothelioma. Radiology 169:145–148

Ros PR (1994) Malignant liver tumors. In: Gore RM, Levine MS, Laufer I (eds) Gastrointestinal radiology. Saunders, Philadephia, pp 1897–1946

Rosai J (1996) Ackerman's Surgical Pathology, 8th ed. Mosby-Year Book, St. Louis, pp 903–913, 919–921

Ryan J, Straus DJ, Lange C, et al (1988) Primary lymphoma of the liver. Cancer 61:370–375

Sanders LM, Botet JF, Straus DJ, et al (1989) CT of primary lymphoma of the liver. AJR 152:973–976

Sherlock S, Dooley J (1993) Diseases of the Liver and Biliary System, 9th edn. Blackwell Scientific Publications, Oxford, pp 44–61

Shirkhoda A, Ros PR, Farah J, et al (1990) Lymphoma of the solid abdominal viscera. Radiol Clin North Am 28:785–799

Silverman FN, Kuh JP (1993) In: Caffey's, Pediatric X-Ray Diagnosis: An Integrated Imaging Approach, 9th edn. Mosby-Year Book, St.Louis, pp 960–967

Siskin GP, Haller JO, Miller S, et al (1995) AIDS-related lymphoma: Radiologic features in pediatric patients. Radiology 196:63–66

Smith WL, Franken EA, Mitros FA (1983) Liver tumors in children. Semin Roentgenol 18:136–148

Stark DS, Bradley WG (1992) Magnetic Resonance Imaging, 2nd edn. Mosby-Year Book, St. Louis, pp 2093–2095

Stephens DH, Johnson CD (1994) Primary malignant neoplasms of the liver. In: Freeny PC, Stevenson GW (eds) Margulis and Burhenne's alimentary tract radiology. Mosby-Year Book, St. Louis, pp 1662–1687

Tavares MH, Saracoca A, Oliveria EA, et al (1979) Thorium dioxide and the liver: updated clinical and biochemical findings. Environ Res 18:173–177

Weissieder R, Stark DD, Elizondo G, et al (1988) MRI of hepatic lymphoma. Magn Reson lmaging 6:675–681

Wheeler DA, Edmondson HA (1985) Cystadenóma with mesenchvrnal stroma (CMS) in the liver and bile ducts. A clinicopathologic study of 17 cases, 4 with malignant change. Cancer 56:1434–1445

Whelan JG, Creech JL, Tamburro CH (1976) Angiographic and radionuclide characteristics of hepatic angiosarcoma found in vinyl chloride workers. Radiology 118:549–557

White PG, Adams H, Smith PM (1993) The computed tomographic appearances of angiosarcoma of the liver. Clin Radiol 48:321–325

Ziegier JL, Beckstead JA, Volberding PA, et al (1984) Non-Hodgkin's lymphoma in 90 homosexual men: relation to generalized adenopathy and the acquired immunodeficiency syndrome. N Engl J Med 311:565–570

11 Epidemiology and Pathology of Liver Metastases

D. Campani, M.A. Caligo, I. Esposito, and G. Bevilacqua

CONTENTS

11.1 Introduction

The liver is one of the organs mostly involved in metastatic disease from a variety of cancers, in particular those of the gastrointestinal tract. The proportion of patients with liver metastases increases with the progression of the neoplasia. Metastatic tumors account for about 98% of all hepatic malignancies and are found in nearly 4% of all liver biopsies (Craig et al. 1989). They develop from both epithelial and mesenchymal tissue, but the epithelial tumors spread more frequently to the liver. In a large series of 10,736 malignant neoplasms, Pickren et al. (1982) reported that the metastatic tumor in the liver was 41 times more frequent than the primary hepatic tumor.

11.2 Epidemiology

In the large Roswell Park Memorial Institute series (Pickren et al. 1982), hepatic involvement by primary tumors was present in 4444 (41.4%) out of 10,736 cases. Lymph nodes were the site with the highest incidence of metastases (57%); the frequency in the lung was 39.7%, 35% in the bone and 20.3% in the adrenal. Since lymph node involvement is by the lymphatic route, the liver appears to be the most frequent site of blood-borne metastases.

No differences are observed between sexes or races in the frequency of liver metastases, but the data suggest a decrease in the incidence of liver metastases as age increases.

The incidence of liver metastases from tumors arising in organs drained by the portal vein is higher than that observed in tumors spreading through the systemic circulation (Table 11.1). Furthermore,

Table 11.1. Distribution of tumors by primary site and incidence of liver metastases (modified from Pickren et al. 1982)

Site	No. (%)	Liver metastases No. (%)
Lung and trachea	1377 (12.8)	593 (43.1)
Bone marrow	1237 (11.5)	643 (52.0)
Breast	1047 (9.8)	635 (60.6)
Lymph nodes	946 (8.8)	525 (55.5)
Uterus	702 (6.5)	200 (28.5)
Oral cavity-pharynx	658 (6.1)	90 (13.7)
Skin	439 (4.1)	160 (36.4)
Colon	426 (4.0)	242 (56.8)
Prostate	403 (3.8)	66 (16.4)
Ovary-fallopian tube	364 (3.4)	177 (48.6)
Upper respiratory	338 (3.1)	59 (17.5)
Bladder-urethra	337 (3.1)	96 (28.5)
Stomach	323 (3.0)	158 (48.9)
Rectum	307 (2.9)	141 (45.9)
Kidney-ureter	284 (2.6)	113 (39.8)
Pancreas	197 (1.8)	148 (75.1)
Central nervous system	192 (1.8)	2(1.0)
Endocrine	181 (1.7)	45 (24.9)
Esophagus	178 (1.7)	38 (21.3)
Testis	119 (1.1)	65 (54.6)
Bone-muscle	116 (1.1)	26 (22.4)
Vagina-external genitalia	61 (0.6)	16 (26.2)
Small intestine	39 (0.4)	21 (53.8)
Gallbladder extra-hepatic bile ducts	38 (0.4)	23 (60.5)
Eye	18 (0.2)	14 (77.8)
Penis	16 (0.1)	1 (6.3)
Anus	14 (0.1)	4 (28.6)
Unknown	137 (1.3)	54 (39.4)
Miscellaneous	242 (2.3)	89 (36.8)
Total	10736 (100.0)	4444 (41.4)

D. Campani, MD; Division of Pathology, Department of Oncology, University of Pisa, Via Roma 57, I-56125 Pisa, Italy
M. A. Caligo, MD; Division of Pathology, Department of Oncology, University of Pisa, Via Roma 57, I-56125 Pisa, Italy
I. Esposito, MD; Division of Pathology, Department of Oncology, University of Pisa, Via Roma 57, I-56125 Pisa, Italy
G. Bevilacqua, MD, Professor and Chairman; Division of Pathology, Department of Oncology, University of Pisa, Via Roma 57, I-56125 Pisa, Italy

tumors from portal organs are more likely to metastasize only to the liver than elsewhere. As shown in Table 11.1, tumors from eye, mammary gland, lymph nodes, testis and bone marrow also have a high frequency of liver metastases.

Tumors of various cell types show differences in liver metastatic involvement (Table 11.2). Leukemias have a high incidence of liver involvement; among the carcinomas, the highest frequency is observed in small cell carcinomas while squamous cell carcinomas produce the lowest percentage of liver metastases. Metastatic sarcomas in the liver are more common than primary hepatic sarcomas, but compared to carcinomas they produce liver metastases less frequently than anaplastic carcinomas, adenocarcinomas and small cell carcinomas, but more frequently than squamous cell and transitional cell carcinomas.

Liver metastases appear as single or multiple foci, the latter being the commonest. Small cell carcinomas, anaplastic carcinomas, transitional cell carcinomas and Hodgkin's disease almost always produce multiple metastases. Breast cancer and tumors of the urinary and endocrine system seldom give rise to single metastatic foci. Squamous cell carcinomas, tumors growing in portal organs and those of the testes and ovaries often show a single metastatic pattern.

Table 11.2. Tumor cell type and incidence of metastases (modified from PICKREN et al. 1982)

Histotype	Liver metastases No. (%)	No. (%)
Adenocarcinoma	4161 (38.8)	1997 (48.0)
Squamous cell carcinoma	2082 (19.4)	362 (17.4)
Leukemia	1056 (9.8)	590 (55.9)
Non-Hodgkin's lymphoma	922 (8.6)	415 (45.0)
Transitional cell carcinoma	343 (3.2)	98 (28.6)
Sarcomas	333 (3.1)	113 (33.9)
Hodgkin's disease	303 (2.8)	185 (61.1)
Malignant melanoma	302 (2.8)	185 (61.3)
Anaplastic carcinoma	267 (2.5)	118 (44.2)
Small cell carcinoma	242 (2.3)	157 (64.9)
Gliomas	188 (1.8)	2 (1.1)
Germ cell tumors	149 (1.4)	82 (55.0)
Carcinosarcoma	56 (0.5)	28 (50.0)
Neuroblastoma	53 (0.5)	33 (62.3)
Others	279 (2.6)	79 (28.3)
Total	10736 (100.0)	4444 (41.4)

11.3 Structural and Molecular Aspects of Liver Invasion by Cancer Cells

Malignant cells have the ability to invade and destroy normal tissue locally and at distant sites. The metastatic process consists of sequential steps including the detachment of cells from the primary tumor, invasion of the surrounding tissue, penetration into the circulating system, implantation into the capillary beds of the target organs, extravasation and invasion into the target tissue, formation of a vascular network, and finally proliferation at the secondary site of implantation (FIDLER 1990; FIDLER and RADINSKI 1990). Each of these steps must be completed to produce clinically relevant metastases. The failure of one of these processes, such as high degree of antigenicity, inability to invade the host stroma or to grow in a distant organ, eliminates the metastatic potential of the neoplastic cells.

Nevertheless, the mechanisms through which metastatic invasion takes place remain unknown. The anatomic localization of the primary tumor can influence in part the site of the secondary implantation. This is particularly true for tumors from portal organs, which metastasize most commonly to the liver. However, the natural pathways of drainage do not wholly explain the distribution of metastases and an organ tropism has also been suggested. In 1889, PAGET observed that different tumors metastasize preferentially to certain organs, suggesting that the organ microenvironment (the "soil") can influence the implantation, invasion, survival, and growth of particular tumor cells (the "seed"). According to this theory, tumor cells need to bind to specific ligands expressed on the endothelial cells and then to recognize and adhere both to the extracellular matrix (ECM) components and to the cells of the target organ (ZVIBEL and KRAFT 1993). Furthermore, target organs secrete paracrine growth stimulatory or inhibitory factors that will affect the growth of tumor cells (RADINSKY 1995). Tumor metastasis in the liver is a complex process in which two different events take place: the invasion of normal tissue by tumor cells on one hand and the anti-invasion mechanisms of host defense systems on the other.

The liver has two afferent blood vessels, the hepatic artery and the portal vein, and receives 1550 ml of blood per minute into its sinusoidal system. The hepatic sinusoids are wide and lined by typical fenestrated endothelial cells; there are three other types of sinusoidal cells: the perisinusoidal cells, located in the space of Disse (between the endothelial cells and the hepatocytes), the Kupffer cells and the liver-associated lymphocytes, which are found on the luminal side of the endothelium. Kupffer cells are the fixed macrophages in the liver with non-specific tumoricidal ability, and are actively involved in the host defense against tumor-cell invasion (Radinsky 1995). Endothelial cells do not form junctions with adjacent cells and have many fenestrae of different sizes, which lack diaphragms, so that they may filter sinusoidal blood. In this way, neoplastic emboli may be retained in the narrowest sites of the sinusoidal bed by mechanic entrapment, also favored by swollen endothelial cells, Kupffer cells and aggregated platelets; then, they may pass through the endothelium into the space of Disse and invade the liver. In 1952 Luke et al. demonstrated that, after intravenous and intraportal injections of tumor cells in experimental animals, there were many more metastatic implants in the liver than in the lung. This striking difference was attributed to the characteristic of liver microcirculation. These results have been confirmed in more recent times (Gjoen et al. 1989; Bagge et al. 1983; Barbara-Guillem et al. 1989), but other aspects should be emphasized in order to explain the process of metastasization.

Adhesion molecules seem to be involved in the detachment of the neoplastic cells from the primary tumor, of which the cadherin family is particularly important. The extracellular domain of cadherins contains several Ca^{2+}-binding domains and these self-associate and cause intercellular adhesion. Several intracellular proteins, α- and β-catenins, participate in linking the cytoplasmic domains of the cadherins to cytoskeletal elements. This is essential for the process of cadherin-mediated adhesion and cell aggregation. The cadherin-catenin complex binds to the cytoskeletal elements and the phosphorylation of catenins appears to regulate the adhesive function of the complex. Several cadherins and cadherin-like molecules have been identified. Of these, E-cadherin has been extensively studied and frequently found deleted or mutated in mammary infiltrating lobular cancer (Berx et al. 1995). Furthermore, the expression of E-cadherin in epithelial cell lines has been regarded as suppressor of invasive potential (Vleminckx et al 1991). Another adhesion molecule involved in the detachment of neoplastic cells is represented by the DCC (deleted in colon cancer) suppressor gene product. This gene is inactivated in colon and gastric cancer (Uchino 1992) and seems to have inhibitory effects on the metastasization of colorectal tumor cells (Levine 1993).

The loss of the intercellular junctions permits the invasion of the extracellular matrix (ECM). The ECM is composed of basement membranes and interstitial connective tissue. Each ECM component is made up of collagens, glycoproteins and proteoglycans. Type IV collagen and laminin represent the major fraction of the collagen proteins and of the glycoproteins, respectively. Laminin interacts with other macromolecules of the basement membrane, such as type IV collagen, heparan sulfate proteoglycans and with itself to provide and preserve the stability of the basement membrane. Furthermore, the laminin is able to recognize specific epithelial cell receptors. Several studies have demonstrated that the expression of the laminin receptor by the monoclonal antibody MLuC5 is associated with poor prognosis in breast cancer patients (Stetler-Stevenson et al. 1993). In addition to laminin-specific receptors, tumor cells also express integrins that can serve as receptors for many components of the ECM, including fibronectin, laminin, collagen and vitronectin (Albelda 1993). CD44 is a transmembrane glycoprotein expressed as one or more isoforms derived from alternative splicing of the RNA and differences in the pattern of glycolysilation. These isoforms have been reported to be expressed differentially between non-metastatic and metastatic tumors of the pancreas. CD44 participates in cellular adhesion and binding to ECM components, which may be mediated by cytoskeletal elements. CD44 promotes adhesion to collagen types I and IV, fibronectin, endothelial cells, and it is the major receptor for the extracellular glycosaminoglycan hyaluronate matrix component . Tumor cells with high levels of CD44 are likely to be adept at extravascular dissemination (Albelda 1993). The capability of the neoplastic cells to adhere to the endothelial wall or to the ECM in a specific way has been demonstrated by in vitro and in vivo models. For example, Hosono et al. (1998) and associates demonstrated that cells derived from pancreatic cancer, which often produce hepatic metastases, expressed a high quantity of sialyl Lewis (a) and sialyl Lewis (x) antigens, CD44H and β-1 integrin and could adhere to human endothelial and mesothelial cells. This adhesion, leading to liver implantation of cancer, was inhibited by antibodies against sialyl Lewis (a) and b-1 integrin, suggesting an important role played by these molecules in the metastatic process (Hosono et al. 1998). Moreover, an in vivo microscopy study of hepatic metastases, performed by Kan et al. (1995), demonstrated the strong tendency of the neoplastic cells to adhere to the endothelial wall in three animal models of liver metastases. The tumor marker carcinoembryonic antigen (CEA) may also play a role in cell adhesion in liver metastasis from colorectal cancer; in fact, intravenous injection of CEA increased the number of liver metastases in an experimental model of colon cancer (Jessup and Thomas 1989).

After attachment, neoplastic cells must create passageways for migration by passive growth pressure and by active enzymatic degradation of the ECM components. Among the enzymes involved in this process are the metalloproteinases, a family of metal-dependent endopeptidases (Stetler-Stevenson 1990), which are able to degrade type IV collagen, type V collagen, gelatin and proteoglycans. They are produced by connective tissue cells, as well as by many tumor cells. Experimental models demonstrated that chemical inhibitors of type IV collagenases greatly reduced metastases. Two natural tissue inhibitors of metalloproteinase (TIMPs) were isolated and their genes cloned: TIMP1e TIMP2 (Stetler-Stevenson et al.1993) greatly reduce both neoplastic invasion and angiogenesis (Stetler-Stevenson et al.1993). Injection of recombinant human TIMP reduced experimentally induced metastases in mice (Schultz et al. 1988). Cathepsin D, a cysteine proteinase, and urokinase-type plasminogen activator, a serine proteinase, are also important in the degradation of ECM. These enzymes act on numerous substrates such as fibronectin, laminin, and proteoglycans. High levels of cathepsin D in the serum are of poor prognostic value in breast cancer patients (Alvarez 1990). Recent studies demonstrated that the organ environment can influence the ability of metastatic cells to degrade the ECM through the production of growth factors and cytokines by stromal cells (Tandon 1990). This explains why in some cases the target tissue may be an unpermissive environment, an unfavorable "soil", for the growth of tumor "seeds"; in fact the presence of protease inhibitors can prevent the establishment of a tumor colony.

Cellular locomotion is the next step of invasion, by propelling tumor cells through the degraded basement membranes and areas of matrix proteolysis. Cellular motility is regulated by microtubule assembly. The NM23 gene seems to be associated with this process because its protein product produces the transphosphorylation of GDP to GTP, which is a fundamental event in microtubule assembly (Radinsky and Ellis 1996). The role of the NM23 gene is complex, as the same protein is involved in metastatic progression and in the control of cellular proliferation and differentiation. The association between a low NM23 gene expression and a high metastatic potential suggests a role of this gene in metastasis suppression. Motility is caused by tumor cell-derived cytokines, such as autocrine motility factors (AMF) (Biggs et al. 1990) or paracrine factors such as the hepatocyte growth factor (HGF). The effect of HGF is mediated by its binding to the tyrosine kinase type receptor protein encoded by the c-met oncogene (Nabi 1992). In addition, cleavage products of the matrix component such as collagen and laminin and some growth factors such as insulin-like growth factors I and II have chemotactic activity for tumor cells.

Once in the target organ, tumor development is allowed by a mixture of growth factors acting in a paracrine and autocrine way. Liver is a rich source of growth factors: for example, transforming growth factor-alpha (TGF-α) is a physiologic regulator of liver regeneration (Direnzo et al. 1995); TGF-α production by hepatocytes may have a paracrine role stimulating the proliferation of adjacent non-parenchymal cells through the epidermal growth factor receptor (EGF-R) (Mead and Fausto 1989). Another mitogen for hepatocytes is the hepatocyte growth factor (HGF) (Michalapoulos 1990), synthesized from liver nonparenchymal cells (endothelial and Kupffer cells). These growth factors, produced by tissue undergoing repair, may also stimulate the proliferation of receptive malignant tumor cells, expressing compatible receptors; this demonstrates that physiological signals can be utilized by neoplastic cells. A modern interpretation of Paget's hypothesis is that organ-specific metastasis results from the proliferation of tumor cells, differentially expressing growth factor receptors. Therefore, the production of metastatic tumors in the liver is determined by the ability of the cells to reach the organ, but also by the ability to proliferate in the hepatic parenchyma. Some experiments have demonstrated that the expression of growth factor receptors by cancer cells directly correlates with their ability to produce hepatic metastases: for example, analysis of the mRNA expression levels of EGF-R in many human colon cancer lines shows that highly metastatic cell lines have higher expression than low metastatic cell lines (Radinsky 1995).

Angiogenesis is another important factor in primary and metastatic tumor growth. Neoplastic cells producing angiogenetic factors, including vascular endothelial growth factor (VEGF), acidic and basic fibroblast growth factor (a and bFGF), tumor-necrosis factor a (TNF-α), TGF-α and TGF-β, angiogenin, angiotropin and platelet-derived endothelial-cell growth factor (PDEGF) are prone to metastasize and to grow in the secondary organ independent of the local blood supply (GHERARDI and STOKER 1991).

11.4 Pathology

Tumor deposits are multiple in the majority of cases. They can be single or confluent, varying from less than 1 mm to many centimeters in diameter. Rarely, there may be diffuse replacement of liver parenchyma such that nodules cannot be identified grossly. The gross features of liver metastases are often typical for some tumors (Figs. 11.1–11.3).

Metastases from colon carcinoma often appear as a few large nodules with central umbilication. The nodules from breast or lung carcinoma are usually medium in size without extensive necrosis or hemorrhage and with early central umbilication. Metastatic lesions of miliary type, simulating cirrhosis, are observed in breast, prostate or stomach metastatic cancer.

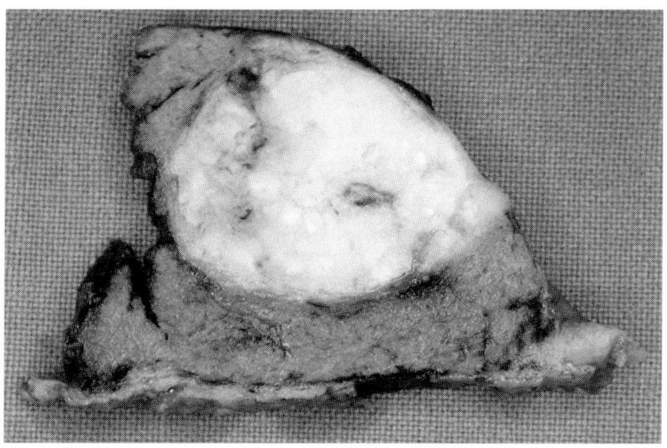

Fig. 11.1. Metastatic carcinoma. This cut surface shows a single large mass from a primary colon adenocarcinoma

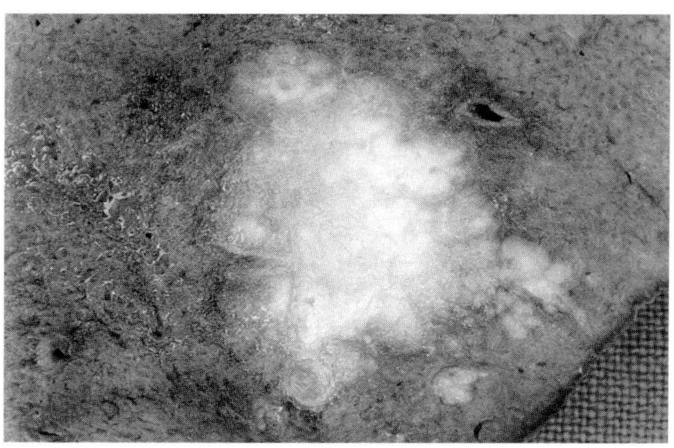

Fig. 11.2. Metastatic carcinoma. This metastatic carcinoma (primary in pancreas) consists of a single mass with numerous small satellites

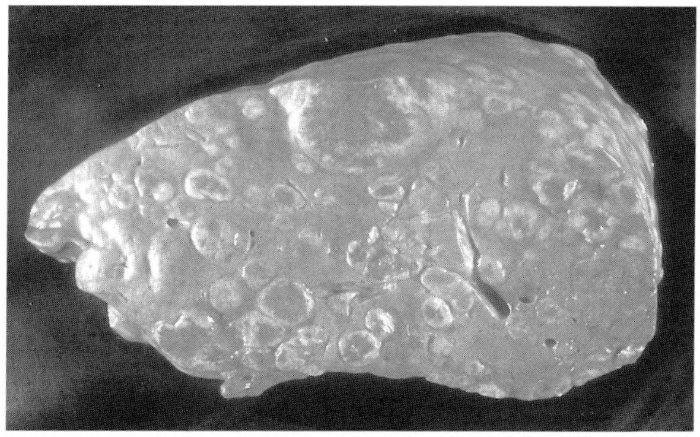

Fig. 11.3. Metastatic carcinoma. Multiple nodules of similar size with central depression and hemorrhage (primary lung bronchogenic carcinoma)

Squamous-cell carcinomas typically have a necrotic center, whereas small-cell carcinoma, sarcoma, seminoma, melanoma or non-Hodgkin's lymphoma often display a fish-flesh appearance (Figs. 11.4–11.6).

Many hepatic lesions may show a gross appearance indistinguishable from metastatic lesions. This happens for adenoma, nodular hyperplasia, bile duct hamartoma, granulomas and, rarely, for hepatocellular carcinoma or cholangiocarcinoma. An unusual growth pattern of metastatic colon carcinoma is represented by spreading throughout the biliary tree along intact basement membranes. This pattern could be mistaken for primary biliary neoplasia (KANAI et al. 1998). Another example of rare growth pattern has been described for neuroendocrine, ovarian and uterine cervical tumors producing

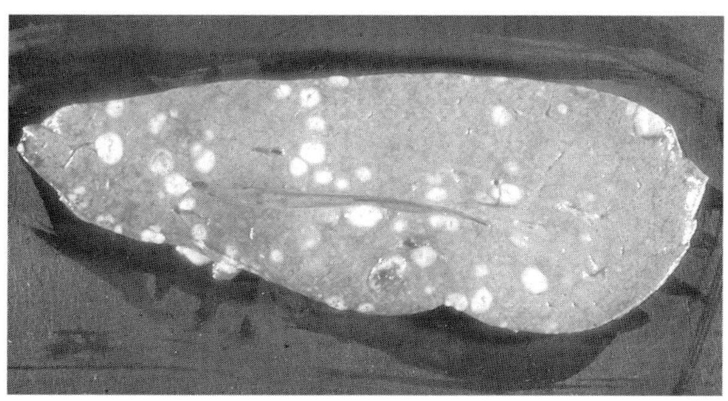

Fig. 11.4. Melanoma. Nodules of metastatic melanoma with a fish flesh appearance

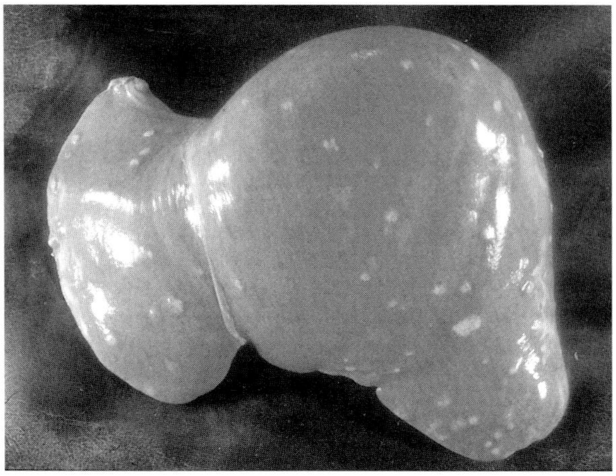

Fig. 11.5. Metastatic carcinoma. Subcapsular multiple nodules of metastatic carcinoma (bladder origin)

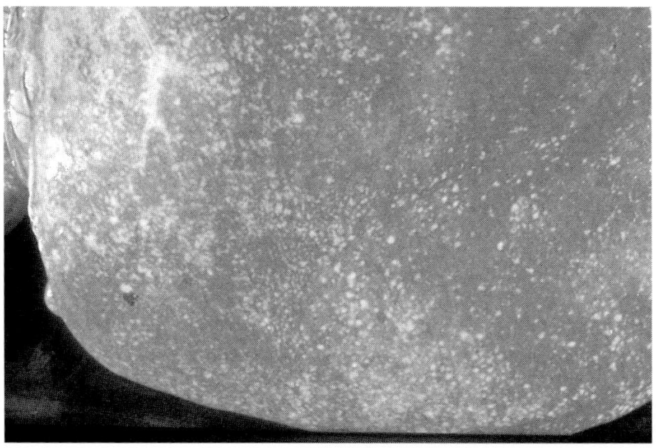

Fig. 11.6. Lymphoma. Miliary spread of non-Hodgkin's lymphoma

pseudocystic liver metastases mimicking polycystic liver disease (Riopel et al. 1997). Cirrhotic and fatty liver is less susceptible to metastatic invasion than normal liver (Estermann et al. 1996; Melato et al. 1989). The reasons for these findings need to be clarified; the alteration of the hepatic architecture could be an explanation.

The microscopic features of metastatic tumors can repeat the histologic aspects of the primary site, including the stromal component, particularly conspicuous in neoplasias from breast, pancreas and stomach, but scant in small cell carcinomas. Other neoplasms do not usually evoke a local reaction and may grow in the sinusoids, simulating hepatocellular carcinoma (HCC). This is the case of small cell carcinomas and melanomas; the latter also grow in a trabecular pattern and have a cytology that may resemble HCC; for these reasons, especially in amelanotic cases, diagnosis is difficult and light microscopy is not sufficient.

Another problem is that of distinguishing HCC from adrenal and renal cell carcinoma, which often have a trabecular pattern of growth and show clear cell features, or from metastatic adenocarcinomas or cholangiocarcinomas. Recognizing primary from metastatic liver carcinomas is often difficult, in particular when they are poorly differentiated. Moreover, approximately 5% of oncologic patients have a diagnosis of unknown primary tumors and among these, according to recent studies, the prevalence of liver metastases is about 30% (Hayashi et al. 1997). A good approach for evaluating these patients is to start with a liver biopsy in order to discover the primary site. Therefore, the pathologist must use special techniques, such as histochemistry, immunohistochemistry and, in some cases, electron microscopy, for a differential diagnosis, which could have prognostic significance.

11.5 Differential Diagnosis

Distinguishing primary hepatocellular carcinoma from metastatic tumors is often difficult, especially when they are poorly differentiated. The periodic acid-Schiff reaction after diastase digestion (dPAS) is useful in the differentiation of mucin-negative HCC from cholangiocellular carcinoma (CCC) or from certain metastatic tumors, which show a positive result in the majority of cases. Van Gieson's stain may help to distinguish the bile pigment in the tumor. Bile production is specific for the hepatocellular origin of the neoplasia.

Many studies have indicated the utility of immunohistochemistry in the differential diagnosis of metastatic neoplasias. It was previously thought that the cytokeratin (CK) expression could be useful in distinguishing HCC, CCC and metastatic carcinoma (Ayoub et al. 1998; Johnson et al. 1988). CK and the epithelial membrane antigen (EMA) are considered useful markers of epithelial origin (Ayoub et al. 1998; Fisher et al. 1987). Hepatocytes express CK8 and CK18, while biliary epithelial cells also express CK7 and CK19 (Balaton et al. 1988; Moll et al. 1982). About 50% of HCC also express bile duct type CKs (CK7, CK19), in addition to CK8 and CK18 (Denk et al. 1992). Different results have been reported by various authors using several monoclonal antibodies to CK with different specificities. CAM 5.2 is a monoclonal antibody which recognizes CK8, CK18, and CK19 and reacts with most HCCs (Ayoub et al. 1998). AE1 recognizes CK10, CK14, CK15, CK16, and CK19 and reacts with the bile duct epithelium but not with hepatocytes. Some authors found no reaction of AE1 with HCCs (Ayoub et al. 1998) and others found that it reacted with many HCCs (van Eyken et al. 1988; Ma et al. 1993). AE3 does not react with normal hepatocytes (Battifora 1988) but it stains none (Tseng et al. 1982) to 30% (van Eyken et al. 1988) of HCCs. These results suggest that the cytokeratin profile may not be a reliable way to distinguish HCCs from cholangiocellular carcinoma or from liver metastases (Christensen et al. 1989; Anthony and Bannasch 1994). Several other antibodies to epithelial antigens have been used in the differentiation of primary and metastatic liver tumors: Leu-M1; tumor-associated glycoprotein-72 (B72.3); human milk fat globule (HMFG-2); BCA-225, a glycoprotein secreted by the T47D breast carcinoma cell line; Ber-EP4, reacting with two glycoproteins present on the surface and in the cytoplasm of all epithelial cells, except the superficial layers of squamous epithelia, hepatocytes and mesothelial cells. Only BCA-225 demonstrated a significant difference between HCCs, generally negative, and metastatic adenocarcinomas, generally positive (Thung et al. 1979). Cholangiocellular carcinomas have a staining profile similar to that of metastatic cancer (van Eyken et al. 1988).

Many studies suggest the usefulness of carcinoembryonic antigen (CEA) in distinguishing HCCs from metastatic carcinomas in the liver, especially those from the gastrointestinal tract. In HCCs, CEA staining, using a monoclonal antibody, is rare (van Eyken and Desmet 1993; Desmet et al. 1990; Ganjei et al. 1988; Ferrandez-Izquierdo and Llombart-Bosh 1987; Brumm et al. 1989) compared to CCCs and metastatic tumors from the gastrointestinal tract, where it is frequently positive. The use of a polyclonal-antibody to CEA produces a typical canalicular stain in HCCs, which is absent in CCCs and in metastatic tumors (van Eyken et al. 1988).

In conclusion, the antibody useful for distinguishing HCC from metastatic carcinomas is pCEA. A bile canalicular staining pattern with pCEA would confirm a diagnosis of HCC, while positive cytoplasmic and negative bile canalicular staining would support a diagnosis of metastatic carcinoma. Furthermore, of the antibodies to cytocheratins, the most useful appears to be the CU-18 which recognizes BCA-225.

Tumors arising from the neuroendocrine system express particular markers such as chromogranin, neuron-specific enolase (NSE), synaptophysin, and sometimes hormones evaluable by immunohistochemistry. Malignancies other than carcinomas such as sarcomas, melanomas, central nervous system neoplasias, lymphomas, leukemias, and multiple myelomas can metastasize to the liver. A panel of monoclonal or polyclonal antibodies has to be employed to identify the primary site. In particular, antibodies to vimentin are able to recognize the mesenchymal origin of the neoplasia; in addition, the positivity of actin or factor VIII-related antigen permits a diagnosis of smooth muscle or endothelial cell origin. Combined S-100 protein and HMB-45 positivity support a melanocytic origin of the neoplasia. NSE and neurofilaments are markers of neuronal cells. The leukocyte-common antigen (LCA) is a panlymphocyte marker. Since immunocytochemical markers often lack specificity, an accurate evaluation of the morphology, together with clinical findings, should be performed to determine the nature of the neoplasia.

References

Albelda SM (1993) Role of integrins and other cell-adhesion molecules in tumor progression and metastasis. Lab Invest 68:4–8

Alvarez OA (1990) Inhibition of collagenolytic activity and metastases of tumor cells by recombinant human tissue inhibitor of metalloproteinases. J Natl Cancer Inst 82:589–594

Anthony PP, Bannasch P (1994) Tumors and tumor-like lesions of the liver and biliary tract. In: MacSween RNM, Anthony PP, Sheuer PJ. (eds) Pathology of the liver. Churchill Livingstone, Edimburgh, pp 635–667

Ayoub JP, Hess KR, Abbruzzese MC, Lenzi R, Raber MN, Abbruzzese JL (1998) Unknown primary tumors metastatic to liver. J Clin Oncol 16:2105–2112

Bagge U, Skolnik G, Ericson LE (1983) The arrest of circulating tumor cells in the liver microcirculation. J Cancer Res Clin Oncol 105:134–140

Balaton AJ, Nehama-Siboni M, Gotheil C(1988) Distinction between hepatocellular carcinoma, cholangiocarcinoma, and metastatic carcinoma based on immunohistochemical staining for carcinoembryonic antigen and for cytocheratin 19 on paraffin sections. J Pathol 156:305–310

Barbara-Guillem E, Alonso-Varona A, Vidal-Vanaclocha F (1989) Selective implantation and growth in rats and mice of experimental liver metastasis in acinar zone one. Cancer Res 49:4003–4010

Battifora H (1988) Diagnostic uses of antibodies to keratins: a review and immunohistochemical comparison of seven monoclonal antibodies. In: Fenoglio CM, Wolff M (eds) Progress in Surgical Pathology, vol 8. Masson, New York, pp 1–5

Berx G, Clenton-Janson AM, Nollet F (1995) E-cadherin is a tumor invasion suppressor gene mutated in human lobular breast cancers. EMBO J 14:6107–6115

Biggs J, Hersperger E, Steeg PS, Liotta LA, Shearn A (1989) Drosophila gene that is homologous to a mammalian gene associated with tumor metastasis codes for a nucleoside diphosphate kinase. Cell 63: 933–940

Brumm C, Schulze C, Charles K (1989) The significance of alpha-fetoprotein and other tumor markers in differential immunocytochemistry of primary liver tumors. Histopathology 14:503–513

Christensen WN, Boitnott JK, Kuhajda FP (1989) Immunoperoxidase staining as a diagnostic aid for hepatocellular carcinoma. Mod Pathol 2:8–12

Craig JR, Peters RL, Edmonson HA (1989) Tumors of the liver and intrahepatic bile ducts. Fascicle 26, 2nd series. Washington, DC: Armed Forces Institute of Pathology

Denk H, Krepler R, Lackinger E (1982) Biochemical and immunohistochemical analysis of the intermediate filament cytoscheleton in human hepatocellular and in hepatic neoplastic nodules of mice. Lab Invest 46:584–596

Desmet VJ, van Eyken P, Sciot R. Cytocheratins (1990) for probing cell lineage relationship in developing liver. Hepatology 12:1249–1251

Direnzo MF, Poulsom R, Olivero M, Comoglio PM, Lemoine NR (1995) Expression of the met hepatocyte growth factor receptor in human pancreatic cancer. Cancer Res 55:1129–38

Estermann F, Thiebault S, Turnani C, Djabri M, Wiedmann, Sondag D (1996) Pseudocystic hepatic metastases from a carcinoma of the uterine cervix mimiking polycystic liver disease. Gastroenterol Clin Biol 20:1125–1128

Ferrandez-Izquierdo A, Llombart-Bosh A (1987) Immunohistochemical characterization of 130 cases of primary hepatic carcinomas. Pathol Res Pract 182: 783–791

Fidler IJ (1990) Critical factors in the biology of human cancer metastasis: twenty-eighth GHA. Clowes Memorial Award Lecture. Cancer Res 50:6130–6138

Fidler IJ, Radinsky R (1990) Genetic control of cancer metastasis. J Natl Cancer Inst 82:166–168

Fisher HP, Altmannsberger M, Weber K, Osborn M (1987) Keratin polypeptides in malignant epithelial liver tumors: differential diagnostic and histogenetic aspects. Am J Pathol 127:530–537

Ganjei P, Nadji M, Albores-Saavedra J, Morakles AR (1988) Histologic markers in primary and metastatic tumors of the liver. Cancer 62:1994–1998

Gherardi E, Stoker (1991) M. Hepatocyte growth factor-scatter factor: mitogen, motogen, and met. Cancer Cells 3:227–232

Gjoen T, Seljelid R, Kolset S (1989) Binding of metastatic colon carcinoma cells to liver macrophages. J Leukoc Biol 45:362–369

Hayashi S, Masuda H, Shigematsu M (1997) Liver metastasis rare in colorectal cancer patients with fatty liver. Hepato-Gastroenterology 44:1069–1075

Hosono J, Narita T, Kimura N (1988) Involvement of adhesion molecules in metastasis of SW1990, human pancreatic cancer cells. J Surg Oncol 67:77–84

Jessup JM, Thomas P (1989) Carcinoembryonic antigen: function in metastasis by human colorectal carcinoma. Cancer Metastasis Rev 1:263–280

Johnson DE, Herndier BG, Medeiros LJ (1988) The diagnostic utility of the keratin profiles of hepatocellular carcinoma and cholangiocarcinoma. Am J Surg Pathol 12:187–197

Kan Z, Ivancev K, Lunderquist A, McCuskey P, McCuskey R, Wallace S (1995) In vivo microscopy of hepatic metastases: dynamic observation of tumor cell invasion and interaction with Kupffer cells. Hepatology 21:487–494

Kanai T, Konno H, Tanaka T (1998) Anti-tumor and antimetastatic effects of human-vascular-endothelial-growth factor-neutralizing antibody on human colon and gastric carcinoma xenotransplanted orthotopically into nude mice. Int J Cancer 77:933–936

Levine AJ (1993) The tumor suppressor genes. Annu Rev Biochem 62:623–651

Luke B (1952) Differential grouth of metastatic tumors in liver and lung. Experiments with rabbit V2 carcinoma. Cancer Res, 12: 734–738

Ma CK, Zarbo RJ, Frierson HF, Lee MW (1993) Comparative immunohistochemical study of primary and metastatic carcinomas of the liver. Am J Clin Pathol 99:551–557

Mead JE, Fausto N (1989) Trasforming growth factor-a may be a physiological regulator of liver regeneration by means of an autocrine mechanism. Proc Natl Acad Sci USA 86:1558–1562

Melato M, Laurino L, Mucli E, Valente M, Okuda K (1989) Relationship between cirrhosis, liver cancer and hepatic metastases. Cancer 64:455–459

Michalopoulos GK (1990) Liver regeneration: molecular mechanisms of growth control. FASB J 4:176–187

Moll R, Franke WW, Schiller DL (1982) The catalogue of human cytocheratins: patterns of expression in normal epithelia, tumors and cultured cells. Cell 31:11–24

Nabi IR (1992) Autocrine motility factor and its receptor: role in cell locomotion and metastasis. Cancer Metastasis Rev 11:5–10

Paget S (1989) The distribution of secondary grouth in cancer of the breast. Cancer Metastasis Rev 8:98–101

Pickren JW, Tsukada Y, Lane WW (1982) Liver Metastasis. Analysis of Autopsy Data. In: Weiss L, Gilbert HA (eds) Liver Metastasis. Hall Medical Publishers, Boston pp 2–18

Radinsky R (1995) Molecular mechanisms for organ-specific colon carcinoma metastasis. Eur J Cancer 31a:1091–1095

Radinsky R, Ellis LM (1996) Molecular determinants in the biology of liver metastasis. Surg Oncol Clin N Am 5:215–229

Riopel MA, Klimstra DS, Godellas CV, Blumgart LH, Westra WH (1997) Intrabiliary growth of metastatic colonic adenocarcinoma. Am J Surg Pathol 21:1030–1036

Schultz RM, Silberman S, Persky B, Bajowski AS, Carmichael DF (1988) Inhibition by recombinant tissue inhibitor of metalloproteinases of human amnion invasion and lung colonization by murine B16-F10 melanoma cells. Cancer Res 48:5539–5545

Stetler-Stevenson WG (1990) Type IV collagenases in tumor invasion and metastasis. Cancer Metastasis Rev 9:289–330

Stetler-Stevenson WG, Aznavoorian S, Liotta LA (1993) Tumor cell interactions with the extracellular matrix during invasion and metastasis. Annu Rev Cell Biol 9:541–573

Tandon AK (1990) Cathepsin D and prognosis in breast cancer. N Engl J Med 322:297–305

Thung SN, Gerber MA, Sarno E, Popper H (1979) Distribution of five antigens in hepatocellular carcinoma. Lab Invest 41:101–105

Tseng SC, Jarvinen MJ, Nelson WG (1982) Correlation of specific keratins with different types of epithelial differentiation: monoclonal antibody studies. Cell 30:361–372

Uchino S (1992) Frequent loss of heterozygosity at the DCC locus in gastric cancer. Cancer Res 52:3099–3104

van Eyken P, Desmet VJ (1993) Cytocheratins and the liver. Liver 13:113–122

van Eyken P, Sciot R, Paterson A (1988) Cytocheratin expression in hepatocellular carcinoma: an immunohistochemical study. Hum Pathol 19:562–568

Vleminckx K, Mareel M, Vakaet LJr, Friers W, van Roy F (1991) Expression of E-cadherin in epithelial cell lines is negatively correlated with invasion. Clin Exp Metastasis 8:17–23

Zvibel I, Kraft A (1993) Extracellular matrix and metastasis. In: Zern MA, Reid LM (eds) Extracellular matrix: its chemistry, biology, and pathobiology, vol 22. Marcel Dekker, New York, pp 559–580

12 Ultrasound and Color Doppler Ultrasound of Liver Metastases

P. Ricci, M. Coniglio, A. Di Filippo, R. Kayal, G. Pizzi, and V. Cantisani

CONTENTS

12.1 Introduction

In western countries metastases are the most common cause of malignant focal liver lesions. Metastases are 18–20 times more common than primary malignant tumors. Sixty percent of patients with newly diagnosed solid tumors (excluding skin cancer other than melanoma) have clinically evident or microscopic metastases, when the primary tumor is diagnosed (Liotta and Stetler-Stevenson 1989). The true prevalence of metastatic disease is unknown. In 1950, Abrams et al. reviewed a series of 1000 autopsy cases of epithelial malignancy in which colorectal, breast, lung and gastric carcinomas accounted for almost two-thirds of the primary tumors. The liver and abdominal lymph nodes were the most common sites involved (49% for both). The liver was the most common organ involved in colorectal carcinoma (65%), in colon carcinoma and in rectal carcinoma (47%). Liver metastases were present in 61% of patients with breast carcinoma and in 45% of patients with gastric carcinoma.

The process of invasion and metastasis of neoplastic cells is extremely complex and not fully understood. The process of metastasis proceeds through a series of sequential steps that involve complex tumor-host interactions. Results of numerous studies have confirmed that metastatic organ involvement is not random and cannot be explained on the basis of blood flow alone (Killion and Fidle 1989). The liver may be fertile soil for the metastatic cell because of the presence of humoral factors that promote cell growth. The specific configuration of the endothelial lining of the liver may make the liver susceptible to metastatic disease. The endothelial cells are perforated by small fenestrae without diaphragms, which creates a sievelike configuration. This morphology serves as a potential open connection between the sinusoids and the extracellular matrix of the space of Disse. Thus the normal barriers to metastatic cells commonly present in most organs are absent or incomplete in the liver.

Detection of liver metastases is a unique challenge for the radiologist, primarily because the liver has a dual blood supply. Some authors estimate that the hepatic artery supplies 20–30% of the total blood flow to the liver, whereas the portal vein supplies 70–80% (Fink and Chaudhuri 1991). Most people assume that the primary mode of metastatic cell delivery in gastrointestinal cancer is the portal vein. Autopsy evidence supports this assumption: tumor emboli are rarely seen in the hepatic artery end vessels and are commonly seen in the portal venules. By the time metastases are clinically evident, however, they usually receive the majority of their blood supply from the hepatic artery, although several studies have shown that many metastases receive substantial blood flow from the portal vein.

There are many methods available for the detection of intrahepatic metastatic disease, including transabdominal, intraoperative and laparoscopic ul-

P. Ricci, MD; Department of Radiology, University of Rome "La Sapienza", Viale Regina Elena 324, I-00161 Rome, Italy
M. Coniglio, MD; Department of Radiology, University of Rome "La Sapienza", Viale Regina Elena 324, I-00161 Rome, Italy
A. Di Filippo, MD; Department of Radiology, University of Rome "La Sapienza", Viale Regina Elena 324, I-00161 Rome, Italy
R. Kayal, MD; Department of Radiology, University of Rome "La Sapienza", Viale Regina Elena 324, I-00161 Rome, Italy
G. Pizzi, MD; Department of Radiology, University of Rome "La Sapienza", Viale Regina Elena 324, I-00161 Rome, Italy
V. Cantisani, MD; Department of Radiology, University of Rome "La Sapienza", Viale Regina Elena 324, I-00161 Rome, Italy

trasound (US), CT and MR imaging, and radionuclide scanning. The role of imaging is to detect all sites of disease in the liver and to select the patients most eligible for cure.

12.2 Conventional Ultrasound

The sonographic appearance of liver metastases is variable, and no definite association exists between the histologic type and the sonographic appearance. Usually they can be divided into nodular and diffuse lesions. Sonographic patterns of nodular metastatic disease include target pattern, hypoechoic, isoechoic, hyperechoic, calcified and cystic (Table 12.1) (Fig. 12.1).

The target pattern or bull's-eye pattern is usually characterized by a central echogenic area and peripheral hypoechoic rim. When the peripheral hypoechoic rim is thin (<3 mm), the appearance has been described as the halo sign, while a thick rim (>3 mm) identifies the target pattern. The hypoechoic peripheral rim is caused by compressed and edematous normal liver parenchyma around the tumor or more likely by a zone of proliferating tumor in the periphery of the lesion. Less often we can see target pattern metastases with a central ipo-anechoic area and hyperechoic rim, generally related to hypervascular lesions with a necrotic central area (Parulekar and Bree 1998). Target pattern is not specific, but is most often seen in malignant tumors, most commonly metastatic lesions in the liver rather than benign tumors. In a study of 100 liver tumors, the target sign was seen in 88% of malignant lesions and only in 14% of benign tumors (Wernecke et al. 1992). Usually this kind of metastases is secondary to gastrointestinal or pancreatic tumors.

Hypoechoic lesions can be secondary to lymphoma, melanoma, breast and lung carcinoma, and, less commonly, related to gastrointestinal malignant tumors.

Isoechoic metastases are uncommon and can be detected by the hypoechoic halo sign or if they displace adjacent vessels.

Hyperechoic metastases frequently arise from gastrointestinal tumors, and most commonly adenocarcinoma of the colon. Sometimes they can be secondary to renal cell carcinoma, islet cell carcinoma of the pancreas, carcinoid and chorioncarcinoma. The echogenicity is related to the vascularity of the tumor: most hypervascular lesions appear hyperechoic and most hypovascular lesions are hypoechoic.

Table 12.1. US patterns of liver metastases

Patterns	Metastasis
Target pattern	Different primary malignant disease
Hypoechoic	Lymphoma, melanoma, breast and lung carcinoma (most common) Gastrointestinal tumors (less common)
Hyperechoic	Colon carcinoma Gastrointestinal tumors Renal cell carcinoma Islet cell carcinoma of the pancreas Carcinoid Chorioncarcinoma
Calcified	Colon carcinoma (mucinous type) Cystadenocarcinoma of the ovary Adenocarcinoma of the stomach Leiomyosarcoma Osteosarcoma Neuroblastoma Breast adenocarcinoma Melanoma
Cystic	Sarcomas (leiomyosarcoma of gastrointestinal origin) Cystadenocarcinoma (pancreas, ovary) Colon carcinoma (mucinous type) Squamous cell carcinoma
Diffuse	Breast carcinoma Different primary malignant tumors

Calcified metastases appear hyperechoic with distal acoustic shadowing. Calcification may be central, peripheral or the entire mass may be calcified. Calcified metastases are commonly due to carcinoma of the colon (mucinous type), cystoadenocarcinoma of the ovary, adenocarcinoma of the stomach, islet cell carcinoma of the pancreas, leiomyosarcoma, osteosarcoma, neuroblastoma, and, rarely, adenocarcinoma of the breast and melanoma.

Cystic metastases are rare and can be secondary to metastatic sarcomas, mainly leiomyosarcoma of gastrointestinal origin. They can also occur in other malignant disease like cystoadenocarcinomas of the ovary and pancreas. Cystic metastases can result from cystic primary tumors or from necrosis of metastatic lesions. Unlike simple hepatic cysts, the cystic metastases usually have irregular margins, a thick wall, mural nodules, multiple septa, or a fluid-fluid level (Parulekar and Bree 1998).

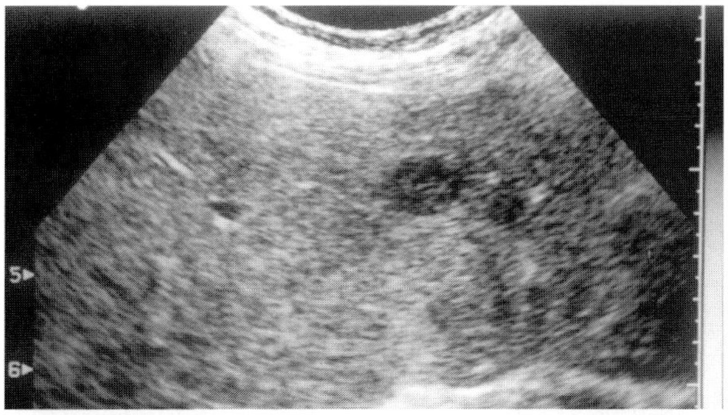

a

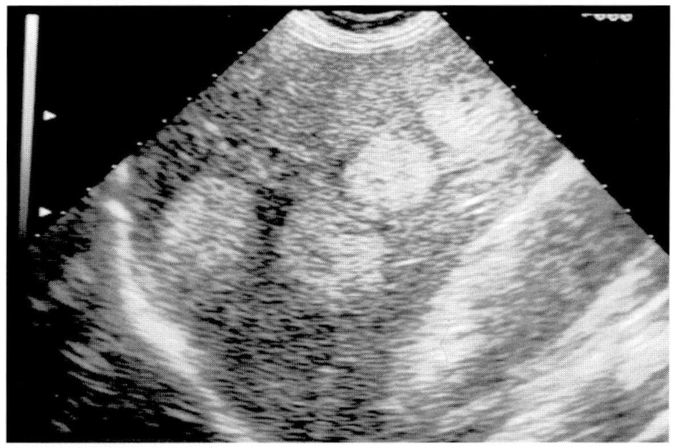

b

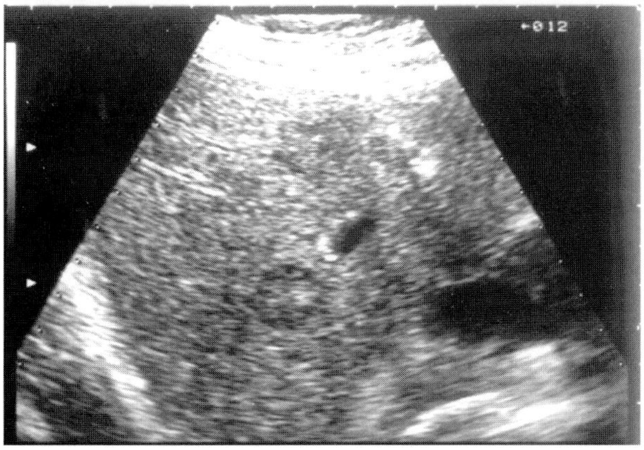

c

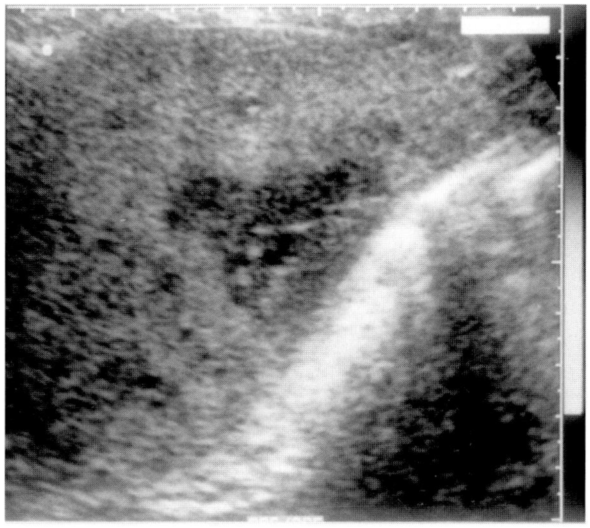

d

Fig. 12.1a–d. Different US patterns of liver metastases: **a** Hypoechoic pattern from pancreatic carcinoma, better evaluable with high-frequency probe (3.5 vs 7.5 MHz). **b** Hyperechoic pattern from colon carcinoma. **c** Target pattern from breast cancer. **d** Hypoechoic pattern with small calcifications from ovarian cancer

The diffuse type of metastatic disease distorts liver parenchyma and produces a diffusely inhomogeneous echo pattern. Frequently there is involvement of the biliary tree responsible for jaundice or of the hepatic veins responsible for Budd-Chiari syndrome. This kind of lesion is rare and may be difficult to differentiate from other hepatic disorders: cirrhosis, diffusely infiltrating hepatocellular carcinoma or focal fatty infiltration. Diffuse infiltration of the liver is frequently seen secondary to metastatic disease from breast carcinoma, but it can also be secondary to other malignant tumors.

12.3 Color Doppler Ultrasound

Color Doppler US is a major advance in sonography of liver lesions, because it enables the pattern of blood flow to be determined within and around such lesions. Liver lesions are, in fact, difficult to differentiate from each other by using conventional sonography.

Color Doppler can aid the differentiation of hepatocellular carcinoma (HCC) from other liver masses on the basis of the patterns of blood flow within and around the lesions on color Doppler flow imaging. Four patterns are commonly described: (a) a fine blood-flow network surrounding the tumor nodule (basket pattern); (b) blood flow that runs into and branches within the tumor (vessel within the tumor); (c) color-stained dots or patches in the central region of the tumor (spot pattern); and (d) a dilated portal vein meandering around the tumor nodules (detour pattern) (Tanaka et al. 1990). The basket and the vessel-within-the-tumor patterns are characteristic of HCC, the spot pattern occurs most frequently in hemangiomas, and the detour pattern can be detected in metastases. However, even though most metastatic lesions are avascular as seen with color-Doppler sonography, internal flow can be seen in 33% of metastatic lesions. Therefore it is difficult to differentiate various hepatic tumors solely on the basis of their color Doppler patterns.

The utility of conventional duplex Doppler sonography for differentiating hepatic tumors has been reported by several authors. A peak systolic flow velocity of 0.40 m/s or greater suggests a malignant hepatic tumor rather than hemangioma, with a sensitivity of 67%, a specificity of 91% and an accuracy of 71%. However, measurement of tumoral peak systolic flow velocity fails to differentiate HCC from hepatic metastases. When considering the Doppler shift, we can check that the mean peak systolic Doppler shift for hepatomas (4.72±1.72 kHz) is significantly higher than that of metastases (1.99±1.63 kHz) and hemangiomas (0.53±0.75 kHz). While the specificity is high, the corresponding sensitivities are low: therefore a negative test is not reliable. The resistive index (quantity difference between peak systole and end diastole divided by peak systole) finally plays no role in differentiating hepatomas from metastases or malignant from benign hepatic lesions. If we look at different lesions, we can obtain a wide range of impedance to flow (Reinhold et al. 1995).

The hepatic tumor index (the ratio of peak systolic velocity in the tumor to that in the hepatic artery) obtained from color Doppler US can be useful in differentiating HCCs from hepatic metastases. The hepatic artery normally tapers and divides. Therefore the peak systolic velocity seen in the distal side of a hepatic branch does not exceed the velocity seen in the proximal side. In hepatic tumors the feeding arteries are directly supplied by hepatic artery branches. However, because tumor vessels have many variations, the peak systolic velocities obtained from the hepatic artery do not necessarily exceed the velocities of tumoral pulsatile flow. The hepatic tumor index represents the ratio of peak systolic velocities obtained from tumoral pulsatile flow and the proximal side of the hepatic artery.

The mean hepatic tumor indexes obtained reported in the current literature are 1.14±0.37 for HCC, 0.63±0.22 for metastases and 0.60±0.17 for hemangiomas (Numata et al. 1997). The hepatic tumor indexes of hepatocellular carcinoma significantly exceed those of metastases and hemangiomas. An hepatic tumor index equal to or greater than 1.0 is associated with 76% sensitivity, 92% specificity and 82% accuracy in distinguishing hepatocellular carcinomas from hepatic metastases. In lesions with a tumoral peak systolic velocity of 0.40 m/s or greater, an hepatic tumor index equal to or greater than 1.0 is associated with 91% sensitivity, 83% specificity and 89% accuracy in distinguishing HCCs from hepatic metastases.

The use of duplex Doppler US to measure hepatic arterial and portal venous blood flow in patients with colorectal carcinoma has been reported by Leen et al. in 1991. By using the ratio of hepatic arterial to total liver blood flow (Doppler perfusion index – DPI), they initially noted that patients with overt liver metastases could be distinguished from control subjects at initial examination. Later, as they followed patients over time, they noted that those with a high DPI (over 0.3) either had liver metastases at initial examination or developed them over the next year. This suggests that the US-guided DPI technique could help detect both overt and occult (very small) liver metastases . The reported DPI sensitivity (100%), accuracy (86%) and negative predictive rate (100%) for liver metastases are very impressive and are substantially better than those observed with either of the imaging modalities or findings at laparotomy.

The main disadvantage of this approach is that the measurements must be performed by an experienced, skillful and meticulous operator to prevent considerable artifactual variability in the results. The evaluation of DPI needs, in fact, the measurement of hepatic artery peak systolic and portal vein main velocities and the correct evaluation of the cross-sectional areas of both artery and vein. We have to consider always that a 1-mm error in cross-sectional area means a 20% error in the evaluation of flow.

One potential deficiency in this technique is that patients with cirrhosis may have similar changes in hepatic perfusion. In fact the DPI values in cirrhotic patients are very high. Patients with cirrhosis can be differentiated from those with metastases by the congestive index, defined as the ratio of the portal vein cross-sectional area to the time average velocity of blood flow in the portal vein.

12.4 Ultrasound Contrast Media

The use of contrast agents in focal liver lesions has also been studied by several investigators. Because of the large variety of focal liver lesions and the dual blood supply of the liver, assessment of liver lesions with contrast-enhanced color Doppler is much more complex, however.

The data in the literature are at times contradictory, but typical features of some pathologies are emerging. Hepatocellular carcinomas are almost invariably hypervascular centrally and peripherally after contrast administration, and any liver lesion displaying these features must be regarded with great suspicion, although some benign lesions, such as focal nodular hyperplasia and adenoma, may behave in a similar fashion. Demonstration of vessels in hemangiomas less than 3 cm in size is rare, while larger hemangiomas usually display peripheral vessels after contrast administration. Most metastases of common tumors, such as colorectal or pancreatic primaries, typically show only a mild degree of peripheral vascularity, whereas hypervascular metastases (neuroendocrine tumor or renal cell carcinoma) often display vascularity throughout after contrast.

Three main patterns of vascular distribution on contrast enhanced US are commonly described:

1. Vessels within the lesions
2. Vessels at the periphery of the lesions
3. Vessels both within and at the periphery of the lesion

Pattern 2 is most frequent in metastases from breast cancer, while pattern 3 is commonly seen in metastases from colorectal carcinoma (Campani et al. 1998) (Fig. 12.2).

Imaging tumor vascularity with contrast-enhanced Doppler US should allow much earlier assessment of treatment response than the conventional imaging criterion of reduced tumor size. Several Italian groups are using contrast-enhanced Doppler of malignant liver lesions to guide and monitor percutaneous ablation procedures (Bartolozzi et al. 1998).

Because microbubble echo-enhancers are blood pool agents, they can be used as intravascular tracers to dynamically study blood flow in body organs or tumors, in order to perform functional kinetic studies of physiological indexes such as transit times and perfusion. Flow in malignant tumor vasculature is known to have considerable spatial and temporal variation. All these features are potentially accessible to dynamic studies with US contrast agents and should be reflected in time/intensity curves. There is a significant difference in the shape of time/intensity curves in different tumors. Normal liver paren-

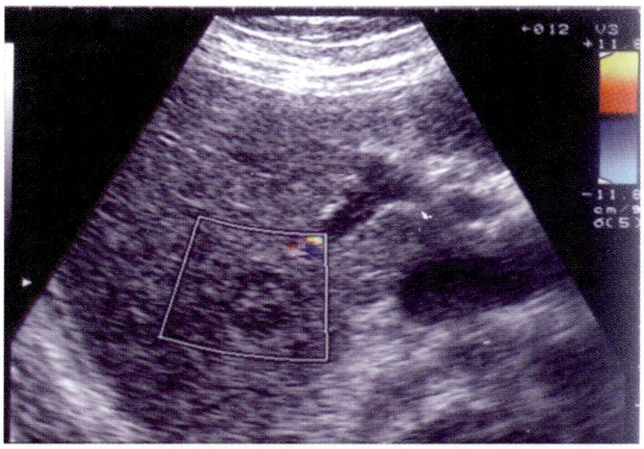
a

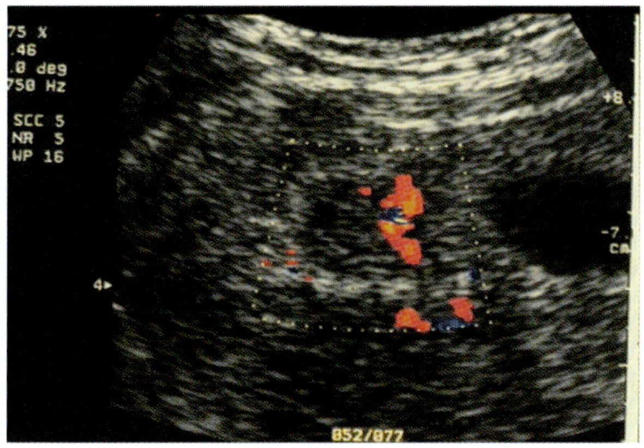
b

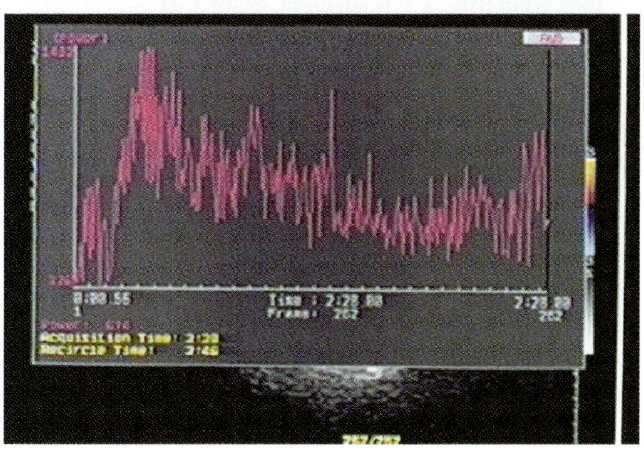
c

Fig. 12.2a–c. Color-Doppler US: hypovascular metastasis from breast carcinoma (**a**). After i.v. injection of Levovist (Schering AG, Berlin, Germany: 4 g, 300 mg/ml, slow injection rate), evidence of flow signals at the periphery of the lesion (**b**). The time/intensity curve reveals only the presence of arterial supply, without evidence of the portal phase (**c**) chyma or a regenerating nodule present a bimodal curve due to the presence of both arterial and portal phases, while the portal phase is quite small in HCCs and completely absent in metastases. These encouraging results seem to indicate that contrast enhanced Doppler US can reliably aid the differentiation of different liver lesions.

Apart from simple backscatter, various effects occur on insonation, including harmonic resonance, microbubble disruption and stimulated acoustic emission. All these phenomena should be considered as non-linear effects, which occur when increasing sound pressure is applied to microbubbles.

Harmonic imaging is a technique which allows the evaluation of echoes coming from microbubbles, while echoes from tissue are relatively suppressed. The result is similar to that of digital subtraction angiography and is related to the production of specific harmonic signal from microbubbles, when insonated with higher sound pressure. Harmonic imaging can be used both in gray-scale and Doppler US and is particularly useful to detect contrast in small vessels, thus enhancing the visualization of the vascularization in small tumors.

The most important non-linear effect for the evaluation of liver metastases is probably the stimulated acoustic emission, which is a specific transient non-linear microbubble response to insonation associated with the display of wide-frequency high-intensity Doppler shift. It appears as superadded wide-frequency signals and on color-Doppler as a characteristic color mosaic effect obtainable from all tissues containing a sufficiently high number of microbubbles. The effect is caused by microbubble disruption or destruction and has been best described with SHU 563 (Schering AG, Germany), a novel encapsulated agent. After an initial blood pool phase, it accumulates in the liver and the spleen, where it is taken up by the RES. It therefore has liver-specific properties with lesions such as metastases standing out as a focal color void against a background diffuse polychromatic stimulated acoustic emission (SAE) signal. This promises to increase the sensitivity of liver detection with US, similar to the recent results with liver-specific MR agents (Albrecht and Blomley 1997). Some data from Hammersmith Hospital (Blomley et al. 1997) indicate that Levovist has also a liver specific late phase during which it also produces SAE. It can be used to improve lesion detection: several cases of previously undetected metastases made visible by SAE with Levovist have in fact been reported.

References

Abrams HL, Spiro R, Goldstein N (1950) Metastases in carcinoma. Cancer 3:74–85

Albrecht T, Blomley M (1997) Contrast agents add new dimension to sonography. Diagnostic Imaging Europe 11:21–33

Bartolozzi C, Lencioni R, Ricci P, et al (1998) Hepatocellular carcinoma treatment with percutaneous ethanol injection: evaluation with contrast-enhanced color Doppler US. Radiology 209:387–393

Blomley M, Albrecht T, Cosgrove D, et al (1997) Stimulate acoustic emission imaging („sonoscintigraphy“) with the US contrast agent Levovist: a reproducible Doppler ultrasound effect with potential clinical utility. Acta Radiol 154:345–351

Campani R, Calliada F, Bottinelli O, et al (1998) Contrast enhancing agents in ultrasonography: clinical applications. Eur J Radiol 27:161–170

Fink S, Chaudhuri K (1991) Physiological considerations in imaging liver metatstases from colorectal carcinoma. Am J Physiol Imaging 6:150–160

Killion JJ, Fidle IJ (1989).The biology of tumor metastasis. Semin Oncol 2:106–115

Leen E, Goldberg JA, Robertson J, et al (1991). Detection of hepatic metastases using duplex color Doppler sonography. Ann Surg 214:599–604

Liotta LA, Stetler-Stevenson WG (1989) Principles of molecular cell biology of cancer. Cancer metastasis. In: De Vita VT jr, Hellman S, Rosenberg SA (eds) Cancer: principles and practice of oncology. Lippincot Philadelphia, pp 98–115

Numata K, Tanaka K, Kiba T, et al (1997) Use of hepatic tumor index on color Doppler sonography for differentiating large hepatic tumors. AJR 168: 991–995

Parulekar SG, Bree RL (1998) Liver. In: McGahan JP, Goldberg BB (eds) "Diagnostic US: a logical approach", Lippincott-Raven Publishers, Philadelphia, chapter 21

Reinhold C, Hammers L, Taylor CR, et al (1995) Characterization of focal hepatic lesions with duplex sonography: findings in 198 patients. AJR 164:1131–1135

Tanaka S, Kitamura T, Fujita M, et al (1990) Color Doppler flow imaging of liver tumors. AJR 154:509–514

Wernecke K, Vassallo P, Bick U, et al (1992) The distinction between benign and malignant liver tumors on sonography: value of the hypoechoic halo. AJR 159:1005–1009

13 Computed Tomography of Liver Metastases

G. Simonetti, M. Pocek, F. Maspes, E. Squillaci, and G. Serafini

CONTENTS

13.1 Introduction

The developments in computed tomograpy (CT) that have taken place over the last 2 decades have dramatically increased the capability to detect and characterize focal liver lesions and have made CT the technique of choice in the evaluation of hepatic metastases. At the same time, advances in the medical and surgical treatment of secondary liver tumors have continued to be a challenge to these advances in radiology. It is clear that a successful outcome depends on knowledge of the size and location of the tumor burden, and accurate radiological assessment is crucial in identifying the subgroups of patients who may benefit from surgery and also in preventing unnecessary radical surgery, with its high morbidity, in those likely to gain only a short term benefit. The correct choice between different CT techniques is crucial to performing an accurate evaluation of liver metastases. The authors focus on specific CT techniques, including bolus dynamic CT, dual and triple phase spiral CT, CT arteriography and arterioportography, delayed CT, high-dose CT and Lipiodol CT. The clinical applications and results of these different techniques are also discussed.

G. Simonetti, MD; Professor and Chairman; Department of Radiology, University of Rome "Tor Vergata", S. Eugenio Hospital, Piazzale dell'Umanesimo 10, I-00143 Rome, Italy

M. Pocek, MD; Professor, Department of Radiology, University of Rome "Tor Vergata", S. Eugenio Hospital, Piazzale dell'Umanesimo 10, I-00143 Rome, Italy

F. Maspes, MD; Department of Radiology, University of Rome "Tor Vergata", S. Eugenio Hospital, Piazzale dell'Umanesimo 10, I-00143 Rome, Italy

E. Squillaci, MD; Department of Radiology, University of Rome "Tor Vergata", S. Eugenio Hospital, Piazzale dell'Umanesimo 10, I-00143 Rome, Italy

G. Serafini, MD; Department of Radiology, University of Rome "Tor Vergata", S. Eugenio Hospital, Piazzale dell'Umanesimo 10, I-00143 Rome, Italy

13.2 Hepatic Contrast Enhancement

Generally, liver malignant tumors present a vascularization mostly sustained by the hepatic artery branches as opposed to the healthy hepatic parenchyma, where 75–80% of blood supply depends on the portal vein and only 20–25% on the hepatic artery. Metastases can be hyper- or hypovascular depending on their arterial blood supply. The great majority of metastases are hypovascular while only certain types of tumors, such as breast and renal cell carcinomas, melanomas, sarcomas, and endocrine tumors present a rich arterial supply.

In CT, scanning with iodinated contrast media (CM) allows the lesions to be better identified by exploiting their differences in blood supply from the hepatic parenchyma.

In fact, the intravenous administration of contrast media increases the differences in CT attenuation between metastases and normal liver. The greater the densitometric difference between tumor and liver parenchyma, the more conspicuous the lesions are. Thus, during the administration of CM, we should attempt to deliver the CM especially to either the liver parenchyma or the liver tumor, but not both (IRIE and KUSANO 1996; SILVERMAN et al. 1995b,d, 1996, 1998). The contrast media is delivered to the hepatic parenchyma through three different phases (Fig. 13.1):

- An early or arterial phase, lasting 24–45 s after the start of infusion of CM, which represents 20–30% of the hepatic parenchyma densitometric increase
- An intermediate or portal venous phase (45–90 s after the start of injection of CM), which accounts for the remaining 70–80% of the liver densitometric increase
- A late or equilibrium phase (90 s–5 min after the initial contrast injection) which corresponds to the time when the contrast media finds its equilibrium within the vascular and extravascular compartments.

Most metastases are of the hypovascular type, and are better detected during the portal venous phase of CM distribution when the hepatic parenchyma enhancement reaches its peak and the difference between parenchyma (hyperdense) and lesion (hypodense) results are highlighted (IKEDA et al. 1996). On the other hand, metastases due to hypervascular tumors, because of their rich arterial blood supply, often become isodense when the hepatic parenchyma is scanned during the portal venous phase, while they may be more easily identified as hyperdense lesions during the arterial phase.

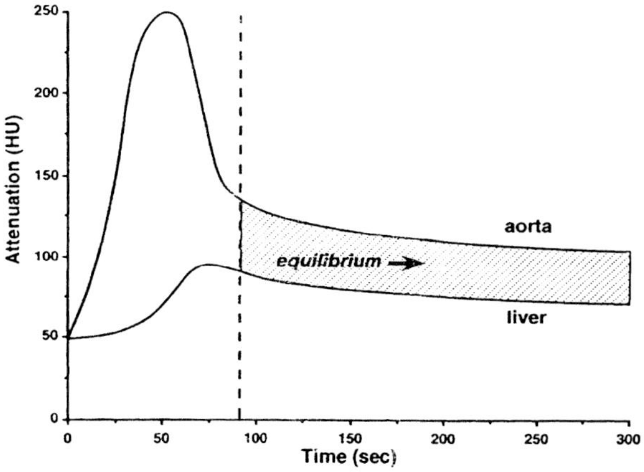

Fig. 13.1. Aortic and hepatic enhancement curves showing times for arterial, portal and equilibrium phases. At approximately 90 s, the curves for the liver and aorta become parallel and this has been defined as the start of the equilibrium phase of enhancement (modified from BLUEMKE et al. 1995a)

The optimal time window to show the presence of focal hepatic lesions ranges from 20 to 90 s after the start of infusion of CM. The correct way to perform a CT scan of the liver is to complete it before the onset of the equilibrium phase of hepatic enhancement (FOLEY 1989; SMALL et al. 1994; SILVERMAN et al. 1995d).

It may happen that during the equilibrium phase, since contrast rapidly diffuses from vessels into the extravascular and interstitial spaces, hypovascular lesions in the liver may become isodense to liver parenchyma and may not be detected. This is the so-called "disappearing lesion" phenomenon, which is quite often observed in conventional CT – where the technical time required to scan the entire liver does not allow the completion of the image acquisition before the beginning of the equilibrium phase (Fig. 13.2).

13.3 Scanning Techniques

CT techniques used in the study of hepatic metastases are as follows:

- Conventional CT: noncontrast CT; bolus dynamic CT (BDCT)
- Spiral CT: dual-phase technique; triple-phase technique
- CT arterial portography (CTAP)
- CT arteriography (CTA)
- Delayed CT
- High-dose CT (HDCT)
- Lipiodol CT

13.3.1 Conventional CT

13.3.1.1 Noncontrast CT

Secondary hepatic lesions can be identified also by performing unenhanced CT because metastases are often characterized by a hypodensity which highlights them against the surrounding hepatic parenchyma. This phenomenon is explained by the glycogen content of normal hepatocytes, which characterizes hyperdensity of the healthy liver but which lacks

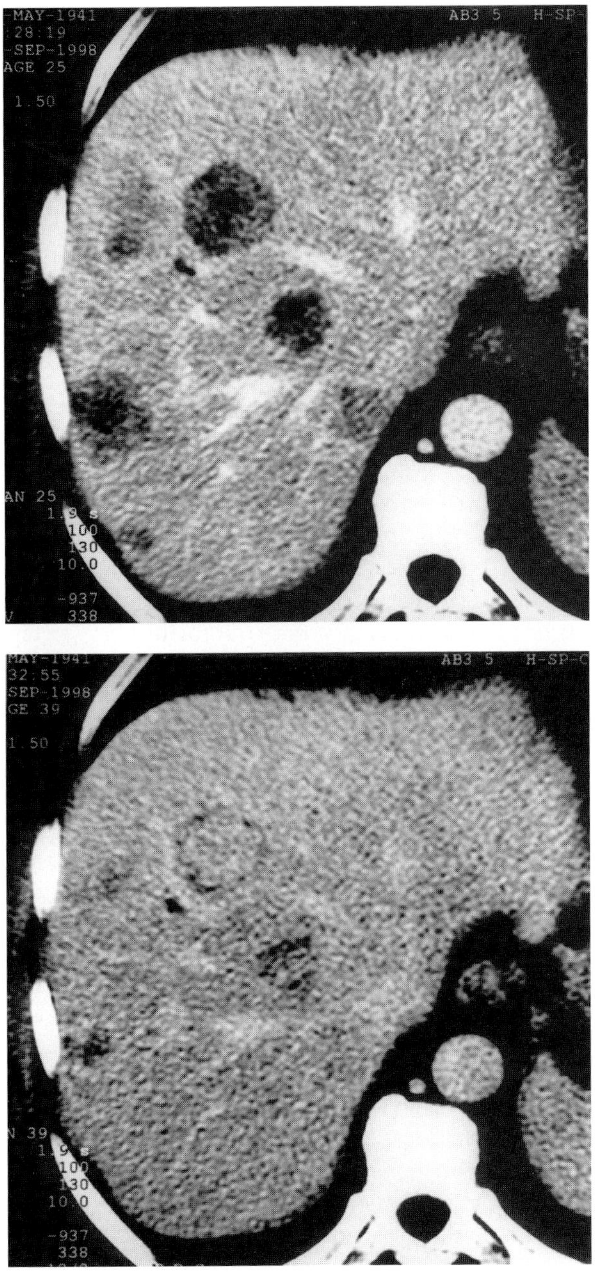

a b

Fig. 13.2a,b. During portal venous phase acquisition, the scan demonstrates the presence of multiple colon carcinoma metastases characterized by hypodensity to the surrounding parenchyma (**a**); in the equilibrium phase, there is an underestimation both of the number and size of lesions ("disap-

in metastases that therefore appear hypodense. Generally, conventional CT is performed by 10-mm slice collimation and 10-mm table speed. Using the current equipment, scanning time for liver imaging is 2–2.5 min. Preliminary noncontrast CT followed by contrast media image acquisition has a significant diagnostic value for many reasons.

Hypovascular metastases are lesions which could remain undetected after the contrast media i.v. administration due to the long technical times of the conventional CT which do not permit the completion of the liver examination before the onset of the equilibrium phase (Fig. 13.3).

Hypervascular metastases are lesions which may become isodense with the hepatic parenchyma after the i.v. CM administration because in conventional CT image acquisition takes place mainly during the portal phase. During this phase the liver progressive enhancement may significantly reduce the attenuation difference from hypervascular lesions that, for this reason, may go undetected. Hypervascular metastases have been reported to be isodense to normal liver with dynamic CT in 25–39% of cases (Bressler et al. 1987). Such a low diagnostic accuracy can be corrected by unenhanced CT, which is currently considered crucial in the study of hypervascular metastases. Furthermore, unenhanced CT is a useful method for evaluating the effectiveness of therapy; in fact the lesion size may be underestimated after contrast administration (Fig. 13.4).

Noncontrast CT allows also the detection of the presence of calcification, which occurs in mucin-producing metastases such as those from the colon and ovary, as well as hemorrhage. Both calcification and hemorrhage may be obscured after CM administration.

The study of different cases shows that sensitivity of noncontrast imaging varies between 14% and 61% (Hollett et al. 1995). The lowest sensitivity value refers to small lesions (1–1.5 cm) because it could be difficult to discriminate between them and the nonopacified vessels (Silverman et al. 1995a).

13.3.1.2 Bolus Dynamic CT

Bolus dynamic CT consists of rapid acquisition of axial images of the liver using automatic table incrementation during simultaneous i.v. injection of a bolus of 150–180 ml of 60% contrast agent. This enables a good visualization of hypovascular metastases because the image acquisition takes place mainly during the portal venous phase of CM distribution and lesions are visualized as hypodense areas within the hyperdense hepatic parenchyma (Freeny 1989).

The study of different cases shows wide-ranging values in dynamic CT sensitivity of metastatic le-

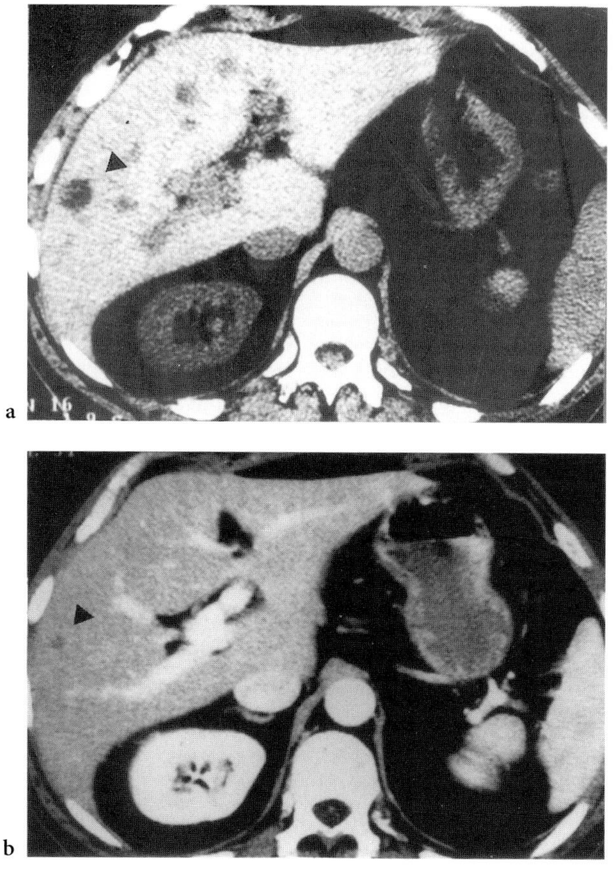

Fig. 13.3a,b. Unenhanced CT shows a small metastatic nodule (*arrowhead*) (**a**); the lesion is less visible on dynamic CT performed during equilibrium phase because of its tendency to become isodense to the liver parenchyma (*arrowhead*) (**b**)

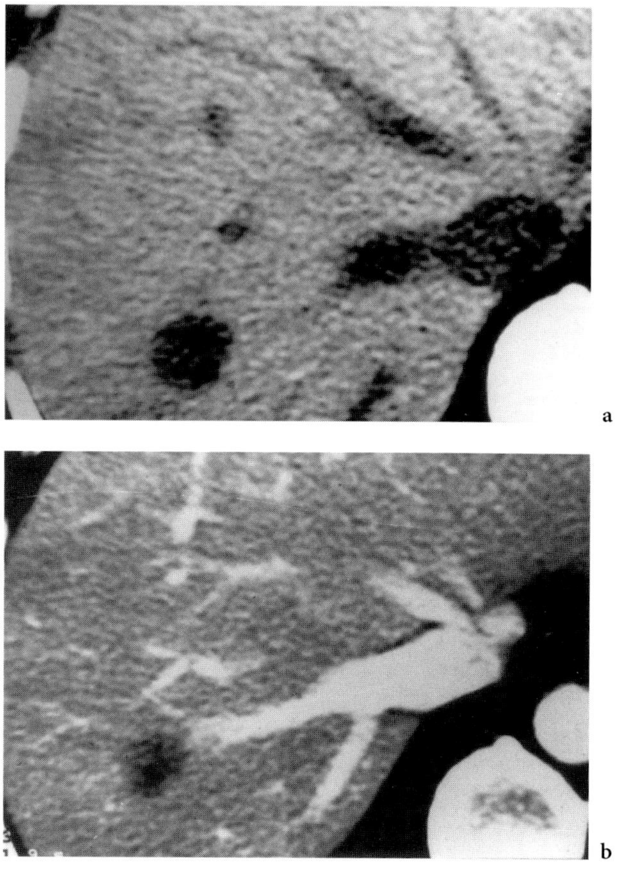

Fig. 13.4a,b. Hypodense metastasis caused by breast cancer is well demonstrated in noncontrast imaging that allows the evaluation of true dimensions of the lesion (**a**); in the images obtained after CM administration the dimensions of the lesion are underestimated (**b**)

sions between 38% and 93%. This great variability is correlated most of all to the size of the lesions observed, to the scanning technique and the equipment used. In fact, only in highly qualified centers, thanks to the employment of an accurate technique, does dynamic CT sensitivity reach 68% in the evaluation of small lesions (1–1.5 cm) exceeding 90% for bigger ones (Chezmar et al.1988; Baron 1994; Dodd and Baron 1993; Platt et al. 1997; Reinig et al. 1987).

13.3.2 Spiral CT

13.3.2.1 Introduction

The technology of spiral, or helical, scanning increases the CT diagnostic sensitivity compared with conventional techniques in the evaluation of hepatic metastases at least by 10% (Bluemke et al. 1995a).

Volumetric acquisition data permits:

- A dramatic reduction in scanning times (20–40 s vs 2–2.5 min for conventional CT)
- An optimal administration of contrast media. By means of the spiral technique, which is characterized by short imaging-acquisition times, we are able to examine the liver both in the arterial and portal venous phase of contrast media distribution (dual-phase technique).

In this way, without disregarding the good outcome of portal venous phase imaging (which allows the detection of most of the hepatic metastases appearing as hypovascular lesions), it is possible to identify the hypervascular lesions characterized by an early hyperdensity during the arterial phase:

- The acquisition of a contiguous set of images, which eliminates the problem of respiratory misregistration, which has important implications in the detection of small focal liver lesions (Fig. 13.5)
- To reconstruct overlapping images retrospectively, which improves the resolution in the *z*-axis direction, reducing the problems caused by partial volume averaging and allowing more accurate characterization of small lesions
- To perform accurate multiplanar and three-dimensional reformats, useful for better localization of the lesions and to demonstrate their relationship with the vascular structures (ZEMAN and SILVERMAN 1995; ZEMAN et al. 1993).

13.3.2.2 Dual-Phase Imaging

13.3.2.2.1 TECHNIQUE

Image acquisition in the arterial phase and later in the portal venous phase is commonly called dual-phase technique. The arterial and portal venous phases take place respectively between 20 and 45 s and 45 and 90 s after the start of contrast media i.v. injection. It is basic to perform a correct scan so that the contrast media is accurately administered taking care of both quantity and flow-rate by observing the appropriate acquisition times for the different phases. Most authors use a 3–6 ml/s injection flow-rate for a 150–180 ml total dose. High flow-rates (4–6 ml/s) make it possible to convey to the liver a more homogeneous bolus which shows a better lesion enhancement.

Recent studies have shown that a 2–3 ml/s flow-rate is inadequate to visualize hepatic metastases, in particular if they are secondary to hypervascular tumors, which are often visible only during the arterial phase (OLIVER and BARON 1996; BONALDI et al. 1995). In fact, dual-phase technique diagnostic sensitivity is impaired most of all by false-negatives caused by an incorrect execution of scanning during the arterial phase due to the employment of low rates of contrast media administration.

Data acquisition times must be well correlated to the contrast media injection rate. For this reason, it is necessary to calculate with extreme accuracy the bolus timing especially in the case of patients with altered cardiac circulation conditions.

New automated computer programs have been developed to monitor the enhancement of either the liver parenchyma, the abdominal aorta, or both dur-

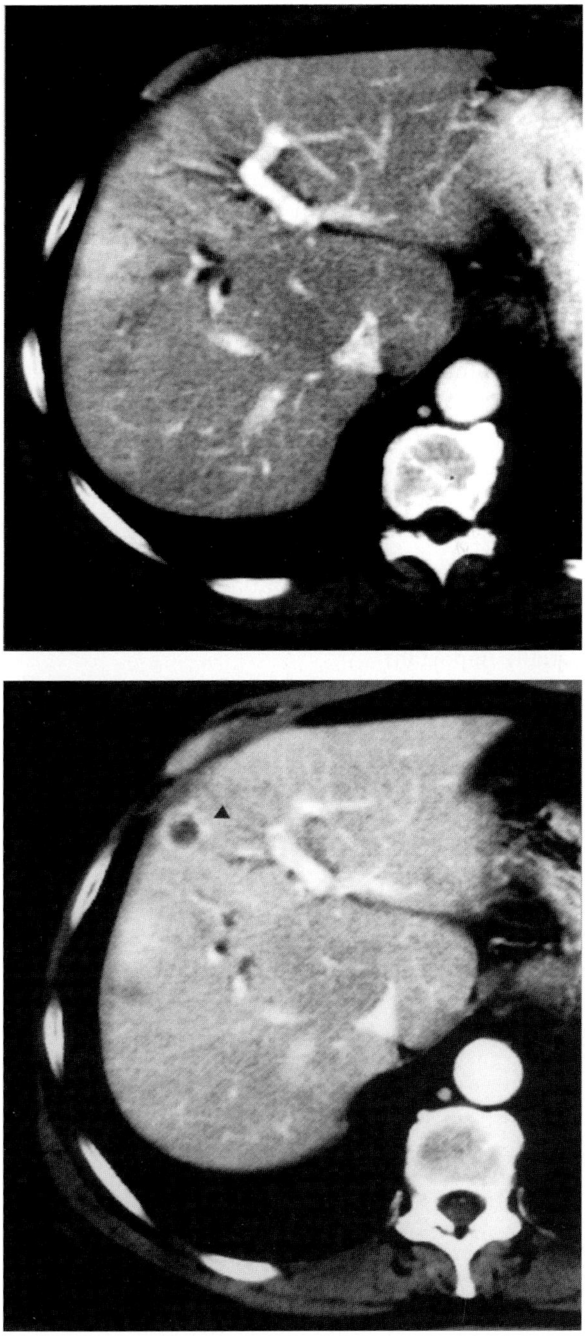
a

b

Fig. 13.5a,b. Scanning performed by conventional CT, because of respiratory misregistration, does not allow the detection of the presence of a colon carcinoma metastasis located in the IV hepatic segment (**a**); imaging by spiral CT during the portal venous phase, instead, demonstrates the lesion well as a 9-mm-diameter hypodense area with a hyperdense perilesional ring (*arrowhead*) (**b**) ing the early stages of injection of CM, and these programs can be used to decide when to start scanning with optimal contrast enhancement characteristics (SILVERMAN et al. 1995c). For arterial phase imaging, this is performed using a test bolus (20 ml of CM) during dynamic acquisition (every 1 s) at zero table index. A region of interest (ROI) is positioned over the abdominal aorta at a level corresponding to the most cephalad extent of the liver and the computer program calculates the time-density curve which determines the correct delay time to start scanning (Fig. 13.6).

Determining the delay time for image acquisition is less complex for the portal phase because of its wider time window. The optimal time window is between 50 and 70 s, depending on the flow-rate adopted.

If contrast media administration methods represent an important aspect of the dual-phase technique, the correct choice of acquisition protocols is equally important.

Currently, most authors employ 7–8 mm slice collimation with 1:1 pitch and a 4 mm reconstruction interval. In this way it is possible to examine a 19.2–25.6 cm portion along the patients' z-axis covering the whole liver in 24–32 s (Table 13.1) (OLSON et al. 1996).

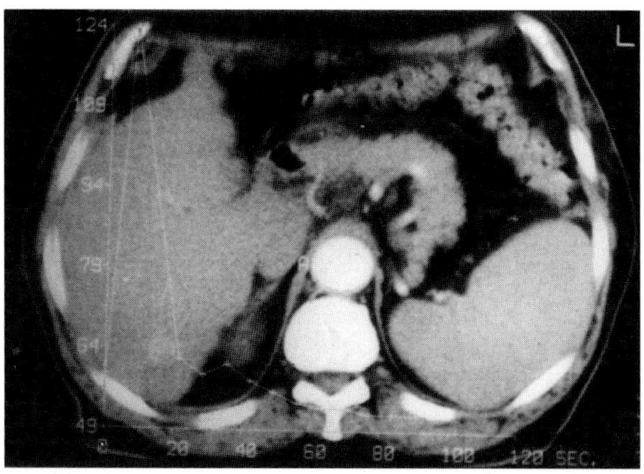

Fig. 13.6. Time-density curve which shows the correct delay time for the performance of arterial phase imaging

Table 13.1. Spiral CT: liver imaging protocol (from BLUEMKE et al. 1995a)

Slice thickness	8 mm
Table incrementation	8 mm
Reconstruction interval	4 mm
Image volume length	19.2–25.6 cm
Imaging time	24–32 s

Diagnostic accuracy can improve without increasing the acquisition time by overlapping-image reconstructions, which enables the reduction of the possible artifacts deriving from partial volume averaging (Fig. 13.7). The role of overlapping reconstruction intervals with spiral CT in the detection of hepatic lesions was evaluated by URBAN et al. (1993). In 42 consecutive patients with lesions less than 4 cm in size, 10% more liver lesions were detected using 4-mm intervals vs 8-mm intervals (251 vs 229 lesions, respectively). Also, radiologists were able to detect lesions with a higher degree of confidence with 4-mm reconstruction intervals. Lesions that were considered "definite" were diagnosed 33% more frequently using 4-mm reconstruction intervals (191 vs 144 lesions).

13.3.2.2.2
Clinical Indications

The use of the dual-phase technique to detect hepatic metastases must be correlated above all to the possibility that scanning during the arterial phase increases spiral CT diagnostic sensitivity in the detection of hypervascular metastases, because they may become isodense in the portal phase (Fig. 13.8) (PATTEN et al. 1993).

Hypervascular metastases are more frequently caused by renal cell carcinoma, breast carcinoma, neuroendocrine tumors (islet cell, carcinoid), sarcomas, thyroid carcinoma and melanomas (Table 13.2). While image acquisition role for hepatocellular carcinoma (HCC) diagnosis during the arterial phase is now widely accepted, a minor number of studies have been initiated to evaluate dual-phase sensitivity in the hypervascular metastases demonstration. However, in the light of preliminary experience, the great majority of authors recommend the dual-phase technique to study hypervascular metastases.

In his study carried out on 23 patients presenting 206 lesions secondary to carcinoma, PAULSON et al. (1998) demonstrated that during the arterial phase there is a 14% increase in the number of visualized nodules and a better enhancement in 35% of cases versus scanning performed in basal conditions and in the portal phase.

In another study, HOLLETT et al. (1995) reported in the arterial phase a 37% diagnostic sensitivity increase in the detection of hypervascular metastases and, generally, of neoplastic lesions with a <1 cm diameter.

Independently of the hypo- or hypervascular nature of the tumor, during the arterial phase the best

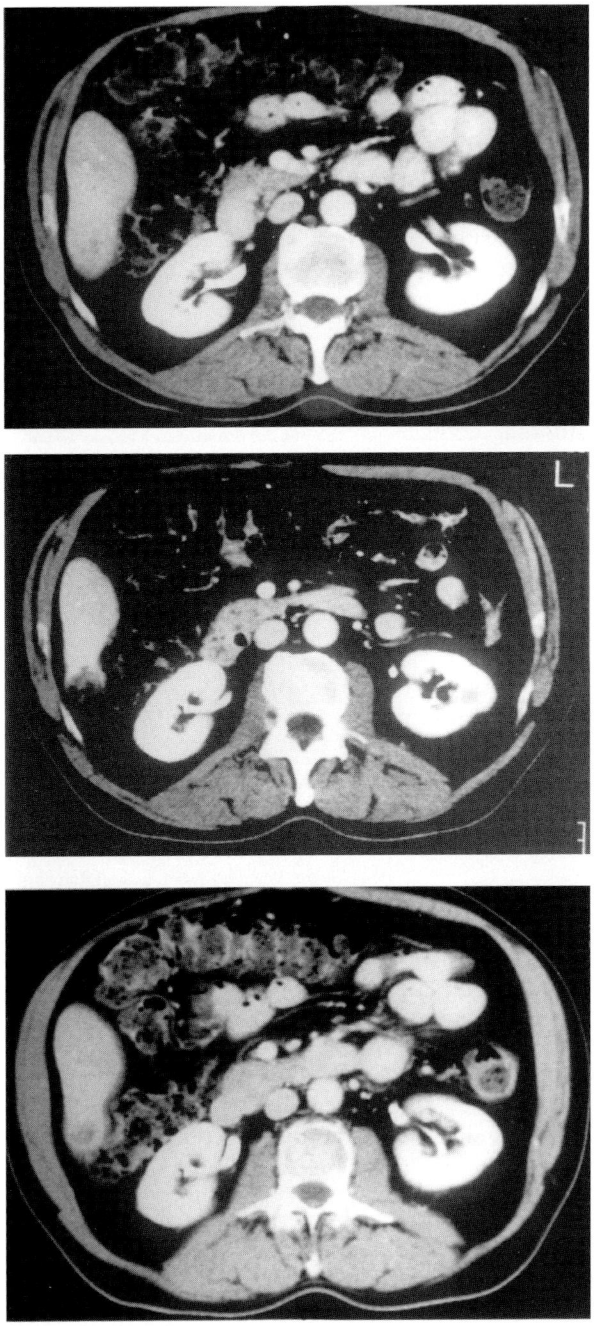

Fig. 13.7a–c. Liver metastasis caused by colon carcinoma. The artifacts deriving from partial volume averaging due to the colon (**a,b**) can be differentiated from liver metastasis with spiral CT by a small reconstruction interval which demonstrates the lesion as a metastasis (**c**)

visualization of all <1 cm metastases is determined by the fact that in small lesions the predominant blood flow is supplied by the hepatic artery. On the other hand, when tumors grow the arterial vascularization spread is determined by the histologic nature of the tumor.

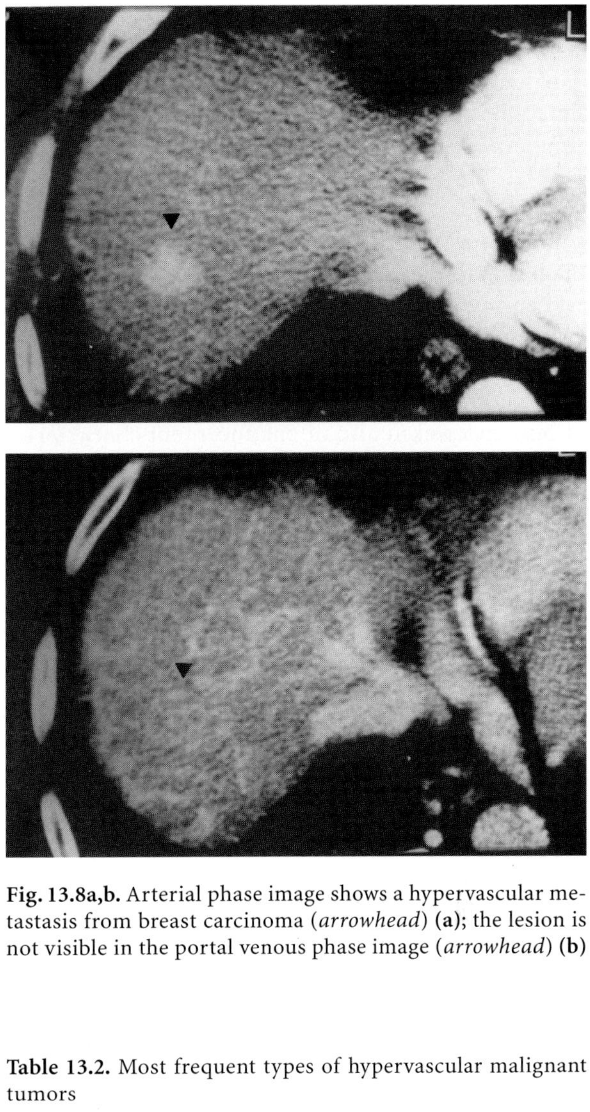

Fig. 13.8a,b. Arterial phase image shows a hypervascular metastasis from breast carcinoma (*arrowhead*) (**a**); the lesion is not visible in the portal venous phase image (*arrowhead*) (**b**)

Table 13.2. Most frequent types of hypervascular malignant tumors

Renal cell carcinoma
Breast carcinoma
Neuroendocrine tumors
Sarcoma
Melanoma
Thyroid carcinoma

In the case of hypervascular lesions detectable also during the portal venous phase, observation during the arterial phase enables the correct evaluation of their dimensions (Oliver and Baron 1996). We know in fact that often during the venous phase hypervascular metastases are totally or partially isodense to the surrounding hepatic parenchyma. Further, while necrotic areas within the tumor are clearly detectable during the portal venous phase, the surrounding neoplastic tissue portion can appear as isodense, thus inducing an underestimation of the true dimensions of the lesion. Since the hepatic enhancement portal venous phase has a wider time window than the arterial one, the same lesion could have contrast enhancement variations and appear a different size if observed at an early or late venous phase. For this reason, the arterial phase becomes important also as a means to correctly assess the lesion dimensions.

The employment of the dual-phase technique has great importance in the after-chemotherapy follow-up screening of metastases. The answer to chemotherapy, in fact, must be evaluated not only in terms of dimensions but also of enhancement characteristics during the arterial phase. Some lesions that before treatment were fairly enhanced in the arterial phase (hypervascular metastases) after chemotherapy may keep the same characteristics or show a decrease or even a total lack of enhancement.

Contrast enhancement decreases also when the size of the lesion remains the same, indicating a positive response to chemotherapy because it demonstrates tumoral tissue replacement by inactive fibrous tissue. Conversely, a lesion which remains unaltered on subsequent checks and presents active foci in the arterial phase imaging indicates disease flare-up.

The dual-phase technique is not employed very much in the evaluation of hypovascular lesions because, generally, arterial phase acquisition does not add any diagnostic information to the scan performed during the portal venous phase (Figs. 13.9, 13.10). Only sometimes can dual-phase imaging be useful in the study of hypovascular lesions, as in the case of colon carcinoma metastases where the presence of the typical hypervascular rim, which is important for lesion characterization, can be better detected in the arterial phase (Ch'en et al. 1997).

The study of hypovascular metastases can be performed only during the portal phase (single-phase acquisition technique) but, as already mentioned, taking care not to reach the equilibrium phase in order to avoid the "disappearing lesion" phenomenon, caused by the contrast media homogenization between intra- and extravascular space.

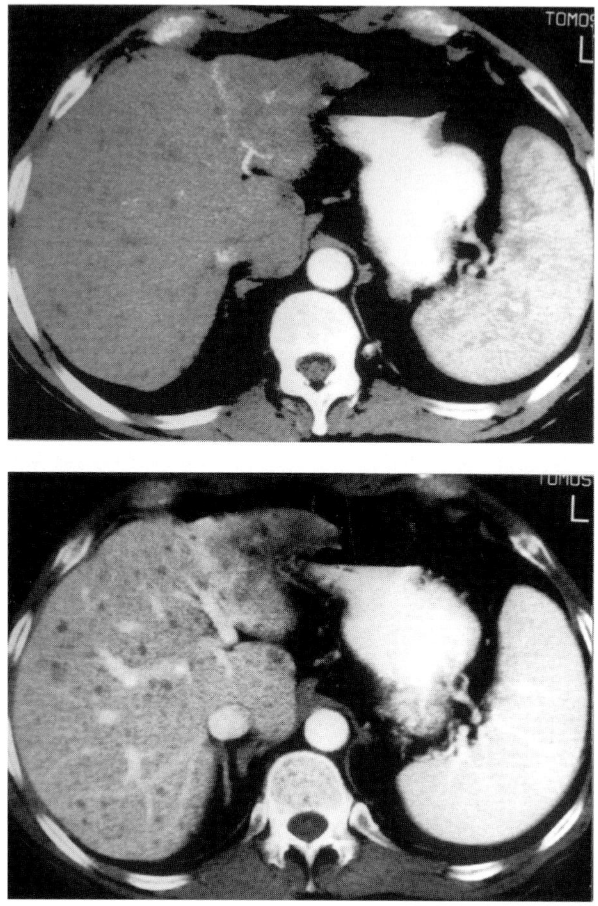

a

b

Fig. 13.9a,b. Multiple metastases smaller than 1 cm caused by colon carcinoma. The lesions are hypovascular and not well detected in the arterial phase image (**a**); conversely, the lesions are well recognizable as nodular low-attenuation areas

13.3.2.2.3 Differential Diagnosis and Pitfalls

The lesions which more often cause problems of differential diagnosis with hypervascular metastases in arterial phase acquisition are small hemangiomas that may present a rapid and homogeneous enhancement just like a hypervascular malignant lesion. Acquisition in the portal venous phase allows differential diagnosis because the metastasis shows a rapid washout becoming iso- or hypodense, while hemangioma keeps its enhancement and presents the same attenuation as the surrounding vascular structures (Fig. 13.11).

Further, in the arterial phase, it is not always possible to make a differential diagnosis between focal nodular hyperplasia (FNH) and hypervascular hepatic metastases, especially if the nodule is small and without the characteristic central hypodense scar. FNH nodules, in fact, similarly to the hypervascular metastases, become isodense in the portal venous phase. In these cases only clinical correlation can clarify the nature of the lesions even though, sometimes, a bioptic examination is necessary.

In the images obtained during the portal venous phase, one of the most common pseudolesions is rep-

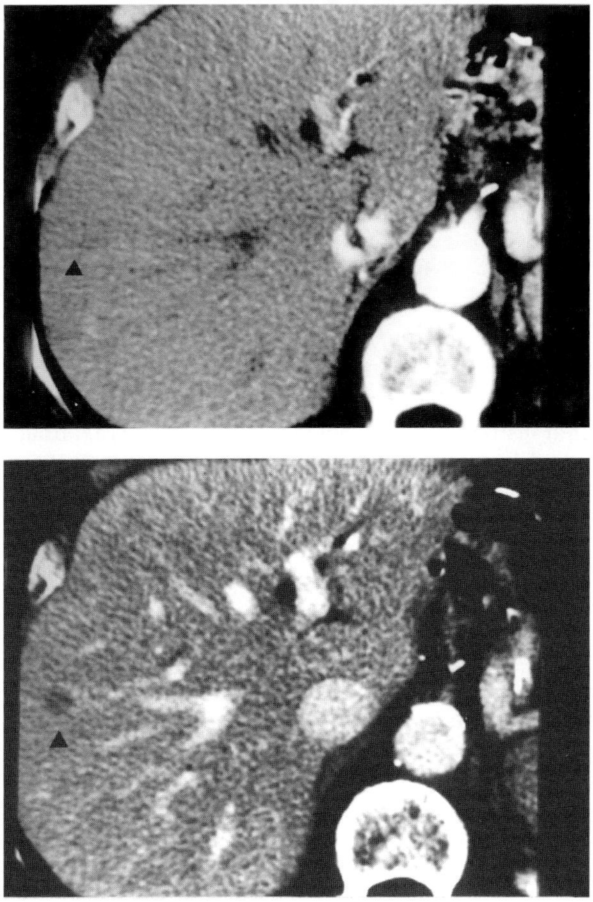

a

b

Fig. 13.10a,b. No liver lesions are visible on a CT scan performed in the arterial phase (*arrowhead*) (**a**); conversely, the subcentimetric lesion is easily demonstrated in the portal venous phase image (*arrowhead*) (**b**)

resented by a low-attenuation area which typically is antero-located in the medial and/or lateral segment of the left lobe surrounding the falciform ligament (Fig. 13.12). Some authors (Ohashi et al. 1995; Bluemke et al. 1995c) have demonstrated that in this area there is an infiltration of fatty tissue secondary to hypoxic phenomena caused by a portal perfusion defect due to an aberrant blood supply in this area.

Furthermore, it is important to know the bolus timing artifacts which may produce differential diagnosis problems. These artifacts come about when scanning is not performed using the correct technique because image acquisition does not observe the appropriate delay times after contrast media administration.

It may happen that during the arterial or portal venous phase, vascular branches of the portal or sovrahepatic veins are mistaken for hypovascular le-

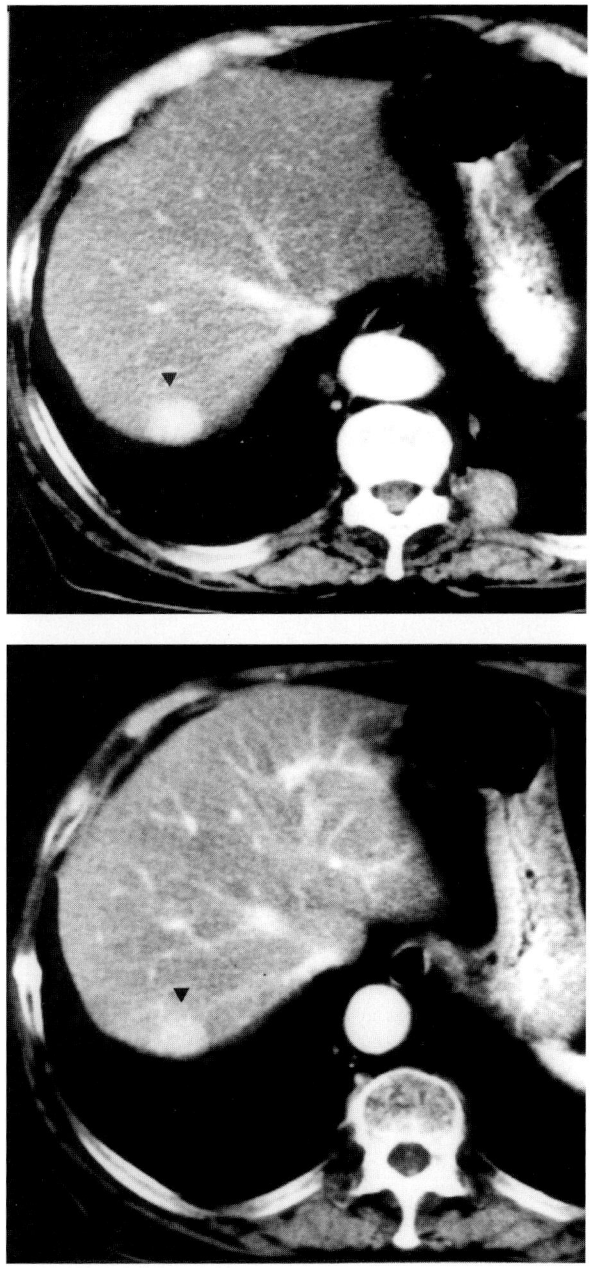

a

b

Fig. 13.11a,b. Differential diagnosis between metastasis and hemangioma. Arterial phase image shows a hypervascular lesion located in the VIII hepatic segment (*arrowhead*) (**a**); in the portal venous image the lesion remains enhanced to a degree equal to that of other liver vessels and this is charac-

sions. Normally, during arterial phase imaging, liver venous structures are not opacified. However, a comparison with the images obtained during the venous phase makes an easy discrimination from possible hypovascular lesions but, if scanning has been performed in the portal venous phase only and too soon

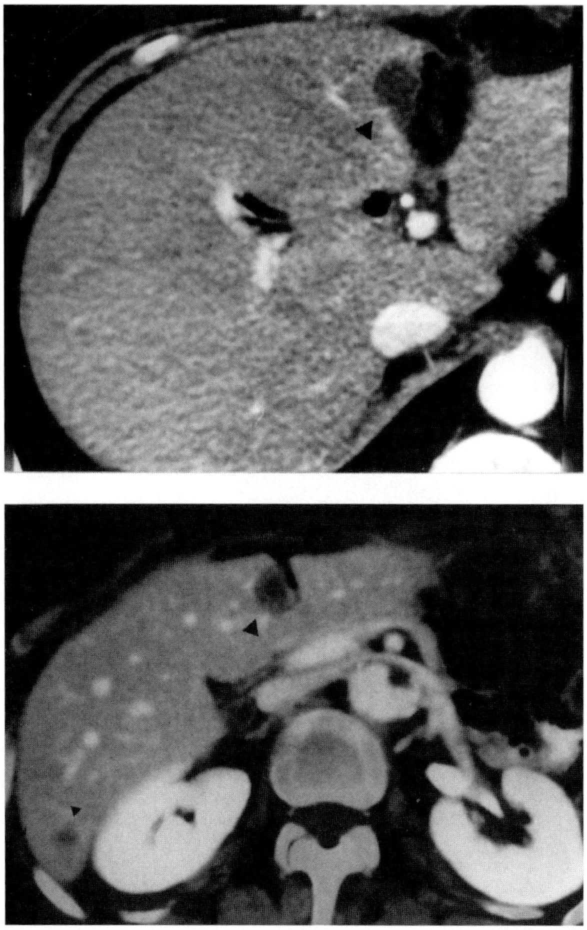

a

b

Fig. 13.12a,b. Differential diagnosis between pseudolesion and metastasis. Portal venous phase image shows a typical pseudolesion located around the falciform ligament (*arrowhead*) (**a**); portal venous phase image shows a nodular lesion located around the falciform ligament (*arrowhead*). In this case the more rounded and less definite margins of the lesion demonstrate that the nodular low-attenuation area is a metastasis. Another smaller metastatic nodule is also visible

after the administration of the CM, a differential diagnosis between venous branches not yet opacified and hypovascular lesions can be difficult (Freeny 1997).

Another source of pitfalls during dual-phase technique image acquisition may be due to the presence of vascular malformations, arterial-venous shunts, fistulas or aneurysms of the hepatic artery, which may produce a difficult discrimination between neoplastic lesions. In the great majority of cases, comparison between the images obtained during the two different phases enables the elimination of any possible doubt even though, sometimes, an investigation by color Doppler imaging may become necessary (Freeny 1997).

13.3.2.3 Triple-Phase Spiral CT

Performing unenhanced CT in addition to dual-phase image acquisition is commonly called triple-phase CT. Noncontrast liver scanning maintains a crucial role for oncologic patients' staging also in spiral CT. As demonstrated by authoritative studies, noncontrast liver scanning is important especially in the evaluation of hypervascular metastases. In their study of the employment of triple-phase spiral CT to detect carcinoid metastases, which are typically hypervascular, Paulson et al. (1998) demonstrated that lesions are better detected in noncontrast imaging than in those obtained by dual-phase technique. If unenhanced scanning does not show any additional nodule it makes it possible, however, to visualize approximately one-third of the lesions.

In a study conducted on 80 women affected by breast carcinoma, Frederick et al. (1997) reported a sensitivity of 61% for unenhanced CT vs 59% for image acquisition during arterial phase and 85% during portal phase. In a study involving 84 patients with biopsy-proved hypervascular hepatic metastases, Oliver et al. (1997) demonstrated a statistically higher increase in the number of lesions detected by means of unenhanced CT plus portal venous phase imaging than the lesions detected with dual-phase technique. In particular, noncontrast images made possible the detection of 28% more lesions during the portal venous phase vs 13% of acquisition during the arterial phase.

Most authors agree on the usefulness of the triple-phase technique in the staging and follow-up of patients with primitive hypervascular tumors (van Leeuwen et al. 1996).

Conversely, unenhanced scanning with spiral CT is not employed to evaluate patients with biopsy-proved primitive hypovascular tumors, because it does not increase the investigation diagnostic sensitivity (Fig. 13.13).

13.3.3 CT Arterial Portography and CT Arteriography

13.3.3.1 Introduction

CTAP and CTA represent the integration of an angiographic technique and a computed tomographic scan. They consist of a CT scan performed by selective administration of CM in the portal

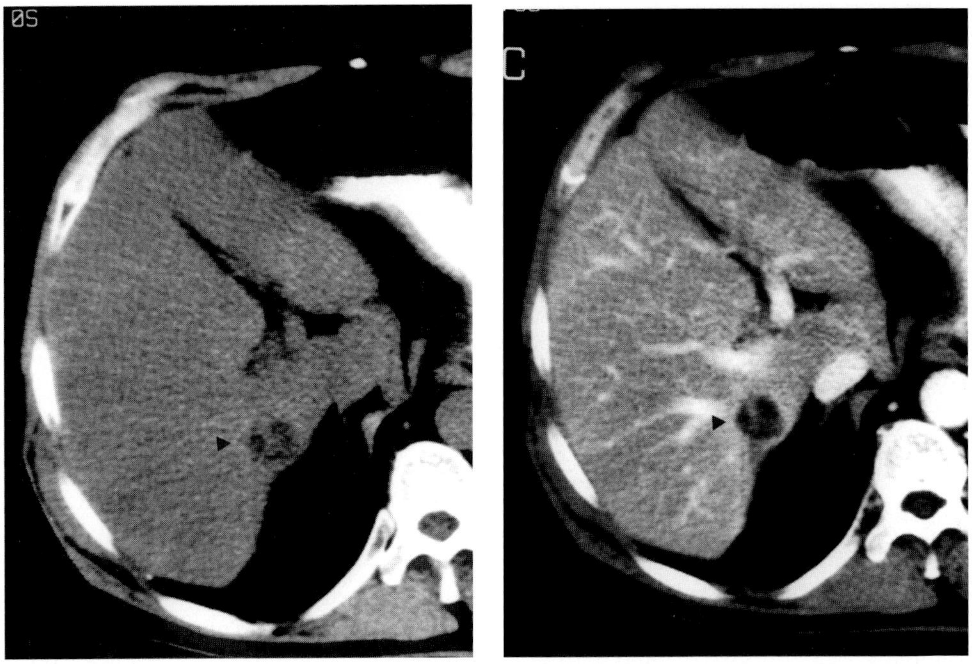

a b

Fig. 13.13a,b. Colon carcinoma metastasis located in the V hepatic segment. The lesion is well detectable as a hypodense area both in noncontrast scans (*arrowhead*) (**a**) and in the portal phase image (*arrowhead*) (**b**)

venous system (CTAP) or in the hepatic arterial tree (CTA) after positioning under angiographic guidance a catheter in the superior mesenteric artery or in the splenic artery in CTAP and in the hepatic artery in CTA.

CTA allows the demonstration of hepatic tumors, most of which receive their blood supply from the hepatic artery, as hyperdense areas with respect to the surrounding hepatic parenchyma, which is not enhanced because of the CM direct distribution at the lesion level (Fig. 13.14). CTAP, on the contrary, uses the full contrasting effect of hepatic parenchyma, perfused by the CM, and lesions are visualized as areas with a lower attenuation value.

CTA and CTAP find their main application in the evaluation of patients with malignant hepatic tumors who will undergo a limited surgical resection which requires a precise lesion localization. However, these invasive and costly investigations are useless for those patients who will not benefit from surgery. CTAP and CTA are the imaging techniques with the greater diagnostic sensitivity for hepatic focal lesion detection. Their sensitivity is especially high for small lesion (<1.5 cm) demonstration. The sensitivities of these two techniques (81–91% using conventional CT and more than 90% using spiral CT) are not significantly different (Freeny 1997; Bluemke et al. 1995b; Kanematsu et al. 1997). Moreover, CTAP is generally used more often than CTA for the following reasons:

- Because most hepatic lesions are hypovascular
- Because the frequent incidence of variations in hepatic arterial anatomy may make selective catheterism difficult or the evaluation of hepatic parenchyma incomplete.

CTA is useful in the evaluation of hypervascular metastases because the visualization of a small hyperdense lesion is easier than that of a hypodense one (Freeny 1990). Both these methods present a low specificity which, associated with their limited accuracy in the evaluation of extrahepatic pathology, contributes to limiting their employment to preoperative patient evaluation (Paley and Ros 1997; Paulson et al. 1992).

13.3.3.2 Techniques

13.3.3.2.1 CTAP

Before the CTAP study, routine angiography of the celiac and superior mesenteric arteries is performed to demonstrate the arterial supply of the liver, to exclude the presence of a replaced right hepatic ar-

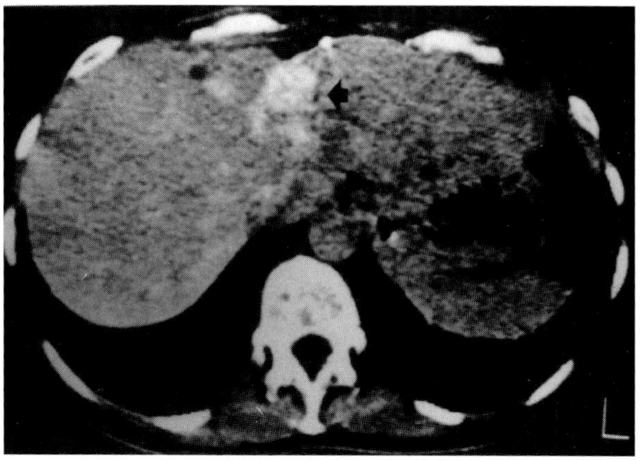

Fig. 13.14. CTA shows a high density metastatic lesion located in the II hepatic segment (*arrow*). A small cyst is also visible

tery and prove the patency of the splenic artery and the splenic, superior mesenteric, and portal veins. The total volume of CM injected should be minimized to prevent tumoral enhancement due to arterial perfusion and a resultant decrease in liver-to-lesion attenuation value differences on CTAP. At the conclusion of angiography, the catheter is positioned in the proximal splenic or superior mesenteric artery and the patient is moved to the CT suite (Kanematsu et al. 1997). According to some authors (Lupetin et al. 1996), it is better to place the catheter in the splenic artery instead of in the superior mesenteric artery because, in this way, during CTAP there is a greater and more homogeneous enhancement of the hepatic parenchyma and fewer nontumorous perfusion defects.

The acquisition protocol recommended by most authors for spiral CT is the same as that advised to examine the liver by intravenous administration of CM. It consists of 8-mm slice collimation and 8-mm/s table speed with a 4-mm reconstruction interval; 150 ml 30% iodinated contrast media is administered at a 3-mm/s infusion rate (Bluemke et al. 1995a). Other authors (Paley and Ros 1997; Freeny 1997) recommend a different protocol with a higher dose of contrast media (150–200 ml at 60%) and 5-mm slice collimation with a pitch able to cover the entire hepatic parenchyma during a single breath-hold.

The most frequently adopted delay time is 24–32 s from the start of CM injection. By employing this delay time to begin scanning, the hepatic parenchyma can be evaluated before the contrast media distribution to the systemic circulation, which begins 60 s after the start of infusion. Further, in this way scanning can be completed during the parenchymal enhancement peak, starting about 18 s after the contrast media initial administration and lasting about 44 s. In this way it is possible to obtain the maximal differentiation in contrast enhancement between parenchyma (hyperdense) and metastases (hypodense) resulting in an optimal lesion detection. However, other authors (Paley and Ros 1997; Freeny 1997) prefer to start scanning at a later time (66–70 s from the start of CM injection) because with this delay time perfusion abnormalities are less frequent.

13.3.3.2.2
CTA

To perform CTA after the preliminary angiography, the catheter is positioned in the common hepatic artery. Generally, 200 ml of contrast media at 15% is administered with a 4-ml/s injection rate, and a 10-s delay-time must be observed to start image acquisition. The collimation, pitch and reconstruction interval employed by the various authors to perform spiral acquisition are the same as those used when scanning is performed by intravenous administration of CM. Generally the contrast media concentration used is not greater than 15% because this has improved the quality of the CTA scans by reducing perfusion abnormalities (Freeny 1990).

13.3.3.3 Clinical Indications, Differential Diagnosis, and Pitfalls

13.3.3.3.1
CTAP

The main role of CTAP consists in the preoperative evaluation of patients. Especially when the spiral technique is used, CTAP makes it possible to evaluate with a high degree of accuracy the effective lesion resectability by defining exactly the metastases segmental localization and their relationships with vascular structures, both crucial in correctly planned surgery.

A recent study (Small et al. 1993) has pointed out that, on the basis of CTAP, surgery can be avoided in 64% of patients. These findings demonstrate the high sensitivity of this technique even though it would seem that it is now progressively less used. This decrease is for several reasons. First, lesion detection with spiral CT performed with peripheral intravenous CM appears to be excellent. Second, CTAP is expensive and, finally, improved surgical techniques, including use of cryotherapy, intraoperative ultrasonography, and laparoscopy, have altered the practice patterns of surgeons in treating patients with liver metastases (Bluemke et al.1995b; Ikeda et al. 1996).

CTAP low specificity in discriminating malignant lesions from benign tumors or perfusion defects is well demonstrated by the high false-positive (15%) and false-negative (9–19%) rates reported in recent studies (Lupetin et al. 1996; Honda et al. 1992; Paulson et al. 1992).

False-negatives are often due to perfusion defects caused by metastases compressing the proximal portal branches. In these cases, a wide hypodense area much bigger than the lesion is visualized and this may easily be mistaken for a nontumoral perfusion defect. The presence of the so-called "straight-line" sign, that is, a linear rim separating the opacified and nonopacified parenchyma, typical of perfusion defects but not of neoplastic lesions, may contribute to engendering diagnostic confusion.

False-positives may be due to focal perfusion defects caused by variations in the perihepatic venous drainage or in the subcapsular portal perfusion. These pseudolesions, demonstrated in approximately 15% of CTAP, may be single or multiple and, in many cases, exhibit characteristic appearances and locations (Lupetin et al. 1996).

The most common and easily recognizable one can be found in the medial segment of the left hepatic lobe (quadrate lobe) and can present a square, round, or ovular configuration. Originally, it was believed that it could be reconducted to a focal steatosis, whilst now it is certain that it relates to a perihepatic venous anomaly. Specifically, in 6–14% of the population, the right gastric vein (pyloric vein) drains directly into the quadrate lobe instead of the portal vein, to which it is normally connected. Since this variation in the venous system predominates, during CTAP this portion of hepatic parenchyma does not present enhancement and is visualized as a hypodense area which can mimic a malignant lesion. Similar pseudolesions can be present around the falciform ligament and are probably caused by other perihepatic venous anomalies (Fig. 13.15).

False-positives may also be caused by a lesion centrally located in the hepatic parenchyma that, thus compressing or infiltrating the portal vein, engenders the defect of subsegmental, segmental or lobar perfusion which can mimic metastases.

All the causes of possible diagnostic pitfalls must be known to be able to reduce to a minimum false-positive and false-negative rates and the ensuing therapeutic disadvantages. Just think that when a pseudolesion is mistaken for a metastasis, a patient may be judged as inoperable with obvious consequences quod vitam and quod valitudinem. Of great help in this sense is the performance of delayed CT scans, which increase this technique's diagnostic accuracy, usually enabling the discrimination between a hypovascular malignant lesion and a perfusion abnormality (Nelson et al. 1992).

a
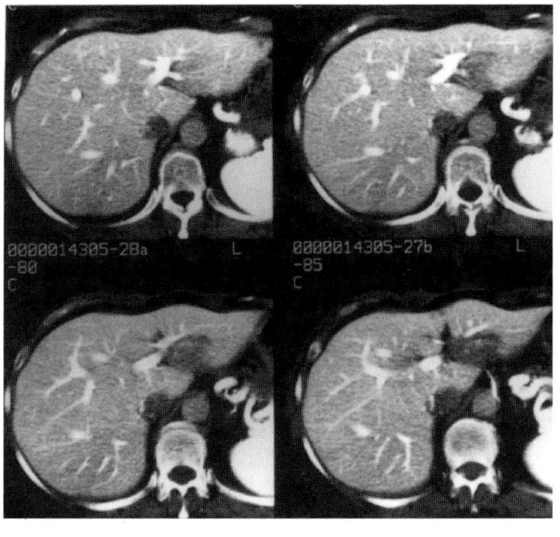

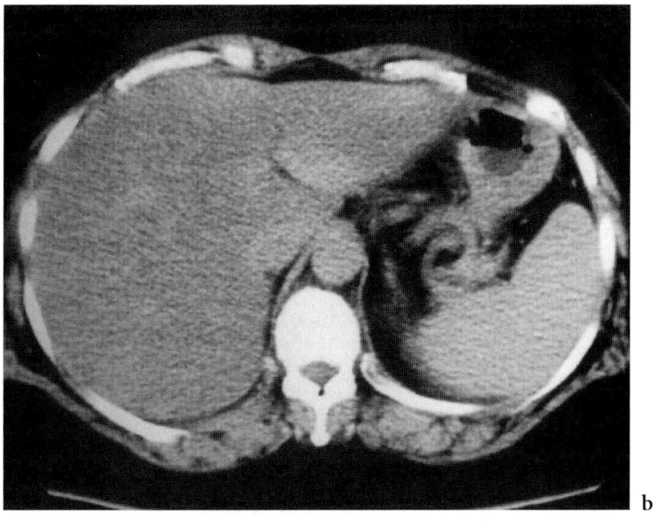
b

Fig. 13.15a,b. Spiral CTAP demonstrates a perfusion defect located in the left hepatic lobe near the falciform ligament (**a**). Delayed CT scan shows enhancement of the defect, a finding indicative of a pseudolesion (**b**)

13.3.3.3.2
CTA

CTA is mainly indicated for the preoperative evaluation of patients presenting hypervascular malignant lesions. Similarly to CTAP, CTA is also less frequently used due to the high sensitivity of standard spiral CT and of other investigating techniques.

The disadvantages of CTA include perfusion abnormalities due to variations in the hepatic arterial anatomy resulting in segmental or lobar nonperfusion, focal areas of hyperfusion due to laminar flow or the siphoning effect of a hypervascular lesion, and an area of increased perfusion, typically adjacent to the gallbladder fossa, which can mimic a lesion. Small tumors may also be poorly visualized, and portal branches can mimic tumor nodules.

13.3.4
Delayed CT

Delayed CT consists of obtaining axial scans of the liver 4–6 h following administration of contrast containing a total iodine dose of at least 60 g. This dose of iodine has been shown to produce an increase in hepatic attenuation of 20 HU over baseline noncontrast enhanced scans. Delayed CT finds the physiopathological bases for its diagnostic sensitivity in the normal hepatocytes' capacity to progressively concentrate the iodinated contrast media after its course from the intravascular compartment into the extravascular one (Perkerson et al. 1985). This brings about an enhancement of the hepatic parenchyma, reaching its peak 4–6 h after contrast media administration. Metastases can thus be demonstrated as areas with low-attenuation values compared to the liver (Fig. 13.16).

In a study performed by Chezmar et al. (1988) by means of delayed CT, 30 out of 93 malignant hepatic lesions (86%) were detected, while dynamic CT detected 86 of them (92%). Delayed CT visualized 6 out of 19 (67%) <1 cm nodules, whilst the dynamic CT detection rate was 68%. Nelson et al. (1989) reported a 73% sensitivity for delayed CT. In a study by Freeny et al. (1990), the rate of nodules detected by delayed CT was 60% vs 57% by dynamic CT (Platt et al. 1997).

Delayed CT represents an easy and noninvasive technique able to provide additional information for lesion characterization. Its main application is as an additional technique to evaluate, after CTAP or CTA, patients who are considered possible candidates for surgical resection. Delayed CT, in fact, provides useful help in solving diagnostic problems related to the presence of the perfusion abnormalities frequently occurring in CTAP and CTA and which often make discrimination from hepatic malignant lesions difficult. Conversely to what happens in metastases, in fact, hepatic parenchymal areas where perfusion defects occur contain normal hepatocytes and, in delayed scans, appear isodense against the normal liver (Bernardino et al. 1986; Heiken et al. 1989; Irie et al. 1995).

13.3.5
High-Dose CT

Computed tomography of hepatic metastases performed by intravenously injecting high doses of contrast media (200 ml with 60–65 g of iodine) increases density differences between a lesion and the healthy surrounding parenchyma. HDCT is indicated in the evaluation of hypovascular metastases, which represent a great many lesions, because it amplifies the contrasting effect of hepatic parenchyma in the portal phase by making a better visualization of the lesion hypodensity.

Recently, Freeny (1997) demonstrated that helical CT carried out using 200 ml of contrast media (64 g iodine) administered i.v. at a 5-ml/s flow-rate can produce hepatic contrast enhancement equal to 86% of that obtained with CTAP.

This degree of hepatic enhancement may be enough to allow a degree of accuracy in detecting lesions just like the CTAP, which is about 90%. These authors are currently using the high dose technique to evaluate patients with potentially resectable hypovascular metastases, first of all colorectal carcinoma, instead of CTAP, and their initial results are encouraging. Nevertheless, further studies are necessary to assess this method's diagnostic accuracy (Choi et al. 1996; Fink and Chaudhuri 1991; Soyer et al. 1994).

13.3.6
Lipiodol CT

Previous studies have shown that CT following intraarterial injection of Lipiodol (Lipiodol CT) has a high detectability rate for small nodules of HCC. In fact, the infusion of a small volume of Lipiodol into the hepatic artery is followed by selective and extended retention of the iodized oil within HCC lesions. Hence, on CT scans obtained 3–4 weeks after the injection, even tiny tumor deposits can be iden-

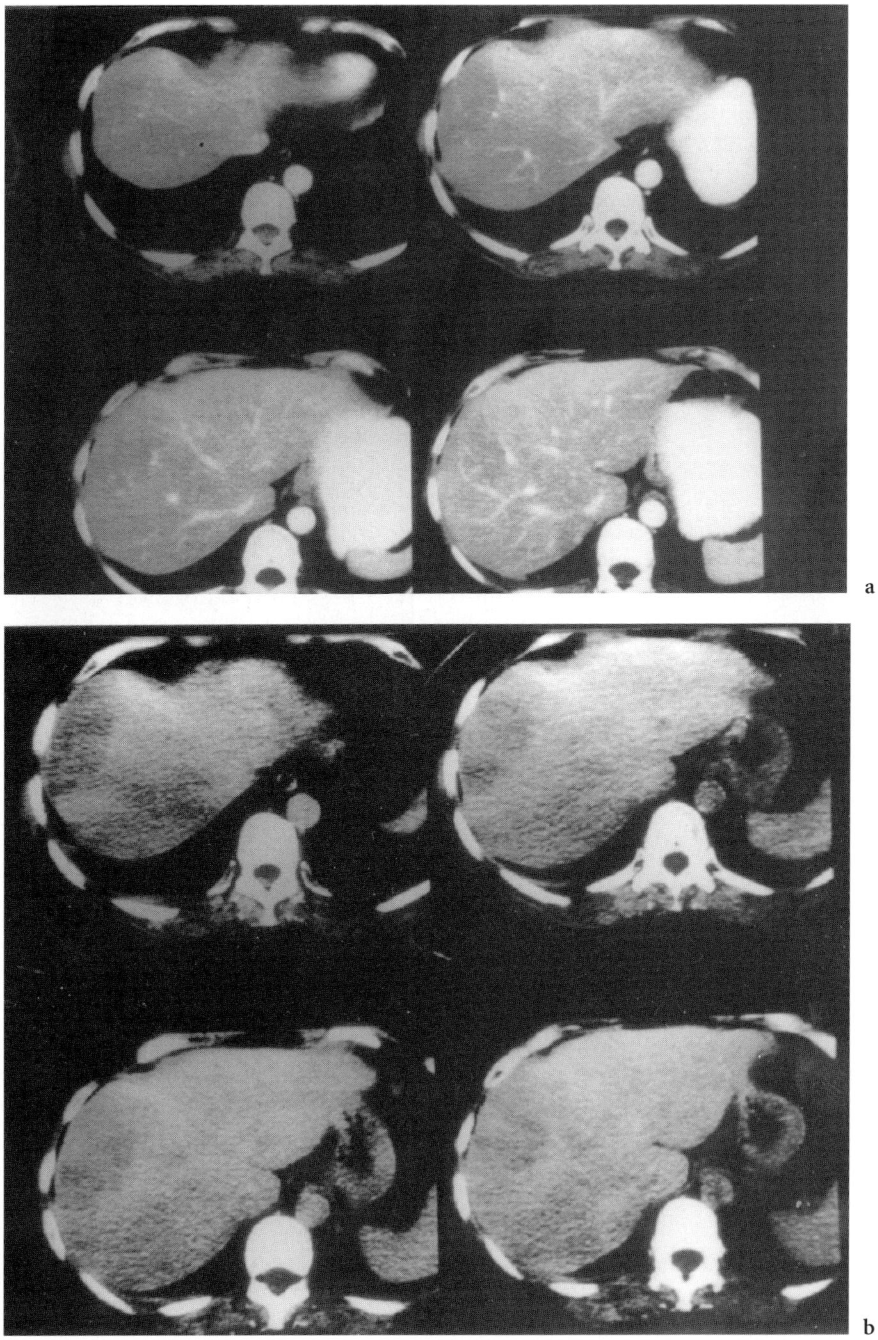

Fig. 13.16a,b. CT scan performed during the portal venous phase demonstrates no evidence of focal liver lesion (a). Delayed CT scan performed after 4 h shows large metastatic lesions from colon carcinoma (b)

tified because they stand out as highly hyperattenuating areas as compared with nontumorous liver tissue.

Various authors have demonstrated that Lipiodol deposit is not specific for HCC but may build up, although with different retention patterns, also in metastases, hemangiomas, and focal nodular hyperplasias. On the basis of these observations, Lipiodol CT has found limited applications for characterizing liver lesions detected with other imaging modalities. However, this method is increasingly used for the preoperative staging of patients with an already proved HCC to demonstrate possible small intrahepatic metastatic nodules (<2 cm) associated with the main lesion (Fig. 13.17). With regard to this point, a study conducted on 32 patients with HCC who had undergone hepatectomy reports 70.4% sensitivity in detecting small intrahepatic metastases, with a 90.5% positive predictive value (Lencioni et al. 1997). In addition, Lipiodol CT does not find any application in the staging of patients with a primitive tumor of another nature.

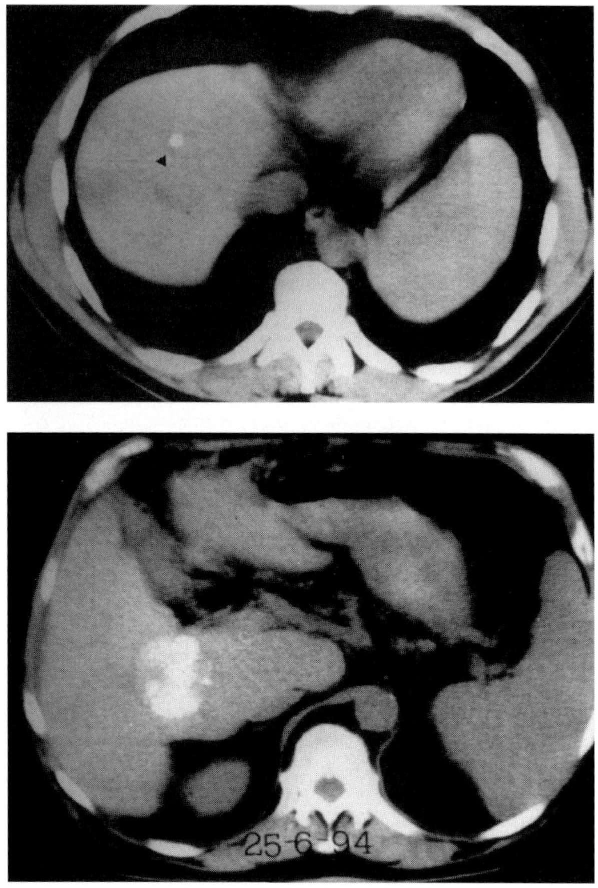

a

b

Fig. 13.17. Lipiodol CT shows a small intrahepatic metastatic nodule of HCC located in the VIII segment (*arrowhead*) **(a)** associated with the main lesion **(b)**

13.4 Conclusions

If the use of CT generally enables the identification of hepatic metastases – especially on the basis of their typical vascularization aspects and ensuing behavior after CM administration – it must be considered that, quite often, diagnosis can become more difficult since metastases may present a great structural polymorphism (both related to the primitive tumor and therapy-induced characteristics) and may be further associated with a pathologic hepatic substrate which contributes to complicating their demonstration.

For instance, it may happen that cystic metastases (e.g. ensuing from ovarian cystoadenocarcinoma) cannot be differentiated by cysts of another nature, or that the presence of intrametastastic calcifications makes difficult the discrimination from lesions of a parasitic or granulomatous type.

Moreover, a diffuse hepatic steatosis, by reducing the liver density, may make metastases isodense and thus undetectable. Instead, focal areas of normal liver may be spared of fat and retain their normal higher CT density and simulating metastatic deposits. Also the presence of regenerative nodules within a cirrhotic liver can mimic the presence of metastases.

A knowledge of the significant clinical data is very important for making a diagnosis, although sometimes, even if the CT scan is performed correctly, only a biopsy can clarify the nature of the lesion.

References

Baron RL (1994) Understanding and optimizing use of contrast media for CT of the liver. AJR 163:323–331

Bernardino M, Erwin B, Steinberg H et, al (1986) Delayed hepatic CT scanning: increased confidence and improved detection of hepatic metastases. Radiology 159:71–74

Bluemke DA, Soyer P, Fishman EK (1995a) Spiral CT evaluation of Liver Tumors. In: Fishman EK, Jeffrey R-B (eds) Spiral CT: Principles, Techniques and Clinical Applications. Lippincott-Raven, New York, pp 25–44

Bluemke DA, Soyer PA, Chan BW, et al (1995b) Spiral CT during arterial portography: technique and applications. RadioGraphics 15:623–637

Bluemke DA, Soyer P, Fishman EK (1995c) Nontumorous low-attenuation defects in the liver on helical CT during arterial portography: frequency, location, and appearance. AJR 164:1141–1145

Bonaldi VM, Bret PM, Reinhold C, et al (1995) Helical CT of the liver: value of an early hepatic arterial phase. Radiology 197:357–363

Bressler EL, Alpern MB, Glazer GM, et al (1987) Hypervascular hepatic metastases: CT evaluation. Radiology 162:49–51

Ch'en IY, Katz DS, Jeffrey RB, et al (1997) Do arterial phase helical CT images improve detection or characterization of colorectal liver metastases? Comput Assist Tomogr 21(3):391–397

Chezmar JL, Rumancik WM, Megibow AJ, et al (1988) Liver and abdominal screening in patients with cancer: CT vs MR imaging. Radiology 168:43–49

Choi BI, Freeny P, Heyano S (1996) High-dose helical CT of the liver with computer automated scan technology: comparison with helical CT arterial portography and conventional helical CT. Radiology 201:145–149

Dodd GD III, Baron RL (1993) Investigation of contrast enhancement in CT of the liver: the need for improved methods. AJR 160:643–646

Fink S, Chaudhuri K (1991) Physiological considerations in imaging liver metastases from colorectal carcinoma. Am J Physiol Imaging 6:150–160

Foley WD (1989) Dynamic hepatic CT. Radiology 170:617–622

Frederick MG, Paulson EK, Nelson RC (1997) Helical CT for detecting focal liver lesions in patients with breast carcinoma: comparison of noncontrast phase, hepatic arterial phase, and portal venous phase. J Comput Assist Tomogr 21:229–235

Freeny PC (1989) Dynamic hepatic CT. Radiology 170:617–622

Freeny PC (1990) Hepatic CT: techniques, applications and results. In: Ferrucci J, Stark D (eds) Liver imaging: current trends and new techniques. Reading Mass, Andover, pp 28–38

Freeny PC (1997) Helical computed tomography of the liver: techniques, applications and pitfalls. Endoscopy 29:515–523

Freeny PC, Crane R, Feldman R, et al (1990) Preoperative hepatic for lesion detection using bolus- dynamic CT, CT angiography, delayed iodine CT, and MR. Radiology 177:227-232

Heiken J, Weyman P, Lee J, et al (1989) Detection of focal hepatic metastases: prospective evaluation with CT, delayed CT, CT during arterial portography, and MR imaging. Radiology 171:47–51

Hollett MD, Jeffrey RB, Nino-Murcia M, et al (1995) Dual-phase helical CT of the liver: value of arterial phase scans in the detection of small (<1.5 cm) malignant hepatic neoplasm. AJR 164:879–884

Honda H, Matsuura Y, Murakami J, et al (1992) Differential Diagnosis of hepatic tumors (hepatoma, hemangioma, and metastasis) with CT: value of two-Phase incremental imaging. AJR 159:735–740

Ikeda A, Freeny P, Ryan J, et al (1996) Preoperative high-dose helical CT of the liver: comparison with surgery, pathology, and intraoperative ultrasound in the detection of hypovascular hepatic neoplasm. Radiology 201:420–426

Irie T, Kusano S (1996) Contrast-enhanced spiral CT of the liver: effect of injection time on time to peak hepatic enhancement. Comput Assist Tomogr 20:633–637

Irie T, Takeshita K, Wada Y, et al (1995) CT evaluation of hepatic tumors: comparison of CT with arterial portography, CT with infusion hepatic arteriography, and simultaneous use of both techniques. AJR 164:1407–1411

Kanematsu M, Imaeda T, Hoshi H, et al. (1997) Methodological assessment of combined spiral CT angiography and CT arterial portography. Abdom Imaging 22:404–409

Lencioni R, Pinto F, Armillotta N, et al (1997) Intrahepatic metastatic nodules of hepatocellular carcinoma detected at Lipiodol-CT: imaging-pathologic correlation. Abdom Imaging 22:253–258

Lupetin AR, Cammisa BA, Beckman I, et al (1996) Spiral CT during arterial portography. RadioGraphics 16:723–743

Nelson RC, Chezmar JL, Sugarbaker PH, el al (1989) Hepatic tumors: comparison of CT during arterial portography, delayed CT, and MR imaging for preoperative evaluation. Radiology 172:27–34

Nelson RC, Thompson GH, Chezmar JL, et al (1992) CT during arterial portography: diagnostic pitfalls. RadioGraphics 12:705–718

Ohashi I, Ina H, Gomi N, et al (1995) Hepatic pseudolesion in the left lobe around the falciform ligament at helical CT. Radiology 196:245–249

Oliver JH, Baron RL (1996) Helical biphasic contrast-enhanced CT of the liver: technique, indications, interpretation, and pitfalls. Radiology 201:1–14

Oliver JH, Baron RL, Federle MP, Jones BC, Sheng R (1997) Hypervascular liver metastases: do unenhanced and hepatic arterial phase CT images affect tumor detection? Radiology 205:709–715

Olson MC, Posniak HV, Demos TC, et al (1996) Helical computed tomography at 1.5:1 pitch reconstructed at 15 mm and 7 mm intervals for examination of patients with suspected metastatic disease. Can Assoc Radiol J 47:54–58

Paley MR, Ros PR (1997) Hepatic metastases: computed tomography versus magnetic resonance imaging in 1997. Endoscopy 29:524–538

Patten R, Byun JY, Freeny PC (1993) CT of hypervascular hepatic tumors: are unenhanced scans necessary for diagnosis? AJR 161:979–984

Paulson EK, Baker ME, Hilleren DJ, et al (1992) CT arterial portography: causes of technical failure and variable liver enhancement. AJR 159:745–749

Paulson EK, McDermott VG, Cheogan MT, de Long DM, Frederick MC, Nelson MC (1998) Carcinoid metastases to the liver: role of triple-phase helical CT. Radiology 206:143–150

Perkerson RB Jr, Erwin BC, Baumgartner BR, et al (1985) CT densities in delayed iodine hepatic scanning. Radiology 155:445-449

Platt JF, Francis IR, Ellis JH, et al (1997) Difference in global hepatic enhancement assessed by dynamic CT in normal subjects and patients with hepatic metastases. Comput Assist Tomogr 21:348–354

Reinig JW, Dwyer AJ, Miller DL, et al (1987) Liver metastases detection: comparative sensitivities of MR imaging and CT scanning. Radiology 162:43-47

Silverman PM, Cooper C, Zeman RK (1995a) Imaging of the liver: a survey update of prevailing techniques for conventional CT scanning. Abdom Imaging 20:348–352

Silverman PM, O'Malley J, Tefft MC,et al (1995b) Detection of hepatic metastases by helical CT: effect of different time delays between contrast administration and scanning. AJR 164:619–623

Silverman PM, Roberts S, Tefft MC, et al (1995 c) Helical CT of the liver: clinical application of an automated computer technique, smartprep, for obtaining images with optimal contrast enhancement. AJR 165:73–78

Silverman PM, Cooper C, Trock B, et al (1995 d) The optimal temporal window for CT of the liver using a time-density analysis: implications for helical (spiral) CT. Comput Assist Tomogr 19:73–79

Silverman PM, Roberts SC, Ducic I, et al (1996) Assessment of a technology that permits individualized scan delays on helical hepatic CT: a technique to improve efficiency in use of contrast media. AJR 167:79–84

Silverman PM, Kohan L, Ducic I, et al (1998) Imaging of the liver with helical CT: a survey of scanning techniques. AJR 170:149–152

Small WC, Mehard WB, Langmo LS, et al (1993) Preoperative determination of the resectability of hepatic tumors: efficacy of CT during arterial portography. AJR 161:319–322

Small WC, Nelson RC, Bernardino ME, et al (1994) Contrast-enhanced spiral CT of the liver: effect of different amounts and injection rates of contrast media on early contrast enhancement. AJR 163:87–92

Soyer P, Bluemke DA, Hruban RH, Sitzmann JV, Fishman EK (1994) Hepatic metastases from colorectal cancer: detection and false-positive findings with helical CT during arterial portography. Radiology 193:71–74

Urban BA, Fishman EK, Kuhlman JE, et al (1993) Detection of focal hepatic lesions with spiral CT: comparison of 4 and 8 mm interscan spacing. AJR 160:783–787

van Leeuwen MS, Noordzij J, Feldberg MAM, et al (1996) Focal liver lesions: characterization with triphasic spiral CT. Radiology 201:327–336

Zeman RK, Silverman PM (1995) Abdomen and Pelvis. In: Pennington J, Ramos Englis M (eds) Helical/Spiral CT: a practical approach. McGraw-Hill, New York, pp153–220

Zeman RK, Fox SH, Silverman PM, et al (1993) Helical (spiral) CT of the abdomen. AJR 160:719–725

14 Magnetic Resonance Imaging of Liver Metastases

G.F. Pistolesi, R. Caudana, and G. Morana

CONTENTS

G.F. Pistolesi, MD, Professor and Chairman; Department of Radiology, University of Verona, Borgo Roma Hospital, Via delle Menetone 10, I-37134 Verona, Italy
R. Caudana, MD; Department of Radiology, University of Verona, Borgo Roma Hospital, Via delle Menetone 10, I-37134 Verona, Italy
G. Morana, MD; Department of Radiology, University of Verona, Borgo Roma Hospital, Via delle Menetone 10, I-37134 Verona, Italy

14.1 Introduction

The presence of liver metastases has a remarkable impact on the survival rate. Such an event is relatively frequent: for instance, hepatic secondaries are found in approximately 40% of patients with colorectal cancer (Ferrucci 1994). In the diagnostic approach to liver metastases, the imaging plays a fundamental role in selecting those patients who can benefit from surgical resection. This treatment, performed with the correct indication, drastically improves the survival rate: 5-year survival rate of 20%–40% for metastases from colorectal carcinoma (Butler et al. 1986; Hughes et el. 1988; Ferrucci and Stark 1990; Fegiz et al. 1991; Scheele et al. 1991; Nakamura et al. 1992) with a risk of morbidity and mortality of 2%–7% (Holm et al. 1989; Scheele et al. 1991; Vetto et al. 1990). Conversely, in untreated colorectal hepatic metastases, the mean survival rate is drastically reduced (Wagner et al. 1984): 21 months for solitary lesions with a 5-year survival of 16% (Greenway 1988), 15 months for multiple metastases confined within a single liver lobe and 10 months for diffuse involvement of the liver.

The imaging role is organized into three diagnostic steps. The first two concern the detection and characterization of the metastases respectively, while the third step evaluates the resectability of the metastases. This chapter considers the contribution of magnetic resonance (MR) in these diagnostic steps, after a preliminary evaluation of the MR features of the metastases.

14.2 MR Features of Metastases

The variation in the gross morphology of liver metastases, their localization and their number is very wide (Semelka and Mitchell 1996; Semelka and

Kelekis 1997). The shape of the lesion is usually roundish (Fig. 14.1–14.2); nevertheless the metastases from colorectal adenocarcinoma larger than 3 cm commonly have a cauliflower aspect (Fig. 14.3). The majority of metastatic lesions have ill defined margins. However, metastases from squamous-cell carcinoma and those from endocrine tumor, often roundish, present sharp margins (Fig. 14.2). The site of the metastases is usually intrahepatic, prevailing within the right lobe; exceptionally the metastases may be localized on the liver capsule, owing to the intraperitoneal spread (ovarian and colonic adenocarcinomas).

The metastases from poorly differentiated adenocarcinomas and from endocrine tumors are usually numerous, <2 cm sized and disseminated to the whole liver (Fig. 14.2).

14.2.1 Signal Intensity

The signal intensity of the metastases differs from that of the liver since their T1 and T2 relaxation times are longer, owing to the higher content of free water molecules. Therefore on T1 weighted images the signal intensity of the metastases is lower (darker) than that of the hepatic tissue (Figs. 14.1, 14.2, 14.3), while it is higher (brighter) on T2 weighted images (Figs. 14.1, 14.2, 14.3). Conversely, on proton density (PD) images the difference of the signal intensity between the metastasis and the hepatic tissue is not significant (Fig. 14.1) because both tissues contain an elevated number of protons.

14.2.2 Peculiar Pathologic Conditions

Some peculiar pathologic conditions can modify the behavior of the signal intensity of the metastases. Whenever colliquative necrosis or infectious edema is present within the metastasis, the signal intensity further increases on T2 weighted images. On the other hand, if coagulative necrosis, fibrous matrix or calcifications are present within the metastasis, the elevated signal intensity on T2 weighted images is decreased. Finally, whenever subacute intralesional hemorrhage or particular substances are produced by metastatic tissue, the signal intensity of T1 weighted images – usually low – is increased.

These different conditions are considered in succession.

14.2.2.1 Colliquative Necrosis

The reduced arterial blood flow within the central area of the metastases may cause colliquative necrosis, which shows a very high signal intensity on T2 weighted images (Fig. 14.4), completely similar to that of fluid content of the cysts (Fig. 14.5), due to the increased amount of free water molecules. The differential diagnosis is obtained with paramagnetic contrast medium (CM), as detailed in the following sections.

14.2.2.2 Infectious Edema

Infectious edema occurs more frequently in metastases from colorectal carcinoma (bacteria originating from intestinal lumen). Infected metastases sometimes simulate liver abscesses (Semelka and Kelekis 1997), showing a central, remarkable increase in signal intensity on T2 weighted images (fluid content) and an irregular border with high signal intensity, but lower than the center of the metastasis. The use of CM is useful for characterization of the infected metastases as better detailed below.

14.2.2.3 Coagulative Necrosis

The sudden interruption of the arterial blood flow within the central area of the metastasis may determine coagulative necrosis, which reduces the signal intensity on T2 weighted images (Fig. 14.6), owing to the denaturation of intracellular proteinaceous macromolecules (Outwater et al. 1991). Conversely, in the peripheral zone of the metastasis (viable tumor cells), the signal intensity remains elevated on T2 weighted images (Fig. 14.6).

14.2.2.4 Fibrous Matrix

The fibrous matrix as well, sometimes recognizable in the metastasis from colorectal cancer, lowers (Semelka et al. 1994) the usually high signal intensity of the lesion (Fig. 14.3). The huge macromolecular complexes forming collagen fibrils behave like solid state structures containing strongly bound protons which decrease the signal intensity.

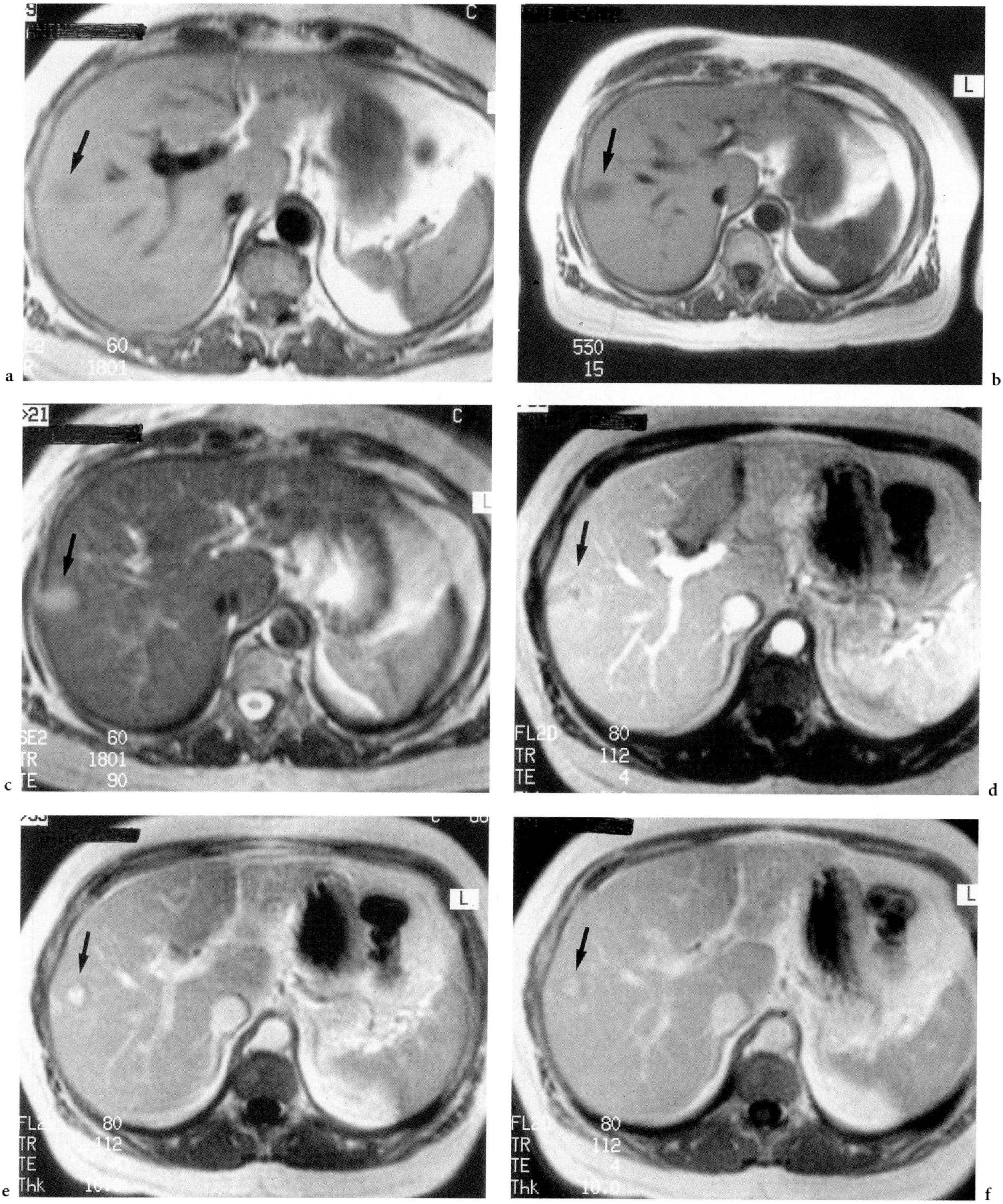

Fig. 14.1a–f. Hypovascular metastasis from breast carcinoma. **a–c** SE sequence. On PD the image (**a**) the lesion (*arrow*) shows a mild hypointensity slightly different to that of the hepatic tissue. On the T1 weighted image (**b**) the lesion shows lower signal intensity than the hepatic tissue; on the T2 weighted image (**c**) higher signal intensity of the lesion than the hepatic tissue. **d–f** Dynamic study with GRE sequence (T1 weighted images) after bolus injection of Gd-DTPA. During the phase of vascular distribution of the CM (**d**), peripheral ring enhancement of the lesion due to the better arterial perfusion compared to the central zone and to the perilesional hepatic tissue. Progressive interstitial pooling of the CM (**e**) with delayed central enhancement of the lesion due to the reduced arterial perfusion compared to the peripheral zone. Interstitial clearance of the CM (**f**) with peripheral hypointense ring of the lesion due to the faster interstitial clearance (peripheral wash-out) compared to the central zone and to the perilesional hepatic tissue

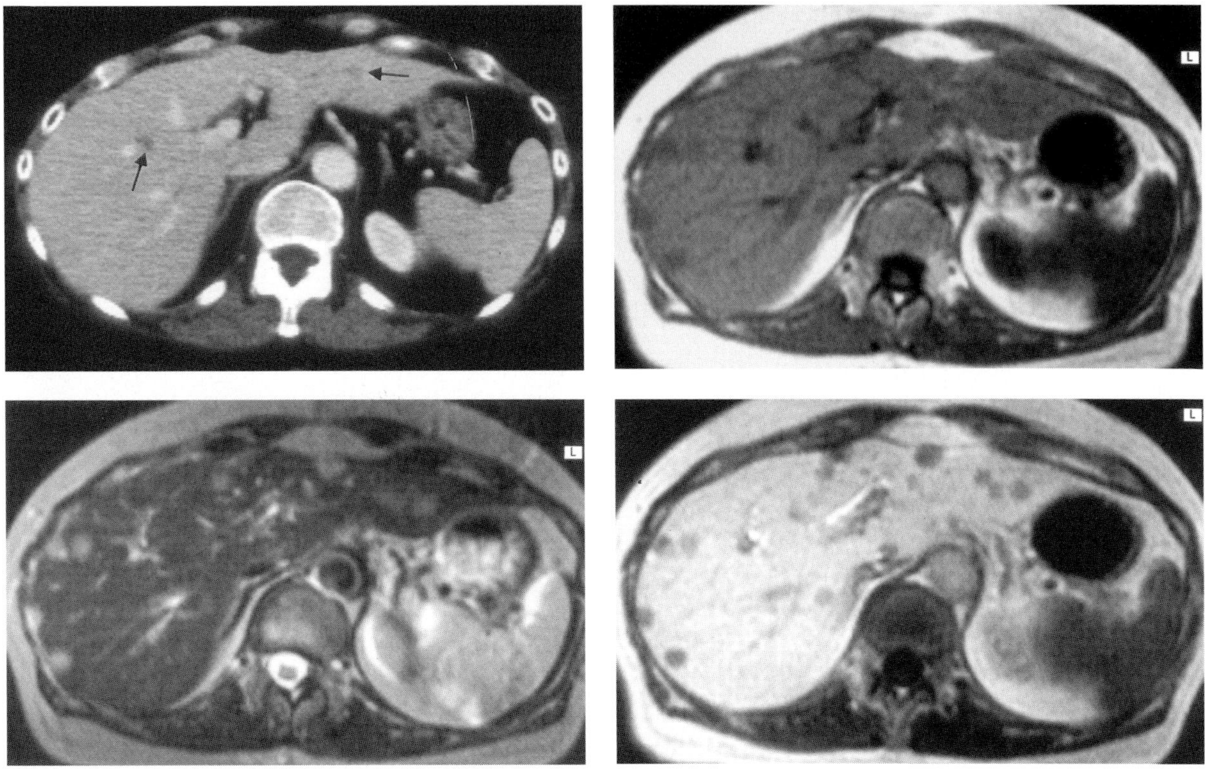

Fig. 14.2a–d. Metastases from intestinal carcinoid. **a** Contrast enhanced CT scan shows two slightly hypodense lesions (*arrows*) within both the liver lobes. On a T1 weighted image with GRE sequence (**b**) some slightly hypointense lesions within the right liver lobe. The hypointensity of the lesions is weaker than usual, due to the production of serotonin. On a T2 weighted image with SE sequence (**c**) numerous slightly hyperintense lesions within both the liver lobes. On a T1 weighted image with GRE sequence (**d**) 60 min after injection of hepatocyte targeted CM (Gd-BOPTA) more confident detection of subcentimeter lesions due to the intense enhancement of the hepatic tissue; the metastases have a round shape with sharp edges

14.2.2.5 Calcifications

The calcifications, rarely present within metastases from colorectal carcinoma, cause a remarkable reduction of signal intensity. Their differentiation from fibrous matrix or coagulative necrosis – easily obtained with CT– is very difficult with MR.

14.2.2.6 Hemorrhage

Metastases may present hemorrhage. Methemoglobin present in the subacute phase may shorten T1 relaxation time, owing to the paramagnetic effect (just as with paramagnetic CM); it follows a remarkable increase of signal intensity on T1 weighted images which enables hemorrhagic foci to be distinguished (Arrive' et al. 1996) in comparison to the metastatic and hepatic tissue (Fig. 14.7).

14.2.2.7 Production of Particular Substances

The production of particular substances by metastatic tissue (melanin, mucin, serotonin) may increase, with varying degrees, their signal intensity on T1 weighted images (Semelka and Kelekis 1997). For instance, the melanin (metastases from melanoma) has paramagnetic properties which increase the signal intensity on T1 weighted images.

The mucin (macrocystic adenocarcinoma of the pancreas or ovarium) induces analogous result (increase in signal intensity on T1 weighted images) but with a different mechanism than melanin. In fact, owing to the binding of water molecules with proteinaceous macromolecules, the content of free-water molecules within the metastatic tissue is reduced, causing an increase in signal intensity on T1 weighted images.

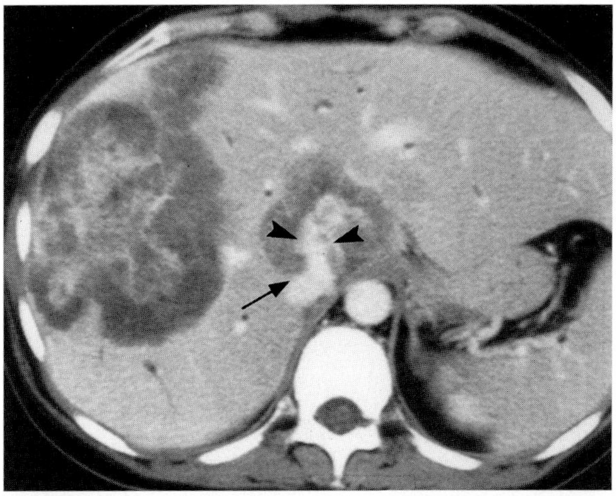

a

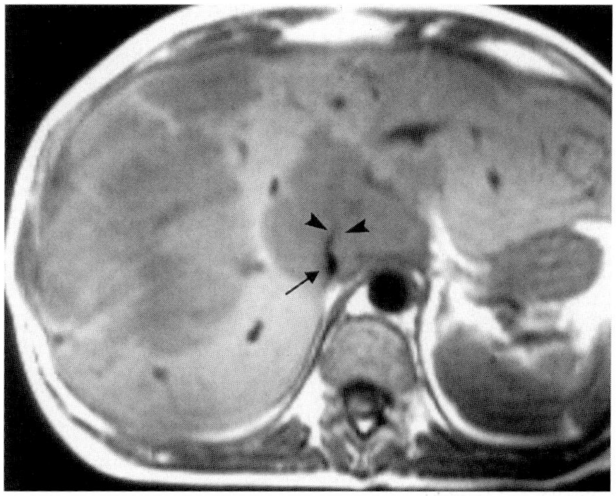

b

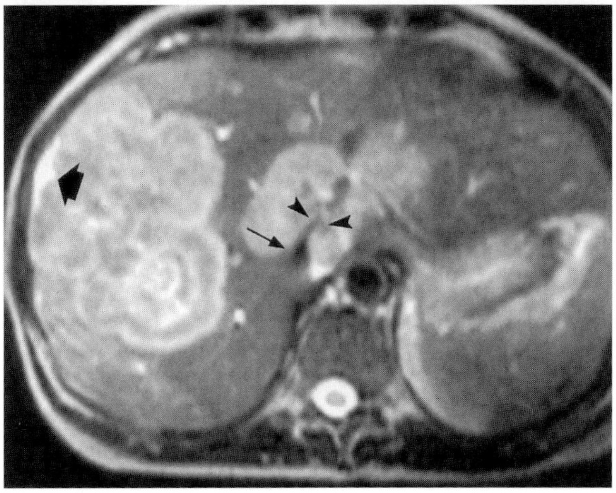

c

Fig. 14.3a–c. Metastases from colorectal carcinoma with involvement of the central hepatic vessels. **a** Contrast enhanced CT scan shows two large cauliflower type lesions infiltrating the inferior vena cava (*arrow*) as well as the hepatic veins (*arrowheads*). Intrahepatic bile ducts are slightly dilated owing to the metastatic involvement of the liver hylum. **b,c** SE sequence. On T1 (**b**) and T2 (**c**) weighted images the lesions are hypointense and hyperintense respectively; the involvement of the central hepatic vessels is well shown in both the images; on a T2 weighted image (**c**) the hypointense areas within the larger lesion represent the fibrous matrix; the subtle subcapsular fluid collection (*large arrow*) and the intrahepatic mildly dilated bile ducts show an elevated signal intensity analogous to that of the CSF surrounding the spinal cord

The serotonin (carcinoid tumor) behaves like mucin (binding of free water molecules with proteinaceous macromolecules within the metastases), increasing the signal intensity on T1 weighted images (Figs. 14.2).

14.3 Guidelines for Detection of Metastases

In diagnostic oncology of the liver, MR evaluation must be first of all focused on detection of the metastatic lesions (Saini and Nelson 1995), which depends on the size threshold of the lesion as well as contrast-to-noise ratio (C/N).

14.3.1 Size Threshold of the Lesion

From the viewpoint of focal liver lesion detection, each imaging modality has a macroscopic size threshold, which mainly depends on the spatial resolution of the machine. On the other hand, detection of as small as possible metastases represents the real goal of all the currently used imaging modalities. A postmortem assessment of the size of liver metastases has shown that the ratio between metastases larger than 1 cm and those smaller than 1 cm is approximately 1:1.6 for metastases of colorectal adenocarcinoma and 1:4 for other liver metastases (Schulz and Borchard 1992). Since it is accepted (Wernecke et al. 1991) that the size threshold of transabdominal ultrasound (US), CT and MR is 1 cm, it follows that for each metastasis seen, there is the possibility of missing at least one

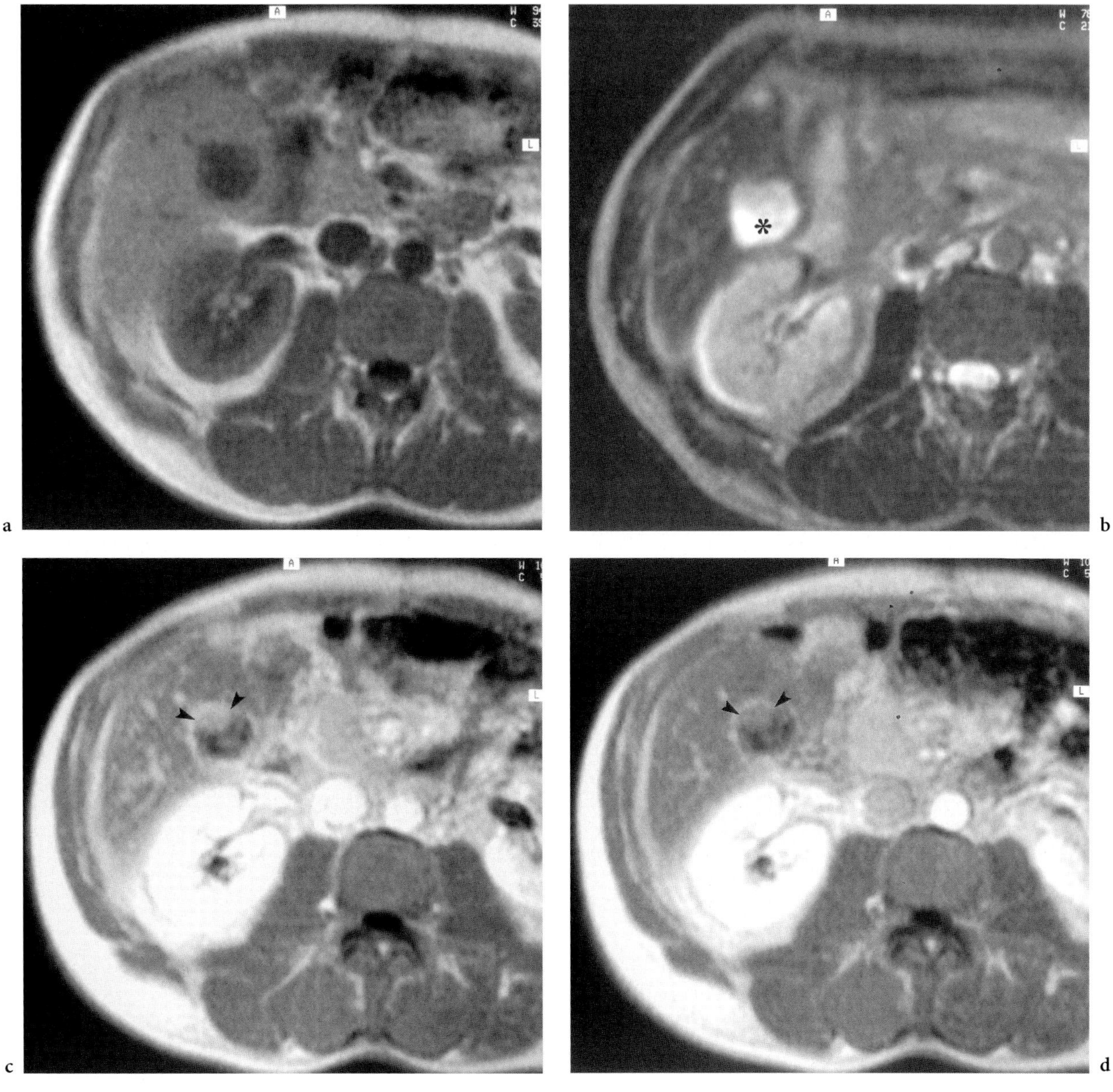

Fig. 14.4a–d. Hypervascular metastasis from colorectal carcinoma with colliquative necrosis. **a,b** T1 (**a**) and T2 (**b**) sequences. On T2 weighted image (**b**) the lesion is hyperintense compared to the hepatic tissue; the colliquative necrosis (*asterisk*) within the central zone of the lesion shows a more elevated signal intensity, identical to that of the CSF around the spinal cord. **c,d** Dynamic study with GRE (T1 weighted images) after bolus injection of Gd-DTPA. During the vascular phase of distribution of the CM (**c**), a thin ring of peripheral enhancement of the lesion with a nodule anteriorly located (*arrowheads*) corresponding to the viable portion of the tumor. During the interstitial pooling of the CM (**d**) absence of enhancement of the central area of the lesion, not perfused owing to the colliquative necrosis

metastasis in the case of colorectal adenocarcinoma and four in the case of other malignant tumors. The size threshold of focal lesion detection is moreover greatly reduced by the sharpness of the edge (Mafhouz et al. 1996).

14.3.2 Contrast-to-Noise Ratio

The contrast-to-noise ratio (C/N) depends on two factors (Hendrick 1988): the difference in signal intensity of the hepatic tissue versus that of the metastasis (contrast:C) and the amount of the image

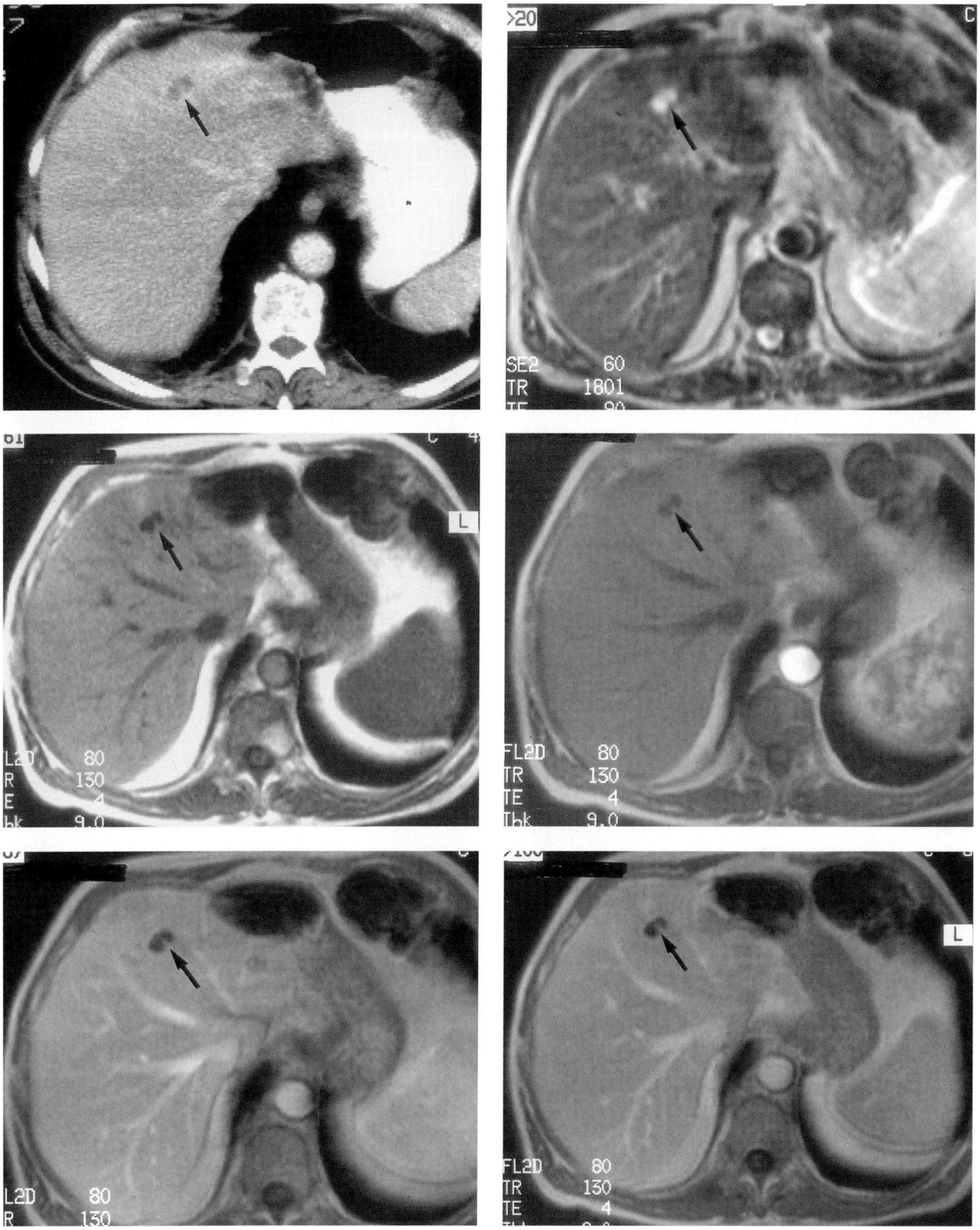

a b c d e f

Fig. 14.5a–f. Cysts (abdominal-perineal resection for rectal carcinoma performed 1 year previously). **a** Contrast enhanced CT scan shows a small bilobate hypodense lesion (*arrow*) with doubtful density values not allowing its characterization. **b,c** SE (**b**) and GRE (**c**) sequences. On T2 (**b**) and T1 (**c**) weighted images the lesion with sharp borders shows hyperintense and hypointense signal respectively, identical to that of the CSF around the spinal cord. **d–f** Dynamic study with GRE sequence (T1 weighted images) after a bolus injection of Gd-DTPA. During the phases of arterial (**d**) and portal (**e**) vascular distribution of CM as well as during the interstitial phase (**f**), no enhancement of the cysts is recognized

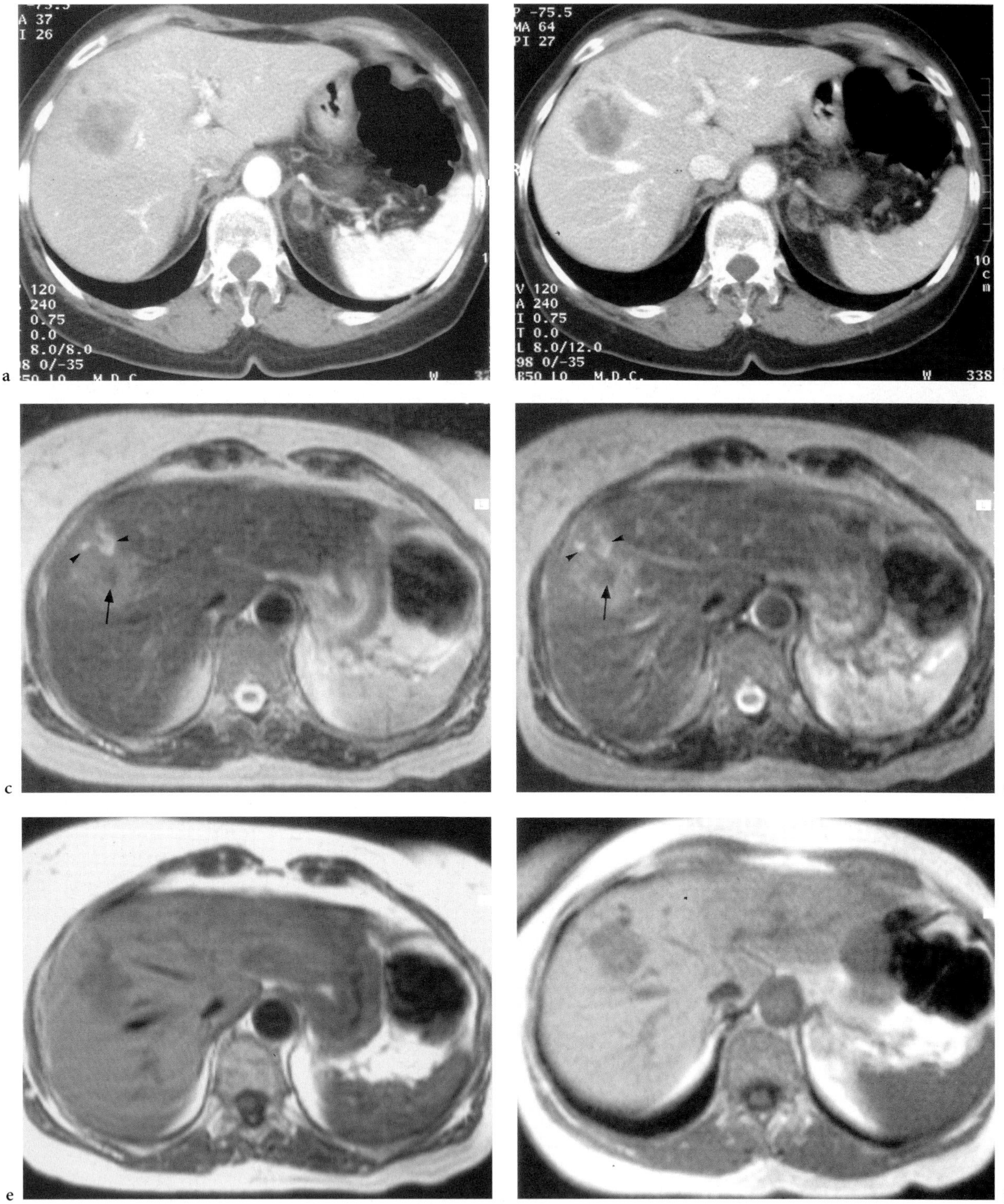

Fig. 14.6a–f. Hypovascular metastasis from colorectal carcinoma with coagulative necrosis. **a,b** Dynamic contrast enhanced CT scans: during the vascular phases of arterial (**a**) and portal (**b**) distribution of the CM the hypodense lesion does not show enhancement. **c,d** On T2 weighted images with SE (**c**) and FSE (**d**) sequences, faint hyperintensity at the periphery of the lesion which shows irregular borders; the central coagulative necrosis (*arrow*) appears hypointense. Dilated hyperintense intrahepatic bile ducts (*arrowheads*) within the hepatic tissue at the periphery of the lesion. **e,f** On T1 weighted images with SE (**e**) and GRE (**f**) sequences, uniform hypointensity of the lesion. A remarkable reduction of motion artifacts is seen on T2 (**d**) and T1 (**f**) weighted fast sequences compared to conventional SE T2 (**c**) and T1 (**e**) weighted sequences

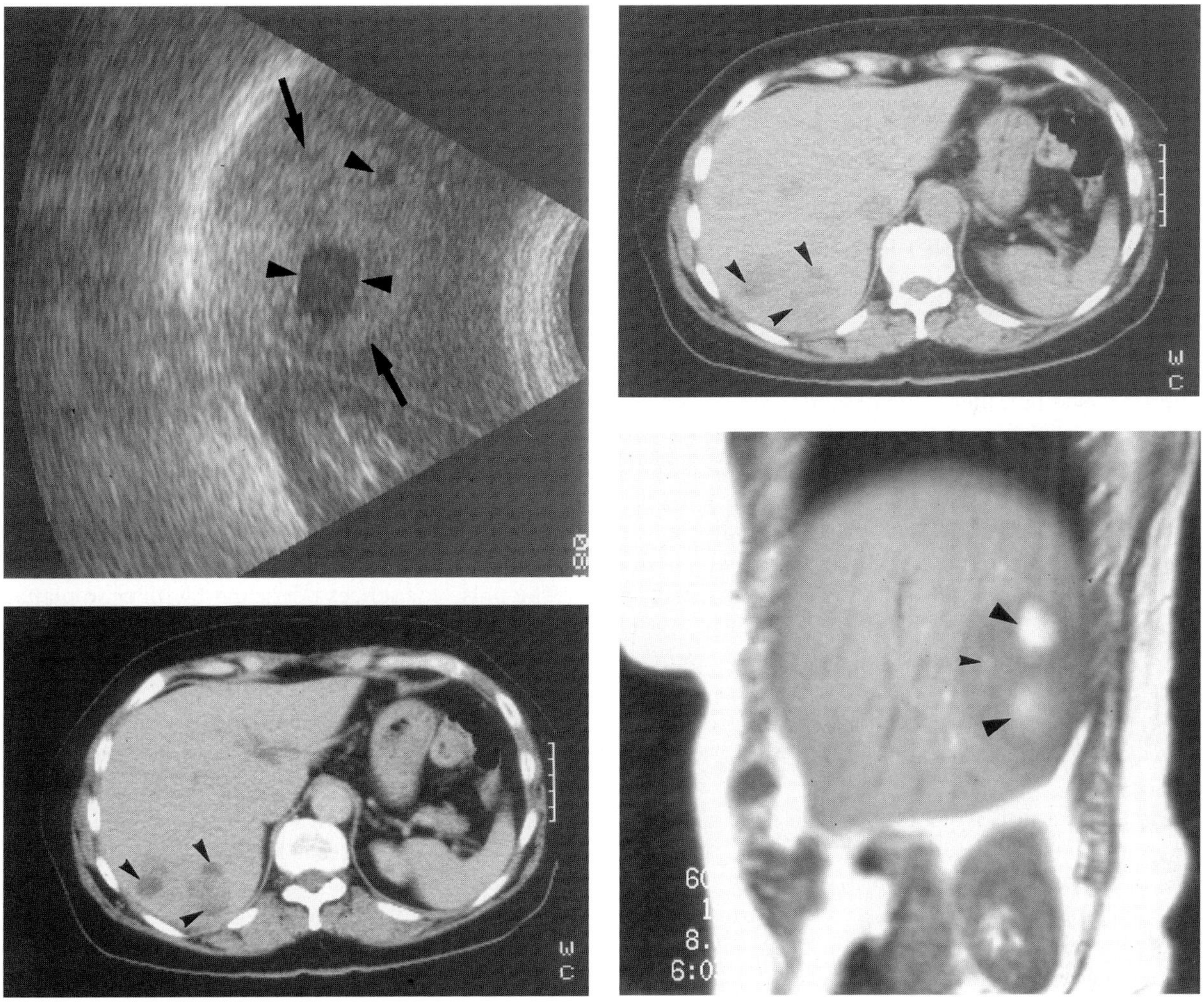

Fig. 14.7a–d. Metastasis from intestinal carcinoid with hemorrhage. **a** Longitudinal US scan shows slightly hyperechoic lesion (*arrows*) with hypoechoic foci with corpuscular fluid content (*arrowheads*). **b,c** Unenhanced (**b**) and contrast enhanced (**c**) CT scans show multiple fluid collections (*arrowheads*) within the lesion, better demonstrated on enhanced scan. T1 weighted sagittal image with SE sequence (**d**) shows the hemorrhagic hyperintense areas (*arrowheads*) within the lesion, due to the presence of methemoglobin

noise (N) respectively. In other words, the difference of the signal intensity between the metastasis and the perilesional liver (parameter C) depends on the tissue's intrinsic characteristics reproduced by PD, T1 and T2 relaxation times with the degrading and unremovable image noise (parameter N). Either the pulse sequences or the CM is able to emphasize the C/N increasing C or reducing N, as discussed below. The more elevated the C/N, the easier the detection of focal lesions, with a consequent decrease in the size threshold of identification.

14.3.2.1 Choice of the Pulse Sequence

The choice of the pulse sequence represents the most important moment for the detection of the metastasis because C/N depends on the intrinsic properties of tissues (normal and metastatic) as well as on the modality of MR image acquisition (Crooks 1991; Grellet et al. 1993; Mitchell 1994; Saini and Nelson 1995; Weisskoff and Edelman 1996). The different pulse sequences allow the emphasis of the C/N, affecting either the parameter C or N: practically speaking, inversion recovery (IR), spin echo (SE) and fat suppression sequences mainly affect parameter C, while fast sequences mainly affect parameter N.

14.3.2.1.1
Increment of Parameter C
Among the pulse sequences allowing the increment of parameter C (contrast) the IR provides a strong T1 weighting (metastases appear very dark in comparison to liver tissue); this sequence, widely used in the past (Stark et al. 1987; Reinig et al. 1989), suffers from motion artifacts. Nowadays, the availability of high performance gradients allows IR sequences to be obtained – in particular, short time IR (STIR) – within a very short acquisition time (20–25 s) with the elimination of motion artifacts, still maintaining a high C/N. The SE sequence has been considered to have the best C/N especially on T2 weighted images (Foley et al. 1987) in which the metastasis appears brighter than the normal tissue; conversely, on PD images the C/N is considerably lower and therefore these images are less often requested. From the practical point of view, T2 weighted images are consequently the best for detection of liver metastases and therefore must be always performed.

Fat suppression sequences increase the C/N, improving the parameter C (Semelka et al. 1992, 1993b; Schwartz et al. 1993; Larson et al. 1994), thus facilitating the detection of metastases (Fig. 14.8). In fact, the fatty infiltration of the liver often associated with metastatic involvement reduces the difference in signal intensity between the lesion and the hepatic tissue on T2 weighted images.

14.3.2.1.2
Reduction of Parameter N
The use of fast sequences (gradient echo, fast spin echo, echo planar imaging) allows the reduction of parameter N (noise) to be obtained thanks to the breathhold, which drastically reduces the respiratory motion artifacts in the images. In fact, considering liver imaging, the main source of image noise is represented by respiratory artifacts which increase parameter N, hence reducing the image C/N. Moreover, the C/N achievable with fast sequences is not only due to the reduction of the parameter N but also to the value of the parameter C, the latter affected by the type of pulse sequence implemented. For instance, fast spin echo (FSE) T2 weighted images show low N (Low et al. 1993; Siewert et al. 1994) owing to the drastic reduction of motion artifacts (Figs. 14.6, 14.8), but since also C is low, the resulting C/N is inferior to that of T2 weighted conventional SE sequences. It turns out that the detection of the metastasis may be more difficult (Outwater et al. 1994; Rydberg et al. 1995; Taupitz et al. 1995) since the metastatic tissue is less bright in comparison to that usually found on conventional SE T2 weighted images (Fig. 14.8). To recover the satisfactory values of parameter C on FSE T2 weighted sequences, the application of fat suppression is necessary (Schwartz et al. 1993) in order to obtain elevated values of C/N, equivalent to those of conventional SE T2 weighted sequences (Fig. 14.8).

T1 weighted images obtained with gradient echo (GRE) sequence implementing a flip angle of 80° allow a high C/N owing to the reduction of parameter N (Semelka et al.1991, 1992, 1994); the metastases appear dark in comparison to the hepatic tissue (Fig. 14.6).

The pulse sequences performed with echo planar imaging (EPI) are even faster and therefore totally free from respiratory artifacts (Saini et al. 1994). T1 and T2 weighted images obtained with EPI show an increased parameter C and a reduced parameter N, both leading to a higher C/N than that of the images achieved with SE pulse sequences (Jung et al. 1997; Ichikawa et al. 1998); however, the clinical experience on liver metastases is limited.

In short, the results of lesion detection obtained with various pulse sequences have not been completely encouraging compared with those of the conventional SE T2 weighted sequence, excluding EPI, which needs, however, more clinical evaluation on liver metastases. For this reason, besides the improvement in the performances of the pulse sequences, research has been focused on the development of CM dedicated to liver imaging.

14.3.2.2 Utilization of Contrast Media

In fact, the utilization of contrast media (CM) plays an important role in the detection of liver metastases since it influences the C/N (Brash 1992; Saini 1992; Grellet et al. 1993; Schuman-Gianpieri 1993; Lauffer 1996), increasing parameter C, in a fashion that depends on both the magnetic properties of the CM (increase or decrease in signal intensity) as well as its pharmacokinetics (selective enhancement of the hepatic tissue and/or of the lesion).

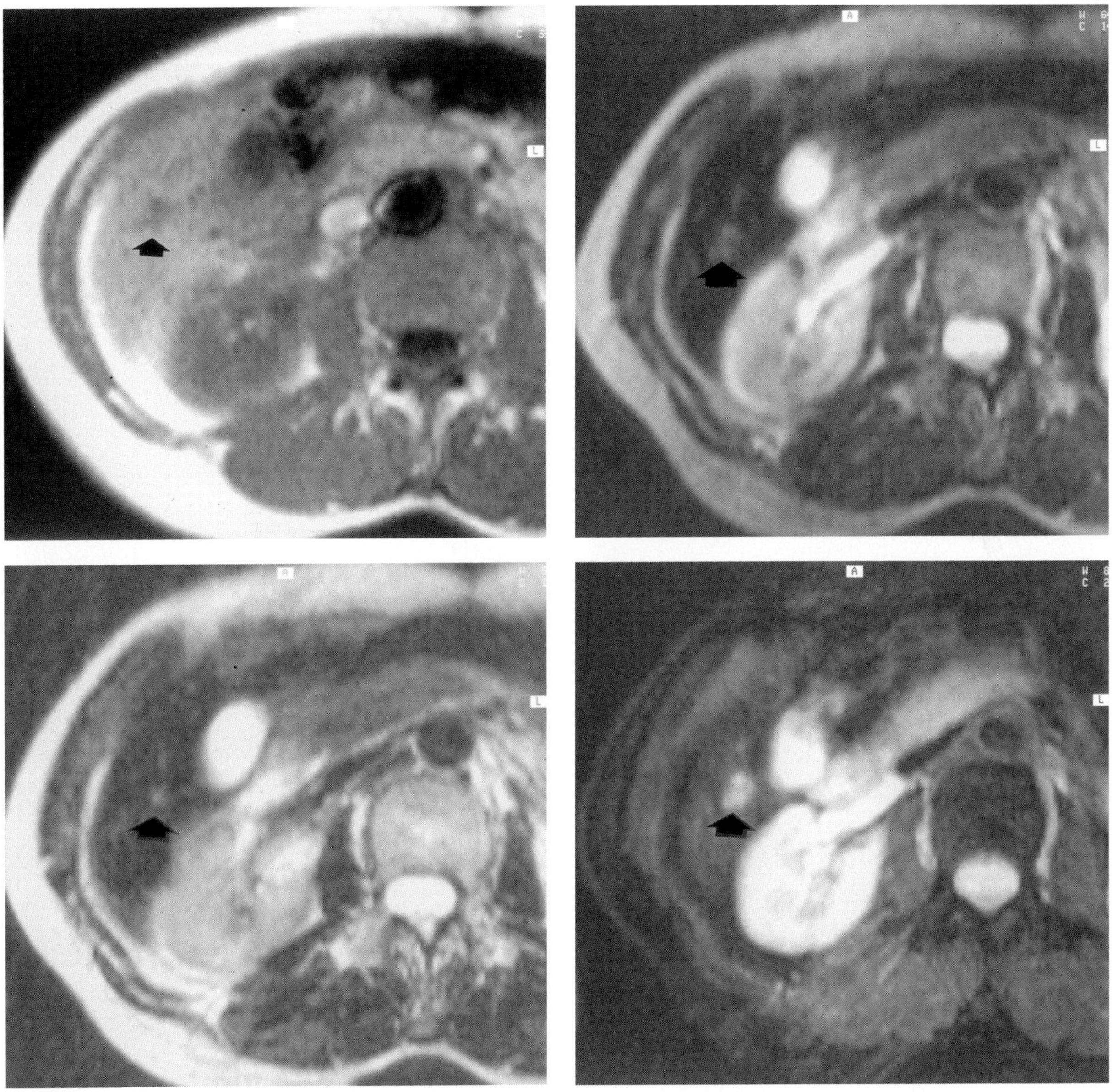

a b c d

Fig. 14.8a–d. Metastasis from breast carcinoma. On a T1 weighted image with GRE sequence (**a**) the lesion (*arrow*) shows faint hypointensity compared to the hepatic tissue (low C/N). **b–d** On T2 weighted images with SE (**b**) and FSE (**c**) sequences the lesion shows a weak signal intensity compared to the hepatic tissue (low C/N) and therefore the metastasis is not confidently detectable. On a T2 weighted image with fat suppression (**d**) the notable hyperintensity of the lesion compared to the hepatic tissue (elevated C/N) allows more confident detection of the metastasis

14.3.2.2.1 Magnetic Properties

With regard to the magnetic properties, the positive CMs, owing to the paramagnetic effect of some chemical elements (Gd, Mn), which drastically shorten the T1 relaxation time of the uptaking tissue, lead to a notable increase in signal intensity on T1 weighted images (Figs. 14.1, 14.2, 14.4, 14.5). The negative CMs, exploiting the superparamagnetic effect of the super paramagnetic iron oxide (SPIO) particles, cause a conspicuous shortening of the T2 relaxation time of the uptaking tissue, thus producing a remarkable decrease in signal intensity on T2 weighted images (Fig. 14.9).

14.3.2.2.2 Pharmacokinetics

The description of the pharmacokinetics of the CM

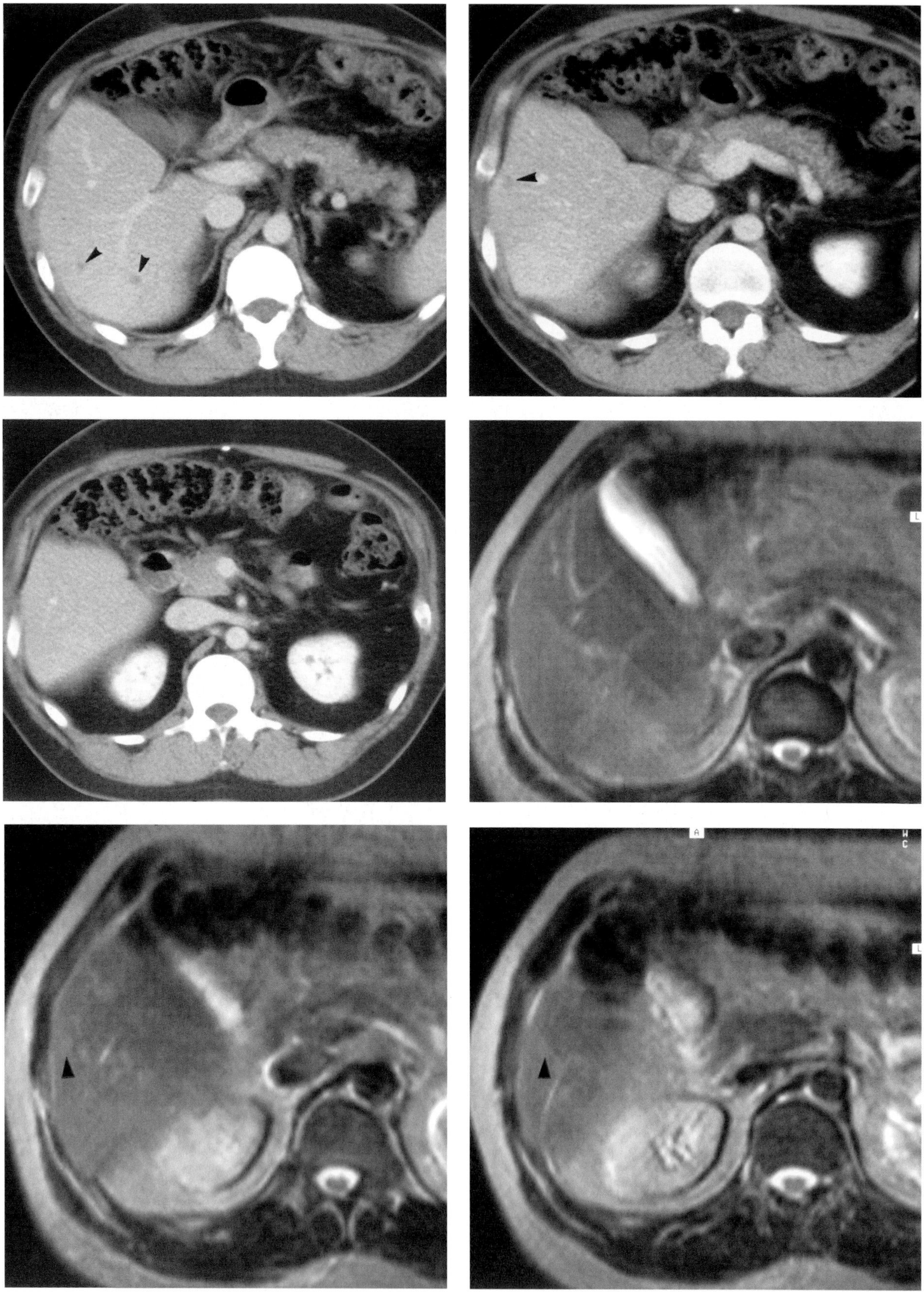

a b c d e f

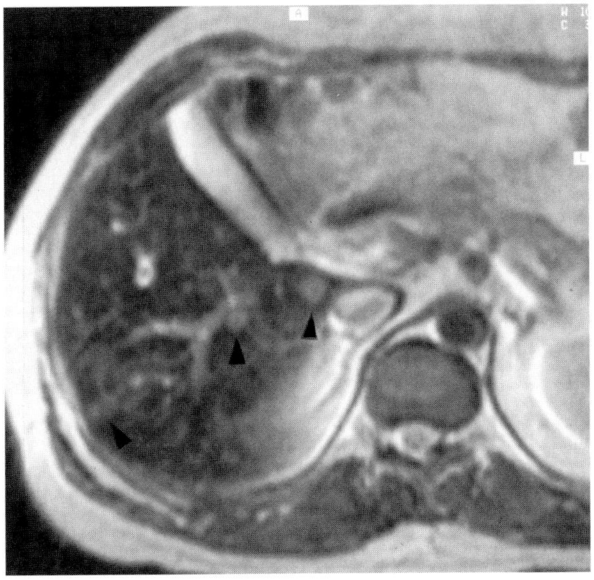

g

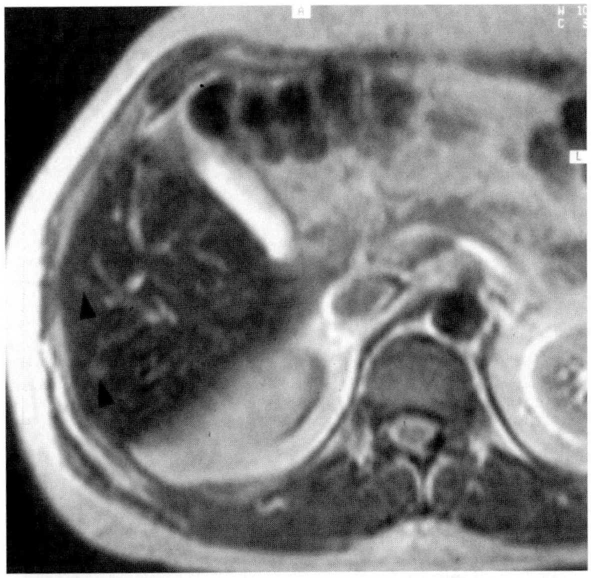

h

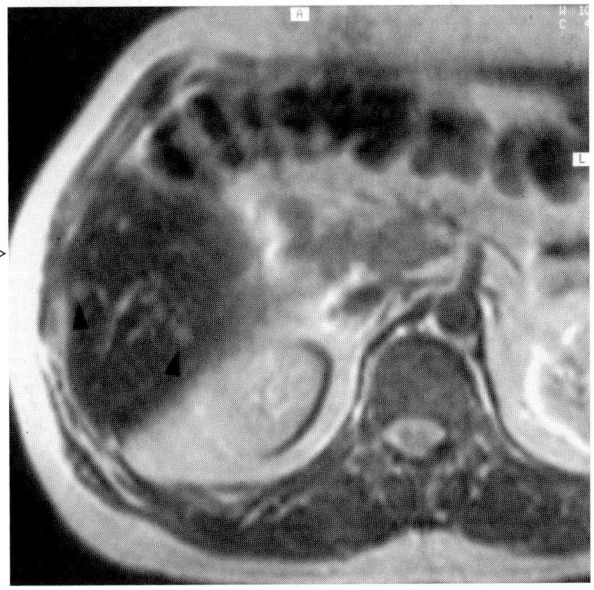

i

Fig. 14.9a–i. Metastases from colorectal carcinoma. **a–c** Cranio-caudal contrast enhanced CT scans show some subcentimeter slightly hypodense lesions (*arrowheads*) within the right liver lobe. **d–i** Same cranio-caudal transaxial MR slices: T2 weighted images with SE sequence before (**d–f**) and 30 min after (**g–i**) injection of reticulo-endothelial targeted CM (SPIO particles). The remarkable negative enhancement of the hepatic tissue, due to the uptake of CM, increases the difference of the signal intensity between the lesions and the hepatic tissue (elevated C/N), leading to a better visualization of the small metastases, more confidently detectable compared to the unenhanced images (low C/N)

requires a preliminary note of some anatomic features of the hepatic and metastatic tissues which influence the uptake as well as the elimination of the CM. The liver has a dual blood supply: blood enters the liver mainly through the portal vein (75%) and, in a lesser amount, through the hepatic artery (25%). At the level of the hepatic lobule the portal and arterial blood blends within the sinusoidal capillaries. The endothelial cells of these sinusoids are separated by pores 100–1000 nm in size, thus allowing the passage of huge molecules and/or small particles. Within the extracellular interstitial space (space of Disse), between the fenestrated sinusoids and the surface of the hepatocyte membrane, are located the reticuloendothelial cells (Kupffer cells) assigned to phagocytosis. The microvilli of the hepatocyte membrane expand the hepatocyte surface available for the passage of the substances coming from the extracellular interstitial space; the substances eliminated with the bile are directly carried into the biliary canaliculi. Conversely, the metastases receive almost exclusively arterial blood, mainly in the periphery of the lesion better perfused than the center.

By exploiting the different pharmacokinetics of the CM (specific tissular distribution and timing), two methods may be followed to increase the C/N operating on the parameter C: to achieve the selec-

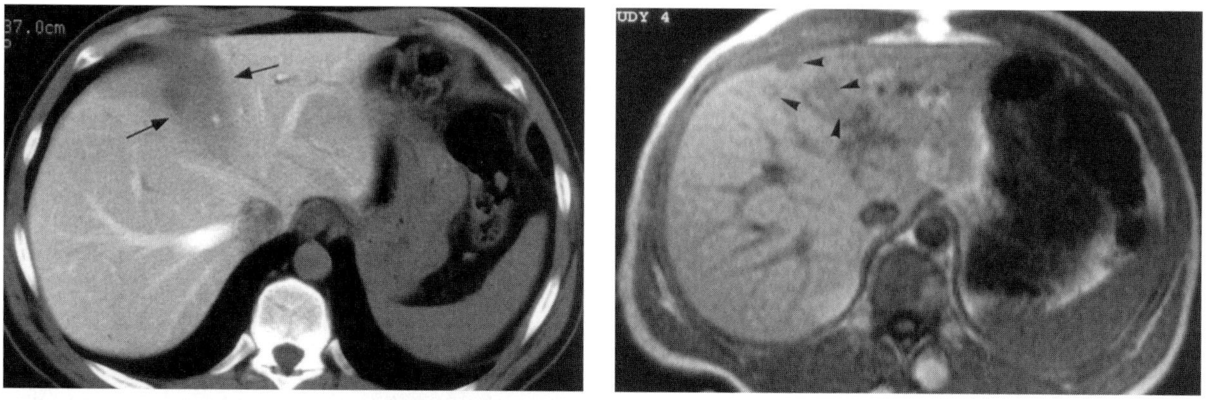

a b

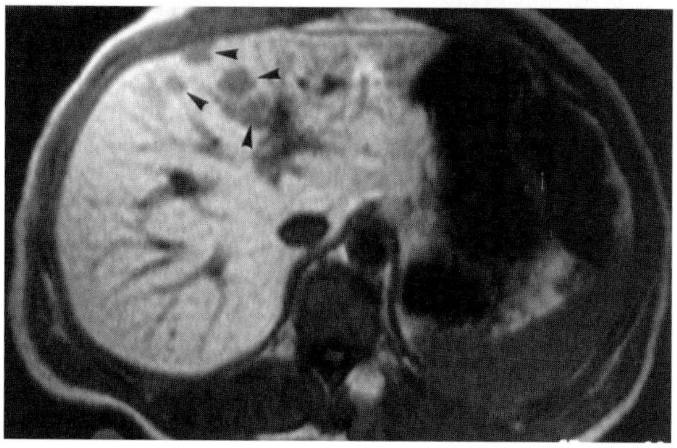

c

Fig. 14.10a–c. Metastases from colorectal carcinoma. **a** CT arterial portography scan shows a triangular area of reduced enhancement of the hepatic tissue at the level of the caudate lobe (*arrows*) consistent either with metastatic involvement or with perfusion defect. **b,c** T1 weighted images with GRE sequence before (**b**) and 60 min after (**c**) the injection of hepatocyte targeted CM (Mn-DPDP). The notable positive enhancement of the hepatic tissue due to the uptake of CM increases the difference of signal intensity between the lesions (*arrowheads*) and the hepatic tissue (elevated C/N) compared to the unenhanced images (low C/N), allowing confident detection of four metastatic lesions (courtesy of Neil Rofsky, MD, Department of Radiology. New York University Medical Center, USA)

tive enhancement of the hepatic tissue or that temporarily selective of the metastasis. In both cases the detection of the metastasis is improved.

14.3.2.2.3
Selective Enhancement of Hepatic Tissue

The selective enhancement of the hepatic tissue is due to the exclusive uptake of the CM by the Kupffer cells (SPIO) or by hepatocytes (Mn-DPDP, Gd-EOB-DTPA, Gd-BOPTA).

14.3.2.2.3.1
Negative Selective Enhancement

The rationale of negative selective enhancement is to eliminate the already low signal intensity of the hepatic tissue on T2 weighted images so that the usual elevated signal intensity of the metastasis becomes significantly different (increase in parameter C). The consequent increment in the C/N improves the detection of the metastases (Fig. 14.9). This result is obtained using the CM targeted to the reticuloendothelial system (SPIO particles), which after i.v. injection quickly cross (plasma half-life: 8 min) the sinusoidal pores passing into the space of Disse' where, owing to their size (60–80 nm), they are recognized and then phagocytosed by the Kupffer cells (80% of the injected dose) while 6%–10% is taken up by the spleen (Weissleder et al. 1989). On the contrary, since metastases do not contain Kupffer cells, the SPIO particles are not taken up by the metastatic tissue. The maximum negative enhancement of the hepatic tissue is obtained in less than 1 h and lasts more than 1 day. The normal signal intensity of the hepatic tissue is recovered in 7 days (Brash 1992). The best imaging window of the SPIO particles ranges between 30 min and 6 h after the injection (Gandon et al. 1991; Ros et al. 1995; Kopp et al. 1997).

14.3.2.2.3.2
Positive Selective Enhancement

The rationale of the positive selective enhancement is to increase the signal intensity of the hepatic tissue, already elevated on T1 weighted images, in order to expand the difference (increase in the parameter C) versus the habitual low signal intensity of the metastasis; the consequent increase in the C/N improves the detection of the metastases (Figs. 14.2, 14.10). This result is obtained using the hepatocyte targeted CMs (Mn-DPDP, Gd-EOB-DTPA, Gd-BOPTA), which accumulate only in the hepatic tissue, since the metastases do not contain hepatocytes.

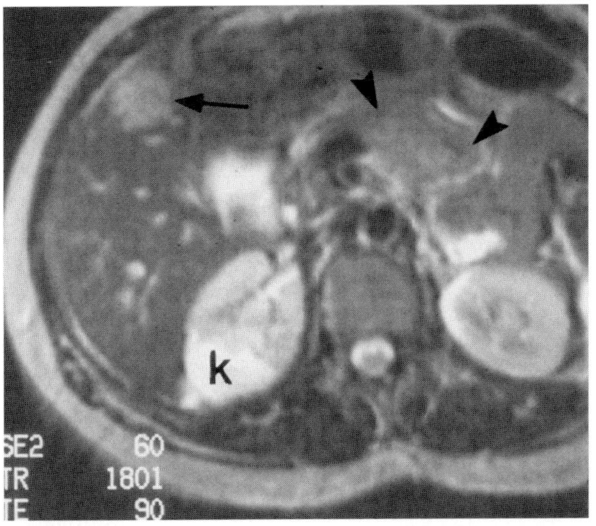

a

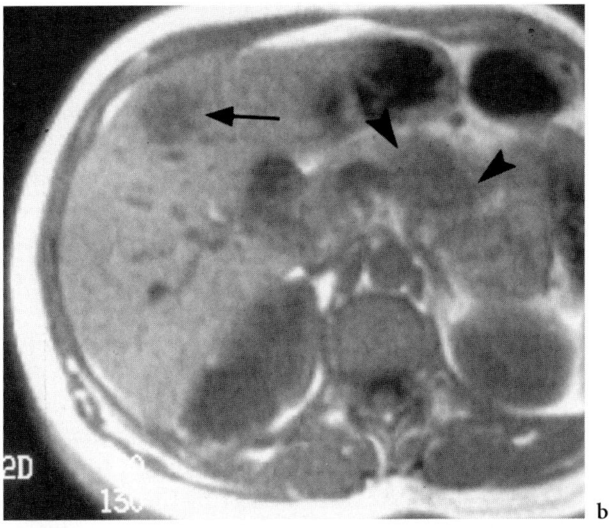

b

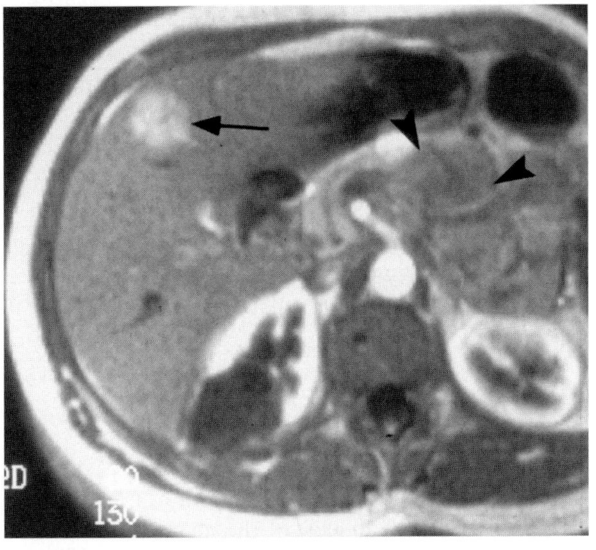

c

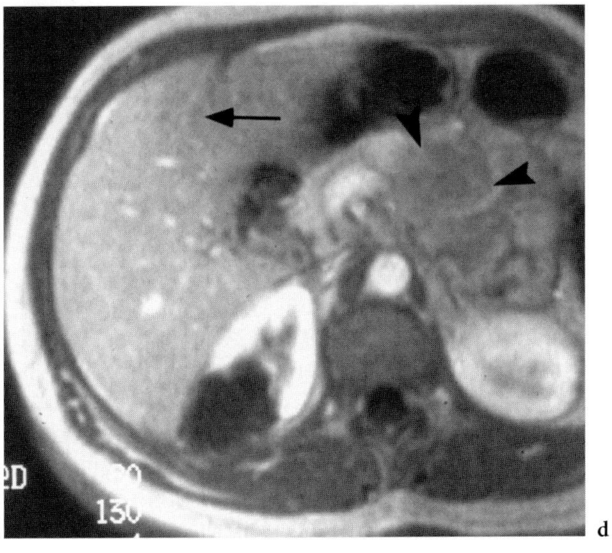

d

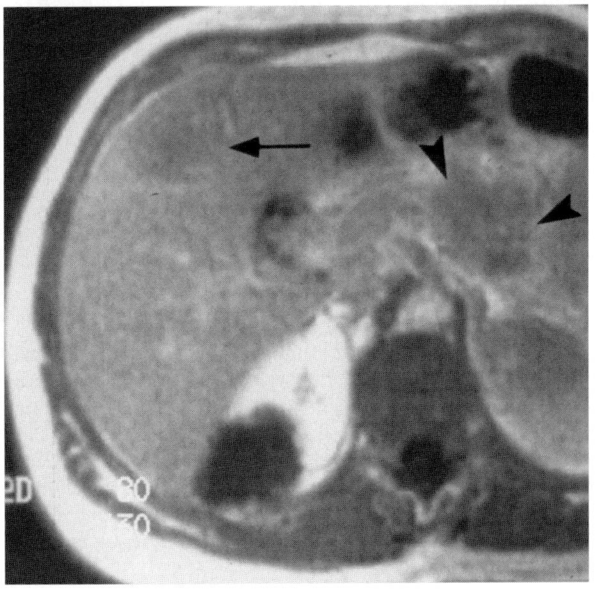
e

Fig. 14.11a–e. Hypervascular metastasis from non-functioning endocrine tumor of the pancreas. **a** On a T2 weighted image with SE sequence the metastasis (*arrow*) is homogeneously more intense than the hepatic tissue, with a signal intensity similar to that of the primary tumor (*arrowheads*) localized within the body of the pancreas. Renal cyst (**k**). **b–e** Dynamic study with GRE sequences (T1 weighted images) before (**b**) and after (**c–e**) bolus injection of Gd-DTPA. On unenhanced image (**b**) the lesion shows a lower signal intensity than the hepatic tissue, identical to that of the primary pancreatic tumor. During the arterial phase of vascular distribution of CM (**c**), the lesion shows a remarkable and homogeneous enhancement (positive contrast). During the portal phase of vascular distribution of CM (**d**) the lesion is not recognizable since the enhancement of the metastasis corresponds to that of the hepatic tissue. During the phase of the clearance of CM (**e**) from the extracellular interstitial space, the lesion shows a moderate reduction of the enhancement compared to the hepatic tissue which is due to the faster interstitial clearance of CM within the better perfused metastatic nodule

For the sake of simplicity a brief description of the two groups of CM is needed.

The chemical similarity of the Mn-DPDP with B_6 vitamin has been indicated as the reason of the hepatocellular uptake of this CM (Brash 1992). After the administration in healthy volunteers, the peak liver enhancement occurs between 15 min and 30 min after the i.v. injection, persisting up to 6 h with a wide imaging window (Lim et al. 1991; Hamm et al. 1992; Reimer et al. 1996; Wang et al. 1998).

Gd-EOB-DTPA and Gd-BOPTA are two gadolinium chelate positive CMs which seem to use the same transport system (organic anion) involved in the hepatocellular uptake of bilirubin (Schumann-Gianpieri 1993). Both CMs present the following two characteristics: the first regards the modality of administration, since the i.v. injection as a bolus of these CMs allows the dynamic study to be performed like conventional CMs, giving positive enhancement (Gd-DTPA, Gd-DOTA) considered in the following section; the second is related to the hepatocellular uptake followed by the biliary excretion of the CM: the peak liver enhancement occurs around 60 min after i.v. injection for both the CMs (Vogl et al. 1992; Hamm et al. 1995; Caudana et al. 1996).

14.3.2.2.4
Selective Enhancement of Metastases

The selective enhancement of the metastasis is obtained with conventional positive CMs (Gd-DTPA, Gd-DOTA), which have the same pharmacokinetics of the water soluble iodinated contrast agents used in conventional radiology and CT (Brasch 1992). After 20–30 s from i.v. injection, the CM reaches the liver through the hepatic artery, where it mainly distributes to the metastasis; meantime the CM immediately passes into the extracellular interstitium, where it accumulates before the elimination through the blood stream. The positive enhancement of the metastasis is temporarily selective since it is limited to the arterial distribution of the CM. In fact, the metastatic tissue receives the CM not diluted by the portal blood (which does not perfuse the metastasis) while, in the same phase, the normal liver tissue receives the CM greatly diluted by the predominant unenhanced portal blood.

After 40–60 s from i.v. injection the venous spleno-mesenteric returning blood stream, which contains the CM, enters the liver through the portal vein and distributes exclusively into the hepatic tissue (where the portal perfusion prevails) but not into the metastasis, which is devoid of portal vasculature.

The mentioned features of the perfusion of the metastatic and hepatic tissues have some implications regards imaging which can be evaluated by the dynamic study. This study – performed with the injection of a compact bolus of gadolinium chelate CM followed by the rapid acquisition of breath hold sets of T1 weighted images – allows the separation of the phases of arterial and portal vascular distribution respectively from those of interstitial accumulation and clearance of the CM. These images facilitate the detection (Larson et al. 1994; Hamm et al. 1997) and the characterization of the metastases (Mirowitz et al. 1991; Hamm et al. 1994; Mafhouz et al. 1996), the latter considered in Sect. 14.4.

In the following sections, a brief description of the dynamic perfusional study (represented by three phases of vasculo-tissular distribution of the CM) is given.

14.3.2.2.4.1
Phase of Vascular Distribution

During the phase of vascular distribution of the CM, the rate of the selective enhancement of the metastasis depends on the degree of the arterial blood supply of the neoplastic tissue, due to the lack of portal venous blood flow (Figs. 14.1, 14.4, 14.11, 14.12, 14.13). Conversely, the following portal enhancement exclusively affects the hepatic tissue (Fig. 14.12); in this phase the potential persistent arterial enhancement of the metastatic tissue may show the same degree as that of the liver, consequently making the detection of the lesion impossible (Fig. 14.11).

Fig. 14.12a–f. Hypovascular metastasis from colorectal carcinoma. **a,b** SE sequence. On T2 weighted image (**a**) the metastasis (*arrow*) is weakly hyperintense compared to the hepatic tissue (low C/N).On PD image (**b**) the metastasis is slightly hypointense compared to the hepatic tissue, being therefore detectable with difficulty. **c–f** Dynamic study with GRE sequence (sagittal T1 weighted images) before (**c**) and after (**d,f**) bolus injection of Gd-DTPA. On unenhanced image (**c**) the lesion is highly hypointense compared to the hepatic tissue (elevated C/N). During the arterial (**d**), portal (**e**) phases of vascular distribution and of pooling of CM (**f**) into the extracellular interstitial space the lesion does not show any enhancement compared to the hepatic tissue (negative contrast) owing to its insufficient perfusion. During the portal phase (**e**) the highest enhancement of the hepatic tissue compared to that of the other phases leads to the more significant difference in signal intensity between the lesion and the healthy tissue (maximum C/N)

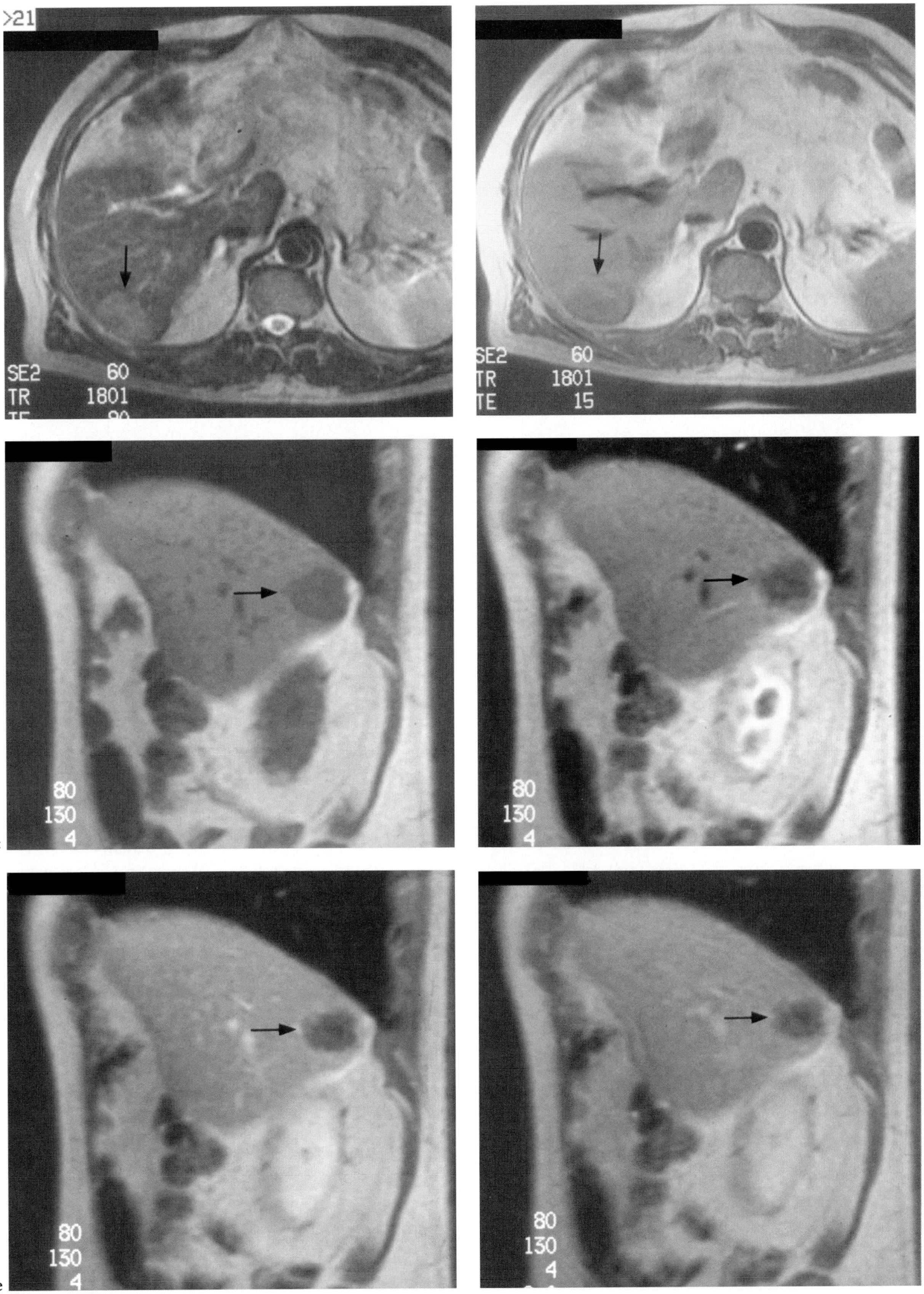
>21
SE2 60
TR 1801
SE2 60
TR 1801
TE 15
80
130
4
80
130
4
80
130
4
80
130
4

a b c d e f

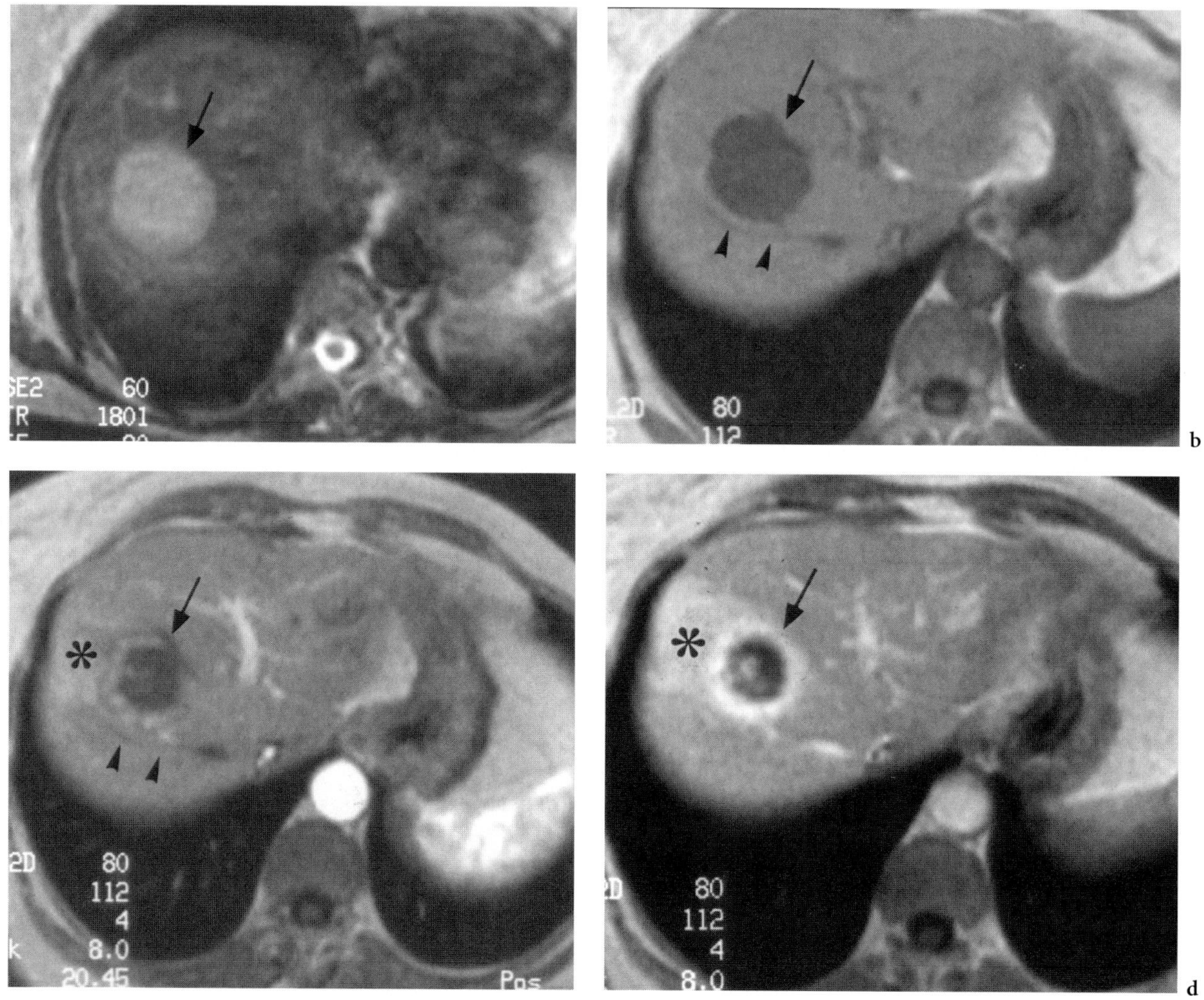

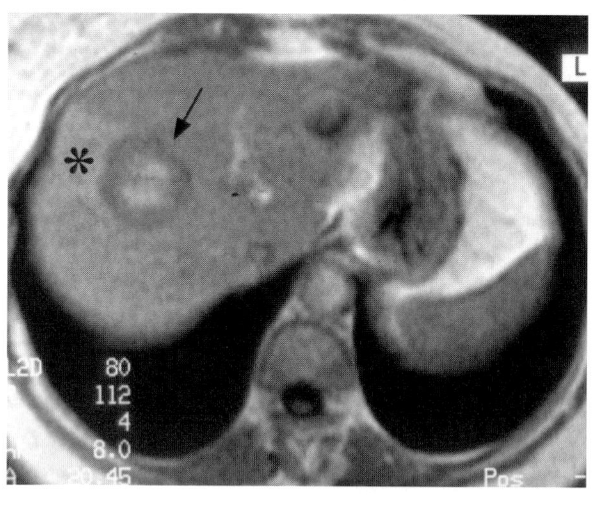

Fig. 14.13a–e. Infected metastasis from colorectal carcinoma. On a T2 weighted image with SE sequence (**a**) the metastasis (*arrow*) is homogeneously more intense than the hepatic tissue. **b–e** Dynamic study with GRE sequence (T1 weighted images) before (**b**) and after (**c–e**) bolus injection of Gd-DTPA. On an unenhanced image (**b**) the metastasis shows a signal intensity notably lower than that of the hepatic tissue; the hepatic vein (*arrowheads*) is slightly displaced. During the arterial (**c**) and portal (**d**) phases of vascular distribution of CM, peripheral ring enhancement due to the better perfusion compared to the central zone of the lesion. During the phase of pooling of CM (**e**) into the extracellular interstitial space, central enhancement of the lesion due to the slow interstitial accumulation of CM; peripheral wash-out due to the faster clearance of CM from the extracellular interstitial space. The ill defined enhancement (*asterisk*) of the perilesional hepatic tissue indicates inflammation due to the infection of the metastasis

14.3.2.2.4.2
Pooling into Extracellular Interstitial Space

The following phase is characterized by the progressive pooling into the extracellular interstitial space of the CM (whatever the arterial or portal afferent supply) up to reaching an interstitial concentration of CM balanced with the intravascular one (2 min).

Within the metastasis the extracellular interstitial pooling of the CM is relatively slower than in the hepatic tissue (Figs. 14.1, 14.4, 14.12, 14.13), therefore favoring not only the detection of the lesion but also its characterization as explained in Sect. 14.4.

14.3.2.2.4.3
Clearance of Extracellular Interstitial Space
In the following phases (5–10 min after i.v. injection) a gradual clearance of the extracellular interstitial space takes place, owing to the return of the CM from the interstitial space into the venous blood stream for its renal excretion; only a minimal amount of the injected CM (1%–2%) is excreted at a late stage by the hepatocytes into the biliary tree. Also in this phase of the dynamic perfusional study, the metastases may show an extracellular interstitial clearance relatively slower than that of the hepatic tissue (Figs. 14.1, 14.11, 14.13), as explained in Sect. 14.4.

From the practical point of view, the stronger enhancement of the metastases during the arterial phase facilitates the detection of the hypervascular ones (Fig. 14.11), while the stronger enhancement of the hepatic tissue during the portal phase would favor the detection of the hypovascular one (Fig. 14.12). On the other hand, either during the arterial and portal vascular phases or in the following interstitial accumulation and clearance, the dynamic patterns of the enhancement become delineated which allow the characterization described in the following paragraph.

14.4 Guidelines for Characterization of Metastases

The evaluation of the dynamic patterns of the enhancement allows the characterization of different types of metastases (hypovascular, hypervascular, infected) as well as the differential diagnosis with benign lesions (cyst, hemangioma, focal nodular hyperplasia), which on unenhanced images may have a signal intensity behavior similar to that of the metastases.

14.4.1 Hypovascular Metastases

These metastases receive a reduced arterial blood supply in comparison to that of the hepatic tissue. Therefore, during the arterial and portal phases of vascular distribution of the CM, the enhancement of the liver is stronger than that of the lesion since the latter receives less arterial blood in comparison to the normal tissue and it does not receive any portal blood. Therefore, the signal enhancement predominates in the hepatic tissue during all the phases of the dynamic perfusional study and the lesion shows negative contrast (Fig. 14.12).

14.4.2 Hypervascular Metastases

During the arterial phase some of these metastases, especially when small sized, show a homogeneous enhancement stronger than that of the hepatic tissue due to uniform perfusion of the tumoral nodule (Ackerman 1974; Lin et al. 1984; Kan et al. 1993). In this phase the lesion shows positive contrast (Fig. 14.11) since the enhancement predominates within the metastatic tissue.

However, the large hypervascular metastases receive arterial blood mainly in the periphery of the lesion than in the worse perfused center. Thus, during the arterial phase of distribution of the CM (Figs. 14.1, 14.13), these metastases show an intense peripheral ring of enhancement (Semelka et al. 1993a; Withney et al. 1993; Larson et al. 1994). In the following phases the enhancement of the periphery and the center of the larger metastases shows the opposite behavior (Larson et al. 1994; Mafhouz et al. 1994). Into the center of the lesion, where either the extracellular interstitial pooling or the clearance of CM is reduced owing to the impaired perfusion of these areas, the CM accumulates (delayed central pooling) with an enhancement which gradually superates that of the hepatic tissue (Figs. 14.1, 14.13). Conversely, at the better perfused periphery of the metastasis, the pooling of CM into the extracellular interstitial space and its clearance are faster than those of both the center of the lesion and the normal perilesional tissue. This behavior, defined peripheral wash-out, appears as a hypointense halo (Figs. 14.1, 14.13) since the enhancement prevails within the central zone of the metastasis and within the perilesional hepatic tissue.

14.4.3 Infected Metastases

These lesions show the typical pattern of hypervascular large metastases (ring enhancement during the vascular phases; central pooling with peripheral wash-out of CM during the following

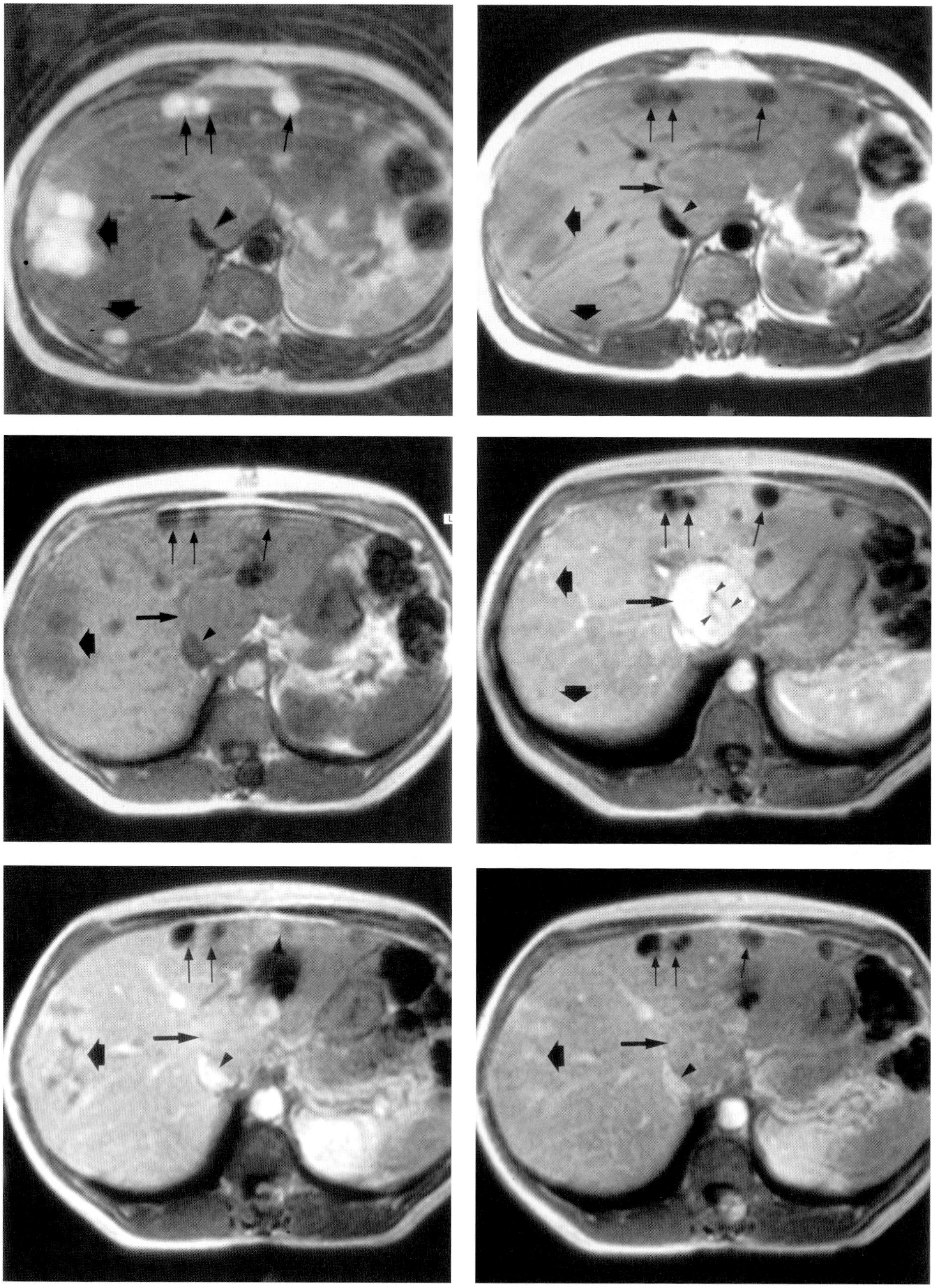

a b c d e f

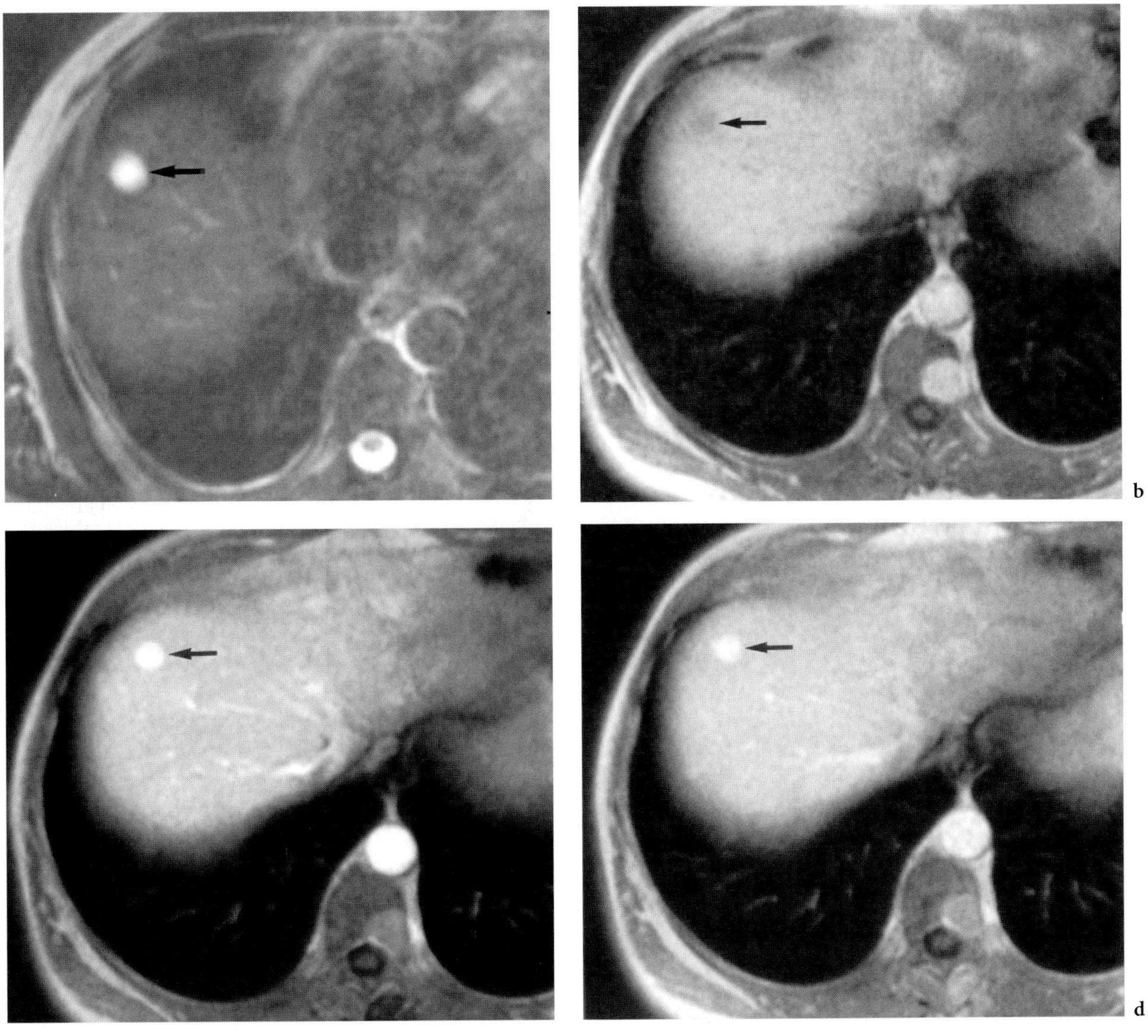

a b c d

Fig. 14.15a–d. Hemangioma. On T2 weighted image **(a)** the lesion (*arrow*) shows sharp borders and hyperintensity analogous to that of the CSF around the spinal cord. On a T1 weighted image **(b)** the signal intensity is lower than that of the hepatic tissue but higher than that of the CSF, owing to the content of blood. **c,d** Dynamic study with GRE sequence (T1 weighted images) after bolus injection of Gd-DTPA. During the arterial phase of vascular distribution of CM **(c)** as well as during the pooling of CM **(d)** into the extracellular interstitial space, intense, homogeneous and prolonged enhancement of the small hemangioma is seen compared to the hepatic tissue (positive contrast)

◁ **Fig. 14.14a–f.** Multiple benign lesions (cysts, hemangiomas, focal nodular hyperplasia). **a,b** T2 and T1 weighted images with SE sequence. **c–f** Dynamic study with GRE sequence (T1 weighted images) before **(c)** and after **(d–f)** bolus injection of Gd-DTPA. The cysts (*small arrows*) show sharp borders and signal intensity behaving identically to the CSF around the spinal cord, with strong hyperintensity on T2 weighted image **(a)** and hypointensity on T1 weighted images **(b,c)**. During the arterial **(d)**, portal **(e)** and interstitial **(f)** phases of distribution of CM no enhancement of the cysts is seen (negative contrast). On T1 weighted images **(b,c)** the hemangiomas (*large arrows*) show a signal intensity higher than that of the cysts due to the content of blood. During the arterial **(d)**, portal **(e)** and interstitial **(f)** phases of distribution of CM progressive enhancement of hemangiomas from the periphery to the center; the peripheral ring of enhancement, due to the arterial perfusion of the lesion, shows a nodular pattern. On unenhanced images **(a–c)**, focal nodular hyperplasia (*arrow*) shows an isointense signal compared to the hepatic tissue; mild compression of inferior vena cava (*arrowhead*). During the arterial phase of distribution of CM **(d)** strong enhancement of the lesion (positive contrast) due to its arterial perfusion; hypointense central scar (*small arrowheads*). During portal **(e)** and interstitial **(f)** phases of distribution of the CM, the lesion is not detectable owing to its enhancement identical to that of the hepatic tissue phases), with an additional ill defined perilesional enhancement (Fig. 14.13d,e), which is due to the inflammatory hyperemia of the surrounding hepatic tissue (Semelka and Kelekis 1997). The differential diagnosis has to be done with liver abscess, which shows a central area of elevated signal intensity on T2 weighted images due to the suppurative colliquation, devoid of enhancement during the dynamic perfusional study.

14.4.4 Benign Lesions

The importance of the characterization of these lesions cannot be ignored considering that they may coexist together with metastases with an incidence ranging between 15.5% and 63.9% (Karhunen 1986; Jones et al. 1992; Bruneton et al. 1998). Also in these cases the evaluation of the dynamic patterns of enhancement allows the differential diagnosis.

14.4.4.1 Cysts

The cysts with a homogeneous fluid content show an elevated signal intensity on T2 weighted images (Figs. 14.5, 14.14), behaving like the metastases (Fig. 14.4) with colliquative necrosis (Wittenberg et al. 1988). The differential diagnosis is achieved on the dynamic study (Semelka and Mitchell 1996; Semelka and Kelekis 1997): in all the phases the cysts do not show any enhancement versus the hepatic tissue constantly appearing sharply delineated, with negative contrast (Figs. 14.5, 14.14); the necrotic metastases conversely show a peripheral enhancement where the neoplastic tissue is viable (Fig. 14.4).

14.4.4.2 Hemangioma

Also hemangiomas, like metastases, receive their blood supply exclusively from the hepatic artery. Therefore, during the arterial phase, the small hemangiomas may show a homogeneous enhancement (Fig. 14.15) higher than that of the hepatic tissue (positive contrast), due to the fast pooling of the CM within the lesion, as hypervascular small metastases (Larson et al. 1994; Mitchell et al. 1994; Katsuyoshi et al. 1996; Semelka and Mitchell 1996). In these small hemangiomas the differential diagnosis is based on the persistence of the homogeneous enhancement, more prolonged (Fig. 14.15) than that of the small hypervascular metastases, which usually does not exceed the minute (Fig. 14.11).

Nevertheless, the majority of hemangiomas, medium or large sized, typically show the gradual fill-in from the periphery to the center of the lesion. As stated before also in these cases the differential diagnosis with the metastases of similar size is based on the dynamic patterns of the enhancement (Hamm et al. 1990; van Beers et al. 1990). In fact, during the arterial-portal vascular phases the intense ring of peripheral enhancement has a nodular aspect which is typical of the hemangioma (Fig. 14.14), while that of the metastasis has a regular thickness (Figs. 14.1, 14.13). Successively, the peripheral wash-out with central pooling of the CM (recognizable during the interstitial pooling and clearance of the CM) is typical of the metastases (Figs. 14.1f, 14.13d), while the hemangioma, during the same phases, shows a more homogeneous enhancement (Fig. 14.14).

14.4.4.3 Focal Nodular Hyperplasia

Finally, also focal nodular hyperplasia (FNH) receives blood supply exclusively from the hepatic artery, showing an intense and homogeneous enhancement (positive contrast) during the arterial phase (Fig. 14.14) like the hypervascular small metastases (Fig. 14.11). Nevertheless, the homogeneous enhancement of the FNH does not exceed the arterial phase (Katsuyoshi 1996) unlike the hypervascular metastasis, which may show prolonged enhancement in the following phases. During the portal phase as well as in the following phases of interstitial pooling and clearance of CM, the behavior of the enhancement of the FNH is identical to that of the hepatic tissue from which the lesion cannot therefore be differentiated (Fig. 14.14). The presence of the central scar (Fig. 14.14) facilitates the differential diagnosis versus the metastasis.

14.5 Resectability of Metastases

At present, the resection of liver metastases represents a unique potentially curative therapy, the alternative treatments (systemic chemotherapy or in hepatic arterial infusion; selective chemoembolization; cryosurgery; termoablation and laser photocoagulation) being exclusively palliative.

14.5.1 Rationale for Resection of Metastases

The therapeutic approach to the hepatic metastases must consider if these lesions were detected at the same time of the primary tumor (synchronous metastases) or, on the other hand, successively (metachronous metastases).

14.5.1.1 Synchronous Metastases

With regard to synchronous metastases, the choice of therapy (surgical excision, alternative treatment) needs to consider some features of the primary tumor (intra- or extraabdominal location, grade of biological aggressiveness, grade of locoregional spread) as well as of the metastases (surgical resectability, grade of response to the alternative treatments, impairment of liver functions).

14.5.1.1.1 Intra- or Extraabdominal Location of the Primary Tumor

The intra- or extraabdominal location of the primary tumor may influence the choice between two possible options (surgical excision, alternative treatment), since the metastasectomy may increase the morbidity and mortality of the surgical treatment, prolonging the operation and increasing the invasiveness: for instance, thoracotomy for the excision of the primary lung cancer and laparotomy for the resection of liver secondaries.

14.5.1.1.2 Grade of Biological Aggressiveness of the Primary Tumor

The grade of biological aggressiveness of the primary tumor affects the choice of therapeutic option (surgical or alternative treatment of the liver metastases), since the surgical approach to metastases is not justified in those tumors which rapidly diffuse locoregionally, giving distant metastases (lung small cell carcinoma, breast cancer, adenocarcinomas of the esophagus, stomach and pancreas).

14.5.1.1.3 Advanced Locoregional Spread of the Primary Tumor

In those cases of advanced locoregional spread of the primary tumor, the surgical option may be still rational for those oncotypes (carcinoid tumor, melanoma) showing a positive prognosis (higher survival rate) after surgical cytoreduction; conversely, the surgical treatment may not be justified for those tumors (colorectal carcinoma) showing an ineffective response to metastasectomy.

14.5.1.1.4 Surgical Resection of Hepatic Metastases

The surgical resection of the hepatic metastases is not achievable when both the liver lobes are involved in more than four focal lesions as well as when the central hepatic vessels (hepatic veins, inferior vena cava, portal vein) are infiltrated or extrahepatic spread from primary tumor is present, either abdominally (peritoneal and/or lymph nodes metastases) or extraabdominally (Sugarbaker 1990; Baker and Pelley 1995).

14.5.1.1.5 Sensitivity to Alternative Treatments

The sensitivity to alternative treatments depends on the biological behavior, the latter related to the oncotype of the primary tumor. In some instances (colorectal carcinoma), the effectiveness of the alternative treatments is very poor; thus metastasectomy, if practicable, is the only therapeutic option. Conversely, in other oncotypes (breast cancer; endocrine tumors of the pancreas), the choice of alternative treatment instead of the surgical one is justified.

14.5.1.1.6 Impairment of Hepatic Function

Serious impairment of the hepatic function, due to the metastatic involvement of the liver, indicated either by the symptomatology (weight loss, jaundice, hepatomegaly, ascites) or by the alteration of the laboratory indices (bilirubin, alkaline phosphatase, lactate acid dehydrogenase, serum albumin), narrows the indications – up to eliminating them completely – of both therapeutic options (surgical or alternative treatment).

14.5.1.2 Metachronous Metastases

With regard to the metachronous metastases, the rationality of their surgical excision follows the same criteria as those just described, when the primary tumor has not been treated with surgery, radiation therapy or chemotherapy. On the other hand, when the primary tumor has been treated (surgical excision, local sterilization with radiotherapy and/or chemotherapy), the criteria expressed in Sects. 14.5.1.1.1 (location of the primary tumor) and 14.5.1.1.3 (locoregional spread of the primary tumor) should not be considered.

14.5.2 MR Evaluation of Surgical Resectability of Metastases

This section considers the contribution of MR to the assessment of surgical resectability (definition of the number of metastases, identification of the involvement of the central hepatic vessels) in the light of the lower reliability of this modality versus US and CT in the detection of extrahepatic abdominal and extraabdominal spread.

14.5.2.1 Number of Metastases

According to comparative evaluation series (Stark et al. 1987; Fretz et al. 1990; Vassiliades et al. 1991; Wernecke et al. 1991; Rummeny et al. 1992; Hagspiel et al. 1995; Seneterre et al. 1996; Zerhouni et al. 1996; Strotzer et al. 1997), MR reliability in the detection of the real number of metastases is higher than that of US and CT, both in terms of sensitivity (44%–78% for MR versus 39%–53% for US and 41%–71% for CT) and in terms of accuracy (91%–97% for MR versus 88%–89% for CT). In spite of these results, CT is still indicated as an approach to the third diagnostic step since this modality is more easily available across institutions than MR; moreover, CT is highly reliable – as MR – in the assessment of the involvement of the central hepatic vascular structures, and superior in the detection of abdominal extrahepatic as well as extraabdominal spread of metastatic disease (Baker and Pelley 1995; Mahfouz et al. 1996). In a prospective study, Steele et al. (1991) evaluated the accuracy of CT in the selection of patients for surgical resection of hepatic metastases of colorectal carcinoma: in only 7% of cases did CT fail to demonstrate the metastases successively found on laparotomy, but in 33% of cases it caused underestimation of the number of lesions detected. This means that at least in 40% of the cases would the evaluation with a more sensitive and accurate imaging modality been able to reduce the quota of CT errors.

Considering the more sensitive imaging modalities, CT arterial portography (CTAP) should be mentioned first. On comparative series (Soyer et al. 1993; Strotzer et al. 1997), CTAP shows a sensitivity (94%–96%) higher than that of MR (64%–78%) but with invasiveness and numerous false-positive diagnoses of metastases. Consequently, MR with hepatocyte and reticuloendothelial targeted CM, owing to the lack of invasiveness and the elevated sensitivity (56%–96%) in the detection of metastases (Fretz et al. 1990; Hagspiel et al. 1995; Caudana et al. 1996; Strotzer et al. 1997), might replace CTAP in the assessment of resectable metastases. However, this hypothesis has to wait for the conclusion of the ongoing trials, testing the efficacy and the tolerance of the liver specific CM. Finally, intraoperative US (IOUS) shows a higher sensitivity (80%–96%) than that of noninvasive modalities (CT, MR) but inferior to that of CTAP (Machi et al.1991; Soyer et al.1992; Hagspiel et al. 1995).

14.5.2.2 Involvement of Hepatic Vessels

The reliability of MR in the detection of the involvement of the central hepatic vessels is very high thanks to the easy demonstration of the intra- and extrahepatic vascular network (flow-void phenomenon: lack of the signal in the lumen of the patent vascular channels). This allows the demonstration of the hepatic veins, inferior vena cava, main portal vein as well as their relationship with the lesions (Figs. 14.13, 14.14), even on unenhanced images. Therefore, the demonstration of the involvement of one of these vessels is accurately achieved on T1 and T2 weighted images (Fig. 14.3), contraindicating surgical excision. However, CT is reliable not only for the evaluation of the involvement of the vascular structures (Fig. 14.3) but also for the detection of peritoneal and/or abdominal lymph-node metastases, whereas MR is less accurate (Baker and Pelley 1995; Mafhouz et al. 1996).

References

Ackermann (1974) The blood supply of experimental liver metastases. IV. Changes in vascularity with increasing tumor growth. Surgery 75:589–596

Arrive' L, Lewin M, Wendum D, et al (1996) Lésions hépatiques hyperintenses sur les séquences d'IRM pondérées en T1. Feuillets de Radiologie 36:205–212

Baker ME, Pelley R (1995) Hepatic metastases: basic principles and implications for radiologists. Radiology 197:329–337

Brasch RC (1992) New directions in the development of MR imaging contrast media. Radiology 183:1–11

Bruneton JN, Raffaelli CH, Maestro C, et al (1998) Pathologie tumorale du foie chez le patient porteur d'un cancer. Feuillets de Radiologie 38:91–96

Butler J, Attiyen FF, Daly JM (1986) Hepatic resection for metastases of the colon and rectum. Surg Gynecol Obstet 162:109–113

Caudana R, Morana G, Pirovano G, et al (1996) Focal malignant hepatic lesions: MR imaging enhanced with gadolinium benzyolxipropionictetra-acetate (BOPTA). Preliminary results of phase II clinical application. Radiology 199:513–520

Crooks LE (1991) Some consideration for MR imaging of the liver. Radiology 180:615–616

Fegiz G, Ramacciato G, Gennari L, et al (1991) Hepatic resection for colorectal metastases: the Italian multicenter experience. J Surg Oncol 2(S):144–154

Ferrucci JT (1994) Liver tumor imaging. Current concepts. Radiol Clin North Am 32:39–54

Ferrucci Jt, Stark DD (1990) Liver Imaging. Current trends and new technique. Andover Medical Publisher Inc.

Foley WD, Kneeland JB, Cates JD, et al (1987) Contrast optimization for the detection of focal hepatic lesions by MR imaging at 1.5 T. AJR 149:1155–1160

Fretz CJ, Stark DD, Metz CE, et al (1990) Detection of hepatic metastases: comparison of contrast-enhanced CT, unenhanced MR imaging, and iron-oxide enhanced MR imaging. AJR 155:763–770

Gandon Y, Heautot JF, Brunet F, et al (1991) Superparamagnetic iron oxide: clinical time response study. Eur J Radiol 12:195–200

Greenway B (1988) Hepatic metastases from colorectal cancer: resection or not? Br J Surg 75:513–519

Grellet J, Bellin MF, Dion E, et al (1993) Techniques d'IRM appliquées au diagnostic des tumeurs hepatiques. J Radiol 74:67–76

Hagspiel KD, Neidl KFW, Eichenberger AC, et al (1995) Detection of liver metastases: comparison of superparamagnetic iron-oxide enhanced and unenhanced MR imaging at 1.5 T with dynamic CT, intra-operative US, and percutaneous US. Radiology 196:471–478

Hamm B, Fischer E, Taupitz M (1990) Differentiation of hepatic hemangiomas from metastases by dynamically contrast enhanced MR Imaging. J Comput Assist Tomogr 14:205–216

Hamm B, Vogl TJ, Branding GM, et al (1992) Focal liver lesions: MR imaging with Mn-DPDP. Initial clinical results in 40 Patients. Radiology 182:167–174

Hamm B, Thoeni RFL, Gould RG, et al (1994) Focal liver lesions: characterization with unenhanced and dynamic contrast enhanced MR Imaging. Radiology 190:417–423

Hamm B, Starks T, Muhler A, et al (1995) Phase I clinical evaluation of Gd-EOB-DTPA as a hepatobiliary MR contrast agent: safety, pharmacokinetics, and MR imaging. Radiology 195:785–792

Hamm B, Mahfouz AE, Taupitz M, et al (1997) Liver metastases: improved detection with dynamic gadolinium-enhanced MR imaging? Radiology 202:677–682

Hendrick RE (1988) Contrast and noise. In: Stark DD, Bradley WG (eds) Magnetic Resonance Imaging. The C.V. Mosby Company, St Louis, pp 66–83

Holm A, Bradley E, Aldrete J (1989) Hepatic resection of metastases from colorectal carcinoma: morbidity, mortality, and pattern recurrence. Ann Surg 209:428–434

Hughes KS, Rosenstein RB, Songhorabody F, et al (1988) Resection of the liver for colorectal carcinoma metastases: a multi-institutional study of indications for resection. Dis Colon Rectum 31:1–4

Ichikawa T, Haradome H, Hachiya J, et al (1998) Diffusion-weighted MR Imaging with a single shot echoplanar sequence: detection and characterization of focal hepatic lesions. AJR 170:397–402

Jones EC, Chezmar JR, Nelson RC, et al (1992) The frequency and significance of small (<15 mm) hepatic lesions detected by CT. AJR 158:535–539

Jung G, Krahe T, Kugel H, et al (1997) Prospective comparison of fast SE and GRASE sequences and Echo Planar imaging with conventional SE sequences in the detection of focal liver lesions at 1.0 T. J Comput Assist Tomogr 21:341–347

Kan Z, Ivancev K, Lunderquist A, et al (1993) In vivo microscopy of hepatic tumors in animal models: a dynamic investigation of blood supply to hepatic metastases. Radiology 187:621–626

Karhunen PJ (1986) Benign hepatic tumors and tumor-like conditions in men. J Clin Pathol 39:183–188

Katsuyoshi I, Kazumitsu H, Takeshi F, et al (1996) Liver neoplasms. Diagnostic pitfalls in cross-sectional imaging. RadioGraphics 16:273–293

Kopp AF, Laniado M, Dammann F (1997) MR Imaging of the liver with Resovist: safety, efficacy, and pharmacodynamic properties. Radiology 204:749–756

Larson RE, Semelka RC, Bagley AS, et al (1994) Hypervascular malignant liver lesions: comparison of various MR imaging pulse sequences and dynamic CT. Radiology 192:393–399

Lauffer RB (1996) MRI contrast agents: basic principles. In: Edelmann RR, Zlatkin MB, Hesselink JR (eds) Clinical Magnetic Resonance Imaging, 2nd ed., vol 1, W.B. Saunders, Philadelphia, pp 177–191

Lim KO, Stark DD, Leese PT, et al (1991) Hepatobiliary MR imaging: first human experience with Mn-DPDP. Radiology 178:79–82

Lin G, Lunderquist A, Hagerstrandt I, et al(1984) Postmortem examination of the blood supply and vascular pattern of small liver metastases in man. Surgery 96:517–526

Low RN, Francis IR, Sigeti JS, et al (1993) Abdominal MR imaging: comparison of T2-weighted fast and conventional Spin-Echo, and contrast-enhanced fast multiplanar spoiled gradient-recalled Imaging. Radiology 186:803–811

Machi J, Isomoto H, Kurohiji T, et al (1991) Accuracy of intraoperative ultrasound in diagnosing liver metastases from colorectal cancer: evaluation with post-operative follow-up results. World J Surg 15:551–557

Mahfouz AE, Hamm B, Wolf KJ (1994) Peripheral wash-out: a sign of malignancy on dynamic gadolinium enhanced MR images of focal liver lesions. Radiology 190: 49–52

Mahfouz AE, Hamm B, Mathieu D (1996) Imaging of metastases to the liver. Eur Radiol 6:607–614

Mirowitz SA, Lee JKT, Gutierrez E, et al (1991) Dynamic Gadolinium-enhanced rapid acquisition spin-echo MR imaging of the liver. Radiology 179:371–376

Mitchell DG (1994) Focal hepatic lesions: the continuing search for the optimal MR imaging pulse sequences. Radiology 193:17–18

Mitchell DG, Saini S, Weinreb J, et al (1994) Hepatic metastases and cavernous hemangiomas: distinction with standard- and triple-dose gadoteridol-enhanced MR imaging. Radiology 193:49–57

Nakamura S, Yokoi Y, Suzuki S, et al (1992) Results of extensive surgery for liver metastases in colorectal carcinoma. Br J Surg 79:35–38

Outwater EK, Tomaszewski E, Daly JM, et al (1991) Hepatic colorectal metastases: correlation of MR imaging and pathologic appearance. Radiology 180:327–332

Outwater EK, Mitchell DG, Vinitski S (1994) Abdominal MR imaging: evaluation of a fast spin echo sequence. Radiology 190:425–429

Reimer P, Rummeny EJ, Shamsi K, et al (1996) Phase II clinical evaluation of Gd-EOB-DTPA: dose, safety, aspects, and pulse sequence. Radiology 199:177–183

Reinig JW, Dwyer AJ, Miller DL, et al (1989) Liver metastases: detection with MR Imaging at 0.5 and 1.5 T. Radiology 170:149–153

Ros PR, Freeny PC, Harms SE, et al (1995) Hepatic MR imaging with ferumoxide: a multicentric clinical trial of the safety and efficacy in the detection of focal hepatic lesions. Radiology 196:481–488

Rummeny EJ, Wernecke K, Saini S, et al (1992) Comparison between high field strenght MR imaging and CT for screening of hepatic metastases: a receiver operating characteristic analysis. Radiology 182:879–886

Rydberg JN, Lomas DJ, Coakley KJ, et al (1995) Comparison of breath-hold fast spin-echo pulse sequences for T2-weighted MR imaging of liver lesions. Radiology 194:431–437

Saini S (1992) Contrast-enhanced MR imaging of the liver. Radiology 182:12–14

Saini S, Nelson RC (1995) Technique for MR imaging of the liver. Radiology 197:575–577

Saini S, Reimer P, Hahn PF, et al (1994) Echo-planar MR imaging of the liver in patients with focal hepatic lesions: quantitative analysis of images made with various sequences. AJR 163:1389–1393

Scheele J, Stangl R, Altendorf-Hofmann A, et al (1991) Indicators of prognosis after hepatic resection for colorectal secondaries. Surgery 110:13–29

Schulz W, Borchard F (1992) Größe der Lebermetastasen bei geringer metasrasenzahl. Eine quantitative studie an postmortalen lebern. Röfo Fortschr Geb Roentgenstr Neuen Bildgeb Verfahr 156:320–424

Schumann-Gianpieri G (1993) Liver contrast media for magnetic resonance imaging: interrelations between pharmacokinetics and imaging. Invest Radiol 28:753–756

Schwartz LH, Seltzer SE, Tempany CMC, et al (1993) Prospective comparison of T2-weighted fast spin-echo, with and without fat suppression, and conventional spin-echo pulse sequences in the upper abdomen. Radiology 189:411–416

Semelka RC, Kelekis NL (1997) Liver. In: Semelka RC, Ascher SM, Reinhold C (eds) MRI of the abdomen and pelvis. Wiley-Liss, New York, pp 19–135

Semelka RC, Mitchell DG (1996) Liver and biliary system. In: Edelman RR, Zlatkin MB, Hesselink JR (eds) Clinical magnetic resonance imaging, Vol 2. WB Saunders, Philadelphia, pp 1466–1512

Semelka RC, Simm FC, Recht M, et al (1991) T1-weighted sequences for MR imaging of the liver: comparison of three techniques for single-breath, whole-volume acquisition at 1.0 and 1.5 T. Radiology 180:629–635

Semelka RC, Shoenut JP, Kroeker MA, et al (1992) Focal liver disease: comparison of dynamic contrast-enhanced CT and T2-weighted fat-suppressed, FLASH, and dynamic gadolinium-enhanced MR imaging at 1.5 T. Radiology 184:687–694

Semelka RC, Cumming MJ, Shoenut JP, et al (1993a) Islet cell tumors: comparison of dynamic contrast enhanced CT and MR imaging with dynamic gadolinium enhancement and fat suppression. Radiology 186:799–802

Semelka RC, Hricak H, Bis KG, Werthmuller C, et al (1993 b) Liver lesion detection: comparison between excitation-spoiling fat suppression and regular spin-echo at 1.5 T. Abdom Imaging 18:56–60

Semelka RC, Bagley AS, Brown ED, et al (1994) Malignant lesions of the liver identified on T1 – but not T2 – weighted MR images at 1.5 T. JMRI 4:315–318

Seneterre E, Taourel P, Bouvier Y, et al (1996) Detection of hepatic metastases: ferumoxide-enhanced MR imaging versus unenhanced MR imaging and CT during arterial portography. Radiology 200:785–792

Siewert B, Muller MF, Foley M, et al (1994) Fast MR imaging of the liver: quantitative comparison of the techniques. Radiology 193:37–42

Soyer P, Levesque M, Elias D, et al (1992) Detection of liver metastases from colorectal cancer: comparison of intraoperative US and CT during arterial portography. Radiology 183:541–544

Soyer P, Levesque M, Caudron C, et al (1993) MRI of liver metastases from colorectal cancer vs CT during arterial portography. J Comput Assist Tomogr 17:67–74

Stark DD, Wittenberg J, Rodney JB, et al (1987) Hepatic metastases: randomized, controlled comparison of detection with MR Imaging and CT. Radiology 165:399–406

Steele G Jr, Bleday R, Mayer R, et al (1991) A prospective evaluation of hepatic resection for colorectal carcinoma metastases to the liver: Gastrointestinal Tumor Study Group protocol 6584. J Clin Oncol 9:1105–1112

Strotzer M, Gmeinwieser J, Schmidt J, et al (1997) Diagnosis of liver metastases from colorectal carcinoma. Comparison of spiral-CTAP combined with intra-venous contrast-enhanced spiral-CT and SPIO-enhanced MR combined with plain MR imaging. Acta Radiol 38:986–992

Sugarbaker PH (1990) Surgical decision making for large bowel cancer metastatic to the liver. Radiology 174:621–626

Taupitz M, Speidel A, Hamm B, et al (1995) T2-weighted breath-hold MR Imaging of the liver at 1.5 T: results with a three-dimensional steady-state free precession sequence in 87 patients. Radiology 194:439–446

van Beers B, Demeure R, Pringot, et al (1990) Dynamic spin-echo imaging with Gd-DTPA: value in the differentiation of hepatic tumors. AJR 154:515–519

Vassiliades VG, Foley WD, Alarcon J, et al (1991) Hepatic metastases: CT versus MR imaging at 1.5 T. Gastrointest Radiol 16:159–163

Vetto JT, Hughes KS, Rosenstein R, et al (1990) Morbidity and mortality of hepatic resection for metastatic colorectal carcinoma. Dis Colon Rectum 33:408–413

Vogl TJ, Pegios W, Mcmahon C, et al (1992) Gadobenate dimeglumine. A new contrast agent for MR imaging: preliminary evaluation in healthy volunteers. AJR 158:887–892

Wagner JS, Adson MA, Van Heerden JA, et al (1984) The natural history of hepatic metastases from colorectal cancer. Ann Surg 199:502–508

Wang C, Ahlstrom H, Ekholm S, et al (1998) Diagnostic efficacy of Mn-DPDP in MR imaging of the liver. A phase III multicentre study. Acta Radiol 38:643–649

Weisskoff RM, Edelman RR (1996) Basic principles of MRI. In: Edelman RR, Zlatkin MB, Hesselink JR (eds) Clinical magnetic resonance imaging, Vol 1. WB Saunders, Philadelphia, pp 3–51

Weissleder R, Stark DD, Engelstad B, et al (1989) Superparamagnetic iron oxide pharmacokinetics and toxicity. AJR 152:167–173

Wernecke K, Rummeny E, Bongartz G, et al (1991) Detection of hepatic masses in patients with carcinoma: comparative sensitivities of sonography, CT, and MR imaging. AJR 157:731–739

Withney WS, Herfkens RJ, Jeffrey RB, et al (1993) Dynamic breath-hold multiplanar spoiled gradient-recalled MR imaging with gadolinium enhancement for differentiating hepatic hemangiomas from malignancies at 1.5 T. Radiology 189:863–870

Wittenberg J, Stark DD, Forman PF, et al (1988) Differentiation of hepatic metastases from hepatic hemangiomas and cysts by using MR imaging. AJR 151:79–84

Zerhouni EA, Rutter C, Hamilton SR, et al (1996) CT and MR imaging in the staging of colorectal carcinoma: report of the Radiology Diagnostic Oncology Group II. Radiology 200:443–451

15 Intraoperative Ultrasound for Hepatic Metastases

G. Di Candio, A. Pietrabissa, and F. Mosca

CONTENTS

15.1 Introduction

The confirmed presence of liver metastases alters the surgical strategy of many abdominal neoplasms. At the time of initial treatment of primary tumor, for which surgery is advisable only in localized cases, such as in pancreatic cancer, even detection of the smallest metastatic nodule involves a poor prognosis and any surgical approach becomes palliative. In the case of colorectal or neuroendocrine tumor metastases, the identification of number and site of nodules is crucial, since the therapeutic role of hepatic resection in the 10% of patients where it is technically allowed is clearly proven (August et al. 1985).

Preoperative diagnosis of synchronous hepatic metastases is routinely achieved with abdominal ultrasound, while for metachronous metastases, especially if a liver resection is planned, ultrasound (US), CT and sometimes MR imaging are used. In this case the staging should be very accurate, in order to avoid unnecessary surgical exploration in unresectable patients. Traditional angiography is used less frequently, due both to its invasiveness and the improved vascular image quality, obtained with CT arterial portography, helical CT and MR imaging. Regardless of the diagnostic work-up that brings the patient to surgery, the following steps should be followed before resection. Abdominal exploration with liver manual palpation, the accurate research of any extrahepatic disease, and the use of intraoperative ultrasound (IOUS). This latter must be considered the "gold standard" in the detection of impalpable liver metastases. With new probes it is possible to recognize metastases with a diameter of less than 3–4 mm. The IOUS advantages are the acquisition of data not available with other techniques (small and deep nodules, not visible or palpable, overlooked by other preoperative imaging modalities), its role combined with or as an alternative to conventional radiology (such as in the study of the biliary tree), for confirmation of surgical radicality and, last but not least, as a guide for diagnostic-therapeutic procedures. Since hepatocellular carcinoma often originates in a cirrhotic liver, the main purposes of resective surgery and IOUS are the identification of cancer, its vascular relations and the consecutive limitation of the percentage of liver to be resected. In the case of colorectal metastases, the problem is apparently more simple. Residual liver is, in the majority of cases, normal, and able to bear even wider resections, but the frequently large number of nodules necessitate, in every case, precise planning of the parenchyma to be taken away. The IOUS helps in avoiding lesions of major vessels and allows, at the same time, at least a safe margin of 1 cm to be maintained.

15.2 Indications

Liver is the frequent site of abdominal cancer metastases, such as gastric, colonic and pancreatic tumors, due to its double blood inflow system (75% portal and 25% from hepatic artery), and its histological structure, which makes it a filter toward the

G. Di Candio, MD; Division of General and Experimental Surgery, Department of Oncology, University of Pisa, Via Paradisa 2, I-56124 Pisa, Italy
A. Pietrabissa, MD; Division of General and Experimental Surgery, Department of Oncology, University of Pisa, Via Paradisa 2, I-56124 Pisa, Italy
F. Mosca, MD, FACS; Professor and Chairman, Division of General and Experimental Surgery, Department of Oncology, University of Pisa, Via Paradisa 2, I-56124 Pisa, Italy

systemic circulus. Hepatic metastases can be detected during colorectal primitive cancer surgery in a range of 8–30% of patients (Finlay and McArdle 1986; Freeny and Marks 1986; Gozzetti and Mazziotti 1989; Saenz et al. 1989). Around 40% of patients will develop, mostly in the following 24 months, a recurrence, which is apparently localized in the liver in 20% of cases (Table 15.1). For this reason colorectal metastases surgery, especially if metachronous, has become, in Western countries, the main indication for hepatic resection.

Neoplastic emboli are commonly identified in the autoptic livers of patients with cancers draining in the portal system. These are possible also for other cancers, such as lymphoma, leukemia, melanoma, connective neoplasia, lung and breast cancer, but there is not much enthusiasm for resecting so-called "nonporta" metastases, since they are rarely localized only in the liver. Nevertheless, some authors have recently focused on this field, raising 5-year survivals also for this group of patients (Harrison et al. 1997; Miyazaki et al. 1997).

Among the various histological patterns, the colorectal and neuroendocrine tumor metastases are those for which liver resection is effective in improving long-term survival and even curative in a limited group of long-term survivors. For these forms, hepatic resection has become routine (Fong et al. 1997; Gayowsky et al. 1994; Jamison et al. 1997; Scheele et al. 1995; Ohlson et al. 1998; Taylor et al. 1997). The operative mortality is inferior to 5%, and, in more recent reports, it is easy to find consecutive series of more than 100 patients treated without mortality. Five-year survival for colorectal metastases has reached 25%, and it must be compared with the 9–10 months of the natural history of the untreated disease (Table 15.2). After curative liver resection, 20%–40% of patients develop a recurrence still limited to the liver. A repeat resection, if technically possible, may also improve long-term survival (Pinson et al. 1996; Tuttle et al. 1997, Fernandez-Trigo et al. 1995; Fong et al. 1994). Recently, Bismuth et al. (1996a,b) presented a study in which lesions, considered unresectable, can be later resected if understaged by neoadjuvant chemotherapy. The

Table 15.1. Staging of liver metastases (Gayowsky et al.1994)

I	Solitary unilobar, of any size
II	Multiple, unilobar, 2 cm or less
III	Multiple, unilobar, >2 cm
IVa	Bilobar involvement
IVb	Nodal involvement, extrahepatic disease

Table 15.2. Overall results in the surgical treatment of colorectal hepatic metastases

Study	Patients	Operative mortality (%)	Survival (5 years)
Gayowosky et al. 1994	204	0	32
Scheele et al. 1995	434	4.4	39
Shirabe et al. 1997	31		39
Taylor et al. 1997	123	0	34
Jenkins et al. 1997	131	3.8	25
Jamison et al. 1997	280		27
Fong et al. 1997	456	2.8	38
Cady et al. 1998	244		30
Ohlson et al. 1998	111	6	25

40% 5-year survival is impressive and rewards this aggressive approach (Table 15.3).

Various determinants of prognosis have been published: number, site and nodule dimensions, presence of extrahepatic disease, level of carcinoembryonic antigen (CEA), primary tumor (T) and N stage, histological grading, metastases synchronicity or amount of disease-free interval before detection, the need for intraoperative blood transfusions, and an adequate surgical margin. Patients with one or two metastases, with a 1-cm surgical margin and low CEA levels, have a 5-year disease-free survival of 30% (Cady et al. 1998; Nakamura et al. 1997). Positive surgical margins are certainly a negative factor, accompanied by many recurrences, often localized in the liver, without influencing significantly the percentage of extrahepatic recurrences (Cady et al. 1992).

From a histological point of view, the neoplastic embolus reaches the liver, and its growth is stimulated by the particular local conditions, the latter fostered by filter function of the hepatic tissue. In this site, the lesion extends thanks to the activation of proteolytic and angiogenetic factors, with the establishment of a real independent vascularity. In contrast to liver cancer, growth is fast and we do not

Table 15.3. Long-term survival for repeat hepatic resection for liver colorectal metastases

Study	Patients	Operative mortality (%)	Survival, 5 years (%)
Fog et al. 1994	25		30
Pinson et al. 1994	10	0	88 (2 years)
Fernandez et al. 1995	170		32
Bismuth et al. 1996	44	0	44
Tuttle et al. 1997	23	0	32

detect the formation of a peripheral pseudocapsule. Margins appear infiltrative at an early stage, with portal and suprahepatic system venule involvement, lymphatic and biliary tree diffusion. Moreover, there are microsatellite lesions. After histological examination of the surgical findings, SHIRABE et al. 1997 detected these aspects within 10 mm from the margin in all the metastatic lesions, in a macroscopically safe parenchyma. For nodules with a diameter of less than 4 cm, these aspects are rare (2/9 of lesions present at least one), while the percentage increases for larger nodules (6/7 of lesions) (SHIRABE et al. 1997).

While in liver cancer surgery in cirrhosis, the main concern is the anatomical removal of the segments, which are a tributary of their own portal pedicle, in surgery of metastases, respect for the free margin is more important. This must be larger, as mentioned above, than 10 mm (CADY et al. 1998). Recently, ELIAS et al. (1998) suggested a tough approach, not applying too rigidly the 10-mm measure, due to the fact that, in his experience, he recorded significant survival values also with smaller margins.

Nevertheless the positive surgical margin must make us consider the surgery as a palliative, such as in the presence of extrahepatic disease: both conditions give a 5-year survival of 0% (JENCKINS et al. 1997). The lymph node involvement at the hepatic hilum must be regarded as extrahepatic disease; it is findable in 28% of patients where liver surgery might seem complete (R0). In this case, as well, the 5-year survival collapses from 48% (negative lymph nodes) to 3% (positive lymph nodes) (BECKURTS et al. 1997). For this reason it is advisable to obtain frozen sections of periportal and celiac lymph nodes before major surgery.

The entity and kind of resection depend on dimensions, number and site of detected lesions. Wedge resections are advised for small metastases (up to 2–3 cm), especially if superficial; segmentary resections in the case of deeper lesions, involving one or two segments; and major hepatectomy (three to four segments) for multiple nodules, but limited to one lobe.

15.3 Methods

Intraoperative ultrasound can be performed through laparoscopy or laparotomy. In the first case, dedicated probes are introduced into the abdomen through 10-mm cannulae, 35–50 cm long, less than 10 mm in caliper and with a 5–10 MHz transducer at the tip, which allows high lateral resolution (<1 mm), and a depth of up to 10 cm. The right length and mobility of the transducer are necessary to obtain a good exploration of the furthest and narrowest abdominal recesses, without the necessity of multiple access. It is the orientation and scanning difficulty that makes this technique more difficult and slightly less accurate with respect to laparotomic ultrasonography (96% vs 79%) (COZZI et al. 1996).

Laparotomic ultrasound is performed with dedicated probes of a particular shape: pen (phased array or mechanical sector scan), bar and T-shaped (linear array or miniconvex) (Fig. 15.1). The frequency must exceed 5 MHz and better results are obtained with at least 7.5 MHz, which gives excellent spatial resolution and penetration. Recently we have used high definition probes with variable frequency (broad-band) from 8 to 13 MHz. Images especially provide the main capacity of ultrasound for the identification of both anatomical structures and micronodules with a diameter of up to 2–3 mm (Figs. 15.2–15.5). So much so that, especially in inhomogeneous livers for chronic hepatopathy or cirrhosis, the number of identified nodules is overwhelming, and most of them do not have a pathological meaning (microcysts, regenerative nodules, microangiomas). It is necessary with the new frequencies, regarding the semeiotics of liver echostructure, to reduce number of false positives (2–4%) (MACHI et al 1991, STONE et al. 1994).

Minor frequencies are used at the beginning of ultrasound exploration to obtain a total view of the liver (Figs. 15.6–15.8), while we use higher frequencies to evaluate more superficial lesions or for specific study of intralesional flow and major vessel compression and/or infiltration (Fig. 15.9). High definition new probes and equipment includes du-

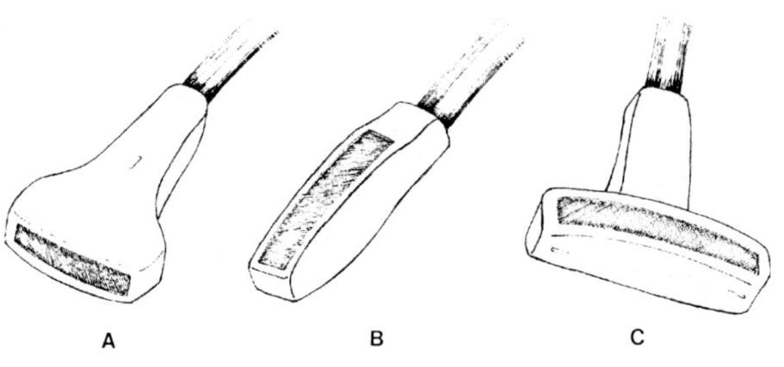

Fig. 15.1A–C. Intraoperative probes: **A** miniconvex, pen shaped; **B** linear, and **C** T shaped

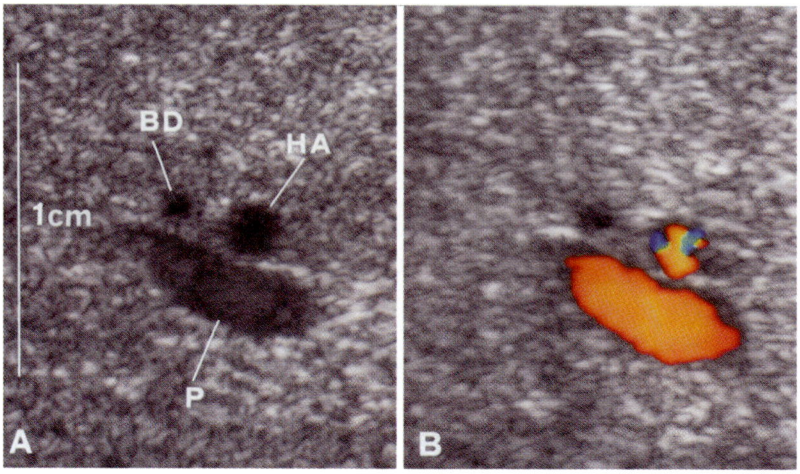

Fig. 15.2. A Intraoperative (13 MHz) scan showing the portal triad at the hepatic fifth segment. *HA*, hepatic artery; *BD*, biliary duct (1 mm or less in diameter); *P*, portal vein. **B** color Doppler study

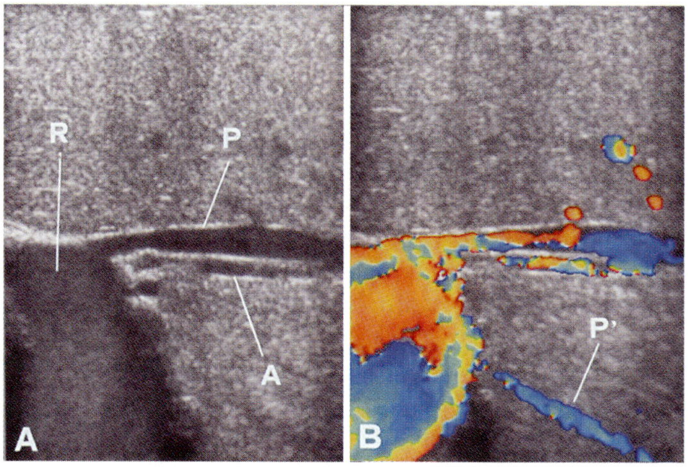

Fig. 15.3. A High definition scan (11 MHz). *R*, cul de sac of the umbilical portion of the left portal venous branch. *P and A*, segment III branches (vein and artery) arising from the cul de sac. **B** The same scan studied with color-Doppler. *P'*, segment II branch originating at the corner of the transverse and umbilical portions of left portal vein

plex and color-Doppler facilities, which are helpful for the less expert operator in vessel identification. It is also possible to perform an analysis of intralesional vascularization with color Doppler and a flow spectral analysis, which are used to differentiate lesions (for example, hemangioma/metastases).

Color-Doppler sensitivity is very high: with the best instruments we can record an intralesional flow starting from a speed of only 5 mm/s. New technology has made obsolete other techniques of image amplification such as hepatic perfusion with perfluorocytlbromide (PFOB, CO_2 microbubbles, or sugar-linked microbubbles). The liver ultrasound exploration is better performed on the organ in situ during resection of the primary lesion and in the case of negative bimanual palpation. On the other hand, it is a good procedure for complete mobilization, if synchronous lesions are visible and/or palpable and in the case of resective surgery for metachronous metastases, to identify occult nodules.

Even if they are precisely located by preoperative CT, the intraoperative localization of metastases can be carried out, especially if they are deep and small. The subsequent liver mobilization and clockwise rotation on the pedicle can make difficult the correlation between the two-dimensional CT image and the new anatomical situation. IOUS allows, on the other

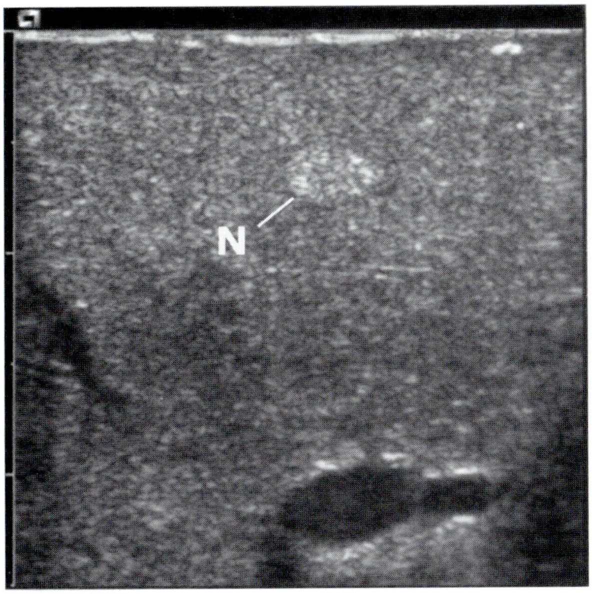

Fig. 15.4. Scan (11 MHz) in a cirrhotic liver: small (3 mm in diameter) hyperechoic satellitosis (*N*) around a large hepatocellular carcinoma

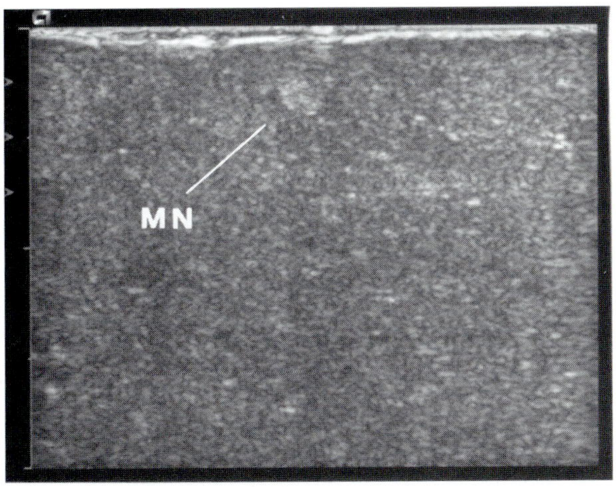

Fig. 15.5. Ultrasonic appearance of a small (1.5–2 mm in diameter) subcapsular adenomatous hyperplasia (*MN*) in a chronic HCV hepatitis

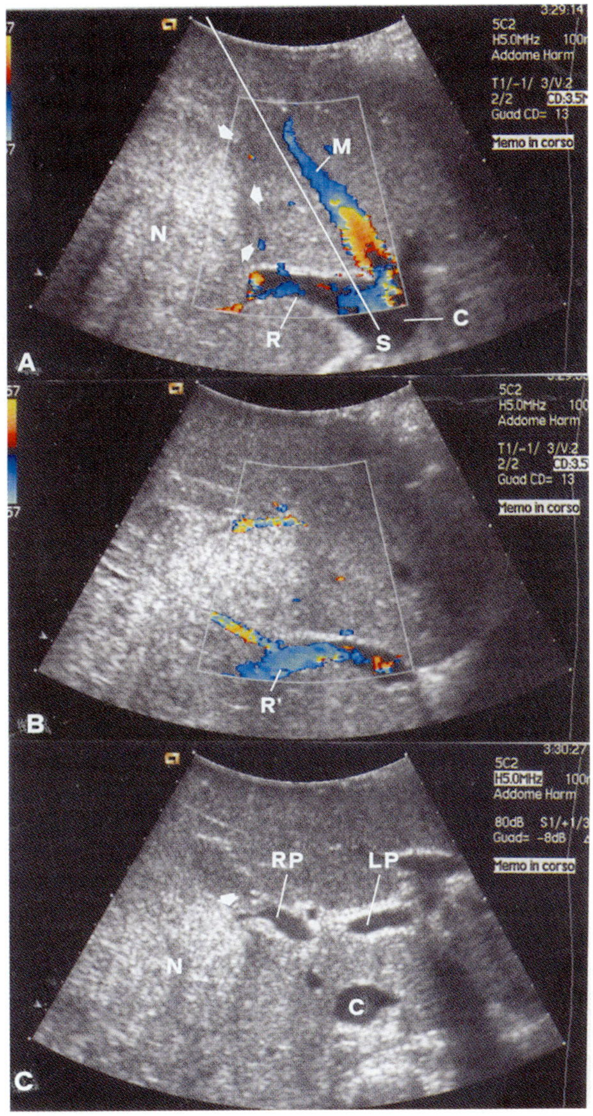

Fig. 15.6A–C. First wide liver survey with a 5-MHz convex probe in a case of metachronous right lobe colorectal metastasis (*N*), more than 8 cm in diameter. The nodule is hyperechoic with an hypoechoic peripheral rim (*arrows*). *M*, middle hepatic vein, 2 cm from the neoplastic margin; *R*, right hepatic vein, completely involved (*R'*) by the tumor; *C*, inferior vena cava, transversely scanned. *S*, hypothetical orientation of the surgical plane to be transected. The neoplasia involves the right posterior branch of the portal vein (*RP*). *LP*, left branch of the portal vein

hand, easy identification of the nodules and, if used in real-time and simultaneously with dissection, we can avoid an accidental lesion of the large suprahepatic and/or portal vessels, or include them in the resection if necessary, nevertheless keeping a free surgical margin. Lesions must all be described on the basis of their segment and of the kind of relationship with the major vessels to disclose technical contraindications, based on the hepatectomy extension needed, and, in the case of chronic hepatitis or cirrhosis, limiting the adequacy of the liver remnant.

Laparotomic and laparoscopic ultrasound examinations are completed within 10–15 min; time depends on the US approach (ultrasound laparoscopy is more difficult in terms of spatial correlation between ultrasound image, probe orientation and

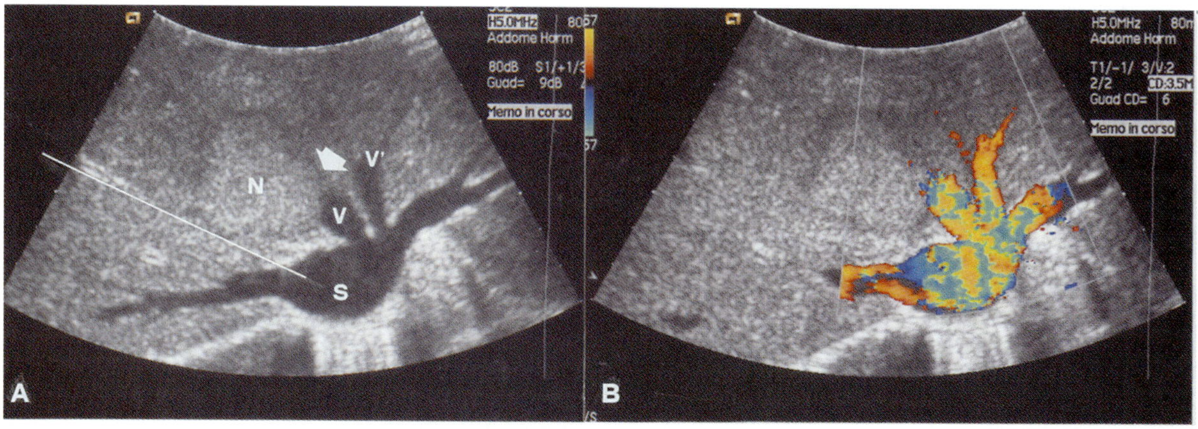

Fig. 15.7. **A** Convex scan (5 MHz) in a case of metachronous colorectal metastasis (*N*) located between the VIII and IV segments. Ultrasonography identifies a double middle hepatic vein (*V and V'*) and the tumor infiltrating the lateral one, *V* (*arrow*). **B** The same scan performed with color Doppler

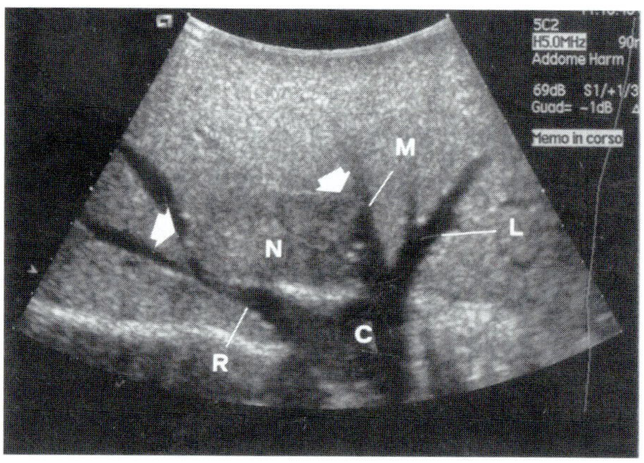

Fig. 15.8. Wide scan (5 MHz) of a solitary colorectal metastasis of the fifth hepatic segment, 4 cm in diameter involving both right and middle hepatic veins (*R and M, arrows*). *L*, left hepatic vein

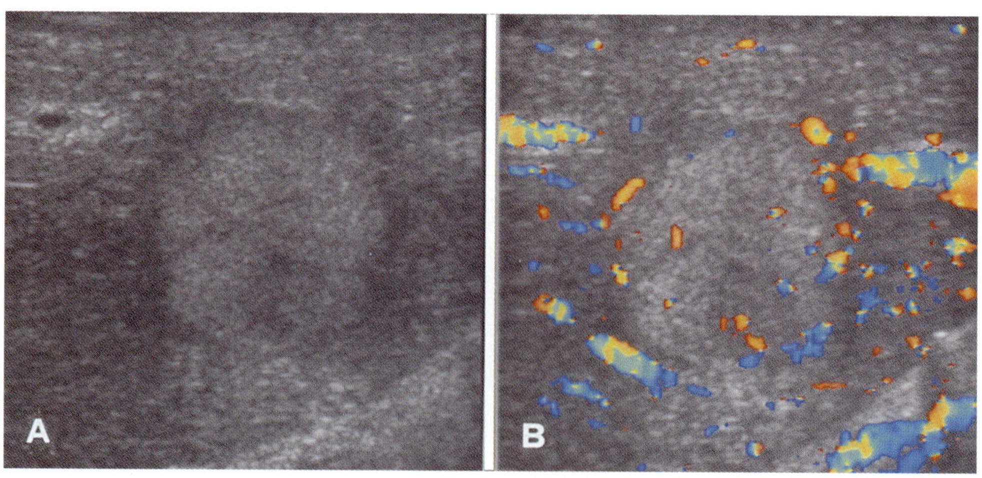

Fig. 15.9. **A** Hepatic scan (11 MHz) of a solitary colorectal metastasis, hyperechoic with halo. **B** Color Doppler performance, showing the prevalently perinodular vascularization with few and irregular vessels inside

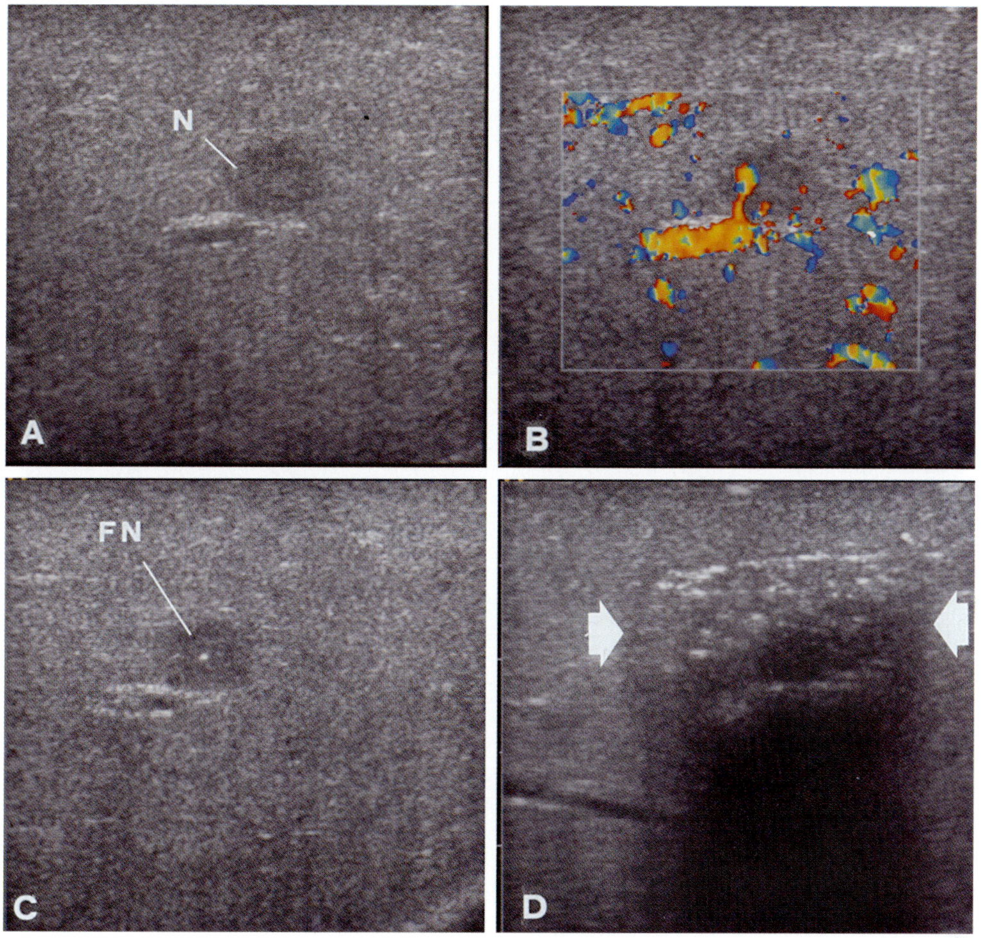

Fig. 15.10. **A** Scan (11 MHz) of a small neuroendocrine metastasis (*N*, 3–4 mm in diameter), isoechoic, residual in the II segment after multiple wedge resections in the contralateral hepatic lobe. **B** Color Doppler study showing a small feeding artery. **C** Echoguided free hands cytology with a Chiba needle (*FN*), 21 gauge. **D** Echoguided alcoholization with 5 cc. Observe the wide and homogeneous diffusion of the alcohol inside and around the lesion (*arrows*)

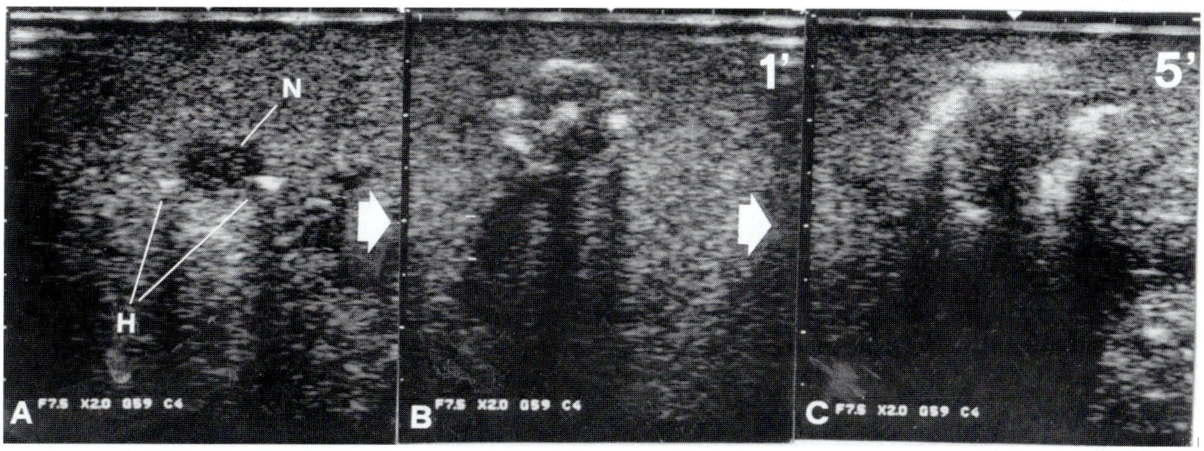

Fig. 15.11. **A** Intraoperative transhepatic US-guided radiofrequency (*RF*) tissue ablation of a small liver metastasis, *N* (6×4 mm), in a patient with duodenal adenocarcinoma. *H*, Echoguided insertion of a monopolar RF expandable needle electrode with four hooks deployed and placed just outside the neoplastic area. RF is applied for 8 min at 95°. **B,C** Progressive nodule heating at the 1st and 5th min of radiofrequency power supply

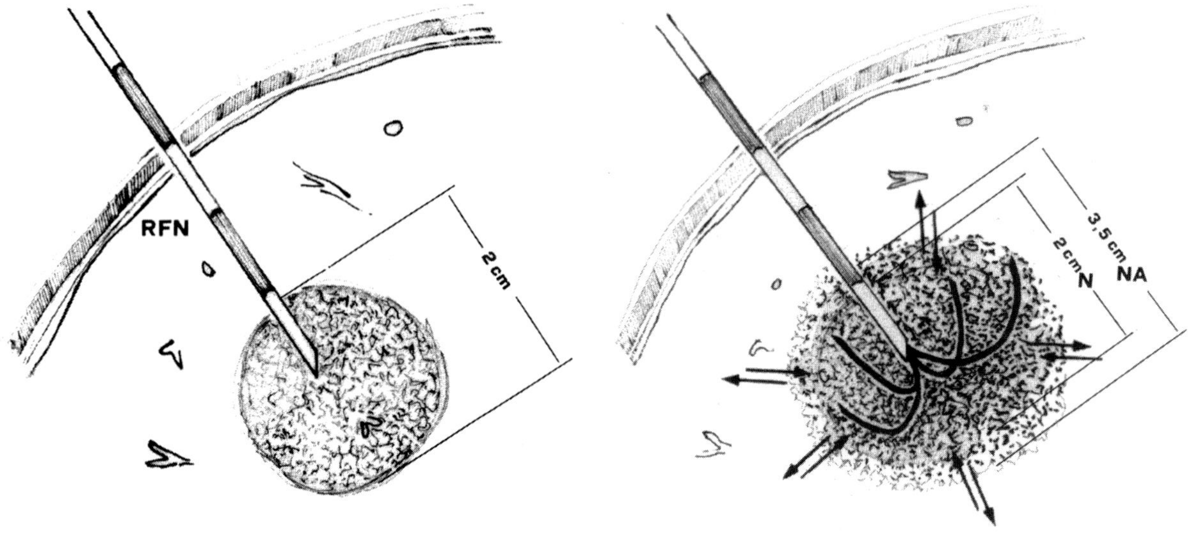

Fig. 15.12. RF thermal ablation with an expandable needle electrode (*RFN*). In the case of metastatic disease the diameter of the lesion (*N*) has to be largely inferior (i.e., 2 cm) to the hypothetical thermal lesion achievable (*NA*, 3, 3.5 cm with monopolar needles)

mind extrapolation of the nodule position, and needs more time than the "open" study) and from operator experience. To facilitate image understanding, it is now possible to use a tridimensional computer reconstruction of the bidimensional images, with a process requiring, in real time, not more than 10 s (Motohide et al. 1998). With ultrasound guidance it is also possible to guide intraoperative procedures: biopsies of nodules missed by preoperative work-up (it is preferable to perform needle core biopsies instead of cytology, which is faster but less accurate), the direct injection of liquid dyes (3–5 ml of indigo carmine) in a portal branch to perform staining of the portal area for anatomic hepatectomy, the transhepatic drainage of biliary tree or the performance of alcoholization, radiofrequency, microwaves and laser thermal ablations, or cryotherapy (Figs. 15.10–15.12).

15.4 Results

The clinical evaluation of any new technology is based on its accuracy and on a comparison with already established methods. This includes the quantity of obtainable information, the confidence level required to modify a previous clinical evaluation, and how much this strategy modification can positively influence the prognosis in defined subgroups of patients. From this viewpoint the IOUS appears to be an examination which will quickly receive a "validity certificate", thanks to its capability to modify the intraoperative strategy in the initial applications and in nonexpert hands. For this reason it has become a routine examination in surgical oncology of the abdomen. With IOUS we can detect 93% of liver lesions, more than CT scans (47%) and surgical exploration (66%) (Machi et al. 1991). Of the lesions discovered with US, 10–40% do not appear during palpation and inspection (Finlay and McArdle 1986; Machi et al. 1987; Olsen et 1990; Charnley et al. 1991), and additional information on the presence and number of metastases is achieved in a percentage ranging from 3 to 23% of cases (Boldrini et al. 1987; Stadler et al. 1991; Paul et al. 1994; Machi and Siegel 1996; Olsen 1990; Stone et al. 1994; Fortunato et al. 1995; Takeuchi et al. 1996) (Figs. 15.4, 15.10, 15.11). This range can be justified with the quality of technical instrumentation and the experience of the operator, but also from the level of preoperative selection of patients and the study of groups with more advanced disease, in which, obviously, the method will appear more effective.

The difference between palpation and IOUS results increases if we exclude metastases appearing in the liver capsule on the clinical examination, but which are frequently missed by preoperative and intraoperative sonography, because of the short distance between the nodule and transducer, so that the nodule falls outside the focal length of the ultrasonic beam. This problem can now be completely overcome using appropriate probes of greater than 10 MHz in frequency with a broad band that tends to make the near field more uniform. For small and deep lesions (<1 cm), the sensitivity increases from 33% of clinical examinations to 83% of IOUS (Knol et al. 1993). Palpation and IOUS become complementary before any surgical approach of the liver, and IOUS should be considered the most accurate instrumental examination we have, influencing surgical strategy in 38–60% of cases (Solomon et al. 1994; Bezzi et al. 1998) (Table 15.4).

Beyond the identification of lesions, the IOUS is useful also to confirm or exclude the presence of nodules detected with conventional CT or with more accurate techniques, such as helical- and porto-CT, which might present false positive results (Haiken et al. 1989). During dissection, adjusted with anatomical "classical" reference points, it is possible that the removed section does not include the nodule, or

Table 15.4. IOUS results in detection of unknown liver metastases of gastrointestinal primary tumors

Study	Patients	IOUS only (%)	FN (%)
Boldrini et al. 1987	86	3.5	–
Machi et al. 1991	189	9.5	13
Charnley et al. 1991	99	9	–
Stone et al. 1993	56	5	17
Solomon et al. 1994	51	13	25

that the latter is facing the section surface. Moreover, we can have more or less important vascular lesions, from which bleeding originates. Cady et al. (1998) demonstrates, in a recent work, that the routine use of intraoperative ultrasound goes together with a significant reduction of resections with positive margins.

The ultrasound aspect of hepatic metastases is extremely variable.

The majority of small metastases are hypoechoic, while the large ones are hyperechoic with a peripheral halo (Figs. 15.9, 15.10). In some cases the lesion is not clearly visible, since the sonographic pattern is isoechoic in respect of surrounding parenchyma and its identification is possible only with the presence of a subtle peripheral hypoechoic halo and thanks to the indirect signs of vascular compression/infiltration. Neoplastic thrombosis in the portal venous system is rare, whereas it is often observed in advanced hepatocellular carcinoma (Fig. 15.13).

High definition ultrasound (10–13 MHz) of enlarged hilar lymph nodes (1 cm or bigger) allows the demonstration, on the basis of sonographic pattern and Doppler study, of their neoplastic involvement.

Reactive lymph nodes are oval, with regular margins, have a well demonstrated germinal center, and marked and regularly diffused vascularization (Fig. 15.14). In the case of metastases we observe an irregular increase in the lymph node, which loses its oval shape to gain a more rounded one with irregular and "rigid" margins. The structure appears strongly with partial or total disappearance of the germinal center. The blood flow appears irregular to color Doppler and absent in some areas (Fig. 15.15).

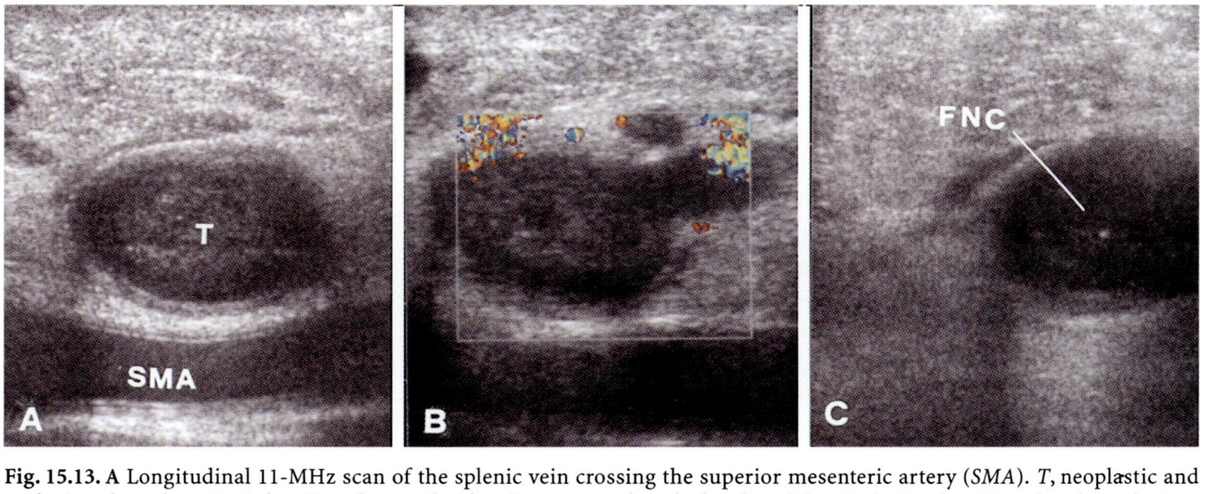

Fig. 15.13. A Longitudinal 11-MHz scan of the splenic vein crossing the superior mesenteric artery (*SMA*). *T*, neoplastic and occlusive thrombus. **B** Color Doppler study showing a complete lack of endoluminal signal. **c** Free hands technique echoguided biopsy of the neoplastic thrombus

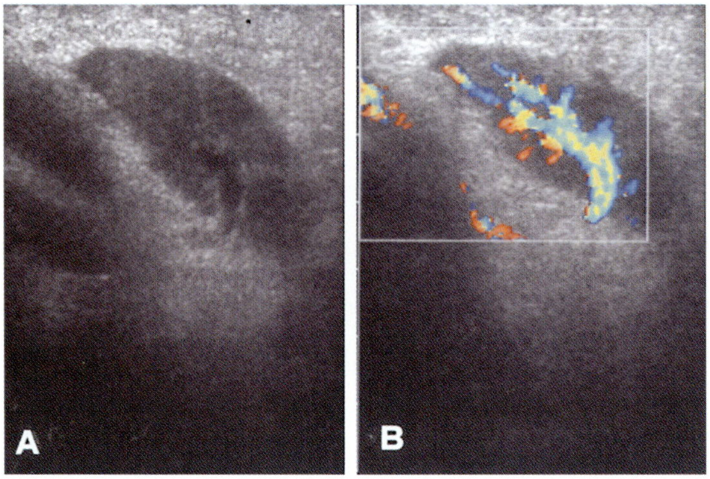

Fig. 15.14. A Scan (13 Mhz) of a large reactive lymph node (15+10 mm) with oval shape in the hepatoduodenal ligament in a case of synchronous metastasic disease from a colorectal primary tumor. **B** Vascular resolution increases using higher Doppler frequencies showing an homogeneous vascularization

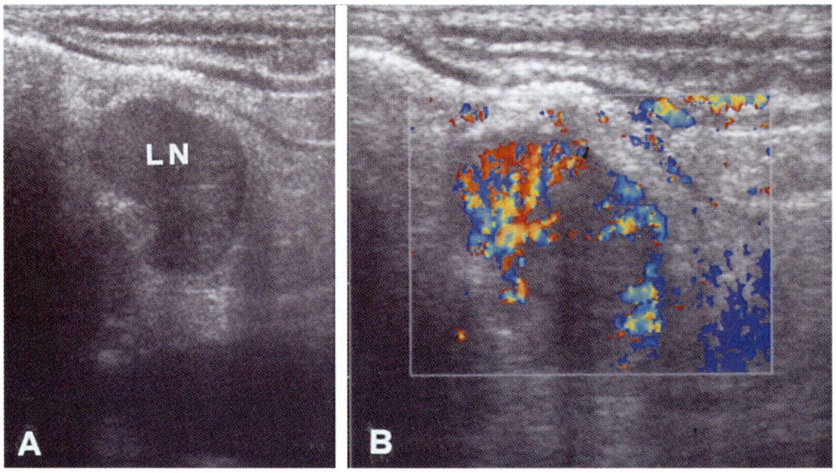

Fig. 15.15. A Scan (13 MHz) of an involved lymph node at the hepatic hilum in a patient with metachronous liver colorectal metastasis. **B** Intense blood flow signals with irregular course and uneven distribution are visible in the lymph node

Studies on clinical and instrumental follow-up of patients with negative IOUS for colorectal metastases have raised much interest. If ultrasound negativity was accompanied with a really low risk of recurrence, this might, theoretically, influence the therapeutic strategies for this patient group, excluding them, for example, from expensive and rigid follow-ups or from adjuvant chemotherapy. If we consider the studies in which only patients are involved with negative ultrasound, the percentage of recurrences varies from 9% to 21% of cases. Probably, the metastases escaping from IO ultrasound require 6–24 months to increase and become visible for the new imaging. Therefore these data do not justify the exclusion of patients with negative IOUS from chemotherapy programs and follow-up.

To understand the value to be attributed to ultrasound negativity, it is possible to refer to recent results obtained by Paul et al. (1996) and Leen et al. (1996): 16–25% of patients with negative IOUS developed an hepatic recurrence within the 24 months following the therapeutic resection.

References

August DA, Sugarbaker PH, Ottow RT, Gianola FJ, Schneider PD (1985) Hepatic resection of colorectal metastases: influence of clinical factors and adjuvant intraperitoneral 5-fluorouracil via Teckhoff catheter on survival. Ann Surg 210:210–218

Beckurts KT, Holscher AH, Thorban S, Bollschweiller E, Siewert JR (1997) Significance of lymph node involvement at the hepatic hilum in the resection of colorectal liver metastases. Br J Surg 84:1081–1084

Bezzi M, Silecchia G, De Leo A, Carbone I, Pepino D, Rossi P (1998) Laparoscopic and intraoperative ultrasound . Eur J Radiol 27:S207–S204

Bismuth H, Adam R, Navarro F, Castaing D, Engerran L, Abascal A (1996 a) Re-resection for colorectal liver metastasis. Surg Oncol North Am 5:353–364

Bismuth H, Adam R, Levi F, et al (1996 b) Resection of nonresectable liver metastases from colorectal cancer after neoadjvant chemotherapy. Ann Surg 224:509–520

Boldrini G, Gaetano AM, Giovannini I, et al (1987) The systematic use of operative ultrasound for detection of liver metastases from colorectal carcinoma: initial experience. World J Surg 11:622–627

Cady B, Stone MD, McDermott WV, et al (1992) Technical and biological factors in disease free survival after hepatic resection for colorectal metastases. Arch Surg 127:561–569

Cady B, Jenkins RL, Steele GD jr, et al (1998) Surgical margin in hepatic resection for colorectal metastases. Ann Surg 227:566–571

Charnley RM, Norris DL, Dennison AR, Amar SS, Hardcastle JD (1991) Detection of colorectal liver metastases using intraoperative ultrasonography. Br J Surg 78:45–48

Cozzi PJ, McCall JL, Jorgensen JO, Morris DL (1996) Laparoscopic vs open ultrasound of the liver: an in vitro study. HPB Surg 10:87–89

Elias D, Cavalcanti A, Sabourin JC, et al (1998) Resection of liver metastases from colorectal cancer: the real impact of the surgical margin. Eur J Surg Oncol 24:174–179

Fernandez-Trigo V, Shamsa F, Sugerbaker PH (1995) Repeat liver resection for colorectal metastasis. Repeat hepatic metastases registry. Surgery 117:296–304

Finlay IG, McArdle CS (1986) Occult hepatic metastases in colorectal carcinoma. Br J Surg 73:732–735

Fong Y, Blumgart LH, Cohen A, Fortner J Brennan MF (1994) Repeat hepatic resections for metastatic colorectal cancer Ann Surg 220:657–662

Fong Y, Cohen AM, Fortner JG, et al (1997) Liver resection for colorectal metastases. J Clin Oncol 15:938–946

Fortunato L, Clair M, Hoffmann J, Sigurdson ER, Sauter ER, Barber LW, Eisenberg B (1995) Is CT portography (CTAP) really useful in patients with liver tumors who undergo intraoperative ultrasonography (IOUS) ? Am Surg 61:560–565

Freeny PC, Marks WM (1986) Patterns of contrast enhancement of benign and malignant hepatic neoplasms during bolus dynamic and delayed CT. Radiology 160:613–618

Gayowsky TJ, Iwatsuki S, Madariaga JR, et al (1994) Experience in hepatic resection for metastatic colorectal cancer: analysis of clinical and pathologic risk factors. Surgery 116:703–710

Gozzetti G, Mazziotti A (1989) Expectations and possibilities of liver resections in the management of secondary liver tumors. In: Lygidakis NJ, Tytgat GNJ (eds) Hepatobiliary and pancreatic malignancies. Georg Thieme Verlag, Stuttgart New York, p 183

Heiken JP, Weiman PJ, Lee JKT, et al (1989) Detection of focal hepatic masses: prospective evaluation with CT, delayed CT, CT during arterial portography, and MR imaging. Radiology 171:47–51

Harrison LE, Brennan MF, Newman E, et al (1997) Hepatic resection for noncolorectal, nonneuroendocrine metastases: a fifteen-year experience with ninety-six patients. Surgery 121:625–632

Jamison RL, Donohue JH, Nagorney DM, Rosen CB, Harmsen WS, Ilstrup DM (1997) Hepatic resection for metastatic colorectal cancer results in cure for some patients. Arch Surg 132:505–510

Jenkins LT, Millikan KW, Bines SD, Staren ED, Doolas A (1997) Hepatic resection for metastatic colorectal cancer. Ann Surg 63:605–610

Knol JA, Marn CS, Francis IR, Rubin JM, Bromberg J (1993) Comparison of dynamic infusion and delayed computed tomography, intraoperative ultrasound and palpation in the diagnosis of liver metastases. Am J Surg 165:81–88

Leen E, Angerson WJ, O'Gorman P, Cooke TG, McArdle CS (1996) Intraoperative ultrasound in colorectal cancer patients undergoing apparently curative surgery: correlation with two year follow up. Clin Radiol 51:157–159

Machi J, Sigel B (1996) Operative ultrasound in general surgery. Am J Surg 172:15–20

Machi J, Sigel B, Donhave PE, et al (1987) Intraoperative Ultrasonography in biliary surgery. In: Makuuchi M (ed) Abdominal intraoperative ultrasonography. Igaku Shoin, Tokio, p 167

Machi J, Isomoto H, Kurohiji T, et al (1991) Accuracy of intraoperative ultrasonography in diagnosing liver metastases from colorectal cancer: evaluation with postoperative follow up results. World J Surg 15:551–557

Miyazaki M, Itoh I, Nagakawa K, et al (1997) Hepatic resection of liver metastases from gastric carcinoma. Am J Gastronterol 92:490–493

Motohide S, Go W, Masahiro O, Hiroshi H, Masaki K (1998) Clinical application of three dimensional ultrasound imaging as intraoperative navigation for liver surgery. Nippon Geka Gakkai Zasshi 99:203–207

Nakamura S, Suzuki S, Baba S (1997) Resection of liver metastases of colorectal carcinoma. World J Surg 21:741–747

Ohlson B, Stenram U, Tranberg KG (1998) Resection of colorectal liver metastases: 25-year experience. World J Surg 22:268–276

Olsen AK (1990) Intraoperative ultrasonography and the detection of liver metastases in patients with colorectal cancer. Br J Surg 77:998–999

Paul MA, Mulder LS, Cuesta MA, Sikkenk AC, Lyesen GKS, Meijer S (1994) Impact of intraoperative ultrasonography on treatment strategy for colorectal cancer. Br J Surg 81:1660–1663

Paul MA, Blonjous AM, Cuesta MA, Meijer S (1996) Prognostic value of negative intraoperative ultrasonography in primary colorectal cancer. Br J Surg 83:1741–1743

Pinson CW, Wright JK, Garrard CL, Blair TK, Sawyers JL (1996) Repeat hepatic surgery for colorectal cancer metastasis to the liver. Ann Surg 223:765–773

Saenz NC, Cady B, McDermott WV, Steele GO (1989) Experience with colorectal cancer metastatic to the liver. Surg Clin North Am 69:361–370

Scheele J, Stang R, Altendorf-Hofman A, Paul M (1995) Resection of colorectal liver metastases. World J Surg 19:59–71

Shirabe K, Takenaka K, Gion T, et al (1997) Analysis of prognostic risk factors in hepatic resection for metastatic colorectal carcinoma with special reference to the surgical margin. Br J Surg 84:1077–1080

Solomon MJ, Stephen MS, Gallinger S, White GH (1994) Does intraoperative hepatic ultrasonography change surgical decision making during liver resection? Am J Surg 168:307–310

Stadler J, Holscher AH, Adolf J (1991) Intraoperative ultrasonographic detection of occult liver metastases in colorectal cancer. Surg Endosc 5:36–40

Stone MD, Kane R, Bothe A jr, Jessup JM, Cady B, Steele GD (1994) Intraoperative ultrasound imaging of the liver at the time of colorectal cancer resection. Arch Surg 129:431–436

Takeuchi N, Ramirez JM, Mortensen NJ, Cobb R, Whuittlestone T (1996) Intraoperative ultrasonography in the diagnosis of hepatic metastases during surgery for colorectal cancer. Int J Colorectal Dis 11:92–95

Taylor M, Forster J, Langer B, Taylor BR, Greig PD, Mahut C (1997) A study prognostic factors for hepatic resection for colorectal metastases. Am J Surg 173:467–471

Tuttle TM, Curley SA, Roth MS (1997) Repeat hepatic resection as effective treatment of recurrent colorectal liver metastases. Ann Surg Oncol 4:125–130

III Interventional Radiology

16 Rationale for Non-surgical Interventional Treatment of Hepatocellular Carcinoma

J. Bruix and C. Bru

CONTENTS

16.1 Introduction

Hepatocellular carcinoma (HCC) is still seen as a neoplasm with a very grim prognosis. This concept was established decades ago, when the diagnosis was almost always achieved at an advanced stage or even after death. However, the availability of ultrasound (US) and its wide use in the conventional clinical setting for the evaluation of patients with suspicion of liver disease has prompted a radical change in the timing of diagnosis. Patients with HCC may be now diagnosed at an early asymptomatic stage (Okuda 1986) when potentially effective therapies can be indicated and this has raised a marked interest in defining the criteria and staging systems that should be used to properly manage HCC patients.

In the present chapter we will review what is the rationale for the strategy applied in our group to detect, stage and treat patients with this neoplasm. It has to be emphasized that most of the treatment options applied in HCC patients have not been evaluated within randomized controlled trials and, thus, the estimated benefits of treatment are dealt with in comparison with the reported natural history of untreated patients supposedly diagnosed at the same evolutionary stage. As we will comment later, this information used to compare outcome may be biased and, thus, the comparison may be misleading.

J. Bruix, MD; Liver Unit, Hospital Clinic, University of Barcelona, Villarroel 170, E-08036 Barcelona, Spain
C. Bru, MD; Department of Radiology, Hospital Clinic, University of Barcelona, Villarroel 170, E-08036 Barcelona, Spain

16.2 Early Detection

The first requirement for applying a radical treatment is to detect the tumor at an early stage when those therapeutic options aiming to be radical may be indicated. In geographic areas with a high HCC incidence, such as China, the screening programs are population based and usually consist of determining alpha-fetoprotein (AFP) concentration in large series of individuals and selecting for specific examination those subjects with increased concentration of this tumoral marker (Okuda et al. 1985; Tang and Yang 1985). This screening policy shows that the majority of patients diagnosed at a subclinical stage in these areas exhibit increased AFP concentration, while the analysis of the patients diagnosed at advanced/symptomatic stages shows a lower sensitivity of this tumoral marker (Tang and Bing-Hui 1989) with values not markedly different from those reported in the Western world (Okuda 1986; Taketa 1990; Bruix et al. 1992; Sherman et al. 1995). In fact, most of the small HCC submitted to radical treatment after intentional screening with US and AFP exhibit normal or almost normal AFP values (Bruix 1993) and, thus, despite isolated cases of increased AFP values due to early HCC, it can be suggested that AFP has a reduced usefulness for early HCC detection. In Western countries the HCC incidence is not as high, and it is known that this tumor is almost restricted to patients with liver cirrhosis (Johnson and Williams 1987; Bruix et al. 1991). If patients with compensated liver cirrhosis are intentionally screened, almost 5% of them may be diagnosed with HCC and this proportion increases to 15–20% when studying patients admitted because of variceal bleeding or with spontaneous bacterial peritonitis (Bruix 1993). Furthermore, follow-up studies from separate countries have shown the 5-year probability of developing an HCC in patients with hepatic cirrhosis may exceed 20% (Colombo et al. 1991; Ikeda et al. 1993; Sato et al. 1993; Tsukuma et al. 1993; Cottone et al. 1994; Takano et al. 1995; Ganne-Carrie et al. 1996; Elizalde et al. 1996). Thus, most Western groups recommend following patients with chronic liver disease at regular intervals to facilitate the early detection of the HCC, which should be considered one of the most frequent complications during the evolution of chronic liver diseases.

Therefore, if a patient is diagnosed with liver cirrhosis, the first question to be raised is if the patient should be treated if diagnosed with HCC. If the answer is negative because of advanced age, severe impairment of the liver function without being a candidate for liver transplantation or the presence of associated diseases, there is no sense in establishing an early detection plan, since it will only prompt an increase in economic cost without a potential benefit in survival. This is an important consideration since some negative assumptions regarding the advantages of regular screening may be due to a low applicability of the available treatments, or even to the non-availability of some of the radical options by the group performing the screening. On the contrary, if the answer is positive, a regular follow-up should be advised. The benefits of this policy are debatable since there are no randomized controlled trials comparing an active screening schedule vs a conventional follow-up. Therefore, the cost-effectiveness of early detection plans has been estimated through analytical models based on several theoretical assumptions regarding incidence, risk factors, applicability of treatments and survival of treated and untreated subjects (Sarasin et al. 1996; Collier and Sherman 1998). Since all these concepts are based on published data from different centers at different periods, it is difficult to translate the findings of these calculations to the clinical setting for a given patient.

HCC screening is based on US and AFP determination (Okuda 1986; Collier and Sherman 1998). The diagnostic efficacy of des-gamma-carboxy-prothrombin is similar to AFP, and other tumor markers are of minor usefulness (Weitz and Liebman 1993). Taking into account that the mean tumor volume doubling time has been estimated to be 3–4 months (Sheu et al. 1985; Ebara et al. 1986; Okazaki et al. 1988; Barbara et al. 1992), the best screening interval should range between 4 and 6 months. However, it should be stressed that AFP is seldom increased above normal values in patients with small solitary HCC (Okuda 1986; Bruix et al. 1992). In addition, patients with chronic viral infection may present fluctuating AFP values related to the necroinflammatory episodes (Liaw et al. 1986; Takano et al. 1995). Thus, the usefulness of AFP for early detection is debatable. It has been shown that persistently increased AFP values imply a higher risk for HCC development and some authors suggest that these patients should be followed more frequently, but again there is no evidence that this is a beneficial policy. However, it should be kept in mind that increased AFP values, as is the case with male sex, viral infection or age above 50 years, constitute markers of increased risk (Poynard et al. 1991; Ganne-Carrie et al. 1996), but they do not imply a faster tumor growth. Thus, the selection of candidates fitting these characteristics would increase the number of HCC detected and, potentially, the cost-effectiveness of the early detection plans (Collier and Sherman 1998), but they should not prompt a different screening schedule. In the daily clinical practice, the presence of a markedly increased and sustained AFP concentration with negative US findings should prompt the realization of a spiral computed tomography (CT) scan to rule out an undetected HCC. If this technique is also negative, the need to perform magnetic resonance imaging (MRI) or hepatic angiography should be considered. Other potential tools to recognize subjects at higher risk are the presence of liver cell dysplasia (Borzio et al. 1995), an abnormal architectural profile (Shibata et al. 1998) or an increased proliferative activity as reflected by proliferating cell nuclear antigen (Mehta 1995).

The US detection of a solid focal lesion within the liver in a patient with long-standing chronic liver disease should raise the suspicion of HCC whatever its echogenic appearance, and additional imaging techniques and a fine needle biopsy of the nodule should be considered to confirm or discard HCC. Upon confirmation of the HCC the physicians attending the patient should decide which is the most adequate treatment approach.

16.3 Patient Evaluation

The evaluation of the patients should take into account the staging of the tumor and the impairment of the liver function, which may be deteriorated as a result of HCC development or be abnormal because of the underlying liver disease. The techniques to apply to stage the neoplasm and to evaluate the liver function should not be the same for all the patients. On the contrary, they should be tailored to each case according to the initial findings and potential therapeutic options to be applied either in the conventional clinical setting or within research trials. In that sense, if the first evaluation by clinical examination and/or US reveals an end-stage liver disease fitting into group C of Child-Pugh's classification (Pugh et al. 1973) with a performance status test ≥ 3 (Sorensen et al. 1993), and the patient has any contraindication for orthotopic liver transplantation (advanced age, severe associated diseases), there may be no sense in carefully evaluating the stage of the HCC in daily clinical practice since no option will have an impact on survival. Thus, this strata of patients should only be further explored and/or treated within the application of specific research protocols. Similarly, if the first approach discloses an advanced tumor stage precluding any potential therapeutic approach, there is no clinical sense in indicating additional examinations. However, there is no consensus in defining this category. In our group, we do not consider for antineoplastic treatment patients belonging to stage 3 of the Okuda classification (Okuda et al. 1985) and/or those with a performance status ≥ 3 (Sorensen et al. 1993). Both methods are useful to identify those patients with a poor life expectancy (less than 3 months) and in our opinion these patients should merely receive symptomatic treatment to avoid unnecessary suffering.

After this initial approach to identify those individuals who will not be treated, the management of the patients will depend on the treatment algorithm of each group since there is no consensus regarding which is the first therapeutic option to be considered in patients with HCC. There are no randomized controlled trials comparing radical options (resection, transplantation, ethanol injection) versus no treatment or even between themselves (Yokoyama et al. 1990). Thus, below we will describe our present treatment schedule, detailing not only the criteria and requirements for each of the therapeutic options, but also the scientific background supporting our policy.

16.4 Therapeutic Approach

16.4.1 Surgical Resection

For most authors the first option to be evaluated should be surgical resection, leaving orthotopic liver transplantation as a second approach. Surgical resection should aim to eliminate the HCC and the surrounding non-tumoral tissue. This neoplasm disseminates at early stages through the invasion of the subsegmentary branches of the portal vein, and the vicinity of the nodule is the most frequent site of dissemination (Nakashima and Kojiro 1987). This has provided the basis for performing anatomical resections (Makuuchi 1995). Their end-point would be to identify the portal vessel supplying the segment or subsegment of the liver where the HCC is located and to resect the tissue margin that bears the highest risk of containing unrecognized microscopic tumor nests. Major lobectomy is contraindicated in patients with cirrhosis and most groups select for surgery patients with well preserved liver function and solitary tumors without vascular invasion or extrahepatic spread. Child-Pugh's classification (Pugh et al. 1973) is widely used to assess the liver function, but this classification is not adequate to provide a proper selection of candidates. A large proportion of patients will develop hepatic decompensation (namely ascites) after the operation and this event is associated with impaired survival. Japanese surgeons take into account the ICG metabolic rate (Makuuchi 1995), but we have recently shown that postoperative decompensation is mainly related to the presence of portal hypertension (Bruix et al. 1996). Accordingly, the criterion for indicating surgical resection is a well preserved liver function with normal portal pressure. Following this policy the 5-year survival may exceed 70%, the main drawback being the high disease recurrence rate, which exceeds 50% at 5 years (Franco et al. 1990; Shirabe et al. 1991; Bismuth et al. 1993; Izumi et al. 1994; Okada et al. 1994; Makuuchi 1995; Fuster et al. 1996). The presence of microscopic vascular invasion or additional nodules in the resected tissue implies a higher recurrence risk (Shirabe et al. 1991; Izumi et al. 1994; Okada et al. 1994, 1995; Fuster et al. 1996). Tumor size constituted a very important predictor some years ago, but the quality of the imaging techniques applied nowadays has reduced the potential risk of unrecognized additional tumor sites despite large tumor size, and this has led to tumor size no longer being such a major determinant of recurrence risk. Accordingly, there is no clear cut limit in terms of diameter. However, large tumors may require larger resections with an increased risk of liver failure. Thereby, the indication of surgery should also take into account the volume of functional liver to be resected (this being the volume of liver to be resected minus the volume corresponding to the HCC) and the functional liver that will remain after resection (Okamoto et al. 1984). Accordingly, the resection of a large solitary HCC occupying all the right lobe may be well tolerated since the proportion of functional liver that will be eliminated is minimal. The aforementioned pathological findings establish the risk of disease recurrence due to tumor cell dissemination prior to surgery. This will prompt most of the recurrences appearing early during follow-up, but the underlying cirrhosis should be considered a premalignant disease and new metachronic tumors may appear during follow-up at early, medium and long term.

Treatment of the tumor with chemoembolization prior to surgery has not shown any benefit (Sudan et al. 1998) and there are studies suggesting that this treatment may lead to more bleeding during the operation and even be associated with a higher recurrence rate (Nagasue et al. 1989).

There is no accepted treatment for preventing recurrence but a recent study has suggested that retinoid administration may be useful in this regard (Muto et al. 1996). Similarly, there is no unequivocal treatment of recurrence. If it appears as a solitary small nodule, the patients may benefit again from surgery (if they satisfy the previously mentioned criteria) or even from liver transplantation or ethanol injection. If radical options are not feasible, palliative options such as chemoembolization may be evaluated, but there are no data showing a potential impact on survival.

16.4.2 Orthotopic Liver Transplantation

At the beginning of the transplantation era, the results of orthotopic liver transplantation for HCC were extremely disappointing. Most of the transplanted patients were treated at an advanced stage and this was associated with a high early mortality, associated with an unacceptably high recurrence rate that impaired the medium to long term survival (Iwatsuki et al. 1985; O'Grady et al. 1988). However, later on it was shown that patients with tumors found incidentally during the orthotopic liver transplantation have a survival indistinguishable from cirrhotics without HCC (Yokoyama et al. 1991; Pichlmayer et al. 1995; Figueras et al. 1997) and it was demonstrated that recurrence rate was related to tumor stage (Ringe et al. 1989; Yokoyama et al. 1991; Bismuth et al. 1993; McPeake et al. 1993; Pichlmayer et al. 1995; Marsh et al. 1997). Therefore, those programs that continued to accept patients with HCC restricted the indication to patients with solitary small tumors, defined by solitary HCC ≤5 cm or up to three nodules each one less than 3 cm. This selection has been shown to provide excellent results in terms of recurrence and survival if the orthotopic liver transplantation is successfully performed (Mazzaferro et al. 1996; Llovet et al. 1998). From a practical point of view the main drawback of orthotopic liver transplantation is its applicability. There is a huge shortage of donors, and while waiting for the liver the HCC may progress and contraindicate the procedure (Pereira and Williams 1998). To avoid this event, some groups treat the patients in the waiting list with chemotherapy, chemoembolization or ethanol injection or other percutaneous approach (Bismuth et al. 1993; Stone et al. 1993; Figueras et al. 1997). Phase II trials have suggested a potential benefit of this policy, but it has been suggested that the main determinant of success is the application of restrictive criteria (Llovet et al. 1998), while treatment by itself would not change the evolution of the disease.

HCC recurrence after orthotopic liver transplantation is related to an advanced tumor stage, mainly reflected by macroscopic vascular invasion and extrahepatic spread. Interestingly, the application of the TNM classification (International Union Against Cancer 1997) has no predictive power since it does not accurately define the evolutionary stage of the HCC (Llovet et al. 1998). For example: a solitary tumor measuring 2 cm and showing vascular invasion would be classified as stage 2, while a patient having two small HCC foci <2 cm located in separate lobes and being potentially synchronic would be classified as stage 4.

Applying the previously mentioned inclusion criteria, the survival at 5 years is around 70%, which compares with the outcome after surgery in selected candidates. However, the recurrence rate after orthotopic liver transplantation is less and this may prompt some physicians to favor orthotopic liver transplantation before resection. Nevertheless, the decision between both options should take into account that the survival may be the same and that there may be differences in terms of quality of life (ZETTERMAN and MCCASHLAND 1995; NAVASA et al. 1996). Furthermore, most of the HCC patients will complicate cirrhosis of viral origin (BRUIX et al. 1989) and this may recur in the implanted liver, which may evolve to cirrhosis again (GANE et al. 1996; ARAYA et al. 1997). Thus, the benefits of orthotopic liver transplantation should be tempered and carefully evaluated.

16.4.3
Percutaneous Therapies

There are several techniques that can be used to treat tumoral nodules percutaneously under US, CT or MRI guidance, but the US guided injection of ethanol is the one that has been more widely used. It has been shown that small solitary nodules will be almost always completely necrosed and the survival of treated patients is the same as the survival of patients submitted to surgical resection if considering old series (CASTELLS et al. 1993; LIVRAGHI et al. 1995). However, since surgery allows the ablation of the main nodule and the surrounding satellites, surgical resection should be considered a better option than percutaneous ethanol injection (PEI) in carefully selected patients (BRUIX et al. 1996). In addition, the use of intraoperative US will prompt the detection and elimination of minute nodules not recognized by the preoperative staging, and this more complete treatment should result in an improvement in the long term results.

PEI is highly useful in tumors less than 3 cm in diameter (VILANA et al. 1992; ISHII et al. 1996). Above this limit, the tumors may have septa and the intratumoral diffusion of the ethanol is impaired. Injection of a larger ethanol volume, even under general anesthesia (LIVRAGHI et al. 1998), or the combination of ethanol injection with prior chemoembolization has been reported to increase the success rate (LENCIONI et al. 1998). However, this suggestion is based on the results of uncontrolled investigations and when critically compared with recent data about the natural history and prognosis of untreated non-surgical HCC (LLOVET et al., 1999), the benefits of the procedure are not evident. Probably, in some patients the treatment is able to completely necrose the HCC, but the evolution of the underlying liver disease and the appearance and progression of new tumor nodules may counteract the effects of the initially successful treatment, thus precluding the identification of a statistically significant benefit in survival. The treatment of patients with more than one tumor site is also controversial. If the nodules are smaller than 3 cm and correspond to synchronic neoplasm, the treatment may be successful, but the failure rate is increased and frequently the follow-up discloses additional tumor nests, while the impact in survival is not evident. PEI requires repeated injections and its success requires the diffusion of the ethanol within the HCC. Other agents such as boiling water (HONDA et al. 1994) or acetic acid (OHNISHI et al. 1998) may have a better tissue penetration. However, the management of boiling water is not as easy as that of ethanol, and the results obtained with acetic acid are not markedly better than those reported by several recognized groups when injecting ethanol. The most promising alternative to ethanol injection is the thermal ablation of the tumors by the use of radiofrequency. This more sophisticated technique does not require an intratumoral diffusion and with only one treatment session it is possible to achieve the complete necrosis of tumors exceeding 3 cm in size. Thus, this technique could substitute ethanol injection. However, it should be stressed that the economic cost of radiofrequency is higher, that tumors located in the vicinity of the gall bladder or near to the diaphragm cannot be treated, and that the complications rate and tolerance may be not as good as with ethanol injection. Accordingly, carefully designed studies should be performed to define its place.

16.4.4
Palliative Treatments

If the patients cannot benefit from radical treatment, they may be considered for therapies that will not eliminate the disease, but are expected to delay the appearance of complications related to tumor growth and to improve the survival of the patients. It is important to note that there is no evidence suggesting that any of the available options really improves survival (BRUIX 1997; TRINCHET and BEAUGRAND 1997) and, in addition, some of the therapeutic approaches will induce the appearance of symptoms in patients in whom the disease has not yet induced any clinical manifestation. Thus, the decision to apply an invasive treatment with unknown impact on survival should be carefully balanced by taking into account the likelihood of inducing transient or persistent side effects that may impair temporarily the quality of life of the patients. This consideration should be applied for any of the interventional therapeutic approaches that can be indicated in patients diagnosed at an advanced stage. This includes the selective injection of Lipiodol, coupled with chemotherapy (Kanematsu et al. 1989; Kalayci et al. 1990) or with I-131 (Raoul et al. 1997), transarterial embolization with (Group d'Etude et de Traitement de Carcinome Hepatocellulaire 1995) or without chemotherapy (Bruix et al. 1998), the external or internal radiation of the liver and even some non-interventional procedures such as conventional chemotherapy (Nerestone et al. 1986; Okada et al. 1992). Therefore, the present approach to the management of patients with HCC not suitable for radical treatment should be based on the careful application of therapeutic investigations aiming to define the usefulness of any of the available options. The value of the data produced by these investigations will depend on the quality of their design and for this purpose it is mandatory to take into account the natural history of the disease of untreated individuals. As stated previously, the time at which the diagnosis is achieved has been progressively advanced and, thus, the survival reported in studies published years ago is no longer useful to estimate the potential survival improvement due to a new therapeutic option. In addition, when defining the prognosis of the patients at HCC diagnosis we cannot use the results derived from the data of these old investigations (Okuda et al. 1985; Attali et al. 1987; Calvet et al. 1990; Stuart et al. 1996) in which most of the patients were diagnosed at advanced stages and/or had decompensated underlying liver disease. When reviewing the outcome of patients with small solitary HCC on compensated cirrhosis (Ebara et al. 1986; Cottone et al. 1989; Barbara et al. 1992; Livraghi et al. 1995), it becomes apparent that the concepts should also be revisited since the reported survival is less than that observed nowadays in patients diagnosed at intermediate stages (Llovet et al. 1998, in press). The observed improvement in survival of the patients diagnosed nowadays with HCC cannot be attributed merely to the advancement of the diagnosis since other major points may be relevant. The identification of the role of non-steroidal anti-inflammatory drugs in the development of renal failure in patients with cirrhosis (Arroyo et al. 1986) has eliminated its use in treating the pain frequently associated with the evolution of the HCC. Simultaneously, the diuretic treatment of sodium and water retention in these patients has been properly defined (Bataller et al. 1998) and in those presenting tense ascites it has been shown that paracentesis followed by albumin infusion is the treatment of choice, not having serious side effects. Similarly, the treatment of spontaneous bacterial peritonitis has also improved (Navasa et al. 1997). Until very recently, this complication was lethal, but with the administration of non-nephrotoxic antibiotics the infective episode may be solved and its recurrence may be prevented by the chronic administration of quinolones. Finally, some years ago variceal bleeding was a major cause of death without an effective treatment. The availability of drugs to control the bleeding episode and the development of endoscopic sclerotherapy has reduced the initial mortality due to bleeding (D'Amico et al. 1995) and, thus, expanded the survival of the patients. All these aspects prompted us recently to reevaluate the natural history of patients with untreated HCC diagnosed at an intermediate stage. As previously described, patients diagnosed at an early stage and amenable for surgery, transplantation or PEI/radiofrequency are not enrolled into randomized placebo controlled trials for obvious ethical reasons, but the lack of effective treatment for patients diagnosed at an intermediate stage prompted us to conduct randomized controlled trials to assess the benefits of transarterial embolization (Llovet et al. 1998) and of estrogen blockade (Castells et al. 1995). The patients included in these trials were selected according to a previously established schedule aiming to have a homogeneous population and to avoid patients with very poor prognosis in whom the treatment is unlikely to have an impact on survival. On the other hand they were not submitted to radical treatment because of their baseline conditions (usually advanced tumor stage) that contraindicated these procedures. Thus, the analysis of these untreated patients has provided not only the outcome that should be expected in patients diagnosed nowadays with HCC at an intermediate stage, but also the minimal survival that should be achieved in patients with HCC at an earlier stage who are submitted to invasive and risky procedures such as transplantation. In that regard, we have found that the 1-, 2- and 3-year survival of these patients is as high as 54%, 40% and 28%, respectively. Furthermore, the analysis of the prognostic factors of these untreated patients disclosed that the main predictors of the outcome are the presence of cancer related symptoms (constitutional syndrome, impairment of the performance status) and the existence of an aggressive tumor phenotype (evidenced by vascular invasion or extrahepatic spread). Therefore, the 3-year survival of the subgroup of patients without any adverse characteristic exceeds

50% while it is less than 10% in the subgroup having at least an adverse factor (LLOVET et al. 1999). It has to be emphasized that the impressive survival of the favorable group is the same or even better than the outcome of some of the published series of unselected patients with a theoretically well compensated liver disease submitted to surgical resection, or the outcome of some cohorts of patients with less advanced tumors submitted to transplantation. Furthermore, these figures also exceed the data of historical series describing the survival of untreated patients with small solitary HCC on compensated cirrhosis. Accordingly, in the present day the evaluation of the survival of patients with HCC at an intermediate stage entered into phase II trials to investigate options such as large volume ethanol injection, transarterial embolization followed by ethanol injection or the use of new antineoplastics should carefully analyze the characteristics of the patients to establish to which strata they belong and, thus, estimate their baseline life expectancy. Similarly, the calculation of the sample size of randomized control trials should be based on these recent survival data. Otherwise, the trials will be hampered by a severe type II error and their conclusions may not be realistic (SIMONETTI et al. 1997).

16.5 Summary

It has to be emphasized that several advances have been made during the last few years: the diagnosis can be achieved at stages at which some potentially useful options may be applied; their indication and application have been refined; and, finally, additional approaches, such as percutaneous treatment, are now available. In the next few years, new therapeutic modalities including gene therapy will be introduced. Their usefulness will have to be defined through well designed clinical trials, which will hopefully demonstrate an unequivocal improvement of the survival of the patients diagnosed with this so far devastating neoplasm.

References

Araya V, Rakela J, Wright T (1997) Hepatitis C after orthotopic liver transplantation. Gastroenterology 112:575–582

Arroyo V, Ginès P, Rimola A, et al (1986) Renal function abnormalities, prostaglandins, and effects of nonsteroidal anti-inflammatory drugs in cirrhosis with ascites. Am J Med 81:104–122

Attali P, Prod'Homme S, Pelletier G, et al (1987) Prognostic factors in patients with hepatocellular carcinoma. Attemps for selection of patients with prolonged survival. Cancer 45:2108–2111

Barbara L, Benzi G, Gaiani S, et al (1992) Natural history of small untreated hepatocellular carcinoma in cirrhosis: a multivariate analysis of prognostic factors of tumour growth rate and patient survival. Hepatology 16:132–137

Bataller R, Sort P, Ginés P, et al (1998) Hepatorenal syndrome: definition, pathophysiology, clinical features and management. Kidney Int 53:S47-S53

Bismuth H, Chiche L, Adam R, et al (1993) Liver resection versus transplantation for hepatocellular carcinoma in cirrhosis. Ann Surg 218:145–151

Borzio M, Bruno S, Roncalli M, et al (1995) Liver cell dysplasia is a major risk factor for hepatocellular carcinoma: a prospective study. Gastroenterology 108:812–817

Bruix J (1993) Diagnostico temprano del carcinoma hepatocellular: implicaciones clinicas. Med Clin (Barc) 100:228–234

Bruix J (1997) Treatment of hepatocellular carcinoma. Hepatology 25:259–262

Bruix J, Barrera JM, Calvet X, et al (1989) Prevalence of antibodies to hepatitis C virus in spanish patients with hepatocellular carcinoma and hepatic cirrhosis. Lancet 1004–1006

Bruix J, Castells A, Bru C (1991) Características clínicas y pronóstico del carcinoma hepatocelular. ¿Existen diferencias geográficas? Gastroenterol Hepatol 14:520–524

Bruix J, Castells A, Bru C (1992) Diagnosis and treatment of hepatocellular carcinoma. A western perspective. Cancer J 5:17–22

Bruix J, Castells A, Bosch J, et al (1996) Surgical resection of hepatocellular carcinoma in cirrhotic patients. Prognostic value of preoperative portal pressure. Gastroenterology 111:1018–1022

Bruix J, Llovet JM, Castells A, et al (1998) Transarterial embolization *versus* symptomatic treatment in patients with advanced hepatocellular carcinoma. Results of a randomizated controlled trial in a single institution. Hepatology 27:1578–1583

Calvet X, Bruix J, Ginés P, et al (1990) Prognostic factors of hepatocellular carcinoma in the West: a multivariate analysis in 206 patients. Hepatology 12:753–760

Castells A, Bruix J, Bru C, et al (1993) Treatment of small hepatocellular carcinoma in cirrhotic patients: a cohort study comparing surgical resection and percutaneous ethanol injection. Hepatology 18:1121–1126

Castells A, Bruix J, Bru C, et al (1995) Treatment of hepatocellular carcinoma with tamoxifen: a double-blind placebo-controlled trial in 120 patients. Gastroenterology 109:917–922

Collier J, Sherman M (1998) Screening for hepatocellular carcinoma. Hepatology 27:273–278

Colombo M, De Franchis R, Del Ninno E, et al (1991) Hepatocellular carcinoma in Italian patients with cirrhosis. N Eng J Med 325:675–680

Cottone M, Virdone R, Fusco G, et al (1989) Asymptomatic hepatocellular carcinoma in Child's A cirrhosis. A comparison of natural history and treatment. Gastroenterology 96:1566–1571

Cottone M, Turri M, Caltagirone M, et al (1994) Screening for hepatocellular carcinoma in patients with Child's A cirrhosis: an 8-year prospective study by ultrasound and alpha-fetoprotein. J Hepatol 21:1029–1034

D'Amico G, Pagliaro L, Bosch J (1995) The treatment of portal hypertension: a meta-analytic review. Hepatology 22:332–354

Ebara M, Ohto M, Shinagawa T, et al (1986) Natural history of hepatocellular carcinoma smaller than three centimeters complicating cirrhosis. A study in 22 patients. Gastroenterology 90:289–298

Elizalde JI, Castells A, Planas R, et al (1996) Prevalencia del carcinoma hepatocelular en pacientes cirróticos portadores de una derivación portosistémica. Análisis de cohortes. Gastroenterol Hepatol 19:189–193

Figueras J, Jaurrieta E, Valls C, et al (1997) Survival after liver transplantation in cirrhotic patients with and without hepatocellular carcinoma: a comparative study. Hepatology 25:1485–1489

Franco D, Capussotti L, Smadja C, et al (1990) Resection of hepatocellular carcinomas. Results in 72 European patients with cirrhosis. Gastroenterology 98:733–738

Fuster J, Garcia-Valdecasas JC, Grande L, et al (1996) Hepatocellular carcinoma and cirrhosis. Results of surgical treatment in a European series. Ann Surg 223:297–302

Gane E, Naoumov N, Qian K, et al (1996) A longitudinal analysis of hepatitis C virus replication following liver transplantation. Gastroenterology 110:167–177

Ganne-Carrie N, Castaign C, Chapel F, et al (1996) Preditive score for the development of hepatocelular carcinoma and additional value of liver large cell dysplasia in Western patients with cirrhosis. Hepatology 23:1112–1118

Group d'Etude et de Traitement de Carcinome Hepatocellulaire (1995) A comparison of lipiodol chemoembolization and conservative treatment for unresectable hepatocellular carcinoma. N Engl J Med 332:1256–1261

Honda N, Guo Q, Uchida H, et al (1994) Percutaneous hot saline injection therapy for hepatic tumors: an alternative to percutaneous ethanol injection therapy. Radiology 190:53–57

Ikeda K, Saitoh S, Koida I, et al (1993) A multivariate analysis of risk factors for hepatocellular carcinoma: a prospective observation of 795 patients with viral and alcoholic cirrhosis. Hepatology 18:47–53

International Union Against Cancer (UICC) (1997) TNM classification of malignant tumours, 5th edn. Sobin LH, Wittekind Ch (eds). New York, Wiley- Liss, pp 74–77

Ishii H, Okada S, Nose H, et al (1996) Local recurrence of hepatocellular carcinoma after percutaneous ethanol injection. Cancer 77:1792–1796

Iwatsuki S, Gordon RD, Shaw BW, et al (1985) Role of liver transplantation in cancer therapy. Ann Surg 202:401– 407

Izumi R, Shimizu K, Ii T, et al (1994) Prognostic factors of hepatocellular carcinoma in patients undergoing hepatic resection. Gastroenterology 106:720–727

Johnson PJ, Williams R (1987) Cirrhosis and the aetiology of hepatocellular carcinoma. J Hepatol 4:140–147

Kalayci C, Johnson PJ, Raby N et al (1990) Intrarterial adriamycin and lipiodol for inoperable hepatocellular carcinoma: a comparison with intravenous adriamycin. J Hepatol 11:349–353

Kanematsu T, Furuta T, Takenaka K, et al (1989) A 5-year experience of lipiodolization: selective regional chemotherapy for 200 patients with hepatocellular carcinoma. Hepatology 10:98–102

Lencioni R, Paolicchi A, Moretti M, et al (1998) Combined transcatheter arterial embolization and percutaneous ethanol injection for the treatment of large hepatocellular carcinoma: local therapeutic effect and long-term survival rate. Eur Radiol 8:439–444

Liaw YF, Tai DI, Chu C, et al (1986) Early detection of hepatocellular carcinoma in patients with chronic type B hepatitis. Gastroenterology 90:263–267

Livraghi T, Bolondi L, Buscarini L, et al (1995) No treatment, resection and ethanol injection in hepatocellular carcinoma: a retrospective analysis of survival in 391 patients with cirrhosis. J Hepatol 22:522–526

Livraghi T, Benedini V, Lazzaroni S, et al (1998) Long term results of single session percutaneous ethanol injection in patients with large hepatocellular carcinoma. Cancer 83:48–57

Llovet JM, Bruix J, Fuster J, et al (1998) Liver transplantation for treatment of small hepatocellular carcinoma: the TNM classification does not have prognostic power. Hepatology 27:1572–1577

Llovet JM, Bustamante J, Castells A, et al (1999) Natural history of untreated non-surgical hepatocellular carcinoma: rationale for the design and evaluation of therapeutic trials. Hepatology 29:62-67

Makuuchi M (1995) Surgical treatment for hepatocellular carcinoma. In: Arroyo V, Bosch J, Rodés J (eds) Treatments in Hepatology. Masson, Barcelona, pp 341–352

Marsh W, Dvorchik I, Subotin M, et al (1997) The prediction of risk of recurrence and time to recurrence of hepatocellular carcinoma after orthotopic liver transplantation: a pilot study. Hepatology 26:444–450

Mazzaferro V, Regalia E, Doci R, et al (1996) Liver transplantation for treatment of small hepatocellular carcinomas in patients with cirrhosis. N Engl J Med 334:693–699

McPeake JR, O'Grady JG, Zaman S, et al (1993) Liver transplantation for primary hepatocellular carcinoma: tumor size and number determine outcome. J Hepatol 18:226–234

Mehta R (1995) The potential for the use of cell proliferation and oncogene expression as intermediate markers during liver carcinogenesis. Cancer Lett 93:85–102

Muto Y, Moriwaki H, Ninomiya M, et al (1996) Prevention of secondary primary tumors by an acyclic retinoid, polyprenoic acid, in patients with hepatocellular carcinoma. N Eng J Med 334:1561–1567

Nagasue N, Galizia G, Kohno H, et al (1989) Adverse effects of preoperative hepatic artery chemoembolization for resectable hepatocellular carcinoma: a retrospective comparison of 138 liver resections. Surgery 106:81–86

Nakashima T, Kojiro M (1987) Hepatocellular Carcinoma. Springer Verlag, Tokyo

Navasa M, Forns X, Sánchez V, et al (1996) Quality of life, major medical complications and hospital service utilization in patients with primary biliary cirrhosis after liver transplantation. J Hepatol 25:129–134

Navasa M, Rimola A, Rodés J (1997) Bacterial infections in liver disease. Sem Liv Dis 17:323–333

Nerenstone SR, Ihde DC, Friedman MA (1986) Clinical trials in primary hepatocellular carcinoma: current status and future directions. Cancer Treat Rev 15:1–31

O'Grady JG, Polson RJ, Rolles K, et al (1988) Liver transplantation for malignant disease. Results in 93 consecutive patients. Ann Surg 207:373–379

Ohnishi K, Yoshioka H, Ito S, et al (1998) Prospective randomized controlled trial comparing percutaneous acetic acid injection and percutaneous ethanol injection for small hepatocellular carcinoma. Hepatology 27:67–72

Okada S, Okazaki N, Nose H, et al (1992) Prognostic factors in patients with hepatocellular carcinoma receiving systemic chemotherapy. Hepatology 16:112–117

Okada S, Shimada K, Yamamoto J, et al (1994) Predictive factors for postoperative recurrence of hepatocellular carcinoma. Gastroenterology 106:1618–1624

Okamoto E, Kyo A, Yamanaka N, et al (1984) Prediction of the safe limits of hepatectomy by combined volumetric and functional measurements in patients with impaired hepatic function. Surgery 95:586–592

Okazaki N, Yoshino M, Yoshida T, et al (1988) Evaluation of the prognosis for small hepatocellular carcinoma based on tumor volume doubling time. Cancer 83:2207–2210

Okuda K (1986) Early recognition of hepatocellular carcinoma. Hepatology 6:729–738

Okuda K (1992) Hepatocellular carcinoma: recent progress. Hepatology 15:948–963

Okuda K, Ohtsuki T, Obata H, et al (1985) Natural history of hepatocellular carcinoma and prognosis in relation to treatment. Cancer 56:918–928

Pereira SP, Williams R (1998) Limits to liver transplantation in the UK. GUT 42:883–885

Pichlmayr R, Weimann A, Oldhafer KJ, et al (1995) Role of liver transplantation in the treatment of unresectable liver cancer. World J Surg 19:807–813

Poynard T, Aubert A, Lazizi Y, et al (1991) Independent risk factors for hepatocellular carcinoma in french drinkers. Hepatology 13:896–90

Pugh RNH, Murray-Lyon IM, Dawson JL, et al (1973) Transection of the oesophagus for bleeding oesophageal varices. Br J Surg 60:646–664

Raoul JL, Guyader D, Bretagne JF, et al (1997) Prospective randomized controlled trial of chemoembolization versus intra-arterial injection of 131-I-labeled iodized oil in the treament of hepatocellular carcinoma. Hepatology 26:1156–1161

Ringe B, Wittekind C, Bechstein WO, et al (1989) The role of liver transplantation in hepatobiliary malignancy. Ann Surg 209:88–98

Sarasin FP, Giostra E, Hadengue A (1996) Cost-effectiveness of screening for detection of small hepatocelular carcinoma in Western patients with Child-Pugh class A cirrhosis. Am J Med 17:422–434

Sato Y, Nakata K, Kato Y, et al (1993) Early recognition of hepatocellular carcinoma based on altered profiles of alphafetoprotein. N Eng J Med 328:1802–1806

Sherman M, Peltekian KM, Lee C (1995) Screening for hepatocellular carcinoma in chronic carriers of hepatitis B virus: incidence and prevalence of hepatocellular carcinoma in a north american urban population. Hepatology 22:432–438

Sheu JC, Sung JL, Chen DS, et al (1985) Growth rate of asymptomatic hepatocellular carcinoma and its clinical implications. Gastroenterology 89:259–266

Shibata M, Morizane T, Uchida T, et al (1998) Irregular regeneration of hepatocytes and risk of hepatocellular carcinoma in chronic hepatitis and cirrhosis with hepatitis C virus infection. Lancet 351:1773–1777

Shirabe K, Kanematsu T, Matsumata T, et al (1991) Factors linked to early recurrence of small hepatocellular carcinoma after hepatectomy:univariate and multivariate analysis. Hepatology 14:802–805

Simonetti RG, Liberati A, Angiolini C, et al (1997) Treatment of hepatocellular carcinoma: a systematic review of randomized controlled trials. Ann Oncol 8:117–136

Sorensen JB, Klee M, Palshof T, et al (1993) Performance status assessment in cancer patients. An inter-observer variability study. Br J Cancer 67:773–775

Stone MJ, Klintmalm GB, Polter D, et al (1993) Neoadjuvant chemotherapy and liver transplantation for hepatocellular carcinoma: a pilot study in 20 patients. Gastroenterology 104:196–202

Stuart KE, Anand AJ, Jenkins RL (1996) Hepatocellular carcinoma in the United States. Prognostic features, treatment outcome, and survival. Cancer 77:2217–22

Sudan D, Sudan R, Schafer D, et al (1998) Without victory there is no survival: transarterial lipiodol chemoembolization and hepatocellular carcinoma. Hepatology 28:270–271

Takano S, Yokosuka O, Imazeki K, et al (1995) Incidence of hepatocellular carcinoma in chronic hepatitis B and C: a prospective study of 251 patients. Hepatology 21:650–655

Taketa K (1990) Alpha-fetoprotein: reevaluation in hepatology. Hepatology 12:1420–1432

Tang ZY, Yang BH (1985) Early detection of subclinical hepatocellular carcinoma. In: Tang ZY (ed) Subclinical hepatocellular carcinoma.Springer Verlag, Berlin, pp 12–21

Tang ZY, Bing-Hui Y (1989) Further evaluation of alpha-fetoprotein as tumor marker for hepatocellular carcinoma – with special reference to subclinical cancer. In: Tang ZY, Wu MC, Xia SS (eds) Primary Liver Cancer. China Academic Publishers, Beijing and Springer Verlag, Berlin, pp 239–246

Trinchet JC, Beaugrand M (1997) Treatment of hepatocellular carcinoma in patients with cirrhosis. J Hepatol 27:756–765

Tsukuma H, Hiyama T, Tanaka S, et al (1993) Risk factors for hepatocellular carcinoma among patients with chronic liver disease. N Eng J Med 328:797–801

Vilana R, Bruix J, Brú C, et al (1992) Tumor sizes determines the efficacy of percutaneous ethanol injection for treatment of small hepatocellular carcinoma. Hepatology 16:353–357

Weitz IC, Liebman HA (1993) Des-gamma-carboxy (abnormal) prothrombin and hepatocellular carcinoma: a critical review. Hepatology 18:990–997

Yokoyama I, Todo S, Iwatsuki S, et al (1990) Liver transplantation in the treatment of primary liver cancer. Hepatogastroenterology 37:188–193

Yokoyama I, Sheahan DG, Carr B, et al (1991) Clinicopathologic factors affecting patient survival and tumor recurrence after orthotopic liver transplantation for hepatocellular carcinoma. Transplant Proc 23:2194–2196

Zetterman RK, McCashland TM (1995) Long-term follow-up of the orthotopic liver transplantation patient. Semin Liv Dis 15:173–180

17 Transcatheter Arterial Chemoembolization of Hepatocellular Carcinoma

A. Roche

CONTENTS

17.1 Introduction

Hepatocellular carcinoma (HCC) is associated with liver cirrhosis in 80% of cases and when the tumor is diagnosed, the very poor hepatic function, due to the underlying liver disease, is so frequent that extended surgical resection is contraindicated in most cases. Because of the poor prognosis of nonresectable HCC, an aggressive approach is justified. Systemic or intraarterial chemotherapy has been used for years but has such a poor objective response rate in any of the large reported series that it has almost been abandoned. At the same time, the treatment of HCC by transcatheter arterial embolization (TAE) of the hepatic artery (Roche 1978) and then by combination of occlusion and regional chemotherapy (transcatheter hepatic arterial chemoembolization, TACE) has been investigated and developed since the 1970s. In the early 1980s, the ability of Lipiodol to selectively target hepatic tumors when injected intraarterially was reported by Japanese authors and developed as a complementary therapeutic tool; and nowadays transcatheter hepatic arterial treatments such as TAE, TACE, Lipiodol-TACE (L-TACE) or Lipiodol chemotherapy (L-TAC) play an important role in the therapeutic management of HCC.

17.2 Rationale

Most of the blood supply to hepatic tumors is derived from the hepatic artery. Consequently, the basic concept of TACE is to deliver a high dose of chemotherapeutic agents directly to the liver, since arterial obstruction results in extensive tumor necrosis caused by ischemia. The advantage of TACE administration of an anticancer agent as compared with its systemic infusion lies in its first pass effect. For this reason, the more elevated the total body clearance of the therapeutic agent is, the more arguments there are to use it intraarterially. Moreover, this advantage is proportional to the extraction coefficient of the drug. Finally, it is also reversely proportional to the blood flow of the artery in which it is infused.

The main goals of TACE are:

- Tumor necrosis after ischemia induced by embolization

A. Roche, MD; Professor, Interventional Radiology Section, Institut Gustav-Roussy, 39 rue Camille Desmoulins, F-94800 Villejuif, France

- Increased drug concentration into the tumor by selective arterial injection intensified by the arterial flow slow-down induced by embolization (decreased washout and increased contact duration). An intraarterial injection may raise up to 20 times the local drug concentration that would be obtained from an i.v. injection and embolization allows a threefold increase in tumoral doxorubicin concentration from an hepatic artery injection (SIGURDSON et al. 1986)
- A theoretically increased efficiency of certain drugs (doxorubicin, mitomycin) in ischemic tumors
- Better hepatic clearance of the drug resulting in a diminution of systemic concentrations. For instance, 5-FU and doxorubicin have extraction rates of 90% and 60% respectively, leading to lower systemic concentrations in spite of an increased tumoral exposure to the anticancer agent (Table 17.1).

Table 17.1. Pharmacokinetic characteristics of the main anticancer drugs

Drug	Total body clearance (l/min)	Hepatic extraction (%)
Adriamycin	0.4	20–60
Cisplatin	0.3–0.5	0
5-FU	2.5	50–80
Mitomycin	0.6	4–18
Fluxoridin	2.8	90
Streprozotocin	0.4	5

17.3 Techniques

17.3.1 Perioperative Management

Good pre- and postoperative i.v. hydration must be carried out to prevent nephrotoxicity from contrast media, chemotherapeutic drugs and uric acid formation from tumoral necrosis. TACE must be done under hemodynamic monitoring. Arterial blood pressure, pulse rate, oxygen saturation and cardioscope monitoring are followed. Neuroleptanalgesia, prior to TACE, may be obtained with i.v. fentanyl and midazolam. Some authors have reported that intraarterial administration of lidocaine, just prior to and during TACE, permitted a marked reduction in the amount of narcotic analgesia (MOLGAARD et al. 1990).

Hospitalization, after chemoembolization, averages 72 h while liver function tests, creatinine and complete blood count are monitored daily. Patients generally receive 3 l of intravenous fluid a day. Analgesics and anti-inflammatory drugs are routinely given to minimize the post-embolization syndrome and broad-spectrum antibiotics are given intravenously during hospitalization, starting just before the procedure and maintained for 5 days. A morphine sulfate drip infusion may be required in some patients to achieve complete postprocedural pain control.

17.3.2 Catheterization and Injections

Initial angiography is performed for each session, in order to evaluate hepatic portal perfusion, arterial feeders of the tumor(s), portal and hepatic vein tumor thrombus, arterio-portal shunt, esophageal varices and portal hypertension signs. After placement of a 5F sheath, hepatic arteriography and superior mesenteric arterial portography are performed with a 4 or 5F catheter. The same catheter is generally used for both angiography and treatment unless technical difficulties prevent selective catheterization, in which case a coaxial 3F micro-catheter system is used. Hydrophilic polymer-coated guidewires and catheters account to a large extent for the success of selective catheterization, whatever the anatomical or hemodynamic situation is.

In each appropriate artery, an emulsion of the anticancer drug in Lipiodol is first injected; the emboles are then pushed until blood flow is at least slowed down. When multiple tumors are disseminated in both lobes, the treatment may be given into the proper hepatic artery, distal to the gastroduodenal artery origin. In the case of single tumor or small HCC, the catheterization and the treatment should be superselective. Whenever the hepatic artery is occluded, an attempt must be made to catheterize extrahepatic collaterals eventually supplying the liver.

Multiple sessions are generally recommended, the rhythm of which differs in the literature from a systematic cure every 2 months to treatment only on request when the tumor grows or markers increase.

17.3.3 Anatomy

17.3.3.1 Variations in Arterial Supply

The high frequency (close to 50%) of *accessory hepatic arteries*, arising from the superior mesenteric artery, the left gastric, as well as from the gastroduodenal or the aorta, is well known. When selective catheterization of such a branch is found to be time consuming, it may be useful to ligate it with coils for redistribution at the end of the first session of TACE. Thus, proximal endovascular ligation of a replaced left hepatic artery originating from the left gastric may be a useful maneuver, as its repeated selective catheterization frequently proves to be uncertain.

When the proper hepatic artery is occluded, hepatic vascularization is assumed by *collateral circulation*, which is to be systematically explored: duodenal pancreatic, inferior phrenic, left gastric, intercostal, lumbar, internal mammary arteries (Fig. 17.1).

When developing in a subcapsular and extraperitoneal area of the liver, hypervascular HCC may be spontaneously partially vascularized by some posterior parietal pedicles (mainly inferior phrenic artery) for the dorsal and internal territory of the right lobe (segments VI or VII) (Xu and Yan 1993), or by the superior phrenic artery (terminal branch of the internal mammary) for the anterior and cranial territories (mainly segments IV and III) (Kim et al. 1995). When the tumor is so located in the liver, these arteries should be systematically assessed each time tumor filling by Lipiodol looks incomplete on CT after L-TACE via the proper hepatic artery (Fig. 17.2). One should also pay attention to these arteries when biological and morphological responses are still incomplete despite apparently complete treatment of the tumor via the hepatic artery alone.

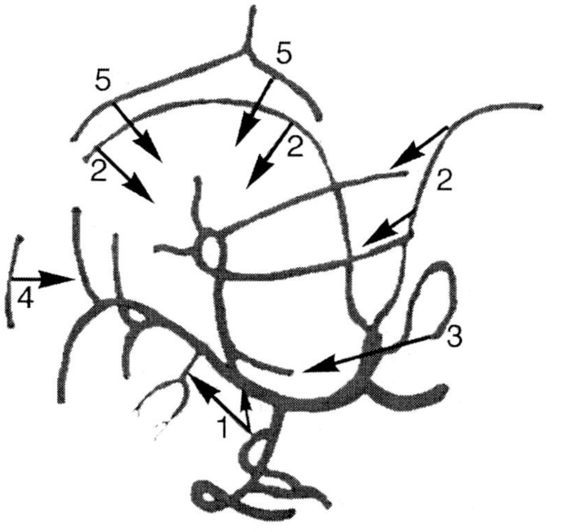

a

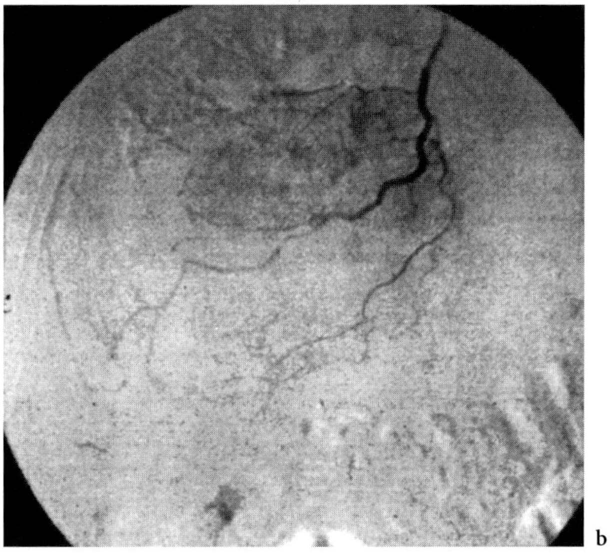

b

Fig. 17.1a,b. Collateral circulations for the liver. **a** Schematic representation of main collateral circulation sources for the liver: duodenal pancreatic (*1*), inferior phrenic (*2*), left gastric (*3*), intercostal and lumbar (*4*), internal mammary (*5*). **b** Right internal mammary artery participating in the vascularization of subcapsular cranial and anterior HCC nodules

17.3.3.2 Extrahepatic Branches of the Hepatic Artery

The hepatic artery gives more or less constant extrahepatic branches. The cystic artery generally arises from the right hepatic, but may also originate from the left hepatic, in almost 10% of cases. The right gastric artery originates from the proper hepatic (50%) or the left or middle hepatic artery (45%), but it originates from the right hepatic artery in 5% of cases. Each time it looks atraumatic to catheterize the hepatic arteries downstream from the cystic and/or the gastric arteries before therapeutic injection, one should do this, in order to totally avoid gallbladder or gastric complication.

In 11% of cases, several duodenal branches originate from the hepatic artery downstream from the origin of the gastroduodenal and the supraduodenal artery; commonly the first main branch of the gastroduodenal originates from the proper or the right hepatic artery in 4% of cases. As it gives important feeders to the common bile duct as well as for the duodenum and the pancreas, TACE must be delivered downstream from its origin.

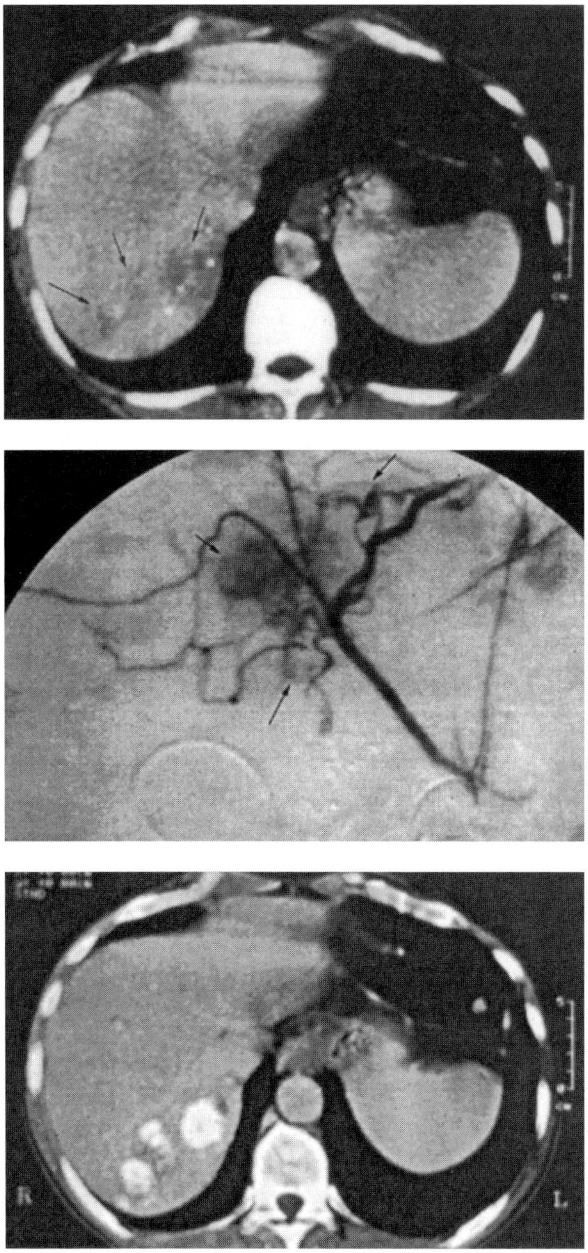

a b c

Fig. 17.2a–c. Subcapsular posterior HCC mainly fed by an extra hepatic artery. The tumor, (*arrows*), presents a very poor Lipiodol uptake on CT control (**a**) 3 weeks after the first L-TACE via the hepatic artery. During the second session, opacification of the right inferior phrenic artery (**b**) showed that it massively participated in tumor vascularization (*arrows*). After complementary L-TACE via the inferior phrenic artery, tumor Lipiodol uptake appeared satisfactory (**c**)

An accessory left gastric artery may originate from the left hepatic artery, at the upper part of the hepatic ligament (Fig. 17.3). This variation occurs in 3% and 15%, respectively, of the Caucasian and Asian population. It explains some gastric complications after TACE despite apparently selective hepatic catheterization. Exceptionally a dilated hepatic falciform artery, arising from the left hepatic artery, may be demonstrated. It should then be ligated by endovascular maneuvers prior to TACE, to prevent a possible supraumbilical skin rash

All these extrahepatic branches (including the gastroduodenal artery) may be protected against adverse effects of TACE by previous endovascular liga-

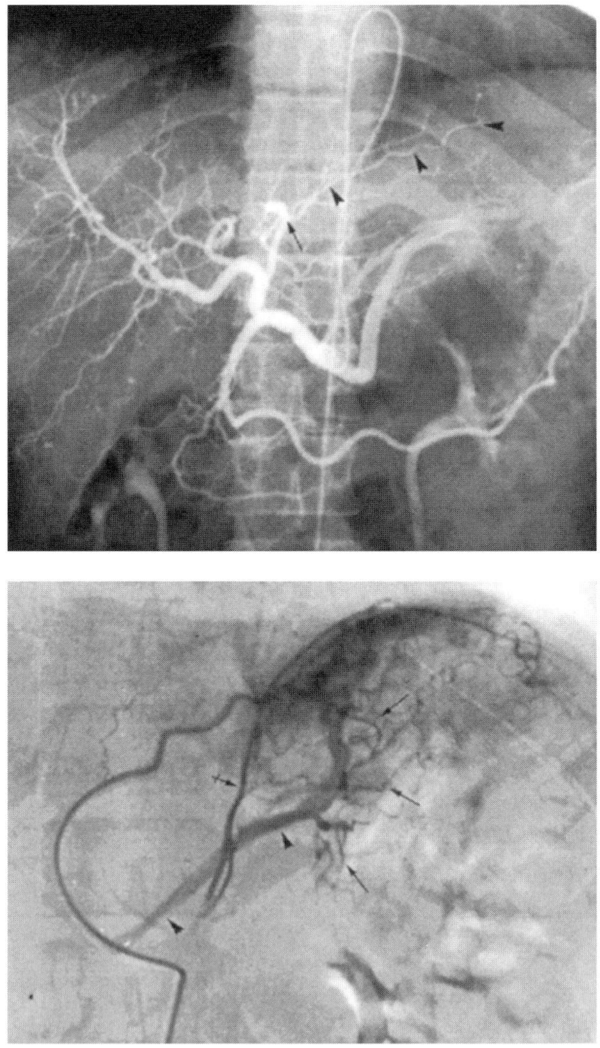

a b

Fig. 17.3a,b. Accessory gastric artery originating from the left hepatic artery. This anatomical variation must be identified before treatment. **a** The gastric accessory artery (*arrowheads*) originates from the distal portion of the left hepatic (*arrow*). Selective opacification (**b**) shows its territory (upper fundus), drainage in the left gastric vein (*arrowheads*), and anastomosis with the left gastric artery territory (*arrows*) and the left inferior phrenic (*crossed arrow*) participating in the vascularization of the cardia tion with coils or microcoils when, for any reason, the therapeutic liver infusion has to be performed upstream to their origin.

17.3.3.3 Hemodynamics

Under various pathologic conditions leading to an increased demand for arterial supply to the liver, such as very hypervascular HCC, arteriovenous shunting, and associated low intrahepatic portal blood perfusion, the direction of flow in the gastroduodenal artery may reverse to a hepatopetal direction, acting as collateral supply to the liver.

Celiac trunk stenosis or compression by the median arcuate ligament is encountered in about 10% of patients. When it occurs, the superior mesenteric artery provides a blood supply to the liver, the stomach and the spleen through the pancreatic vessels and there is a reversal of blood flow in the common hepatic artery as well as in the gastroduodenal artery.

In these situations, catheterization with coaxial microcatheters, generally via the superior mesenteric artery, is mandatory for safely and selectively treating the liver (Okazaki et al. 1993) (Fig. 17.4).

17.3.4 Segmental Lipiodol Chemoembolization

Segmental or subsegmental L-TACE is confined to the tumoral area after selective catheterization. It is considered more efficacious upon the tumor, mainly because – due to more or less wedge therapeutic injections – Lipiodol-induced ischemia and chemotherapy concern the local portal radicles as well as the feeding arteries. Drug delivery to the tumor and portal filling may be enhanced by simultaneous temporary occlusion of the corresponding hepatic vein with a balloon catheter (Okazaki et al. 1997). Complete tumor filling with Lipiodol can be achieved along subsegmental L-TACE in more than 70% of patients, which is much more than after conventional transcatheter treatment, where it is obtained in about one-third of cases. It presents very few short term complications and none of liver function deterioration that may be associated with administration of L-TACE in the whole liver (Matsui et al. 1993; Ohno et al. 1994). Nevertheless, its indications are limited to small and still asymptomatic tumors that are discovered along systematic screening programs, and are broadly the same as those of segmental resection and percutaneous ablation techniques.

17.3.5 Drugs

Regardless of regimen, systemic chemotherapy very rarely gives in excess of a 30% response rate and does not affect survival. It has also been reported that doxorubicin, one of the potentially most active drugs in HCC under i.v. administration, led to fatal complications due to cardiotoxicity in 18% of patients. Lack of effects of chemotherapy might be caused by the expression of multidrug resistance gene, abnormal p53 function, tumor heterogeneity and/or poor delivery of the drug to the target. Consequently, TACE has to deal with poor effective chemotherapeutic tools and must take care of possibly severe general and hepatic adverse effects. Doxorubicin and cisplatin are the two most frequently used drugs for TACE. In the literature, doxorubicin has been reported as being associated with less necrosis and survival than cisplatin (Kasugai et al. 1989; Majno et al. 1997), and for these authors, cisplatin is routinely preferred, except when renal failure is present. To minimize the general side-effects, the recommended dose/session and total maximum dose are generally the same as for systemic administration. Some have used higher doses (Nakamura et al. 1990) that were well-tolerated but did not significantly improve the results.

The rationale for adding chemotherapy to embolization is theoretically evident. However, a randomized study failed to demonstrate any enhancement of the therapeutic effect when adding cisplatin to TAE (Chang et al. 1994).

17.3.6 Embolization

Many embolic materials are available but Gelfoam fragments are generally preferred because a beneficial recanalization occurs after 3–4 weeks, allowing repeated sessions by the same main pedicles. Ivalon causes more durable vascular occlusion and is responsible for flow redistribution into collateral vessels. Considering the so-called "normal" parenchyma, the less it is perfused by the portal vein, the less aggressively it should be embolized via the artery. Regarding the intensity of the induced ischemia, the most important parameter of the embolization material is the particle size. The smaller it is,

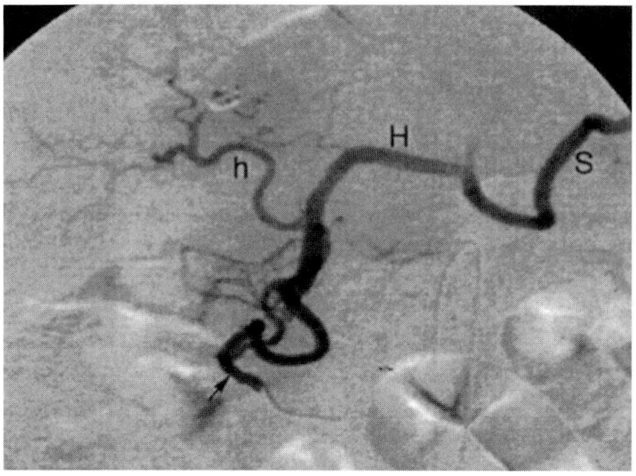

a

Fig. 17.4a–e. L-TACE in a patient with celiac trunk stenosis due to the arcuate ligament. **a** The superior mesenteric artery provides blood supply to the liver and the spleen; catheterization of a duodenal pancreatic artery (*arrow*) (*S*, splenic artery; *H*, common hepatic artery; *h*, right hepatic artery); hypervascular HCC of the right lobe (**b**) (*arrows*). **c** Selective catheterization of the right hepatic artery via a duodenal-pancreatic arcade with a coaxial microcatheter. Initial CT showing the tumor (*arrows*) (**d**) and control 8 years later (**e**)

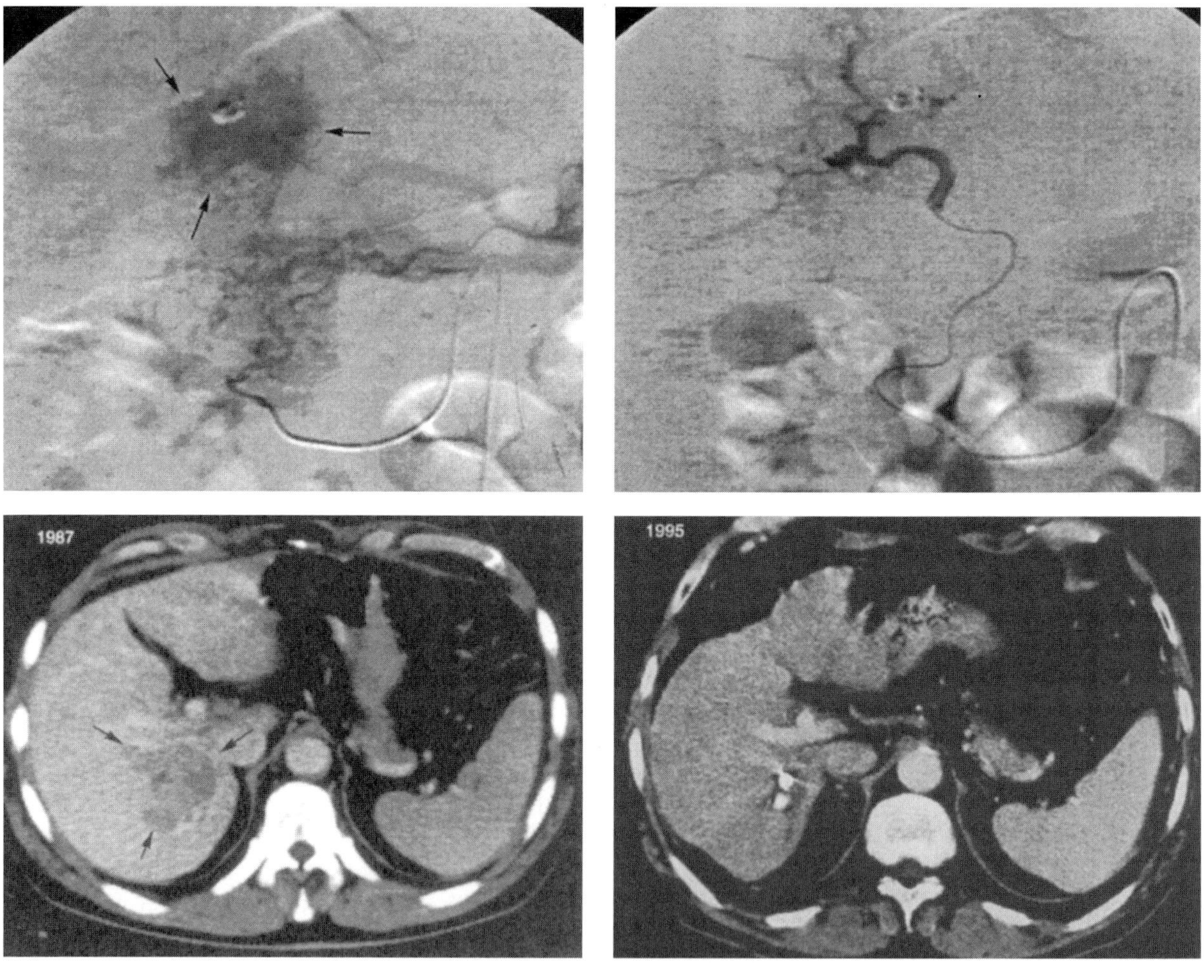

b c d e

the more distally the occlusion will be located and the less the collateral circulation will develop. One- to 5-mm Gelfoam particles, which have been soaked in contrast medium, are embolized into the artery until a markedly diminished flow is observed. Particle size and arterial slow-down intensity (as evaluated under fluoroscopy) are adapted to the status of the hepatic portal perfusion, being less aggressive (larger particles and lesser degree of arterial slow-down) in cases of poor hepatic portal perfusion. Consequently, Gelfoam powder is generally avoided for embolizing the whole liver in cirrhotic patients, in whom it is responsible for a 17% early mortality rate (Stuart et al. 1993). On the other hand,

Gelfoam powder may – or even should – be used when hyperselective catheterization of the tumor feeders can be achieved, so that the nontumoral parenchyma will not be affected by ischemia. In patients with advanced cirrhosis, some authors have proposed using autologous clot as an embolizing agent, in order to minimize the adverse effects of ischemia upon the liver parenchyma (GUNJI et al. 1992).

Coils are generally used to perform endovascular ligations, either to protect an extra-hepatic branch from TACE or to redistribute the liver arterial supply. Coils are generally contraindicated as embolic material for TACE itself since it produces proximal ligation of the hepatic artery, which induces almost no ischemia but massive development of collateral pathways that will impede later sessions (as well as surgical ligation).

Embolization has been considered to be an efficient treatment in HCC since the 1970s (ROCHE et al. 1978). Recently, in a prospective trial, the 1-year survival rate after L-TACE (86.3%) proved to be superior to survival after L-TAC (65.9%) (HATANAKA et al. 1995). BRUIX et al. (1998) assessed the effects of transarterial embolization (Gelfoam particles ± proximal coils) on the survival of patients with nonresectable HCC. Patients were randomized to embolization or symptomatic treatment. Fifty-five percent of the embolized group exhibited a partial response, resulting in a significantly lower probability of tumor progression during follow-up. Each time the patient does not present any of the contraindications for embolization, it should therefore be part of the transcatheter arterial treatment.

17.3.7 Lipiodol and Emulsions

17.3.7.1 Lipiodol

Fixation of Lipiodol in hypervascular tumors after intraarterial injection has been demonstrated for many years. It was first used as a diagnostic tool, due to this property of targeting and remaining fixed in tumors. Its kinetics have been studied by MILLER et al. (1987), who demonstrated Lipiodol deposition in tumoral and peritumoral vessels as well as its migration across the vessel wall to come and persist into close contact to the tumoral cells. The increased permeability of neoplastic vessels, and the absence of reticulo-endothelial cells inside the tumors, may explain these phenomena.

When injected into the arteries of the liver, Lipiodol has *four major effects*:

1. Lipiodol is preferentially uptaken in tumor tissue with ratios between Lipiodol in tumor/Lipiodol in healthy liver equal to 4.3–3.6 in hepatocarcinoma (RAOUL et al. 1988). This fixation lasts much longer in the tumor than in the healthy liver, with Lipiodol penetrating the tumor cells
2. Lipiodol slows down the arterial circulation. Indeed, Lipiodol acts as a plastic embolic agent, adjusting itself to the size of the vessels it must go through, to such an extent that it enters the portal circulation. This embolic effect is temporary, so that any Lipiodol which is not fixed in the tumor tissue finally exits via the capillaries into the hepatic vein system
3. Through the presinusoidal arterio-portal anastomosis, the Lipiodol reaches the portal veins (KAN et al. 1993), and its pharmacokinetic benefit and efficacy are at least partially ascribed to this ability to penetrate both the arterial and the portal supply of tumors (KAN 1996). As it reaches the portal system, it induces transient portal hypertension (SATO et al. 1993), and particular attention should be paid to cirrhotic patients with a potential risk of bleeding due to grade III or IV esophageal varices
4. It has a vascular selectivity for large (and mainly tumoral) arteries (DE BAÈRE et al. 1995).

When injected into arteries, emulsions of Lipiodol and anticancer drugs have demonstrated a pharmacokinetic benefit as compared to drug alone (NAKAMURA et al. 1989; FUKUSHIMA et al. 1992).This benefit can be due to either of the effects of Lipiodol. The slowing down of the blood flow definitely increases the duration of contact between drug and tumors. The associated portal infusion as well as the tumor selectivity of Lipiodol might also favorably influence drug targeting. Most authors claim that the addition of Lipiodol contributes to prolonging survival (UCHIDA et al. 1993). Clinically, the 1-year survival rate of hepatocarcinomas treated with a Lipiodol/doxorubicin emulsion is correlated with Lipiodol uptake in tumors (VAN BEERS et al. 1989) although Lipiodol has not been demonstrated to have any antitumor properties (TAKAYASHU et al. 1987). Massive uptake of Lipiodol by the tumor seems to be associated with a lower local recurrence rate (MATSUI et al. 1993; MURAKAMI et al. 1994). In a randomized trial, YOSHIKAWA et al. (1994) demonstrated that infusion of Lipiodol/drug emulsion for treatment of HCC was significantly more effective on response rate and survival than the drug alone. The 4-year survival of HCC is higher for patients treated with L-TACE (13%) than with TACE (3.4%) (NAKAMURA et al. 1994). Nevertheless, some reports are conflicting, showing equal survival in patients who do not receive Lipiodol (HATANAKA et al. 1995).

17.3.7.2
Emulsions

Anticancer agents can be theoretically mixed with Lipiodol under three main categories: suspension, solution or emulsion. Manual suspension of drug powder into Lipiodol does not allow homogeneous and safe repartition of drug in the mixture. Very few anticancer drugs are liposoluble and efficient drugs against HCC cannot be easily solubilized in Lipiodol. Consequently, emulsion is generally preferred and intraarterial injection of emulsions of Lipiodol with drugs is nowadays widely used for the treatment of liver tumors.

Selectivity and hemodynamic properties of Lipiodol depend on the type of emulsion one uses. For instance, the ratio between uptake in the lung and in the lung plus liver is 49% and 19% respectively for pure Lipiodol and water-in-oil emulsions (DE BAÈRE et al. 1996a). On the basis of experimental studies (DE BAÈRE et al. 1995, 1996a), one should be warned about the use of small-droplet oil-in-water emulsions that have a low embolic effect, high lung uptake and a low ratio of tumor to nontumorous liver uptake. On the contrary, large-droplet water-in-oil emulsions provide the best uptake of iodized oil by the tumor and induce a massive slow-down of the arterial flow. It is also to be noted that water-in-oil emulsions produce the strongest and, from a therapeutic point of view, the most attractive embolic effect on the portal system (DE BAÈRE et al. 1998).

Moreover, in water-in-oil emulsions, drug droplets are protected in the Lipiodol until they are released from Lipiodol when they reach arteries of an equivalent size. Consequently, a certain degree of vascular targeting for the drug can be expected from the emulsion when the size of the drug droplets corresponds to the diameter of targeted vessels (DE BAÈRE et al. 1995).

When mixing the two phases (oil and drug) without any particular precaution, one obtains a random direction of emulsion (either water-in-oil or oil-in-water) and no definite droplet size. Some precautions are needed to *prepare the most efficient emulsion* for TACE with the conventional pumping method, drug-in-Lipiodol with a size of drug droplets from 30 to 120 μm:

1 Water phase volume must be smaller than oily phase volume. Most drugs present as powders; the needed quantity (in mg) must be diluted in a smaller volume of water than the volume of Lipiodol: for example, 8 ml of drug (in water phase) for 10 ml of Lipiodol
2 Begin the pumping by firmly pushing all the drug in the Lipiodol (and not Lipiodol in the drug); maneuvers 1+2 will establish the water-in-oil direction of the emulsion
3 Then perform 20 complete and vigorous pushes and pulls (from one syringe to the other) through the stopcock; this allows the preparation of droplets of drug ranging from 30 to 120 μm (>70% being between 70–100 μm).

17.3.7.3
Dose

The generally recommended dose of Lipiodol is <10 ml for each session. Some recommend using a dose of Lipiodol (in ml) equal to 1–1.5 times the tumor diameter (expressed in cm) (NAKAO et al. 1994). One author recommends using a higher dose of oil (>15 ml) (OI et al. 1994) to induce massive overflow of iodized oil (and of the supposed link drug) from the hepatic artery into the portal vein through the arterioportal communications. Nevertheless, it has been demonstrated that severe pulmonary complications related to intraarterial injection of Lipiodol were correlated to the dose and appeared for doses close to 20 ml (CHUNG et al. 1993).

17.4
Contraindications

As normal liver parenchyma is supplied both by hepatic artery and portal vein, it does not necrose following arterial embolization if its portal supply is normal. Consequently, when the main portal vein is occluded, or presents a reversal of flow due to portal hypertension or porto-caval surgical shunting, complete hepatic artery occlusion is contraindicated. Nevertheless, it does not contraindicate Lipiodol injection, the oil being a very transient occluding agent for the normal liver tissue.

Pericholangitis and parenchymal focal necroses have been experimentally described after injection of Lipiodol alone in the hepatic artery, and up to 12.5% of bile duct injuries have been reported after L-TACE, as a result of microvascular damage to the peribiliary capillary plexus. Local drug toxicity is probably amplified by the transient embolic effect of Lipiodol in the peribiliary plexus. As a consequence of this toxicity of L-TACE upon the bile ducts, TACE should be avoided in any liver territory presenting dilated bile ducts, except after drainage.

Transcatheter treatments may progress to irreversible hepatic failure in patients with severe hepatic dysfunction. So high is this risk that Child's C and Okuda III patients are broadly considered as contraindicated for intravascular locoregional treatments. Elevated total bilirubin (>50 μmol/l), serum GOT/AST more than 200 U/l, or ascites are predicting factors for severe complications and should be considered as contraindications in cirrhotic patients as well.

Esophageal varices need care because they may rupture immediately after treatment. If there is any risk of rupture, it is recommended that endoscopic sclerotic therapy be conducted before treatment.

Pulmonary contraindications for lymphography must be respected when using Lipiodol intraarterially, as the oil that is not retained in the tumor will also block the lung capillaries.

17.5 Side-Effects and Complications

The normal post-embolization response of nonspecific symptoms such as nausea, fever, and pain can be associated with significant leukocytosis and increase in liver enzymes. This syndrome may be difficult to differentiate from infection; it is related to tissular necrosis and experienced to a variable degree by all patients. Clinical symptoms last 48–72 h in most cases. Biologic cytolysis is invariably present but recedes within 7–10 days. The syndrome is treated symptomatically and, in most cases, decreases in severity with subsequent chemoembolizations. The overall treatment mortality, highly dependent on the severity of the associated cirrhotic liver disease, is generally reported as 2% to 7%.

The normal organs, such as liver parenchyma, gallbladder and bile ducts, stomach, duodenum, or even pancreas, located in the distribution of the hepatic artery, are – or may be – also infused in addition to the tumor. Complications from local ischemic and/or drug toxicity include hepatitis, cholecystitis, sclerosing cholangitis, gastroduodenal ulcerations and hemorrhage. In order to achieve the maximum effect of chemotherapy and minimize the local complications of TACE, the vascular anatomy and hemodynamics of the liver and its adjacent organs should be carefully evaluated before treatment. Infarction of these organs is a rare complication, but prevention of passage of embolus and drug into the cystic artery is frequently impossible and cholecystitis occurs in 10%; it should be treated conservatively.

Severe symptoms related to pulmonary oil embolism are very rare. It has been only reported in patients who had received more than 20 ml of Lipiodol; these patients suffered from cough, hemoptysis, dyspnea, and decrease in arterial partial pressure of oxygen, that developed 2–5 days after treatment and generally cleared 1–4 weeks later.

Passage of the embolus or chemotherapy into gastroduodenal, splenic or superior mesenteric arteries is prevented by highly selective catheterization and slow injection. If reflux occurs, the patient may respectively experience ischemic pancreatitis, splenic infarction or subacute intestinal obstruction.

Vasculitis occurs along the courses of TACE in 15–20% of patients. It may result either from intimal damage secondary to catheter manipulations or as a consequence of the chemotherapy injection. This drug toxicity for the endothelium accelerates degradation of the main hepatic arteries and might therefore reduce the feasibility of further chemoembolizations unless suitable collaterals are available for catheterization. In an experimental study we demonstrated that adriamycin was more aggressive against arteries than cisplatin; other authors reported that, in TACE sessions, vasculitis was correlated to cisplatin and associated embolization.

Renal failure is a frequent complication if a very active pre- and postoperative i.v. hydration is not carried out. Hepatic failure, demonstrated by jaundice and ascites, may occur in all patients with associated cirrhotic disease.

Tumor rupture, over the hours or days following TACE, has been reported and is generally responsible for fatal complications.

Tumor necrosis is desirable but, in huge tumors, it can sometimes also injure the surrounding bile ducts, leading to biloma formation (Inoue et al. 1991a) (Fig. 17.5).

Necrosis and liver abscess of the liver parenchyma occur in less than 1% of cases, but are among the more severe complications encountered after TACE. Bile contamination, associated bile duct inju-

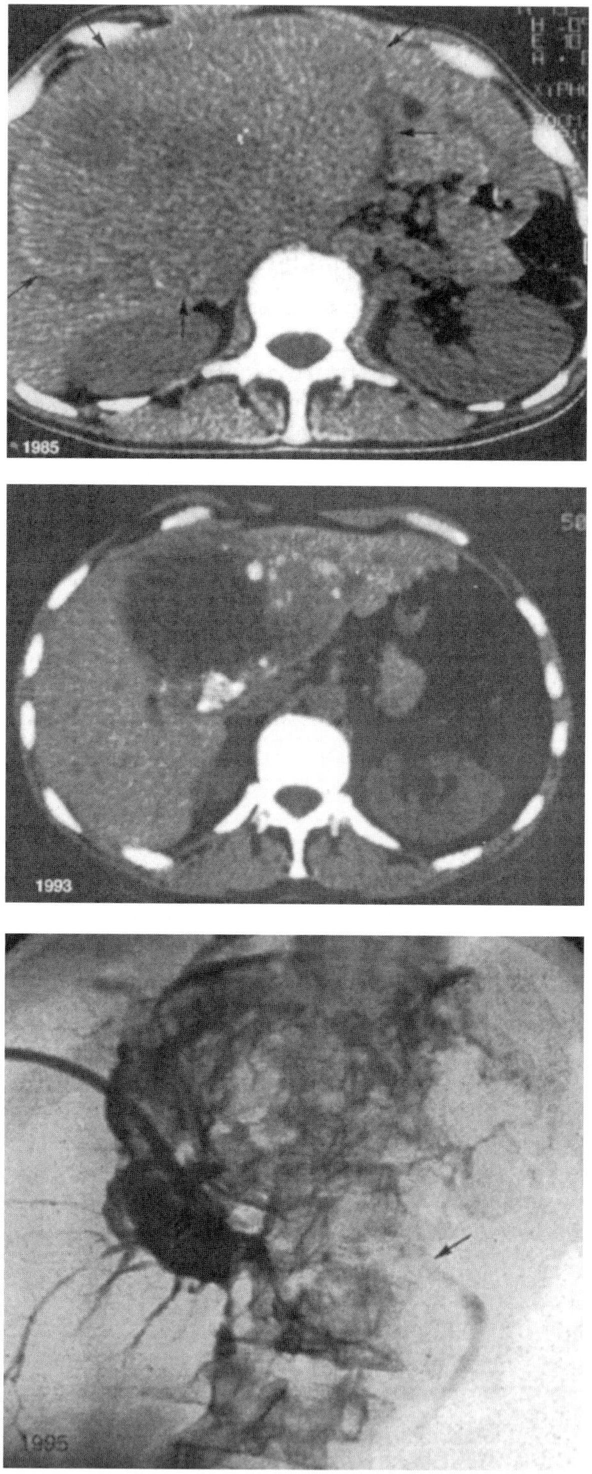

Fig. 17.5a–c. Massive tumor necrosis, with bile duct damage, after ten sessions of L-TACE to control a huge HCC (10-year survival). **a** Huge, single but nonresectable tumor (*arrows*). Excellent response at 8-year follow-up (after ten sessions along 4 years) (**b**). At 10-year follow-up, the tumor is controlled but the patient presents tumor necrosis communicating with bile ducts (biloma) and hepatic duct stenosis (*arrow*) (later treated by metallic stenting) (**c**)

ries and, above all, bilio-enteric anastomoses should be considered as major risk factors for liver abscess formation after TACE (De Baère et al. 1996b). Retrograde enteric bacterial contamination in most of these patients transforms TACE from a clean procedure to a contaminated one, which indicates antibiotic therapy as treatment, as opposed to prophylaxis. Cephalosporin with cefazolin, or amoxicillin/clavulanate, has yielded good results in this field.

17.6 Indications and Results

17.6.1 Response

In the different series, transcatheter arterial treatments lead to about 50% of complete responses and 25% of partial responses on elevated alphafetoprotein level. Complete morphological response is exceptional on the basis of the World Health Organization standard criteria, as some scar image nearly always persists. In the literature, complete plus partial morphological responses are reported in about 45% of cases (25–60%) and, interestingly, most of the responses occur before the third session of treatment (Bismuth et al. 1992).

Tumor necrosis after transcatheter arterial treatments has been reported through series of operated patients (Table 17.2), and the corresponding data apply mainly to small tumors.

The treatment appears to be most efficacious for HCC forming single nodules and presenting an expanding growth pattern, as opposed to the replacing and massive growth types where complete necrosis was not encountered (Hashimoto et al. 1995).

Table 17.2. Reported percentage of tumor necrosis after transcatheter arterial treatments

Study	Treatment regimen	95–100% necrosis	50–94% necrosis
Tanaka et al. 1992	L-TACE	20%	–
Bismuth et al. 1992	L-TACE	26%	48%
Spreafico et al. 1994	L-TACE or -TAC	36%	–
Higuchi et al. 1994	TAE	Small HCC: 70%	20%
		Large HCC: 44%	35%

In small HCC, complete necrosis is much more frequent and is correlated with the intensity of Lipiodol uptake by the tumor (SPREAFICO et al. 1994) (Fig. 17.6). When necrosis is incomplete, residual viable cells are found mainly in the extracapsular zone of small tumors, whereas in large HCC they are located in the tumor interior (HIGUCHI et al. 1994).

17.6.2 Survival

In nonrandomized studies (Table 17.3), transcatheter arterial treatments improve survival. As an example, in a comparative multicenter trial in which each treated patient was matched with an untreated one, the 1-, 2- and 3-year probabilities of survival were respectively 64%, 38% and 27% in the treated group and respectively 18%, 6% and 5% in the untreated one (BRONOWICKI et al. 1994).

Table 17.3. Survival after transcatheter arterial treatments in nonrandomized studies

Nonrandomized studies	Survival (%)			
	1 year	2 years	3 years	4 years
NAKAMURA et al. 1989				
L-TACE	54	33	18	–
VETTER et al. 1991				
L-TACE	59	30	–	–
Control	0	0	–	–
YOSHIMI et al. 1992				
Child's A L-TACE	78	65	65	65
Resection	78	61	47	42.5
Child's B L-TACE	89	71	43	21.5
Resection	79	55	37	27.5
BISMUTH et al. 1992				
L-TACE	44	–	–	–
NGAN et al. 1993				
L-TACE	53	38	–	–
MATSUI et al. 1993[a]				
L-TACE	100	–	67	–
BRONOWICKI et al. 1994				
L-TACE	64	38	27	27
Control	18	6	5	
HATANAKA et al. 1995				
L-TACE	86	–	–	–
TACE	80	–	–	–
L-TAC	66	–	–	–

[a]All patients with small HCC and treated with subsegmental L-TACE

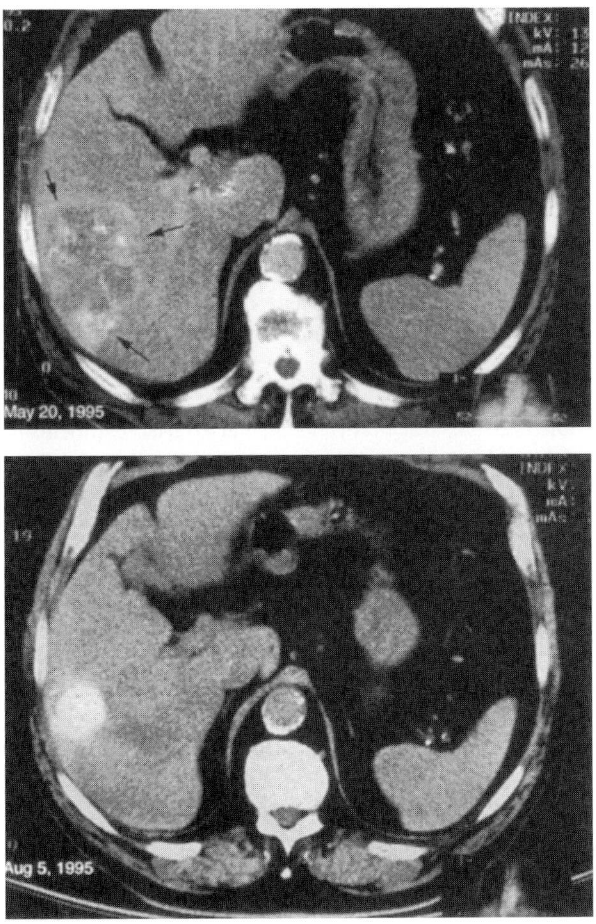

a
b

Fig. 17.6a,b. HCC of the right lobe (**a**). Partial response 2.5 months after the first session of L-TACE, correlated with a very intense uptake of Lipiodol (**b**)

When considering results in nonrandomized (as well as in randomized) studies, one should pay careful attention to patient selection, which greatly modifies spontaneous and post-therapeutic survival; as demonstrated in Tables 17.3 and 17.4, survival after L-TACE may be 5–7 times higher in HCC suitable (or almost suitable) for surgery as compared with survival in treated patients with unresectable tumors.

Lipiodol accumulation pattern has been correlated to 1-year survival (VAN BEERS et al. 1989) and to rate of local recurrence (MURAKAMI et al. 1994); the more complete the accumulation is, the better the prognosis.

Considering the high risk of fatal complications, it is widely admitted that HCC associated with severe cirrhotic liver disease (Child's C or Okuda III)

Table 17.4. Five-year survival after L-TACE

Studies	5-year survival (%)
Yamada et al. 1985[a]	6
Roche 1991[a]	7.5
Uchida et al. 1993[a]	9
Nakamura et al. 1994[a]	8
Bronowicki et al. 1996[b]	
L-TACE	47
Resection	43
Transplantation	48
Untreated	0

[a]Patients with unresectable tumors
[b]All patients with anatomically operable tumors

should not be treated by transcatheter arterial approaches. Nevertheless, promising results have been reported in patients with advanced cirrhosis, in whom Gelfoam was replaced by autologous clot, with a 2-year survival of 100% and 50% respectively in Child's B and C (Gunji et al. 1992).

Surprisingly, randomized studies have failed to show statistically significant gain in the treated groups (Table 17.5). Despite a 33% response rate, survival was not improved in a group of patients treated by TACE with doxorubicin and Gelfoam powder (Pelletier et al. 1990). In another randomized trial, the 1-year survival after L-TACE was higher than in a control group but the difference was not significant (Groupe d'étude et de traitement de l'hépatocarcinome 1995). In a study comparing TAE with symptomatic treatment there were no differences in survival at 2 and 4 years (Bruix et al. 1998). Pelletier et al. (1998) recently compared L-TACE (Gelfoam particles, Lipiodol-lecithin-cisplatin emulsion) + tamoxifen with tamoxifen alone. An objective tumoral response was more frequently observed in the treated group (24% vs 5.5%); the relative risk of death in the treated group as compared with the tamoxifen group was 0.92; but L-TACE caused two deaths, and it induced signs of liver failure in 51% of the patients. No difference in survival was noted between the two groups.

These disappointing results, despite a proved reduction of tumor growth, might be related to the rather aggressive approaches adopted in these protocols, which accounted for deterioration of liver function, and even early liver failure in some patients. Differences from these European studies and Asian series might also be due to the high prevalence of alcoholic liver disease in Europe, as compared with Asia, where posthepatitic disease is predominant.

17.6.3 Prognostic Factors

Predicting factors for success of transcatheter arterial treatments have been studied by multiple teams (Ngan et al. 1993; Bronowocki et al. 1994; Mondazzi et al. 1994; Taniguchi et al. 1994; Urata et al. 1994; Hatanaka et al. 1995) and the results are summarized in Table 17.6. In practice, there are no rigid criteria today for excluding transcatheter treatments on the basis of adverse factors, but the greater the risk for the patient, the more careful selection must be.

17.6.4 Treatment of Life-Threatening Complications

Peritoneal bleeding due to *tumor rupture* is a fatal complication in 7.5% of HCC. It may occur either spontaneously or be a complication of minimal trauma or biopsy. Spontaneous ruptures seem more frequent in African and Asian patients and in HCC developing in patients with primary biliary cirrhosis. Extravasation of the contrast medium is frequently diluted by ascites and is also difficulty differentiated from tumor staining on anteroposterior view. Consequently, if direct visualization of contrast medium leakage in the peritoneal cavity is a reliable sign, it is found in only 10–15% of cases (Roche 1996). Successful hemostasis is initially achieved in all patients after emergency embolization (Okazaki

Table 17.5. Survival after transcatheter arterial treatments in randomized studies

Controlled studies	Survival (%)		
	1 year	2 years	4 years
Pelletier et al. 1990			
TACE	24	–	–
Control	31	–	–
Groupe d'étude... 1995			
L-TACE	62	–	–
Control	43,5	–	–
Pelletier et al. 1998			
L-TACE	51	24	–
Control	55	26	–
Bruix et al. 1998			
TAE	–	49	13
Control	–	50	27

Table 17.6. Prognostic factors for survival after transcatheter arterial treatments

Study	Treatment regimen	Significant predictive factors for survival
TANIGUCHI et al. 1994	TAE	Nonadvanced cirrhosis and uninodular tumor
URATA et al. 1994	L-TAC	Patient >50 years old Nodular type Tumor size <5 cm Negative tumor invasion of the portal vein <10 intrahepatic mets AFP <400 ng/ml Okuda stage I
MONDAZZI et al. 1994	L-TACE or L-TAC	Age Child-Pugh or Okuda grade Total serum bilirubin Tumor size before treatment Degree of Lipiodol accumulation in the tumor Gelfoam use Changes in tumor size and AFP after treatment
Other main reported factors		Encapsulated tumor Well-differentiated HCC

et al. 1991; SOYER et al. 1993); there is a correlation between serum bilirubin level (<3 mg/dl) and survival (OKAZAKI et al. 1991); the mean length of survival after embolization has been reported to be from 5.5 to 7 months in patients with low bilirubin level.

Paraneoplastic syndrome is not unfrequent in HCC but life-threatening manifestations are exceptional. Hypercalcemia is one, which may need emergency treatment and can benefit from TAE in selected cases. TAE has proved to be immediately efficacious in controlling circulating calcium level when hypercalcemia was due to tumoral secretion of humoral mediators which release calcium from bones (ROCHE et al. 1979). This rare indication (less than 1% of HCC and 10% of HCC with hypercalcemia) must be differentiated from hypercalcemia due to bone metastases, which are much more frequent in HCC.

17.6.5 Preoperative Treatment

Transcatheter arterial treatments have been proposed as adjunctive therapy with surgical therapies in an attempt to shrink the tumor before resection or to control tumor growth before liver transplantation, but its benefit is still controversial.

For some authors its disadvantages are: increased peroperative technical difficulties related to perihepatic adhesions or decrease in peroperative sonographic detectability of nodules, earlier recurrence after resection, or even decreased survival for patients in whom preoperative TACE had induced partial necrosis (NAGASUE et al. 1989; ADACHI et al. 1993). Malignant hepatocytes are less sensitive to hypoxia than normal hepatocytes; this reduced sensitivity is also mediated through p53 and is less frequently abnormal in well-differentiated HCC (WANG et al. 1997). Consequently, when inducing incomplete necrosis, embolization might leave in place poorly differentiated cells and exhibit an aggressive behavior as compared with untreated patients where these more advanced clones might be partially impeded by the surrounding tumoral tissue (BRUIX et al. 1998). In the same way, some have shown that incomplete tumor necrosis after TACE could be a predisposing factor to lung metastases (LIOU et al. 1995).

For other groups, for whom preoperative TACE is considered as beneficial, it takes place in staging of the patients (Lipiodol CT) and represents the first palliation (SAVASTANO et al. 1994); it induces morphological downstaging in about 30% of cases (BISMUTH et al. 1992), with a mean reduction in tumor size of 32% (that is about 2.5 cm) (YU et al. 1993) that permits liver resection in some patients who, otherwise, had been unresectable; it is an effective treatment in patients awaiting liver transplantation (SPREAFICO et al. 1994).

In large series (HARADA et al. 1996) there is no difference in survival of resected patients, either they have undergone preoperative TACE or not. Recently, MAJNO et al. (1997) found a subgroup of patients (those who had downstaging after preoperative TACE) in whom the disease free interval and 1- and 5-year survival were markedly improved when compared with those who did not receive preoperative TACE or were not downstaged by TACE.

On basis of these reports, it might be reasonable to reserve "preoperative" treatment to unresectable tumors in an attempt to permit resection in some cases. In patients with resectable lesions or those who are planned for transplantation, preoperative

TACE might be beneficial as far as downstaging could considerably improve long-term survival; but, previously, it would be important to select candidates by defining predictive factors for significant tumor necrosis and shrinking after TACE.

Fibrolamellar HCC tends to affect younger patients without underlying liver disease. Prolonged survival for patients with advanced tumor stage is not exceptional, and curative liver resection supports a more favorable prognosis than in HCC. Nevertheless, some tumors are so large at the time of diagnosis that surgical resection is contraindicated. In a series of four patients treated with L-TACE we obtained stabilization in one case, and a decrease in tumor size in two allowing for subsequent hepatic resection (Soyer et al. 1992).

17.6.6 Combined Treatments

In order to achieve complete necrosis of the tumor, *combined arterial and portal venous embolization* has been proposed (Nakao et al. 1986; Yamakado et al. 1994). This very aggressive approach induced severe parenchymal infarction besides complete tumor necrosis, so that it indicated segmental surgical resection in 40% of the reported cases. Considering these side-effects, it should be reserved for very selected (and infrequent) cases with a small tumor located near the surface of the liver but nevertheless unresectable.

Transcatheter arterial treatments *combined with percutaneous ethanol injection* (PEI) have also been evaluated. In one trial, patients had single encapsulated large HCC (more than 3 cm) and were treated either with one session of L-TACE alone or pretreated with L-TACE and submitted 2 weeks later to PEI (Tanaka et al. 1992); the combination of L-TACE and PEI significantly increased the morphological response rate, the frequency of complete necrosis and the 1-, 2- and 3-year survival. In a randomized trial, the results of combined L-TACE and PEI were compared with repeat L-TACE procedures (Bartolozzi et al. 1995) in large HCC (3–8 cm) with no more than two daughter nodules; complete response rate, tumor recurrence and survival without recurrence were significantly better in the L-TACE/PEI group, which also appeared to have fewer adverse effects on liver function.

17.6.7 Treatment of Postoperative Recurrent Hepatocellular Carcinoma

In recent years, and thanks to systematic screening, HCC could be more frequently diagnosed at an early stage and operated upon. However, it is quite clear that recurrence often occurs in residual liver, even if curative hepatectomy is performed. Re-resection is desirable in recurrent HCC if it can be completely resected; nevertheless, recurrent HCC presents as multiple metastatic foci in more than 54% of cases (Park et al. 1993), which dramatically limits the indications for surgery. The usefulness of transcatheter arterial treatments has been evaluated in such cases by different Asian groups, whose results are summarized in Table 17.7.

Table 17.7. Postoperative recurrences: survival after transcatheter arterial treatments

Studies	No. pts.	Survival (%)				
		1 year	2 years	3 years	4 years	5 years
Nakao et al. 1991						
L-TACE	66	88	57	42	27	–
Oral chemotherapy	15	80	27	18	–	–
Nagashima et al. 1992						
L-TACE or L-TAC	86	82	–	29	–	7.7
Park et al. 1993						
L-TACE	87	74.7	55	–	–	–
Imai et al. 1995						
L-TACE	61	69	41	21	17	8

It appears that 1- and 2-year survival rates of patients treated by TAE or L-TACE do not differ from those of a control group of patients with Child's A primary HCC treated with L-TACE alone (PARK et al. 1993). It is also suggested that L-TACE is more effective than oral chemotherapy (NAKAO et al. 1991), that survival is better in small and single tumors, and that it is correlated to the absence of distant metastasis or portal vein involvement (IMAI 1995). Thus, transcatheter arterial treatments may be recommended as efficient tools for palliative control of tumor growth when postoperative recurrences occur.

17.6.8 Hepatocellular Carcinoma with Extended Portal Vein Thrombosis

Endoluminal portal and/or hepatic vein invasion by a tumor cast is found by the pathologist in more than respectively 70% and 40%. During arteriography, the thrombus appears hypervascular in 2/3 to 3/4 of cases. Progressive retrograde invasion of intrahepatic portal radicles may lead to the complete occlusion of the main portal vein division, then its trunk and even sometimes its infra-hepatic tributaries. The intra-luminal evolution of hepatic vein invasion may be similarly extensive towards the inferior vena cava, the right atrium and even the pulmonary artery. Extended portal or hepatic vein invasion is a situation one has frequently to deal with in most non-Asian or African countries. In alcoholic liver cirrhosis, it is encountered at the time of diagnosis in 50% of patients who were not known to belong to a high risk group for HCC and, thus, who could not enter a systematic screening program.

Extended portal vein tumor thrombus is associated with poor spontaneous survival. Nevertheless, L-TACE or L-TAC (contraindications for embolization depending on the thrombus extension and the remaining hepatic portal perfusion) may be efficient treatments for controlling tumor growth. Lipiodol accumulation in the tumor thrombus has been documented, as well as necrosis of the thrombus after treatment was demonstrated (DERHY et al. 1990; KATSUMORI et al. 1993). As portal vein thrombosis is generally considered as contraindicating extended surgery, patients whose tumor thrombus disappears after treatment may sometimes be operated on (KATSUMORI et al. 1993).

Even if prognosis of this type of HCC is still poor when compared with tumors that do not involve the portal vein or its first branches, L-TAC and/or L-TACE may influence survival very positively. In the literature the 6-month survival was demonstrated to be as high as 100% despite endovenous tumor occlusion of the portal vein (KATSUMORI et al. 1993). Some series report more than 7-year survival of patients with portal vein occlusion treated by transcatheter approaches (INOUE et al 1991b) (Fig. 17.7).

In a large series of 110 patients with HCC invading major portal branches and classified as Child's A or B, treated either by L-TAC or L-TACE, the cumulative survival rates at 6 months, 1 year, 2 years and 3 years were respectively 48%, 30%, 18% and 9% (CHUNG et al. 1995). In this series, it appeared that limitation of parenchymal tumor extension to one or two segments was a much more significant predicting factor for absence of complications and efficacy of therapy than extension of the tumor thrombus. In the corresponding group of patients the median time of survival was significantly longer (22 months) than in the other (5 months). In a prospective controlled study in patients with main portal vein obstruction (LEE et al. 1997), L-TAC(E) appeared as a safe modality when patients had good liver function and hepatopetal collateral portal circulation in the porta hepatis; a beneficial effect on survival was only observed for nodular-type HCC. In some cases, L-TACE may also control hepatic vein tumor thrombus, even with inferior vena cava or right atrium extension (DAZAI et al. 1989). These data indicate that when the tumor is limited in extent and hepatic function is preserved, L-TAC(E) is probably effective and safe for the palliation of HCC with major portal vein invasion.

17.7 Conclusions: A Pragmatic Approach

Indications for L-TACE in HCC must consider the type of tumor and the severity of the underlying liver disease. Schematically, one can consider three main different situations from the best prognosis to the worst: (a) small tumor and Child's A cirrhosis, (b) unresectable tumors on Child's A or B, and (c) massive HCC or Child's C cirrhosis. Furthermore, some patients present a thrombosis of the main portal vein, most of them being in the group c but some belonging to group b or even group a (Table 17.8).

In *group a*, indications of L-TACE are still controversial:

- Its efficiency, as compared to surgery or percutaneous ablation, is not clearly demonstrated

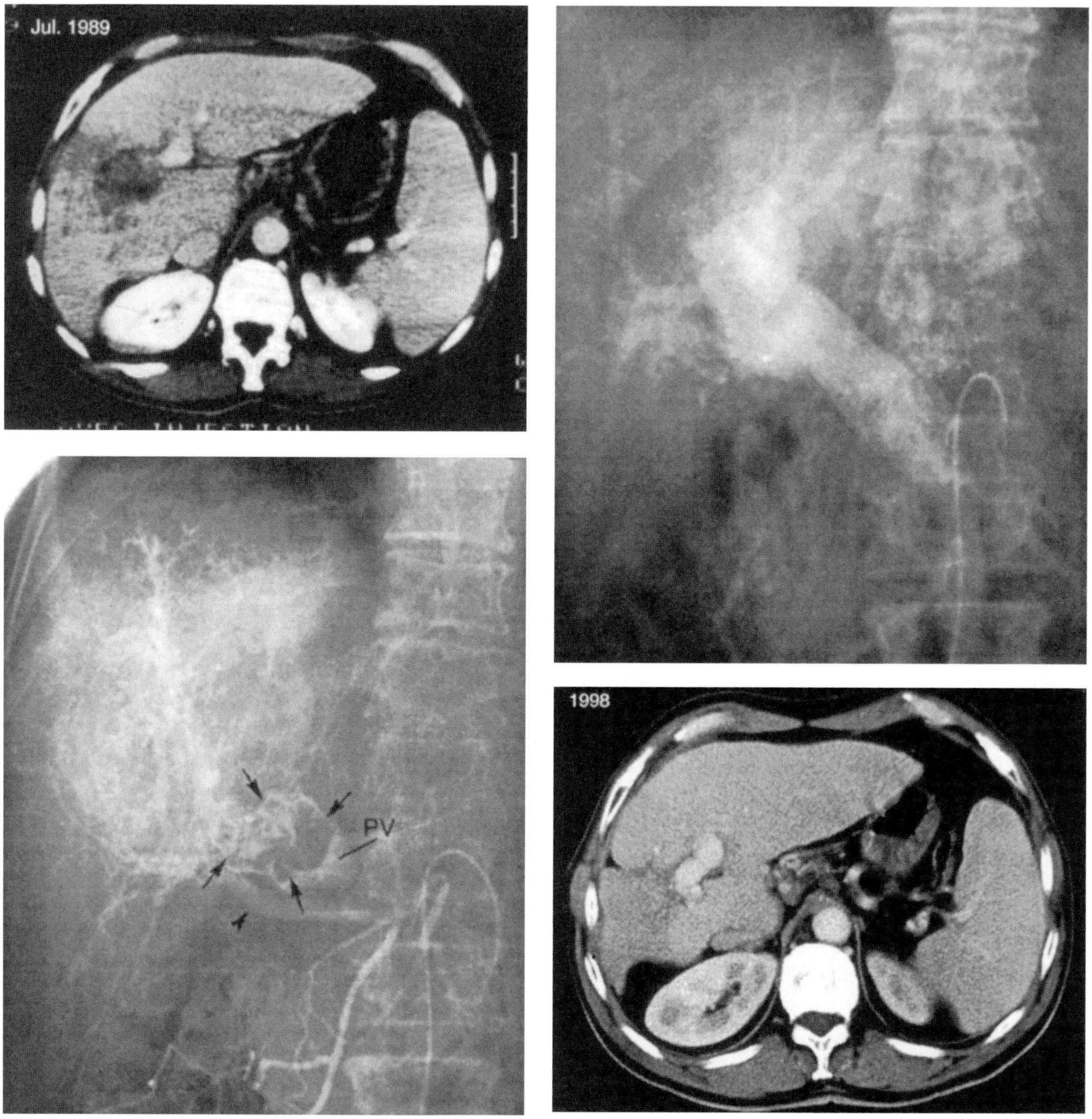

a b c d

Fig. 17.7a–d. HCC with tumor thrombus in the portal vein. Still under complete response 9 years after treatment by L-TAC and then L-TACE. **a** Tumor of the right lobe surrounded by daughter nodules. **b** Large hypervascular tumor thrombus (*arrows*) occluding the main portal vein (*PV*) and contraindicating embolization (*arrowhead,* hepatic artery); treated with L-TAC alone. The patients recovered a patent portal vein 1 month after the first session (**c**) and could then be treated by L-TACE over three complementary sessions. Nine years after this treatment, the patient is still in complete remission; CT (**d**) proves tumor disappearance and shrinkage of the surrounding liver

- Advantages of preoperative TACE are still debated. In a subgroup of patients responding to preoperative L-TACE, the prognosis after resection or transplantation seems to be improved; but the predicting factors for the response are still unclear
- A combination of L-TACE with percutaneous ablation techniques seems better than L-TACE alone, but is not demonstrated to be better than percutaneous ablation alone, particularly since radiofrequency ablation is available

Table 17.8. Place of L-TACE in HCC treatments

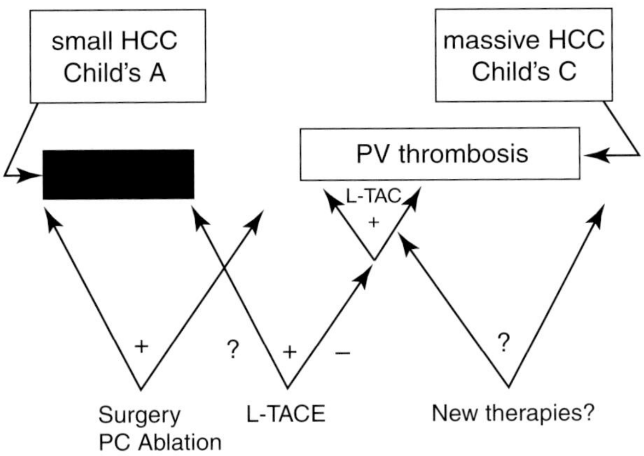

In conclusion, for this group, it should certainly be recommended to carry out complementary studies, likely to be randomized.

In *group b*, since no treatment, except TACE, has proved any efficacy upon tumor growth, the disappointing results of randomized studies are not a definitive argument for abandoning transcatheter arterial treatments. These studies have certainly demonstrated that the mean survival of Western patients could not be dramatically improved by TACE; but all experienced teams in transcatheter arterial treatments have also seen patients with advanced HCC who had been obviously improved for years by this treatment. On one hand, predictive factors for efficacy of the treatment are still unclear. On the other hand, one should consider that only responders can expect prolonged tumor control and a benefit in survival, and finally that the response nearly always occurs before the third session. Consequently the treatment can be logically proposed to any patient of this group, but subject to termination if the tolerance is poor or if the patient still has not responded after the second session. When the treatment is maintained, the time interval between each cure is then determined according to the biological, morphologic and symptomatic responses as well as to the clinical tolerance to chemoembolization.

Some patients with a tumor thrombus occlusion of the main portal vein enter groups b or a. Only those who present a limited parenchymal tumor extension should be submitted to transcatheter arterial treatments: L-TAC (without embolization) for the first or the two first sessions, and then L-TACE if they respond and the portal vein has reopened.

In *group c*, it is broadly recommended not to perform any transcatheter arterial treatment:

- L-TACE has proved to be more dangerous than efficacious when more than 60% of the liver is infiltrated by the tumor, or when the underlying liver disease is severe
- When a patient presents with a small HCC developed on a Child's C cirrhosis, percutaneous ablation seems preferable with regard to its better tolerance

Consequently, in this group of patients the initiation of new protocols and new therapies under phase I trials should be recommended.

References

Adachi E, Matsumata T, Nishizaki T, Hashimoto H, Tsuneyoshi M, Sugimachi K (1993) Effects of preoperative transcatheter hepatic arterial chemoembolization for hepatocellular carcinoma. The relationship between postoperative course and tumor necrosis. Cancer 72:3593–3598

Bartolozzi C, Lencioni R, Caramella D, et al (1995) Treatment of large HCC: transcatheter arterial chemoembolization combined with percutaneous ethanol injection versus repeated transcatheter arterial chemoembolization. Radiology 197:812–818

Bismuth H, Morino M, Sherlock D, et al (1992) Primary treatment of hepatocellular carcinoma by arterial chemoembolization. Am J Surg 163:387–394

Bronowicki JP, Vetter D, Dumas F, et al (1994) Transcatheter oily chemoembolization for hepatocellular carcinoma. A 4-year study of 127 French patients. Cancer 74:16–24

Bronowicki JP, Boudjema K, Chone L, et al (1996) Comparison of resection, liver transplantation and transcatheter oily chemoembolization in the treatment of hepatocellular carcinoma. J Hepatol 24:293–300

Bruix J, Llovet JM, Castells A, et al (1998) Transarterial embolization versus symptomatic treatment in patients with advanced hepatocellular carcinoma: results of a randomized, controlled trial in a single institution. Hepatology 27:1578–1583

Chang JM, Tzeng WS, Pan HB, Yang CF, Lai KH (1994) Transarterial embolization with or without cisplatin treatment of hepatocellular carcinoma. Cancer 74:2449–2453

Chung JW, Park JH, Im JG, Han JK, Han MC (1993) Pulmonary oil embolism after transcatheter oily chemoembolization of hepatocellular carcinoma. Radiology 187:689–693

Chung JW, Park JH, Han JK, Choi BI, Han MC (1995) Hepatocellular carcinoma and portal vein invasion: results of treatment with transcatheter oily chemoembolization. AJR 165:315–321

Dazai Y, Katoh T, Katoh I, Sueda S, Yoshida R (1989) A rare case of chemoembolization therapy for metastatic right atrial tumor thrombus associated with hepatocellular carcinoma. Chest 96:434–436

De Baère T, Dufaux J, Roche A, Counnord JL, Berthault MF (1995) Circulatory modifications induced by intra-arterial injections of iodized oil and emulsions of iodized oil and doxorubicin. Radiology 194:165–170

De Baère T, Zhang X, Aubert B, et al (1996a) Quantification of tumor uptake of iodized oils and emulsions of iodized oils: experimental study. Radiology 201:731–735

De Baère T, Amenabar J, Lagrange C, Roche A (1996b) Severe infectious complications after hepatic locoregional therapy. Hepatology 23:1436–1440

De Baère T, Denys A, Briquet R, Chevallier P, Laurent A, Roche A (1998) Modifications of arterial and portal hemodynamic after injection of iodized oils and emulsions of iodized oil in the hepatic artery: experimental study. J Vasc Interv Radiol 9:305–310

Derhy S, Bessis L, Atallah R, Ajavon Y, Eisele G, Roche A (1990) Repermèabilisation portale après chimiothérapie Lipiodolée intra-artérielle au cours d'un hépatocarcinome. A propos de 3 cas. Gastroenterol Clin Biol 14:893–895

Fukushima S, Kubota M, Kojima T, et al (1992) Preparation and evaluation of two formulations: cisplatin suspension in Lipiodol and polylactic acid microspheres containing aclarubicin hydrochloride for hepatic arterial administration therapy for hepatocellular carcinoma. Reg Cancer Treat 1–2:36–39

Groupe d'étude et de traitement du carcinome hépatocellulaire (1995) A comparison of Lipiodol chemoembolization and conservative treatment for unresectable hepatocellular carcinoma. N Engl J Med 332:1256–1261

Gunji T, Kawauchi N, Ohnishi S, et al (1992) Treatment of hepatocellular carcinoma associated with advanced cirrhosis by transcatheter arterial chemoembolization using autologous blood clot: a preliminary report. Hepatology 15:252–257

Harada T, Matsuo K, Inoue T (1996) Is preoperative hepatic arterial chemoembolization safe and effective for hepatocellular carcinoma. Ann Surg 224:4–9

Hashimoto T, Nakamura H, Hori S, et al (1995) Hepatocellular carcinoma: efficacy of transcatheter oily chemoembolization in relation to macroscopic and microscopic patterns of tumor growth among 100 patients with partial hepatectomy. Cardiovasc Intervent Radiol 18:82–86

Hatanaka Y, Yamashita Y, Takahashi M, et al (1995) Unresectable hepatocellular carcinoma: analysis of prognostic factors in transcatheter management. Radiology 195:747–752

Higuchi T, Kikuchi M, Okazaki M (1994) Hepatocellular carcinoma after transcatheter hepatic arterial embolization. A histopathologic study of 84 resected cases. Cancer 73:2259–2267

Imai Y (1995) Transcatheter arterial chemoembolization for postoperative recurrent hepatocellular carcinoma: therapeutic results in correlation with radiologic findings and treatment methods. Nippon Igaku Hoshasen Gakkai Zasshi 55:395–401

Inoue Y, Nakamura H, Takashima S, Yamazaki K, Toyoshima H, Iwasaki M (1991a) Biloma following transcatheter oily chemoembolization. Radiat Med 9:57–60

Inoue K, Akaji H, Nakamura H (1991b) Transcatheter oily chemoembolization for the treatment of large hepatocellular carcinoma with an accompanying tumor thrombus in the right main branch of the portal vein and arterioportal shunting: report of one patient still surviving after more than seven years. Radiat Med 9):105–107

Kan Z (1996) Dynamic study of iodized oil in the liver and blood supply to hepatic tumors: an experimental investigation in several animals species. Acta Radiol 37(S):257-258

Kan Z, Ivancev K, Hägerstrand I, et al (1993) In vivo microscopy of hepatic tumors in animal models: a dynamic investigation of blood supply to hepatic metastases. Radiology 187:621–626

Kasugai H, Kojima J, Tatsuta M, et al (1989) Treatment of hepatocellular carcinoma by transcatheter arterial embolization combined with intraarterial infusion of a mixture of cisplatin and ethiodized oil. Gastroenterology 97:965–971

Katsumori T, Fujita M, Satoh O, et al (1993) Transcatheter hepatic segmental chemo-Lipiodol-embolization against hepatocellular carcinoma accompanied by tumor thrombosis in the portal vein. Nippon Igaku Hoshasen Gakkai Zasshi 25:713–715

Kim JH, Chung JW, Han JK, Park JH, Choi BI, Han MC (1995) Transcatheter arterial embolization of the internal mammary artery in hepatocellular carcinoma. J Vasc Interv Radiol 6:71–74.

Lee HS, Kim JS, Choi IJ, Chung JW, Park JH, Kim CY (1997) The safety and efficacy of transcatheter arterial chemoembolization in the treatment of patients with hepatocellular carcinoma and main portal vein obstruction. Cancer 79:2087–2093

Liou TC, Shih SC, Kao CR, Chou SY, Lin SC, Wang HY (1995) Pulmonary metastasis of hepatocellular carcinoma associated with transarterial chemoembolization. J Hepatol 23:563–568

Majno PE, Adam R, Bismuth H, et al (1997) Influence of preoperative transarterial lipiodol chemoembolization on resection and transplantation for hepatocellular carcinoma in patients with cirrhosis. Ann Surg 226:688–703

Matsui O, Kadoya M, Yoshikawa J, et al (1993) Small hepatocellular carcinoma: treatment with subsegmental transcatheter arterial embolization. Radiology 188:79–83

Miller D, O'Leary T, Girton M (1987) Distribution of iodized oil within the liver after hepatic arterial injection. Radiology 162:849–852

Molgaard CP, Teitelbaum GP, Pentecost MJ, et al (1990) Intraarterial administration of lidocaine for analgesia in hepatic chemoembolization. J Vasc Interv Radiol 1:81–85

Mondazzi L, Bottelli R, Brambilla G, et al (1994) Transarterial oily chemoembolization for the treatment of hepatocellular carcinoma: a multivariate analysis of prognostic factors. Hepatology 19:1115–1123

Murakami R, Yoshimatsu S, Yamashita Y, Sagara K, Arakawa A, Takahashi M (1994) Transcatheter hepatic subsegmental arterial chemoembolization therapy using iodized oil for small hepatocellular carcinomas. Correlation between Lipiodol accumulation pattern and local recurrence. Acta Radiol 35:576–580

Nagashima T, Kikuchi T, Yamamoto H, Asano T, Isono K (1992) The treatment for recurrent hepatocellular carcinoma in residual liver. Reg Cancer Treat 1–2:40–42

Nagasue N, Galizia G, Kohno H, et al (1989) Adverse effects of preoperative hepatic artery chemoembolization for resectable hepatocellular carcinoma: a retrospective comparison of 138 liver resections. Surgery 106:81–86

Nakamura H, Hashimoto T, Oi H, Sawada S (1989) Transcatheter oily chemoembolization of hepatocellular carcinoma. Radiology 170:783–786

Nakamura H, Hashimoto T, Inoue Y, Inoue K, Akaji H, Sawada S (1990) Transcatheter oily chemoembolization with high doses of adriamycin in the treatment of large hepatocellular carcinoma (10 cm or more in diameter). Radiat Med 8:188–190

Nakamura H, Mitani T, Murakami T, et al (1994) Five-year survival aftervtranscatheter chemoembolization for hepatocellular carcinoma. Cancer Chemother Pharmacol 33(Suppl):89–93

Nakao N, Miura K, Takahashi H, et al (1986) Hepatocellular carcinoma: combined hepatic arterial and portal venous embolization. Radiology 161:303–307

Nakao N, Kamino K, Miura K, et al (1991) Recurrent hepatocellular carcinoma after partial hepatectomy: value of treatment with transcatheter arterial chemoembolization. AJR 156:1177–1179

Nakao N, Uchida H, Kamino K, et al (1994) Determination of the optimum dose level of Lipiodol in transcatheter arterial embolization of primary hepatocellular carcinoma based on retrospective multivariate analysis. Cardiovasc Intervent Radiol 17(2):76–80

Ngan H, Lai CL, Fan ST, Lai EC, Yuen WK, Tso WK (1993) Treatment of inoperable hepatocellular carcinoma by transcatheter arterial chemoembolization using an emulsion of cisplatin in iodized oil and gelfoam. Clin Radiol 47:315–320

Ohno K, Yamada K, Nakamura T, et al (1994) Usefulness and safety of segmental-subsegmental TAE for hepatocellular carcinoma in cases of liver hypofunction. Nippon Igaku Hoshasen Gakkai Zasshi 54:798–800

Oi H, Kim T, Kishimoto H, Matsushita M, Tateishi H, Okamura J (1994) Effective cases of transcatheter arterioportal chemoembolization with high-dose iodized oil for hepatocellular carcinoma. Cancer Chemother Pharmacol 33(Suppl): S69-S73

Okazaki M, Higashihara H, Koganemaru F, et al (1991) Intraperitoneal hemorrhage from hepatocellular carcinoma: emergency chemoembolization or embolization. Radiology 180:647–651

Okazaki M, Higashihara H, Ono H, et al (1993) Chemoembolization for hepatocellular carcinoma via the inferior pancreaticoduodenal artery in patients with celiac artery stenosis. Acta Radiol 34:20–25

Okazaki M, Higashihara H, Shijo H (1997) Chemoembolization. In: Livraghi T, Makuuchi M, L Buscarini (eds) Diagnosis and treatment of hepatocellular carcinoma. Greenwich Medical Media, London, pp:307–326

Park JH, Han JK, Chung JW, Han MC, Kim ST (1993) Postoperative recurrence of hepatocellular carcinoma: results of transcatheter arterial chemoembolization. Cardiovasc Intervent Radiol 16:21–24

Pelletier G, Roche A, Ink O, et al (1990) A randomized trial of hepatic arterial chemoembolization in patients with unresectable hepatocellular carcinoma. J Hepatol 11:181–184

Pelletier G, Ducreux M, Gay F, et al (1998) Treatment of unresectable hepatocellular carcinoma with Lipiodol chemoembolization: a multicenetr randomized trial. J Hepatol 29:129–134

Raoul JL, Bourguet P, Bretagne JF, Duvauferrier R (1988) Hepatic artery injection of I-labeled Lipiodol: biodistribution study results in patients with hepatocellular carcinoma and liver metastases. Radiology 168:541–545

Roche A (1991) Chemoembolization of liver malignancies. In: Ferrucci JT, Mathieu DG (eds) Advances in Hepatobiliary Radiology. CV Mosby Company, Baltimore, pp 295–305

Roche A (1996) Angiography in hepatocellular carcinoma. In Livraghi T, Makuuchi M, Buscarini L (eds) Diagnosis and treatment of hepatocellular carcinoma. Greenwich Medical Media, London, pp 129–139

Roche A, Doyon D, Harry G, Weingarten A, Edouard A (1978) L'embolisation artérielle hépatique: à propos de 35 cas. Nouvelle Presse Médicale 7:633–637

Roche A, Franco D, Dhumeau D, Bismuth H, Doyon D (1979) Emergency hepatic arterial embolization for secondary hypercalcemia in hepatocellular carcinoma. Radiology 133:315–316

Sato M, Yamada R, Uchida B, Hedgepeth P, Rösch J (1993) Effects of hepatic artery embolization with Lipiodol and gelatine sponge particles on normal swine liver. Cardiovasc Intervent Radiol 16:348–354

Savastano S, Feltrin GP, Miotto D, Chiesura-Corona M, Casarrubea G, Cecchetto A (1994) The preoperative chemoembolization of hepatocarcinoma due to cirrhosis. Radiol Med 88:620–624

Sigurdson E, Ridge J, Daly J (1986) Intra-arterial infusion of doxorubicin with degradable starch microspheres. Arch Surg 121:1277–1281

Soyer P, Roche A, Rougier P, Levesque M (1992) Nonresectable fibrolamellar hepatocellular carcinoma: outcome of 4 cases treated by intra-arterial chemotherapy. J Belge Radiol 75:463–468

Soyer P, van Beers B, Goffette P, Zeitoun G, Pringot J, Levesque M (1993) The role of embolization and chemo-embolization in the emergency treatment of hemoperitoneum caused by spontaneous rupture of hepatocellular carcinoma. Gastroenterol Clin Biol 17:643–648

Spreafico C, Marchiano A, Regalia E, et al (1994) Chemoembolization of hepatocellular carcinoma in patients who undergo liver transplantation. Radiology 192:687–690

Stuart K, Stokes K, Jenkins R, Trey C, Clouse M (1993) Treatment of hepatocellular carcinoma using doxorubicin/ethiodized oil/gelatin powder chemoembolization. Cancer 72:3202–3209

Takayasu K, Shima Y, Muramatsu Y, et al (1987) Hepatocellular carcinoma: treatment with intraarterial iodized oil with and without chemotherapeutic agents. Radiology 162:345–351

Tanaka K, Nakamura S, Numata K, et al (1992) Hepatocellular carcinoma: treatment with percutaneous ethanol injection and transcatheter arterial embolization. Radiology 185:457–460

Taniguchi K, Nakata K, Kato Y, et al (1994) Treatment of hepatocellular carcinoma with transcatheter arterial embolization. Cancer 73:1341–1345

Uchida H, Matsuo N, Nishimine K, Nishimura Y, Sakaguchi H, Ohishi H (1993) Transcatheter arterial embolization for hepatoma with Lipiodol. Sem Intervent Radiol 10:19–26

Urata K, Matsumata T, Kamakura T, Hasuo K, Sugimachi K (1994) Lipiodolization for unresectable hepatocellular carcinoma: an analysis of 205 patients using univariate and multivariate analysis. J Surg Oncol 56:54–58

van Beers B, Roche A, Jamart J, Cauquil P, Pariente D, Derhy S

(1989) Iodized oil retention of hepatocellular carcinoma on CT after transcatheter chemotherapy. Acta Radiol 30:415–418

Vetter D, Wenger JJ, Bergier JM, Doffoel M, Bockel R (1991) Transcatheter oily chemoembolization in the management of advanced hepatocellular carcinoma in cirrhosis: results of a western comparative study in 60 patients. Hepatology 13:427–433

Wang XW, Jia L, Sun Z, Harris C (1997) Interactive effects of p53 tumor suppressor gene and hepatitis B virus in hepatocellular carcinoma. In: Arroyo V, Bosch J, Bruguera M, Rodes J (eds) Therapy in liver diseases. The pathophysiological basis of therapy. Masson, Barcelona, pp 471–478

Xu HB, Yan XQ (1993) Diagnosis and therapy for primary hepatic carcinoma: transcatheter inferior phrenic arteriography and chemoembolization. J Tongji Med Univ 13:186–189

Yamada R, Sato M, Nomura S, Yamada T, Nakatsuka H (1985) Transcatheter arterial embolization of hepatocellular carcinoma: results of 519 cases in 7 years 9 months. J Jpn Soc Cancer Ther 20:1627

Yamakado K, Hirano T, Kato N, et al (1994) Hepatocellular carcinoma: treatment with a combination of transcatheter arterial chemoembolization and transportal ethanol injection. Radiology 193:75–80

Yoshikawa M, Saisho H, Ebara M, et al (1994) A randomized trial of intraarterial infusion of 4'-epidoxorubicin with Lipiodol versus 4'-epidoxorubicin alone in the treatment of hepatocellular carcinoma. Cancer Chemother Pharmacol 33 (Suppl):S149-S152

Yoshimi F, Nagao T, Inoue S, et al (1992) Comparison of hepatectomy and transcatheter arterial chemoembolization for the treatment of hepatocellular carcinoma: necessity for prospective randomized trial. Hepatology 16:702–706

Yu YQ, Xu DB, Zhou XD, Lu JZ, Tang ZY, Mack P (1993) Experience with liver resection after hepatic arterial chemoembolization for hepatocellular carcinoma. Cancer 71:62–65

18 Percutaneous Ethanol Injection of Hepatocellular Carcinoma and Borderline Lesions

R. Lencioni, D. Cioni, A. Paolicchi, M. Moretti, A. Cicorelli, and C. Bartolozzi

CONTENTS

18.1 Introduction

Hepatocellular carcinoma (HCC) is one of the most common neoplasms worldwide and occurs in association with cirrhosis in over 90% of patients (Colombo et al. 1991). Presently, many patients with cirrhosis undergo screening procedures that permit the early detection of HCC. As a result of widespread screening programs, the detection of HCC while it is small and unifocal has increased significantly (Bartolozzi et al. 1995b; Lencioni et al. 1996). Unfortunately, many patients with HCC are not suitable candidates for hepatic resection. Surgery is often precluded because of hepatic dysfunction secondary to underlying cirrhosis. These patients have little functional reserve and would be at high risk for postoperative hepatic failure. Also, because of the associated cirrhosis, these patients are at high risk for the development of future tumors (Bartolozzi and Lencioni 1996; Colombo et al. 1991; Trevisani et al. 1993). That is, the initial lesion may be the prelude to other lesions. The metachronous nature of HCC in patients with cirrhosis must be considered when treatment options are weighted. Because of the significant underlying hepatic disease, treatment methods that result in minimal damage to uninvolved hepatic parenchyma are best for the majority of patients with HCC (Lin et al. 1997; Imamura et al. 1998; De Sanctis et al. 1998).

Percutaneous ethanol injection (PEI) is a percutaneous technique aimed at achieving nonsurgical ablation of small liver tumors, particularly HCC. PEI has proven to be a safe, effective, and inexpensive treatment option for patients with cirrhosis and small HCC (Bartolozzi and Lencioni 1996; Lencioni and Bartolozzi 1997; Shiina et al. 1987, 1990a; Sugiura et al. 1983; Livraghi and Vettori 1990; Livraghi et al. 1986; Ebara et al. 1990). Absolute ethanol destroys tumor tissue mainly because of the dehydrating and denaturating effects it has on protein. In addition, ethanol has a thrombotic effect on tumor vascularity. Ethanol exerts tumoricidal and thrombotic effects locally, and usually does not damage noncancerous liver parenchyma (Bartolozzi and Lencioni 1996; Lencioni and Bartolozzi 1997). Although initially performed in patients with unresectable HCC lesions only, PEI is

R. Lencioni, MD; Division of Diagnostic and Interventional Radiology, Department of Oncology, University of Pisa, Via Roma 67, I-56125 Pisa, Italy
D. Cioni, MD; Division of Diagnostic and Interventional Radiology, Department of Oncology, University of Pisa, Via Roma 67, I-56125 Pisa, Italy
A. Paolicchi, MD; Division of Diagnostic and Interventional Radiology, Department of Oncology, University of Pisa, Via Roma 67, I-56125 Pisa, Italy
M. Moretti, MD; Division of Diagnostic and Interventional Radiology, Department of Oncology, University of Pisa, Via Roma 67, I-56125 Pisa, Italy
A. Cicorelli, MD; Division of Diagnostic and Interventional Radiology, Department of Oncology, University of Pisa, Via Roma 67, I-56125 Pisa, Italy
C. Bartolozzi, MD, Professor and Chairman; Division of Diagnostic and Interventional Radiology, Department of Oncology, University of Pisa, Via Roma 67, I-56125 Pisa, Italy

now used with a curative aim also in some operable patients, following the impressive long-term survival curves recently reported (Bartolozzi and Lencioni 1996; Lencioni and Bartolozzi 1997).

With the increase in experience, however, limitations of PEI have also emerged. Treatment with PEI alone, in particular, has been proved to be insufficient in patients with large HCC, because alcohol diffusion within the tumor mass was incomplete and residual viable neoplastic tissue often persisted along the periphery of the treated lesion (Vilana et al. 1992; Lencioni et al. 1995a; Livraghi et al. 1992). To overcome these drawbacks of PEI, newer treatment schedules, such as single-session PEI under general anesthesia (Livraghi et al. 1993; Giorgio et al. 1996), or combined therapeutic approaches, such as transcatheter arterial chemoembolization (TACE) followed by PEI have been recently developed and clinically tested (Allgaier et al. 1998; Bartolozzi et al. 1995a; Lencioni et al. 1994c, 1998d; Tanaka et al. 1998).

In this chapter, we critically reviewed indications and contraindications, technique, adverse effects and complications, follow-up protocol, local therapeutic effect and long-term survival after PEI treatment. On the basis of our 11 years of experience, we attempted in this paper to clarify the present role of PEI in the treatment of HCC and borderline lesions. Hence, the relationship of PEI to other currently available interventional therapies was also analyzed.

18.2 Indications and Contraindications

Eligibility for treatment with PEI depends on many factors, including patient age and performance status; presence and severity of liver cirrhosis; histology, site, size and number of lesions.

18.2.1 General Eligibility Criteria

To be considered eligible for treatment by PEI, patients must have some general characteristics. First, as PEI is a local treatment, disease must be confined to the liver, without evidence of vascular invasion or extrahepatic metastases. In addition, the tumor to treat by PEI must be a nodular lesion with well-defined borders. The presence of a clear and easy-to-detect target for injections is crucial for the outcome of PEI. Finally, the tumor nodule must be preferentially solitary and smaller than 3–4 cm.

A careful evaluation of the clinical status of the patient is necessary to establish the indication for PEI. Patients with severe liver dysfunction (Child-Pugh class C cirrhosis) should be excluded from PEI since in these cases treatment of the tumor would probably result in no benefit for survival (Livraghi et al. 1992). A prothrombin time ratio (normal time/patient's time) greater than 40–50% and a platelet count higher than 40 000–50 000/μl are required to prevent bleeding.

18.2.2 Hepatocellular Carcinoma

The rationale for PEI in the treatment of HCC is based on the following points: (a) ultrasound (US) screening in patients with liver cirrhosis allows detection of small HCC lesions in a preclinical stage; (b) ethanol shows a selective diffusion in HCC, because it is a soft tumor surrounded by hard cirrhotic liver; (c) PEI is effective and safe, being associated with negligible complication rates; (d) unlike surgery, PEI does not involve loss of noncancerous parenchyma, which is important because in cirrhotic patients hepatic function is already compromised and any intervention that worsens it further hastens the onset of liver failure; (e) local recurrences or new HCC lesions emerged during the follow-up can be treated again with PEI.

PEI may be considered a viable therapeutic approach for patients with Child-Pugh A or B liver cirrhosis and single, nodular-type HCC lesions smaller than 3 cm. Surgical resection, however, is still recommended in lesions emerged in noncirrhotic livers or in the case of superficially located lesions in patients with extremely well compensated cirrhosis. In the presence of multiple tumor nodules, in contrast, intraarterial treatment such as chemoembolization remains the treatment of choice, although PEI can be proposed as an alternative choice when the patient has up to three lesions smaller than 3 cm each. For patients with HCC tumors exceeding 3 cm (single lesion or main lesion associated with one or two daughter nodules), PEI can be profitably combined with chemoembolization, as discussed in the relevant chapter.

18.2.3 Borderline Lesions

As a result of careful US studies performed in patients with liver cirrhosis for early diagnosis of HCC, an increasing number of small hepatocellular nodular lesions arising in cirrhotic livers and lacking histopathological features of definite cancer have been increasingly detected over the past few years. These lesions, known as macroregenerative nodules or adenomatous hyperplasia (AH), are currently termed dysplastic nodules or borderline lesions, although various nomenclatures have been proposed. These nodules are now considered an intermediate step between a simple regenerative nodule and an overt HCC (Nakanuma et al. 1993): the emergence of HCC within AH nodules and the transformation of AH into HCC after serial observation, in fact, have been reported (Arakawa et al. 1986; Takayama et al. 1990; Lencioni et al. 1994a), and the monoclonal origin of these lesions has been ascertained by molecular biological studies (Tsuda et al. 1988). Aggressive treatment of these borderline lesions, therefore, has been recommended (Takayama et al. 1990; Lencioni et al. 1993a). While chemoembolization has no therapeutic effect on this pathologic entity, because it lacks the hypervascular arterial supply of HCC (Takayasu et al. 1993), the small size makes this lesion suitable for treatment by PEI (Lencioni et al. 1993a, 1994b; Livraghi et al. 1989).

18.3 Technique

18.3.1 Pretreatment Work-up

Number, location, and size of all tumor deposits in the liver must be accurately defined to establish eligibility for PEI. A standard staging protocol should include at least US combined with spiral CT or multislice dynamic MRI. Invasive procedures for further imaging the liver parenchyma, such as digital subtraction angiography, CT during arterial portography, or Lipiodol CT may be reserved for patients considered to be potential surgical candidates.

Chest radiography and bone scintigraphy are employed to exclude extrahepatic metastases. Besides routine hematologic tests, the serum level of alphafetoprotein (AFP) has to be determined.

18.3.2 Materials

PEI is best administered with US guidance, because this real-time control allows for a faster procedure time, precise centering of the needle in the target,

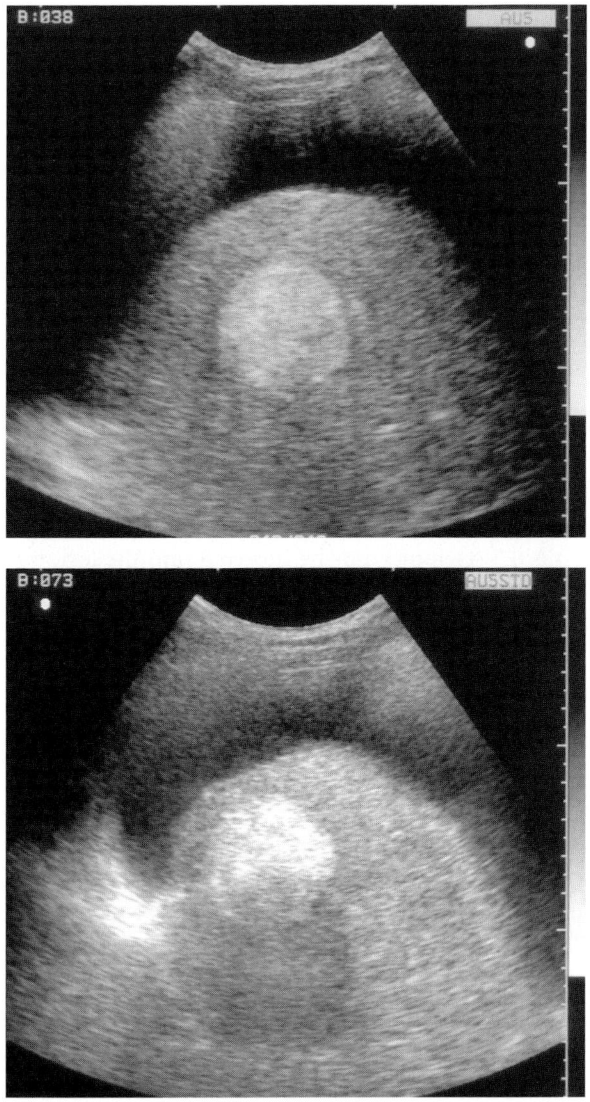

a

b

Fig. 18.1a,b. Percutaneous ethanol injection of hepatocellular carcinoma. Ultrasound image acquired before treatment shows a 4-cm hyperechoic tumor in patient with liver cirrhosis and ascites (**a**). Treatment with ethanol injection is selected, despite tumor size, in view of poorly compensated (Child Pugh class B) cirrhosis. On administration of 10 ml ethyl alcohol with a multihole needle, the lesion is completed embended by the ethanol (**b**)

and continuous monitoring of the procedure (Fig. 18.1). The latter is the most important point for PEI, since the evaluation of the distribution of the injected ethanol within the tumor is crucial to achieving a complete perfusion of the lesion or to identifying unperfused areas to treat in the following sessions. Moreover, real-time monitoring of the injection allows the prevention of excessive alcohol leakage into vessels or bile ducts, which can cause complications and reduce the degree of necrosis.

A one end-hole 22G spinal needle or a multiple side-hole 21G needle with a closed conical tip are commonly used for PEI (Akamatsu et al. 1993; Sheu et al. 1987). The first needle allows a more precise injection in small targets; the second one permits perfusion of larger volumes of tissue in one session (Fig. 18.1). We routinely use the free-hand technique for US guidance and the color Doppler mode to select the most appropriate track for the needle (Bartolozzi et al. 1998; Lencioni et al. 1995b; Ueno et al. 1998). The lack of lateral guide attachment allows scanning at multiple planes during the procedure, which may be useful to better evaluate the diffusion of the injected ethanol. As in some cases lesions treated by PEI may change their echopattern and become hardly depictable on US during the course of treatment, metal micromarkers (steel coils 0.5 cm long) may be inserted into the lesion to facilitate detection (Sheu et al. 1987; Elgidy et al. 1996; Ishizaka et al. 1997; Redvanly and Chezmar 1993; Seki et al. 1989).

18.3.3 Methods

As a rule, PEI does not need hospitalization of the patient and may be performed under local anesthesia. Patients should remain fasting because some may experience nausea. Premedication for analgesia and sedation may be given in selected cases (i.e., patients experiencing severe pain after the first injections).

In the first session, the needle is usually placed in the center of the lesion. The site of the following injections should be chosen in order to ensure perfusion of areas not fully treated during the previous sessions. During each treatment session, one to two injections are performed, and 2–10 ml sterile 95% ethyl alcohol is injected, depending on the size of the lesion and the distribution of the injected ethanol within the tumor. Ethanol injection is generally stopped when homogeneous alcohol perfusion of the lesion is accomplished or when ethanol leaks outside the lesion are repeatedly observed despite changing the site of alcohol injection. In the case of multiple lesions, the nodules can be treated in either the same session or in different sessions, depending mainly on the patient's compliance (Fig. 18.2).

In early reports on PEI, it has been suggested to calculate the total amount of alcohol to inject according to the formula $V=4/3\pi(r+0.5)^3$ where V (in ml) is the volume of ethanol and r (in cm) is the radius of the lesion; 0.5 is added to provide a safety margin, which is based on the concept that a certain amount of the surrounding tissue at the periphery of the lesion as well as the lesion itself must be destroyed to ensure cure of the tumor (Shiina et al. 1990b). However, this formula is not reliable. The amount of alcohol needed to ablate a lesion, in fact, depends on several factors, such as tumor consistency (in soft tumors, ethanol diffuses and is retained by far better than in hard lesions), degree of

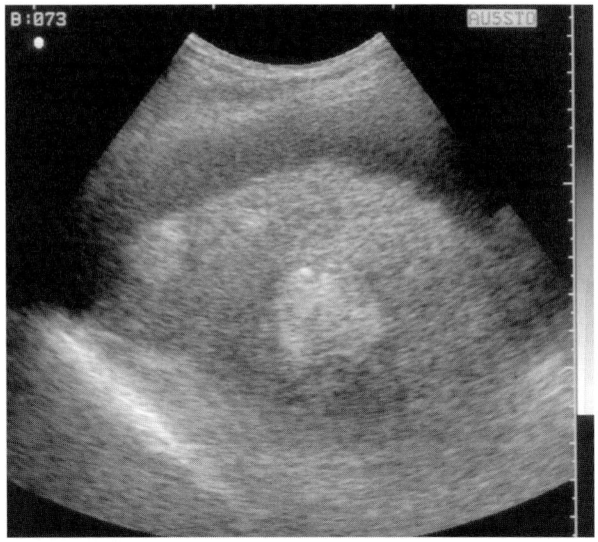

a

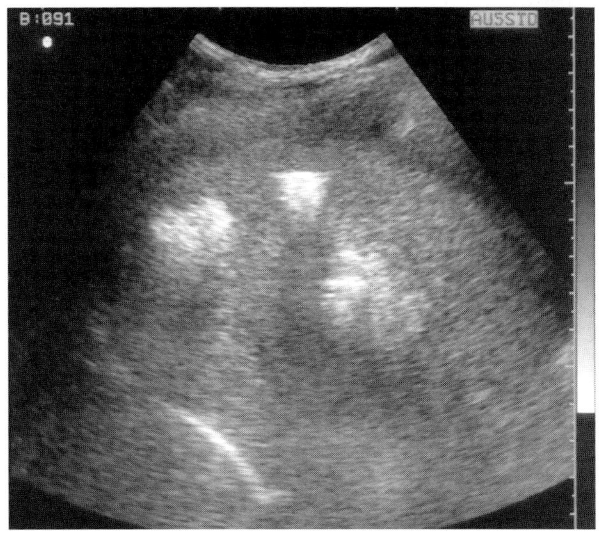

b

Fig. 18.2a,b. Percutaneous ethanol injection in multinodular hepatocellular carcinoma. Ultrasound image acquired before treatment shows three nodular lesions ranging from 1.5 to 3.5 cm in a patient with liver cirrhosis and ascites (**a**). Treatment with ethanol injection is selected, despite the number of lesions, in view of poorly compensated (Child Pugh class B) cirrhosis. After the procedure, the three lesions appear to be completely perfused by the ethanol (**b**) vascularization (hypervascularity enhances washout of the injected ethanol but also makes the lesion more responsive to alcohol-induced thrombosis of tumor vessels), internal septa (which favor segmental distribution of alcohol and may circumscribe unperfused areas), areas of spontaneous necrosis (which provide preferential paths of drainage for alcohol), and tumor capsule (which contain the alcohol but may also protect areas of extracapsular tumor invasion from the ethanol). In fact, this formula has not found wide acceptance and is actually not used in most centers.

Using gray-scale US as imaging guidance, it is not possible to evaluate the necrotic area produced by the previous treatment sessions, owing to the similar appearance of necrosis and viable neoplastic tissue. Therefore, according to the treatment protocol commonly used for PEI, four to eight sessions are scheduled, depending mainly on the size of the lesions, and the outcome of treatment is then checked by means of spiral CT or dynamic MRI (Bartolozzi et al 1994; Lencioni et al. 1993b).

Recently, following advances in Doppler US technology and the introduction of US contrast agents, a new treatment protocol has been proposed, in which response of the tumor during the course of treatment is monitored with color Doppler US. A color Doppler US study of the lesion is performed immediately before each PEI session: intratumoral color signals will be used to target the viable portions of the tumor during the injection. When no intratumoral blood flow signals are found with the unenhanced color Doppler US, a contrast-enhanced color Doppler US study can be performed to search for residual viable tumor areas undetected by the unenhanced study and to target these viable portions of the tumor during the injection (Fig. 18.3).

When no intratumoral enhancing areas are depicted with contrast-enhanced color Doppler US, further evaluation with spiral CT or dynamic MR imaging will be scheduled to confirm the favorable outcome of treatment and rule out possible false-negative results (Bartolozzi et al. 1998; Lencioni et al. 1995b).

This new treatment protocol has a number of distinct advantages in the treatment of HCC with PEI: (a) ethanol injections that follow the first PEI sessions are targeted solely to the residual viable portion of the tumor, which may avoid retreatment of areas already destroyed by previous procedures, thus shortening treatment times; (b) patients can be spared from either too early a suspension of the treatment or the administration of an excessive amount of ethanol; and (c) more expensive imaging examinations – such as spiral CT or dynamic MR imaging – needed to show up the areas of residual viable tumor during the course of treatment can be avoided.

To achieve a more homogeneous perfusion of large lesions, ethanol may be injected into several sites in one session. This also may reduce the overall number of sessions needed. In this case, it is useful to insert two or three needles before starting injection rather than positioning additional needles during the procedure. In fact, guidance of additional needles may be obscured by the hyperechoic appearance of the ethanol previously injected.

After the injection, the needle should be left in place for 1–2 min to reduce reflux through the puncture track into the peritoneal cavity, which may cause significant pain. At the end of the procedure, patients must be kept under medical observation for at least 2 h. Rescanning before leaving the Radiology Department is recommended to detect post-procedure complications.

To expand the use of PEI to larger and more numerous lesions a single-session technique (also termed "one-shot" technique) was recently proposed (Livraghi et al. 1993, 1998; Lencioni et al. 1998c; Giorgio et al. 1996). This technique permits the administration of larger amounts of alcohol compared with conventional PEI. Technique and results are described in the relevant chapter.

18.4 Adverse Effects and Complications

Common side effects after PEI include local pain lasting a few minutes and slight or moderate fever (37–39°C) on the day of injection. Fever is usually observed after the first PEI sessions, which induce the greatest amount of necrosis of tumorous tissue. These side effects are usually tolerated by patients and subside with symptomatic treatment.

Unlike other treatments, PEI has minimal or no negative effects on liver function, although a mild and transient rise of serum transaminase levels may sometimes be observed. In a few patients, a chemical thrombosis of the portal vein branches located in the vicinity of the tumor may occur as a consequence of the endothelial cell injury caused by ethanol leaks into the vessels. Chemical thrombi, however, usually have a minor clinical impact since they tend to disappear spontaneously within a few months of detection (Lencioni et al. 1995c; Seki et al. 1998). Other

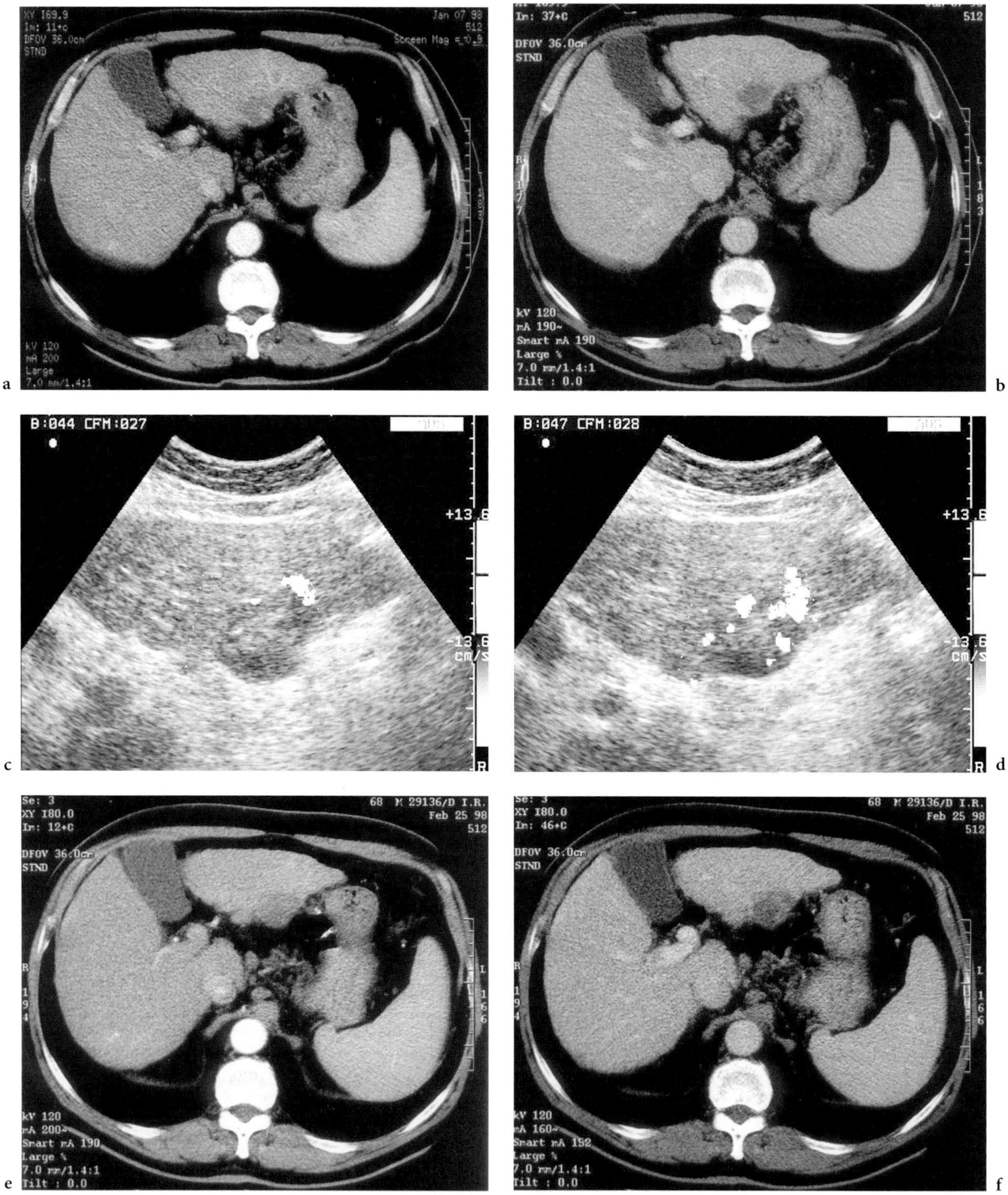

Fig. 18.3a–f. Percutaneous ethanol injection of small hepatocellular carcinoma. After treatment, a small area of residual viable enhancing tumor is depicted by spiral CT (arterial phase, **a**; portal phase, **b**). The viable portion of the tumor is also nicely depicted by color Doppler ultrasound due to clear-cut enhancement (unenhanced color Doppler image, **c**; contrast-enhanced color Doppler image, **d**). After additional treatment performed with contrast-enhanced color Doppler US guidance, complete tumor necrosis is seen on spiral CT (arterial phase, **e**; portal phase, **f**)

minor complications such as pleural effusion, pneumothorax, ascites, decreased hematocrit, vasovagal reaction, myoglobinuria, and transient hypotension are quite uncommon at the usual dosages of alcohol (REDVANLY et al. 1993).

Major treatment-related complications are extremely rare. A case of fatality following PEI of an HCC was described in a patient who died of a myocardial infarct probably caused by cardiovascular imbalance following massive hepatic necroses occurring both close and distant from the injection site (TAAVITSAINEN et al. 1993). Other severe complications reported in the literature include hepatic infarction, intraperitoneal bleeding, and injury of the bile duct (KODA et al. 1992). In addition, some cases of neoplastic seeding have been recently described (CEDRONE et al. 1992; ISHII et al. 1998; SAMMAKE et al. 1998; ZERBEY et al. 1994). Lesions which are superficially located and that are treated with a high number of PEI sessions seem to be particularly at risk for this complication. Considering all the unpublished patients treated with PEI, however, the occurrence of severe complications seems to be low.

18.5 Follow-up Protocol

After the end of the PEI cycle (i.e., when contrast-enhanced color Doppler US shows no residual enhancing areas within the tumor) (BARTOLOZZI et al. 1998; LENCIONI et al. 1995b), evaluation of the outcome of therapy is performed by spiral CT or dy-

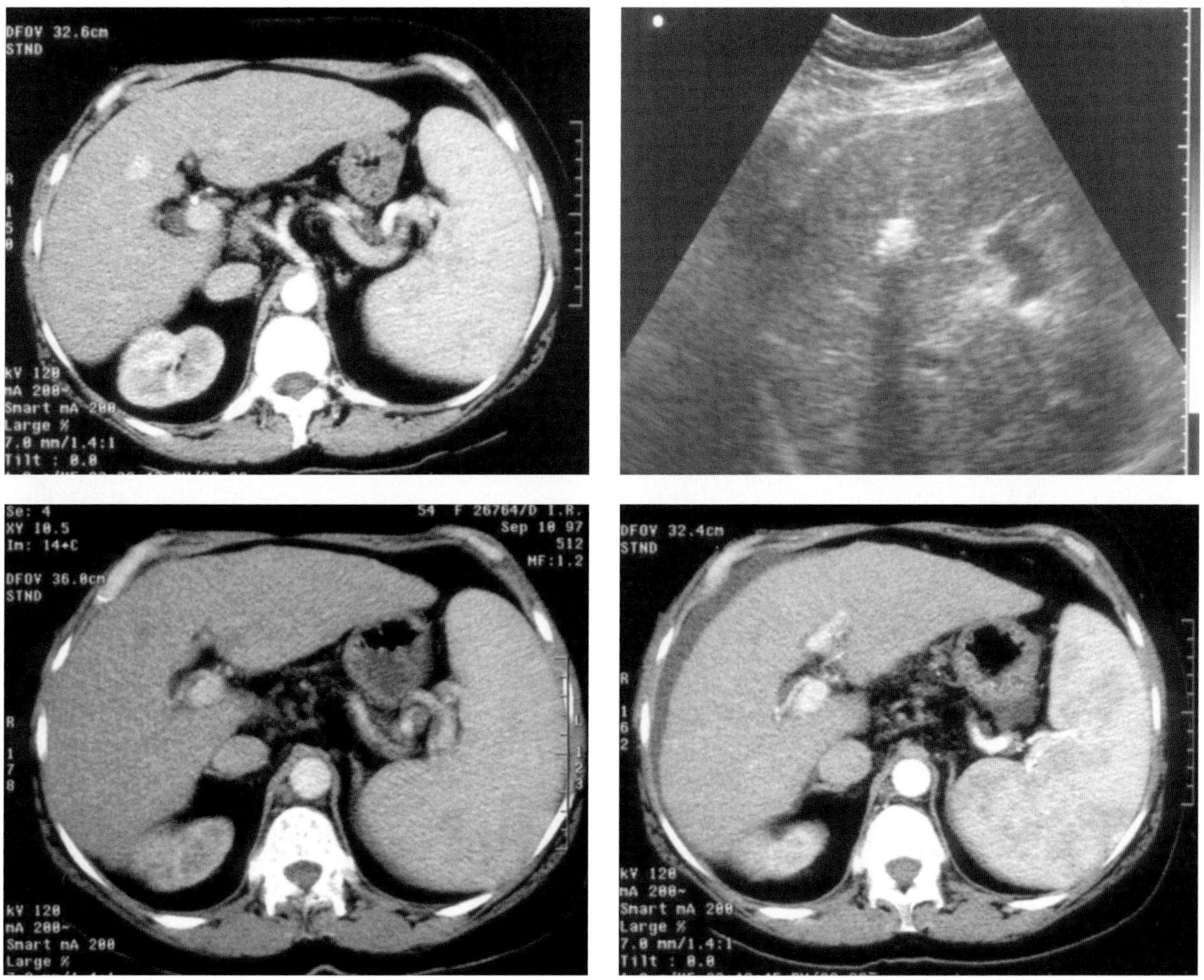

a b c d

Fig. 18.4a–d. Percutaneous ethanol injection of small hepatocellular carcinoma. Before treatment, the small lesion shows hyperattenuation on arterial-phase spiral CT image (**a**). Ultrasound image acquired immediately after ethanol instillation demonstrates homogeneous perfusion of the lesion (**b**). Arterial-phase CT image acquired 1 month (**c**) and 1 year (**d**) after treatment shows complete tumor response namic MRI (Fig. 18.4). Spiral CT and dynamic contrast-enhanced MRI, in fact, are recognized as the standard imaging modalities for evaluating the response of HCC to PEI (Lencioni et al. 1993b).

With spiral CT, lesions ablated by PEI appear as hypoattenuating, nonenhancing areas in both the arterial and the portal venous phases (Fig. 18.5). On the contrary, in the case of partial necrosis, the areas of residual viable neoplastic tissue can be easily recognized as they stand out in the arterial phase against the faintly enhanced normal liver parenchyma and the unenhanced areas of coagulation necrosis (Ebara et al. 1995; Joseph et al. 1993; Yoshikawa et al. 1995). With unenhanced MR imaging, alcohol-induced necrosis is usually shown as a markedly hypointense area on spin-echo T2 weighted images. This peculiar feature is due to the strong dehydrating effect of alcohol, which results in a coagulative necrosis of the tumor. Conversely, viable neoplastic tissue that persists after treatment maintains the high signal intensity shown on spin-echo T2 weighted images obtained before treatment and can therefore be recognized as a hyperintense area. To enhance the diagnostic accuracy of MR imaging, the use of dynamic studies after the administration of a paramagnetic contrast agent is to be recommended. Dynamic contrast-enhanced MR imaging, like spiral CT, may clearly show the presence of residual viable tumor because of the early arterial uptake of contrast resembling that of native lesions. Necrotic tumor, in contrast, fails to enhance throughout the entire dynamic study (Bartolozzi et al. 1994; Fujita et al. 1998; Ito et al. 1995; Lencioni et al. 1995d; Nagel and Bernardino 1993; Shinmoto et al. 1997; Sironi et al. 1991, 1993, 1994).

The post-treatment follow-up protocol for patients who underwent PEI includes: US and assays for AFP serum level at 3-month intervals, and spiral CT or dynamic MRI at 6-month intervals. Patients must be studied to diagnose either recurrences of the treated tumors or recurrences caused by the emergence of new nodular lesions. Complete response is considered to be obtained when no enhancing areas are seen at the level of the treated lesion at contrast-enhanced CT or dynamic MRI, reduction in size persists during the follow-up, and AFP level does not increase.

a b
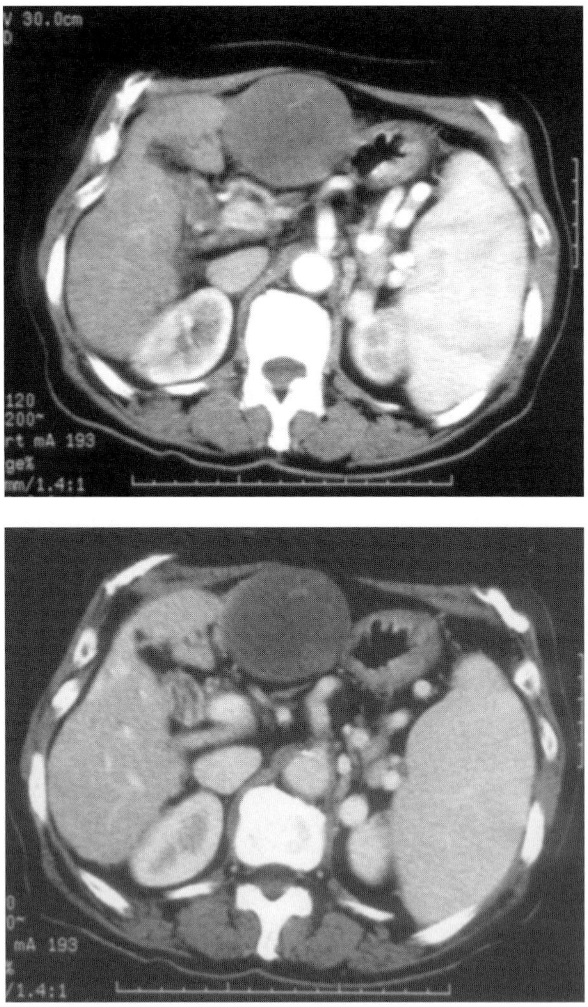

Fig. 18.5a,b. Dual phase spiral CT performed after single-session percutaneous ethanol injection of large hepatocellular carcinoma. The lesion fails to enhance in both the arterial (a) and the portal phase (b), suggesting complete response

18.6 Local Therapeutic Effect

18.6.1 Hepatocellular Carcinoma

The results of PEI in the treatment of HCC have been analyzed from two different points of view: (a) by evaluating the short-term results of treatment, that is by assessing the local effect of PEI through histopathologic examination of lesions resected after the procedure or follow-up imaging studies of the treated tumors; and (b) by evaluating the long-term survival of the treated patients.

At the beginning of the experience with PEI, some patients were resected after treatment. Pathologic examination of the specimens showed that PEI was able to destroy the lesion completely in most cases. Shiina et al. (1991) examined 23 treated lesions of

HCC histopathologically and found that the lesion was completely necrotic in 16 cases, 90% necrotic in six, and 70% necrotic in the remaining case. LIVRAGHI et al. (1988) reported that no viable tumor cells were detected in four patients who underwent surgery after PEI. Interestingly, histopathologic examinations showed that the capsule and some of the surrounding tissue were necrotic in addition to the tumor itself. This suggests that, unlike chemoembolization, PEI can also be effective against intercapsular and extracapsular invasions if they are located in areas the injected ethanol can reach (SHIINA et al. 1991). In cases of incomplete necrosis, viable HCC tissue remained along the edge of the tumors, in portions isolated by septa, or in small daughter nodules located in the vicinity of the main lesion (SHIINA et al. 1991).

More recently, imaging studies performed on a larger number of lesions treated by PEI confirmed that complete tumor necrosis can be achieved with a high probability if proper patient selection has been performed. In one series of 105 patients with 125 HCC lesions smaller than 5 cm treated by PEI, a complete tumor necrosis was shown by CT in 111 of 125 nodules (89%), whereas tumor persistence was seen in 14 of 125 (11%). Twelve of the 14 lesions which were still viable after PEI were larger than 3 cm, thus showing that the size of the nodule plays a key role in determining the outcome of treatment (LENCIONI et al. 1995a).

18.6.2 Borderline Lesions

PEI offers an effective therapeutic option in the management of dysplastic nodules (borderline lesions). In the published series, in fact, this treatment was always able to induce complete necrosis of these tiny nodules, safely preventing their evolution towards HCC (LENCIONI et al. 1993a, 1994b; LIVRAGHI et al. 1989). It has to be considered that surgical removal of these lesions, which are not unequivocally neoplastic, is not readily accepted either by the patient or the surgeon, as it entails the same surgical risk as that of resection of a small HCC. On the other hand, chemoembolization is not effective against borderline lesions, as they lack the typical hypervascular arterial supply of HCC (TAKAYASU et al. 1993).

The mere surveillance of these lesions with US may result in the untimely detection of malignant change, which will occur in up to 90% of cases after 4 years follow-up (LENCIONI et al. 1994b). Nevertheless, it has to be considered that HCC may of course develop in different hepatic segments with respect to the dysplastic nodule treated with PEI (LENCIONI et al. 1994b). Therefore, even if PEI proved to be able to prevent the malignant transformation of the treated lesions, patients with borderline lesions must be considered at high risk for developing HCC and carefully followed. Indeed, the occurrence of HCC bypassing the intermediate step of dysplastic nodule cannot be overlooked, considering that more paths in hepatocarcinogenesis are possible.

18.7 Long-Term Survival

The long-term efficacy of PEI has been demonstrated by the analysis of survival curves of treated patients (Table 18.1). In the Far East, EBARA et al. (1992) reported that in 112 patients in whom there were three or fewer lesions and all lesions were 3 cm or less in diameter, the 3- and 5-year survival rates were 63% and 39%, respectively. In a series of 98 HCC patients treated with potentially curative aim, SHIINA et al. (1993) obtained a 3-year survival of 62% and a 5-year survival of 52%.

In the West, few data are still available concerning the long-term results of PEI. LIVRAGHI et al. (1992) collected the data from five Italian centers and obtained 3-year survival rates of 63% and 31%, respectively, in patients with single or multiple HCC lesions smaller than 5 cm. CASTELLS et al.(1993) reported a 3-year survival of 55% in 30 patients with single lesions smaller than 4 cm, who, however, had severely impaired liver function. We recently investigated the long-term outcomes of PEI-treated cases in our single-institution study of 184 cirrhotic patients in Child Pugh class A or B with either a single tumor 5 cm or less in diameter or multiple (up to 4) HCC nodules smaller than or equal to 3 cm each. In our study, we obtained 3-, 5-, and 7-year survival rates of 67%, 41%, and 19%, respectively. Survival reached 78% at 3 years, 54% at 5 years, and 28% at 7 years in patients with a single HCC 3 cm or less; 61% at 3 years, 32% at 5 years, and 16% at 7 years in patients with a single HCC of 3.1–5 cm; and 51% at 3 years, 21% at 5 years, and 0% at 7 years in patients with multiple lesions (LENCIONI et al. 1997). In a recent multicenter trial which included 746 Italian patients, the 3- and 5-year survival rates of patients with single HCC smaller than or equal to 3 cm were 68%

Table 18.1. Long-term survival rates of patients with small HCC who underwent treatment with PEI

Series	No. of patients	Type of tumor: Size (cm)	Type of tumor: No.	Child-Pugh class	Survival rates (%): 1-year	3-year	5-year
Ebara et al (1992)	60	<3	s+m	A	96	72	51
	33	<3	s+m	B	90	72	48
	19	<3	s+m	C	94	25	0
Livraghi et al (1992)	162	<5	s	A+B+C	90	63	NA
	45	<5	m	A+B+C	90	31	NA
Shiina et al (1993)	98	<6.5	s+m	A+B+C	85	62	52
Castells et al (1993)	30	<4	s	A+B+C	83	55	NA
Lencioni et al (1995a)	64	<5	s+m	A	100	87	55
	41	<5	s+m	B	91	53	13
	52	<3	s	A+B	100	81	54
	30	3.1–5	s	A+B	92	60	21
	23	<3	m	A+B	94	54	0
Livraghi et al (1995)	293	<5	s	A	98	79	47
	149	<5	s	B	93	63	29
	20	<5	s	C	64	0	0
	121	<3	m	A	94	68	36
	63	<3	m	B	93	59	0
Lencioni et al (1997)	127	<5	s+m	A	98	79	53
	57	<5	s+m	B	88	50	28
	94	<3	s	A+B	100	78	54
	50	3.1–5	s	A+B	90	61	32
	40	<3	m	A+B	91	51	21
	70	<3	s	A	100	89	63

s, single; m, multiple (up to three); NA, not available

and 40%, respectively; the 3- and 5-year survival rates of patients with single HCC of 3.1–5 cm were 57% and 37%, respectively; and the 3- and 5-year survival rates of patients with multiple lesions were 47% and 26%, respectively (Livraghi et al. 1995). These similar survival figures reported by different Eastern and Western centers consistently demonstrate the reliability and the reproducibility of PEI.

The long-term outcome of PEI, however, depends on several factors. The severity of the underlying liver cirrhosis according to the classification of Child-Pugh represents one of the most important predictive factors for survival. In our series, in fact, 5-year survival reached 55% in HCC patients classified in Child-Pugh class A, while it was only 13% in those classified in Child-Pugh class B (Lencioni et al. 1995a). In addition, AFP levels on diagnosis are of prognostic significance. In our experience, patients with baseline AFP levels of 200 ng/ml or less had a significantly longer survival than patients with AFP levels exceeding 200 ng/ml. The latter, however, showed a dichotomous behavior, with a very short or a very long survival. This seems to suggest that AFP-secreting tumors may have different biological behaviors, some of them showing a rapid growth, and the others being associated with a lower aggressiveness. The type of tumor is another important prognostic factor. In our experience, patients with uninodular tumors in the range 3.1–5 cm and those with multinodular tumors showed similarly unsatisfactory long-term survival rates (21% and 0% at 5 years, respectively): in contrast, the prognosis of patients with uninodular HCC less than or equal to 3 cm in size was significantly better (5-year survival rate, 54%), thus suggesting that PEI is a highly effective nonsurgical treatment for these cases (Lencioni et al. 1995a.

The efficacy of each treatment modality for HCC must be balanced against the survival of untreated patients (LLOVET et al. 1989). Previous studies, however, demonstrated that even in the case of small nodular lesions detected by US screening, untreated patients show extremely poor long-term survival rates. In the series of EBARA et al. (1986), while 90.7% of 22 patients with HCC lesions smaller than 3 cm receiving no treatment lived for 1 year, only 12.8% lived as long as 3 years. Recently, BARBARA et al. (1992) confirmed that in 39 Caucasian patients with a total of 59 untreated HCC tumors arising from cirrhosis, survival was only 21% at 3 years, despite the fact that 37 of the 39 patients were in Child-Pugh class A or B, that all lesions were smaller than 5 cm, and that 24 of 39 had a solitary lesion. Therefore, considering the severity of the natural history of the disease, treatment with PEI can be assumed to definitely improve patients' survival.

18.8 Tumor Recurrences

Recurrence of HCC may be frequently observed after PEI. Most recurrences, however, are caused by new nodular lesions emerged remotely from the treated tumor. Therefore, they are probably unrelated to the original lesion. In contrast, recurrence at the level of the lesions treated by PEI is extremely rare (CASTELLANO et al. 1997; POMPILI et al. 1997; SHIBATA et al. 1996). In our series of PEI-treated patients with a follow-up of 2–78 months (mean, 22.5 months), recurrence of the tumor was demonstrated in 47 of 91 patients (51.6%) in whom initial treatment had been successful (LENCIONI et al. 1997). In 44 of 47 patients (94%), however, recurrence was represented by the emergence of new nodular lesions in other hepatic segments with respect to the treated tumor or by the development of a diffuse, infiltrative-type HCC. Recurrence of the tumor treated by PEI was found in only 3 of 47 cases (6%). Similar data were reported by Eastern investigators: in the series of SHIINA et al. (1993), the 3-year recurrence rates were 51% in 98 patients treated with a curative aim, while EBARA et al. (1992) reported that new HCC lesions appeared in 90% of patients after 5-year follow-up. Such a high rate of tumor recurrence, however, does not represent a specific drawback of PEI, being also found in cirrhotic patients with HCC treated with any kind of therapy, including surgery (BELGHITI et al. 1992). To improve the prognosis of patients with recurrence, it is important to detect new HCC lesions as early as possible in order to perform new PEI treatments (BARTOLOZZI and LENCIONI 1996; TANIKAWA and MAJINA 1993).

18.9 Ethanol Injection Versus Other Treatment Modalities

18.9.1 Surgical Resection

We found long-term results of PEI equivalent to those of patients treated by hepatic resection. In a recent review including 1272 Child-Pugh class A patients with HCC lesions 5 cm or smaller who underwent resection, the mean 5-year survival rate was 49% (LENCIONI et al. 1997). In our series, survival of Child-Pugh class A patients was 53% at 5 years and 32% at 7 years. According to the Liver Cancer Study Group of Japan, the 5-year survival rate of 347 patients with HCC lesions smaller than 2 cm treated by hepatic resection reached 60% (The Liver Cancer Study Group of Japan 1994). In our study, we obtained 5- and 7-year survival rates of 63% and 42%, respectively, by restricting the analysis to a selected group of 70 patients with single tumor smaller than or equal to 3 cm and Child-Pugh class A cirrhosis. The long-term outcomes of PEI-treated patients seemed to be at least equivalent to those of matched patients submitted for surgical resection also in recent prospective studies comparing PEI and hepatic resection: in one study, there was no difference in long-term survival, despite the fact that patients in the PEI group had significantly worse liver function (LENCIONI et al. 1995a). Similarly, KOTOH et al. (1994) found no difference between long-term prognosis of PEI-treated patients and that of resected cases. Hence, although no randomized trials comparing PEI versus surgery have been performed, the long-term results of the two treatments seem to be quite similar (BELGHITI et al. 1992; CASTELLS et al. 1993; KAWASAKI et al. 1995; LAI et al. 1995; MAZZIOTTI et al. 1998).

18.9.2 Transcatheter Arterial Chemoembolization

No randomized trial to compare survival rates of patients with small HCC treated by PEI with those of patients treated with transcatheter arterial chemoembolization (TACE) have been conducted yet. Long-term management of patients with small HCC with chemoembolization, however, has not been entirely satisfactory (Stefanini et al. 1995). The problems associated with conventional chemoembolization include incomplete tumor necrosis and the adverse effect on liver function induced by repeated procedures (Hashimoto et al. 1995). Comparison of historical data shows that survival after PEI is superior to that after conventional TACE. The mean 5-year survival rate in 556 patients carrying HCC lesions smaller than 5 cm treated with conventional TACE, however, was only 14% (Lencioni and Bartolozzi 1997). The effectiveness of conventional TACE, in fact, is limited in the case of small hypovascular HCC, nonencapsulated HCC, or HCC with extracapsular invasion of tumor cells. Repeated TACE procedures, therefore, must be performed to control the growth of the tumor. However, repeated TACE may cause liver function to worsen because noncancerous liver parenchyma is also damaged (Lencioni and Bartolozzi 1997).

More recently, segmental and subsegmental TACE were introduced (Matsui et al. 1993). In segmental and subsegmental TACE, a microcatheter is inserted into the more distal branches of the hepatic artery, and the drug as well as the embolic material is injected solely in the feeding artery of the tumor. This allows a stronger anticancer effect, sparing at the same time noncancerous liver parenchyma (Matsui et al. 1993). The preliminary results of segmental and subsegmental TACE are encouraging. Matsui et al. (1993) obtained a 3-year survival rate of 78% in a series of 82 Child-Pugh A or B patients with HCC lesions 4 cm or less in diameter treated with subsegmental TACE, which is equivalent to that obtained in our study in patients with single HCC smaller than or equal to 3 cm who underwent PEI. Hence, on the basis of the data now available, the results of subsegmental TACE seem to be comparable to those of PEI. It has to be considered, however, that in nearly 20% of cases selective catheterization distal to the subsegmental artery fails or is anatomically impossible (Matsui et al. 1993).

18.9.3 Radiofrequency Thermal Ablation

Radiofrequency (RF) thermal ablation is a percutaneous technique that has been developed during the past few years in an attempt to overcome the limitations of ethanol injection, particularly in the treatment of hepatic metastases (Rossi et al. 1996, 1998; Solbiati et al. 1997a,b; Lencioni et al. 1998a; Goldberg et al. 1998a,b). With this technique, RF waves are used to induce thermal ablation of small hepatic malignancies. Until a few years ago, RF treatment performed with a single, unmodified monopolar electrode was capable of producing cylindrical lesions no greater than 1.6 cm in diameter. Recent improvements in the RF technique included the development of expandable electrode needles with multiple retractable lateral exit jackhooks on the tip, and the introduction of high-power generators coupled with dual-lumen, cooled-tip electrode needles (Rossi et al. 1996, 1998; Solbiati 1998; Solbiati et al. 1997a,b; Lencioni et al. 1998a; Goldberg et al. 1998a,b). With these advances, the extent of coagulation necrosis that can be obtained with a single-probe insertion has substantially increased. These generators, in fact, are capable of producing spherical or nearly spherical volumes of thermal necrosis up to 3–4 cm in diameter with a single-probe insertion (Solbiati 1998; Solbiati et al. 1997a,b; Lencioni et al. 1998a; Rossi et al. 1998; Goldberg et al. 1998a,b).

In the first clinical experience, 39 patients with a single HCC nodule not more than 3 cm in diameter were treated with monopolar and bipolar methods. The tumoral destruction was achieved in all cases, with normalization of AFP levels in cases where it was increased. The mean number of sessions needed to obtain tumor destruction was 3.3 (range, 1–8). During the follow-up, the treated HCCs slowly diminished in size, becoming not detectable by US or appearing as small hyperechoic areas or as isoechoic areas with a hyperechoic rim. During a mean follow-up of 23 months (range 3–66), 16 of 39 (41%) patients had recurrences: local recurrences, however, occurred in only 5% of cases, whereas 36% of recurrences were due to the emergence of new lesions in other hepatic segments. Most recurrent tumors underwent new courses of RF treatment. Overall, 54 HCC nodules in 39 patients were treated during the study. Median survival time was 44 months (Rossi et al. 1996).

Another group of 23 patients with either a single tumor nodule of not more than 3.5 cm or multiple (up to three) tumor nodules, none of which exceeded 3.0 cm in diameter, was treated by using expandable needle electrodes with four hooks. In this study, 26 tumor nodules were apparently ablated in a mean of 1.5 sessions (1.1 for tumors less than 2.5 cm; 1.7 for the others). Twenty-one patients were followed up for at least 6 months (mean 10 months; range 6–19 months): one patient showed local recurrence, two had new tumor nodules, three had multicentric disease, and 15 remained apparently disease-free (Rossi et al. 1998).

In a third experience, 12 patients with HCC lesions with diameters from 3.8 to 6.5 cm were treated with RITA (expandable needle electrode) after segmental transarterial embolization. In all cases complete ablation was achieved in a mean number of 1.2 sessions. During a mean follow-up of 11 months (range 6–17) two patients died from unrelated causes, and four patients had recurrences. Two cases were treated with a new course of RF ablation, while one was submitted for surgical resection. Thus, nine patients were alive and apparently disease free.

In two recent randomized studies the efficacy of RF thermal ablation and PEI for the treatment of small HCC was compared. Both studies showed that treatment time is significantly shorter by using RF than by using PEI; the radicality of the RF treatment appeared to be higher, being the percentage of cases with complete necrosis greater or the number of recurrences less (Fig. 18.6); no major complications with either of the treatments were observed in one study (Lencioni et al. 1998b); complication rate was higher for RF treatment than that of PEI in the other (Livraghi et al 1999).

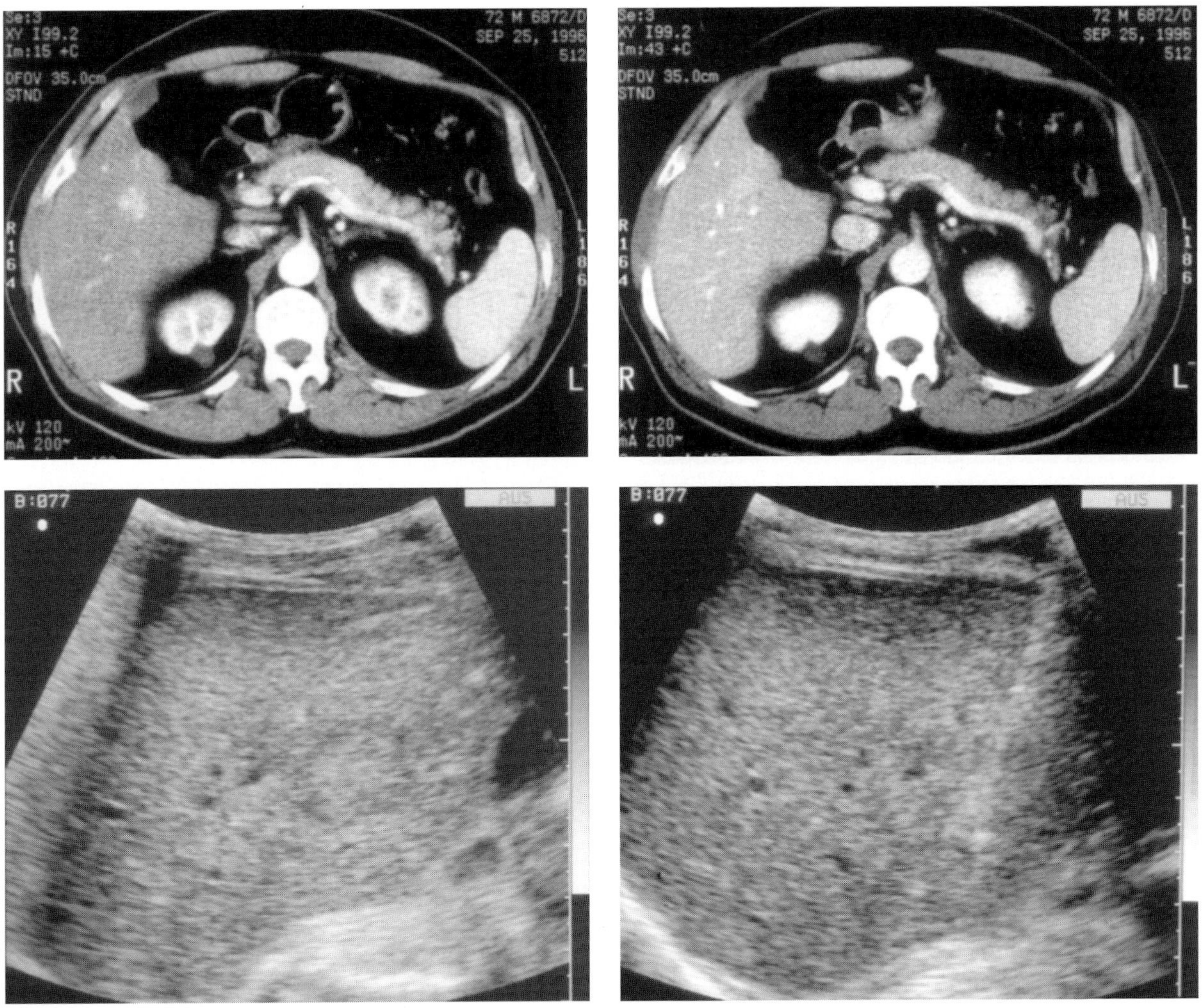

Fig. 18.6a–d. Radiofrequency thermal ablation of small hepatocellular carcinoma. Before treatment, the lesion is hyperattenuating in the arterial phase (**a**) and isoattenuating in the portal phase (**b**). Ultrasound images obtained before (**c**), at the time of the insertion of the electrode needle (**d**), (continued next page)

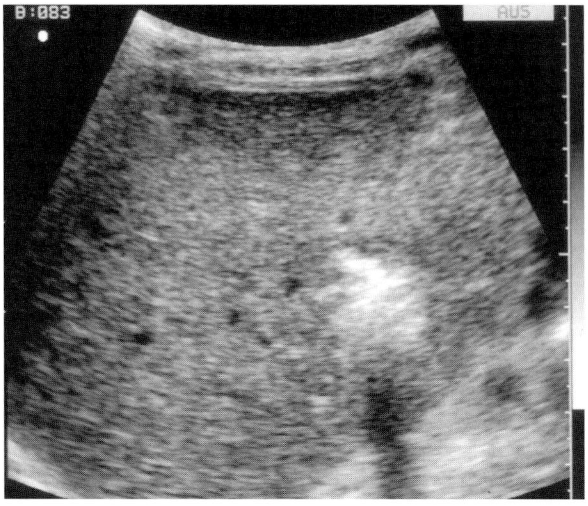
e

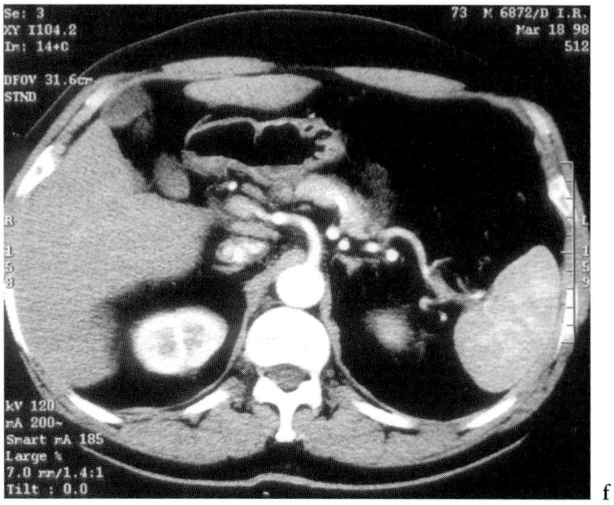
f

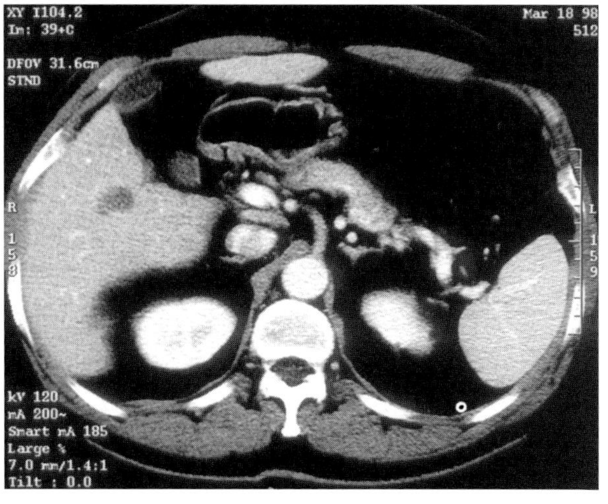
g

Fig. 18.6e–g (Continued). Radiofrequency thermal ablation of small hepatocellular carcinoma. Before treatment, the lesion is hyperattenuating in the arterial phase and immediately after the end of ablation (**e**). Note the typical hyperechoic area due to gas microbubbles caused by the high temperature. Eighteen month later, a complete tumor response is seen on dual phase spiral CT (arterial phase, **f**; portal phase, **g**) with no signs of recurrence

18.10 Conclusions

In conclusion, the summary of the available study demonstrates PEI to be an effective treatment for HCC. Not surprisingly, both the degree of liver dysfunction (according to the classification of Child-Pugh) and the type of the tumor (number and size of HCC lesions) significantly affect survival of PEI-treated patients. Impressive long-term survival rates, indeed, can be obtained in patients with Child-Pugh class A cirrhosis and single HCC smaller than or equal to 3 cm in diameter.

Our current policy is to consider PEI as the treatment of choice for borderline lesions and single HCC lesions smaller than 3 cm. In these cases, in fact, PEI is almost always able to induce complete necrosis of the lesion. Since HCC is a neoplasm that, even when the resection has been radical, will ineluctably recur within 5 years, then a local therapy like PEI, which is not associated with mortality or serious complications, may be preferable. Surgical resection, however, is still recommended in lesions emerged in noncirrhotic livers or subcapsular lesions in patients with extremely well-compensated cirrhosis.

In patients carrying single HCC larger than 3 cm, in contrast, the survival curve after PEI is significantly lower. Recent studies, however, showed that in these cases the efficacy of PEI may be greatly enhanced by pretreatment of the tumor with TACE (Tanaka et al. 1992, 1998; Bartolozzi et al. 1995a). TACE, performed before the beginning of PEI, facilitates alcohol diffusion, by making the texture of the tumor necrotic. Therefore, greater amounts of ethanol can be injected, and larger tumors can be effectively treated (Bartolozzi et al. 1995a; Lencioni et al. 1994c; Tanaka et al. 1991). Combined TACE and PEI is presently the treatment of choice for large (>3 cm) HCC at our institution (Bartolozzi et al. 1995a; Bartolozzi and Lencioni 1996; Lencioni et al. 1994c).

For patients with multinodular HCC, the results obtained in our study with PEI are hardly comparable with those of other treatments, particularly TACE. Treatment with PEI, in fact, was restricted to patients with no more than four lesions smaller than or equal to 3 cm each. In contrast, patients treated with TACE frequently had larger and more numerous lesions. Undoubtedly, some limitations exist in PEI therapy for multinodular HCC. In fact, it is practically impossible to treat more than four lesions because of the number of necessary treatment sessions. Moreover, it is very likely that patients with multiple lesions have also some tiny intrahepatic metastatic nodules undetectable with imaging modalities (Belghiti 1992). TACE, therefore, remains the treatment of choice for the majority of these patients, although PEI can be proposed as a viable alternative in selected cases.

References

Akamatsu K, Miyauchi S, Ito Y, Onkubo K, Maruyama M (1993) Development and evaluation of a needle for percutaneous ethanol injection therapy. Radiology 186:284–286

Allgaier HP, Deibert P, Olschewski M, et al (1998) Survival benefit of patients with inoperable hepatocellular carcinoma treated by a combination of transarterial chemoembolization and percutaneous ethanol injection a single-center analysis including 132 patients. Int J Cancer 79:601–605

Arakawa M, Kage M, Suguhara S, Nakashima T, Suenaga M, Okuda K (1986) Emergence of malignant lesions within an adenomatous hyperplastic nodule in a cirrhotic liver: observations in five cases. Gastroenterology 91:198–208

Barbara L, Benzi G, Gaiani S, et al (1992) Natural history of small untreated hepatocellular carcinoma in cirrhosis: a multivariate analysis of prognostic factors of tumor growth rate and patient survival. Hepatology 16:132–137

Bartolozzi C, Lencioni R (1996) Ethanol injection for the treatment of hepatic tumors. Eur Radiol 6:682–696

Bartolozzi C, Lencioni R, Caramella D, Mazzeo S, Ciancia EM (1994) Treatment of hepatocellular carcinoma with percutaneous ethanol injection: evaluation with contrast-enhanced MR imaging. AJR 162:827–831

Bartolozzi C, Lencioni R, Caramella D, et al (1995a) Treatment of large hepatocellular carcinoma: transcatheter arterial chemoembolization combined with percutaneous ethanol injection versus repeated transcatheter arterial chemoembolizations. Radiology 197:812–818

Bartolozzi C, Lencioni R, Caramella D, Palla A, Bassi AM, Di Candio G (1995b) Small hepatocellular carcinoma: detection with US, CT, MR imaging, DSA and Lipiodol-CT. Acta Radiol 37:69–74

Bartolozzi C, Lencioni R, Ricci P, et al (1998) Hepatocellular carcinoma treatment with percutaneous ethanol injection: evaluation with contrast-enhaced color Doppler US. Radiology 209:387–393

Belghiti J, Panis Y, Farges O, Benhamou JP, Fekete F (1992) Intrahepatic recurrence after resection of hepatocellular carcinoma complicating cirrhosis. Ann Surg 214:114–117

Castellano L, Calandra M, Del Vecchio Blanco C, De Sio I (1997) Predictive factors of survival and intrahepatic recurrence of hepatocellular carcinoma in cirrhosis after percutaneous ethanol injection: analysis of 71 patients. J Hepatol 27:862–870

Castells A, Bruix J, Bru C, et al (1993) Treatment of small hepatocellular carcinoma in cirrhotic patients: a cohort study comparing surgical resection and percutaneous ethanol injection. Hepatology 18:1121–1126

Cedrone A, Rapaccini GL, Pompili M, Grattagliano A, Aliotta A, Trombino C (1992) Neoplastic seeding complicating percutaneous ethanol injection for treatment of hepatocellular carcinoma. Radiology 183:787–788

Colombo M, De Franchis R, Del Ninno, et al (1991) Hepatocellular carcinoma in Italian patients with cirrhosis. N Engl J Med 325:675–680

De Sanctis JT, Goldberg SN, Mueller PR (1998) Percutaneous treatment of hepatic neoplasms: a review of current techniques. Cardiovasc Intervent Radiol 21:273–296

Ebara M, Ohto M, Shinagawa T, et al (1986) Natural history of minute hepatocellular carcinoma smaller than three centimeters complicating cirrhosis. Gastroenterology 90:259–266

Ebara M, Ohto M, Sugiura N, Okuda K, Kondo F, Kondo K (1990) Percutaneous ethanol injection for the treatment of small hepatocellular carcinoma: study of 95 patients. J Gastroenterol Hepatol 5:616–626

Ebara M, Kita K, Yoshikawa M, Sugiura N, Ohto M (1992) Percutaneous ethanol injection for patients with small hepatocellular carcinoma. In: Tobe T, Kameda H, Okudaira M, et al (eds) Primary liver cancer in Japan. Springer-Verlag, Tokyo, pp 291–300

Ebara M, Kita K, Sugiura N, et al (1995) Therapeutic effect of percutaneous ethanol injection on small hepatocellular carcinoma: evaluation with CT. Radiology 195:371–377

Elgindy NM, Lindholm HB, Gunven PM, Ohlsen HL (1996) A modified technique for ethanol injection of liver tumors: preliminary results. Eur Radiol 6:494–501

Fujita T, Honjo K, Takano K, et al (1998) Dynamic MR follow-up of small hepatocellular carcinoma after percutaneous ethanol injection therapy. J Comput Assist Tomogr 22:379–386

Giorgio A, Tarantino L, Francica G, et al (1996) One-shot percutaneous ethanol injection of liver tumors under general anesthesia: preliminary data on efficacy and complications. Cardiovasc Intervent Radiol 19:27–31

Goldberg SN, Gazelle GS, Solbiati L, et al (1998a) Ablation of liver tumors using percutaneous RF therapy. AJR 170:1023–1028

Goldberg SN, Hahn PF, Tanabe KK, et al (1998b) Percutaneous radiofrequency tissue ablation: does perfusion-mediated tissue cooling limit coagulation necrosis? J Vasc Interv Radiol 9:101–111

Hashimoto T, Nakamura H, Hori S, et al (1995) Hepatocellular carcinoma: efficacy of transcatheter oily chemoembolization in relation to macroscopic and microscopic pattern of tumor growth among 100 patients with partial epatectomy. Cardiovasc Intervent Radiol 18:82–86

Imamura M, Shiratori Y, Sato S, et al (1998) Percutaneous hepatic infarction therapy for hepatocellular carcinoma. AJR 171:1031–1035

Ishii H, Okada S, Okusaka T, et al (1998) Needle tract implantation of hepatocellular carcinoma after percutaneous ethanol injection. Cancer 82:1638–1642

Ishizaka H, Ishijima H, Katsuya T, Koyama Y (1997) Percutaneous ethanol injection therapy: use of a directable needle guide. AJR 168:1563–1564

Ito K, Honjo K, Fujita T, Awaya H, Mastumoto T, Mastunaga N (1995) Enhanced MR imaging of the liver after ethanol treatment of hepatocellular carcinoma: evaluation of areas of hyperperfusion adjacent to the tumor. AJR 164:1413–1417

Joseph FB, Baumgartner DA, Bernardino ME (1993) Hepatocellular carcinoma: CT appearance after percutaneous ethanol ablation therapy. Radiology 186:553–556

Kawasaki S, Makuuchi M, Miyagawa S,et al (1995) Results of hepatic resection for hepatocellular carcinoma. World J Surg 19:31–34

Koda M, Okamoto K, Miyoshi Y, Kawasaki H (1992) Hepatic vascular and bile duct injury after ethanol injection therapy for hepatocellular carcinoma. Gastrointest Radiol 17:167–169

Kotoh K, Sakai H, Sakamoto S, et al (1994) The effect of percutaneous ethanol injection therapy on small solitary hepatocellular carcinoma is comparable to that of hepatectomy. Am J Gastroenterol 89:194–198

Lai EC, Fan ST, Lo CM, Chu KM, Liu CL, Wong J (1995) Hepatic resection for hepatocellular carcinoma. An audit of 343 patients. Ann Surg 221:291–298

Lencioni R, Bartolozzi C (1997) Nonsurgical treatments of hepatocellular carcinoma. The Cancer J 10:17–23

Lencioni R, Bartolozzi C, Caramella D, Di Coscio G (1993a) Management of adenomatous hyperplastic nodules in the cirrhotic liver: US follow-up or percutaneous alcohol ablation? Abdom Imaging 18:50–55

Lencioni R, Caramella D, Bartolozzi C (1993b) Response of hepatocellular carcinoma to percutaneous ethanol injection: CT and MR evaluation. J Comput Assist Tomogr 17:723–729

Lencioni R, Caramella D, Bartolozzi C, Di Coscio G (1994a) Long term follow-up study of adenomatous hyperplasia in liver cirrhosis. Ital J Gastroenterol 26:163–168

Lencioni R, Caramella D, Bartolozzi C, Mazzeo S, Di Coscio G (1994b) Percutaneous ethanol injection therapy of adenomatous hyperplastic nodules in cirrhotic liver disease. Acta Radiol 35:138–142

Lencioni R, Vignali C, Caramella D, Cioni R, Mazzeo S, Bartolozzi C (1994c) Transcatheter arterial embolization followed by percutaneous ethanol injection in the treatment of hepatocellular carcinoma. Cardiovasc Intervent Radiol 17:70–75

Lencioni R, Bartolozzi C, Caramella D, et al (1995a) Treatment of small hepatocellular carcinoma with percutaneous ethanol injection. Analysis of prognostic factors in 105 Western patients. Cancer 76:1737–1746

Lencioni R, Caramella D, Bartolozzi C (1995b) Hepatocellular carcinoma: use of color Doppler US to evaluate response to treatment with percutaneous ethanol injection. Radiology 194:113–118

Lencioni R, Caramella D, Sanguinetti F, Battolla L, Falaschi F, Bartolozzi C (1995c) Portal vein thrombosis after percutaneous ethanol injection for hepatocellular carcinoma: value of color Doppler sonography in distinguishing chemical and tumor thrombi. AJR 164:1125–1130

Lencioni R, Mascalchi M, Paolicchi A, Zampa V (1995d) Breath-hold spin-echo MR imaging for evaluation of dynamic enhancement of native and treated hepatocellular carcinoma after intravenous Gd-DTPA administration. MAG*MA 3:151–156

Lencioni R, Pinto F, Armillotta N, Bartolozzi C (1996)Assessment of tumor vascularity in hepatocellular carcinoma: comparison of power Doppler US and color Doppler US. Radiology 201:353–358

Lencioni R, Pinto F, Armillotta N, et al (1997) Long-term results of percutaneous ethanol injection therapy for hepatocellular carcinoma in cirrhosis: a european experience. Eur Radiol 7:514–519

Lencioni R, Goletti O, Armillotta N, et al (1998a) Radio-frequency thermal ablation of liver metastases with a cooled-tip electrode needle: results of a pilot clinical trial. Eur Radiol 8:1205–1211

Lencioni R, Cioni D, Paolicchi A, et al (1998b) Percutaneous treatment of small hepatocellular carcinoma: radio-frequency thermal ablation versus percutaneous ethanol injection: prospective, randamized trial. Radiology 209 (P): 174

Lencioni R, Cioni D, Uliana M, Bartolozzi C (1998c) Fatal thrombosis of the portal vein following single-session percutaneous ethanol injection therapy of hepatocellular carcinoma. Abdom Imaging 23:608–610

Lencioni R, Paolicchi A, Moretti M, et al (1998d) Combined transcatheter arterial chemoembolization and percutaneous ethanol injection for the treatment of large hepatocellular carcinoma: local therapeutic effect and long-term survival rate. Eur Radiol 8:439–444

Lin DY, Lin SM, Liaw YF (1997) Non-surgical treatment of hepatocellular carcinoma. J Gastroenterol Hepatol 12:S319-S328

Livraghi T, Vettori C (1990) Percutaneous ethanol injection therapy of hepatoma. Cardiovasc Intervent Radiol 13:146–152

Livraghi T, Festi D, Monti M, Salmi A, Vettori C (1986) US-guided percutaneous alcohol injection of small hepatic and abdominal tumors. Radiology 161:309–312

Livraghi T, Salmi A, Bolondi L, et al (1988) Small hepatocellular carcinoma: percutaneous alcohol injection – results in 23 patients. Radiology 168:313–317

Livraghi T, Sangalli G, Vettori C (1989) Adenomatous hyperplastic nodules in the cirrhotic liver: a therapeutic approach. Radiology 170:155–157

Livraghi T, Bolondi L, Lazzaroni S, et al (1992) Percutaneous ethanol injection in the treatment of hepatocellular carcinoma in cirrhosis. Cancer 69:925–929

Livraghi T, Lazzaroni S, Pellicanò S, Ravasi S, Torzilli G, Vettori C (1993) Percutaneous ethanol injection of hepatic tumors: single-session therapy with general anesthesia. AJR 161:1065–1069

Livraghi T, Giorgio A, Marin G, et al (1995) Hepatocellular carcinoma and cirrhosis in 746 patients: long-term results of percutaneous ethanol injection. Radiology 197:101–108

Livraghi T, Goldberg SN, Lazzaroni S, et al (1999) Small hepatocellular carcinoma: treatment with radio-frequency ablation versus ethanol injection. Radiology 210:655–661

Livraghi T, Benedini V, Lazzaroni S, Meloni F, Torzilli G, Vettori C (1998) Long term results of single session percutaneous ethanol injection in patients with large hepatocellular carcinoma. Cancer 83:48–57

Llovet JM, Bustamante J, Castells A, et al (1999) Natural history of untreated nonsurgical hepatocellular carcinoma: rationale for the design and evaluation of therapeutic trials. Hepatology 29:62–67

Matsui O, Kadoya M, Yoshikawa J, et al (1993) Small hepatocellular carcinoma: treatment with subsegmental transcatheter arterial embolization. Radiology 188:79–83

Mazziotti A, Grazi GL, Cavallari A (1998) Surgical treatment of hepatocellular carcinoma on cirrhosis: a Western experience. Hepatogastroenterology 45:S1281-S1287

Nagel HS, Bernardino ME (1993) Contrast-enhanced MR imaging of hepatic lesions treated with percutaneous ethanol ablation therapy. Radiology 189:265–270

Nakanuma Y, Terada T, Ueda K, Terasaki S, Nonomura A, Matsui O (1993) Adenomatous hyperplasia of the liver as a precancerous lesion. Liver 13:1–9

Pompili M, Rapaccini GL, De Luca F, et al (1997) Risk factors for intrahepatic recurrence of hepatocellular carcinoma in cirrhotic patients treated by percutaneous ethanol injection. Cancer 79:1501–1508

Redvanly RD, Chezmar JL (1993) Percutaneous ethanol ablation therapy of malignant hepatic tumors using CT guidance. Semin Intervent Radiol 10:82–87

Redvanly RD, Chezmar JL, Strauss RM, Galloway JR, Boyer TD, Bernardino ME (1993) Malignant hepatic tumors: safety of high-dose percutaneous ethanol ablation therapy. Radiology 188:283–285

Rossi S, Di Stasi M, Buscarini E, et al (1996) Percutaneous RF interstitial thermal ablation in the treatment of hepatic cancer. AJR 167:759–768

Rossi S, Buscarini E, Garbagnati F, et al (1998) Percutaneous treatment of small hepatic tumors by an expandable RF needle electrode. AJR 170:1015–1022

Sammak B, Yousef B, Abd El Bagi M, et al (1998) Needle track seeding following percutaneous ethanol injection for treatment of hepatocellular carcinoma. Hepatogastroenterology 45:1097–1099

Schwartz ME, Sung M, Mor E, et al (1995) A multidisciplinary approach to hepatocellular carcinoma in patients with cirrhosis. J Am Coll Surg 180:596–603

Seki T, Nonaka T, Kubota Y, Mizuno T, Sameshima Y (1989) Ultrasonically-guided percutaneous ethanol injection therapy for hepatocellular carcinoma. Am J Gastroenterol 84:1400–1407

Seki T, Wakabayashi M, Nakagawa T, et al (1998) Hepatic infarction following percutaneous ethanol injection therapy for hepatocellular carcinoma. Eur J Gastroenterol Hepatol 10:915–918

Sheu JC, Huang GT, Chen DS, Sung JL, Yan PM, Wei TC (1987) Small hepatocellular carcinoma: intratumor ethanol treatment using new needle and guidance system. Radiology 163:43–48

Shibata T, Sakahara H, Kawakami S, Konishi J (1996) Sonographic characteristics of recurrent hepatocellular carcinoma. Eur Radiol 6:443–447

Shiina S, Yasuda H, Muto H, et al (1987) Percutaneous ethanol injection in the treatment of liver neoplasms. AJR 149:949–952

Shiina S, Tagawa K, Unuma T, et al (1990a) Percutaneous ethanol injection therapy of hepatocellular carcinoma: analysis of 77 patients. AJR 155:1221–1226

Shiina S, Tagawa K, Unuma T, Terano A (1990b) Percutaneous ethanol injection therapy for the treatment of hepatocellular carcinoma. AJR 154:947–951

Shiina S, Tagawa K, Unuma T, et al (1991) Percutaneous ethanol injection therapy for hepatocellular carcinoma: a histopathologic study. Cancer 68:1524–1530

Shiina S, Tagawa K, Niwa Y, et al (1993) Percutaneous ethanol injection therapy for hepatocellular carcinoma: results in 146 patients. AJR 160:1023–1028

Shinmoto H, Mulkern RV, Oshio K, Silverman SG, Colucci VM, Jolesz FA (1997) MR appearance and spectral features of injected ethanol in the liver: implication for fast MR-guided percutaneous ethanol injection therapy. J Comput Assist Tomogr 21:82–88

Sironi S, Livraghi T, Del Maschio A (1991) Small hepatocellular carcinoma treated with percutaneous ethanol injection: MR imaging findings. Radiology 180:333–336

Sironi S, Livraghi T, Angeli E, et al (1993) Small hepatocellular carcinoma: MR follow-up of treatment with percutaneous ethanol injection. Radiology 187:119–123

Sironi S, De Cobelli F, Livraghi T, et al (1994) Small hepatocellular carcinoma treated with percutaneous ethanol injection: unenhanced and gadolinium-enhanced MR imaging follow-up. Radiology 192:407–412

Solbiati L (1998) New applications of ultrasonography: interventional ultrasound Eur J Radiol 27:S200-S206

Solbiati L, Goldberg SN, Ierace T, et al (1997a) Hepatic metastases: percutaneous radio-frequency thermal ablation with cooled-tip electrodes. Radiology 205:367–373

Solbiati L, Ierace T, Goldberg SN, et al (1997b) Percutaneous US guided radio-frequency tessue ablation of liver metastases: Treatment and follow-up in 16 patients. Radiology 202:195–203

Stefanini GF, Amorati P, Biselli M, et al (1995) Efficacy of transarterial targeted treatments on survival of patients with hepatocellular carcinoma: an Italian experience. Cancer 75:2427–2434

Sugiura N, Takara K, Ohto M, Okuda K, Hirooka N (1983) Treatment of small hepatocellular carcinoma by percutaneous injection of ethanol into tumor with real-time ultrasound monitoring. Acta Hepatol Jpn 24:920 (in Japanese).

Taavitsainen M, Vehmas T, Kauppila R (1993) Fatal liver necrosis following percutaneous ethanol injection for hepatocellular carcinoma. Abdom Imaging 18:357–359

Takayama T, Makuuchi M, Hirohashi S, et al (1990) Malignant transformation of adenomatous hyperplasia to hepatocellular carcinoma. Lancet 336:1150–1153

Takayasu K, Wakao F, Moryiama N, et al (1995) Response of early-stage hepatocellular carcinoma and border-line lesions to therapeutic arterial embolization. AJR 160:301–306

Tanaka K, Okazaki H, Nakamura S, et al (1991) Hepatocellular carcinoma: treatment with combination therapy of transcatheter arterial embolization and percutaneous ethanol injection. Radiology 179:715–717

Tanaka K, Nakamura S, Numata K, et al (1992) Hepatocellular carcinoma: treatment with percutaneous ethanol injection and transcatheter arterial embolization. Radiology 185:457–460

Tanaka K, Nakamura S, Numata K, et al (1998) The long term efficacy of combined transcatheter arterial embolization and percutaneous ethanol injection in the treatment of patients with large hepatocellular carcinoma and cirrhosis. Cancer 82:78–85

Tanikawa K, Majima Y (1993) Percutaneous ethanol injection therapy for recurrent hepatocellular carcinoma. Hepatogastroenterology 40:324–327

The Liver Cancer Study Group of Japan (1994) Predictive factors for long term prognosis after partial hepatectomy for patients with hepatocellular carcinoma in Japan. Cancer 74:2772–2803

Trevisani F, Caraceni P, Bernardi M, et al (1993) Gross pathologic types of hepatocellular carcinoma in Italian patients. Cancer 72:1557–1263

Tsuda H, Hirohashi S, Shimosato Y, Terada M, Hasegawa H (1988) Clonal origin of atypical adenomatous hyperplasia of the liver and clonal identity with hepatocellular carcinoma. Gastroenterology 95:1664–1666

Ueno N, Tomiyama T, Tano S (1998) Color Doppler sonography-guided ethanol injection therapy for hepatocellular carcinoma. AJR 170:515–519

Vilana R, Bruix J, Bru C, Ayuso C, Solé M, Rodés J (1992) Tumor size determines the efficacy of percutaneous ethanol injection for the treatment of small hepatocellular carcinoma. Hepatology 16:353–357

Yoshikawa J, Matsui O, Kadoya M, et al (1995) Hepatocellular carcinoma: CT appearance of parenchimal changes after percutaneous ethanol injection therapy. Radiology 194:107–111

Zerbey AL, Mueller PR, Dawson SL, Hoover HC (1994) Pleural seeding from hepatocellular carcinoma: a complication of percutaneous alcohol ablation. Radiology 193:81–82

19 Single-Session Percutaneous Alcohol Ablation of Hepatocellular Carcinoma

T. LIVRAGHI

CONTENTS

19.1 Introduction

Percutaneous ethanol injection (PEI) has become one of the most widely used procedures for treating hepatocellular carcinoma (HCC) in cirrhotic patients. Proposed in the international literature in 1986 (LIVRAGHI et al. 1986), PEI spread rapidly thanks to ease of execution, safety, low cost, repeatability, therapeutic efficacy and survival rates comparable to those of surgical resection (KOTOH et al. 1994; ONODERA et al. 1994; LIVRAGHI et al. 1995a,b). The procedure, performed in several sessions, as a rule in the outpatient clinic, is by consensus indicated for HCC up to 3–5 cm in diameter, and up to three nodules (LIVRAGHI et al. 1995b; SEKI et al. 1989; EBARA et al. 1990; GIORGIO et al. 1992; TANIKAWA 1992; VILANA et al. 1992; SHIINA et al. 1993). A larger quantity of neoplastic tissue would require an inordinate number of injections and hence an unduly long course of treatment, with no guarantee that the whole lesion would be treated.

T. LIVRAGHI, MD; Department of Radiology, General Hospital, Via C. Battisti 23, I-20059 Vimercate, Milan, Italy

To overcome these limitations, i.e., for treating large HCC (>5 cm), a new version of the procedure, known as "single-session" PEI, designed to allow the injection of ethanol as required under general anesthesia, was proposed in 1993 (LIVRAGHI et al. 1993). After these preliminary results, other studies reported greater numbers of patients and long-term results (GIORGIO et al. 1996; FILIPPELLI et al. 1998; LIVRAGHI et al. 1998).

19.2 Technique

We use a commercially available US scanner with 3.5-MHz convex probes that have an incorporated or a lateral needle guide. The procedure is done under general anesthesia, endotracheal intubation and mechanical ventilation. This technique complies with the operative requirement as it allows a period of apnea or respiratory standstill with partial pulmonary inflation, if necessary. During the procedure patients receive fructose 1.6-diphosphate 7500 mg and glutathione-SH 1200 mg by i.v. drip to quicken the metabolism of alcohol and so reduce its unintended systemic effects. After local skin preparation with iodized alcohol, also used as contact medium, the optimal approach is chosen. Any lesion detected by US can be treated by PEI, though some locations are more accessible than others. For lesions in the right lobe an intercostal approach with the patient lying on the left side is often preferred. To instill the alcohol we usually use a 21-gauge needle with closed conical tip and three terminal side-holes (PEIT needle; Hakko, Tokyo, Japan). The perfused area is clearly seen as a patch of hyperechogenicity. Ethanol is injected slowly (1 ml in 5–10 s) and its diffusion checked in real time on the monitor. Ethanol usually spreads within a radius of 2–3 cm around the tip of the needle to the periphery of the lesion except in the case of the focal confluent multinodular form in which diffusion is not homogeneous because of the interposed fibrotic tissue. Injection is stopped when significant leakage outside the lesion is detected or when diffusion is not clearly visible, and then resumed when conditions are right. Leakage is unusual, however, because the surrounding cirrhotic tissue is harder and ethanol tends to remain within the tumor. Ethanol is easily washed out by the rich neoplastic blood supply; as long as ethanol is seen to disappear rapidly, injection is continued intermittently with small boluses until the ethanol pools in the lesion. Care is taken to inject first the deepest portion of the lesion, then the central and lastly the superficial portion, the aim being to prevent any initial superficial spillage of ethanol from spoiling the view for subsequent injections. Care is also taken not to inject ethanol into the hepatic veins, because too high and too sudden a concentration of ethanol in the blood could lead to prolonged hypoxemia (see later). Treatment ends when the tumor appears entirely hyperechogenic on the monitor (Fig. 19.1). Treatment of neoplastic thrombosis, performed with the aim of stopping its progression along the vessel to the main branch, is achieved by targeting the tip of the needle on the thrombus; with one or more injections the alcohol usually diffuses selectively along it. The patient is kept hydrated on the day of treatment and the following day.

Usually, the total volume of alcohol administered per patient ranges from 20 to 100 ml, according to the size. The total volume of ethanol is always smaller than that of the lesion. The number of injections generally ranges from 8 to 20, depending on ethanol distribution, lesion size and degree of vascularization. Time required for the procedure is medially 30 min. The hospital stay is 3–4 days, in the absence of complications.

19.3 Evaluation of Therapeutic Efficacy

During the first years of the procedure, the therapeutic efficacy was evaluated by dynamic CT and US. In the last few years we have used spiral CT (scans performed 25 and 60 s after 4 ml/s of contrast medium injection).

Necrosis of the tumor tissue is considered to be complete when the CT scans show no areas of enhancement within the lesion at 1 month, confirmed on subsequent scans (every 4-6 months), and no growth of neoplastic tissue at the periphery (Fig. 19.1).

Also alpha-fetoprotein (AFP) and des-gamma-carboxi-prothombin (DCP) assay is done before treatment and 4–6 months after, at the same time as CT scanning. However, we do not use these levels to assess the response to treatment, because they may return to normal even when the scans do not show a complete necrosis (due to near-total necrosis of the tumor tissue) or may rise when the scans do show a complete necrosis (due to the presence of intra- or extra-hepatic lesions not detected or as yet undetectable).

19.4 Patients

In our study, we reported the results of 108 consecutive patients. Of these, 80 were men and 28 women (2.8:1), with mean age of 67.3 years (range, 31–87). Ninety-eight had Child's class A disease, 8 class B and 2 class C. Hepatitis B surface antigen and antibody to C virus were positive in 15 (13.8%) patients and 85 (78.7%), respectively; 4 (3.7%) were positive for both. Eight patients (7.4%) without viral infection reported high alcohol consumption. The patients fell into three groups: 24 had a single HCC with intact capsule on imaging, diameter >5 cm (from 5 to 8.5 cm; mean, 6.8) and had been rated inoperable or had refused surgery (group A); 63 had a single infiltrating HCC, diameter 5–10 cm (mean, 7.6) or multiple HCC, encapsulated or infiltrating, from three to six nodules, the largest measuring at least 4 cm (group B); 21 had advanced disease, hepatic (Child's C) or neoplastic (infiltrating HCC) with diameter from 10 cm to a size large enough to be locally symptomatic or with thrombosis of the second branch of the portal vein (group C). The treatment of group A patients was to be curative (i.e., radical, and so five of them with residual areas of viable tissue rated still treatable received additional treatment with conventional PEI); in group B treatment was palliative (debulking to retard neoplastic growth) while the group C patients received compassionate treatment and for trial purposes.

In all, 128 treatments were given, 20 patients receiving single-session PEI more than once due to the onset of new lesions or regrowth of the treated lesion. In 57 patients the AFP level was <20, in 21 patients 21–200 and in 30>200 ng/ml. Patients whose prothombin activity was under 40%, platelet count under 40×10^3/mm^3 or abnormal (more than 10%) values of partial thromboplastin time, were excluded.

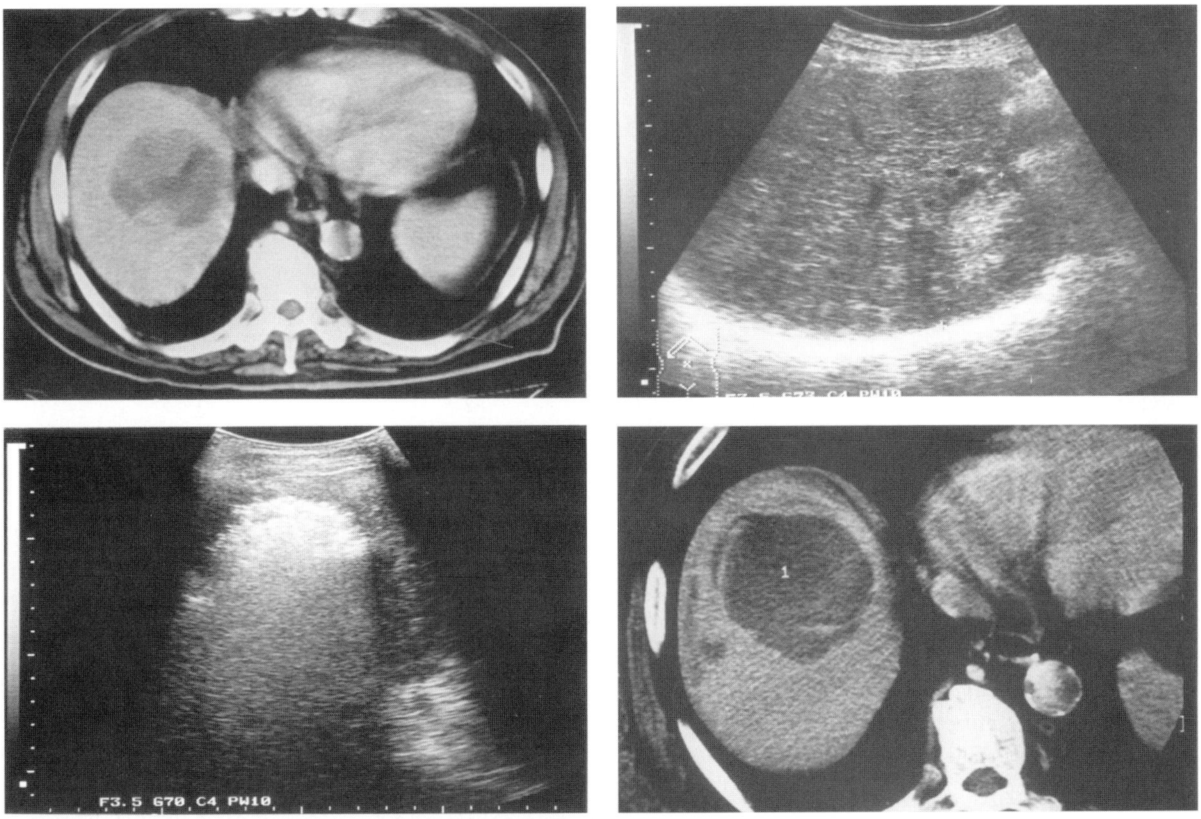

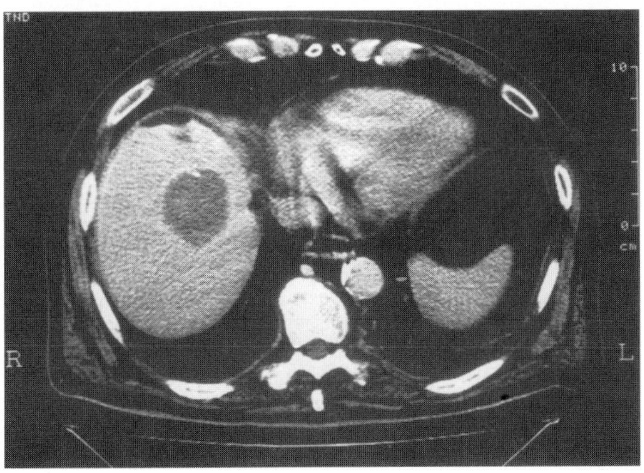

Fig. 19.1a–d. a CT scan during portal phase shows an encapsulated 7 cm HCC of segment 8 before PEI. **b** Subcostal US scan shows the same tumor before PEI. **c** Immediately after "single-session" PEI, intercostal US scan shows the tumor completely filled by ethanol, as an hyperechogenic patch. **d** One month after PEI, on CT scan the tumor appears completely hypodense with zero enhancement, because of the ablation of neoplastic vascular supply. **e** At 5-year follow-up, CT scan confirms complete necrosis of the tumor, reduced in size

19.5 Results

19.5.1 Biochemical Changes

In our study, after the procedure, we observed the following biochemical changes. Blood alcohol levels immediately after treatment were 10–229 mg/dl (mean, 82 mg/dl) and 4 h later 3–142 mg/dl (mean, 47 mg/dl). The value normalized within 20 h in all patients. Statistically significant changes were found in the following laboratory data: arpino transferase, total and unconjugated bilirubin, lactic dehydrogenase, hemoglobin, red cells, white cells, platelets, fibrinogen, prothombin activity, haptoglobin and d-dimer. Table 19.1 shows the mean variation, time of maximum variation (in hours after treatment) and the maximum value recorded. Red cells, platelets and hemoglobin presented a three-phase trend of variation: in the hours immediately after treatment there was a fall, followed by a partial recovery the

Table 19.1. Laboratory data with significant changes after single-session PEI

	Test	Mean variation	Time of maximum variation (in hours)	Maximum change recorded
AST	IU	+457	20	6,026
ALT	IU	+227	20–44	1,728
GGT	IU	+76	20	717
Total bilirubin	mg/dl	+0.95	44	4.8
Unc. bilirubin	mg/dl	+0.7	44	3.6
LDH	IU	+827	20	4500
Hemoglobin	g/dl	-1.4	68	7.8
Red cells	mm^3	-375,000	68	2,600,000
White cells	mm^3	+2,200	44	16,000
Platelets	mm^3	-32,000	68	41,000
Fibrinogen	mg/dl	-60	4	85
PT	%	-60	4–92	20
D-dimer	ng/ml	+2,800	4	8,000
Haptoglobin	mg/dl	-40	20	2
Ammonia	ng/dl	+40	20	177

AST, aspartate aminotransferase; ALT, alanine aminotransferase; GGT, gamma glutamyltranspeptidase; LDH, lactic dehydrogenase; PT, prothrombin activity.

next day and then on day 3 by an even greater reduction from the baseline values. All these values normalized within 10 days.

19.5.2 Side Effects

We observed the following side effects. For a few days patients often reported slight discomfort in the right hypochondrium, in some cases radiating to the epigastrium or to the right shoulder; analgesics were given in the event of severe pain.

Especially in cases in which more than 50 ml was injected, patients presented hyperpyrexia (max 40°C) lasting for a few days. Since the fever was not of septic origin but due to intratumoral necrosis, clearly demonstrated by the presence of gas on the CT and US scans, antibiotics were not given. Only antipyretics were administered as necessary. In a few cases the fever and gas persisted for up to a month. Some patients, especially not drinkers, exhibited drunkenness symptoms, persisting for several hours. Hemoglobinuria, almost always microscopic, was present in 74% of patients. There was a fall in mean blood pressure, systolic by 27 and diastolic by 11 mmHg, 4 and 8 h after treatment. The portal flow rate decreased in 14 patients (63%) by a mean of 1.9 cm/s, returning to the baseline values within a month.

19.5.3 Complications

The following complications were observed in our study. One Child's C patient died (0.7%). This patient, with esophageal varices at risk of bleeding, received 70 ml ethanol for a single tumor 8 cm in diameter. On day 4 he had heavy bleeding complicated by hepatorenal syndrome.

Major complications occurred in six patients (4.6%). One patient with altered coagulation values (prothombin time=45%, platelets=$45\times10^3/mm^3$) and a 7.5-cm tumor of the left lobe, protruding from the ventral margin, presented a peritoneal hemorrhage, which required several blood transfusions. One Child's B patient presented severe liver failure and had to stay in hospital for a month. One patient with five lesions and slightly altered blood creatinine level (1.7 mg/dl) had mild renal insufficiency (2.7 mg/dl), prompting two sessions of dialysis. The fourth, who had a poorly differentiated HCC, presented seeding in the parietal peritoneum, detected 6 months after treatment. Two patients had severe pain in the right hypochondrium lasting 3–4 days; this complication was due to necrosis of a segment of the liver adjacent to the one bearing the tumor, resulting from vascular damage.

In addition, there were some minor complications, requiring no specific treatment: eight slight bleedings into the peritoneum (appearance of fluid effusion, with decrease of 3–4 g/dl of hemoglobin), eight mild hepatic insufficiencies (appearance of small and transient amount of abscitis), seven chemical thromboses of the portal branch feeding the tumor, which cleared spontaneously within 3–4 months, and one case of prolonged hypoxemia which lengthened the assisted ventilation time at the end of treatment by 1 h (this patient received 55 ml in all, some of which was injected accidentally into the suprahepatic veins). No complications were due to general anesthesia.

In 27 patients, Giorgio et al. (1996) reported another death in a Child's C patient with a 7-cm tumor, due to bleeding of esophageal varices. They also reported some minor complications, such as pain, and delayed awakening (8 h after the end of the procedure) in a patient in whom 210 ml of ethanol was delivered.

In 44 patients, Filippelli et al. (1998) reported only some minor complications, such as one slight intraperitoneal bleeding, one cholecystitis and one small hepatic necrosis outside the tumor treated.

19.5.4 Efficacy

In group A 14 patients presented complete necrosis (58.3%); in 5 of these complete necrosis was achieved only after a few outpatient sessions of conventional PEI targeted on the residual areas. The other 10 presented at least 70% necrosis. The neoplastic tissue was replaced by necrotic tissue first and later by fibrotic tissue. The last named, having no blood supply, was easily distinguished from neoplastic tissue, since it presented no enhancement after iodized contrast administration. The largest lesion to show complete necrosis measured 8.2 cm. Tumor diameter, even in the cases of complete necrosis, remained unchanged immediately after treatment, to diminish in different measure after a few months (Fig. 19.1).

In group B complete necrosis was achieved only in encapsulated lesions, that is, in some of the multiple lesions. In the infiltrating lesions of groups B and C 100% necrosis was rarely obtained, but 50% or more was obtained in all cases and near complete necrosis.

In some group C patients shrinkage of the portal thrombus for over 2 years was obtained. In patients whose cancer was already symptomatic the response obtained does not seem to have affected the natural history.

On the AFP front 6-month follow-up revealed the following data. One of the 57 patients with <20 ng/ml presented an increase. Two of those with 21–200 ng/ml showed an increase, 6 a decrease and 13 a normalization. Two of the 30 with >200 ng/ml showed an increase, 25 a decrease and 3 a normalization.

19.5.5 Survival

One-, 2-, 3-year survival rates overall were 68, 56, 41%. The corresponding rates by group were: for A 72, 65, 57%; for B 73, 60, 42% and for C 46, 25, 5%. The longest survivor is alive after 70 months of follow-up.

19.6 Discussion

19.6.1 Biochemical Changes

While conventional PEI, which involves small doses of ethanol at a time, causes no noteworthy changes, single-session PEI causes changes that, though temporary, must be known, because they may give rise to complications.

In our study, the mean of blood alcohol levels observed (82 mg/dl) did not cause any trouble, intoxication symptoms usually appearing over 150 mg/dl. Only in cases over these values were some intoxications lasting 2–4 h observed, above all in abstemious patients. These patients regained consciousness more easily and quickly when treated with drugs during PEI, as observed in our preliminary trial or demonstrated in controlled studies (De Bernardis et al. 1988; Gobbi et al. 1988).

The blood count changes presented three phases. The slight fall in red cells, platelets and hemoglobin immediately after treatment is to be attributed to the initial slight hemolysis induced directly by the ethanol combined with dilution of the blood through i.v. hydration, and to traumatic microhemorrhage. The partial recovery on day 2 is due to an intermediate mobilization of reserves from the spleen and to compensatory diuresis. The more marked fall on day 3 is due to increased intrasplenic hemolysis (especially in the damaged cells) secondary to the increase in portal hypertension; in the case of platelets there was also wear-and-tear due to microvascular thrombosis. The increase in white cells on day 2 is attributable to inflammatory phenomena connected with repair of the tissues and vessels.

Given the initial intravascular hemolysis, there was also an increase in unconjugated bilirubin and a decrease in haptoglobin. The latter, which binds to hemoglobin, is often consumed completely, in part because the baseline values in cirrhotics are lower than in normals. Any free hemoglobin, being small enough to cross the glomerular filter, gives rise to hemoglobinuria. The passage of hemoglobin into the tubules may cause transient obstruction, which has no consequences in normal patients but which may give rise to slight and transient renal insufficiency in those whose blood creatinine levels are raised.

Intravascular clotting immediately after hemolysis leads to an increase in d-dimer and a decrease in fibrinogen, in prothombin activity and, to a lesser degree, in antithrombin III activity. The activation of the ethanol-induced blood coagulation cascade normalizes within a few days. Destruction of hepatic cells (mainly in the non-neoplastic parenchyma) is reflected in the increased transaminases; the fact that the mean increase in aspartate aminotransferase is almost twice that in alanine aminotransferase, and occurs 24 h earlier, suggests early damage to the mitochondria, which precedes the hepatic damage secondary to microvascular thrombosis. Other biochemical changes due to hepatic cell and red cells damage are: an increase in lactic dehydrogenase and, though not to a significant degree, in potassium. The increase in gamma glutamyl transpeptidase argues for an intraparenchymal cholestasis.

19.6.2 Complications

The death of a Child's C patient after heavy bleeding of esophageal varices, complicated by hepatorenal syndrome, is probably to be attributed to the further increase in portal hypertension that occurred in 63% of patients after treatment. Another death from bleeding was reported, due to the same circumstance (Giorgio et al. 1996). While in a Child's class A patient or one without esophageal varices at risk of bleeding, this rise carries no consequences, in a patient with advanced cirrhosis (Child's C or even B, if a high dose of ethanol is planned) or with F3 or F2 varices with red spots we consider the treatment to be contraindicated (administration of nitroglycerin and beta blockers might reduce the risk).

The peritoneal bleed occurred in a patient with several concomitant risk factors, namely superficial location of the tumor, large size involving several punctures, and severe coagulation disorders. Other patients in similar circumstances did not have this complication. We further think it is wise to exclude patients with hyperfibrinolysis or a chronic disseminated intravascular coagulation from treatment, because cirrhotics anyway have a precarious blood coagulation pattern, thrombocyte deficiency, erythrocyte and microvascular fragility and anatomical changes (esophageal varices, congestive gastritis) that are potentially hemorrhagic. Necrosis of hepatic tissue located in another segment was not foreseeable but does not seem to have been a major problem for the patient, the only complaint being pain.

The case of prolonged mild hypoxemia raised no particular problems apart from an extra hour of assisted ventilation at the end of treatment. Hypoxemia did not depend on the amount of injected ethanol. Most probably it was due to pulmonary vascular dilatation and/or arteriovenous communication, and functional right-to left intrapulmonary shunting ensuing from it. Many factors might be involved in the pathogenesis of this alteration: nitric oxide, platelet activating factor, prostglandin E_2, prostacyclin, orthosympathetic reflex, acidosis. Pulmonary interstitial edema, resulting from an increase in vascular permeability (activated macrophages) or cardiac insufficiency may be present (Yakes et al. 1993; Randin et al. 1995; Umans and Levi 1995; Krowka 1995; Castro and Krowka 1996; Chang and Ohara 1996; Riegler et al. 1995; Panos and Baker 1996). The practical upshot of the foregoing remarks is that injection should be stopped as soon as an ethanol leakage into the hepatic venous circulation is detected and that treatment should not be offered to patients with major pulmonary hypertension and heart disease.

Table 19.2 lists the situations considered at risk. In this table, in addition to the above-mentioned contraindications, we included obstructive jaundice. In fact, in our series of metastatic patients submitted

Table 19.2. "Single session" PEI: conditions considered at risk

Marked portal hypertension
Marked pulmonary hypertension
Major heart disease
Risk esophageal varices
Hyperfibrinolysis
Chronic disseminated intravascular coagulation
Chronic renal insufficiency
Obstructive jaundice
Superficial tumors with severe coagulation disorders

to the same procedure, a case of peritoneal bile leak occurred in the presence of biliary dilatation.

19.6.3 Survival

In the light of current knowledge the treatment options open to patients with HCC not at an advanced stage, that is with a single tumor or at most 2–3 unilobar nodules, up to 5 cm in diameter, are four, namely: surgical resection, liver transplantation, PEI and segmental TACE, the choice depending on a number of prognostic factors and on the local social and medical facilities (Livraghi et al. 1995b). For a single HCC of greater size, even if a diameter >5 cm is a relatively adverse prognostic factor on univariate analysis, surgery remains a valid option, subject to stringent selection of patients for a variety of other factors (presence of a capsule, compensated cirrhosis, age not too advanced, AFP not elevated, etc.). For more advanced cases, when surgery is not an option, that is, for an infiltrating tumor or bilobar multifocal presentation, conventional (nonsegmental) TACE is often the only possible treatment. However, even with the recent introduction of more stringent criteria and the consequent considerable reduction of the complication rate, the greatest problems of TACE remain its modest efficacy in large or infiltrating tumors and the poor predictability of results, which may vary widely from patient to patient and even from lesion to lesion in the same patient.

The 3 year survival rate among patients with 5–10 cm HCC reported by the Liver Cancer Study Group of Japan was 45%, though it has to be remembered that their series included patients treated surgically as far back as 1982 (The Liver Cancer Study Group of Japan 1994). More recent series (Nagasue et al. 1993; Sugioka et al. 1993; Izumi et al. 1994; Kim and Kim 1994; Kawarada et al. 1994) report survival rates from 23% to 63%, which are thus similar or lower than those attained in group A patients with single-session PEI, i.e., 57%. This is not easy to explain, for resection should have ensured complete ablation whereas PEI in this study achieved complete necrosis in 58% of cases. The explanation is probably to be sought in the fact that the lower success rate obtained with PEI is counterbalanced by the lower peroperative mortality, i.e., 0.8% vs 4–11% for surgery (Nagasue et al. 1993; Sugioka et al. 1993; Izumi et al. 1994; Kim and Kim 1994; Kawarada et al. 1994) and by the reduced damage to healthy tissue, which in some resections may prove excessive and lead to liver failure; another factor could be that the amount of necrosis, high also in partial responses, was able to greatly slacken the neoplastic growth and so improve survival.

Thus, as PEI is a satisfactory alternative to surgery, no longer the only treatment available, patients can be more accurately selected for surgery with better chances of success in terms both of complications and of survival rates.

Comparison with TACE is less straightforward, because of the diversity and insufficient stratification of patients. The series of patients with HCC >5 cm reported by Taniguchi et al. (1994), Urata et al. (1994) and by Yamada et al. (1995) yielded 3-year survival rates of 17, 18 and 0%, while Nakamura et al. (1994) and the Groupe d'etude et de traitment du carcinome hepatocellulaire (1995) in two series of generically inoperable cases cited 28 and 30%. The series of Bronowicki et al. (1994), stratified according to the Okuda staging, comprising 59 stage I patients (main tumor 5 cm or more in 20, 5–8 cm in 20, 11–15 cm in 9; single in 14 and multiple in 35 cases; 47 Child's A and 2 Child's B; mean age 65 years), yielded a survival rate of 57%. The 3-year survival rate in our group B patients with single-session PEI was 42% and so comparable with that for TACE. The choice should definitely go to PEI when patients are at risk of complications, as in those identified in a study of Chung et al. (1996) and especially when the diameter exceeds 6 cm, since 24% of their patients developed a severe post-embolization syndrome or acute liver failure.

Group C patients have until now not been offered any treatment or at most chemotherapy or hormone therapy, but without appreciable results (Carr 1997; Castells et al. 1995). In some group C patients, that is, those with advanced but not symptomatic cancer and not presenting the risk factors cited above, PEI yielded reasonably good results: a remarkable reduction of diseased tissue and arrest of neoplastic growth for more than a year.

19.7 Conclusions

While aware of the limitations of comparison based on historical data, we feel that single-session PEI has proved to be a valid alternative to patients so far treated surgically or with TACE who present adverse prognostic factors or risks for these therapies. Further, it may be an option for some patients with advanced disease who previously could not benefit from any therapy. The risk of complications nonetheless requires the exclusion of patients presenting situations likely to be risky and solid experience of conventional PEI.

References

Bronowicki J, Vetter D, Dumas F, et al (1994) Transcatheter oily chemoembolization for hepatocellular carcinoma. Cancer 74:16–24

Carr BI (1997) Chemotherapy. In: Livraghi T, Makuuchi M, Buscarini L (eds) Diagnosis and treatment of hepatocellular carcinoma. Greenwich Medical Media, London pp 367–392

Castells A, Bruix J, Bru C, et al (1995) Treatment of hepatocellular carcinoma with tamoxifen: a double-blind placebo-controlled trial in 120 patients. Gastroenterology 109:917–922

Castro M, Krowka MJ (1996) Hepatopulmonary syndrome: a pulmonary complication of liver disease. In: Chang S, Ohara N (eds) Clinics in chest medicine: the lung in liver disease. Vol 17. Saunders Comp, Philadelphia, pp 35–48

Chang S, Ohara N (1996) Pulmonary intravascular phagocytosis in liver disease. In: Chang S, Ohara N (eds) Clinics in chest medicine: the lung in liver disease. Vol 17. Saunders Comp, Philadelphia pp 137–150

Chung JW, Park JH, Han K J, Choi IB, Chung H M,Lee H (1996) Hepatic tumors: predisposing factors for complications of transcatheter oily chemoembolization. Radiology 198:33–40

De Bernardis E, Di Stefano A, Carlino S, Rizza V (1988) Effetti del fruttosio-1,6-difosfato sulle concentrazione ematiche dell'alcool nell'uomo. Recenti Progressi in Medicina 79:28–32

Ebara M, Otho M, Sugiura N, Okuda K, Kondo F, Kondo K (1990) Percutaneous ethanol injection for the treatment of small hepatocellular carcinoma: study of 95 patients. J Gastroenterol Hepatol 5:616–626

Filippelli G, Biamonte R, Conforti S, et al (1998) Alcolizzazione percutanea ecoguidata (PEI) tradizionale e in one shot in 71 pazienti affetti da carcinoma epato cellulare (HCC). Giornale Italiano di Ecografia 1:9–15

Giorgio A, Tarantino L, Francica G, Scala V, Mariniello N, Aloisio T (1992) Percutaneous ethanol injection under sonographic guidance of hepatocellular carcinoma in compensated and decompensated cirrhotic patients. J Ultrasound Med 11:587–595

Giorgio A, Tarantino L, Francica G, et al (1996) One-shot percutaneous ethanol injection of liver tumor under general anesthesia: preliminary data on efficacy and complications. Cardiovasc Intervent Radiol 19:27–31

Gobbi G, Pina P, Fabbrini G, Bonollo L, Martini A (1988) Il fruttosio-1,6-difosfato nel trattamento dell'ebbrezza alcolica acuta. Rif Med 103:175–178

Groupe d'etude et de traitement du carcinome hepatocellulaire (1995) A comparison of lipiodol chemoembolization and conservative treatment for unresectable hepatocellular carcinoma. N Engl J Med 332:1256–1261

Izumi R, Shimizu K, Tohru II, et al (1994) Prognostic factors of hepatocellular carcinoma in patients undergoing hepatic resection. Gastroenterology 106:720–727

Kawarada Y, Ito F, Sakurai H, et al (1994) Surgical treatment of hepatocellular carcinoma. Cancer Chemother Pharmacol 33(S):12–17

Kim ST, Kim KP (1994) Hepatic resections for primary liver cancer. Cancer Chemother Pharmacol 33(S):18–23

Kotoh K, Sakai H, Sakamoto S, et al (1994) The effect of percutaneous ethanol injection therapy on small solitary hepatocellular carcinoma is comparable to that of hepatectomy. Am J Gastrenterol 89:194–198

Krowka MJ (1995) Hepatopulmonary syndrome. What are we learning from interventional radiology, liver transplantation and other disorders ? Gastroenterology 109:978–983

Livraghi T, Festi D, Monti F, Salmi A, Vettori C (1986) US-guided percutaneous alcohol injection of small hepatic and abdominal tumors. Radiology 161:309–312

Livraghi T, Vettori C, Torzilli G, Lazzaroni S, Pellicanò S, Ravasi S (1993) Percutaneous ethanol injection of hepatic tumors: single session therapy under general anesthesia. AJR 161:1065–1069

Livraghi T, Bolondi L, Buscarini L, et al (1995a) No treatment, resection et ethanol injection in hepatocellular carcinoma: a retrospective analysis of survival in 391 cirrhotic patients. J Hepatol 22:522–526

Livraghi T, Giorgio A, Marin G, et al (1995b) Hepatocellular carcinoma and cirrhosis in 746 patients: long-term results of percutaneous ethanol injection. Radiology 197:101–108

Livraghi T, Benedini V, Lazzaroni S, Meloni F, Torzilli G, Vettori C (1998) Long term results of single session PEI in patients with large hepatocellular carcinoma. Cancer 83:48–57

Nagasue N, Kohno H, Chang Y, et al (1993) Liver resection for hepatocellular carcinoma: results of 229 consecutive patients during 11 years. Ann Surg 217:375–384

Nakamura H, Mitani T, Murakami T, et al (1994) Five-year survival after transcatheter chemoembolization for hepatocellular carcinoma. Cancer Chemother Pharmacol 33(S):89–92

Onodera H, Ukai K, Nakano N, et al (1994) Outcomes of 116 patients with hepatocellular carcinoma. Cancer Chemother Pharmacol 33(S):103–108

Panos RJ, Baker SK (1996) Mediators, cytokines and growth factors in liver-lung interactions. In: Chang S, Ohara N (eds) Clinics in chest medicine: the lung in liver disease. Vol 17. Saunders Comp, Philadelphia pp 151–162

Randin D, Vollenweider P, Tappy L, Jequier E, Nicod P, Sherrer U (1995) Suppression of alcohol-induced hypertension by dexamethasone. N Engl J Med 322:1733–1737

Riegler JH, Lang KA, Johnson SP, Westerman JH (1995) Tranjugular intrahepatic portosystemic shunt improves oxygenation in hepatopulmonary syndrome. Gastroenterology 109:978–983

Seki T, Nonaka T, Kubota Y, Mizuno T, Sameshima Y (1989) Ultrasonically guided percutaneous ethanol injection therapy for hepatocellular carcinoma. Am J Gastroenterol 84:1400–1407

Shiina S, Tagawa K, Niwa Y, et al (1993) Percutaneous ethanol injection therapy for hepatocellular carcinoma: results in 146 patients. AJR 160:1023–1028

Sugioka A, Tsuzuki T, Kanai T (1993) Postresection prognosis of patients with hepatocellular carcinoma. Surgery 113:612–618

Taniguchi K, Nakata K, Kato Y, et al (1994) Treatment of hepatocellular carcinoma with transcatheter arterial embolization. Cancer 73:1341–1345

Tanikawa K (1992) Multidisciplinary treatment of hepatocellular carcinoma. In: Tobe T, Kameda H (eds) Primary liver cancer in Japan. Springer, Tokyo pp 327–334

The Liver Cancer Study Group of Japan (1994) Predictive factors for long term prognosis after partial hepatectomy for patients with hepatocellular carcinoma. Cancer 74:2272–2280

Umans JG, Levi R (1995) Nitric oxide in the regulation of blood flow and arterial pressure. Annu Rev Physiol 57:771–775

Urata K, Matsumata T, Kamakura T, Hasuo K, Sugimachi K (1994) Lipiodolization for unresectable hepatocellular carcinoma: an analysis of 205 patients using univariate and multivariate analysis. J Surg Oncol 56:54–58

Vilana R, Bruix J, Bru C, Ayuso C, Solè M, Rodès J (1992) Tumor size determines the efficacy of percutaneous ethanol injection for the treatment of small hepatocellular carcinoma. Hepatology 16:353–357

Yakes W, Englewood C, Bakot R (1993) Cardiopulmonary collapse: sequelae of ethanol embolotherapy. Radiology 189 (P):145

Yamada R, Kishi K, Sato M, Sonomura T, Nishida N, Tanaka K (1995) Transcatheter arterial chemoembolization (TACE) in the treatment of unresectable liver cancer. World J Surg 19:795–800

20 Radiofrequency Thermal Ablation of Hepatocellular Carcinoma

L. Buscarini, R. Lencioni, E. Buscarini, D. Cioni, and C. Bartolozzi

CONTENTS

20.1 Introduction

In this chapter, the principles of radiofrequency (RF) thermal ablation and the techniques currently used in the treatment of hepatocellular carcinoma (HCC) are discussed. Our group was the first to propose, in 1990, the possibility of employing interstitial hyperthermia to percutaneous ablation of liver tumors. In the last few years, technological improvements have been introduced in order to obtain a larger volume of necrosis, to make the procedure more effective, to shorten the time required for the therapy, to enhance the patient's compliance and to reduce the economic cost. Particularly, new types of needle electrodes, such as expandable electrodes and cooled tip electrodes have entered into clinical use. With recent experience, association of radiofrequency thermal ablation with segmental transcatheter arterial embolization has also been used for treatment of large HCC lesions. Currently, with the use of expandable needles, most HCC tumors up to 3.5 cm can be ablated in a single session. By combining RF thermal ablation and arterial embolization, tumors up to 6.5 cm can be effectively treated.

L. Buscarini, MD; Chief, Department of Gastroenterology, General Hospital, Cantone del Cristo 40, I-29100 Piacenza, Italy
R. Lencioni, MD; Division of Diagnostic and Interventional Radiology, Department of Oncology, University of Pisa, Via Roma 67, I-56125 Pisa, Italy
E. Buscarini, MD; Department of Gastroenterology, General Hospital, Cantone del Cristo 40, I-29100 Piacenza, Italy
D. Cioni, MD; Division of Diagnostic and Interventional Radiology, Department of Oncology, University of Pisa, Via Roma 67, I-56125 Pisa, Italy
C. Bartolozzi, MD; Professor and Chairman, Division of Diagnostic and Interventional Radiology, Department of Oncology, University of Pisa, Via Roma 67, I-56125 Pisa, Italy

20.2 Radiofrequency Thermal Ablation

Surgical resection can be performed in a minority of patients with either primary or metastatic liver tumors. Therefore, today, minimally invasive percutaneous therapies such as percutaneous ethanol injection (Lencioni et al. 1995, 1997; 1998d; Bartolozzi et al. 1995; Bartolozzi and Lencioni 1996; Livraghi et al. 1995), radiofrequency interstitial thermal ablation (Buscarini et al. 1992; Lencioni et al. 1998b,c), interstitial laser photocoagulation (Amin et al. 1993), and percutaneous microwave coagulation therapy (PMCT) (Seki et al. 1994a) have been introduced.

RF waves applied for tissue thermal ablation have a frequency energy of about 480–500 kHz. RF waves are a band of electromagnetic radiation subdivided according to the frequency into low frequency energy (up to 300 kHz), intermediate (up to 3 MHz), high frequency energy (up to 300 MHz) and microwaves, which have a wavelength to 1 mm and a frequency up to 2500 MHz. The human body becomes an element of the RF circuit when terminal outputs of the RF generator are connected to electrodes placed/inserted on the body itself. In the monopolar system, the active electrode is represented by a small area where the heat lesion is made, and the dispersive electrode by a large area where heating production is minimal and without discomfort on behalf of the patient.

RF thermal lesion results from a tissue coagulation around the non-insulated tip of a needle electrode. RF heating is due to ionic agitation produced by a flux of a high frequency alternating current into the tissue. This ionic movement provokes a heating defined as resistive heating, directly proportional to the square of current density, which is in turn inversely proportional to the distance from the electrode. Therefore, resistive heating involves a very thin layer of tissue, while a larger tissue destruction is due to heat diffusion. The dimensions of RF thermal lesions are related to the current intensity, to the size of the needle electrode, to heat conduction, and to heat lost via the circulation (convection).

An experimental work, performed on guinea pigs and pigs, showed that the volume of liver thermal lesions induced by RF needle electrodes was related to the temperature, to the exposure time (up to 120 s) and to the needle caliber and the length of the exposed tract of the needle (Rossi et al. 1990). The same results were obtained by using an experimental model in vitro; the authors observed that ultrasound (US) could monitor the thermal lesion as an hyperechoic zone (McGahan et al. 1990); its dimensions showed a good correlation between the diameter of the lesion observed histopathologically (Bosman et al. 1991).

Convection is an important limiting factor of the necrosis volume: in fact, vessels act as a heat sinker. Experimental observations showed that RF coagulation obtained in normal ex vivo pig liver had a diameter about double the coagulation area in normal in vivo pig liver, under the same technical conditions; and that in normal pig liver RF application performed during balloon portal occlusion or during portal vein and hepatic artery clamp induces larger coagulation necrosis areas than RF applied with uninterrupted hepatic blood flow (Goldberg et al. 1998; Patterson et al. 1998).

A crucial point for percutaneous treatments is the size of the necrosis achievable. In RF ablation, the use of high current intensity is limited by tissue carbonization around the needle tip, with a sudden increase in tissue impedance causing interruption of RF wave flow. On the other hand, by prolonging exposure time, the lesion diameter can be increased until a point of thermal balance. The caliber of the non-insulated needle tip (which is the real source of RF waves) is limited by safety reasons to not more than 2 mm. Moreover, heat diffusion is related to the characteristics of the tissue and the loss of heat is bound to the tissue vascularization, which can reduce or impede tissue necrosis.

From a practical point of view the strategies for enlarging thermal lesions are represented by: (a) expansion of radiating area; (b) control of impedance; and (c) tumor devascularization to reduce heat loss. Expansion has been obtained by using multiple needles and expandable needles (Buscarini et al. 1996b; Le Veen 1997; Lencioni et al. 1998b); the control of impedance has been attempted by infusion through the needle electrode of saline during RF ablation (cooled tip needle electrode) (Lorentzen 1996; Solbiati et al. 1997; Lencioni et al. 1998c); reduction of heat loss, by transarterial embolization (Buscarini 1998; Lencioni et al. 1998a) or by portal vein occlusion during the time of RF application (Goldberg et al. 1998). These procedures have been used in clinical practice.

20.2.1 Equipment

The RF delivery systems used in the published papers are RF-current generators (Radionics, Burlington, Massachusetts; and Rita Medical Systems, Mountain View, California) with an active needle electrode and a dispersive electrode.

The generators have 480–500 kHz frequency with a maximum power from 26 to 100 W. The active electrodes have an insulated (by 0.1 mm thick plastic) stainless steel shaft of 24–30 cm length, a caliber ranging from 1.2 to 1.9 mm, and an exposed tip of 1–3 cm length. The tips contain one or two thermistors that allow temperature monitoring in the tissue around the needle tip.

In recent experiences, modified needles have been applied: expandable needles of 1.9 mm in caliber, with retractable lateral hooks of 1.5 cm in length, aimed at obtaining an enlargement of radiating area (Buscarini et al. 1996b; Rossi et al. 1998; Lencioni et al. 1998b); cooled tip needle of 1.2 mm in caliber, where an internal circulation of cold saline maintains a low temperature in a thin tissue layer around the needle tip, in an attempt to avoid charring phenomena even with the use of high power (Solbiati et al. 1997, Lencioni et al. 1998c).

20.2.2
Technique

The monopolar procedure is carried out by connecting the patient to the RF generator via a dispersive electrode. The active electrode needle tip is introduced into the chosen area of the tumor under US guidance using a 3.5-MHz convex probe with a lateral biopsy apparatus. Local anesthesia is performed from the insertion point on the skin to the peritoneum along the puncture line. The power necessary to keep the temperature at the needle tip at 90°C for 2–6 min is delivered. If an expandable needle is used, the hooks are advanced after needle placement and retracted before withdrawing it; with this procedure, the temperature, as measured by thermistors sited at the tip of each hook, ranges between 100 and 115°C for 8–16 min (Buscarini and Rossi 1997; Lencioni et al. 1998b). Needle access may be intercostal, subcostal, or epigastric.

With the bipolar procedure, two active needle electrodes directly connected to the RF generator are inserted into the tumor in parallel 2 cm apart, via the multihole lateral guide apparatus, under US guidance.

With both monopolar and bipolar procedures, the tip of the needle/s is/are placed at each insertion in the deepest part of the tumor. Multiple thermal lesions are created along the major axis of the needle electrode by simply withdrawing the needle and reactivating the RF generator. In case of large masses, multiple insertions of the needle electrode may be performed in different areas of the tumor.

Monopolar procedure produces a single thermal lesion with a volume that ranges from 1.0 to 1.8 cm^3 (Rossi et al. 1990). Bipolar technique generates a thermal lesion of about 8.0 cm^3, that is more than double that of the single lesion performed by the single needle electrode (Rossi et al. 1996). With modified monopolar procedure (cooled needle and expandable needles) it is possible to obtain a lesion with a diameter of about 3–3.5 cm (Buscarini and Rossi 1997; Solbiati et al. 1997; Lencioni et al. 1998b,c).

20.2.3
Ultrasound Monitoring

As experimentally shown, a homogeneous hyperechoic area, often with posterior acoustic shadow, appears around the needle tip when temperature reaches 90°C. This US structural change is visible at every thermal lesion and is independent of the tumor histotype. It usually disappears within 12 h. At the end of the treatment, the US patterns are modified: usually the hypoechoic lesions become isoechoic or hyperechoic areas; the iso-hyperechoic lesions with hypoechoic rim become iso-hyperechoic, iso-hypoechoic, or hypo-hyperechoic areas (Fig. 20.1).

20.2.4
Assessment of Therapeutic Efficacy

The therapeutic efficacy of RF ablation has been documented by serial dosage of serum alpha-fetoprotein (AFP), US guided fine needle biopsies performed after the procedure, and imaging techniques such as dynamic or spiral CT, MR imaging, and selective angiography. If post-treatment investigation reveals residual tumor, additional treatment is administered (Buscarini and Rossi 1997; Lencioni et al. 1998c). Currently, angiography is considered no longer necessary, and can be substituted by color-power Doppler study, completed by US contrast media, and by spiral CT or dynamic MR imaging. Moreover, post-treatment biopsy is no longer recommended routinely, but can be used in case of questionable imaging findings. In fact, even multiple biopsies can miss residual tumoral foci, because the information pertains to a very limited volume of liver. Moreover, biopsy can give a false positive result since areas of non-vital hyperthermia induced apoptosis may mimic viable cancer tissue on light microscopy (Solbiati et al. 1994, 1997).

The timing of therapeutic assessment is controversial: some authors prefer an early examination (within 3 days from the end of therapy), which, however, may be impaired by the presence of a peripheral halo of contrast enhancement caused by reactive inflammation. In later studies, this feature usually disappears and interpretation of images is easier (Figs. 20.2, 20.3).

Follow-up protocol includes dosage of AFP, US, and CT or MR imaging at 3–4 month intervals.

20.2.5
Results

In the first clinical study, 39 patients with single HCC nodule not more than 3 cm in diameter were treated with the monopolar and bipolar methods.

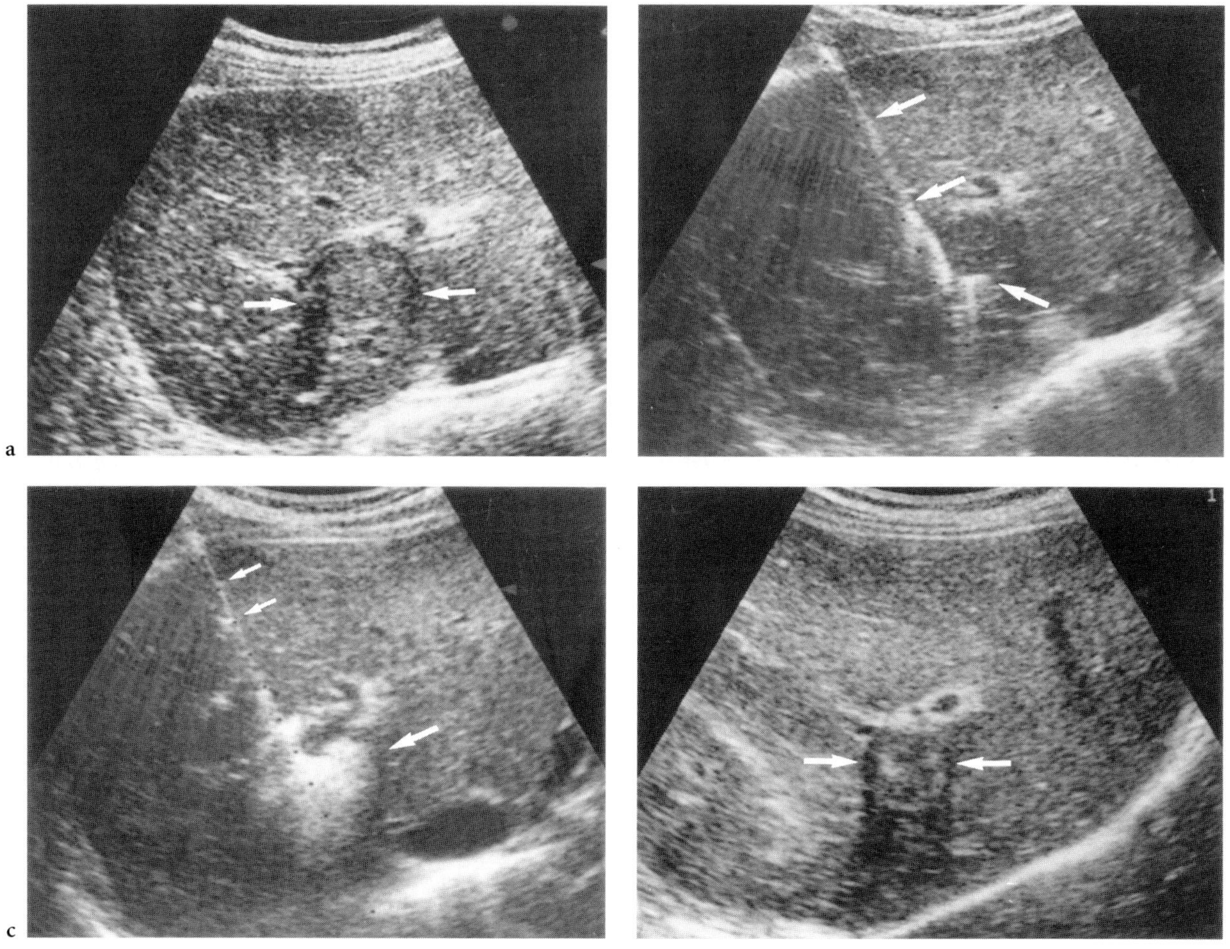

Fig. 20.1a–d. **a** Sonography shows isoechoic hepatocellular carcinoma nodule (*arrows*) with hypoechoic halo and lateral shadows, located in segment VII of liver. **b** The expandable needle (*arrows*) is positioned within the lesion and the hooks are deployed (*arrow*). **c** At the end of treatment an hyperechoic area (*arrow*) appears around the needle hooks: this is the sonographic feature of thermal lesion. **d** Sonogram obtained 3 months after the end of RF interstitial thermal ablation shows that structure of the nodule has completely changed (*arrows*), it is smaller than before the treatment, and it has posterior shadowing

The tumoral destruction was achieved in all cases, with normalization of AFP levels in cases where it was increased. The mean number of sessions needed to obtain tumor destruction was 3.3 (range, 1–8). During the follow-up, the treated HCCs slowly diminished in size, becoming not detectable by US or appearing as small hyperechoic areas or as isoechoic areas with hyperechoic rim. During a mean follow-up of 23 months (range 3–66), 16 of 39 (41%) patients had recurrences: local recurrences, however, occurred in only 5% of cases, whereas 36% of recurrences were due to the emergence of new lesions in other hepatic segments. Most recurrent tumors underwent new courses of RF treatment. Overall, 54 HCC nodules in 39 patients were treated during the study. Median survival time was 44 months (Rossi et al. 1996).

Another group of 23 patients with either single tumor nodule of not more than 3.5 cm or multiple (up to three) tumor nodules, none exceeding 3.0 cm in diameter, were treated by using expandable needle electrodes with four hooks. In this study, 26 tumor nodules were apparently ablated in a mean of 1.5 sessions (1.1 for tumor less than 2.5 cm; 1.7 for the others). Twenty-one patients were followed up for at least 6 months (mean 10 months; range 6–19 months): one patient showed local recurrence, two had new tumor nodules, three had multicentric disease, and 15 remained apparently disease-free (Rossi et al. 1998).

In a third experience, 12 patients with HCC lesions with diameter from 3.8 to 6.5 cm were treated with RITA (expandable needle electrode) after segmental transarterial embolization. In all cases com-

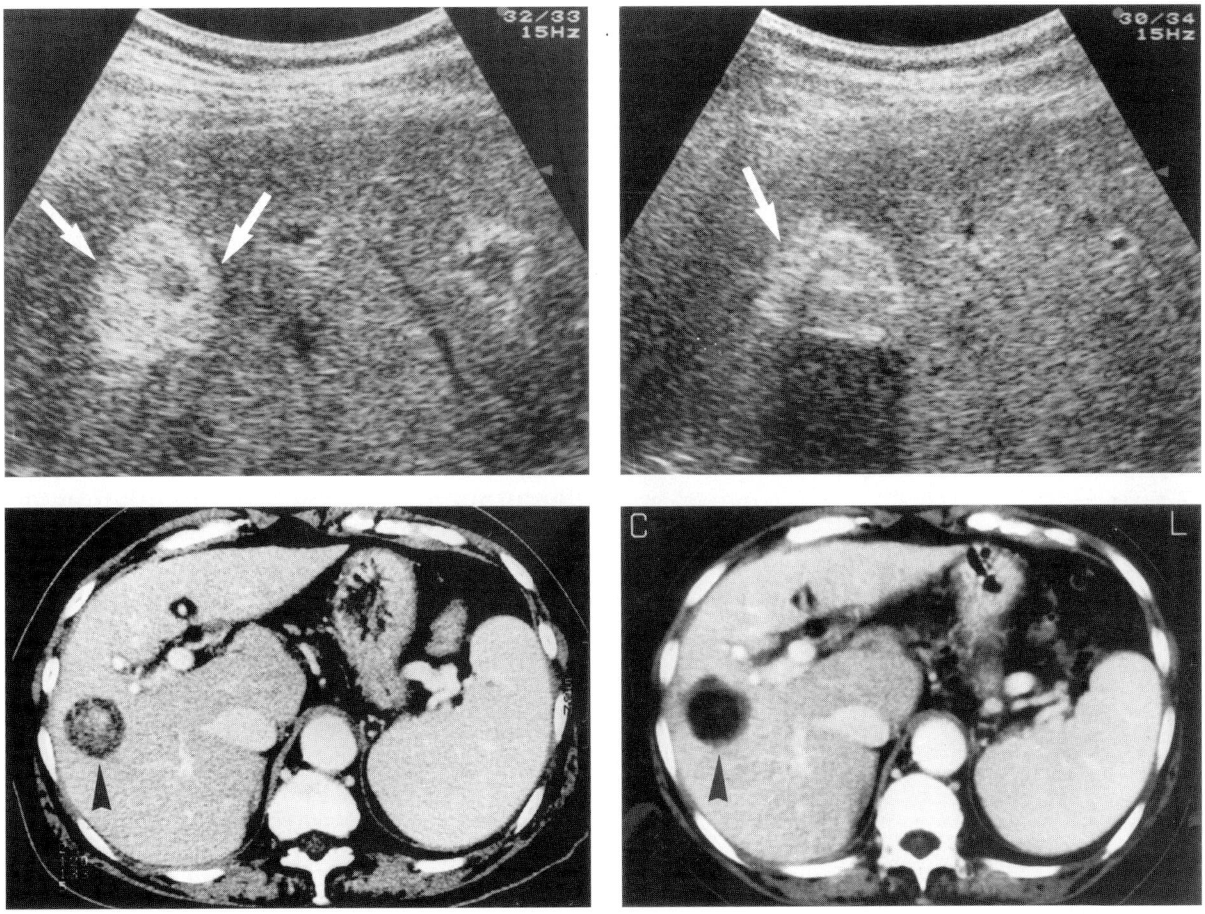

a b c d

Fig. 20.2a–d. a A 3-cm nodule of hepatocellular carcinoma (*arrows*) hyperechoic, located in segment VI. **b** Sonogram obtained 9 months after the end of RF interstitial thermal ablation demonstrates that the nodule (*arrow*) is isoechoic with hyperechoic rim and it has posterior shadowing. **c** Dynamic CT scan obtained before RF interstitial thermal ablation shows hyper- to hypodense tumor (*arrow*). **d** Dynamic CT scan obtained after the end of treatment demonstrates a non-enhancing area (*arrow*) larger than the treated tumor

plete ablation was achieved in a mean number of 1.2 sessions. During a mean follow-up of 11 months (range 6–17) two patients died of unrelated causes, and four patients had recurrences. Two cases were treated with a new course of RF ablation, while one was submitted to surgical resection. Thus, 9 patients were alive and apparently disease free (Buscarini 1998).

In two recent prospective studies the efficacy of RF thermal ablation and percutaneous ethanol injection (PEI) for the treatment of small HCC was compared. Both studies showed that treatment time is significantly shorter by using RF than by using PEI; the radicality of the RF treatment appeared to be higher, being the percentage of cases with complete necrosis greater or the number of recurrences less; no major complications with both the treatments were observed in one study (Lencioni et al. 1998b); complication rate was higher for RF treatment than that of PEI in the other (Livraghi et al. 1999).

Three patients with five HCC nodules treated with the conventional monopolar method died of causes other than HCC. Autopsy was performed and the five treated tumoral lesions were analyzed. Total necrosis was observed in two nodules ranging from 2 to 2.5 cm in diameter; two nodules ranging from 1 to 2.1 cm were no longer detected; in only one HCC nodule of 2 cm in diameter, treated 13 months before, was a tiny viable tumor of few millimeters in size observed (Rossi et al. 1996). Two patients treated with expandable needle electrodes underwent surgery: in one nodule 100% necrosis was found; in the second, 90% necrosis was seen (Rossi et al. 1998).

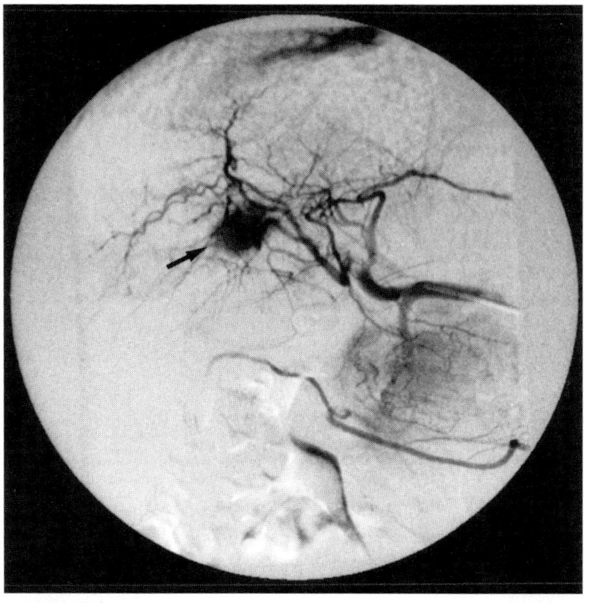

a

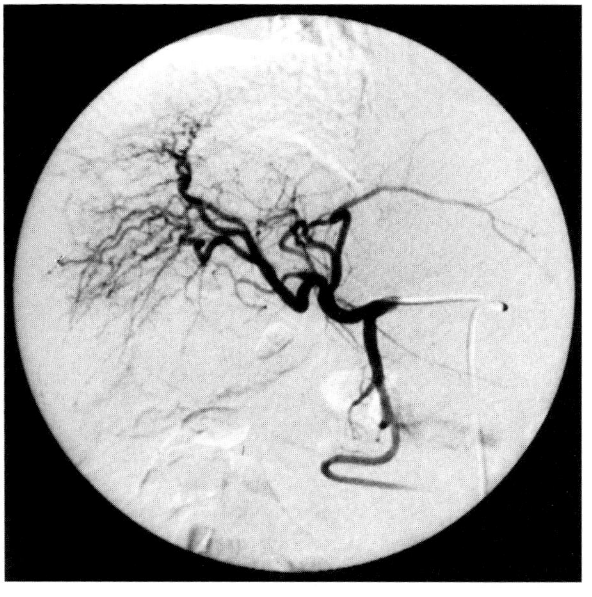

a

Fig. 20.3a,b. a Selective hepatic angiogram obtained before RF interstitial thermal ablation shows tumor vascularity (*arrow*) in right hepatic lobe. **b** After RF interstitial thermal ablation, angiography demonstrates complete disappearance of tumoral stain

20.2.6 Complications

In the first group of treated patients only mild pain in a minority of cases was observed (Rossi et al. 1996). In patients treated with expandable needle electrode, 6 patients experienced mild pain, which required minor analgesia; one patient, who was asymptomatic during the procedure, suffered from intense abdominal pain 2 h after the end of the RF application, requiring analgesia with morphine chloride 10 mg and 0.5 mg of atropine; dynamic CT showed capsular necrosis. One patient had fever the day after that did not require therapy (Rossi et al. 1998). In 5/12 patients treated with association TAE-RF application, fever was observed in the post-treatment period; in one case a colliquative aseptic necrosis arisen in the site of ablated tumor was effectively treated by percutaneous drainage (Buscarini 1998).

20.3 Percutaneous Microwave Coagulation

The wavelength of microwave is small relative to human body size. The tissue behaves mainly as a dielectric material. Because dielectric is not uniform, the field distribution inside the tissue is not predictable and therefore the heating of the tissue is not as predictable as with conduction heating. Tissue coagulation around the electrode has a spindle shape, and the necrosis volume is less than that obtained by using RF waves.

The technique is similar to that described for RF but the needle electrode is inserted through a guiding needle 14 gauge. Percutaneous microwave coagulation was employed in two small series of patients with HCC. In the first study, 18 patients with HCC not more than 2 cm were treated. The treatment was considered to be effective on the basis of US change, confirmed by disappearance of contrast enhancement at CT and/or decreased intensity of the tumor at MR imaging. In all the patients, the treatment required a mean number of 2.8 sessions. In one case the complete necrosis was confirmed at surgery. During a follow-up ranging between 11 and 33 months recurrences occurred in 3 patients who were retreated with microwave coagulation (Seki et al. 1994a).

In the second series (9 patients with HCC measuring 35–67 mm in diameter, who had previously undergone unsuccessful embolization), multiple punctures and multiple microwave emissions were performed in various parts of the tumor; the sessions were two per week. The treatment obtained a complete tumor necrosis evaluated on the basis of dynamic CT in all patients, but after a mean follow-up of 6 months radiological evidence of complete necrosis persisted only in five lesions (Murakami et al. 1995). No complications are cited in either paper.

In an interesting case report, microwave therapy was used in a case of HCC proliferating in the bile duct. The microwave electrode was placed with a guide wire under fluoroscopic guidance obtaining a complete destruction of the intraductal mass. In a follow-up of 12 months no recurrence was observed (Seki et al. 1994b).

20.4 Conclusions

Interstitial hyperthermia can easily destroy liver tumors as demonstrated by US, US guided biopsy, dynamic and spiral CT, MR imaging, selective angiography, pathologic studies and follow-up. The primary goal of this technique is to achieve the largest necrosis in the shortest time. The results obtained by modified monopolar technique (expandable needles and cooled tip needles) or by association of segmental embolization and RF treatment in HCC represent a clear improvement with respect to the previous results, making it possible to destroy large tumors in 1 or 2 sessions.

Compared to other currently available liver tumor treatments, RF interstitial thermal ablation has an acceptable medical cost, which could range from 700 to 1000 $; this cost is similar to that reported for PEI (Livraghi et al. 1995).

RF ablation seems to be a safe technique. The danger of bleeding is reduced by the coagulative power of interstitial hyperthermia. No tumor seeding along the needle track has up to now been seen. In any way we believe that caution is needed to treat superficially located tumors.

References

Amin Z, Donald JJ, Masters A, et al (1993) Hepatic metastases: interstitial laser photocoagulation with real-time US monitoring and dynamic CT evaluation of treatment. Radiology 187:339–347

Bartolozzi C, Lencioni R (1996) Ethanol injection for the treatment of hepatic tumours. Eur Radiol 6:682–696

Bartolozzi C, Lencioni R, Caramella D, et al (1995) Treatment of large hepatocellular carcinoma: transcatheter arterial chemoembolization combined with percutaneous ethanol injection versus repeated transcatheter arterial chemoembolization. Radiology 197:812–818

Bosman S, Phoa SSK, Bosma A, Van Gemert MJC (1991) Effect of percutaneous interstitial thermal laser on normal liver of pigs: sonographic and histopathological correlations. Br J Surg 78:572–575

Buscarini L (1998) Percutaneous RF interstitial thermal ablation (RITA) after transarterial embolization for treatment of large hepatic tumors. Radiology; 209 (P): 329

Buscarini L, Rossi S (1997) Technology for radiofrequency thermal ablation of liver tumors. Seminars Laparoscopic Surg 4:96–101

Buscarini L, Fornari F, Rossi S (1992) Interstitial radiofrequency hyperthermia in the treatment of small hepatocellular carcinoma: percutaneous guidance of electrode needle. In Anderegg A, Despland PA, Henner H, Otto R, eds. Proceedings of Ultraschall Diagnostik 91. Springer-Verlag, Heidelberg, pp 218–222

Buscarini L, Rossi S, Fornari F, Di Stasi M, Buscarini E (1995) Laparoscopic ablation of liver adenoma by radiofrequency electrocautery. Gastrointest Endoscopy 41:68–70

Buscarini L, Di Stasi M, Buscarini E, et al (1996a) Clinical presentation, diagnostic work-up and therapeutic choices in two consecutive series of patients with hepatocellular carcinoma. Oncology 53:204–209

Buscarini L, Rossi S, Di Stasi M, et al (1996b) Percutaneous radio-frequency interstitial thermal ablation of hepatocellular carcinoma. Radiology 201(P):267.

Goldberg SN, Hahn PF, Tanabe KK, et al (1998) Percutaneous radiofrequency tissue ablation: does perfusion-mediated tissue cooling limit coagulation necrosis? JVIR 9:101–111

Lencioni R, Bartolozzi C (1997) Nonsurgical treatment of hepatocellular carcinoma. Cancer J 10:17–23

Lencioni R, Bartolozzi C, Caramella D, et al (1995) Treatment of small hepatocellular carcinoma with percutaneous ethanol injection: analysis of prognostic factors in 105 Western patients. Cancer 76: 1737–1746

Lencioni R, Pinto F, Armillotta N, et al (1997) Long-term results of percutaneous ethanol injection therapy for hepatocellular carcinoma in cirrhosis: a European experience. Eur Radiol 7: 514–519

Lencioni R, Armillotta N, Cioni D, Petruzzi P, Paolicchi A, Bartolozzi C (1998a) Combined segmental arterial embolization and radiofrequency thermal ablation: a new therapeutic approach for large hepatocellular carcinoma. Radiology 209 (P): 565

Lencioni R, Cioni D, Paolicchi A, Armillotta N, Donati F, Bartolozzi C (1998b) Percutaneous treatment of small hepatocellular carcinoma: radiofrequency thermal ablation versus percutaneous ethanol injection: a prospective, randomized trial. Radiology 209 (P): 174

Lencioni R, Goletti O, Armillotta N, et al (1998c) Radio-frequency thermal ablation of liver metastases with a cooled-tip electrode needle: results of a pilot clinical trial. Eur Radiol 8:1205–1211

Lencioni R, Paolicchi A, Moretti M, et al. (1998d) Combined transcatheter arterial chemoembolization and percutaneous ethanol injection for the treatment of large hepatocellular carcinoma: local therapeutic effect and long-term survival rate. Eur Radiol 8:439–444

Le Veen RF (1997) Laser hyperthermia and radiofrequency ablation of hepatic lesions. Sem Intervent Radiol 14:313–324

Livraghi T, Giorgio A, Marin G, et al (1995) Hepatocellular carcinoma and cirrhosis in 746 patients: long-term results of percutaneous ethanol injection. Radiology 197:101–108

Livraghi T, Goldberg SN, Lazzaroni S, et al (1999) Small repatocellular carcinoma: treatment with radio-frequency ablation versus ethanol injection. Radiology 210:655-661

Lorentzen T (1996) A cooled needle electrode for radiofrequency tissue ablation: thermodynamic aspects of improved performance compared with conventional needle design. Acad Radiol 3:556–563

McGahan JP, Browning PD, Brock JM, Tesluk H (1990) Hepatic ablation using radiofrequency electrocautery. Invest Radiol 25:267–270

Murakami R, Yoshimatsu S, Yamashita Y, Matsukawa T, Takahashi M, Sagara K (1995) Treatment of hepatocellular carcinoma: value of percutaneous microwave coagulation. AJR 164:1159–1164

Patterson EJ, Scudamore CH, Owen DA, Nagy AG, Buczkowski AK (1998) Radiofrequency ablation of porcine liver in vivo. Effects of blood flow and treatment time on lesion size. Ann Surg 227:559–565

Rossi S, Fornari F, Paties C, Buscarini L (1990) Thermal lesions induced by 480 KHz localized current field in guinea pig and pig liver. Tumori 76:54–57

Rossi S, Di Stasi M, Buscarini E, et al (1996) Percutaneous radiofrequency interstitial thermal ablation in the treatment of liver cancer. AJR 167:759–768

Rossi S, Buscarini E, Garbagnati F, et al (1998) Percutaneous treatment of small hepatic tumors by an expandable RF needle electrode. AJR 170:1015–1022

Seki T, Wakabayashi M, Nakagawa, et al (1994a) Ultrasonically guided percutaneous microwave coagulation therapy for small hepatocellular carcinoma. Cancer 74:817–825

Seki T, Kubota Y, Wakaba M, et al (1994b) Percutaneous microwave coagulation therapy for hepatocellular carcinoma proliferating in the bile duct. Dig Dis Sci 39:663–666

Solbiati L, Ierace T, Goldberg SN, et al (1994) Percutaneous US-guided radio-frequency tissue ablation of liver metastases : treatment and follow-up in 16 patients. Radiology 202:195–203

Solbiati L, Goldberg SN, Ierace T, et al (1997) Hepatic metastases: percutaneous radio-frequency ablation with cooled-tip electrodes. Radiology 205:367–373

The Liver Cancer Study Group of Japan (1994) Predictive factors for long term prognosis after partial hepatectomy for patients with hepatocellular carcinoma in Japan. Cancer 74:2772–2780

21 Interstitial Laser Photocoagulation of Hepatocellular Carcinoma

F.S. Ferrari, F. Burresi, G. Poggianti, and P. Stefani

CONTENTS

21.1 Introduction

Hepatocellular carcinoma (HCC) is the most frequently occurring type of primary liver tumor. It may appear ex novo in an apparently healthy liver without previous evidence of macro regeneration nodules or, more frequently, in cases of chronic liver disease, especially cirrhosis (Franco 1990). In Italy HCC is found to occur in approximately 3% of cirrhotic patients, while the liver tumors most frequently observed in oncology are metastatic. Autopsy-based research performed between 1905 and 1973 confirmed the presence of hepatic metastases in 24–36% of patients deceased due to malignancies (Bengmark and Hafstrom 1969; Wilkes 1973; Colombo et al. 1991; Wolf et al. 1991).

Surgical intervention is considered the most suitable therapeutic approach since it permits long periods of remission (Steele and Ravikumar 1989; Steele et al. 1991; Vetto et al. 1990). Its application is however greatly limited, since most patients presenting HCC are cirrhotic: limiting the loss of parenchymal volume is of vital importance in order to best conserve hepatic functional capacity (Pommier et al. 1987). This limitation, in addition to the fact that HCC is often multifocal, considerably reduces the number of patients eligible for surgical resection (Livraghi et al. 1997).

Alternative palliative treatments such as radiation and embolization, applied either singly or in association with the locoregional intra-arterial injection of chemotherapeutic agents, have not improved rates of survival. Of the various percutaneous locoregional treatments, transcatheter arterial chemoembolization (TACE) has failed to successfully treat various types of HCCs due to their extensive vascularization: tumor cells, particularly when extracapsular, may be nourished both by branches of the hepatic artery and branches of the portal vein (Lang and Brown 1993; Coldwell et al. 1994).

Percutaneous intrahepatic alcohol injection (PEI) is a technique which allows rapid, relatively safe, low-cost ablation treatment of tumoral masses. It may also be repeated and normally does not result in significant loss of healthy parenchyma. Ultimately, it offers considerably therapeutic efficiency thanks partly to the fact that the ultrasound screening of a cirrhotic population allows HCC to be diagnosed while the nodules are still small (Livraghi et al. 1987, 1991; Sironi et al. 1991).

Unfortunately, PEI may fail to eliminate all tumoral tissue, since the shape and volume of the lesion created depend on the way in which the alcohol spreads throughout it. Distribution may be made inhomogeneous by vascular patterns and the macroscopic histology of the nodules. Therefore the resulting necrosis is neither predictable or replicable (Nolsøe et al. 1993). Furthermore, the systemic effects of ethanol make it possible to treat only a limited volume in each session, making serial treatment sessions lasting from 1 to 8 weeks necessary. Finally, the injection of ethanol, especially in encapsulated lesions, produces an increase in pressure which may

F.S. Ferrari, MD; Department of Radiology, University of Siena, Le Scotte Hospital, Viale Bracci 2, I-53100 Siena, Italy
F. Burresi, MD; Department of Radiology, University of Siena, Le Scotte Hospital, Viale Bracci 2, I-53100 Siena, Italy
G. Poggianti, MD; Department of Radiology, University of Siena, Le Scotte Hospital, Viale Bracci 2, I-53100 Siena, Italy
P. Stefani, MD; Professor and Chairman, Department of Radiology, University of Siena, Le Scotte Hospital, Viale Bracci 2, I-53100 Siena, Italy

provoke an expulsion of alcohol from the HCC to the hepatic capsule, causing pain (Buscarini and Stasi 1996). Such a backflow of ethanol may also permit neoplastic cells to spread along the path of the needle used in the treatment (seeding). Since precise data are lacking, this probability is difficult to estimate but has been calculated as a risk of 0.5% for HCC cases (Cedrone et al. 1991; Zerbey et al. 1994). It would be reasonable to suppose that such a risk is greater in the case of metastasis, which is normally more aggressive (Kaiser 1989).

Considerable interest has recently been directed toward two percutaneous methods based on the generation of total tissue necrosis as a result of local hyperthermia: radiofrequency (RF) and interstitial laser photocoagulation (ILP) (Masters et al. 1992). The idea of using heat to treat tumors is actually ancient, and it seems that even the ancient Romans used cauterization to treat superficial tumors (Hornback 1989). Research by Coley demonstrated in 1893 that tumor cells are in fact more vulnerable to heat damage than healthy tissue. Experimental attempts to treat deeply seated tumors using external heat sources were performed toward the end of the 1970s and during the 1980s.

The research done by LeVeen and other Authors in 1980 confirmed the particular sensitivity of neoplastic tissue to heat damage, partly due to its inability to dissipate heat through increased blood flow as occurs in the healthy surrounding tissue. Nonetheless, the use of locoregional or total body hyperthermia was limited by the lack of instruments capable of making such therapy safe and manageable (Solbiati et al. 1997). It was impossible to hit the target precisely and accurately predict the extent of the lesion. Temperatures of approximately 42° were required to limit damage to the healthy tissue surrounding the tumor while there was no way to monitor the temperature generated within the lesion. Furthermore, tumors exposed to sublethal temperatures proved to become resistant to subsequent heat therapy treatments (Gerner et al. 1980).

Now, with the use of modern cross-sectional imaging, interventional radiology techniques and constantly developing technology it has become possible to treat deep-seated lesions using local hyperthermia by means of a simple percutaneous needle-prick thanks to RF, which uses needle probes placed within the lesion, and ILP, which uses energy provided by a laser and carried by a quartz optical fiber (LeVeen 1987).

21.2 Technique

21.2.1 Biological Effects of Laser Radiation

The laser employed in ILP acts simply as a source of electromagnetic radiation. The main characteristics of laser radiation are monochromaticity, collimation and the production of a coherent band of photons. These characteristics allow energy to be transmitted to extremely limited focal diameters, producing incredibly high levels of power density. The biological response and the extent of the tumor necrosis produced by laser hyperthermia are dependent on the power employed (in Watts), lesion exposure time, the light wavelength used and the absorption characteristics of each tissue.

The laser most widely used in gastroenterology and endoscopy is the neodymium-aluminum-garnet (Nd:YAG) laser which emits a band of light with a wavelength of 1,064 nm (van Eyken et al. 1991; Nolsøe et al. 1993). Much experimental research on the effects of heat therapy with Nd:YAG lasers on normal liver tissue and concerning the hyperthermic ablation of liver tumors in animals has been carried out in the last ten years (Bown 1983; Pacella et al. 1993).

In 1987 Matthewson et al. conducted a study of interstitial laser therapy on rat livers. They applied uncoated 0.4 mm fibers to the hepatic parenchyma of rats during laparotomy and concluded that ILP produces areas of coagulative necrosis which are clearly defined, predictable, reproducible and proportional in size to power and exposure time. They observed that even power levels greater than 1000 J failed to produce areas of necrosis with a diameter larger than 16 mm.

In 1990 Dachman et al. experimented with the effects of this laser technique on live pigs, using ultrasound to position uncoated fiber tips and sacrificing the pigs after various lengths of time in order to evaluate the anatomical and pathological evolution of the lesions. The findings repeatedly displayed areas of coagulative necrosis characterized by vaporization, carbonization and acute flogosis around the fiber tip, while there was no apparent damage to surrounding tissue (Rossi et al. 1990; Steger et al. 1991).

In 1992 Steger et al. experimented with a system employing the parallel insertion of quartz fibers in a dog liver and the use of a splitter to simultaneously deliver power to four fibers in order to obtain larger areas of necrosis. This trial attempted to verify the applicability of ILP in treating lesions of considerable dimensions.

The present protocols for the treatment of liver neoplasms normally require exposure times ranging from 100 to 400 s and power outputs of up to 10 W. The electromagnetic radiation is conveyed by means of a quartz optical fiber (0.2–0.6 mm diameter) fitted into a Chiba needle positioned in the lesion under ultrasound guidance and subsequently retracted 4–5 mm so as to leave the tip of the fiber in direct contact with the neoplasm. The characteristics of the radiation allow it to penetrate the tissues considerably. The collimated band expands in all directions (scattering phenomenon), illuminating a volume of tissue in correspondence with the band's point of incidence. The photons are absorbed as energy by the molecules composing the hepatic tissue, and they consequently enter a state of excitement. Since such a state is unstable, the molecules tend to lose energy through various mechanisms, notably photothermally: as such, the energy is dissipated as heat.

Thus, energy absorption by tissues is followed by rapid heat accumulation which exerts different effects on biological systems depending on the temperature reached. These effects may be reversible (such as acute flogosis caused by a local temperature increase) or irreversible, such as coagulative necrosis, which results in regeneration and fibrosis with a central scar, or instantaneous vaporization, which brings about total tissue destruction.

It is important to note that these alterations are simultaneously present in each lesion produced. The diffusion of the band and thermal conduction produce a elliptic lesion dependent on the level of energy absorbed by the tissues which decreases proportionally to the increase in distance from the tip of the optical fiber. The area nearest to the point of contact with the laser band receives the most energy and undergoes vaporization and carbonization; the peripheral layers undergo coagulative necrosis which results in cellular regeneration or fibrosis; even more peripherally, a perilesional area characterized by acute inflammatory response may be observed. In other words, temperature decreases as the distance from the optical fiber increases, and the various temperatures correspond to various effects.

Temperatures of 43–45°C produce reversible damage to cellular enzymes which may become irreversible if exposure time exceeds 25 min (Steger et al. 1989). Beyond 55–60°C, a macroscopically pale lesion resulting from coagulative necrosis, collagen hyalinization and cellular wrinkling may be observed. At 100°C tissues vaporize and beyond 100°C carbonization takes place. At this point it must be underlined that the effectiveness of this treatment depends on the ability to monitor the position of the fiber with respect to the lesion and to evaluate the extent of the lesion induced in real time (Amin et al. 1993; Livraghi et al. 1997).

21.2.2 Clinical Application

The research reported in the international literature is fundamentally in agreement with regard to the main aspects of the various protocols. Patients are selected according to precise parameters for admission based on their coagulative capacity, a biopsy testing positive for neoplasm, an absence of extrahepatic diffusion of the disease and the number and size of lesions (Pacella et al. 1996). For this final parameter the various protocols are dishomogeneous, with different case studies accepting patients with a maximum number of tumors ranging from 3 to 5 and with diameters not exceeding 6 cm (Jaffe et al. 1968). This disagreement is probably a result of the greatest limitation of ILP, that is, its inability to generate an area of necrosis larger than 16 mm. Undoubtedly, once the splitter method becomes easier to perform and more widespread it will substitute the monofiber, making these size limitations much less restrictive.

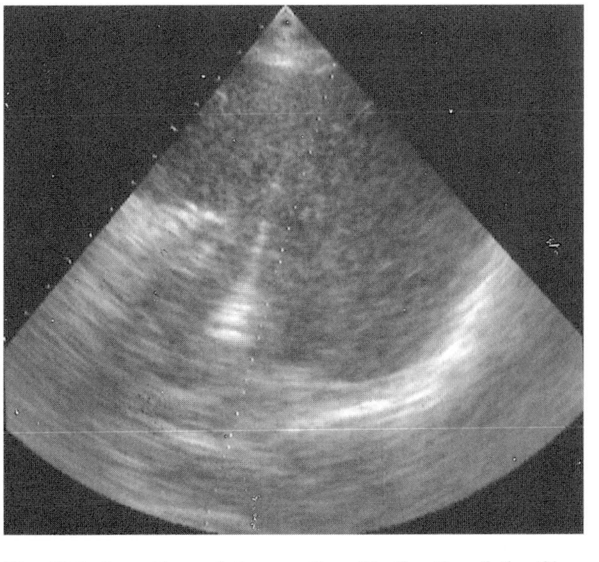

Fig. 21.1. Insertion of the needle with the tip of the fiber displayed

All the patients we studied underwent ultrasound and CT examination, with and without contrast medium, both before and after the laser treatment at intervals determined by their individual cases. The pre-treatment preparation and post-ILP check-ups were no different from those performed in normal liver biopsies: ultrasound was used to locate the neoplasms, the point of percutaneous access was selected, local anesthesia was administered, a Chiba needle (18–22G) was introduced to reach the neoplasm and ultrasound was used to identify the tip of the needle with biplanar scans (Fig. 21.1)(Nolsøe et al. 1993). At this point the stylet was substituted with an optical fiber with an uncoated final portion and the protective needle was retracted (4–5 mm) so that the tip of the fiber was in direct contact with the neoplasm.

Activation of the laser begins the thermal ablation therapy. During the procedure ultrasound monitoring visualizes the modifications in the hypoechoic echostructural pattern typical of small HCCs (Malone and Wyman 1992; Sheu et al. 1984). It should be underlined that the above-mentioned hypoechoic aspect represents the most typical, but not the only, possible pattern of small HCCs: whatever echoic structure is displayed by the malignant nodule, ILP treatment replaces it with an area of dishomogeneous hyperechogeneity with irregular, ill-defined margins around the tip of the optical fiber. This modification of the pattern is due to the phenomena of carbonization and vaporization accompanied by a secondary formation of gas microbubbles.

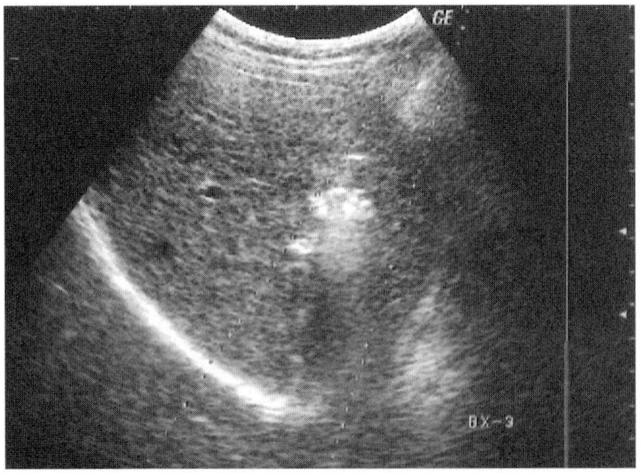

Fig. 21.2. The fiber is heated and tissue evaporation takes place after about 40 s

More peripherally, radially arranged hyperechoic strias represent the emission of gas produced by hyperthermia through the perilesional veins, ultimately illustrating echogeneic spots due to gas present in the hepatic veins. The hyperechogenicity of the nodule expands after approximately 20 s from the start of the treatment, reaching a plateau after 4 min (Fig 21.2). These echostructural modifications impair visibility of the nodule, making it difficult to identify during the course of the treatment (Malone and Wyman 1992). However, these modifications are the only (and somewhat imprecise) means available for evaluating the volume of tissue treated in real time.

A sonogram performed 24 h later would typically display a central hyperechoic area resulting from carbonized tissue surrounded by a hypoechoic ring associated with coagulated tissue. Later sonograms revealed nodules with completely aspecific echostructural characteristics, typically distinguished by an irregular alternation of hypo- and hyperechoic areas but without a discernable distinction between the necrotic tissue and the still-vital tumor mass (Pacella et al. 1995). This demonstrates why the role of sonography must be limited to the staging, directional guidance and real-time evaluation of the treatment and why it is not useful in following up patients treated with ILP (LeVeen 1997; LeVeen et al. 1980; McGahan et al. 1990).

21.3 Treatment Follow-up

The international literature has cited computerized tomography (CT) as the method of choice for the follow-up of ILP. CT examination must not, however, be performed closely following the treatment: after 48 h a halo of perilesional enhancement due to acute heat-induced flogosis is evident, making a differential diagnosis from residual vital neoplastic tissue impossible. Various sources have agreed on performing the first CT examination 15–20 days after treatment, in order to allow observation of the consolidated ILP outcome without flogistic reaction and thus evaluate the entity of the induced necrosis (Amin et al. 1993) (Fig. 21.3).

This enables identification of the areas of complete necrosis as areas which are clearly hypodense in comparison with the healthy parenchyma and prove to be avascular and lacking in enhancement upon administration of contrast medium, while the

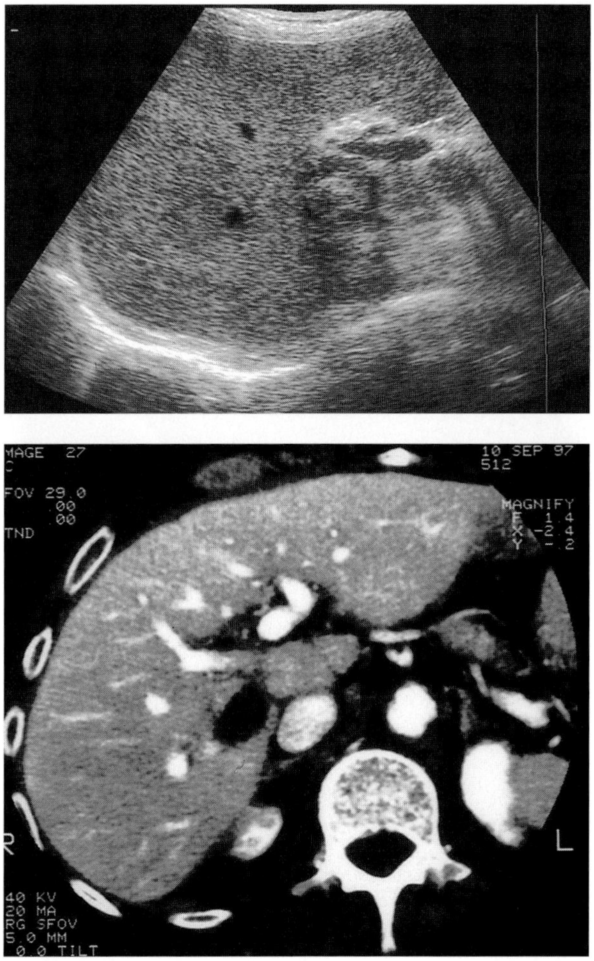

a

b

Fig. 21.3a,b. a HCC in segment I. **b** Complete response following three treatments with ILP. The necrotic area tends to implode

areas of residual vital tumor tissue conserve enhancement and display densitometric values which are between those of necrotic areas and those of healthy parenchyma in a portal phase and equal to those of healthy parenchyma when in equilibrium.

The effectiveness of the treatment is rated with different methods in the various studies. Two or three categories are usually created: some case studies simply distinguish between complete and incomplete necrosis while others distinguish a complete necrosis of a nodule as *grade one*, necrosis of more than 50% of nodular tissue as *grade two* and necrosis of less than 50% of the initial nodule as *grade three*. We have found such distinctions to be unproductive: the objective of ILP is total ablation of the neoplasm, given the biological nature of residual neoplastic tissue. In fact, a considerable cytoreduction (as occurs in treatment of metastatic neoplasms) is insufficient: total eradication of the HCC is imperative. Therefore all lesions displaying incomplete necrosis, irrespective of its extent, must necessarily be retreated until total necrosis is attained (Cecconi and Caspani 1996). At this point, in order to evaluate the feasibility of retreatment, the arrangement of the residual tissue or eventual relapse becomes important (Fig. 21.4). If the neoplastic tissue is irregularly arranged, treatment may be repeated until complete necrosis is achieved. If instead the neoplastic tissue is concentrically arranged around the laser-induced lesion, retreatment is geometrically impossible (McGahan et al. 1990).

As to treatment follow-up, in addition to the fundamental role of CT, new possibilities are emerging thanks to continuing improvements in technique and research on new drugs. The use of sonographic contrast media capable of increasing the sensitivity of echo color Doppler with slower flows is becoming commonplace (Burns et al. 1992, 1993). Understandably, the fact that color Doppler enables the visualization of blood flow (and thus of residual vital tissue) by means of a technique which is replicable, economical and accessible immediately aroused interest among researchers.

A great deal of research has been done on the vascularization of tumor tissue and new insight into the structure and arrangement of neoplastic vessels has been gained which is in correlation with the information obtained thanks to imaging: numerous vascular structures are located peripherally, and in fact, evidence of flow is more easily discerned here than at the center of the tumor. The vessels are irregularly winding and thin-walled, without a muscular tunic, implying reduced resistence and justifying such minimal systo-diastolic variations. Finally, numerous arterio-venous shunts are responsible for a flow of elevated velocity.

Nonetheless, color Doppler analysis of HCCs is often complicated by various factors: the size and location of the nodules, a lack of patient collaboration and, in particular, the low sensitivity of Color Doppler in recognizing the slower flows of small, newly formed vessels. In fact, sonographic contrast media were introduced in an effort to overcome this shortcoming. The initial results of research still in progress on their use with HCCs are promising and imply that during follow-up sonographic contrast media are able to reveal neoplastic tissue which is still vascularized and consequently vital (Angeli et al. 1994).

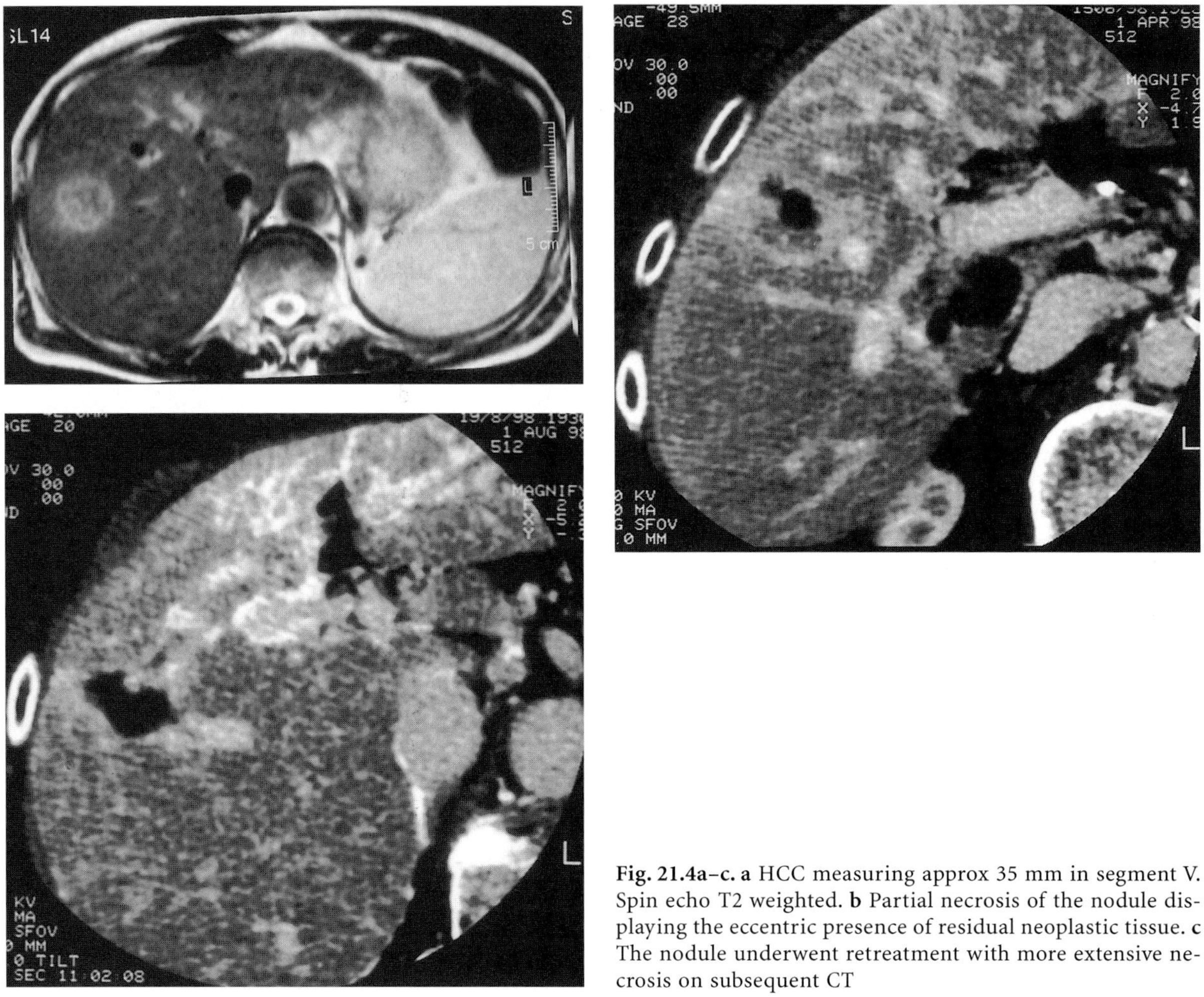

Fig. 21.4a–c. **a** HCC measuring approx 35 mm in segment V. Spin echo T2 weighted. **b** Partial necrosis of the nodule displaying the eccentric presence of residual neoplastic tissue. **c** The nodule underwent retreatment with more extensive necrosis on subsequent CT

21.4 Safety

In general the treatment has been shown to be well tolerated. The adverse effects most frequently reported in the literature include slight abdominal discomfort, sometimes radiating toward the right shoulder or the epigastric area, easily treated with mild analgesics, a slight temperature (37.5–38°C) and nausea. More serious complications have included pleural effusion (when treating nodules near the hepatic cupule) and intrahepatic hematomas (Cecconi and Caspani 1996). A case of injury of the diaphragm and hemipericardium during ILP treatment would suggest avoiding this type of laser hyperthermia in treating nodules located near the major vessels and pericardium in order to avoid the danger of serious complications.

One initial fear was that of venous thrombosis of the vessels surrounding the lesion, which in reality is only a rare possibility. On the contrary, the perilesional vessels play an important role in dispersing heat and protecting the surrounding healthy tissue from heat damage. Another possible danger encountered in all percutaneous treatments is that of spreading neoplastic cells along the path of the needle (seeding) (Cedrone et al. 1992). We have already mentioned seeding as a possible complication during PEI, particularly likely due to the increase of pressure inside the nodule caused by the injection of ethanol, which, as it flows back, carries neoplastic cells with it. Supplying power to the optical fiber during withdrawal affords sterilization of the exit path, thus preventing seeding (van Eyken 1991).

21.5 Results

Our experience is based on the ILP treatment of 18 patients presenting HCCs from December 1995 to November 1996. Twelve patients were classified as belonging to Child's class A and six as belonging to class B. Surgery was contraindicated for all patients due to the multiplicity of foci, insufficient liver function or particular locations of the nodules which made surgical resection especially difficult.

The criteria for exclusion from the case study was that normally used in the international literature and previously mentioned: the presence of extrahepatic disease, the presence of more than 5 liver tumors, a single tumor larger than 6 cm in diameter or altered coagulative capacity. In all 24 nodules were treated and 204 treatment sessions were conducted. The average diameter of the nodules treated was 2.9 cm (1.2–4.8 cm range). The results achieved were evaluated by means of CT examination 20 days following treatment, which revealed 16 nodules with complete necrosis and 6 with incomplete necrosis. Two patients were excluded from follow-up: one of these underwent surgical treatment since ILP failed to effectively treat the nodule; the other failed to participate in the follow-up program and was excluded from our results.

None of the serious adverse effects mentioned in the literature was observed (one patient experienced minor pleural effusion which healed spontaneously), while some pain, eliminated with mild analgesics, and a slight fever were temporarily encountered following practically all treatments. Ultimately, as reported in the international literature, there was no evidence of neoplastic seeding along the needle path.

21.6 Conclusions

The data reported in the international literature clearly demonstrate that the results achieved with ILP depend on accurate centering of the nodule, real-time monitoring of the treatment, accurate evaluation of the induced necrosis and, in particular, the attainment of a necrosis which encompasses the entire volume of the tumor. The body of the international literature universally cites sonography as the most effective imaging technique for accurately centering the nodule and monitoring the necrotic process in real time (MALONE and WYMAN 1992). Instead, CT with contrast medium has been recognized as the gold standard for evaluating the extent of the induced necrosis in follow-up, given that it clearly distinguishes avascular tissue (resulting from complete necrosis) from still-vital residual tumor 15–20 days following treatment. The parameters to be evaluated with CT are the dimensions of the tumor and the relative extent of the induced necrosis. A nodule with a high necrotic volume and which collapses will presumably undergo an involution; that is, a reduction in size is a sign of a favorable progression. All case studies have confirmed the possibility of inducing necrosis in all tumors treated with ILP (AMIN et al. 1993).

At present, the outcome of this treatment is contingent on the dimensions of the nodule and its configuration. The vast majority of small HCCs are encapsulated and grow by means of expansion. This capsule prevents heat from escaping, affording particularly fruitful results with negligible damage to healthy surrounding tissues (Sheu et al. 1984; Pacella et al. 1995). Non-encapsulated HCCs, which grow by means of infiltration, and liver metastases likewise, do not undergo the same phenomena and require greater quantities of energy in order to attain similar therapeutic results, at the same time subjecting the nearby healthy perilesional tissue to greater damage. With regard to nodule dimensions, we have found that the optimal results, in terms of complete necrosis, are obtained with HCCs of less than 3 cm in diameter, due to the intrinsic characteristics of lesions produced by laser hyperthermia, which never exceed a maximum diameter of 16 mm when measured from the tip of a single optical fiber.

An ulterior advantage of ILP treatment is its repeatibility for the treatment of eventual local or distant relapses. These latter are in fact inevitable, illustrating the typical progression of a HCC. They may also be successfully treated with ILP, partly due to the fact that regular ultrasound screening of cirrhotic patients usually permits nodules to be diagnosed while they are still small (Sheu et al. 1984). In contrast, local relapses and areas of residual tumor tissue are likely to be treated without success. Depending of the arrangement of such neoplastic tissue, they may also prove impossible to retreat. If this tissue is arranged concentrically around an induced lesion, ILP treatment is in fact not possible. This again emphasizes the present limitation of laser tissue ablation: the size of the induced necrotic lesion, which is too small to ensure the attainment of a complete necrosis in every tumor during a single session.

The possibility of generating larger necrotic areas would offer the multiple advantages of reducing the number of necessary sessions, diminishing the risk of complications, bringing down costs, decreasing patient discomfort and, most importantly, reducing the chance of non-retreatable local relapses. Research is being done on variations of this technique which foresee the simultaneous application of multiple needles and multiple fibers during a single session, precisely with the goal of increasing the volume of the treated area and consequently of the area of induced necrosis (splitter technique).

References

Amin Z, Donald JJ, Master A, et al (1993) Hepatic metastases: interstitial laser photocoagulation with real-time US monitoring and dynamic CT evaluation of treatment. Radiology 187:339–347

Angeli E, Carpanelli R, Crespi G, et al (1994) Efficacia del SH U 508 A (Levovist) nella valutazione con color-Doppler della vascolarizzazione dell'epatocarcinoma. Radiol Med 87(S):24–31

Bengmark S, Hafstrom L (1969) The natural history of primary and secondary malignant tumors of the liver. Cancer 23:198–202

Bown SG (1983) Phototherapy of tumors. World J Surg 7:700–709

Burns PN, Powers JE, Fritzsch T, et al (1992) Harmonic imaging: a new imaging and Doppler method for contrast enhanced ultrasound. Radiology 185(P):142–147

Burns PN, Powers JE, Hope Simpson D, et al (1993) Harmonic contrast enhanced Doppler as a method for the elimination of clutter. In vivo duplex and color studies. Radiology 189:285–290

Buscarini E, Di Stasi M (1996) Alcolizzazione del carcinoma epatocellulare. In: Buscarini E, Di Stasi M (eds) Complicanze della ecografia operativa addominale. Poletto Ed., Milano, pp 93–100

Cecconi P, Caspani B (1996) Fotocoagulazione interstiziale con laser nel trattamento delle lesioni neoplastiche del fegato. Esperienza preliminare. Radiol Med 92:105–109

Cedrone A, Rapaccini GL, Pompili M, et al (1992) Neoplastic seeding complicating percutaneous ethanol injection for treatment of hepatocellular carcinoma. Radiology 183:787–788

Coldwell DM, Stokes KR, Yakes WF (1994) Embolotherapy: agents, clinical application, and techniques. Radiographics 14:623–643

Coley WB (1893) The treatment of malignant tumors by repeated inoculations of erysipelas with a report of ten original cases. Am J Med Sci 105:487–490

Colombo M, De Franchis R, Del Ninno E, et al (1991) Hepatocellular carcinoma in italian patients with cirrhosis. N Engl J Med 325:675–680

Dachman AH, McGehee JA, Beam TE, et al (1990) US-guided percutaneous laser ablation of liver tissue in a chronic pig model. Radiology 176:129–133

Franco D (1990) Malignancy of the liver. Curr Opin Gastroenterol 6:447–453

Gerner EW, Cross AE, Stickney DG, et al (1980) Factors regulating membrane permeability alter thermal resistance. Ann NY Acad Sci 335:215–233

Hornback NB (1989) Historical aspects of hyperthermia in cancer therapy. Radiol Clin North Am 27:481–488

Jaffe BM, Donegan WL, Watson F, et al (1968) Factors influencing survival in patients with untreated hepatic metastases.Surg Gynecol Obstet 127:1–11

Kaiser HE (1989) Overview of metastatic spreading. In: Gorelik E (ed) Metastases dissemination. Kluver, Dordrecht, pp 1–20

Lang EK, Brown CL (1993) Colorectal metastases to the liver: selective chemoembolization. Radiology 189:417–422

LeVeen HH, Ahmed N, Piccone VA, et al (1980) Radiofrequency therapy: clinical experience. Ann NY Acad Sci 335:362–371

LeVeen RF (1997) Laser hyperthermia and radiofrequency ablation of hepatic lesions. Semin Intervent Radiol 14:313–324

Livraghi T, Festi D, Monti F, et al (1987) US-guided percutaneous alcohol injection of small hepatic and abdominal tumors. Radiology 161:309–312

Livraghi T, Vettori C, Lazzaroni S (1991) Liver metastases: results of percutaneous ethanol injection in 14 patients. Radiology 179:709–712

Livraghi T, Makuuchi M, Buscarini L (1997) Epatocarcinoma. Poletto Editore, Milano

Malone DE, Wyman DR (1992) Sonographic changes during hepatic interstitial laser photocoagulation. Invest Radiol 27:804–813

Masters A, Steger AC, Lees WR, et al (1992) Interstitial laser hyperthermia: a new approach for treting liver metastases. Br J Cancer 66:518–522

Matthewson K, Coleridge-Smith P, O'Sullivan JP, et al (1987) Biological effects of intrahepatic Neodimium: Yttrium-Aluminium-Garnet Laser photocoagulation in rats. Gastroenterology 93:550–557

McGahan JP, Browning PD, Brock JM, et al (1990) Hepatic ablation using radiofrequency electrocautery. Invest Radiol 25:267–270

Nolsøe CP, Torp-Pedersen S, Andersen PH, et al (1993) Ultrasound-guided percutaneous Nd: YAG laser diffuser tip hyperthermia of liver metastases. Semin Intervent Radiol 10:113–124

Nolsøe CP, Torp-Pedersen S, Burchart F, et al (1993) Interstitial hyperthermia of colorectal liver metastases with a US-guided Nd:YAG laser with a diffuser tip: a pilot clinical study. Radiology 187:333–337

Pacella CM, Rossi Z, Bizzarri G, et al (1993) Ultrasound-guided percutaneous laser ablation of liver tissue in a rabbit model. Eur Radiol 3:26–32

Pacella CM, Rossi Z, Bizzarri G, et al (1995) Ultrasound-guided percutaneous laser tissue ablation of small HCC: clinical experiences in ten cases. Eur Radiol 5(5):795

Pacella CM, Bizzarri G, Ferrari FS, et al (1996) La fotocoagulazione interstiziale con laser nel trattamento delle metastasi epatiche. Radiol Med 92:438–447

Pommier RF, Woltering EA, Campbell JR, et al (1987) Hepatic resection for primary and secondary neoplasm of the liver. Am J Surg 153:428–433

Rossi S, Fornari F, Paties C, et al (1990) Thermal lesion induced by 480 Khz localized current field in guinea pig and pig liver. Tumori 76:54–57

Sheu JC, Sung JL, Cheng DS, et al (1984) Ultrasonography of small hepatic tumors using high-resolution linear-array real-time instruments. Radiology 150:797–802

Sironi S, Livraghi T, Del Maschio A (1991) Small hepatocellular carcinoma treated with percutaneous ethanol injection: MR imaging findings. Radiology 180:333–336

Solbiati L, Ierace T, Goldberg SN, et al (1997) Percutaneous US-guided radio-frequency tissue ablation of liver metastases: treatment and follow-up in 16 patients. Radiology 202:195–203

Steele G Jr, Ravikumar TS (1989) Resection of hepatic metastases from colorectal cancer: biologic perspectives. Ann Surg 210:127–138

Steele G Jr, Bleday R, Mayer R, et al (1991) A prospective evaluation of hepatic resection for colorectal carcinoma metastases to the liver: Gastrointestinal tumor study group protocol 6584. J Clin Oncol 9:1105–1112

Steger AC, Lees WR, Walmsley K, et al (1989) Interstitial laser hyperthermia: a new approach to local destruction of tumors. Br Md J 299:362–365

Steger AC, Lees WR, Shorvon P, et al (1992) Multiple-fibre low-power interstitial laser hyperthermia: studies in the normal liver. Br J Surg 79:139–145

Van Eyken P, Hiele M, Fevery J, et al (1991) Comparative study of low-power neodymium-YAG-laser interstitial hyperthermia versus ethanol injection for controlled hepatic tissue destruction. Lasers Med Sci 6:35–41

Vetto JT, Hughes KS, Rosenstein R, et al (1990) Morbidity and mortality of hepatic resection for colorectal carcinoma. Dis Colon Rectum 33:400–413

Wilkes SA (1973) Secondary tumors of the liver. Butterworths, London, England pp 175–183

Wolf RF, Goodnight JE, Krag DE, et al (1991) Results of resection and proposed guidelines for patient selection in instances of non colorectal hepatic metastases. Surg Gynecol Obstet 173:454–460

Zerbey AL, Mueller PR, Dawson SL, et al (1994) Pleural seeding from hepatocellular carcinoma: a complication of percutaneous ethanol ablation. Radiology 193:81–82

22 Combination of Interventional Treatments in Hepatocellular Carcinoma

C. Bartolozzi, S. Rossi, F. Garbagnati, A. Paolicchi, M. Di Giulio, and R. Lencioni

CONTENTS

22.1 Introduction

Hepatocellular carcinoma (HCC) is one of the most common malignancies in the world, with an estimated incidence of about 1,000,000 cases per year worldwide (Lencioni and Bartolozzi 1997). This tumor represents the seventh most common cancer in men and the ninth most common cancer in women. HCC shows considerable differences among the various geographic areas with respect to incidence, etiology, and clinico-pathologic features. While this neoplasm is very common in Southeast Asia and in sub-Saharan Africa, it is relatively rare in the United States and in the north of Europe. The south of Europe is characterized by a medium-to-high incidence of HCC.

In Western countries, as well as in Japan, HCC emerges in cirrhotic livers in more than 90% of cases. Patients with liver cirrhosis, in fact, have long been identified as being a high-risk group for the development of HCC. Yearly incidence of HCC in cirrhotic patients may reach 3–5%, and HCC is recognized as the principal cause of death for these patients (Lencioni and Bartolozzi 1997). Since the mid-1970s, the recognition of the close association of HCC with cirrhosis has stimulated the development of clinical programs for the early detection of HCC in cirrhotic patients. Extensive screening for HCC was made possible by the application of sensitive and specific diagnostic methods, such as assays for serum alpha-fetoprotein (AFP) and real-time ultrasonography (US). Early detection programs have led to the identification of an increasing number of early-stage, asymptomatic tumors, potentially suitable for surgical resection.

Most patients with HCC, however, are not suitable candidates for surgical resection despite early tumor detection. Exclusion from surgery is usually due to either a severe liver dysfunction caused by the coexisting cirrhosis or the presence of multiple tumor nodules at diagnosis. More recently, following unsatisfactory reports on long-term survival rates after surgical resection for HCC, the indications for partial hepatectomy were further restricted. Resective surgery in cirrhotic patients, in fact, remains associated with nonnegligible morbidity and mortality, despite the advances in surgical techniques. Moreover, partial hepatectomy necessarily involves loss of noncancerous parenchyma: this is a crucial point because in cirrhotic patients hepatic function is already compromised and any intervention that worsens it further hastens the onset of liver failure. Finally, because of the underlying cirrhosis, patients with HCC had a high tendency to develop new HCC lesions after removal of the first tumor, with disease-free rates as low as 0% after 5 years (Bartolozzi et al. 1995; Lin et al. 1997; Llovet et al. 1999).

C. Bartolozzi, MD, Professor and Chairman; Division of Diagnostic and Interventional Radiology, Department of Oncology, University of Pisa, Via Roma 67, I-56125 Pisa, Italy
S. Rossi, MD; Department of Gastroenterology, General Hospital, Cantone del Cristo 40, I-29100 Piacenza, Italy
F. Garbagnati, MD; Department of Radiology, National Cancer Institute, Via Venezian 1, I-20100 Milan, Italy
A. Paolicchi, MD; Division of Diagnostic and Interventional Radiology, Department of Oncology, University of Pisa, Via Roma 67, I-56125 Pisa, Italy
M. Di Giulio, MD; Division of Diagnostic and Interventional Radiology, Department of Oncology, University of Pisa, Via Roma 67, I-56125 Pisa, Italy
R. Lencioni, MD; Division of Diagnostic and Interventional Radiology, Department of Oncology, University of Pisa, Via Roma 67, I-56125 Pisa, Italy

As a result of the limitations of surgical resection, and because of the shortage of donor organs for liver transplantation, nonsurgical interventional therapies are currently used to treat the large majority of patients with HCC.

22.2 Interventional Treatments for Hepatocellular Carcinoma

Many interventional techniques aimed at providing local destruction of the tumor have been developed and clinically tested over the last decade. Among these procedures, percutaneous ethanol injection (PEI) has been shown to be effective for the treatment of small, nodular-type HCC (Lencioni et al. 1995, 1997; Livraghi et al. 1995). PEI is able to induce complete or almost complete necrosis of lesions 3 cm or less in greatest dimension, without any adverse effects on the noncancerous liver parenchyma. Moreover, the survival figures reported in several studies indicate that the long-term outcomes of patients with small HCC treated with PEI are almost the same as those of patients who underwent resection.

More recently, interstitial hyperthermia created by radiofrequency (RF) needle electrodes (Lencioni et al. 1998c; Buscarini and Rossi 1997; Goldberg et al. 1998a), laser fibers (Vogl et al 1995), or microwave electrodes (Murakami et al. 1995) has also been used for percutaneous ablation of small HCC. RF thermal ablation, in particular, attracted a great deal of attention as it underwent a very rapid technical evolution over the past few years. Currently, thermal necrosis volumes up to 3–4 cm in diameter can be obtained with a single-probe insertion, thereby enabling ablation of small hepatic tumors in a single session (Buscarini and Rossi 1997; Lencioni et al. 1998b; Goldberg et al. 1998c). When compared with PEI in prospective, randomized trials, RF treatment was found to ensure a more reliable necrosis of HCC lesions smaller than 3 cm, at the same time substantially reducing the number of sessions needed to ablate the tumor (Lencioni et al. 1998b; Livraghi et al. 1998).

If small HCC lesions can be currently ablated successfully in most instances, treatment of large HCC tumors remains problematic. In large tumors, in fact, alcohol diffusion results are inhomogeneous and incomplete, being impeded by the texture of the tumor and by intratumoral septa (Bartolozzi and Lencioni 1996). As a result, viable neoplastic tissue often persists after treatment along the periphery of the lesion. On the other hand, with RF treatment, it is almost impossible to create confluent thermal necrosis volumes covering large neoplastic masses, even if repeated needle insertions are carefully guided with combined US and spiral CT guidance (Lencioni et al. 1998c).

Large HCC lesions are usually treated with transcatheter arterial chemoembolization (TACE), by using various combinations of chemotherapeutic drugs and embolic agents (Florio et al. 1997; Colombo 1997; Matsui et al. 1993). TACE, however, was rarely proved to result in complete necrosis of large HCC lesions. Repeated procedures over time, therefore, are necessary to control the growth of the tumor. Repeated TACE sessions, however, frequently cause a substantial worsening of the liver function, since they damage also noncancerous liver parenchyma. Therefore, despite the fact that an objective response of the tumor was often seen, the real benefit of this treatment for survival has been questioned (Groupe D'Etude de Traitment du Carcinome Hepatocellulaire 1995).

In view of the limitations of each interventional therapy, there is currently a focus on a multimodality strategy for the treatment of HCC. In particular, combinations of different interventional procedures have been tested in attempts to ensure a more effective treatment of large HCC.

22.3 Combined Transcatheter Arterial Chemoembolization and Ethanol Injection

Combined TACE and PEI is a therapeutic option that has been recently proposed to overcome the weakness of each of the two procedures in the treatment of large HCC (Lencioni et al. 1994; Bartolozzi et al. 1995; Tanaka et al. 1992). The rationale for the combination of the two treatments relies on the fact that after TACE tumor consistency is markedly decreased and intratumoral septa are usually disrupted, as a result of the necrotic phenomena induced by the procedure. These histopathologic changes make subsequent treatment with PEI easier, as they provide enhanced ethanol diffusion within the tumor mass. Consequently, higher doses of ethanol with respect to those used in conventional PEI (up to 30–40 ml/session) can be injected, enabling complete and homogeneous perfusion even of large lesions. Moreover, treatment with PEI is facilitated by the TACE-derived fibrous wall around the lesion, which favors a better retention of the injected ethanol within the tumor. Finally, after arterial embolization, the normal wash-out of ethanol is more difficult in the tumorous area, resulting in longer retention of the substance.

The ideal indication for combined TACE and PEI is represented by patients with compensated cirrhosis and a large, solitary, encapsulated HCC. In our experience, nearly 80% of such lesions can be successfully ablated by a single TACE followed by a cycle of 4–8 ethanol injections (Fig. 22.1) (Lencioni et al. 1998d).

On the contrary, in patients with more than one huge tumor or with a main tumor associated with a number of satellite nodules, combined treatment would require an inordinate number of ethanol injections and hence an unduly long course of treatment. Moreover, such patients tend rapidly to develop new HCC lesions as time goes on, and, therefore, a targeted treatment of each lesion would not be possible in whatever manner. In selected cases with a large HCC and a limited number of daughter nodules, PEI can be performed after TACE solely at the level of the main tumor, which is usually the most difficult lesion to control by TACE alone, or in lesions with unsatisfactory response after TACE (Fig. 22.2).

Of interest, no major treatment-related complication was observed following combined TACE and PEI in all published series (Lencioni et al. 1998d; Bartolozzi et al. 1995; Koda et al. 1994; Allgaier et al. 1998; Tanaka et al. 1998; Tateishi et al. 1994). As in most cases a single TACE session was performed; no significant worsening in liver function was observed during the follow-up (Bartolozzi et al. 1995). PEI was not associated with any major adverse effect, despite the larger amounts of alcohol injected with respect to those commonly used for treatment of small lesions. In a few patients, the chemical thrombosis of segmental branches of the portal vein adjacent to the lesion treated by PEI was observed (Lencioni et al. 1998d). This complication, which is not uncommon even after conventional PEI, had only a minor clinical impact, as thrombi disappeared spontaneously within a few months.

We recently reported the long-term outcome of patients treated with combined TACE and PEI (Lencioni et al. 1998d). We obtained 3- and 5-year survival rates of 69% and 47%, respectively, in a population of cirrhotic patients with compensated chronic liver disease and a large (3–9 cm) HCC tumor, occurring singly or in association with no more than two daughter nodules. Not surprisingly, the degree of liver dysfunction (according to the classification of Child-Pugh) significantly affected survival of treated patients. Impressive long-term survival rates, indeed, were obtained in patients with Child-Pugh class A cirrhosis, who had a survival of 75% at 3 years and of 59% at 5 years (Lencioni et al. 1998d).

The survival figures obtained in patients treated with combined TACE and PEI are far higher than those reported for matched patients treated by either TACE or PEI alone. The results of this combination therapy, in fact, have been compared with those obtained with the standard TACE protocol commonly used for treating large HCC in two prospective, randomized studies (Bartolozzi et al. 1995; Tanaka et al. 1992). In both series, therapeutic response and disease-free survival rates were shown to be significantly better in patients treated with combined TACE and PEI than in those submitted to repeated TACE alone. In our trial, in particular, after combined TACE and PEI the median disease-free period was more than doubled and the rates of survival without recurrence were significantly enhanced: while more than 50% of patients treated with TACE and PEI were alive and free of disease after 3 years, tumor recurrence occurred in more than 50% of patients submitted to repeated TACE alone within the 1st year (Bartolozzi et al. 1995). No randomized trial aimed at comparing the combination of TACE and PEI versus PEI alone has been published. However, in retrospective series, treatment was with PEI alone of patients with large HCC resulted in survival rates of only 53% at 3-year and 30% at 5-year (Livraghi et al. 1995).

On the strength of the data now available, combined TACE and PEI should be considered the nonsurgical treatment of choice for cirrhotic patients with large HCC. Long-term survival of patients treated with combined TACE and PEI seems to be comparable, or even better, than that reported in published series of matched patients submitted to surgical resection. Comparisons based on historical data, however, may be biased by several factors. Hence, further prospective, possibly randomized trials investigating the long-term outcomes of patients treated with combined TACE and PEI versus those submitted to surgical resection would be warranted to clarify whether this combination treatment could replace resective surgery even in operable patients.

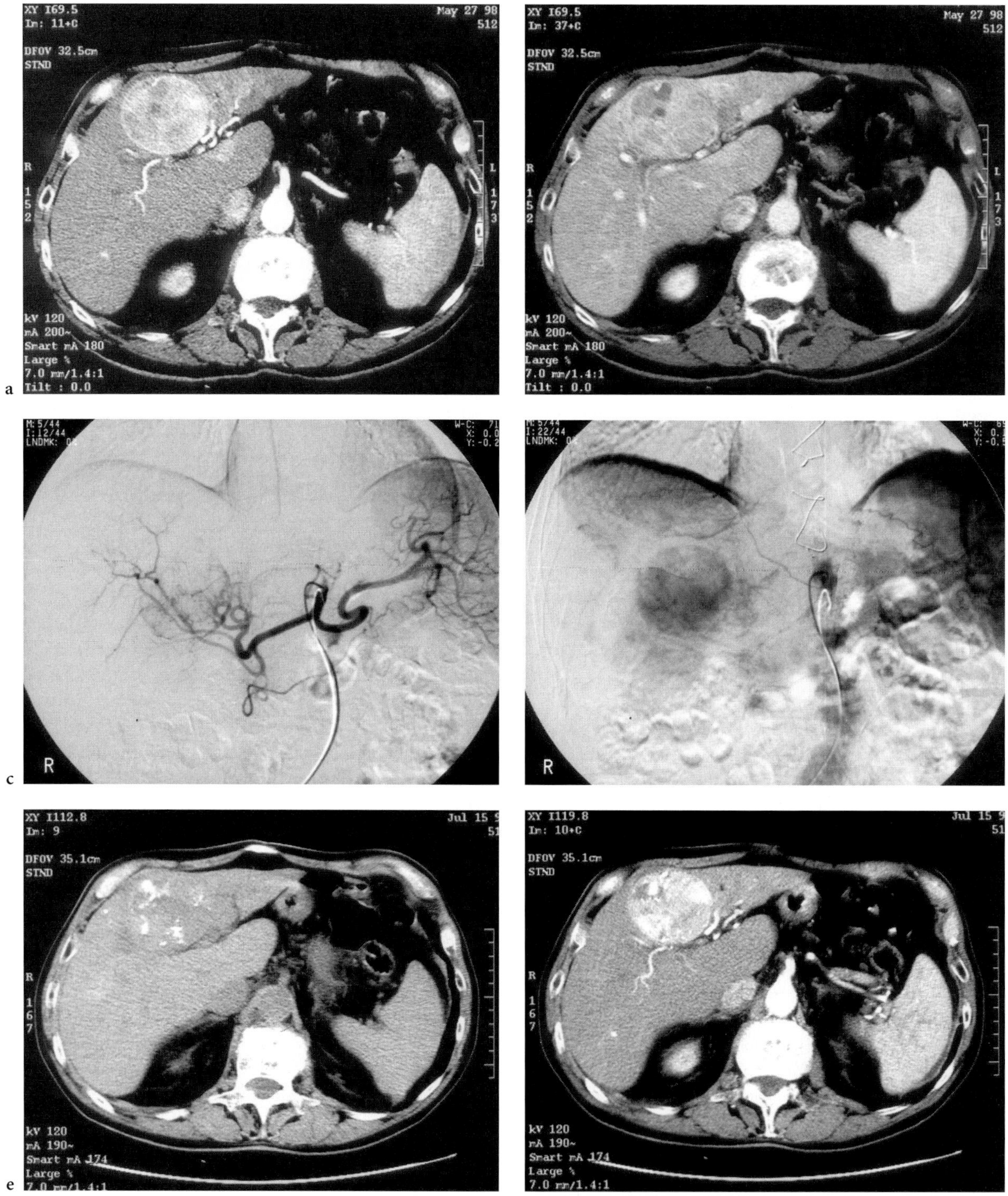

Fig. 22.1a–i. Large hepatocellular carcinoma treated with combined transcatheter arterial chemoembolization and ethanol injection. Before treatment, spiral CT in the arterial (**a**) and portal phase (**b**) shows large, hypervascular tumor. Digital subtraction angiography (arterial phase, **c**; parenchymal phase, **d**) confirms uninodular tumor. CT performed 4 weeks after chemoembolization shows minimal retention of iodized oil (**e**) with persistent enhancement (arterial phase, **f**; portal phase, **g**). After completion of treatment with ethanol injection, the lesion is markedly reduced in size and no longer enhances in both the arterial (**h**) and the portal phase (**i**)

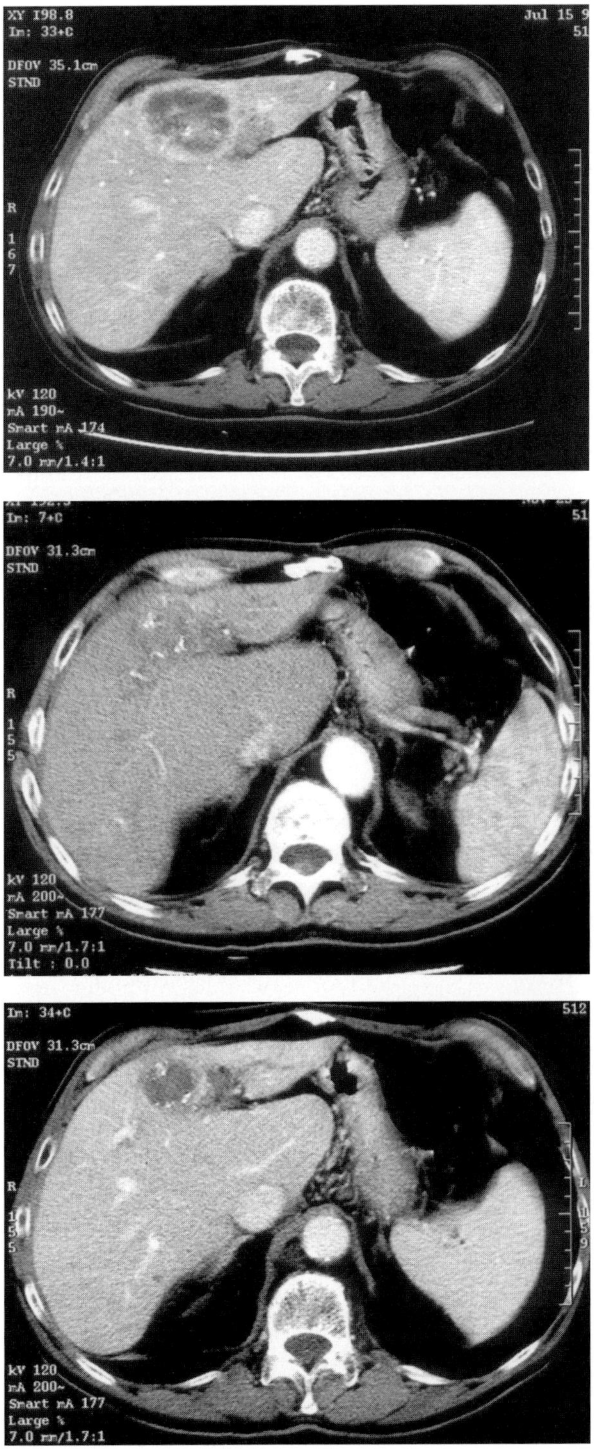

g h i

Fig. 22.1g–i (Continued)

22.4 Combined Transcatheter Hepatic Arterial Balloon Occlusion/Embolization and Radiofrequency Thermal Ablation

The goal of RF interstitial thermal ablation for hepatic tumors is to offer a chance of efficacious and safe treatment for many patients without surgical prospects. Ablation of neoplastic tissue is achieved through creation of thermal lesions around the noninsulated tip of a radiofrequency electrode which is percutaneously inserted into the tumor nodule (Rossi et al. 1993). Thermal lesions are areas of coagulative necrosis surrounded by a band of reactive-regenerative cells with focal vascular neogenesis evolving into fibrosis (Rossi et al. 1990; McGahan et al. 1991). They are caused by the resistive heat which is generated in a core of tissue adhering to the noninsulated needle electrode tip through the ionic "friction" induced by RF energy, and by the diffusion of this heat by conduction to the surrounding tissue (Organ 1976; Cosman et al. 1983).

The final size of the thermal lesions depends upon the total heat deposition in the tissue, the thermal conductivity of the tissue, and the heat loss through convection by tissue blood flow which acts as a heat sink (Organ 1976; Cosman et al. 1983). The heat deposition in the tissue depends in turn on the RF energy delivered (power and exposure time), the active exposed electrode tip, and the temperatures achieved in the tissue (Organ 1976; Cosman et al. 1983).

In early experimental and clinical studies using an RF generator which delivered only 30 W maximum power in monopolar mode combined with a 14G maximum caliber needle electrode, the volume of thermal necrosis created for each activation of the system was about 1.8 cm^3. This meant that in order to achieve ablation of tumor nodules smaller than 3.0 cm in diameter multiple electrode insertions and RF sessions were necessary (Rossi et al. 1993, 1996; Solbiati et al. 1997a). The need to create a large volume of thermal necrosis at each activation of the RF generator, thus avoiding multiple electrode insertions and simplifying the procedure, became evident. To this end, industries focused their attention on the possibility of increasing the energy delivered to the tissue.

A new generation of RF generators capable of greater power output was produced and the extra power available was exploited through two new kinds of electrodes. These were expandable electrodes in which the noninsulated surface was en-

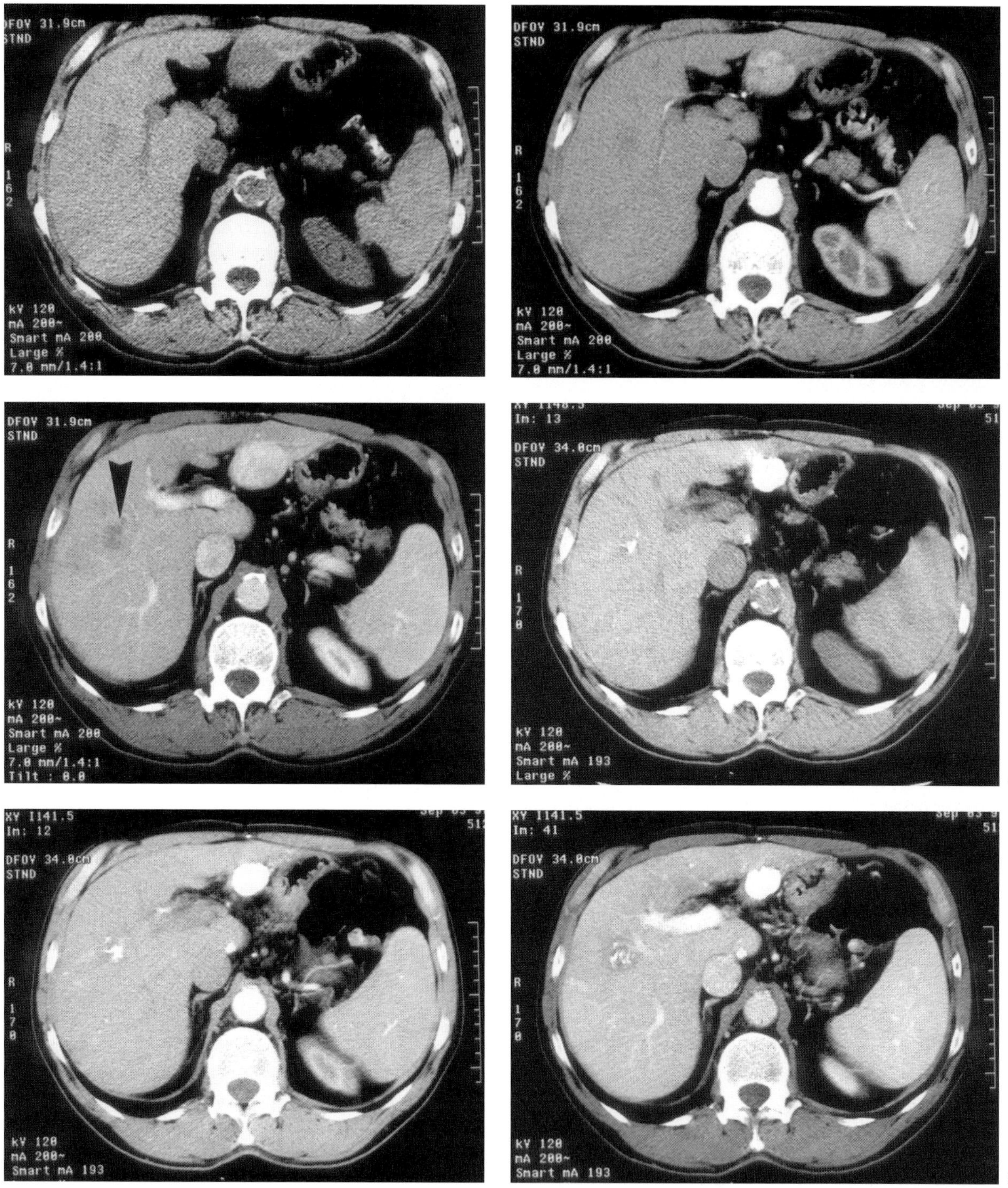

a b c d e f

Fig. 22.2a–i. Hepatocellular carcinoma treated with combined transcatheter arterial chemoembolization and ethanol injection. Before treatment, spiral CT in the precontrast (**a**), arterial (**b**), and portal phase (**c**) demonstrate large, hypervascular tumor in left liver lobe and small, hypovascular lesion in right lobe (*arrow in* **c**). On CT performed 4 weeks after transcatheter arterial chemoembolization, complete and homogeneous retention of iodized oil is depicted within the main tumor, suggesting complete response (baseline scan, **d**; arterial phase, **e**; portal phase, **f**). The small lesion shows incomplete accumulation of Lipiodol, with persistent viable tissue along the periphery. After completion of treatment with ethanol injection at the level of the small lesion, CT demonstrates a hypoattenuating area of coagulation necrosis replacing the lesion, which still contains some Lipiodol droplets inside (baseline scan, **g**; arterial phase, **h**; portal phase, **i**)

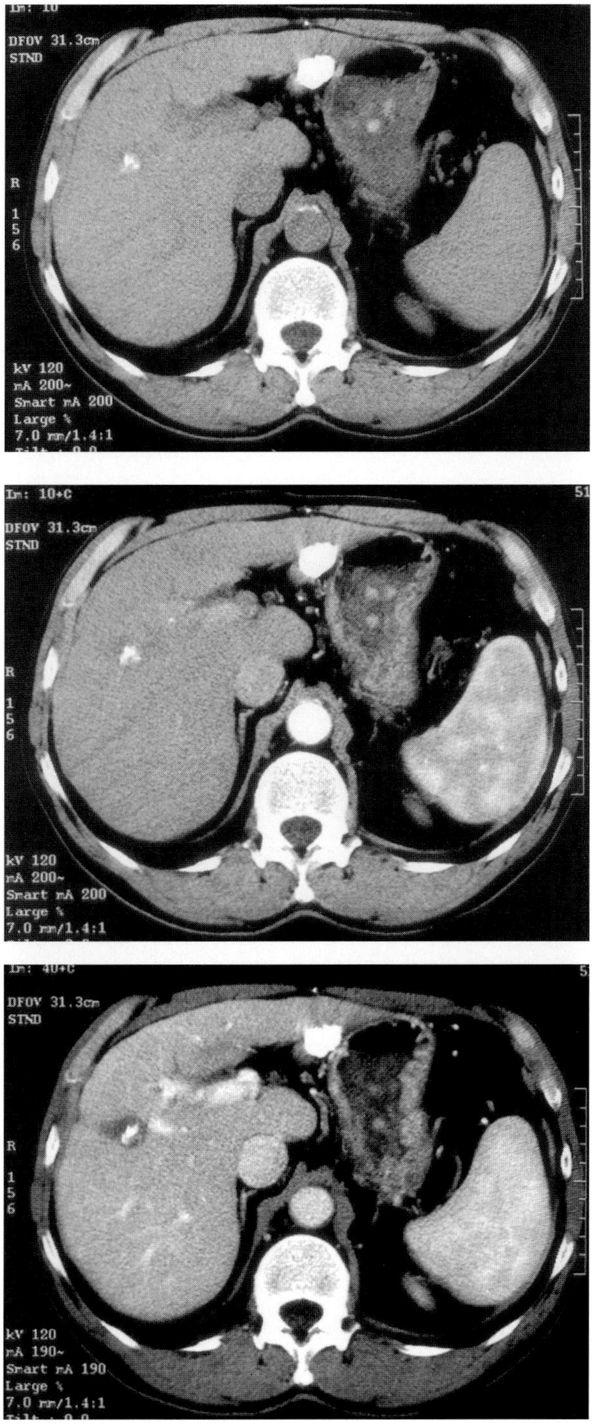

Fig. 22.2g–i (Continued)

larged by hooks that could be deployed from the tip at an angle of 90° to each other with a maximum deployment diameter of 3.0 cm (Rossi et al. 1998; Lencioni et al. 1998a), and cooled-tip electrodes in which the noninsulated tip was cooled with circulating water to allow deposition of a greater amount of energy by reducing the impedance in the adhering tissue (Lorenzen 1996; Solbiati et al. 1997a; Lencioni et al. 1998b). These new electrodes produced an area of necrosis ranging from about 2.8 cm to 3.2 cm in diameter for each activation of the RF generator and permitted successful treatment of tumor nodules less than 2.5 cm in diameter in a single session sometimes with a single electrode insertion (Rossi et al. 1998; Solbiati et al. 1997b). Nevertheless, heat loss by convection due to tissue vascularization still limited the size of the thermal lesions thereby preventing treatment of tumor nodules larger than 2.5 cm with a single needle electrode insertion. Besides, the thermal lesions created was sometimes irregular in shape owing to the presence of large vessels near the electrode resulting in early local recurrences (Fig. 22.3) (Rossi et al. 1998; Solbiati et al. 1997b).

In order to widen the use of RF interstitial thermal ablation for management of hepatic tumors, therefore, it is necessary to create larger thermal lesions, that are predictable in size and regular in shape. For this reason attention has now shifted to the relationship between the size and shape of thermal lesions and hepatic blood flow. Two experimental studies have been published in which a series of thermal lesions was created in pig livers after reduction or elimination of the tissue blood flow by occlusion of either the hepatic nourishing vessels or both the nourishing and draining vessels to eliminate the heat loss by convection (Goldberg et al. 1998b; Rossi et al. 1999). One study evaluated the thermal lesions obtained with an 18G cooled-tip electrode in explanted calf liver and in vivo either in normally perfused pig liver or during balloon catheter occlusion of hepatic vessels. Eight lesions created in normal pig liver and nine lesions after hepatic vessels occlusion were analyzed. Five of these latter were made during portal vein occlusion, two during hepatic artery occlusion and two during celiac artery occlusion. Impedance value in the system and an exposure time of 12 min were used as constant parameters. A significant increase in the diameter of the thermal lesions obtained during reduction of portal blood flow compared with those obtained in normally vascularized liver and during occlusion of the hepatic artery was reported (Goldberg et al.

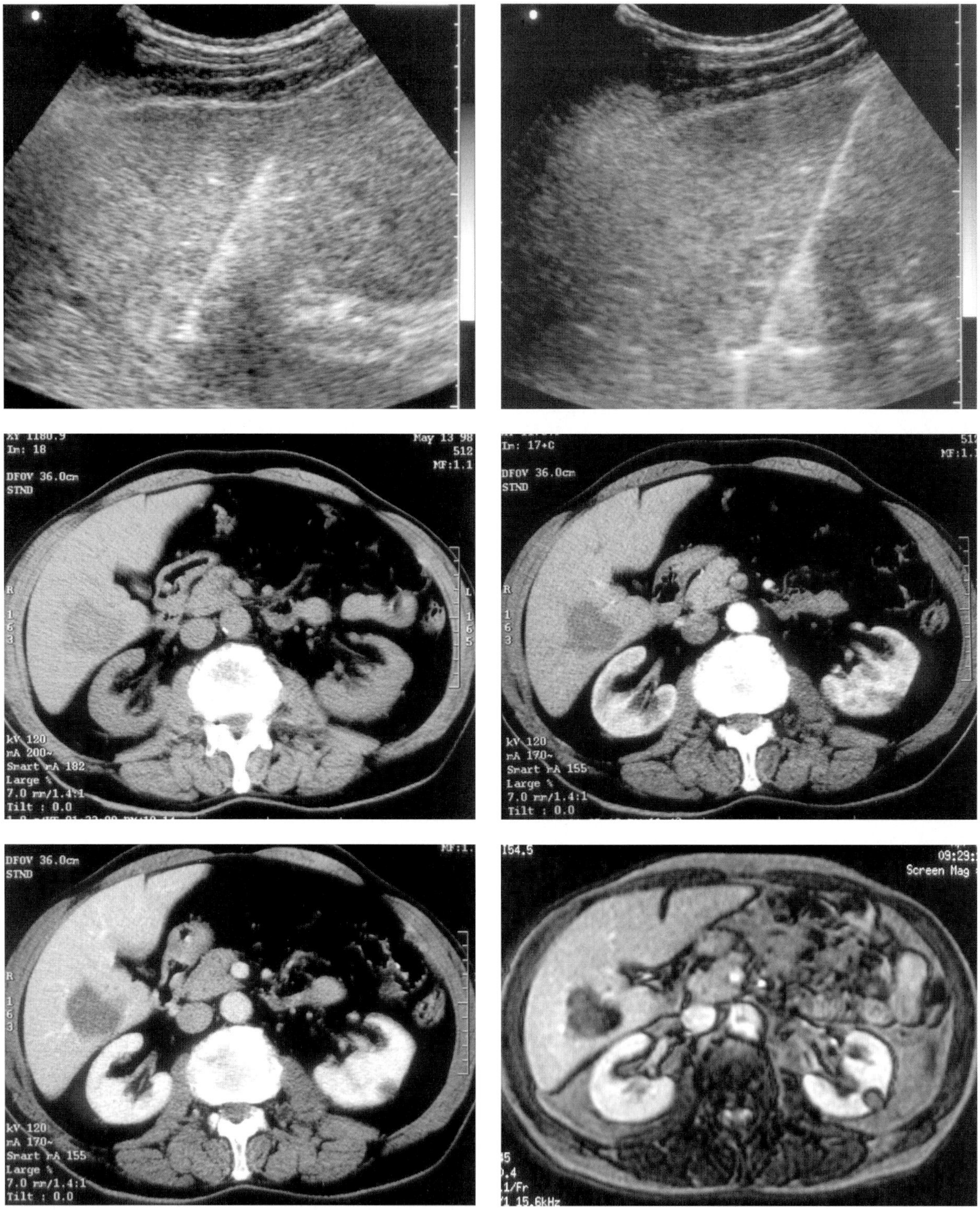

a b c d e f

Fig. 22.3a–f. Hepatocellular carcinoma treated with radiofrequency thermal ablation. US images show insertion of the needle (**a**), and deployment of the hooks within the lesion (**b**). After creation of two thermal lesions with a single needle insertion, a large area of coagulation necrosis is depicted at spiral CT (baseline scan, **c**; arterial phase, **d**; portal phase, **e**) and dynamic contrast-enhanced MR imaging (**f**). However, the shape of the thermal lesion is irregular and a small area of residual viable tumor tissue is detected in the antero-medial aspect of the tumor. The incompleteness of necrosis was caused by the adjacency of the antero-medial portion of the tumor to arterial and portal vessels

1998b). In the second study the thermal lesions were achieved through a 14G expandable electrode and always using the same constant parameters as regards the temperatures and exposure times applied. Series of four lesions were made in explanted calf liver and in vivo in pig liver in conditions of normal hepatic blood flow, during surgical occlusion of the hepatic artery, the portal vein, or both the hepatic artery and the portal vein and during occlusion of the hepatic vein by balloon catheter. This study demonstrated that tissue vascularity contributes significantly both to the final size and to the shape of the thermal lesions. The final diameter increased more or less proportionally as the blood flow decreased. Lesions obtained during occlusion of the hepatic artery had a slightly but not significantly larger diameter than those created in normally vascularized liver, while lesions with a significantly larger diameter were achieved during occlusion of the portal vein. These findings are in agreement with the dual vascularization of the liver: hepatic artery flow contributes less than 20% to the overall hepatic blood flow while portal vein flow supplies the remaining 80% (LAUTT and GREENWAY 1987). Besides, the presence of residual patent large vessels resulted in irregularities of the margins of the thermal lesions in both cases. The thermal lesions obtained with the Pringle maneuver as well as those obtained during subtotal occlusion of the hepatic veins equaled those seen in explanted liver in diameter and were always regular in shape. The low impedance values detected during RF procedures performed after subtotal occlusion of the hepatic vein compared with all the other experimental situations suggested that abrupt occlusion of the hepatic vein leading to sudden tissutal stasis with hyperhydration could result in modifications of tissue conductivity which could contribute to the size of the lesions obtained (ROSSI et al. 1999).

Although tumor vascularization is known to differ profoundly from that of normal hepatic tissue, the findings in these preliminary studies supported the idea that occlusion of the vessels supplying the tumor tissue during the RF procedure, by avoiding heat loss by convection, might result in ablation of a large volume of tissue at each activation of the generator. It would thus be possible to treat large tumor nodules with a single electrode insertion. Mechanical occlusion of the hepatic artery, of the portal vein and of the hepatic vein in clinical practice has already been performed routinely in patients without major complications (YAMADA et al. 1983). The addition of the RF procedure during or soon after vascular occlusion will add difficulties but these are easily surmountable by interventional radiologists.

On this basis, since hepatocellular carcinomas (HCC) are known to be supplied almost completely by vessels arising from the hepatic artery (BREDIS and YOUNG 1954) in preliminary clinical studies, HCC nodules up to 8.5 cm in diameter were treated by RF interstitial thermal ablation during arrest of hepatic artery blood flow (Fig. 22.4) (GARBAGNATI et al 1998; LENCIONI et al 1998a).

Occlusion of the hepatic artery was achieved by Gelfoam embolization or by balloon catheter occlusion and RF treatment was performed under local anesthesia by using a multistep technique (Fig. 22.5).

In these series, apparently complete necrosis was observed at radiological imaging in treated HCC nodules without major complications (GARBAGNATI et al. 1998). In all cases thermal necrosis reproduced the tumor nodule shape because intact portal blood flow outside the tumor nodule acted as a heat sink and prevented diffusion of heat. This was clearly demonstrated in 10 patients in whom remote thermometry was performed by placing one thermistor just inside and one just outside the tumor nodules during the RF procedure. A temperature gradient was detected with killing temperatures inside the tumor nodule and nonkilling outside (S. ROSSI, F. GARBAGNATI, and R. LENCIONI, unpublished data). In addition, since low impedance values were detected during the RF procedures and the thermal lesions were larger than expected, stopping the arterial supply in HCC most likely leads to modification in tissue conductivity.

In fact, it is known that tissue impedance values reflect the degree of tissue hydration and its ability to transfer heat (ORGAN 1976; COSMAN et al. 1983; DJAVAN et al. 1997; RING et al. 1989). These low tissue impedance values might be the cause of such large thermal lesions because tissue displaying a low impedance value tends to produce larger thermal lesion than tissue displaying a high impedance value (ORGAN 1976; COSMAN et al. 1983; DJAVAN et al. 1997; RING et al. 1989). When hepatic artery occlusion is achieved by balloon catheter, the procedure can be completed with subsequent embolization with Lipiodol to destroy daughter nodules outside the main tumor or near its capsule (Fig. 22.6) as shown in preliminary clinical studies (S. ROSSI, F. GARBAGNATI, and R. LENCIONI, unpublished data).

Metastatic nodules supplied by vessels arising from the portal vein will require either portal vein occlusion or the Pringle maneuver during the RF procedure. In a preliminary report, GOLDBERG et al.

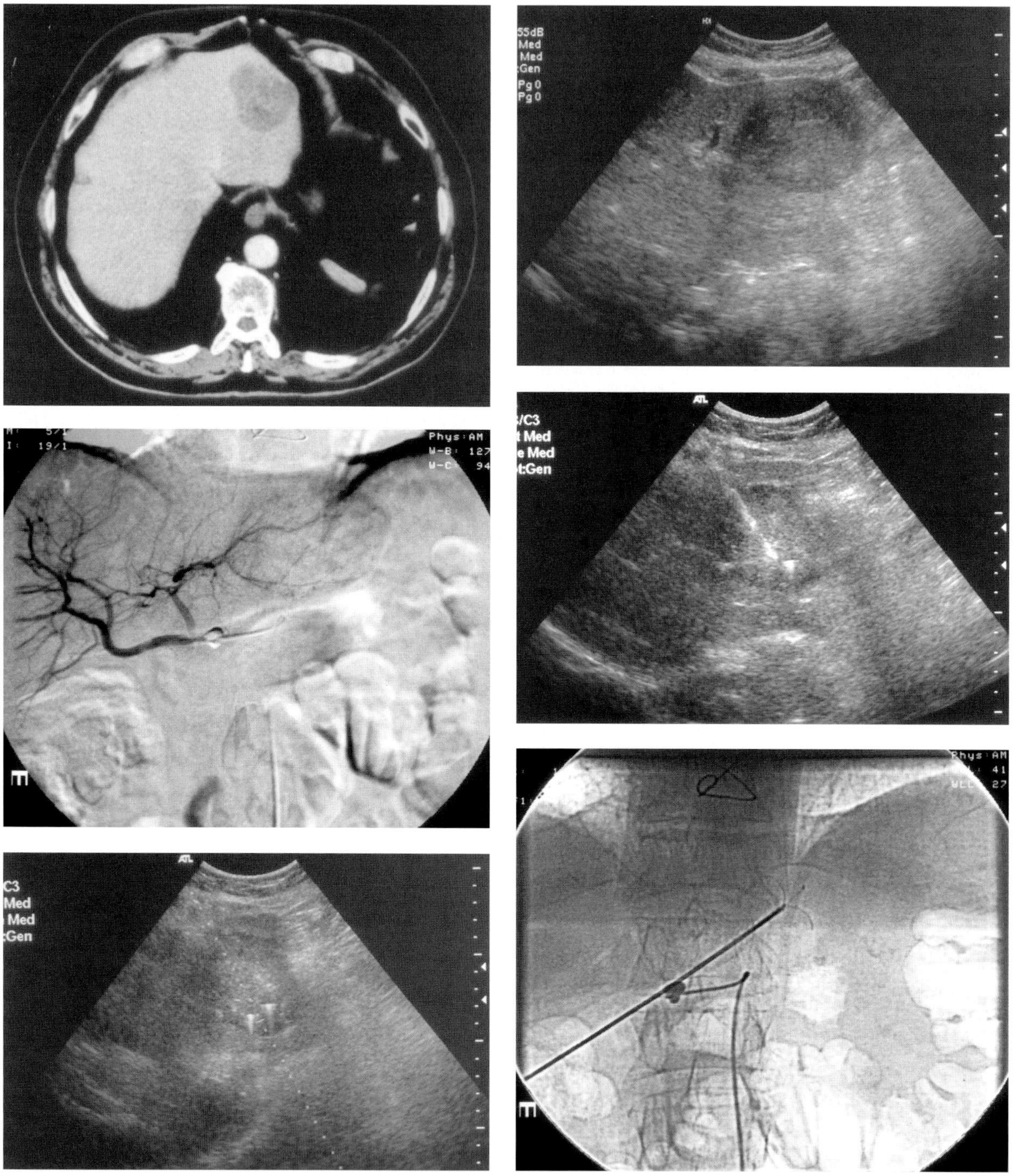

Fig. 22.4a–l. Hepatocellular carcinoma treated with radiofrequency thermal ablation during balloon catheter occlusion of the arterial vessel supplying the tumor-bearing area. Pretreatment CT (**a**), US (**b**), and angiography (**c**) show large, solitary tumor of the left hepatic lobe. The expandable electrode needle is placed within the lesion under US guidance (**d**) and the hooks are deployed (**e**). The balloon catheter is then inflated and the arterial flow to the tumor is stopped (**f**). The creation of the thermal lesions is monitored by US, by analyzing the typical hyperechoic image produced by heat (**g,h**). At the end of the procedure, a hyperechoic rim is detected at the periphery of the mass (**i**), and angiography shows devascularization of the tumor (**j**). An anticancer-in-oil emulsion is then injected to treat any possible satellite lesion located in the portal territory of the tumor (**k**). CT obtained after treatment shows hypoattenuating tumor with massive Lipiodol retention in surrounding hepatic parenchyma (**l**)

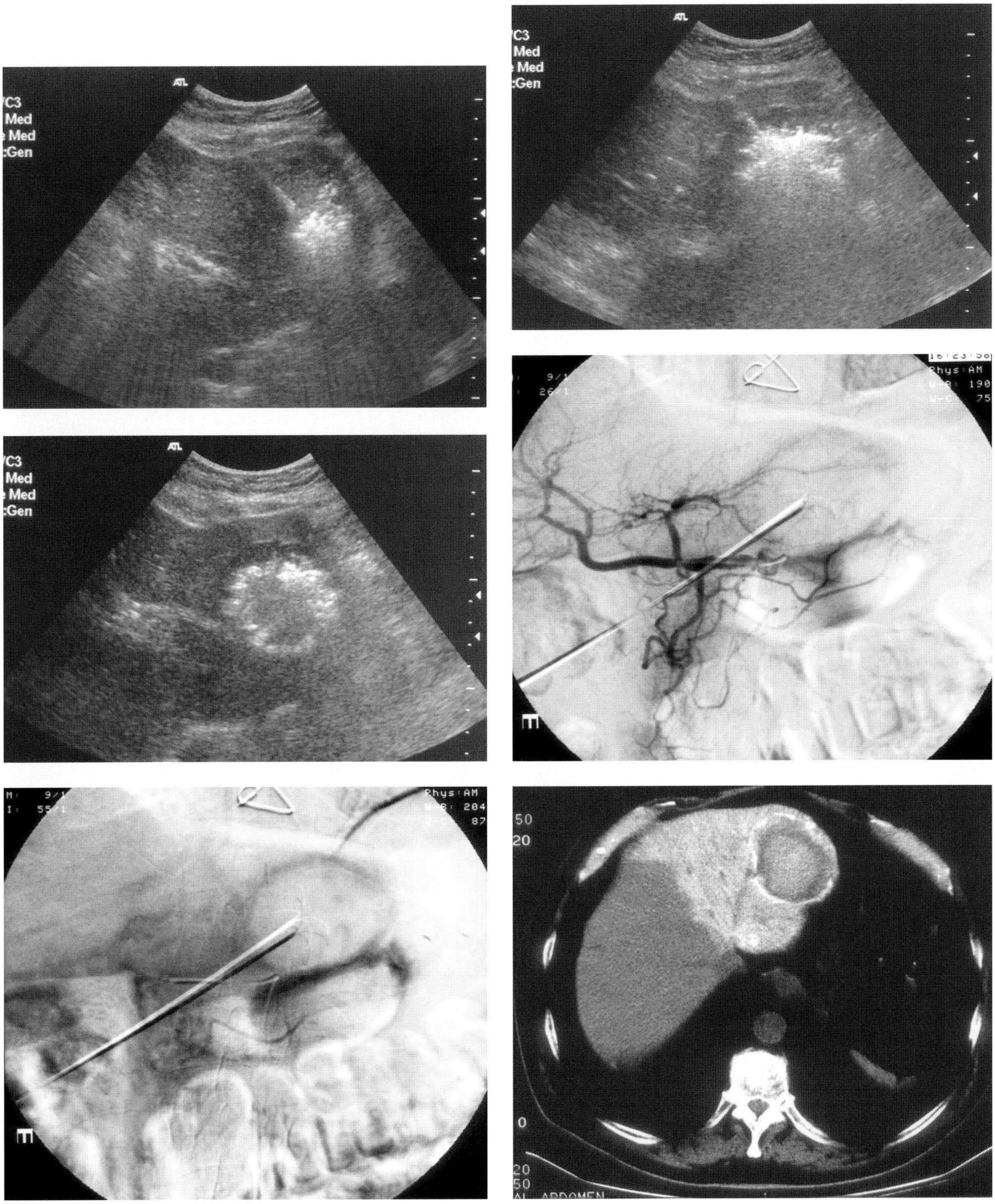

g h i j k l

Fig. 22.4g–i (Continued)

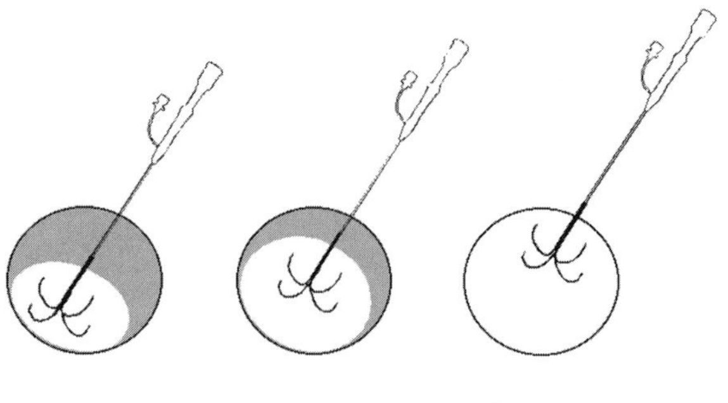

Fig. 22.5. Single-session multi-step RF ablation technique used for the treatment of large HCC lesions. After creation of the first thermal necrosis, the hooks are retracted and the electrode needle is withdrawn 1.5 cm along its major axis. The hooks are then redeployed, and the RF generator is reactivated. Three to five thermal lesions are created, depending on the size of the tumor

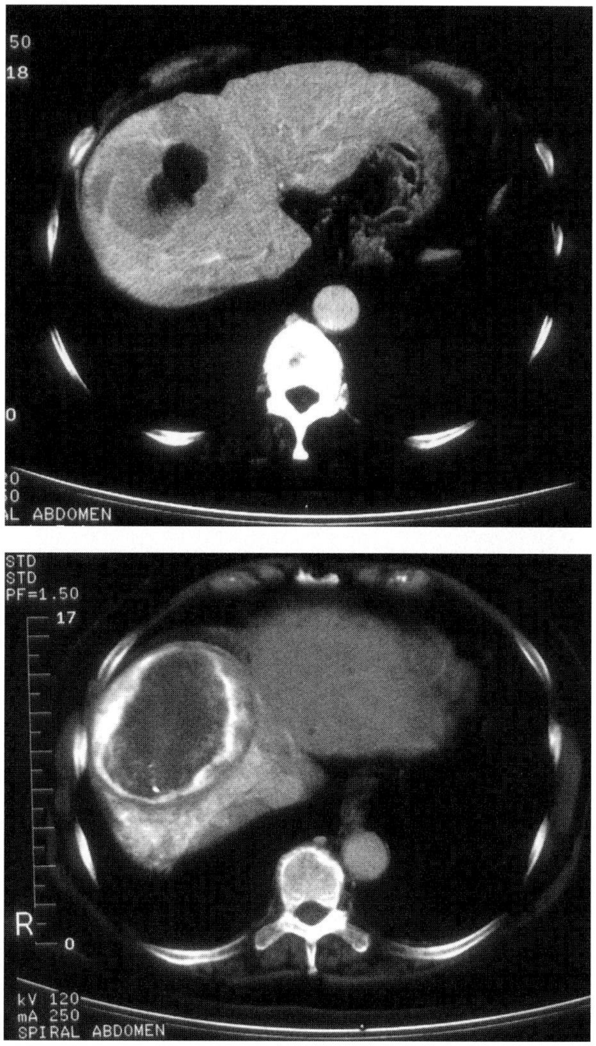

a

b

Fig. 22.6a,b. Hepatocellular carcinoma treated with radiofrequency thermal ablation. After the first treatment session, performed according to the conventional technique, only a limited central area of necrosis is detected at CT (a). After repetition of radiofrequency thermal ablation during balloon catheter occlusion of the arterial vessel supplying the tumor-bearing area, a much larger area of necrosis is observed (b). Note Lipiodol accumulation at the periphery of the tumor

(1998b) obtained a large volume of necrosis in three metastatic nodules treated during occlusion of portal flow compared with other three metastatic nodules treated with unaltered blood flow.

In conclusion, occlusion of the blood flow to avoid heat loss by convection results in the creation of RF-induced thermal lesions larger in diameter than those obtained in normally vascularized tissue using the same needle electrodes and the same exposure time and temperatures or impedance. This technique showed promise in preliminary clinical trials and could reasonably be applied in the treatment of large tumor nodules in patients without surgical prospects to achieve large volumes of thermal necrosis, thus shortening treatment time and reducing costs. Occlusion of the hepatic artery seems to be appropriate for HCC and for metastatic nodules with a similar vascular pattern while either occlusion of the portal vein or the Pringle maneuver is most suitable for metastatic nodules. Occlusion of the hepatic vein could probably be useful for all tumor nodules irrespective of their vascular supply. However, further studies are needed because both tumor vascularity and tumor tissue characteristics such as hydration and impedance differ substantially from those of normal liver tissue and are poorly known. Besides, debulking of tumor mass does not necessarily prolong the patient's survival.

References

Allgaier HP, Deibert P, Olschewski M, et al (1998) Survival benefit of patients with inoperable hepatocellular carcinoma treated by a combination of transarterial chemoembolization and percutaneous ethanol injection a single-center analysis including 132 patients. Int J Cancer 79:601–605

Bartolozzi C, Lencioni R (1996) Ethanol injection for the treatment of hepatic tumours. Eur Radiol 6:682–696

Bartolozzi C, Lencioni R, Caramella D, et al (1995) Treatment of large hepatocellular carcinoma: transcatheter arterial chemoembolization combined with percutaneous ethanol injection versus repeated transcatheter arterial chemoembolization. Radiology 197:812–818

Bredis C, Young G (1954) The blood supply of neoplasms in the liver. Am J Pathol 30:969–85

Buscarini L, Rossi S (1997) Technology for radiofrequency

thermal ablation of liver tumors. Semin Laparoscopic Surg 4:96–101

Colombo M (1997) Treatment of hepatocellular carcinoma. J Viral Hepat 4:S125–S130

Cosman ER, Nashold BS, Badenbaugh P (1983) Stereotactic radiofrequency lesion making. Appl Neurophysiol 46:160–166

Djavan B, Zlotta AR, Susani M, et al (1997) Transperineal radiofrequency interstitial tumor ablation of the prostate: correlation of magnetic resonance imaging with histopatologic examination. Urology 50:986–993

Florio F, Nardella M, Balzano S, Caturelli E, Siena D, Cammisa M (1997) Treatment of hepatocellular carcinoma: a single-center experience. Cardiovasc Intervent Radiol 20:23–28

Garbagnati F, Rossi S, Di Tolla G, Di Stasi M (1998) Percutaneous treatment of large hepatocellular carcinoma by radiofrequency interstitial thermal ablation during hepatic artery stop flow. Min Inv Ther 7:32

Goldberg SN, Gazelle GS, Solbiati L, et al (1998a) Ablation of liver tumors using percutaneous RF therapy. AJR 170: 1023–1028

Goldberg SN, Hahn PF, Tanabe KK, et al (1998b) Percutaneous radiofrequency tissue ablation: does perfusion-mediated tissue cooling limit coagulation necrosis? JVIR 9:101–111

Goldberg SN, Solbiati L, Hahn PF, et al (1998c) Large-volum tissue ablation with radiofrequency by using a clustered, internally cooled electrode technique: loboratory and clinical experience in liver metastases. Radiology 209: 371–379

Groupe d'Etude et de Traitement du Carcinome Hepatocellulaire (1995) A comparison of Lipiodol chemoembolization and conservative treatment for unresectable hepatocellular carcinoma. N Engl J Med 332:1256–1261

Koda M, Okamoto K, Miyoshi Y, et al (1994) Combination therapy with transcatheter arterial embolization and percutaneous ethanol injection for advanced hepatocellular carcinoma. Hepatogastroenterology 41:25–29

Lautt WW, Greenway CV (1987) Conceptual review of the hepatic vascular bed. Hepatology 7:952–963

Lencioni R, Bartolozzi C (1997) Nonsurgical treatment of hepatocellular carcinoma. Cancer J 10:17–23

Lencioni R, Vignali C, Caramella D, et al (1994) Transcatheter arterial embolization followed by percutaneous ethanol injection in the treatment of hepatocellular carcinoma. Cardiovasc Intervent Radiol 17:70–75

Lencioni R, Bartolozzi C, Caramella D, et al (1995) Treatment of small hepatocellular carcinoma with percutaneous ethanol injection: analysis of prognostic factors in 105 Western patients. Cancer 76:1737–1746

Lencioni R, Pinto F, Armillotta N, et al (1997) Long-term results of percutaneous ethanol injection therapy for hepatocellular carcinoma in cirrhosis: a European experience. Eur Radiol 7:514–519

Lencioni R, Armillotta N, Cioni D, et al (1998a) Combined segmental arterial embolization and radiofrequency thermal ablation: a new therapeutic approach for large hepatocellular carcinoma. Radiology 209 (P):565

Lencioni R, Cioni D, Paolicchi A, et al (1998b) Percutaneous treatment of small hepatocellular carcinoma: radio-frequency thermal ablation versus percutaneous ethanol injection: prospective, randamized trial. Radiology 209 (P): 174

Lencioni R, Goletti O, Armillotta N, et al (1998c) Radio-frequency thermal ablation of liver metastases with a cooled-tip electrode needle: results of a pilot clinical trial. Eur Radiol 8:1205–1211

Lencioni R, Paolicchi A, Moretti M, et al (1998d) Combined transcatheter arterial chemoembolization and percutaneous ethanol injection for the treatment of large hepatocellular carcinoma: local therapeutic effect and long-term survival rate. Eur Radiol 8:439–444

Lin DY, Lin SM, Liaw YF (1997) Non-surgical treatment of hepatocellular carcinoma. J Gastroenterol Hepatol 12:S319-S328

Livraghi T, Giorgio A, Marin G, et al (1995) Hepatocellular carcinoma and cirrhosis in 746 patients: long-term results of percutaneous ethanol injection. Radiology 197:101–108.

Livraghi T, Goldberg SN, Meloni F, et al (1998) Percutaneous ablation of small hepatocellular carcinoma (HCC): a prospective comparison between percutaneous ethanol instillation (PEI) and radiofrequency (RF) ablation therapy. Radiology 209 (P): 175

Llovet JM, Bustamante J, Castells A, et al (1999) Natural history of untreated nonsurgical hepatocellular carcinoma: rationale for the design and evaluation of therapeutic trials. Hepatology 29:62–67

Lorenzen T (1996) A cooled needle electrode for radiofrequency tissue ablation: thermodynamic aspects of improved performance compared with conventional needle design. Acad Radiol 3:556–563

Matsui O, Kadoya M, Yoshikawa J, et al (1993) Small hepatocellular carcinoma: treatment with subsegmental transcatheter arterial embolization. Radiology 188:79–83

McGahan JP, Browning PD, Brock JM, Tesluk H (1990) Hepatic ablation using radiofrequency electrocautery. Invest Radiol 25:267–270

Murakami R, Yoshimatsu S, Yamashita Y, Matsukawa T, Takahashi M, Sagara K (1995) Treatment of hepatocellular carcinoma: value of percutaneous microwave coagulation. AJR 164:1159–1164

Organ LW (1976) Electrophysiologic principles of radiofrequency lesion making. Appl Neurophysiol 39:69–76

Ring ME, Huang SKS, Gorman G., Graham AR (1989) Determinants of impedance rise during catheter ablation of bovine myocardium with radiofrequency energy. PACE 12:1502–1513

Rossi S, Fornari F, Paties C, Buscarini L (1990) Thermal lesions induced by 480 kHz localized current field in guinea pig and in pig livers. Tumori 76:54–57

Rossi S, Fornari F, Buscarini L (1993) Percutaneous ultrasound-guided radiofrequency electrocautery for the treatment of small hepatocellular carcinoma. J Intervent Radiol 8: 97–103

Rossi S, Di Stasi M, Buscarini E, et al (1996) Percutaneous RF interstitial thermal ablation in the treatment of liver cancer. AJR 167:759–768

Rossi S, Buscarini E, Garbagnati F, et al (1998) Percutaneous treatment of small hepatic tumors by an expandable RF needle electrode. AJR 170:1015–1022

Rossi S, Garbagnati F, De Francesco I, et al (1999) Relationship between shape and size of radiofrequency induced thermal lesions and hepatic vasculariszation. Tumori 85:128–132

Solbiati L, Goldberg SN, Ierace T, et al (1997a) Hepatic metastases: percutaneous radio-frequency thermal ablation with cooled-tip electrodes. Radiology 205:367–373

Solbiati L, Ierace T, Goldberg SN et al. (1997b) Percutaneous US-guided RF tissue ablation of liver metastases: long term follow-up. Radiology 202:195–203

Tanaka K, Nakamura S, Numata K, et al (1992) Hepatocellular carcinoma: treatment with percutaneous ethanol injection and transcatheter arterial embolization. Radiology 185:457–460.

Tanaka K, Nakamura S, Numata K, et al (1998) The long term efficacy of combined transcatheter arterial embolization and percutaneous ethanol injection in the treatment of patients with large hepatocellular carcinoma and cirrhosis. Cancer 82:78–85

Tateishi H, Kinuta M, Furukawa J, et al (1994) Follow-up study of combination treatment (TAE and PEIT) for unresectable hepatocellular carcinoma. Cancer Chemother Pharmacol 33:19–23

Vogl TJ, Muller PK, Hammerstingl R, et al (1995) Malignant liver tumors treated with MR imaging-guided laser-induced thermotherapy: technique and prospective results. Radiology 196:257–265

Yamada R, Sato M, Kawabata M, Nakasuka H, Nakamura K, Takashima S (1983) Hepatic artery embolization in 120 patients with unresecable hepatoma. Radiology 148:397–401

23 Rationale for Treatment of Metastatic Disease of the Liver

P. F. CONTE, A. FALCONE, and E. PFANNER

CONTENTS

23.1 Introduction

Several primary tumors, such as breast cancer, bronchogenic carcinoma, and malignant melanoma, frequently develop liver metastases; however, the incidence of liver metastases is particularly high in case of tumors arising from the gastrointestinal tract, mainly colorectal cancer. Nearly 20% of patients with colorectal cancer already have liver metastases at the time of diagnosis of primary tumor, while an additional 30 to 40% of patients will develop liver metastases subsequently. Other tumors frequently develop liver metastases in the course of their natural history, such as pancreatic cancer (60%), breast cancer (55%), gastric cancer (50%), melanoma (22%), lung cancer (45%), kidney cancer (30%), and bladder cancer (20%). However, in these cases the presence of liver metastases is synchronous with widespread hematogenous metastases.

Some years ago oncologists were so pessimistic about the outcome of liver metastases that no treatment was recommended; on the contrary, at the present time impressive improvements in diagnostic and therapeutic procedures have been made and a substantial fraction of patients with liver metastases can experience a prolonged survival or even cure.

P.F. CONTE, MD; Chief, Division of Medical Oncology, Department of Oncology, University of Pisa, Via Roma 57, I-56125 Pisa, Italy
A. FALCONE, MD; Division of Medical Oncology, Department of Oncology, University of Pisa, Via Roma 57, I-56125 Pisa, Italy
E. PFANNER, MD; Division of Medical Oncology, Department of Oncology, University of Pisa, Via Roma 57, I-56125 Pisa, Italy

The choice of the most appropriate treatment for a patient with liver metastases requires knowledge of the natural history of the disease and an accurate staging of the primary tumor and metastatic deposits.

For several reasons, systemic chemotherapy represents the modality most frequently used in the treatment of hepatic metastases. In fact although hepatic metastases are often present, the liver is rarely the sole site of metastatic disease. Therefore the application of systemic chemotherapy represents in the vast majority of patients the most convenient, cost-effective, and efficient approach.

This chapter will examine the most frequent tumors which develop liver metastases, focusing on the rationale for interventional procedures in the treatment of liver metastatic lesions.

23.2 Metastases from Colorectal Cancer

Liver metastases are most frequently seen in colorectal cancer. Data reported by the NIH Consensus Conference (1990) show that about 150,000 Americans are diagnosed with colorectal cancer every year, and over 60 000 of these will die from this tumor. The corresponding figures in Italy are 40 new cases every 100 000 people/year with 11 000 deaths/year. Over 20% of patients show hepatic metastases at the time of diagnosis, and about 30–40% will develop metastases after resection of their primary tumor. About half of the patients with colorectal cancer will die secondary to metastatic disease and for many of these patients the involvement of the liver is the major and often the only determinant of survival (NIH Consensus Conference 1990; WOOD et al. 1976; LISE et al. 1990; AUGUST et al. 1985). Colorectal cancer cells spread from primary tumor to the liver through the portal circulation. Liver metastases develop a rich blood supply, and both the hepatic artery and the portal vein can supply blood to these lesions. These lesions tend to grow rapidly and the natural progression of these metastases depends on several factors, including histologic type of primary tumor, extent of hepatic involvement, physiologic status of the liver parenchyma and growth properties of the tumor cells. Again, the overall survival of patients is also affected by the extent of the primary lesion and by the prevention of local recurrences, especially for rectal tumors (Gennari et al. 1986; Hughes et al.1989; Steele et al. 1991; Cady et al. 1970; Goslin et al. 1982).

If untreated, liver metastases from colorectal cancers show a very poor prognosis: median survival ranges from 3 to 20 months (Steele et al. 1991; Cady et al. 1970: Goslin et al. 1982; Scheele et al. 1990; Finan et al. 1985; Wagner et al. 1984; Lahr et al. 1983) although long-term survivors have occasionally been reported. The standard chemotherapeutic agent for advanced colorectal cancer is 5-fluorouracil (5-FU), but tumor response rates are only 10–15% and median survival is only 6 to 12 months. In the past 15 years, biomodulation of 5-FU by leucovorin (LV) or by methotrexate (MTX) has been extensively explored. The meta-analysis with 5-FU + LV was based on 1381 patients and demonstrates that tumor response rate with the addition of LV to 5-FU improves from 13% to 40% (P=0.51) while survival was not affected. The meta-analysis with MTX + 5-FU was based on 1178 patients included in 8 randomized clinical trials and showed that tumor response rate improved from 10% for 5-FU alone to 19% for 5-FU/MTX (P=0.04) (Advanced Colorectal Cancer Meta-Analysis Project 1994). Moreover, survival was significantly prolonged and median overall survival was 9.1 months in the 5-FU group, and 10.7 months in the 5-FU/MTX groups (P=0.024) (Advanced Colorectal Cancer Meta-Analysis Project 1994).

Another approach to improve 5-FU efficacy is the administration of 5-FU as a continuous infusion. Concerning this point, a meta-analysis has been recently published (Meta-Analysis Group in Cancer 1998) based on 1219 patients included in six randomized trials comparing the administration of 5-FU by continuous intravenous infusion (CI) versus the bolus administration in advanced colorectal cancer. Tumor response rate was 22% in patients assigned to 5-FU CI and 14% in patients assigned to 5-FU bolus (95% CI=0.41–0.75) (P=0.0002). The median survival time was 12.1 months in the 5-FU CI group compared with 11.3 months in the 5-FU bolus group (P=0.04). Locoregional infusional chemotherapy in the treatment of colorectal hepatic metastases has also been investigated. Although promising results have been reported in terms of response rate (42–50%) (Kemeny et al. 1987; Rougier et al. 1992), no definitive advantage over systemic treatment in terms of survival has been demonstrated (Meta-Analysis Group in Cancer 1996).

Liver resection is the standard treatment for limited and technically resectable hepatic metastases from colorectal carcinoma: 5-year survival rate is about 37% in patients with completely resected solitary liver metastases (Hughes et al. 1986; Registry of Hepatic Metastases 1988; Nordlinger et al. 1996). Even if randomized trials are lacking, the evidence in favor of surgical resection for solitary metastases is strong: two studies have compared the survival of patients who underwent resection with that of patients with unresected solitary liver metastasis; of interest none of the unresected patients survived more than 3 years (Scheele et al. 1990; Wilson and Adson 1976).The indications for resection of multiple hepatic lesions are more controversial. Many studies have shown that patients who undergo resection of two or three hepatic lesions have a survival similar to that observed after resection of a solitary metastasis (Hughes et al. 1988; Doci et al. 1991; Schlag et al. 1990; Cady et al. 1992). In case of four or more lesions, the role of surgical resection is questionable; however, even in these situations, some studies report good results (Doci et al. 1991; Schlag et al. 1990; Cady et al. 1992; Elias et al. 1991). In particular, in the study from Milan among 100 patients with resected hepatic metastases, eighteen had three or more lesions; the median survival for the patients with solitary lesions was 36 months versus 28 months for patients with four or more lesions, while 5-year survival was identical in both groups (Doci et al. 1991). From these studies the prognostic indicators of long term survival after resection of liver metastases are: number of metastatic lesions (less than four), diameter of the lesions (less than 5 cm), no extrahepatic disease, long disease free interval after resection of primary tumor (more than 2 years) and low carcino-embryonic antigen (CEA) level (<5 mg/ml). The possibility of obtaining long term survivors after resection of liver metastases indicates that metastatic colorectal carcinoma to the liver is not always a disseminated disease; it is therefore rational to offer to patients who cannot undergo surgery for technical or medical reasons, alternative interventional procedures in an attempt to destroy all metastatic lesions. Alternative treatment strategies for patients with unresectable liver metastases include systemic chemotherapy, loco-regional (intraarterial or intraportal) chemotherapy, cryosurgery, radio-frequency tissue ablation, percutaneous ethanol injection, arterial embolization and chemo-embolization and external radiotherapy (KUVSHINOFF 1998; DURAND-ZALESKI et al. 1998).

23.3 Metastases from Other Primary Malignancies

Excluding the above mentioned tumors, other tumors that frequently develop liver metastases are breast cancer, lung cancer, gastric cancer and pancreatic cancer. A common characteristic of these tumors is that at the time of liver metastases appearance there is generally a systemic extrahepatic involvement. Therefore, in these cases, the only therapeutic choice is systemic chemotherapy. Pancreatic and gastric adenocarcinomas represent the two other common gastrointestinal malignancies that frequently metastasize to the liver as well as to multiple other sites. Response rates to systemic chemotherapy for hepatic metastases in these diseases are low (25%) and are associated with a short survival of 3–4 months. However, in a selected subgroup of patients, such as patients with a long progression free survival or patients with solitary liver metastases, in some cases a surgical approach is offered and sometimes long-term survivals have been reported. Therefore also in these patients with tumors which usually develop disseminated metastatic disease but with an "uncommon" natural history it is rational to evaluate the role of interventional procedures alternative to surgery.

References

Advanced Colorectal Cancer Meta-Analysis Project (1994) Meta-analysis of randomized trials testing the biochemical modulation of 5-fluorouracil by methotrexate in metastatic colorectal cancer. J Clin Oncol 12:960–969

August DA, Sugarbaker PH, Ottow RT, Gianola FJ, Schneider PD (1985) Hepatic resection of colorectal metastases. Influence of clinical factors and adjuvant intraperitoneal 5-fluorouracil via Tenckhoff catheter on survival. Ann Surg 201:210–218

Cady B, Monson DO, Swinton NW (1970) Survival of patients after colonic resection for carcinoma with simultaneous liver metastases. Surg Gynecol Obstet 131:697–700

Cady B, Stone MD, Mc Dermott WV Jr, et al (1992) Technical and biological factors in disease-free survival after hepatic resection for colorectal cancer metastases. Arch Surg 127:561–569

Doci R, Gennari L, Bignami P, Montalto F, Morabito A, Bozzetti F (1991) One hundred patients with hepatic metastases from colorectal cancer treated by resection: analysis of prognostic determinants. Br J Surg 78:797–801

Durand-Zaleski I, Earlam S, Fordy C, Davies M, Allen-Mersh TG (1998) Cost-effectiveness of systemic and regional chemotherapy for the treatment of patients with unresectable colorectal liver metastases. Cancer 83:882–888

Elias D, Lasser P, Stambuck J, et al (1991) Nouvel échec dans la tentative de définition des indications d'exerèse des métastases hépatiques d'origine colo-rectales. Gastroenterol Clin Biol 15:3–9

Finan PJ, Marshall RJ, Cooper EH, Giles GR (1985) Factors affecting survival in patients presenting with synchronous hepatic metastases from colorectal cancer: a clinical and computer analysis. Br J Surg 72:373–377

Gennari L, Doci R, Bignami P, Bozzetti F (1986) Surgical treatment of hepatic metastases from colorectal cancer. Ann Surg 203:49–54

Goslin R, Steele G Jr, Zamcheck N, Mayer R, MacIntyre J (1982) Factors influencing survival in patients with hepatic metastases from adenocarcinoma of the colon and rectum. Dis Colon Rectum 25:749–754

Hughes KS, Simon R, Songhorabodi S, et al (1986) Resection of the liver for colorectal carcinoma metastases: a multi-institutional study of patterns of recurrence. Surgery 100:278–284

Hughes KS, Rosenstein RB, Songhorabodi S, et al (1988) Resection of the liver for colorectal carcinoma metastases. A multi-institutional study of long-term survivors. Dis Colon Rectum 31:1–4

Hughes K, Scheele J, Sugarbaker PH (1989) Surgery for colorectal cancer metastatic to the liver. Optimizing the results of treatment. Surg Clin North Am 69:339–359

Kemeny N, Daly J, Reichman B, Geller N, Botet J, Oderman P (1987) Intrahepatic or systemic infusion of fluorodeoxyuridine in patients with liver metastases from colorectal carcinoma. A randomized trial. Ann Intern Med 107:459–465

Kuvshinoff BW (1998) Cost-effectiveness of hepatic artery infusion chemotherapy. Cancer 83:837–838

Lahr CJ, Soong SJ, Cloud G, Smith JW, Urist MM, Balch CM (1983) A multifactorial analysis of prognostic factors in patients with liver metastases from colorectal carcinoma. J Clin Oncol 1:720–726

Lise M, Da Pian PP, Nitti D, Pilati PL, Prevaldi C (1990) Colorectal metastases to the liver: present status of management. Dis Colon Rectum 35:688–694

Meta-Analysis Group in Cancer (1996) Reappraisal of hepatic arterial infusion in the treatment of non-resectable liver metastases from colorectal cancer. J Natl Cancer Inst 88:252–258

Meta-Analysis Group in Cancer (1998) Efficacy of intravenous continuous infusion of fluorouracil compared with bolus administration in advanced colorectal cancer. J Clin Oncol 16:301–308

NIH Consensus Conference (1990) Adjuvant therapy for patients with colon and rectal cancer. JAMA 264:1444–1450

Nordlinger B, Guiguet M, Vaillant JC, et al (1996) Surgical

resection of colorectal carcinoma metastases to the liver. Cancer 77:1254–1262

Registry of Hepatic Metastases (1988) Resection of the liver for colorectal carcinoma metastases: a multi-institutional study of indications for resection. Surgery 103:278–288

Rougier P, Laplanche A, Huguier M, et al (1992) Hepatic arterial infusion of floxuridine in patients with liver metastases from colorectal carcinoma: long-term results of a prospective randomized trial. J Clin Oncol 10:1112–1118

Scheele J, Stangl R, Altendorf-Hofmann A (1990) Hepatic metastases from colorectal carcinoma: impact of surgical resection on the natural history. Br J Surg 77:1241–1246

Schlag P, Hohenberger P, Herfarth C (1990) Resection of liver metastases in colorectal cancer-competitive analysis of treatment results in synchronous versus metachronous metastases. Eur J Surg Oncol 16:360–365

Steele G Jr, Bleday R, Mayer RJ, Lindblad A, Petrelli N, Weaver D (1991) A prospective evaluation of hepatic resection for colorectal carcinoma metastases to the liver: Gastrointestinal Tumor Study Group Protocol, 6584. J Clin Oncol 9:1105–1112

Wagner JS, Adson MA, Van Heerden JA, Adson MH, Ilstrup DM (1984) The natural history of hepatic metastases from colorectal cancer. A comparison with resective treatment. Ann Surg 199:502–507

Wilson SM, Adson MA (1976) Surgical treatment of hepatic metastases from colorectal cancers. Arch Surg 111:330–334

Wood CB, Gillis CR, Blumgart LH (1976) A retrospective study of the natural history of patients with liver metastases from colorectal cancer. Clin Oncol 2:285–288

Young JL Jr, Percy CL, Asire AJ, et al (1981) Cancer incidence and mortality in the United States, 1973–77. Natl Cancer Inst Monogr 57:16–19

24 Radiofrequency Thermal Ablation of Liver Metastases

L. Solbiati, T. Ierace, S.N. Goldberg, M. Dellanoce, L. Cova, and G.S. Gazelle

CONTENTS

24.1 Introduction

Percutaneous image-guided ablative therapies using thermal energy sources have received much recent attention as minimally invasive strategies to treat either benign or malignant diseases. Radiofrequency (RF) induced tissue coagulation has been used in early clinical trials for the treatment of intracranial lesions (Anzai et al. 1995; Cosman et al. 1983), osteoid osteomas (Rosenthal et al. 1995) and hepatocellular carcinomas (HCCs) (Rossi et al. 1993, 1996). Subsequently, the treatment of primary and secondary liver tumors has become the most interesting field of application of radiofrequency, mostly due to the advantages compared to surgical resection, e.g., reduced morbidity and mortality, low cost, and suitability for real-time image guidance. However, for some years the treatment of colorectal metastases using RF ablation alone has been promising, but less efficacious than that observed for HCCs: this has to be related to differences in histopathology and technical limitations.

Histopathologically, most HCCs are surrounded by a fibrous capsule and have a softer consistency than the perilesional densely fibrotic liver. When HCCs undergo treatments with thermal energy sources, like RF, these two characteristics account for optimal heat diffusion within the nodule, while the surrounding liver working as "refractory material" is thoroughly spared (so called "oven effect") (Fig. 24.1).

On the contrary, liver metastases are not capsulated and tend to infiltrate the surrounding, usually non-cirrhotic liver. As a consequence, the amount of energy to be deposited with RF to treat a liver metastasis is much greater than that needed to treat an HCC of the same size, since heating diffuses also throughout the surrounding liver and furthermore a 0.5–1.0 cm thick portion of perilesional liver has to be necrotized, in order to reduce the risk of neoplastic recurrence in a short time (Fig. 24.1) (Goldberg et al. 1997a; Solbiati et al. 1997). In the past, a key limitation of RF ablation was the extent of coagulation produced for a single application of energy (1.6 cm diameter for a single conventional electrode) (Goldberg et al. 1995a; McGahan et al. 1992a,b; Rossi et al.1990), meaning that only tiny metastases (less than 1 cm in size) could be confi-

L. Solbiati, MD; Department of Radiology, General Hospital, Piazzale Solaro 3, Busto Arsizio, I-21052 Varese, Italy
T. Ierace, MD; Department of Radiology, General Hospital, Piazzale Solaro 3, Busto Arsizio I-21052 Varese, Italy
S.N. Goldberg, MD; Department of Radiology, Beth Israel Deaconess Hospital, Harvard Medical School, 330 Brookline Avenue, Boston, MA 02215, USA
M. Dellanoce, MD; Department of Radiology, General Hospital, Piazzale Solaro 3, Busto Arsizio, I-21052 Varese, Italy
L. Cova, MD; Department of Radiology, General Hospital, Piazzale Solaro 3, Busto Arsizio, I-21052 Varese, Italy
G.S. Gazelle, MD; Professor, Department of Radiology, Massachusetts General Hospital, Boston, MA 02214, USA

a b

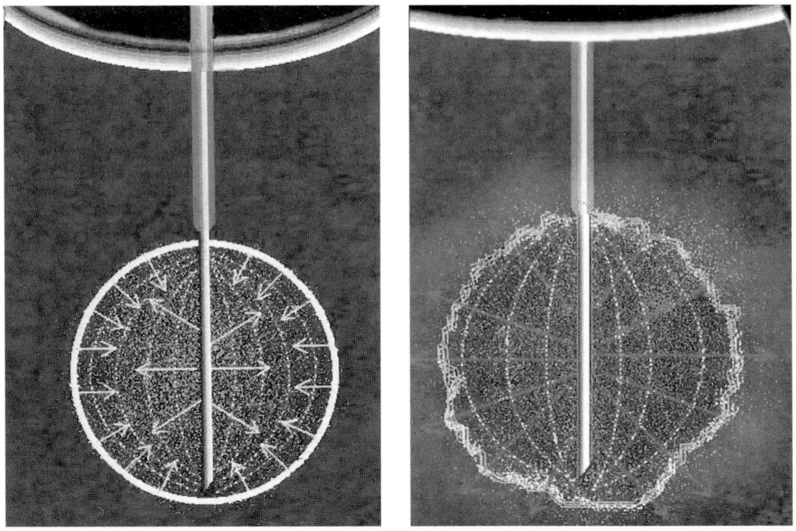

Fig. 24.1a,b. Schematic representation of RF ablation of hepatocellular carcinoma (**a**) and liver metastasis (**b**). In **a** the presence of tumor capsule and the hard consistency of the perilesional cirrhotic account for the mostly intratumoral heating diffusion ("oven effect"). In **b** heating diffuses out from the non-capsulated metastasis, to the normal perilesional liver parenchyma in order to create the peritumoral "safety halo"

dently treated. Because most potentially treatable tumors are larger than this, extended time and labor intensive treatment schedules, with repetitive electrode placements have traditionally been required to treat all but the smallest metastases (Rossi et al. 1996, 1998; Solbiati et al. 1997). This can explain why in the early period of application of RF to liver tumors only one paper specifically dealing with the treatment of liver metastases has been published: Solbiati et al. (1997) have treated 31 tumors in 16 patients with metastatic gastrointestinal carcinomas measuring 1.5–7.5 cm in diameter using conventional monopolar technique with and without multiprobe arrays. In 33% of treated lesions either growth progression or post-treatment recurrence were observed.

Thus, the aim for much subsequent development has been directed at enlarging the zone of necrosis produced from a single application of energy (Fig. 24.2).

24.2 Technique

24.2.1 General Principles of Radiofrequency

RF energy is delivered to the tissue by an electrode (14–20G needle) that is electrically insulated along all but the distal 1–4 cm of the shaft (so called "ex-

a b

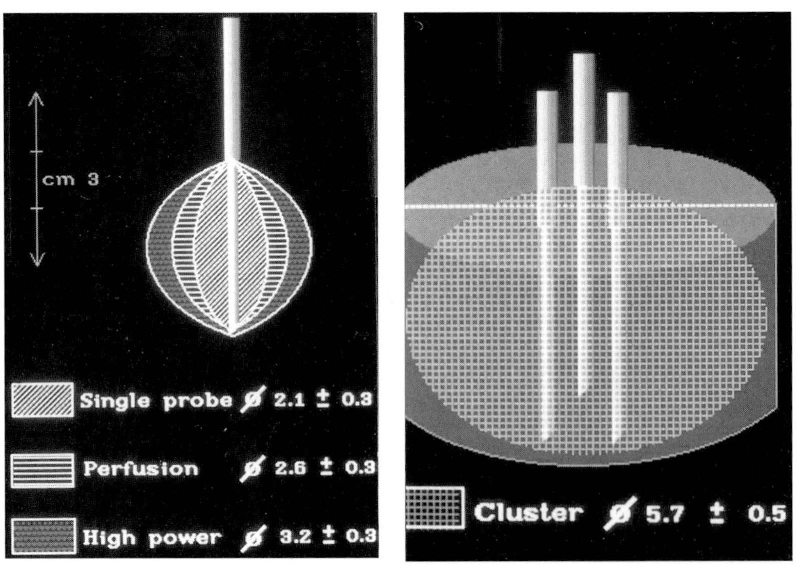

Fig. 24.2a,b. Schematic representation of the progressive increase in size of coagulation necrosis areas achieved with different RF technologies. Mean diameter of necrotic areas is 2.1±0.3 cm with conventional monopolar RF technology, 2.6±0.3 cm with internally cooled electrodes and 3.2±0.3 cm with high RF power combined with cooled electrodes (**a**). With clustered electrodes (**b**) the mean size increases to 5.7±0.5 cm

posed tip" which emits RF current) (Fig. 24.3). The optimal exposed tip length can be selected case by case by the operator according to the size of the lesion to be treated. The electrode is placed directly into the tumor using sonographic, computed tomography (CT) or magnetic resonance (MR) guidance. The electrode is attached to a 500-kHz monopolar RF generator that not only provides the necessary energy to induce coagulation necrosis but also incorporates circuitry that measures the generator output, tissue impedance, and electrode tip temperature. Monitoring of these parameters is necessary to achieve optimal results. As the current attempts to find its path to the grounding pad (placed on the patient's back or thigh), ion agitation is produced within the tissues surrounding the electrode. This agitation is converted by friction into heat, inducing cellular death through coagulative necrosis (Cosman et al. 1984, 1988).

Coagulation diameters larger than 1.6 cm cannot be achieved using conventional electrodes with increased energy deposition because the higher energy results in tissue vaporization and charring near the electrode. This process, in turn, increases local tissue impedance and decreases RF deposition, heat diffusion and coagulation necrosis. Several other approaches have therefore been proposed to overcome these limitations including: the use of multiprobe arrays (Goldberg et al. 1995b), hooked electrodes (Rossi et al. 1998) and bipolar arrays (McGahan et al. 1992b), saline injection during RF application (Livraghi et al. 1997), and the use of internally cooled RF electrodes without and with pulsed or clustered technique (Goldberg et al. 1996a, 1997a,b, 1998; Lorentzen 1996; Solbiati et al. 1997).

24.2.2 Bipolar Electrodes

For bipolar RF ablation, a second, ground electrode is placed in close proximity to (usually within 4 cm) the active electrode. In these systems, heat is generated not only about the active electrode, but also the ground, resulting in larger, elliptiform zones of coagulation necrosis (up to 4.0 cm in long axis) (McGahan et al. 1992a,b). This represents a volume increase compared to conventional monopolar RF; however, because the shape of the induced necrosis does not conform to that of most tumors, the real gain in treatment effect is less significant. Thus even with bipolar RF techniques, multiple treatment sessions are often required to treat large lesions.

24.2.3 Multiprobe Arrays

Goldberg et al. (1995b) have demonstrated that RF can be simultaneously applied to multiple monopolar electrodes in an array. In their study, up to 40

a

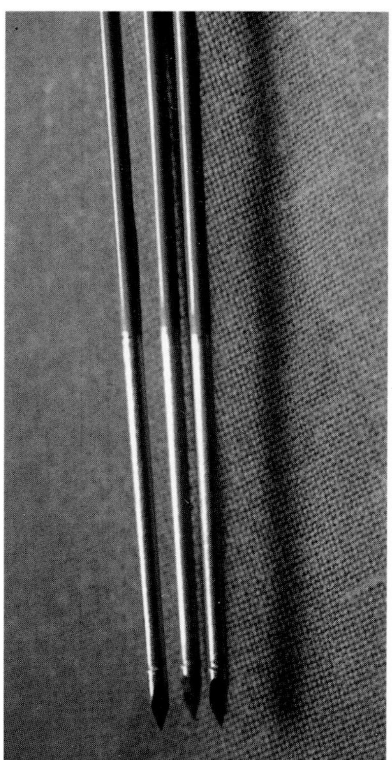

b

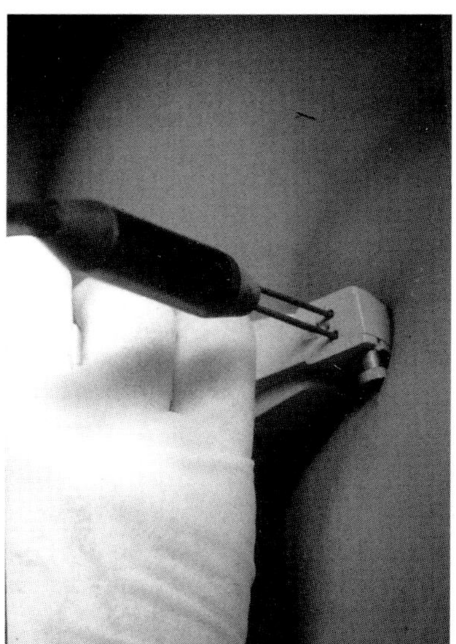

Fig. 24.3a,b. a 2.5 cm long exposed tips of clustered electrode. **b** Clustered electrode inserted into guidance device of US probe during RF ablation procedure

cm^3 (cube of approximately 3.5 cm/side) of ex vivo tissue was coagulated during a single RF application using a four-probe array. Unfortunately, this strategy has been difficult to implement in clinical practice given the technical challenge of precisely positioning multiple needles simultaneously (Solbiati et al. 1997).

24.2.4 Saline Injection during Radiofrequency Ablation

Another strategy used to increase the extent of coagulation using a single electrode insertion is that of injecting normal saline into the tumor through tiny holes at the distal end of the electrode, during RF application (Livraghi et al. 1997). Using this technique, Livraghi et al. (1997) reported coagulation of up to 4.1 cm in diameter. Possible explanations for the increase in coagulation include higher local ion concentration from saline injection, reduced effects of tissue vaporization (i.e., allowing for probe to tissue contact despite the formation of electrically insulating gases), or possibly diffusion of boiling saline into the tissues. Unfortunately, clinical results have been somewhat disappointing with this technique. In their series of 14 patients with tumors up to 4.5 cm in diameter, Livraghi et al. (1997) reported that coagulation volume was unpredictable, that areas of coagulation were irregularly shaped, and, more importantly, that partial necrosis was observed in some lesions smaller than 3 cm.

The most promising techniques, RF application to hooked electrodes or internally cooled electrodes (single or cluster), offer the potential of large-volume coagulation necrosis for clinical tumor ablation therapy. These technologies have become available from commercial vendors (Radionics Inc., Burlington, MA, USA; RITA Inc., Mountain View, CA, USA; and RadioTherapeutics Inc., Mountain View, CA, USA).

24.2.5 Hooked Radiofrequency Systems

The hooked systems allow the deployment of an array of multiple, curved stiff wires in the shape of an umbrella from a single 14- or 16-G cannula (Rossi et al. 1998). Using a 12-hook array in in-vivo porcine liver, Le Veen (1997) has applied RF at 50 W for 5 min with a sequential 8% power increase up to 80 W for a total of 10–12 min to produce spherical regions of coagulation necrosis measuring up to 3.5 cm in diameter. Similar results were found by Siperstein et al. (1997), who applied 30–50 W for 15 min to a four pronged electrode. Reduction of blood flow by clamping of the porta hepatis, or repositioning of the electrodes (turning the electrode catheter 45° for a second insertion), were necessary to achieve reproducible 3.5–4.0 cm of coagulation in in-vivo porcine liver. These investigators further treated 13 neuroendocrine tumors in 6 patients. Preliminary results suggest complete ablation of these tumors.

24.2.6 Internally Cooled Electrodes

Two hollow lumens within an electrode enable internal cooling of the tip with chilled perfusate. As a result, heating of tissues nearest to the electrode is reduced. This allows for greater current deposition without tissue charring or impedance rises. Resultant coagulation necrosis is significantly greater than that achieved without electrode cooling (Fig. 24.2). Experimentally, Goldberg et al. (1996a) found that coagulation volume increased progressively as treatment duration increased to 40 min, but did not increase with longer treatments. Maximum diameter of coagulation measured 2.5±0.2 cm, 3.0±0.1 cm, 4.5±0.2 cm, and 4.4±0.3 cm for the 1 cm, 2 cm, 3 cm, and 4 cm electrode tips, respectively. Reducing either the RF current or treatment duration resulted in smaller volumes of coagulation necrosis for any given tip temperature.

Pathologic analyses demonstrated zones of continuous coagulation necrosis measuring up to 3.6 cm in diameter when RF deposition was greater than 850 mA. Similar results have been reported by Lorentzen (1996), who applied RF to ex vivo calf liver using a 14-G internally cooled electrode and 20°C perfusate.

24.2.7 Pulsed Radiofrequency

If high peak RF currents are applied to internally cooled electrodes in a pulsed fashion, greater local current density can be deposited into tissues in a shorter time, while preventing tissue boiling near the electrode by allowing for heat dissipation in this region (Goldberg et al. 1997a). It is currently unknown what duration of either peak energy or reduced energy deposition, or length of the duty cycle chosen, is optimal for inducing the greatest volume of coagulation necrosis.

24.2.8 Cluster Radiofrequency

Experimentally in ex vivo livers, simultaneous RF application to arrays of three internally cooled electrodes spaced equidistantly at 0.5 (Fig. 24.3) or 1 cm apart was demonstrated to be able to produce uniform circular cross-sectional areas of coagulation necrosis measuring 4.1±0.2 cm in diameter, without internal areas of non-necrosis which can be caused by a larger spacing of the electrodes (Goldberg et al. 1998). In ex vivo livers, simultaneous RF application to internally cooled electrode clusters for 15, 30 and 45 min produces 4.7±0.1 cm, 6.2±0.1 cm, and 7.0±0.2 cm of coagulation, respectively, with an approximately 80% increase in diameter compared to the results of single internally cooled electrodes.

When cluster electrodes are employed, multiple (2–4) standard grounding pads are needed on the patient's thigh with a total surface area of at least 400 cm^2.

24.3 Treatment Protocol

24.3.1 Patient Selection

Preliminary evaluation of patients includes: liver sonography (since most treatments are performed under ultrasound real-time guidance), contrast-enhanced helical CT of the upper abdomen and blood tests (liver function tests and coagulation tests). If obstructive jaundice is present, the treatment cannot be performed due to the risk of bilomas or biliary fistulae. From the oncologic side, only patients with a maximum of 4–5 liver metastases (and no other neoplastic deposits elsewhere depicted by imaging modalities) can be reasonably treated, each of them not exceeding 4–4.5 cm in size. Since, in fact, a peripheral margin of at least 0.5–1.0 cm of apparently healthy hepatic tissue should be ideally treated with the goal of minimizing the risk of local recurrence, currently available technology cannot guarantee adequate treatment of lesions larger than 4.0–4.5 cm. If adequate "safety" margins are not obtained, peripheral tumor growth may occur and have unfavorable geometry for retreatment. Histologically, the metastases most suitable for RF treatment are those originating from tumors with marked liver tropism (mostly colorectal) and hypovascular, compared to the surrounding liver parenchyma (e.g., metastases from colorectal, pancreatic, gastric, renal and breast cancers). Flowing blood, of both the neoplasm and perilesional large vessels functions as a heat sink, severely affected the efficacy of treatment (Solbiati et al. 1997). For safety reasons, only lesions at least 1 cm distant from gallbladder and liver hilum can be treated, due to the possibility of inducing thermal cholecystitis or stenosis of the main bile ducts with obstructive jaundice.

24.3.2 Procedure

According to the amount of energy which has to be given (related to the size of the tumor) and the anatomical location of the target, either local or general anesthesia is administered. Lesions smaller than 2 cm, usually not requiring more than 1000 mA of energy, and located at least 2–3 distant from the liver Glisson's capsule can be treated with local anesthesia. In all the other occurrences, general anesthesia is mandatory. For local anesthesia under conscious sedation, usually fentanyl and droperidol (or benzodiazepam) are administered, following application on the skin of anesthetic cream (Livraghi et al. 1997; Solbiati et al. 1997; Goldberg et al. 1998). For general anesthesia, with or without intubation, propofol is mostly administered as the main drug.

If the target is adequately visible with sonography (US), real time US is the guidance method of choice, using probes with biopsy devices for electrode insertion (Fig. 24.4). When sonographic visualization is poor, either helical CT or open MR is the mandatory guidance method.

The choice of RF technology (electrodes) is mostly based on the size of each target: for lesions smaller than 2.0–2.5 cm, single insertion of hooked electrode or of 3 cm exposed tip, internally cooled needle is mostly performed. Lesions 2.5–3.5 cm in size can be treated with multiple (usually 2) insertions of hooked electrodes or 3.0–4.0 cm exposed-tip internally cooled electrodes or single insertion of clustered electrode. Currently lesions exceeding 4.0 cm in maximum diameter can only be treated with 1–2 insertions of clustered electrode (Goldberg et al. 1998) (Fig. 24.5) or a combination of clustered and single electrode insertions.

With any technology, each insertion lasts 10–15 min, since after this time the impedance rise induced by coagulation necrosis progressively blocks the heat diffusion in the tumor. Depending on the technology and generator used, RF power is either titrated to achieve a specified current or electrode tip temperature. For hooked electrodes, up to 100 W of RF energy is applied for up to 15 min with energy titrated to 90°C tip temperatures.

When cooled-tip electrodes are used, a peristaltic pump infuses 2–3°C distilled water into the cooling lumen at a rate sufficient to maintain a tip temperature of 10–20°C (Goldberg et al. 1996a; Lorentzen 1996). The applied energy is variable, depending on overall tip exposure, but usually does not exceed 1500 mA or 1800 mA for single electrodes of 2 cm or 3 cm tip, respectively, or 2000 mA for a cluster of three electrodes of 2.5 cm tip exposure. Following the procedure, patients are admitted to a clinical or surgical department for a 24–48 h observation period.

Follow-up is by history, clinical examination and diagnostic imaging. Follow-up contrast enhanced CT or MR scans are performed within one week of the procedure. Further CTs will be obtained at 3, 6, 12, 18 and 24 month follow-up visits, and as is deemed clinically necessary. Residual tumor observed at the initial or 1 month CT scan is retreated if at all possible. If tumor progression is noted at 3 month follow-up, additional treatment sessions with radiofrequency tissue ablation are suggested if technically feasible and performed with the consent of the patient and a consensus decision between interventional radiologist and oncologist. No more than three sessions of tumor ablation are performed for any given lesion. The decision to administer simultaneous chemotherapy, other anti-neoplastic regimens, or administer only palliative care are determined by the oncologists, in agreement with the patient.

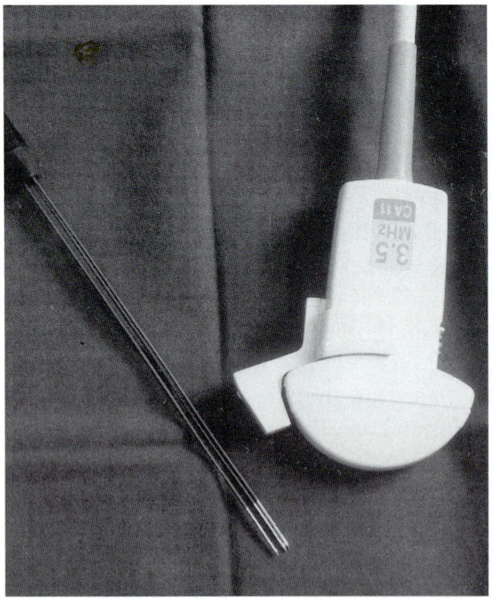

Fig. 24.4. Complete "kit" for RF ablation procedure: electrode (clustered) and US 3.5 MHz convex probe with guidance device

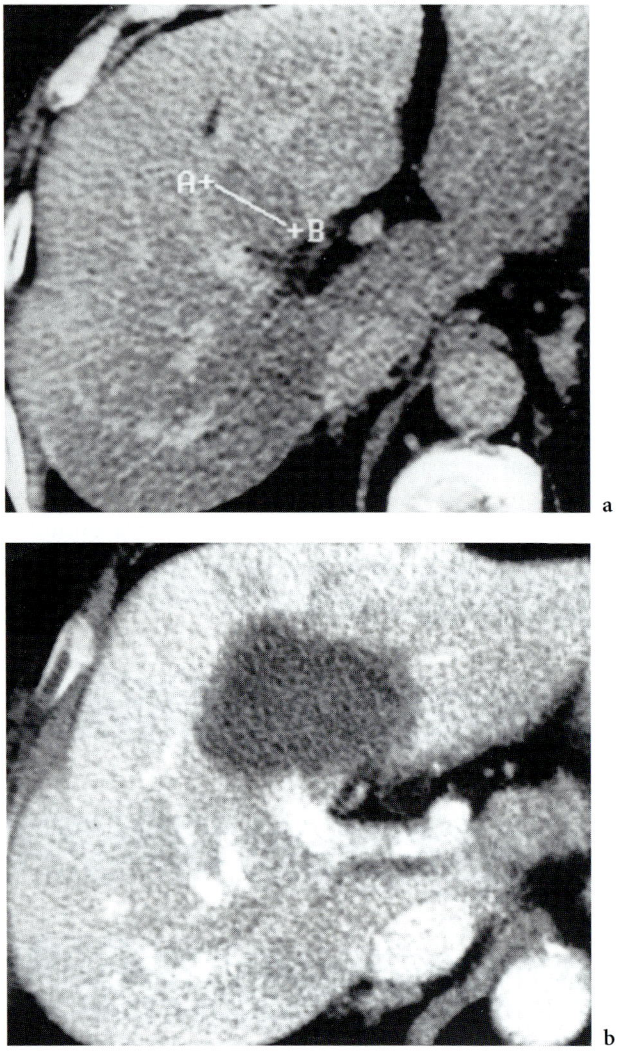

a

b

Fig. 24.5a,b. Complete response of RF ablation procedure. **a** Large (3.8 cm) metastasis from colorectal cancer in segment 4 (markers). **b** At 3-month follow-up, large (5.6 cm in diameter) unenhancing area of coagulative necrosis, involving both the tumor and a peripheral portion of normal liver ("safety halo")

24.4 Histologic Changes Induced by Radiofrequency

Histologic demonstration of tissue changes induced by RF has been achieved in surgical specimens obtained at variable time intervals from RF application (Solbiati et al. 1997). Formalin-fixed, paraffin-embedded tissue from surgical specimens can be stained with conventional hematoxylin-eosin or with peculiar stains for the assessment of cellular death: immunostaining with monoclonal anti-carcinoembryonic antigen antibodies, methods for the demonstration of the activity of cytochrome-c oxidase and succinic dehydrogenase (Hunt 1966) and terminal deoxynucleotidil dUTB-biotin nick end labeling (TUNEL) for staining DNA strand breaks and detecting apoptotic cell nuclei.

Histopathologic findings show that the main change induced by RF application is coagulative necrosis, characterized by homogeneous eosinophilia with preservation of tumor cell outlines. Necrotic areas are separated from peripheral normal liver or residual viable tumor by a 2–3 mm thick halo of granulation tissue with hemorrhagic changes, corresponding to the enhancing peripheral rim at CT and MR imaging (Fig. 24.6).

The size of coagulative necrosis in histopathologic specimens corresponds precisely to the size of unenhancing areas seen at CT and MR imaging. Following the introduction of hooked electrodes and internally cooled electrodes, central areas of char induced by treatments with the single-probe technique are no longer found. Inside the necrotic areas, usually at the periphery, small foci of apparently viable tumor tissue with fully preserved architecture are found. The cells of these foci display cytoplasmic shrinkage and densification, as well as a variable degree of chromatin condensation with focal formation of apoptotic-like bodies. Even when thoroughly morphologically preserved, however, the cells of these foci (areas of "apoptosis" induced by heating) show no enzymatic activity and a completely positive response to TUNEL staining (suggesting extensive fragmentation of DNA chains).

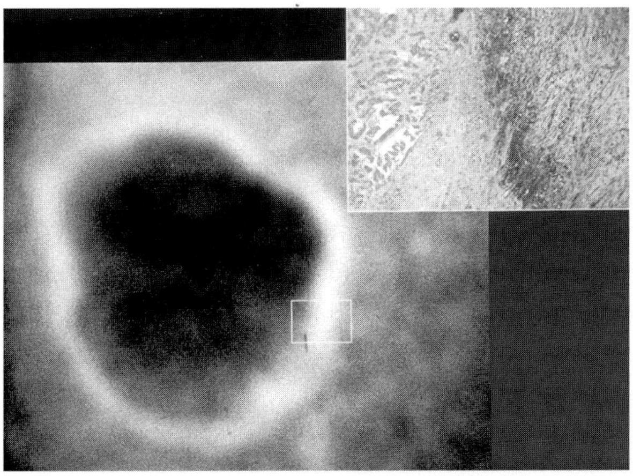

Fig. 24.6. T1-weighted, gadolinium enhanced MRI scan showing a hypointense area of post-RF ablation (3 months before) coagulation necrosis, surrounded by a hyperintense rim representing granulation tissue, as confirmed in the histologic specimen (*top right corner*) including coagulative necrosis (*left*), granulation tissue (*middle*) and unablated perilesional tumor (*right*)

24.5 Follow-up Imaging

24.5.1 Ultrasound

US is now the best imaging method to guide the positioning of the RF electrodes, but B-mode US findings are not helpful in predicting the extent of coagulation necrosis (Livraghi et al. 1997; Rossi et al. 1996; Solbiati et al. 1997). A hyperechoic focus of variable size and shape enlarging during the procedure is seen surrounding the distal portion of the electrode (Fig. 24.7). The size of this bright area overestimates by approximately 10–20% the real size of induced coagulative necrosis, but can be used as an indicator of the amount of necrosis achieved.

If the size of the hyperechoic focus seems apparently smaller than expected, after few minutes, during the same treatment session, US blood pool contrast agents such as Levovist (microbubbles) can be intravenously administered and color Doppler, power Doppler or B-mode contrast harmonic imaging studies can be performed in order to differentiate untreated tumor from avascular coagulation necrosis (Goldberg et al. 1997b; Solbiati et al. 1996, 1999). The detection of residual intratumoral vascularity or of perilesional displacement of liver blood vessels allow the confident assessment of either the completeness of the treatment or the need for further RF application (Fig. 24.8).

The hyperechoic area can, however, obscure the electrode and tumor, and make it relatively difficult to reposition the electrode for further treatment. Follow-up imaging 15–60 min after the procedure often demonstrates complete resolution of this

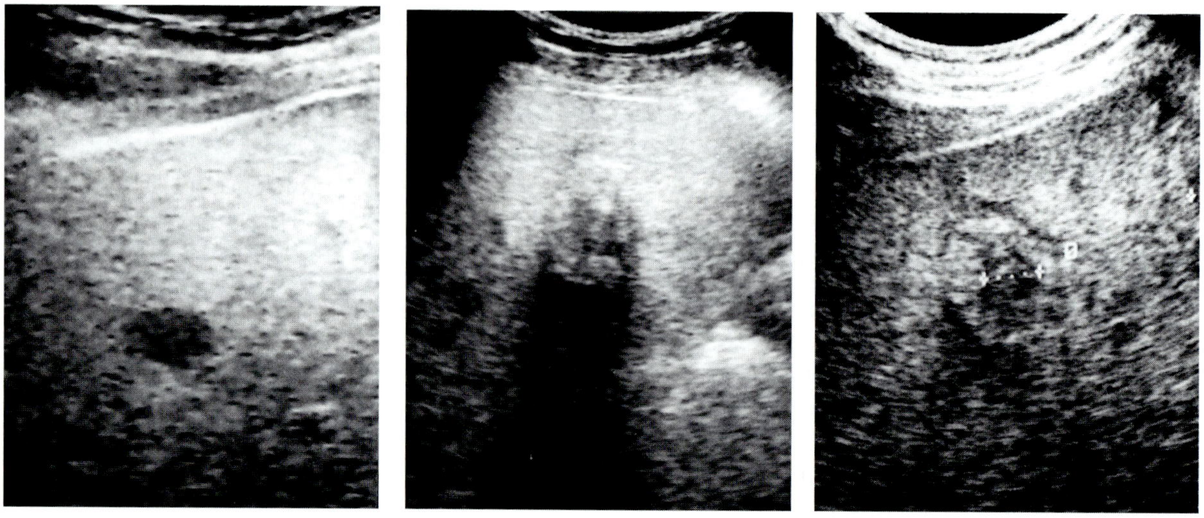

a,b c

Fig. 24.7a–c. a 1.4 cm hypoechoic colorectal metastasis before RF ablation. **b** Immediately at the end of the procedure the lesion is no longer visible and replaced by a wide (2.5 cm) hyperechoic area casting a posterior acoustic shadow. **c** At 7-day US follow-up the area of coagulative necrosis is hardly detectable, being nearly isoechoic and surrounded by an incomplete and thin hypoechoic halo

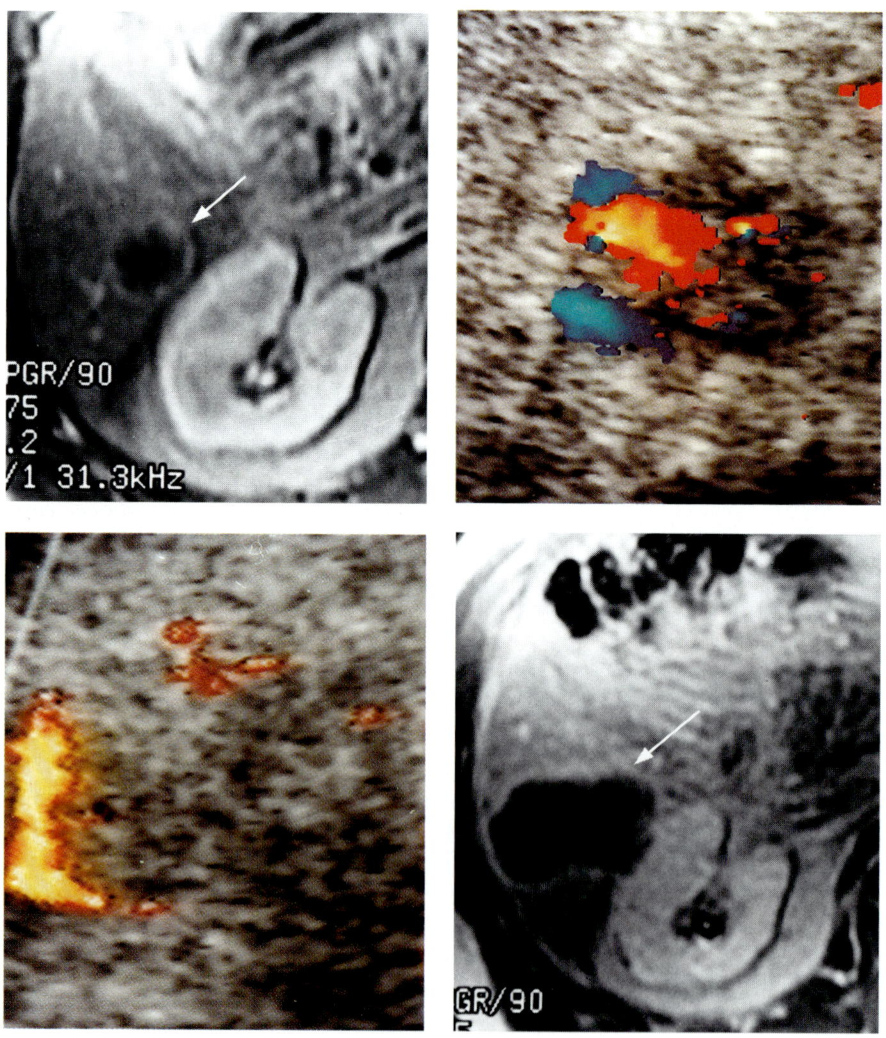

a,b c,d

Fig. 24.8a–d. a T1-weighted, gadolinium enhanced MRI scan shows a hypointense, single, 2 cm colorectal metastasis in segment 6 (*arrow*). **b** Blood flow signals which were undetected on unenhanced color Doppler scans, are seen following drip infusion of Levovist. **c** Fifteen minutes after the end of RF ablation, the actual extent of coagulation necrosis area is not clearly assessed with US. A second administration of Levovist followed by color Doppler study shows a wide (3.5+3.0) avascular area with peripheral displacement of liver blood vessels and no evidence of vascularized residual tumor. **d** At 7-day follow-up, contrast-enhanced MRI confirms a corresponding area of necrosis (*arrow*) hyperechogenicity, which is thought to represent the gas microbubbles forming in the heated tissue. At 3 days to 4 weeks after the procedure, the characteristic peritumoral halo has often disappeared and the ablated tumor cannot be differentiated from normal liver (Fig. 24.7).

24.5.2
CT and MR Imaging

Immediately after RF ablation, treated areas appear on contrast enhanced CT as regions of hypoattenuation devoid of characteristic parenchymal enhancement (Livraghi et al. 1997; Rossi et al. 1996; Solbiati et al. 1997, 1998). These regions are more conspicuous and their margins are better defined 3–14 days after treatment; they can be differentiated from hypoattenuating tumor on delayed opacification images, where hypoattenuation persists in coagulated tissues but not in viable tumor (Fig. 24.9). Radiological-pathological correlations in both experimental and clinical studies have demonstrated that CT findings predict the region of coagulation to within 2 mm (Goldberg et al. 1996; Solbiati et al. 1997).

Follow-up CT and/or MR at 1–3 months has been reported (Solbiati et al. 1997, 1998; Sironi et al. 1996) to be useful for confirming treatment success and for detecting residual peripheral tumor which is often amenable to additional RF sessions. A bulky, irregular rim at the edge of a treatment site is the most common appearance of an incompletely treated lesion. Peripheral tumor regrowth missed at 3-month CT/MR could, however, become apparent only later, at 6–9 months follow-up (Fig. 24.10).

CT/MR follow-up at 6 months in successfully treated lesions demonstrates tumor regression and a smaller coagulation necrosis area (Fig. 24.11). MR signal characteristics of treated tumors can be variable as foci of high, low or heterogeneous T1- and T2-weighted signals can be seen (Sironi et al. 1996). The signal characteristics can vary over time with decreased signal observed on T2-weighted images in most treated lesions by 3 months following treatment. Changes in the signal intensity likely correspond to the altered protein content of the coagulated tissues. Regions of tumor that have been treated do not demonstrate enhancement following the intravenous administration of Gd-DTPA (Sironi et al. 1996; Solbiati et al. 1997). In some cases, images obtained 3 days to 6 months following ablation demonstrate a densely enhancing peripheral rim of fairly uniform thickness surrounding the region of coagulation necrosis (Fig. 24.6). This finding has been demonstrated in experimental animals and in clinical studies to represent an inflammatory reaction to the thermal necrosis.

24.6
Indications for Radiofrequency Ablation

At the very beginning of the clinical experience in the treatment of liver metastases (mostly from colorectal cancer) with RF ablation, four major indications were followed: (1) development of new lesions on follow-up imaging studies in patients already undergoing one or more prior surgical metastasectomies; (2) recurrence of tumor tissue along the margins of previous surgical resection (Fig. 24.12); (3) technically inoperable metastases and (4) metastases in patients refusing surgical resection. The impressive technological improvement of RF in a very short time, the increasing clinical experience, the closer and closer relationships between interventional radiologists and oncologists and, mostly, the demonstration of the promising results achieved with a negligible rate of complications have led to a progressive increase in the number of indications, such as: (1) subsequent detection (once-twice per year) with imaging methods of new small liver metastases in patients with or without history of prior resections (Fig. 24.13); (2) small metastases which would require, for technical or anatomical reasons, large resections; and (3) residual viable tumor following other non-surgical treatments, e.g. metastases from breast cancer surviving after chemotherapy or from neuroendocrine tumor after chemoembolization.

24.7
Results

The rationale for local treatment of hepatic metastases is based primarily on the success achieved using a surgical approach. Without resection, the prognosis for patients with hepatic metastases from colorectal carcinoma is dismal, with 5-year survival reported to be less than 1% and median survival estimated at 9.6 months (3.8–21.3 month range) (Lehnert et al. 1995; Stangl et al. 1994; Steele and Ravikumar 1989). Unfortunately, at least for the

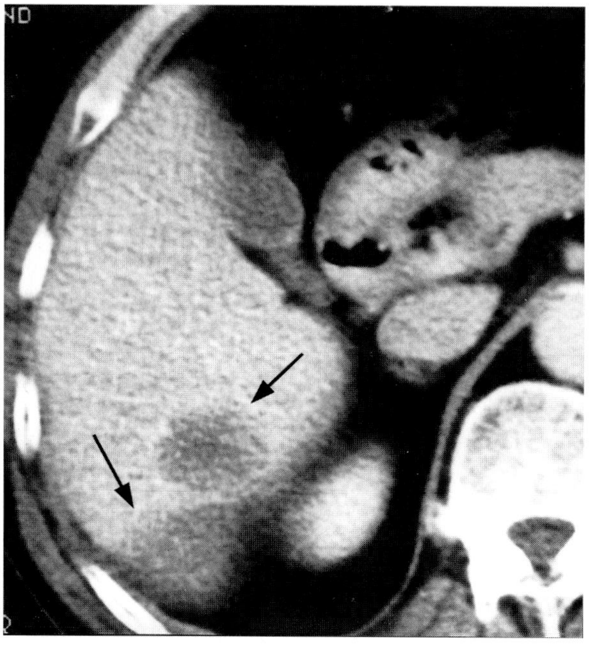
a

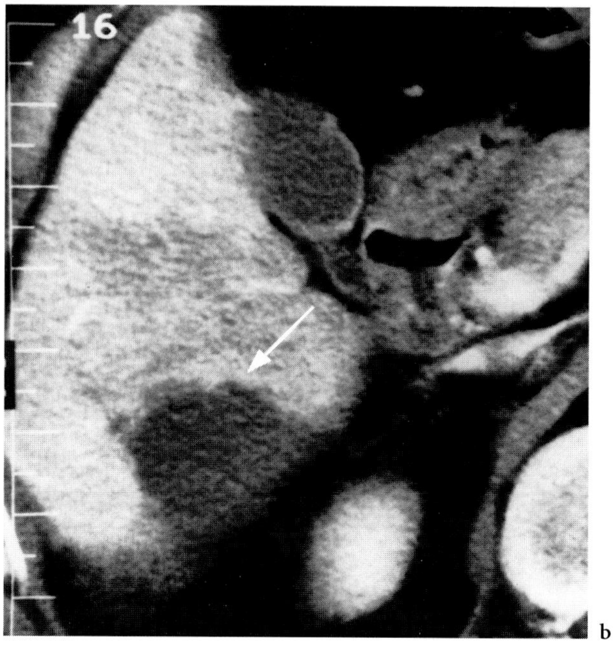

b

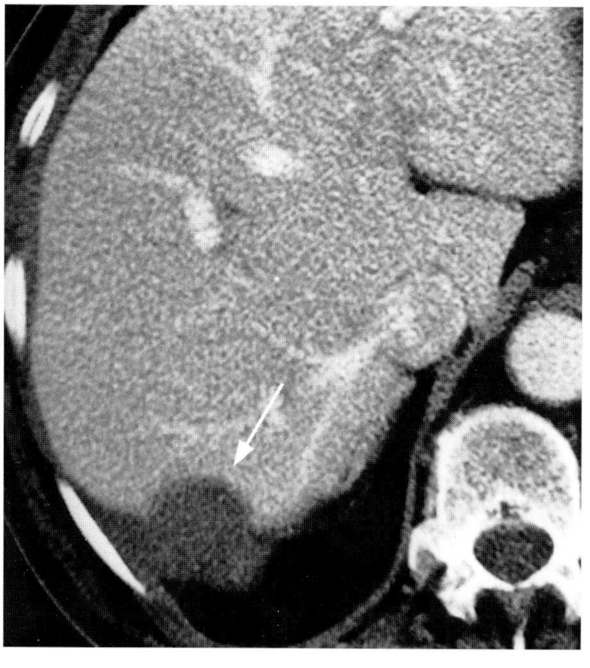
c

Fig. 24.9a–c. Successful RF ablation of two contiguous liver metastases (*arrows*) (**a**) from clear-cell carcinoma of the left kidney. At 6-month follow-up, CT scans (**b,c**) show wide unenhancing areas of coagulative necrosis (*arrows*) with no evidence of residual unablated tumor

most consistent group of liver metastases (from colorectal cancer), systemic chemotherapy, radiation therapy, and PEI have been relatively unsuccessful in significantly improving patient outcomes. In a recent review of the literature, Tellez et al. (1998) has showed that favorable (even though always transient) responses to chemoembolization of colorectal metastases occur only in 63% of cases. As a result, hepatic resection (metastasectomy) is the only widely available curative treatment for these patients. With resection, survival rates of 85–91% at 1-year, 35–43% at 3-year and 21–37% at 5-year follow-up and overall median survival of 33 months have been reported with proper patient selection (Cady and Stone 1991; Gayowski et al. 1994; Lehnert et al. 1995; Petrelli et al. 1991; Saenz et al. 1989). However, despite its success in improving overall patient survival, metastasectomy is associated with significant morbidity (5–18%), as well as a perioperative mortality rate of 2–10% (Cady and

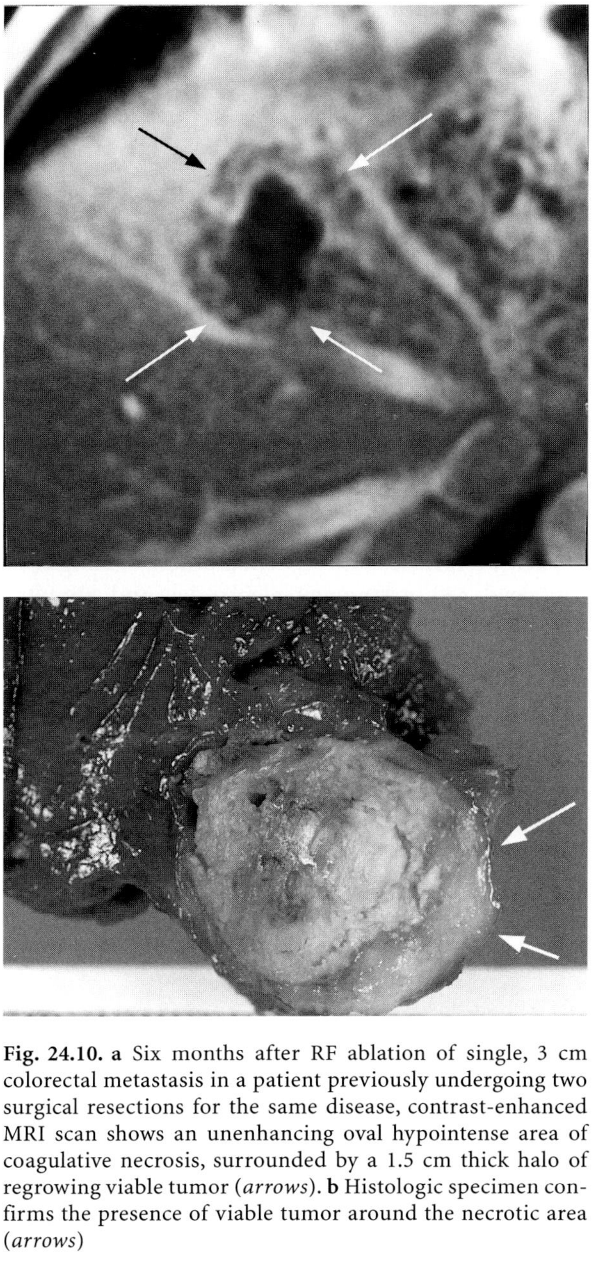

Fig. 24.10. a Six months after RF ablation of single, 3 cm colorectal metastasis in a patient previously undergoing two surgical resections for the same disease, contrast-enhanced MRI scan shows an unenhancing oval hypointense area of coagulative necrosis, surrounded by a 1.5 cm thick halo of regrowing viable tumor (*arrows*). **b** Histologic specimen confirms the presence of viable tumor around the necrotic area (*arrows*)

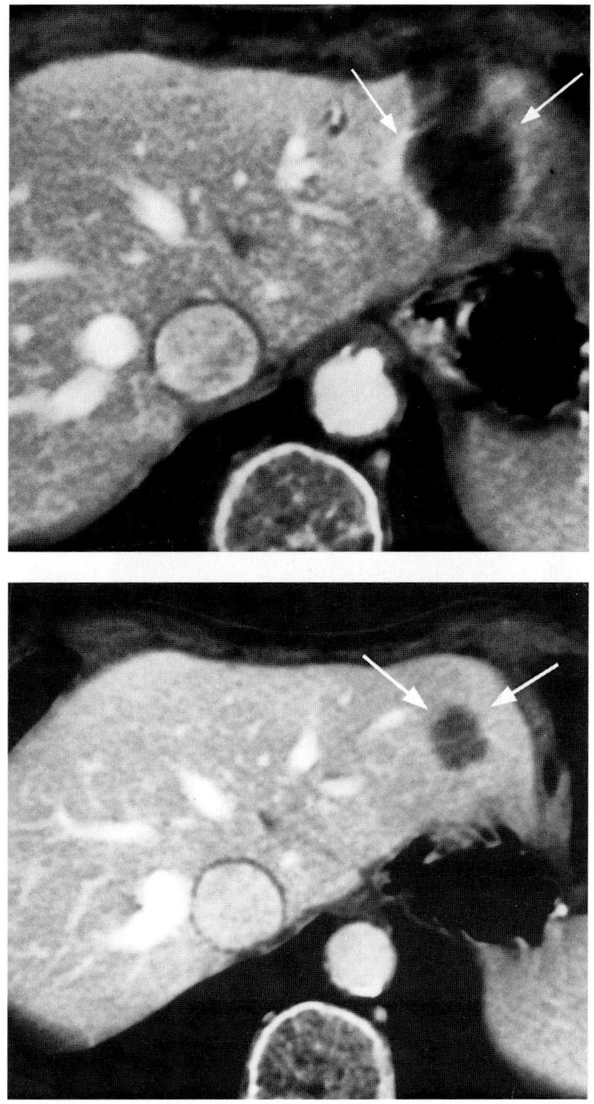

Fig. 24.11a,b. Long-term follow-up of RF-ablated metastasis. **a** 3×2 cm hypodense area of coagulative necrosis in the left lobe (*arrows*) following RF ablation of 2.0 cm metastasis from gastric cancer. **b** At 2-year follow-up, marked decrease in size of the necrotic area (*arrows*), with no evidence of residual viable tumor

Stone 1991; Doci et al. 1991; Gayowski et al. 1994; Lehnert et al. 1995; Saenz et al. 1989; Sugihara et al. 1993). Unfortunately, surgery is actually curative in only 10% of patients (Hemming and Langer 1994; Hughes et al. 1998), with tumor recurrence in the liver occurring in 53–68% of patients at a mean interval of 17 months post primary resection (Doci et al. 1991; Harned et al. 1994; Lehnert et al. 1995; Sugihara et al. 1993). Reresection of new metastases can only be performed in a minority of patients and is associated with higher mortality (up to 9%) and morbidity (up to 50%) than the initial resection (Griffith et al. 1990; Hemming and Langer 1994). Median survival time following reresection is 22 months (Griffith et al. 1990; Hemming and Langer 1994).

For noncolorectal hepatic metastases, only resection of metastases from Wilms' tumors and carcinoids is associated with prolonged survival (Wolf et al. 1991).

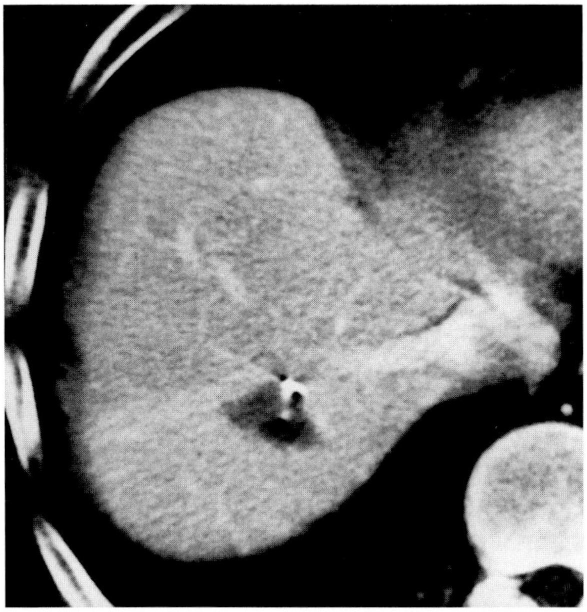

Fig. 24.12. Hypodense area of coagulative necrosis at 1-year follow-up after RF ablation of recurrence of liver colorectal metastasis grown along the margins of previous surgical resection (6 months before) (see adjacent surgical metallic clips)

Furthermore, only a small fraction of patients with hepatic metastases can actually undergo metastasectomy as they are either deemed poor surgical risks, or the number and distribution of their tumors does not permit complete resection while at the same time leaving behind an adequate volume of normal liver to support life.

To date, five series using different methods of radiofrequency application for the treatment of hepatic metastases have been reported as peer-reviewed, full length articles (Livraghi et al. 1997; Rossi et al. 1996; Siperstein et al. 1997; Solbiati et al. 1997, 1998). Abstract presentation of other series of RF treatment for hepatic malignancy have begun to appear (Dodd et al. 1997; Goldberg et al. 1997a).

Rossi et al. (1996) treated 11 patients with 13 hepatic metastases using multiple insertions of conventional monopolar and bipolar radiofrequency electrodes over multiple treatment sessions. Only one patient was alive without evidence of tumor at one year, while local recurrence was evident at CT or pathology in 55% of patients.

Solbiati et al. (1997) have treated 31 tumors in 16 patients with metastatic gastrointestinal carcinomas measuring 1.5–7.5 cm in diameter using conventional monopolar technique with and without multiprobe arrays. Complete treatment, defined as no evidence of local tumor growth by CT and MR imaging at 6-month follow-up was achieved in 66.6% of the lesions, all of which were less than 3 cm in diameter. Disease free survival was achieved in 50% of patients with mean follow up of 16.6 months. Overall survival was 100% at one year and 61.5% at two years. Solbiati et al. (1997) have also reported a series of 29 patients with 44 hepatic metastases from colorectal and other gastrointestinal malignancies measuring 1.5–4.5 cm in diameter, treated using internally cooled electrodes. No more than two treatment sessions were required for any patient. No evidence of local recurrence was seen in 84% of these lesions with a mean follow-up of 7.9 months (range 3–15 months) and disease free survival was seen in 66.7% of patients.

Livraghi et al. (1997) treated 14 patients with 24 hepatic metastases (1.2–4.5 cm diameter) using conventional radiofrequency electrodes and simultaneous intraparenchymal saline infusion. Complete necrosis of the tumor at 6-month follow-up was achieved in 52% of the lesions, all of which were smaller than 3.5 cm in diameter.

Siperstein et al. (1997) treated 13 neuroendocrine liver metastases from 1.5–8.0 cm in diameter in 6 patients using a laparascopic approach to deploy a hooked-electrode system. One to eight applications of RF were used to apply 30–50 W for 5–15 min. Procedure duration lasted from 1:45 to 7:05 h. Preliminary results were encouraging as 3-month CT fol-

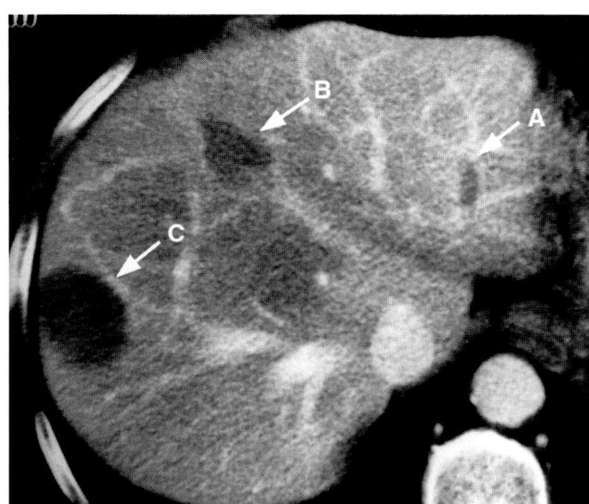

Fig. 24.13. Follow-up CT scan of patient undergoing subsequent RF ablation treatments for colorectal metastases. Presence of hypodense, unenhancing areas of coagulative necrosis from RF ablations performed 18 months (A), 12 months (B) and 6 months (C) previously

low-up for 11 lesions suggested complete ablation of these tumors, and the authors reported "symptomatic improvement in patients with secreting tumor". However, the extremely short duration of follow-up (less than the 6 months) necessary to visualize residual tumor by CT for 2/3 of the patients and the use of subjective patient symptoms over "incomplete" biochemical data as an endpoint strongly suggest that further follow-up is necessary before firm conclusions can be reached about this technique.

Currently, in our group 220 liver metastases (169 from colorectal cancer) have been treated with RF ablation. Of these, 101 colorectal lesions have been followed for 6–40 months (long before the introduction of clustered electrodes): local post-treatment regrowth was found in only 19% of lesions originally smaller than 3 cm and in 43% of lesions larger than 3 cm. In this group of patients with colorectal metastases long term follow-up has been presented (Solbiati et al. 1998) with an overall survival of 92%, 56%, and 32% and a disease-free survival of 56%, 29% and 14% observed respectively at 1-, 2-, and 3-year follow-up. With the increasing technical possibility of achieving large areas of coagulative necrosis and a better imaging follow-up, current (unpublished) survival rates seem to progressively improve (62% at 2 years and 41% at 3 years). These data, apparently slightly less successful than the results of surgical resection reported in the literature (see above), are actually to be considered at least equivalent (if not better) than the surgical data, being mostly obtained in patients assessed as non-surgical candidates.

24.8 Complications

Few complications have been reported for RF ablation in the liver (less than 2% of procedures). Rossi et al. (1996) and Siperstein et al. (1997) reported no complications in their combined series comprising over 100 patients. Solbiati et al. (1997) observed two cases of self-remitting intra-peritoneal bleeding, one each using conventional and cooled-tip electrodes over 100 patients (250 treatments). Transfusions were not required in either case. One case of transient ascites was reported by Livraghi et al. (1997), and attributed to the saline infusion. Livraghi has also orally communicated the occurrence of one case of peritonitis, presumably from a breakdown of sterile technique. Given the limited number of complications weighing against the potential of tumor eradication, the risk-benefit ratio of this procedure is highly favorable.

The primary risks potentially involved with this procedure include: hemorrhage, damage to contiguous structures, potential burns from inadequate grounding of the system, incomplete removal of living tumor, and creation of a "dead space" which may serve as a potential nidus for infection. Damage to nearby structures such as arteries, nerves and the biliary tract will be avoided by appropriate selection of patients, and by precise electrode placement under ultrasound guidance. Burns have been reported as a consequence of inadequate grounding while using a single needle as the ground or while using clustered electrodes without adequately large grounding pads, as occurred in two cases in our experience, both of them patients with unilateral hip prosthesis applied many years before. These 1×2 cm second degree burns healed in 6 weeks with only Silividine application and no other sequelae.

The risk of devitalized tissue serving as a nidus for infection is considered remote for several reasons. Necrotic tumor is common, yet infection is a rare complication. Furthermore, it has been clearly demonstrated that over time resorption of necrotic tissue occurs.

24.9 Conclusions

Percutaneous image-guided application of radiofrequency is a relatively new strategy for inducing thermally mediated coagulation necrosis. As such, RF ablation may ultimately prove beneficial as a minimally invasive method for treating liver metastases. Because the goal of tumor eradication necessitates ablating the entire tumor and a 0.5–1 cm peripheral margin of grossly normal tissue, complete ablation of the entire neoplasm requires the induction of large volumes of coagulation necrosis. Several recent technical innovations, including RF application to multiple and/or internally cooled electrodes, enable increased energy deposition into tissues with a resultant increase in the volume of induced coagulation necrosis. These advances are timely because many sequential, overlapping applications of RF to a single electrode are required to treat all but the smallest of tumors using conventional monopolar electrodes, which is difficult to accomplish in clinical practice. The use of clustered electrodes may therefore allow the treatment of larger metastases with a single application of radiofrequency.

Optimization of RF energy delivery and/or modulation of tumor or organ biology may allow tailoring of induced tissue destruction, thereby enabling adequate and predictable treatment of tumors. However, perfusion mediated tissue cooling limits both tissue heat deposition and the extent of coagulation necrosis induced by RF tumor ablation in vascular tissues and tumors. Development of strategies to reduce blood flow during RF tumor ablation may ultimately allow for an improved treatment effect (Goldberg et al. 1996b), encouraging optimism about the future of RF ablation techniques.

References

Anzai Y, Lufkin R, DeSalles A, et al (1995) Preliminary experience with MR-guided thermal ablation of brain tumors. AJR 16:39–48

Cady B, Stone MD (1991) The role of surgical resection of liver metastases in colorectal carcinoma. Sem Oncol 18:399–406

Cosman ER, Nashold BS, Bedenbaugh P (1983) Stereotactic radiofrequency lesion making. Appl Neurophysiol 46:160–166

Cosman ER, Nashold BS, Ovelman-Levitt J (1984) Theoretical aspects of radiofrequency lesions in the dorsal root entry zone. Neurosurg 15:945–950

Cosman ER, Rittman WJ, Nashold BS, et al (1988) Radiofrequency lesions generation and its effect on tissue impedence. Appl Neurophysiol 51:230–242

Doci R, Gennari L, Bignami, et al (1991) One hundred patients with hepatic metastases from colorectal cancer treated by resection: analysis of prognostic determinants. Br J Surg 78:797–801

Dodd GD III, Halff GA, Rhim H, et al (1997) Radiofrequency thermal ablation of hepatic tumors. Radiology 205(P):723

Gayowski TJ, Iwatsuki S, Madariaga JR, et al (1994) Experience in hepatic resection for metastatic colorectal cancer: analysis of clinical and pathologic risk factors. Surgery 116:703–711

Goldberg SN, Gazelle GS, Dawson SL, et al (1995a) Tissue ablation with radiofrequency: Effect of probe size, gauge, duration, and temperature on lesion volume. Acad Radiol 2:399–404

Goldberg SN, Gazelle GS, Dawson SL, et al (1995b) Radiofrequency tissue ablation using multiprobe arrays: greater tissue destruction than multiple probes operating alone. Acad Radiol 2:670–674

Goldberg SN, Gazelle GS, Solbiati L, et al (1996a) Radiofrequency tissue ablation: increased lesion diameter with a perfusion electrode. Acad Radiol 3:636–644

Goldberg SN, Hahn PF, Schima S, et al (1996b) Percutaneous radiofrequency tissue ablation in the liver: increased coagulation necrosis with portal venous occlusion. Radiology 201(P):250

Goldberg SN, Gazelle GS, Solbiati L, et al (1997a) Large volume radiofrequency tissue ablation: increased coagulation with pulsed technique. Radiology 205(P):258

Goldberg SN, Livraghi T, Solbiati L, et al (1997b) In situ ablation of focal hepatic neoplasms. In: GS Gazelle, S Saini, and PR Mueller (eds) Hepatobiliary and pancreatic radiology: imaging and intervention. Thieme Medical Pub, New York, pp 470–502

Goldberg SN, Solbiati L, Hahn PF, et al (1998) Large-volume tissue ablation with radiofrequency by using a clustered, internally cooled electrode technique: laboratory and clinical experience in liver metastases. Radiology 209:371–379

Griffith KD, Sugarbaker PH, Chang AE (1990) Repeat hepatic resections for colorectal metastases. Surgery 107:101–104

Harned RK, Chezmar JL, Nelson RC (1994) Recurrent tumor after resection of hepatic metastases from colorectal carcinoma: location and time of discovery as determined by CT. AJR 163:93–97

Hemming AW, Langer B (1994) Repeat resection of recurrent hepatic colorectal metastases. Br J Surg 81:1553–1554

Hughes KS, Simon R, Songhorabodi S, et al (1988) Resection of the liver for colorectal carcinoma metastases: a multi-institutional study of indications for resecting. Surgery 103:278–288

Hunt RD (1966) Microscopic histochemical methods for the demostration of enzymes. In: Thompson SW (ed) Selected histochemical and histopathological methods. Charles C. Thomas, Springfield, pp 615–748

Lehnert T, Otto G, Herfarth C (1995) Therapeutic modalities and prognostic factors for primary and secondary liver tumor. World J Surg 19:252–263

Le Veen RF (1997) Laser hyperthermia and radiofrequency ablation of hepatic lesions. Semin Int Rad 14:313–324

Livraghi T, Goldberg SN, Monti F, et al (1997) Saline-enhanced radiofrequency tissue ablation in the treatment of liver metastases. Radiology 202:205–210

Lorentzen T (1996) A cooled needle electrode for radiofrequency tissue ablation: thermodynamic aspects of improved performance compared with conventional needle design. Acad Radiol 3:556–563

McGahan JP, Brock JN, Tessluk H, et al (1992a) Hepatic ablation with use of radiofrequency electrocautery in the animal model. JVIR 3:291–297

McGahan JP, Wei-Zhong G, Brock JM, et al (1992b) Hepatic ablation using bipolar radiofrequency electrocautery. Acad Radiol 3:418–422

Petrelli NJ, Gupta B, Piedmonte M, et al (1991) Morbidity and survival of liver resection for colorectal adenocarcinoma. Dis Colon Rectum 34:899–904

Rosenthal DI, Springfield DS, Gebhart MC, et al (1995) Osteoid osteoma: percutaneous radiofrequency ablation. Radiology 197:451–454

Rossi S, Fornari F, Pathies C, et al (1990) Thermal lesions induced by 480 KHz localized current field in Guinea pig and pig liver. Tumori 76:54–57

Rossi S, Fornari F, Buscarini L (1993) Percutaneous ultrasound-guided radiofrequency electrocautery for the treatment of small hepatocellular carcinoma. J Interv Radiol 8:97–103

Rossi S, Di Stasi M, Buscarini E, et al (1996) Percutaneous RF interstitial thermal ablation in the treatment of hepatic cancer. AJR 167:759–768

Rossi S, Buscarini E, Garbagnati F, et al (1998) Percutaneous treatment of small hepatic tumors by an expandable RF needle electrode. AJR 170:1015–1022

Saenz NC, Cady B, McDermott WV, et al (1989) Experience with colorectal carcinoma metastatic to the liver. Surg Clin North Am 69:361–70

Siperstein AE, Rogers SJ, Hansen PD, et al (1997) Laparoscopic thermal ablation of hepatic neuroendocrine tumor metastases. Surgery 122:1147–1155

Sironi S, Vanzulli A, De Cobelli F, et al (1996) Percutaneous US-guided radiofrequency ablation of liver metastases: dynamic MR imaging follow-up. Radiology 201(P):250

Solbiati L, Ierace T, Crespi L, et al (1996) Three-dimensional power Doppler with an intravascular echo enhancement agent and second harmonic imaging in RF ablation of liver metastases. Radiology 201(P):196

Solbiati L, Goldberg SN, Ierace T, et al (1997) Hepatic metastases: percutaneous radio-frequency ablation with cooled- tip electrodes. Radiology 205:367–374

Solbiati L, Goldberg SN, Ierace T, et al (1998) Long-term follow-up of liver metastases treated with percutaneous US-guided radiofrequency ablation using internally-cooled electrodes. Radiology 209(P):449

Solbiati L, Goldberg SN, Ierace T, et al (1999) Radiofrequency ablation of hepatic metastases: post-procedural assessment with a US microbubble contrast agent – early experience. Radiology 211:643–649

Stangl R, Altendorf-Hofmann A, Charneley RM, et al (1994) Factors influencing the natural history of colorectal liver metastases. Lancet 343:1405–1410

Steele G Jr, Ravikumar TS (1989) Resection of hepatic metastases from colorectal cancer: biologic perspectives. Ann Surg 210:127–138

Sugihara K, Hojo K, Moriya Y, et al (1993) Pattern of recurrence after hepatic resection for colorectal metastases. J Surg 80:1032–1035

Tellez C, Benson AB, Lyster MT, et al (1998) Phase II trial chemoembolization for the treatment of metastatic colorectal carcinoma to the liver and review of the literature. Cancer; 82:1250–1259

Wolf RF, Goodnight JE, Krag DE, et al (1991) Results of resection and proposed guidelines for patient selection in instances of noncolorectal hepatic metastases. Surg Gynecol Obstet 173:454–459

25 Transcatheter Arterial Chemotherapy and Chemoembolization of Liver Metastases

R. Roversi

CONTENTS

25.1 Introduction

Since the early 1960s, the use of percutaneous Seldinger's technique has enabled any visceral arterial tree to be easily reached with low invasivity for diagnostic purposes. Therapy then became the extension of angiography, and arterial infusion chemotherapy (AIC) for liver cancer was first used by Sullivan (1963). Arterial embolization of liver tumors was also performed to reduce pain in large expansive masses or for emergency hemostasis in acute blood loss, and was applied to palliative treatment of the hepatocellular carcinoma by Doyon (1974) and by Goldstein et al. (1987).

Single or multiple localized liver metastases are mainly treated with hepatectomy; however, hepatectomy may not be possible in high-risk patients or when patients refuse to undergo surgery. It may be considered doubtful in any case whether surgery is really the best therapeutic option or not if cost, invasivity, time of hospitalization and rate of recurrences are evaluated. I believe that US-guided thermoablation, laser therapy and cryotherapy will probably replace resective surgery, as already stated for small hepatocellular carcinoma, also for localized metastatic lesions because of lower invasivity, cost and time of hospitalization: encouraging even if not yet established clinical results have been reported (Vogl et al. 1997; Nagata et al. 1997; Maeda 1994; Nakamura 1994).

In multifocal or localized not surgically suitable liver metastases locoregional intraarterial treatments are now extensively used, mainly as a further step of the programmed therapy: systemic chemotherapy still remains in most patients the first step. Anticancer drugs may be delivered mainly using arterial infusion through indwelling catheters or chemoembolizations: hypoxia (Theicher et al. 1981; Roversi et al. 1997) and/or hyperthermia (Tanaka et al.1992; Nagata et al. 1997) may be also associated.

Some techniques employed for AIC of hepatic liver metastases are actually no longer used in clinical practice as surgical dearterialization, even if Nobin et al. (1989) reported 60% good clinical results treating liver metastases from carcinoid with temporary dearterialization and Kimoto et al. (1995) used repeated hepatic dearterialization for unresectable liver metastases from gastric cancer in five cases. Isolated embolization should also be no longer used. Long-term perfusion with indwelling catheters, already extensively employed for at least 20 years, has been now renewed by the technique of percutaneous placement of the device.

Chemoembolizations with DSM or Lipiodolization adds to the effect of the intraarterial drug perfusion the occlusive ischemia obtained with oily contrast media or with reabsorbable materials such as gelatin sponge or microspheres, adding hypoxia and a prolonged contact time to the increased drug delivery and higher concentration in the neoplastic tissue (Wallace et al. 1990).

More invasive and technically complex procedures such as hypoxic hepatic perfusion (Roversi et al. 1997), isolated hepatic perfusion (Ravikumar and Dixon 1996) or isolated hepatic perfusion with tumor necrosis factor (Hafstrom et al. 1994) have

R. Roversi, MD; Chief, Department of Diagnostic Imaging and Interventional Radiology, Bellaria-Maggiore Hospital, Via Altura 3, I-40100 Bologna, Italy appeared in the last few years. Their clinical results are still to be evaluated in randomized trials.

A summary of the most used techniques of AIC derived from the authors is reported in Table 25.1.

The first target of AIC is to treat diffuse metastatic liver disease. Data support the use of adjuvant chemotherapy following complete surgical resection of the primary lesion (Saltz 1991); patients who undergo hepatic resection for colorectal metastases should also be considered for postoperative adjuvant chemotherapy, to decrease the likelihood of recurrence and to improve survival (Curley et al. 1993).

Table 25.1. Summary of the reported AIC techniques

Authors	Source	Technique of treatment
De Dycker RP	Reg Cancer Treat 3/6 (302–304) 1991	Degradable starch microspheres
Civalleri et al.	Br J Surg 76/7 (699–703) 1989	Degradable starch microspheres
Fujimoto et al.	Reg Cancer Treat 6/1 (7–11) 1993	Degradable starch microspheres
Koike et al.	Jpn J Cancer Chemother 15/8 li (2601–2605) 1988	Degradable starch microspheres
Koike et al.	Jpn J Cancer Chemother 16/8 Ii (2818–2821) 1989	Degradable starch microspheres
Mavor et al.	Nucl Med Commun 8/12 (1011–1018) 1987	Degradable starch microspheres
Sakamato et al.	Reg Cancer Treat 6/1 (12–18) 1993	Degradable starch microspheres
Teder et al.	Anticancer Res 13/6A (2161–2164) 1993	Degradable starch microspheres
Kobayashi et al.	Acta Radiol 28/3 (275–280) 1987	Adriamycin/mitomycin c lipiodol suspension
Inoue et al.	Acta Radiol 30/6 (603–608) 1989	Adriamycin/mitomycin c lipiodol suspension
Links et al.	Reg Cancer Treat 6/3 (121–124) 1993	Lipiodol–Adriamycin
Suzuki et al.	Jpn J Cancer Chemother 19/3 (323–326) 1992	Adriamycin4 Ipiodot suspension
Coldwell DM, Mortimer JE	Reg Cancer Treat 3/6 (298–301) 1991	Hepatic artery embolization
Kimoto et al.	Hpb Surg 8/3 (175–180) 1995	Hepatic dearterialization
Wallace et al.	Cardiovasc Intervent Radiol 13/3 (153–160) 1990	Infusion and chemoembolization
Uekado et al.	Jpn J Cancer Chemother 21/10 (1673–1676) 1994	Chemoembolization
Luo et al.	Adv Ther 14/4 (192–198) 1997	Chemoembolization
Lang EK, Brown CL Jr	Radiology 189/2 (417–422) 1993	Selective chemoembolization
Konno et al.	Acta Oncol 33/2 (133–137) 1994	Targeted chemotherapy (CEAT)
Kameyama et al.	Jpn J Cancer Chemother 15/8 Ii (2510–2513) 1988	Lipiodol cisplatin sandwich therapy
Sugimoto E	J Saitama Med Sc IL 21/3 (185–191) 1994	Arterial embolization using Lipiodol
Yamashita et al.	Cancer 64/12 (2437–2444) 1989	5-Fluoro-2-deoxyuridine-c8 in lymphographic agent
Sugimoto et al.	Jpn J Cancer Chemother 1997; 24/12 (1753–1756)	Isolated liver chemoperfusion using cisplatin
Sato et al.	Jpn J Cancer Chemother 19/4 (537–539) 1992	Large doses mitomycin c and 5-fluorouracil
Allen-Mersh et al.	Lancet 344/8932 (1255–1260) 1994	Continuous hepatic-artery floxuridine infusion
Yamamoto et al.	Reg Cancer Treat 6/3 (125–130) 1993	Continuous infusion of IL-2 and intermittent doxorubicin
Nakayama et al.	Jpn J Cancer Chemother 20/11 (1504–1506) 1993	Continuous infusion of 5-fluorouracil
Nakamura K	Jpn J Nucl Med 29/3 (377–383) 1992	Continuous infusion
Mori et al.	Jpn J Cancer Chemother 20/11 (1547–1550) 1993	Continuous infusion of CDDP
Shida et al.	Jpn J Cancer Chemother 22/2 (221–225) 1995	Continuous infusion of 5-fluorouracil plus leucovorin
Arai et al.	Jpn J Cancer Chemother 20/11 (1527–1530) 1993	Intermittent infusion of 5-FU
Arai et al.	Cancer Chemother Pharmacol 40/6 (526–530) 1997	Intermittent infusion of high-dose 5-FU
Tsuji et al.	Jpn J Cancer Chemother 20/11 (1520–1523) 1993	Intermittent high dose 5-FU
Stephens FO	Reg Cancer Treat 5/34 (146–153) 1992	Hepatic artery 5-FU infusion followed by portal vein FUDR
Ichikawa et al.	Reg Cancer Treat 5/34 (154–158) 1992	intra-arterial infusion
Maruyama et al.	Jpn J Cancer Chemother 1997; 24/13 (2011–2014)	Cisplatin/5-fluorouracil intraperitoneal
Ekberg et al.	J Surg Oncol 37/2 (94–99) 1988	Intraperitoneal infusion of 5-FU
Curley et al.	Am J Surg 166/6 (743–748) 1993	Hepatic infusion
Yamamura et al.	Jpn J Cancer Chemother 20/11 (1516–1519) 1993	Infusion of 5-FU and leucovorin
Nakagawa et al.	Jpn J Cancer Chemother 23/6 (783–785) 1996	Infusion of low dose cisplatin and oral administration of high dose doxyfluridine
Tsujitani et al.	Eur J Surg Oncol 17/5 (526–529) 1991	Low-dosage intraportal 5-FU infusion

Table 25.1. Summary of the reported AIC techniques (Continued)

Authors	Source	Technique of treatment
KOHNO et al.	Jpn J Cancer Chemother 22/5 (695–698) 1995	5-FU, leucovorin, etoposide, and cisplatin (FLEP)
DAZZI et al.	Tumori 80/3 (204--208) 1994	High-dose intra-arterial plus intraperitoneal chemotherapy
ICHIKAWA et al.	Reg Cancer Treat 5/34 (154–158) 1992	Balloon occluded arterial infusion
TANADA et al.	Jpn J Cancer Chemother 23/11 (1440–1442) 1996	Arterial embolization chemotherapy – arterial infusion chemotherapy
NOBIN et al.	Acta Oncol 28/3 (419–424) 1989	Dearterialization and embolization
HANSSEN et al.	Acta Oncol 30/4 (523–527) 1991	Interferon with or without hepatic artery embolization
ONOGAWA et al.	Jpn J Cancer Chemother 1997; 24/12 (1804–1808)	Hepatic arterial infusion chemotherapy and systemic endocrine therapy
GOLDBERG et al.	Br J Cancer 63/2 (308–310) 1991	Angiotensin II and cytotoxic microspheres
IWASAKI et al.	Jpn J Cancer Chemother 23/11 (1558–1560) 1996	Hypertensive chemotherapy with angiotensin II
CURLEY et al. tive resection	Am J Surg 166/6 (743–748) 1993	Arterial infusion chemotherapy after cura-
OZEKI et al.	J Jpn Soc Cancer Ther 31/2 (157–162) 1996	Hepatectomy after neoadjuvant chemotherapy
KITADA et al.	Jpn J Cancer Chemother 20/11 (1601–1604) 1993	Thermocoagulation combined with selective intraarterial infusion
AJLOUNI et al.	Am J Clin Oncol Cancer Clin Trials 13/6 (532–535) 1990	Radiation therapy and infusion FUDR
WILEY et al.	Cancer 64/9 (1783–1789) 1989	Hepatic artery 5-fluorouracil and irradiation
HAFSTROM et al.	Reg Cancer Treat 7/34 (172–176) 1994	Isolated regional liver perfusion with tumor necrosis factor-alpha followed by hyperthermic melphalan perfusion
RAVIKUMAR TS DIXON K	Surg Oncol Clin North Am 5/2 (443-449) 1996	Isolated liver perfusion
ROVERSI et al.	Radiologia Medica 93:410–417, 1997	Hepatic hypoxic perfusion

25.2 Intraarterial Perfusion with Port-a-Cath

The technique of implanting an arterial indwelling catheter using a percutaneous subclavian, axillary or femoral approach was first introduced by ARAI (1994) and then used by other groups (WACKER et al. 1997; GROSSO et al. 1997; MORANDI et al. 1998). The percutaneous approach allows a strong increase in the number of the procedures compared to a surgical implant, moreover avoiding long hospitalization and surgical risks. Any difference between the clinical results may be suggested.

A US-guided subclavian percutaneous approach has been suggested by ARAI (1994) and GROSSO et al. (1997) (Fig. 25.1). The femoral approach (Fig. 25.2) could also be used as in the first part of personal experience, involving, however, some discomfort to the patient (SAWADA et al. 1992). The axillary approach (Fig. 25.3) is preferred by us, which combines the advantages of subclavian placement without the need for a US-guided puncture and facilitates replacement and/or removal.

An accurate angiographic understanding of the hepatic vascular anatomy is mandatory before starting the placement of a surgical or percutaneous Port-a-Cath. The most important factor for a successful infusion therapy is a single feeding artery to the liver. In the case of multiple hepatic arteries, one must be selected and the others embolized. Vascular anomalies of the hepatic arteries (Fig. 25.4) can be found in about 37% of cases (DAVITTI et al. 1992), the most frequent being the right hepatic artery arising from the superior mesenteric artery (SMA). The right hepatic artery from the SMA should not be used for the placement, to avoid the risk of distal embolization in the mesenteric territory or retrograde thrombosis: the middle-left hepatic artery arising from the celiac axis should then be used.

Collaterals such as right gastric (RAG), gastroduodenal (GD), and seldomly left gastric artery should also be embolized before the indwelling cath-

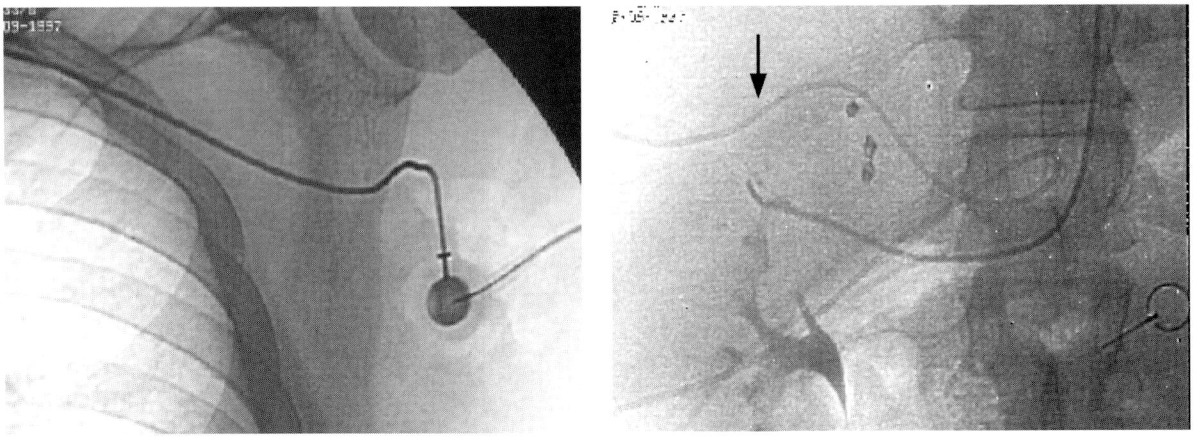

a b

Fig. 25.1a,b. Liver metastases from colorectal cancer treated with AIC through percutaneous Port-a-Cath. Previous ineffective surgical Port-a-Cath (*arrow*). **a** US guided subclavian approach. **b** Catheter's tip pulled into the proper hepatic artery with lateral hole in common hepatic artery. Coils were used for arterial redistribution. Gastroduodenal artery previously ligated

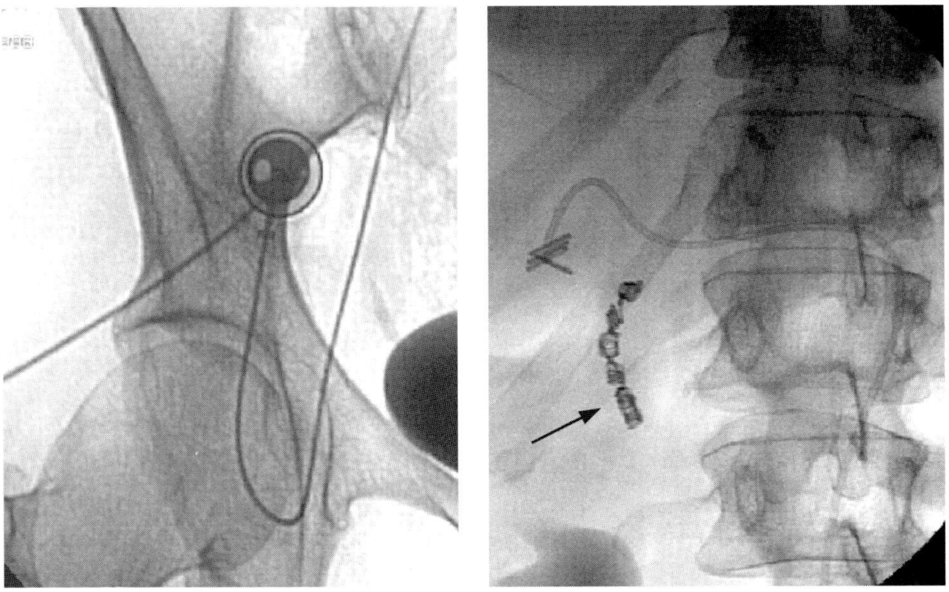

a b

Fig. 25.2a,b. Liver metastases from colorectal cancer treated with AIC through percutaneous Port-a-Cath. **a** Catheter introduced by right femoral approach. Device over the inguinal ligament. **b** Catheter pulled distally into the right hepatic artery with lateral hole cut in the common hepatic artery. Gastroduodenal artery embolized with coils (*arrow*)

eter is placed to avoid the passage of the drug into undesirable areas (Fig. 25.5).

It has been reported by Arai (1994) that if perfusion is performed without a complete redistribution the therapeutic effect decreases and complications occur. A whole liver perfusion cannot be obtained without entirely deriving the hepatic blood flow to a single hepatic artery in the case of multiple vessels, and the embolization of GD cannot be avoided; but I believe it unnecessary to routinely embolize as suggested by Arai (1994) the RAG. We have never observed drug-related gastric symptoms in patients with embolization of only the GD: moreover, a case of large gastric ulcer in our personal experience appeared in a patient with previous embolization of the RAG using acrylic glue.

In surgically implanted Port-a-Caths the catheter is introduced through the GD and pulled into the hepatic artery and the tip is fixed with a surgical stitch. Using the percutaneous approach, the tip can be

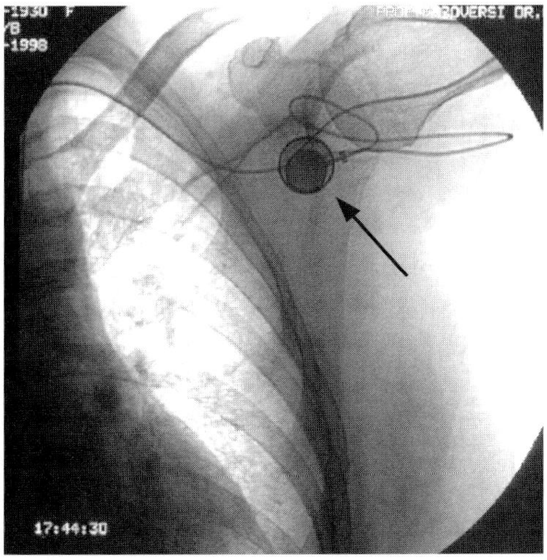

Fig. 25.3. Percutaneous Port-a-Cath. Axillary approach. Device under the external third of the clavicle (arrow)

fixed in the GD with a single bolus of bucrylate (Arai 1994) cutting a lateral hole in the catheter at the level of the proper common hepatic artery. In the experience of Grosso et al. (1997), the distal part of the catheter has been, however, placed freely in the common hepatic artery permitting an easy removal, but with an obviously higher risk of displacement.

In cases with a short proper hepatic artery it may be preferable to pull the catheter subselectively into the hepatic arterial system, previously embolizing GD and cutting a large lateral hole in the catheter at the level of the proper hepatic artery (Fig. 25.5). The

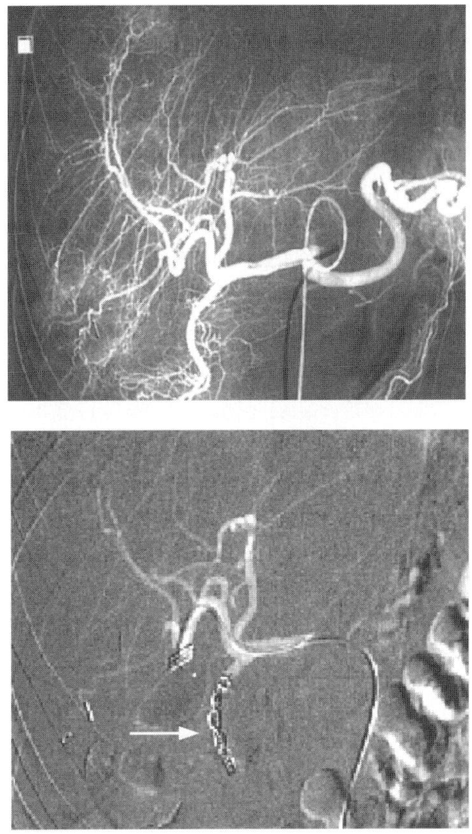

a

b

Fig. 25.5a,b. Liver metastases from colorectal cancer treated with AIC through percutaneous Port-a-Cath. Femoral approach. **a** Hepatic subselective DSA before the procedure: hypervascular lesions in the right lobe. **b** Distal tip pulled into the right hepatic artery with lateral hole in common hepatic artery. Gastroduodenal artery embolized with coils (*arrow*)

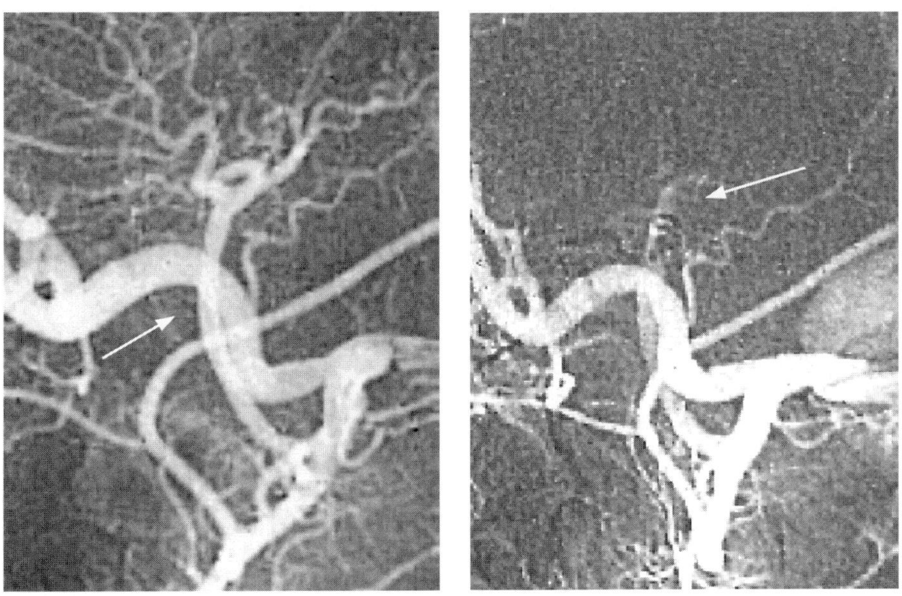

a

b

Fig. 25.4a,b. Redistribution of the hepatic arterial system. **a** Middle hepatic artery arising from gastroduodenal artery (*arrow*). **b** Embolization with coils (*arrow*) of the middle hepatic artery to derive the whole flow to the proper hepatic artery

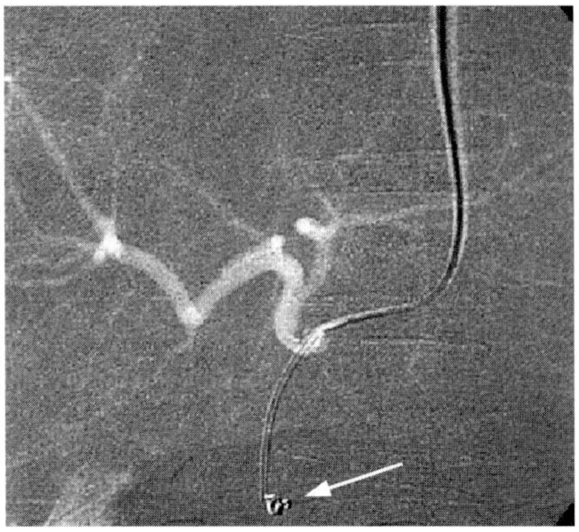

Fig. 25.6. Hepatic subselective DSA femoral percutaneous Port-a-Cath. Good perfusion of the liver

catheter may also be pulled into the GD (Figs. 25.6, 25.9), embolizing with coils the proximal right gastroepiploic artery and cutting a lateral hole in the common hepatic artery. Abnormalities of the liver perfusion not infrequently occur during Port-a-Cath infusion.

Among 51 patients with unresectable metastatic liver tumors who had implanted port systems, 49 perfusion abnormalities were detected in 32 patients (Seki et al. 1996; Hoefer et al. 1990). A correct delivery of the drug to the whole liver and a correct placement of the catheter's tip should always be controlled with CT (Roth et al. 1989; Seki et al. 1996; Miller et al. 1989; Sidibe et al. 1989) through an injection in the device (Figs. 25.7, 25.8, 25.10).

In 25% (122/33) of the procedures we performed positioning the distal tip in the proper hepatic artery without fixation with IBC, a displacement occurred, requiring the immediate repositioning or changing of the catheter (Fig. 25.11).

Arai's technique of fixation with isobutyl-2-cyanoacrylate avoids in almost all cases the displacement, enabling, however, the catheter to be changed if necessary.

The reported mean duration of AIC with percutaneously inserted ports ranges from 27 weeks (Wacker et al. 1997) to the rather optimistic 20.9 months (Arai et al. 1997): the therapy drop-out rate due to catheter-associated complications was very

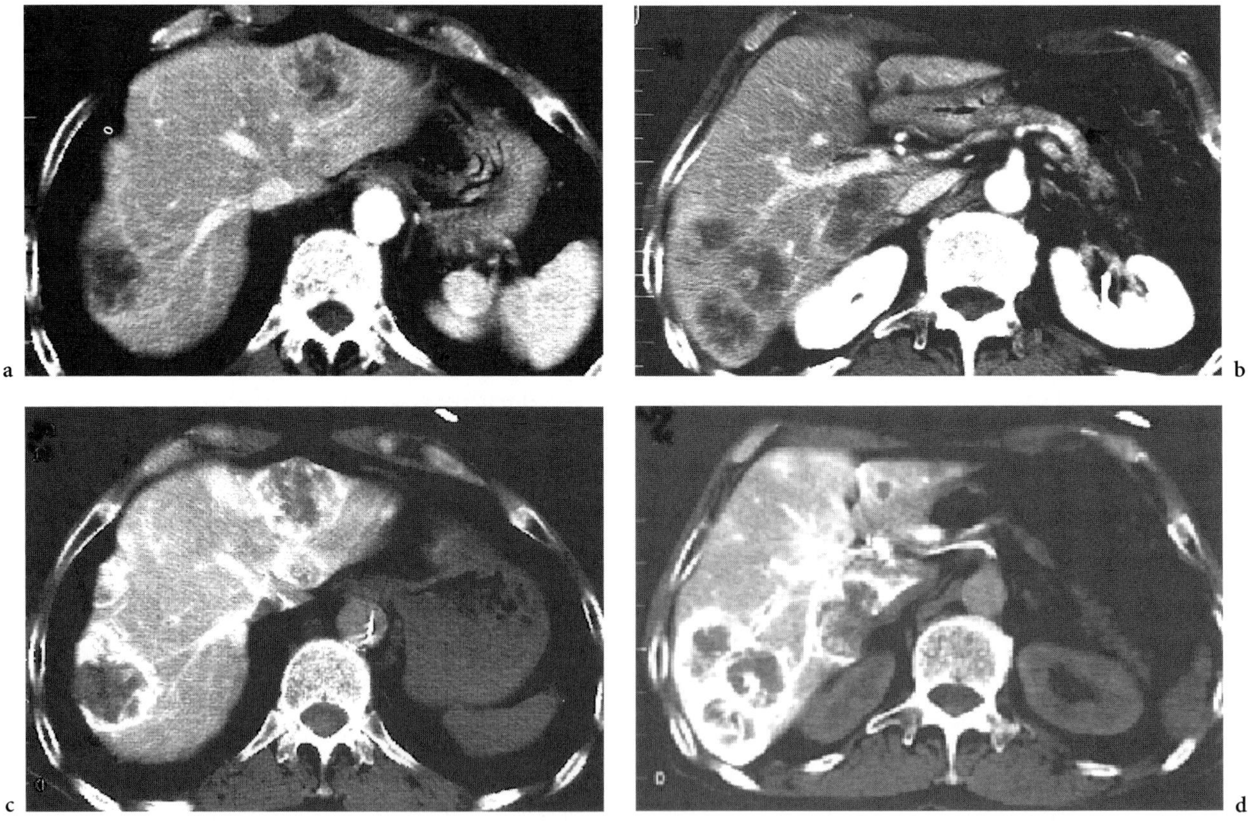

Fig. 25.7a–d. Colorectal liver metastases treated with AIC through percutaneous Port-a-Cath. **a,b** CT before the treatment: lesions in the upper right and left (**a**) and low (**b**) liver lobes, centrally necrotic. **c,d** CT control through the device 24 h after: proper perfusion of the liver; high perfusion of the outer wall of the lesions, well demonstrating the increased drug delivery

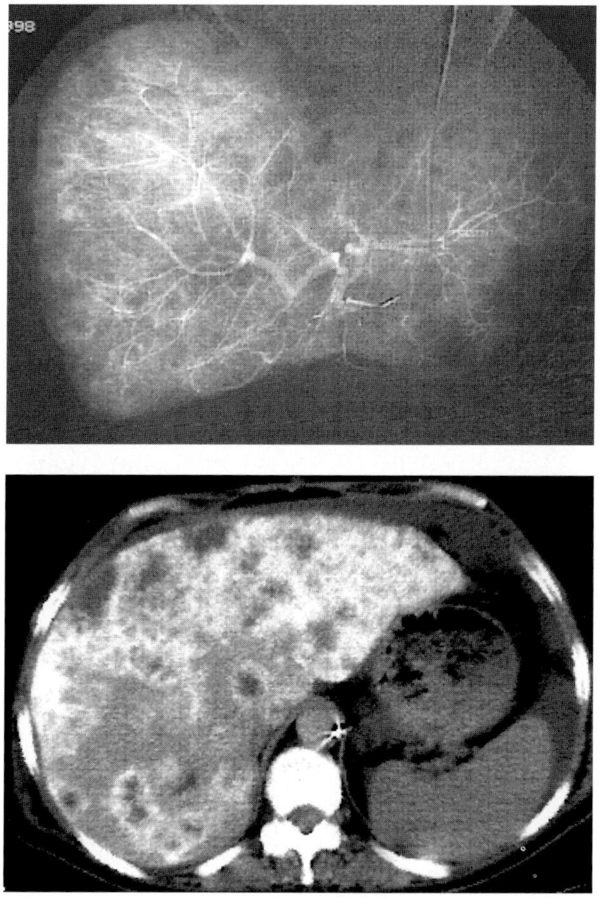

Fig. 25.8a,b. Perfusion controls immediately (**a**, DSA) and 24 h after (**b**, CT)

low (9%) for Arai et al. (1997). In surgical implants the median length of active treatment of 78 patients receiving a port during laparotomy for colon resection or for port implantation was 11 months (Davitti et al. 1992).

Twenty-five complications of surgically implanted port-catheter systems on 78 patients were found by the same group (4 skin necrosis, 3 pocket infections, 2 seromas, 7 extravasation in the area of the chamber with transient local inflammation, 2 ruptures of the catheter and one of the port, 2 hepatic artery thrombosis, 1 artery-biliary fistula, 2 gastric ulcers).

Intrahepatic bilomas (Aoki et al. 1993), pseudothrombosis of the common hepatic artery (Wacker et al. 1995), marked atrophy of the liver (Kameoka et al. 1995), hepatic artery-biliary (Noda et al. 1996) and common bile duct fistulas (Ohori et al. 1996), major upper gastrointestinal hemorrhages (Ross et al. 1996), gastro-duodenal ulcers (Itano et al. 1993), bile duct strictures (Clark and Gallant 1987),

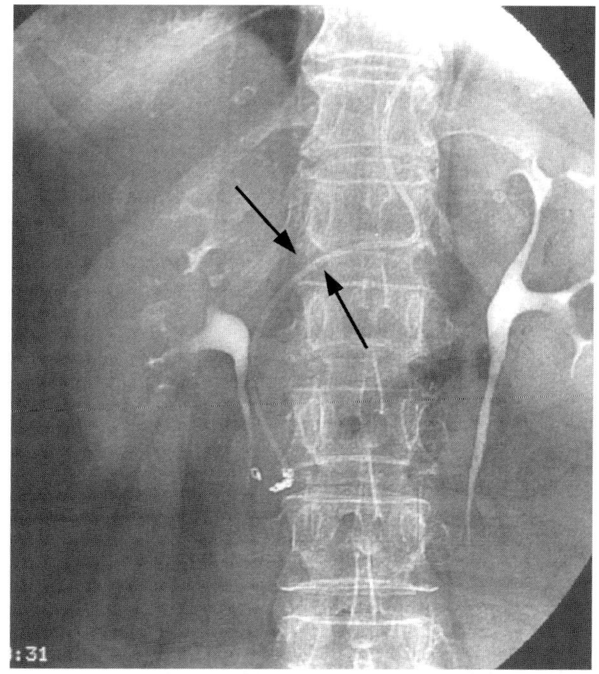

Fig. 25.9. Percutaneous Port-a-Cath by axillary approach. Catheter pulled into the gastroduodenal artery with lateral hole cut in the common hepatic artery. Right gastroepiploic artery embolized (*arrow*) with coils to avoid the passage of drug in the vessels of the gastric wall

progressive arterial perfusion abnormalities (Roth et al. 1989), and fatty metamorphosis in the overperfused liver segment after FUDR therapy (Zeiss et al. 1990) are also reported. Extravasation of 5-fluorouracil (5-FU) following thrombosis of the gastroduodenal artery may perforate into the hepatic artery, portal vein, duodenum or biliary tree causing hepatic artery pseudo-aneurysms (Ross et al.1996).

In the personal still unpublished experience of 122 cases of percutaneously inserted Port-a-Caths, we observed a complication rate of 31% (chiefly pocket infections, ruptures of the catheter and hepatic artery thrombosis) forcing in 33/122 the withdrawal of the device (Fig. 25.10). The incidence of technical problems should certainly decrease along with technical advances, especially new materials.

The reported rate of required hospitalization during the infusion treatment with percutaneous Port-a-Cath has been reported to be 4.3%, 3.9% and 6.5% in cases with colorectal cancer, gastric cancer and breast cancer, respectively, and with an overall rate of 5.1% (Arai 1994).

Using surgical or percutaneous long-term Port-a-Cath infusion, many schedules for the choice of drugs, doses and delivering have been selected by

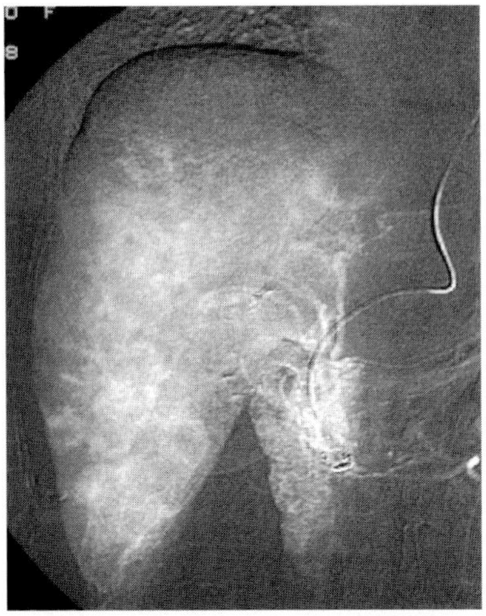

a

Fig. 25.10a–f. Same case as in Fig. 25.9. **a** DSA control: nonproper liver perfusion sparing the left lobe, with passage of contrast medium in duodenal vessels. **b–d** CT control: perfusion of the right lobe. Hyperperfusion of the lesion in the outer wall, suggesting a high-dose delivery of the drug. **e** Later CT control: no perfusion of the right lobe; contrast medium in the left gastric artery with perfusion of the left lobe as well as of the gastric wall. **f** DSA control two weeks later: complete thrombosis of the gastrohepatic artery; patency of the left gastric and splenic arteries. Thrombi around the catheter (*arrows*), despite previous therapy with calciparine

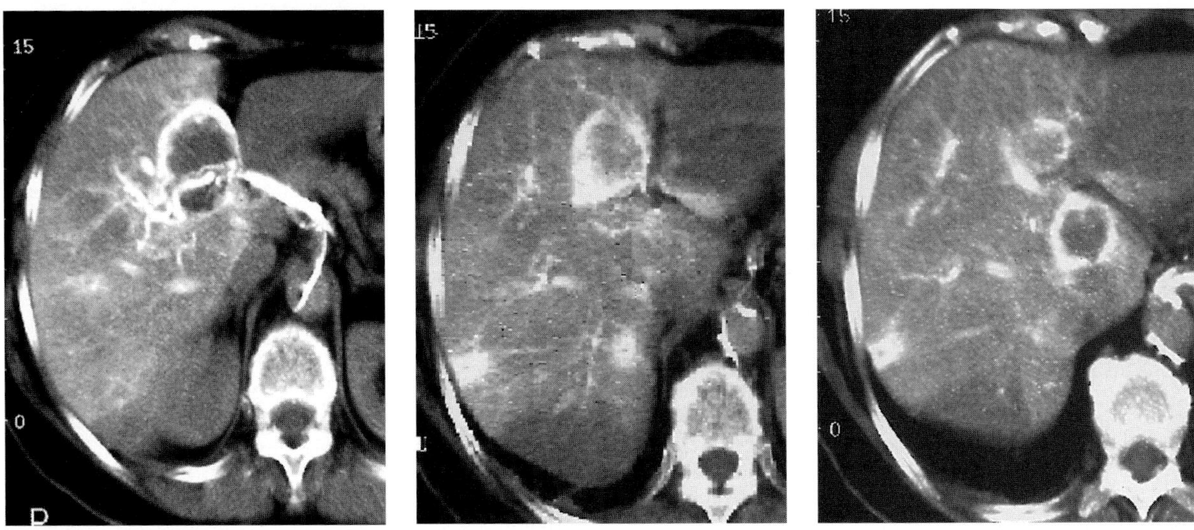

b,c d

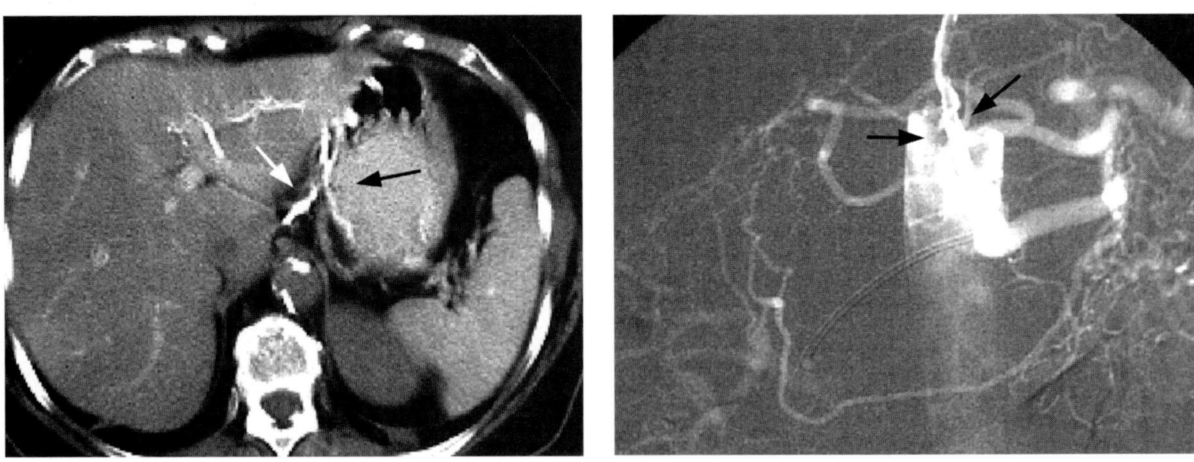

e f

the authors. The most often used drugs have been isolated 5-fluorouracil (Nakayama et al. 1993; Arai et al. 1993,1997), combined mitomycin C and 5-fluorouracil (Sato et al. 1992), 5-fluorouracil plus leucovorin (Shida et al. 1995; Yamamura et al. 1995), platin derivates (Sugimoto et al. 1997; Mori et al. 1993), floxuridine (Allen-Mersh et al. 1994), IL-2 and doxorubicin (Yamamoto et al. 1993), and 5-FU,

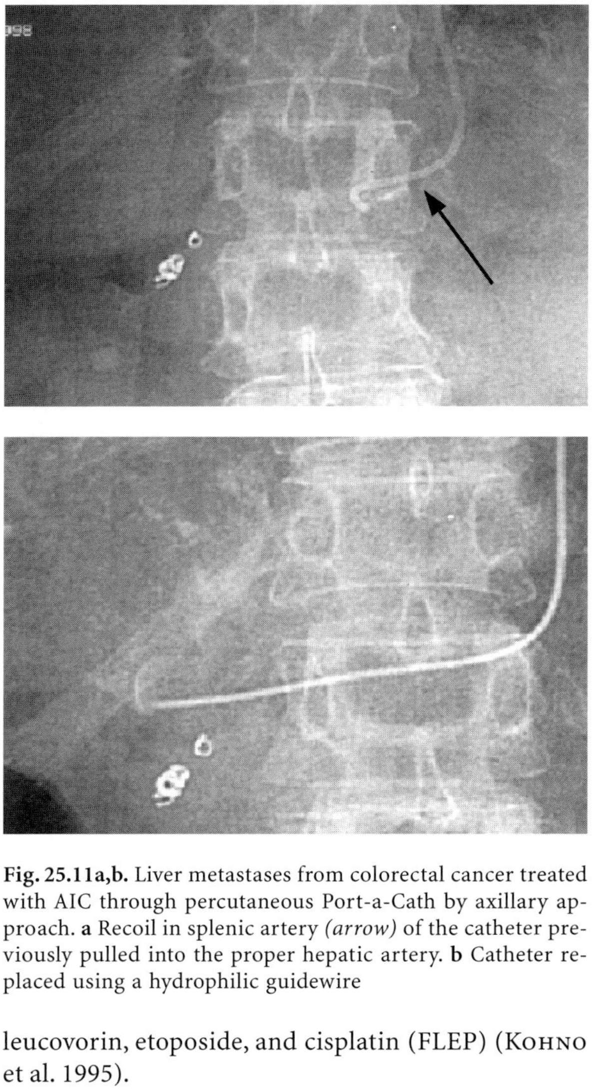

Fig. 25.11a,b. Liver metastases from colorectal cancer treated with AIC through percutaneous Port-a-Cath by axillary approach. **a** Recoil in splenic artery *(arrow)* of the catheter previously pulled into the proper hepatic artery. **b** Catheter replaced using a hydrophilic guidewire

leucovorin, etoposide, and cisplatin (FLEP) (Kohno et al. 1995).

Drugs have been given by continuous infusion in large doses (Sato et al. 1992), by continuous infusion (Yamamoto et al. 1993; Nakayama et al. 1993; Nakamura 1992; Mori et al. 1993; Shida et al. 1995), by weekly intermittent infusion at high doses (Arai et al. 1993,1997; Tsuji et al. 1993), by hepatic artery infusion followed by portal vein infusion (Stephens 1992), by infusion of low dose cisplatin and oral administration of high dose doxyfluridine (Nakagawa et al. 1996), by low-dosage intraportal infusion of 5-FU (Tsujitani et al. 1991) and finally by high-dose intra-arterial infusion plus intraperitoneal chemotherapy (Dazzi et al. 1994). In intermittent hepatic arterial infusion of high-dose 5-FU on a weekly schedule suggested by Arai et al. (1997), 1000 mg/m^2 of 5-FU is administered over 5 h once a week on an outpatient basis.

The frequency of morphological positive response to AIC with Port-a-Caths ranges from 86% for liver metastases from breast cancer to 19% for colorectal metastases treated with low-dose perfusion (Koyanagi 1994). In other reports colorectal metastases showed a higher frequency of response, ranging from 78% (Arai et al. 1997) to 36% (Sidibe et al. 1989) (the last obtained in hypovascular lesions, when in hypervascular 64% of responses was observed by the same group) (Fig. 25.12).

As for survival, 75% at 1 year and 38% at 2 years have also been reported (Iwasaki et al. 1996; Ichikawa et al. 1992; Kondo 1994; Shuto et al. 1997) for colorectal metastases. The maximum reported overall survival was 25 months in colorectal metastases (Arai et al. 1997) and 27 months in breast metastases (Schneebaum et al. 1994; Kitada et al. 1993). Responses obtained using AIC with indwelling catheters are reported in Table 25.2.

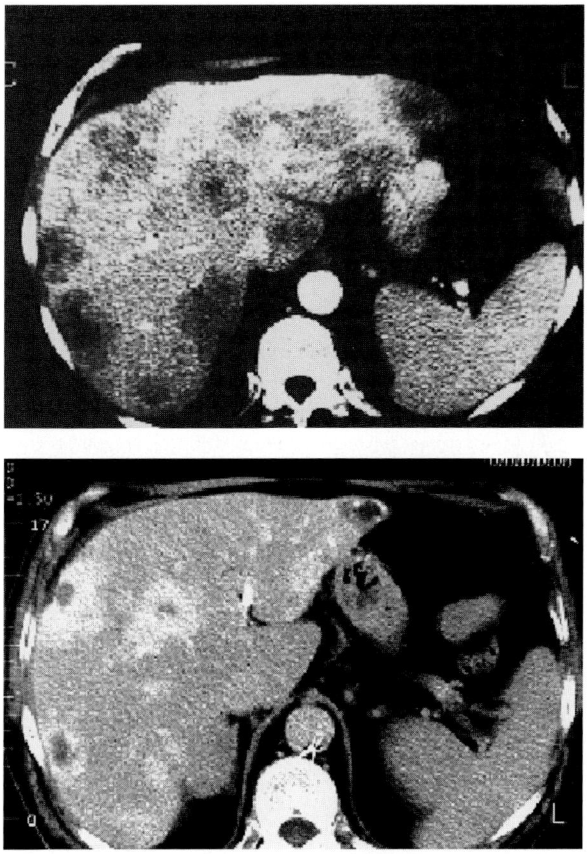

Fig. 25.12a,b. Colorectal liver metastases treated with AIC through percutaneous Port-a-Cath. **a** CT before the treatment: diffuse metastatic lesions in the right and left liver, centrally necrotic and with hypoperfused middle zone. **b** Three months after the start of the AIC decrease of the lesions, together with perifocal hypervascular halo probably expressing reactive granulomatosis

Table 25.2. Morphological and clinical results of AIC through indwelling catheters (surgical and percutaneous implant)

Authors	Year	Primitive	Technique	Response (%)	Overall survival (months)	Survival
ALLEN-MERSH et al.	1994	Colorectal	HAI		13.5	
ARAI	1994	Breast	HAI	81	12.5	
ARAI	1994	Gastric	HAI	72	15	
ARAI	1994	Colorectal	HAI	62		
ARAI et al.	1997	Colorectal	HAI	78	25	
CURLEY et al.	1993	Colorectal	HAI		39	
			Post su. r.			
IWASAKI et al.	1996	Gastric	HAI	66.7		
			Angiotensin II			
SIDIBE et al.	1989	Colorectal	HAI	64		
				Hyperv.		
DAZZI et al.	1994	Colorectal	HAI	59		
			High dose			
ICHIKAWA et al.	1992	Colorectal	HAI	20		2 years: 38%
KOYANAGI	1994	Combined	HAI	52		
			Low dose			
KOYANAGI	1994	Colorectal	HAI	19		
			Low dose			
KOYANAGI	1994	Breast	HAI	86		
			Low dose			
KOYANAGI	1994	Gastric	HAI	33.3		
			Low dose			
SAKAMOTO et al.	1993	Colorectal	HAI	76.6	14.8	
SAWADA et al.	1992	Colorectal	HAI	39		
SCHNEEBAUM et al.	1994	Breast	HAI		27	
SHIDA et al.	1995	Colorectal	HAI	67		1 year: 75%
SIDIBE et al.	1989	Colorectal	HAI	36		
				Hypov.		
Tanada et al.	1996	Colorectal	HAI		15.6	1 year: 54%

HAI, Hepatic arterial infusion

25.3 Transcatheter Arterial Embolization

Transcatheter arterial embolization (TAE) is the first applied technique of angiography by Seldinger's method for the therapy of tumors, and COLDWELL and MORTIMER (1991) believed that liver metastases can be treated by TAE. TAE should, however, be considered out-of-date for the treatment of hepatic metastases except in the case of emergency hemorrhage in order to obtain sudden hemostasis.

For TAE many embolic materials are available, gelatin sponge such as Gelfoam and Spongel, microcapsules of anticancer drugs, albumin microspheres, Lipiodol Ultrafluid, Ivalon, magnetic particles, steel coils, isobutyl-2-cyanoacrylate (IBC), ethanol, and degradable starch microspheres (DSM) (KOIKE et al. 1988, 1989; MAVOR et al. 1987). Gelatin sponge is the most frequently used in liver embolization (Fig. 25.13). It embolizes arteries up to relatively peripheral sites, but it is reabsorbed and then the arteries are reopened.

Microcapsules, albumin microspheres and Lipiodol produce micro-embolization in even more peripheral arteries and are used in DS-TACE and Lp-TACE. Ivalon, magnetic particles, IBC and steel coils are not reabsorbed. The former three agents embolize peripheral arteries, but are only seldom used for hepatic embolization. Coils is routinely employed to occlude proximal arteries during redistribution before the placement of an indwelling catheter or a procedure of hepatic hypoxic perfusion.

Despite its weak rationale, the reported results of isolated TAE in liver metastases are not despicable. A

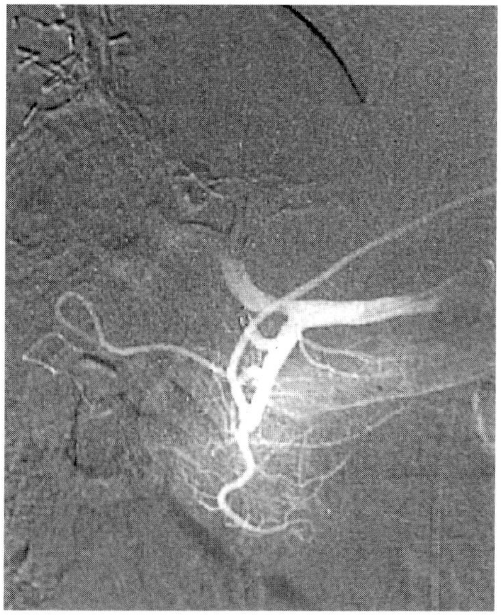

Fig. 25.13. Embolization with gelatin sponge of the whole arterial hepatic system

mean duration of survival of 11.5 months in patients treated with TAE was reported by CHUANG and WALLACE (1981). KURODA et al. (1989) evaluated histologically the effect of TAE in metastatic liver tumors from gastrointestinal cancer resected at surgery or removed at autopsy (TANADA et al. 1997). Three tumors of five were found to be completely necrotized and approximately 80% of the remaining were necrotic.

Extensive thrombosis of the portal system, unusual in liver metastases, is an absolute contraindication for TAE. Embolization can be used, however, in the case of segmental thrombosis. In the case of serum bilirubin levels of higher than 5 mg% or serum cholinesterase levels below 1000 u/ml, embolization procedures should be done in selected cases or using a subselective approach according to GORICH et al. (1993). In our opinion, in patients with metastatic diffuse liver disease showing an increasing progressive level of serum bilirubin, TAE, as TACE or other AIC techniques, should never be used because of their therapeutic uselessness.

Because non-cancerous tissues are also affected, transient hepatic dysfunction may be associated with TAE. GOT, GPT, LDH, and total bilirubin usually increase immediately after, and return to pre-treatment levels about 10 days later. Cholinesterase and serum albumin fall gradually after the treatment, reach the lowest levels about 2 weeks later, and return to pre-treatment levels after about 4 weeks.

These changes depend on the dose of embolic materials and may occasionally progress to unexpected hepatic failure. It is, however, highly uncommon to observe a hepatic failure in TAE-treated patients with previous demonstrated portal venous patency.

25.4 Transcatheter Arterial Chemoembolization

In transcatheter arterial chemoembolization (TACE), the injection of embolic particles follows the intraarterial infusion of chemotherapeutic agents (PENTECOST 1993). TACE may be considered as the most powerful one-shot intraarterial therapy with a high rate of morphological responses for hepatic liver tumors: improvements in long-term survival for patients with metastatic colon cancer have, however, been only suggested but not proven (SOULEN 1997).

Of all the AIC treatments, TACE has been reported to produce the most efficient local tumor control (HOOGEWOUD 1994) and is mainly proposed for the treatment of patients with colorectal metastases to the liver, a resectable primary tumor, and no evidence of other metastatic disease (LANG and BROWN 1993) or for palliation of carcinoid liver metastases (THERASSE et al. 1993).

TACE is typically a two-stage therapy, the first an intraarterial drug infusion, the last a vascular occlusion. The antitumor effect depends on a synergy between the actions of chemotherapy and ischemia, where the occlusion of the tumor arterial supply advantageously follows the controlled infusion of chemotherapeutic drug(s).

Two main procedures are actually employed: DSM-TACE, where reabsorbable microspheres are used as embolizing material: Lp-TACE, so called "targeted therapy" (KONNO 1994), based on the use of oily contrast medium as embolizing material and carrier of antiblastic drugs.

25.4.1 DSM-Chemoembolization

DSM is a suspension of starch microspheres – mean diameter 0.045 mm – obtained through emulsification and polymerization of hydrolyzed potato starch, and suspended in normal saline at 60 mg/ml.

DSM have been in most reports injected together with the intraarterial infusion of the drug, or seldom directly charged with mitomycin C. They have been used experimentally and clinically in the treatment of liver cancer (TEDER and JOHANSSON 1993; MAVOR et al. 1987) to produce a transient vascular occlusion and to slow the blood stream. The potent antitumor effects of DSM-TACE seemed then to derive from the synergistic action of the drug cytotoxicity and retention by DSM (SAKAMOTO et al. 1993). The increase of both the drug's concentration and the time of contact between tissue and drugs improves the efficacy of the drugs inducing a better tumor response (LORENZ et al. 1989). Intraarterially injected DSM also reduce the systemic drug concentration (STARKHAMMAR and HAKANSSON 1987), the temporary blockage of arterioles trapping the co-injected drug in the tumor (STARKHAMMAR et al. 1987). DSM remains in the vascularized liver metastases more than 24 h, resulting in prolonged local delivery of chemotherapeutic agents (PIPERKOVA et al. 1994).

The median biological half-time of the particles within the whole liver was 2.4 days (range 1.5–11.7 days), but was longer in tumors than in normal liver (GOLDBERG et al. 1991b). Based on the mitomycin C levels in the peripheral blood after combined infusion with DSM and mitomycin C, occlusion of intrahepatic vessels with DSM persisted for at least 60 min (FUJIMOTO et al. 1993).

Observations showed a wide range of required DSM dose. Seventy-five percent of the DSM dosage inducing reversed flow in the common hepatic artery should be used for treatment (LORENZ et al. 1989): therefore, each individual dose must be determined by digital subtraction angiography (DSA). A dose of 12.5 mg/kg DSM was found to give an effective tumor targeting as well as a lower regional toxicity.

Vascularity is a major prognostic factor for DSM-TACE as for all techniques of AIC. It is well known that the frequency of hypervascular liver metastases showing complete and partial responses to locoregional treatments is higher if compared to hypovascular metastases.

A reversal of tumor vascularity has been observed by CIVALLERI et al. (1989) after intraarterial injection of DSM: a flow redistribution towards hypovascular areas appeared, showing not previously appreciated cold lesions. A similar effect may also be obtained using intraarterial hypertensive drugs such as angiotensin II or noradrenaline. A postembolization syndrome presenting with transient upper abdominal pain, nausea and vomitting can be expected in nearly two-thirds of treated patients. The observed results of DSM-TACE are reported in Table 25.3.

The highest frequency of positive response for DSM-TACE was 76.2% in colorectal metastases (FUJIMOTO 1994; FUJIMOTO et al. 1993). Forty-two percent of responses in colorectal and 60% in breast metastases, respectively, were observed by LORENZ et al. (1989) and DE DYCKER and TIMMERMANN (1991). Hypervascularization improves the responses of DSM-TACE as of other AIC techniques: 56% of responses occurred in hypervascular lesions, only 12% in hypovascular lesions (CIVALLERI et al. 1989). Hyperthermia has been associated with DSM-TACE by TANAKA et al. (1992) with 40% of responses. Overall survival after DSM-TACE was 12 months for breast and 12±5.9 months for colorectal metastases (FUJIMOTO et al. 1993).

25.4.2 Lipiodol Chemoembolization

In Lp-TACE oily lymphographic agents are used as carriers to convey the anticancer drug to a hypervascular tumor tissue, enabling a simple but effective "targeted chemotherapy": the combination between oily agent and drug is termed "oily anticancer agent" (KONNO 1994). A mean survival time of

Table 25.3. Morphological and clinical results of chemoembolization with detachable starch microspheres (DSM-TACE)

Authors	Year	Primitive	Technique	% Response	Overall survival
CIVALLERI et al.	1989	Combined	DSM-TACE	56 (hyper.)	
CIVALLERI et al.	1989	Combined	DSM-TACE	12 (hypo.)	
DE DYCKER et al.	1991	Breast	DSM-TACE	60	12 months
FUJIMOTO et al.	1993	Colorectal	DSM-TACE	76.2	12.6±5.9 months
LORENZ et al.	1989	Colorectal	DSM-TACE	42	
TANAKA et al.	1992	Combined	DSM-TACE plus hyperthermia	40 (if more than 42°)	

15.8 months and a 2-year survival rate of 23.3% have been reported by SATOH et al. (1990) in metastatic liver cancers treated with chemoembolization using a mixture of an anticancer drug with Lipiodol plus Gelfoam, considered more effective than a mixture of an anticancer drug with Gelfoam alone.

Lipiodol, the most used oily agent in Western countries, is given in Lp-TACE by intraarterial injection: to achieve the targeting, newly formed vessels should be present in the lesion together with evidence of neovascularity, and the tumor should be stained. If there is no vascularity in the tumor, Lipiodol will not flow into it, explaining the high efficacy of Lp-TACE in the treatment of hypervascularized metastases from carcinoid and the low effect in hypovascular colorectal metastases.

Lipiodol should be injected in the proper hepatic artery: in cases with occlusion of the celiac trunk or thrombosis of the hepatic arterial system following multiple procedures Lp-TACE is possible in any case with modern coaxial catheters via tortuous segments of the pancreaticoduodenal arcades (GORICH et al. 1996; BILBAO-JAUREGUIZAR et al. 1991), superior phrenic arteries or hepatic collaterals (Figs. 25.14, 25.15).

Hyperselective Lp-TACE may be used (if associated with percutaneous ethanol injection) for the treatment of single small hepatocellular carcinoma, but in multiple liver metastases only a whole-liver therapy should be performed and the mixture must be injected into the proper hepatic artery.

Lipiodol is delivered proportionally to tumor and normal hepatic tissue depending on the degree of vascularization. It is eliminated from the normal tissue relatively quickly, usually disappearing after 24 h but stays longer in hypervascular tumor tissues, so indicating the efficacy of tumor targeting. Tumor to liver ratios of dose delivered ranged from 1.21:1 to 4.7:1 (median 3.1:1) (PERRING et al. 1994) in cases of hypervascular lesions.

Non-cancerous tissues are also affected by Lipiodol embolization. It is recommended therefore to strictly determine the minimum necessary volume of Lipiodol to inject. In the whole-liver treatment needed for diffuse metastatic disease it is not possible to limit the effect on non-cancerous normal tissues by superselective catheterization. A case is reported where hyperselective Lp-TACE was performed in the left lobe, due to the need to spare the normal liver tissue after a right lobe resection for breast liver metastases (Figs. 25.16, 25.17).

For a successful Lp-TACE targeted therapy, the anticancer drug should be homogeneously suspended in oil droplets and must be stable in the oil,

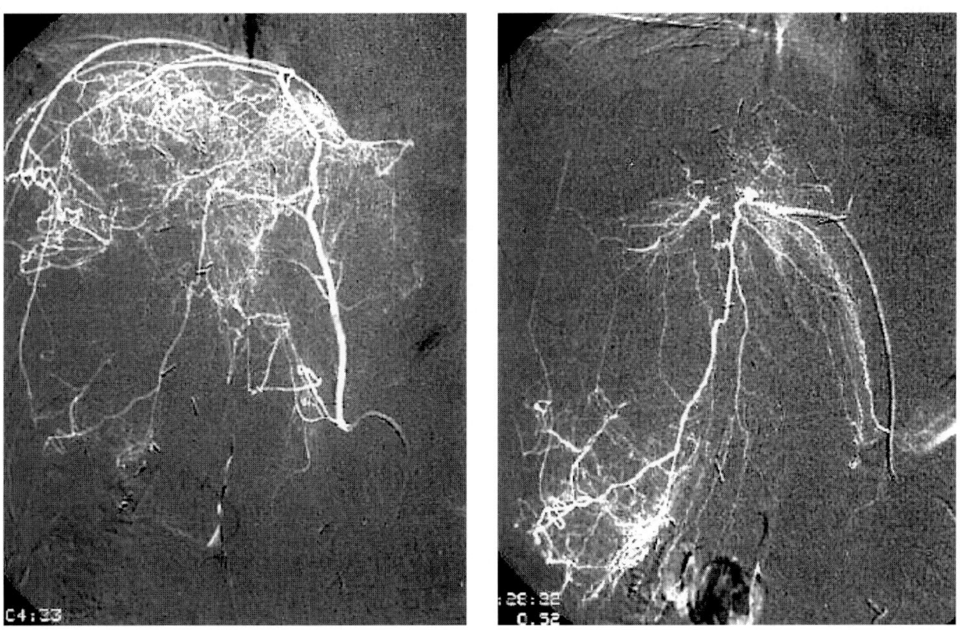

a b

Fig. 25.14a,b. Liver metastases from colorectal cancer treated with Lp-TACE performed through collateral vessels. Complete thrombosis of the hepatic artery after two sessions of HHP and one session of Lp-TACE. Inferior right phrenic artery used for the treatment. **a** Proximal subselective catheterization used to treat the upper segments of the right lobe. **b** Distal hyperselective catheterization to perfuse the caudal segments. A 4F hydrophilic catheter has been used

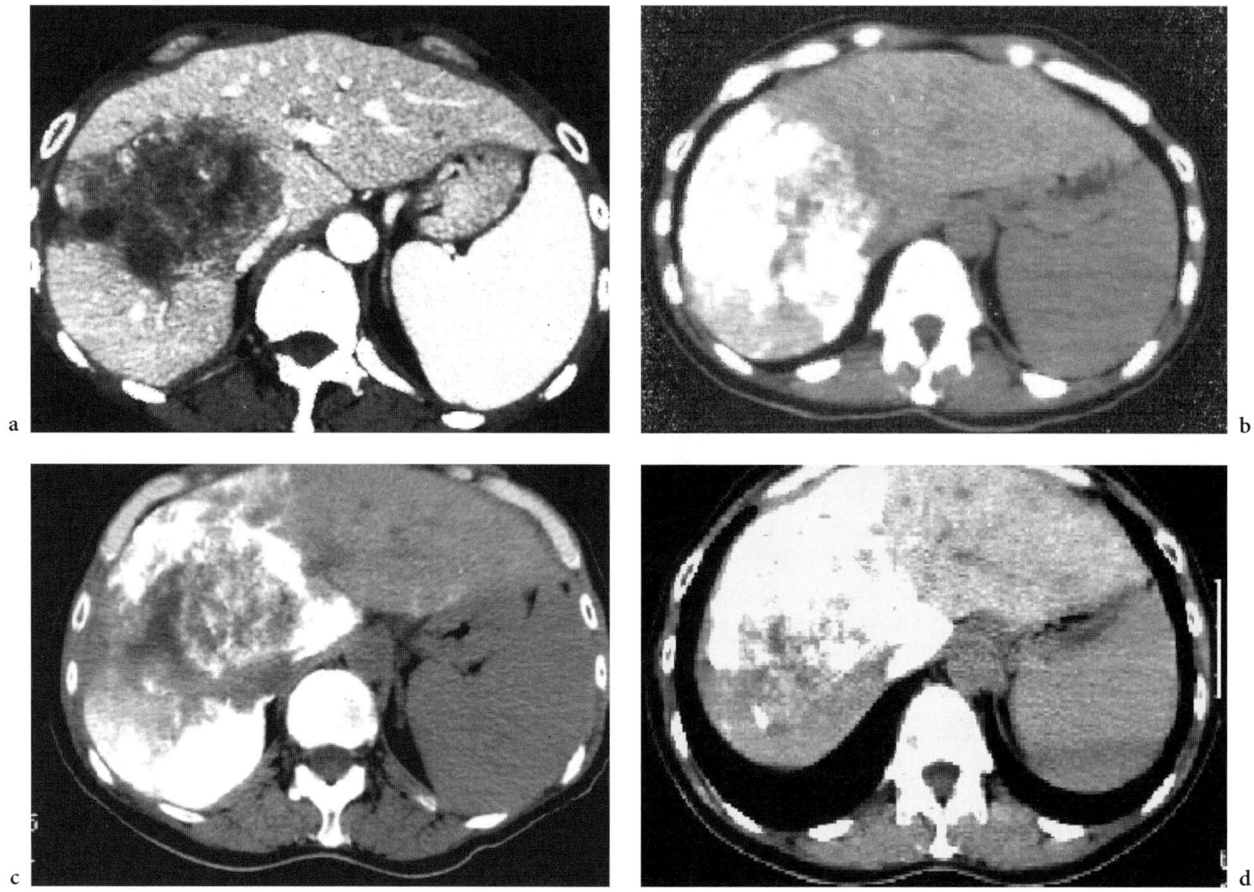

Fig. 25.15a–d. Same patient as in Fig. 25.14. CT controls. **a** Large lesion in the central right lobe before the treatment. **b** Lipiodol after the first session of Lp-TACE with hypertensive induced therapy through the hepatic artery. **c,d** Lipiodol uptake after a further session of Lp-TACE. Infusion in the inferior right phrenic artery. Hypertensive treatment unnecessary because of the small caliber of the feeding vessels to the tumor ensuring a forced infusion of the oily contrast medium

gradually diffusing from the droplets to the surrounding cancer tissues. Lipiodol will act as a reservoir for the anticancer agent (Konno 1994).

The mixture between Lipiodol and drug is usually done dissolving the drug in hydrosoluble contrast medium and mixing the solution with Lipiodol with a 3-way stopcock. Relatively stable mixtures can be prepared if anticancer drugs are dissolved in 60% Urografin, a water soluble contrast medium with distilled water at 1/5 the volume of Urografin: the specific gravity is equivalent to that of Lipiodol and stable mixtures (i.e., water-in-oil emulsion) can be obtained. However, prolonged delivery, which is the biggest advantage of the Lp-TACE, is partially lost in this case because Lipiodol is separated from the drug contained in the hydrosoluble contrast medium, easily washed out leaving the Lipiodol alone in the tissue (Konno 1994). Water soluble anticancer agents should then be used in Lp-TACE if directly dissolved in Lipiodol.

The patterns of Lipiodol uptake in liver metastases were classified into 4 types: homogeneous accumulation (20%) (Fig. 25.18), heterogeneous accumulation (16%), accumulation with a central defect (57%), and no accumulation (7%) (Fig. 25.19) (Inoue et al. 1989).

An obvious correlation was observed between tumor vascularity and Lipiodol accumulation (Sugimoto 1994). The Lipiodol was found to deposit on the periphery of metastases of less than 10 cm diameter (Perring et al. 1994) and to remain in hepatic metastases during the first month in 94%, after 2 months in 31%, and after 3 months in 17% (Kobayashi et al. 1987). An improved targeting of Lipiodol in hypovascular lesions may be achieved using the intraarterial infusion of hypertensive drugs as angiotensin II or noradrenaline (Fig. 25.20).

Adverse events following Lp-TACE such as liver infarction, necrosis of the biliary ducts, bile cysts

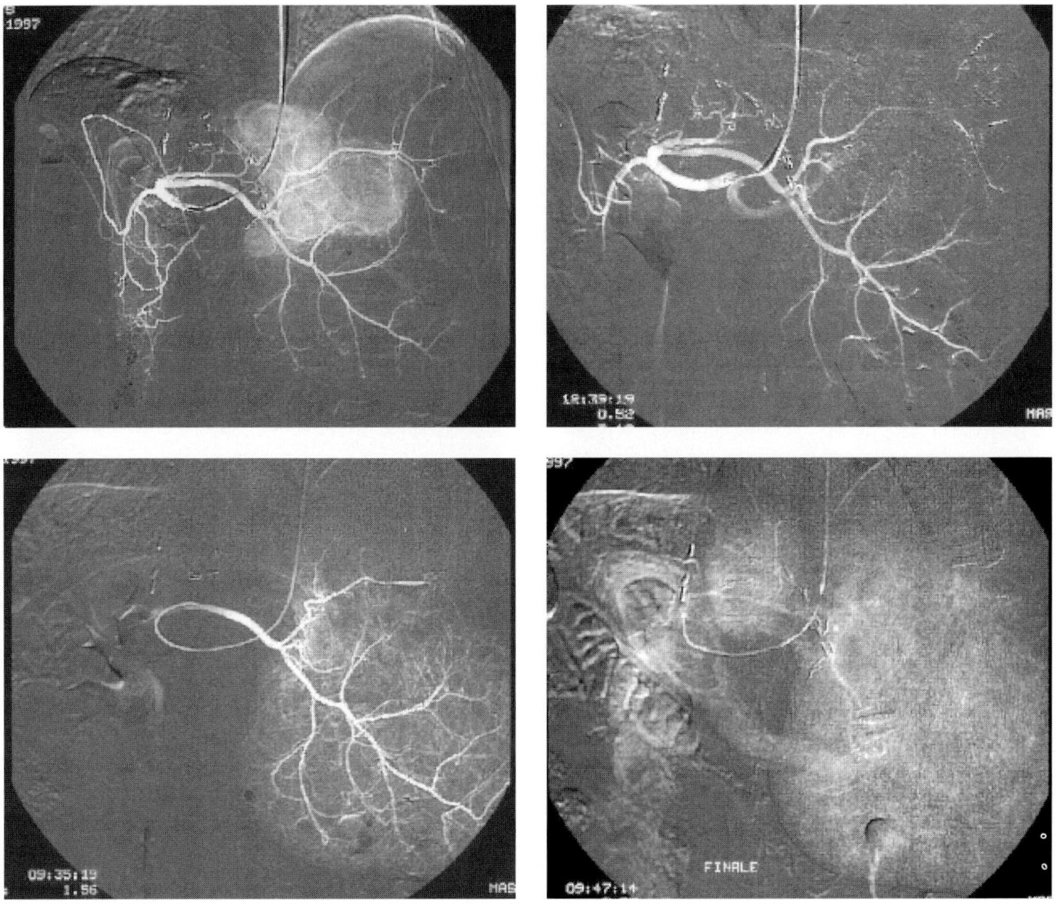

Fig. 25.16a–d. Liver metastases from breast cancer in the left lobe appeared five months after resective surgery of the right lobe. **a** Proximal subselective DSA of the residual hepatic artery : hypervascularized lesion. Lp-TACE performed hyperselectively with coaxial catheters to treat only the affected segments, sparing the normal tissue. **b** Final result. **c,d** DSA control three months later: no revascularization found

(Tsuruta et al. 1990), sclerosing cholangitis (Richardet et al. 1994), bilomas (Inoue et al. 1991), gastroduodenal ulcerations, etc., are below 5% (Gorich et al. 1993). No similar cases were observed in our personal experience, where a high frequency of hepatic arterial thrombosis appeared in patients undergoing multiple sessions of Lp-TACE.

Morphologic changes in the gallbladder after Lp-TACE have been observed in 45.9% of cases due to transient ischemic damage by inflow of Lipiodol with anticancer agent into the cystic artery, which is almost inevitable.

Postembolization syndrome with upper abdominal pain, nausea and vomiting can be expected in nearly two-thirds of patients. A major portal vein obstruction, a compromised hepatic functional reserve, an excessive amount (>20 ml) of iodized oil and a biliary obstruction were considered (Chung et al. 1996) as important predisposing factors to post-embolization syndrome, even if they should rather be considered as true contraindications to Lp-TACE.

Hepatic arterial occlusion after repeated procedures (Chung et al. 1996) not infrequently occurs after multiple Lp-TACE treatments such as after Port-a-Cath infusion or hypoxic hepatic perfusion. Collateral pathways such as inferior phrenic artery or GD may be used to continue the transcatheter treatment (Duprat et al. 1988).

As in TAE, thrombosis of the main or right portal vein should be considered as an absolute, and of the left portal vein as a relative, contraindication: if serum bilirubin levels exceed 5 mg/ml, Lp-TACE as all embolization and chemoembolization procedures should not be performed, except in selected cases or with a hyperselective approach (Gorich et al. 1993).

Pulmonary oil embolism was reported by Chung et al. (1993) if more than 20 ml of iodized oil is used

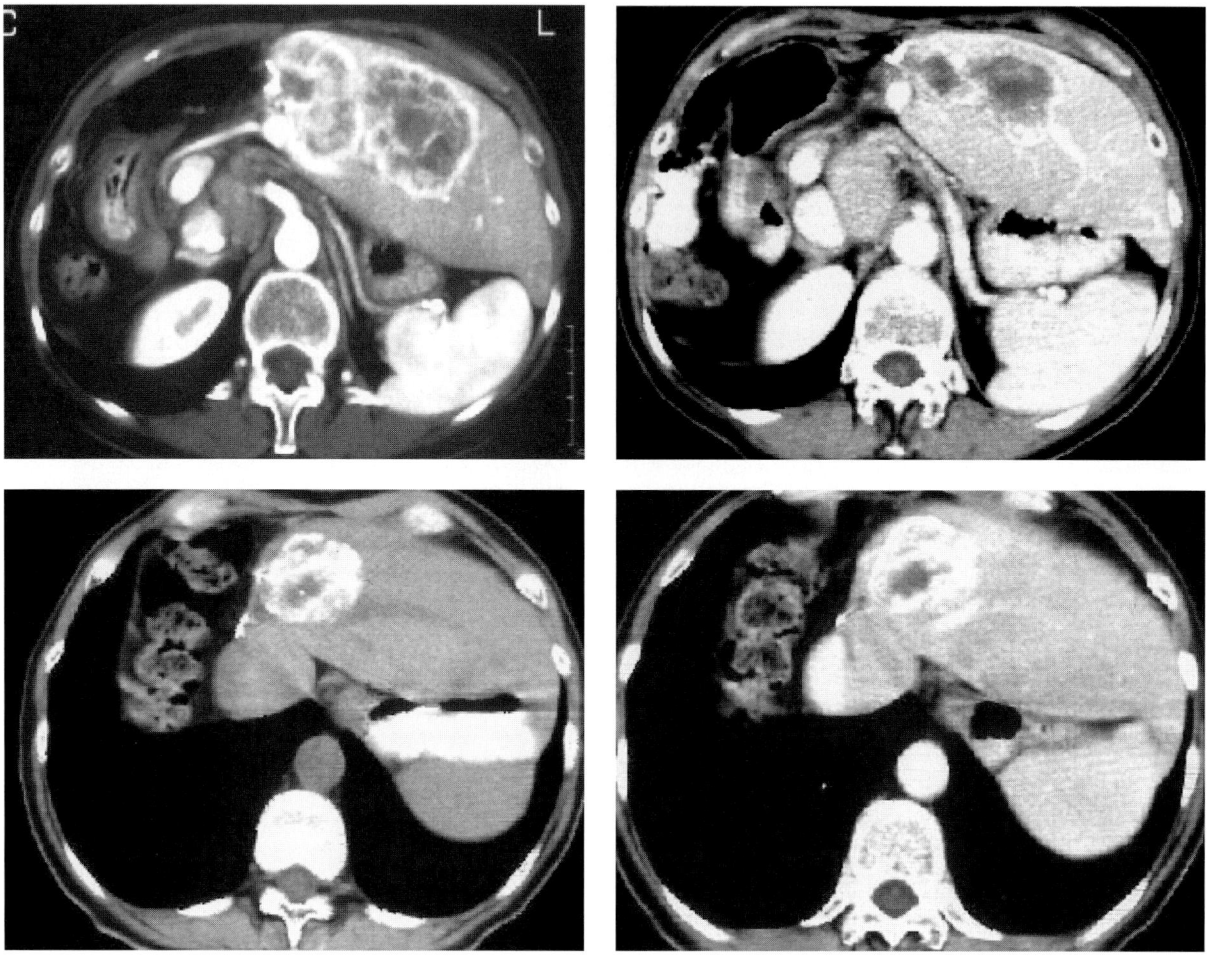

a b c d

Fig. 25.17a–d. Same case as in Fig. 25.16. **a** CT before the treatment: two large highly vascularized masses in the left lobe. **b** CT control three months after hyperselective Lp-TACE: strong reduction in size of the lesions with slight residual peripheral staining. **c** Direct CT three months after the treatment: uptake of Lipiodol. **d** Enhanced CT: no change of the lesion during the enhanced phase, suggesting no recurrence

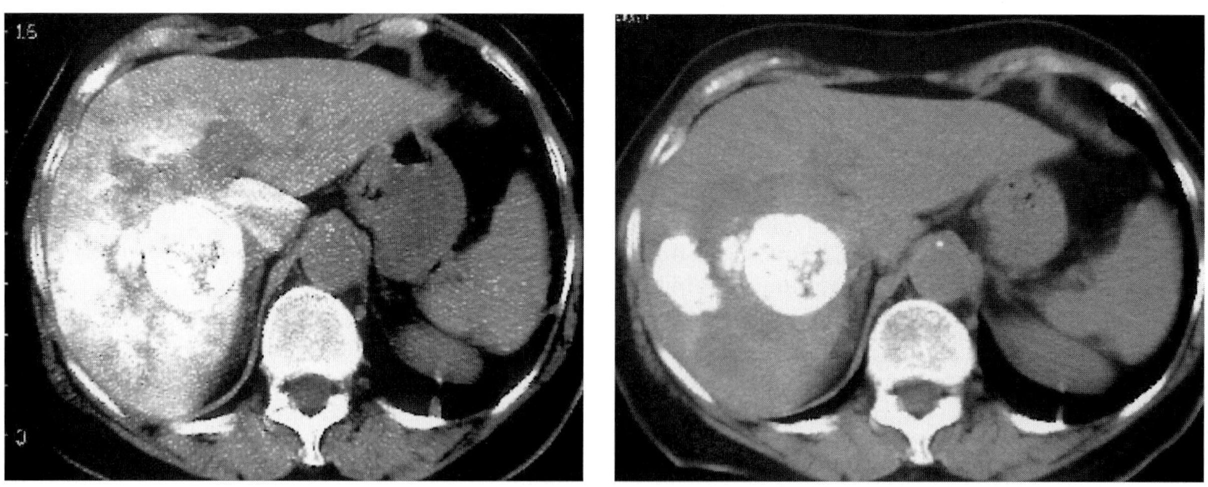

a b

Fig. 25.18a,b. Liver metastases from ovarian cancer treated with Lp-TACE. **a** CT control 24 h after the treatment: strong Lipiodol uptake in a large lesion of the right lobe with satellites around it. Lipiodol partially opacifies the normal liver tissue. **b** CT control two months later: Lipiodol remains in the lesions, when normal tissue is completely washed

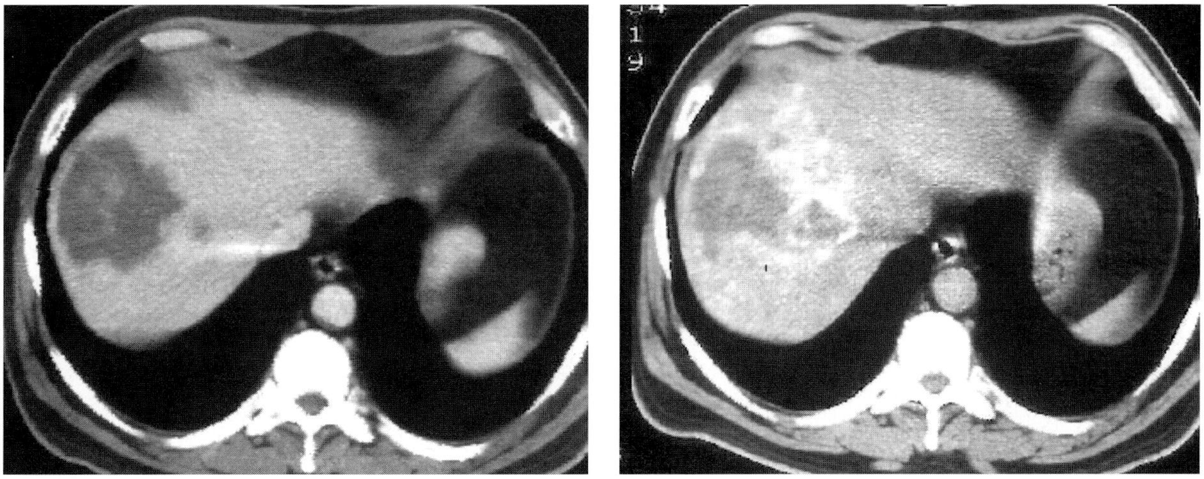

a b

Fig. 25.19a,b. Liver metastases from colorectal cancer treated with Lp-TACE. **a** CT before the treatment: large lesion in the central right lobe with satellites. **b** CT control two weeks later: poor uptake of Lipiodol in the lesion, suggesting a low therapeutic effect

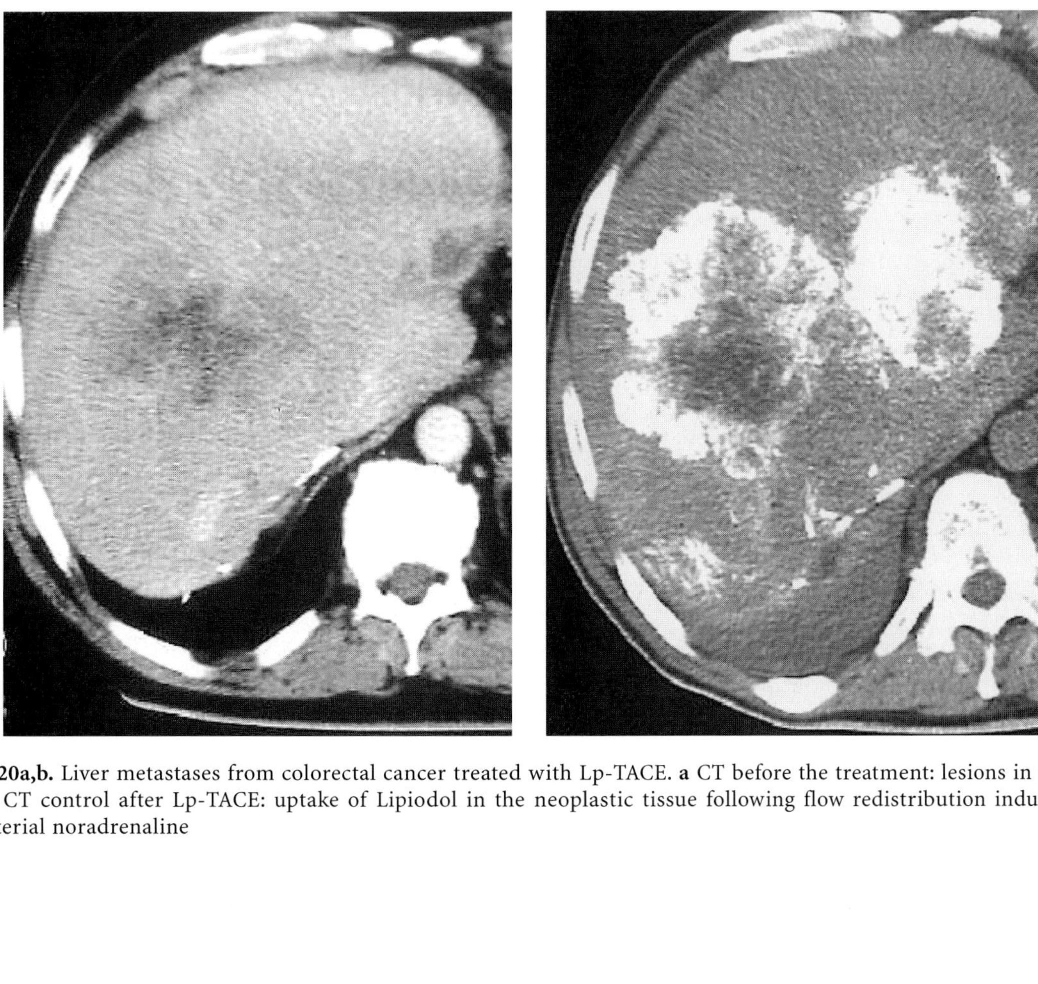

a b

Fig. 25.20a,b. Liver metastases from colorectal cancer treated with Lp-TACE. **a** CT before the treatment: lesions in the right lobe. **b** CT control after Lp-TACE: uptake of Lipiodol in the neoplastic tissue following flow redistribution induced with intraarterial noradrenaline for Lp-TACE: one death occurred 10 days after the treatment because of a respiratory arrest with progression of the pulmonary infiltrate. A total dose of 15 ml of Lipiodol should therefore never be exceeded (Takayasu et al. 1987).

The most often used drugs for Lp-TACE have been adriamycin combined with mitomycin C (Kobayashi et al. 1987; Inoue et al. 1989; Links et al. 1993; Konno et al. 1994), isolated Adriamycin (Suzuki et al. 1992), cisplatin (Kameyama et al. 1988. Araki et al. 1989) and 5-fluoro-2-deoxy-uridine-C8 (Yamashita et al. 1989). Doses commonly employed have been 20–60 mg for doxorubicin (Chung et al. 1996), 40–80 mg for adriamycin (Links et al. 1993), 10 mg for mitomycin C (Sanz Altamira et al. 1997), and 100 mg for cisplatin (Sasaki et al. 1994). In our personal experience 1 mg/kg of doxorubicin dissolved in 15 ml of Lipiodol was routinely delivered. The summary of responses obtained by Lp-TACE is reported in Table 25.4.

Positive responses occurred with a frequency of 60% in hypervascular carcinoid metastases (Nobin et al. 1989; Hanssen et al. 1991). In colorectal metastases, response ranged from 59% in hypervascular to 17% in hypovascular (Kameyama et al. 1993). An overall survival of 13.83 months in colorectal metastases has been observed by Tanada et al. (1996). The maximum 1-year survival for colorectal metastases has been 70% (Yamashita et al. 1989); a 5-years survival of 75% is reported by Hanssen et al. (1991) for carcinoid metastases.

In our personal experience (Roversi 1996) with 27 cases of hepatic metastases from colorectal cancer treated with Lp-TACE with Lipiodolized doxorubicin, positive responses occurred in 43%. In 70% of the patients lost during the follow-up the reason of death was intrahepatic progression, suggesting a low control of Lp-TACE on the hepatic disease. Fifty percent of cases of post-procedure syndrome were also seen by us according to Gorich et al. (1993), with 48% of WHO-based toxicity.

25.5 Hypoxic Hepatic Perfusion

It has been demonstrated (Kameyama et al. 1989, 1993) and previously reported for chemoembolizations with DSM and Lipiodol that a delayed washout of intratumor blood flow with stagnation is associated with the highest concentration of the drug in the hepatic tissue, due to the lack of washout and to a strong increase of the time of contact between the tumor and the drug, with a better extraction during the first pass in the liver.

The occlusion with a balloon catheter of the proper hepatic artery has been initially used to prevent chemoembolic agents from flowing into the gastric branches, redirecting blood flow toward the liver to protect against gastric complications (Nakamura et al. 1991). AIC after the occlusion of hepatic arterial flow has been used for hepatocellular carcinoma (Une et al. 1993) to increase the intrahepatic drug concentration, resulting in response rates higher than those with free-flow infusion

Table 25.4. Morphological and clinical results of chemoembolization with Lipiodolized drugs (Lp-TACE)

Authors	Year	Primitive	Technique	% Response	Overall survival	% Survival
Gorich et al.	1993	Colorectal	TACE	60–80%		
Jacobsen et al.	1995	Carcinoid	TAE	39%		5 years: 71.4%
Hanssen et al.	1991	Carcinoid	TAE	60%		5 years: 75%
Inoue et al.	1989	Colorectal	TACE	59%	11.1 months	1 year: 43%
Kameyama et al.	1993	Colorectal	TACE	50% hyperv.		
Kameyama et al.	1993	Colorectal	TACE	17% hypov.		
Konno et al.	1994	Combined	TACE			1 year: 61%
Nobin et al.	1989	Carcinoid	TAE/DEART	60%		
Sugimoto et al.	1994	Colorectal	TACE	56%	12 months	1 year: 46.8%
Tanada et al.	1996	Colorectal	TACE		13.83 months	1 year: 63%
Yamashita et al.	1989	Colorectal	TACE	46%		1 year: 70%

methods (KAMEYAMA et al. 1989, 1993). A modified stop-flow whole-liver technique of AIC was then developed expressly for the treatment of hepatic metastases (ROVERSI et al. 1997).

A 5-French catheter is percutaneously introduced in the proper hepatic artery: the femoral approach has been used at first, but we actually believe that the brachial or axillary approach should be preferred because of an easier subselective hepatic catheterization. The first step of the hypoxic hepatic perfusion (HHP) is DSA control of the patency of the portal system, which is mandatory also in embolization procedures such as TAE, Lp-TACE or DSM-TACE. A complete redistribution of the arterial flow to achieve a single vessel hepatic inflow must also be performed if necessary according to the criteria proposed for AIC with Port-a-Cath.

The embolization of the RGA to avoid the passage of the drug in the gastric vessels is unnecessary before HHP because of the reversal of flow in RGA following the balloon inflation. GD should be embolized only when the balloon must be inflated in the gastrohepatic artery, due to a short proper hepatic artery (Fig. 25.21). In those cases GD embolization prevents the washout effect by the reversed flow from GD in the arterial hepatic system. The diagnostic catheter is then changed on an hydrophilic guide wire with a 5F balloon catheter (Fig. 25.22). The balloon is placed proximally up to the hepatic bifurcation distally to GD, and the main lumen is connected with a peristaltic pump system. The balloon is then inflated with contrast medium diluted in saline and the hepatic arterial stop-flow is fluoroscopically controlled (Fig. 25.23). Next 250–300 ml of saline with 20–30 mg of MMC are infused by the peristaltic system in 10 min, the infusion starting 5 min after the inflation of the balloon. MMC is used in our protocol because of the strengthening of the cytoreductive effect of alkylating drugs that occlusive ischemia induces on tumor tissues, with a ratio of 10:1 if compared to normoperfused tissues (THEICHER et al. 1981). After the infusion and before the deflation of the balloon a forced embolization of the arterial hepatic system is performed, to obtain a gelatin sponge cast in the arterial system (Fig. 25.24). The balloon catheter is then removed.

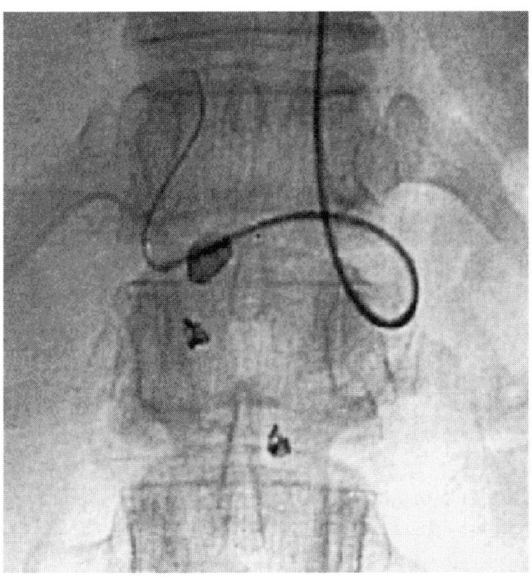

Fig. 25.21. Axillary approach for HHP. Gastroduodenal artery embolized with coils. Balloon inflated in the gastrohepatic artery at the level of GD. Embolization of GD to avoid the reversal of flow in GD toward the hepatic arterial system, limiting the stop-flow effect and washing the drug out of the liver

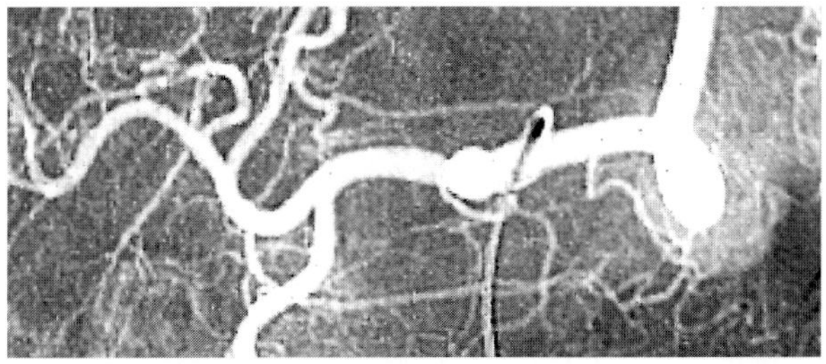

a

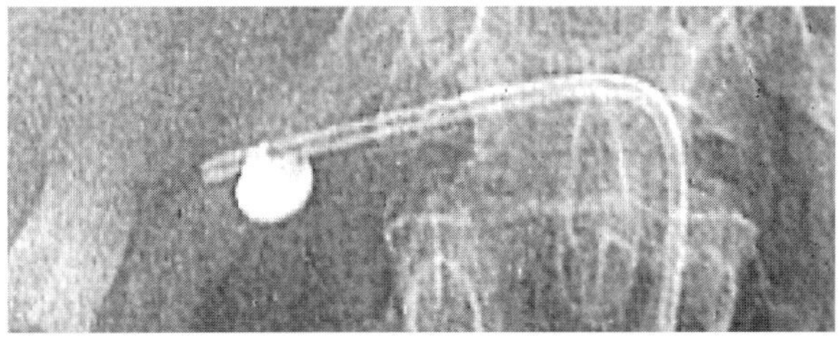

b

Fig. 25.22. a Selective DSA of the celiac axis. b 5F balloon catheter inflated in the proper hepatic artery before HHP

It should be emphasized that a free-flow intraarterial hepatic injection of a drug is followed by an only transient increase of its plasmatic concentration due to the washout effect, if compared to a stop-flow injection. The cessation of the hepatic arterial stream in HHP highly reduces or eliminates the washout effect, so extending the drug-tissue contact. It has been reported that tumors with a free-flow washout time of the drug of less than 80 s are not very responsive to locoregional treatments (KAMEYAMA et al. 1993). A prolonged time of contact between drug and neoplastic tissue obtained with the hepatic arterial occlusion may therefore amplify the cytoreductive effect, which is also improved by the complete first passage extraction and by the ischemic enhancement.

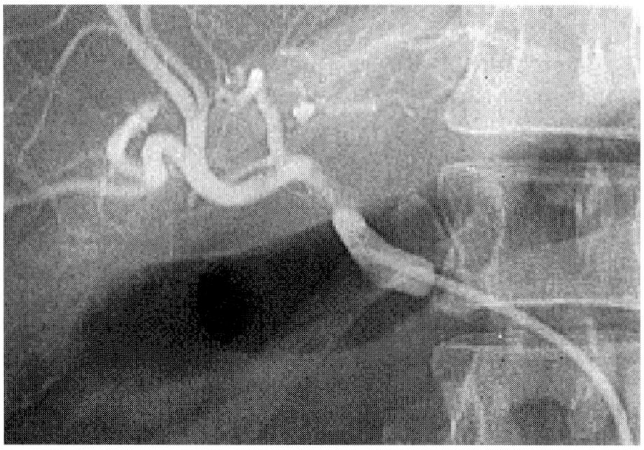

Fig. 25.23. DSA unsubtracted control of the intraarterial stop-flow immediately before HHP. Staining of the contrast medium in proximal hepatic artery. Balloon lengthening along the arterial axis, probably due to overinflation, carefully to avoid to prevent hepatic arterial thrombosis

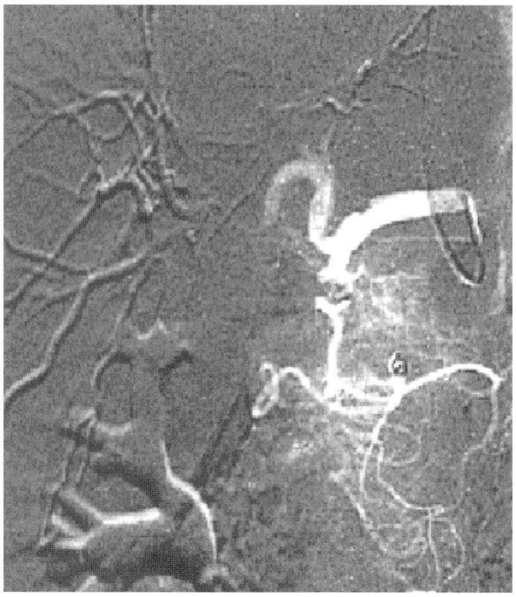

Fig. 25.24. TAE with gelatin sponge after HHP

The balloon occlusion during intraarterial drug perfusion of a volume of solution large enough then achieves a whole-liver perfusion, with a plasmatic concentration of the drug equal to the drug's concentration of the injected solution, and a drug-tissue time of contact maintained for the length of the balloon inflation.

Patient posture should also be considered in HHP, because of the changes of the liver perfusion observed during free-flow intraarterial infusion (Sone et al. 1993).

A selective cytoreductive effect should also be expected using HHP: it is well known (Wallace et al. 1990) that arterial perfusion of liver tumors accounts for more than 90% whereas the portal system contributes two-thirds to the perfusion of normal liver parenchyma (Fig. 25.25).

Hypoxia following hepatic arterial occlusion will then shoot mainly tumor cells, with a selective increase of the cytoreductive effect of MMC (Theicher et al. 1981), lower in the normal liver tissue from which arises the major part of the blood flow from the portal venous system.

The morphologic responses of HHP observed in 98 patients treated for hepatic metastases (mainly from colorectal cancer) are reported in Table 25.5. Apparently complete morphologic responses after HHP (complete necrosis with absence of enhanced viable tissue) occurred in 48% of our patients (Figs. 25.26, 25.27) and responses more than 50% in 80% (Figs. 25.28–25.31). Progression of the disease or no change appeared in 20%. The reported frequency of positive responses for HHP is similar to the frequency obtained using long-term Port-a-Cath infusion (78%) (Arai et al. 1997). CT controls, however, were performed much sooner in our experience (35–40 days). A post-procedure syndrome occurred in 55% of the patients and in 9% an ischemic cholecystitis was observed at CT control (Fig. 25.32). Death also occurred in one patient with a normal portal system, showing a massive hepatic necrosis together with a hepatorenal syndrome four days after a HPP.

Thrombosis of the proper hepatic artery occurred in about 20% of the cases treated with a single session of HHP, probably due both to the overinflation of the balloon with following intimal lesion and to intimal damage by hyperconcentrated drug. In cases in which HHP has been repeated, the frequency of thrombosis of the proper hepatic artery increased up to 60% or more (Fig. 25.33).

No cases of toxicity after HHP occurred; 66% of the patients were symptomatic before the treatment: in 67% of them symptoms disappeared with improvement of the performance status.

Table 25.5. Morphological results of hypoxic hepatic perfusion (Roversi R, unpublished data)

	No of cases	%
Total	98	100
Complete responses	47	48
Partial responses	32	33
No change or progression	19	19

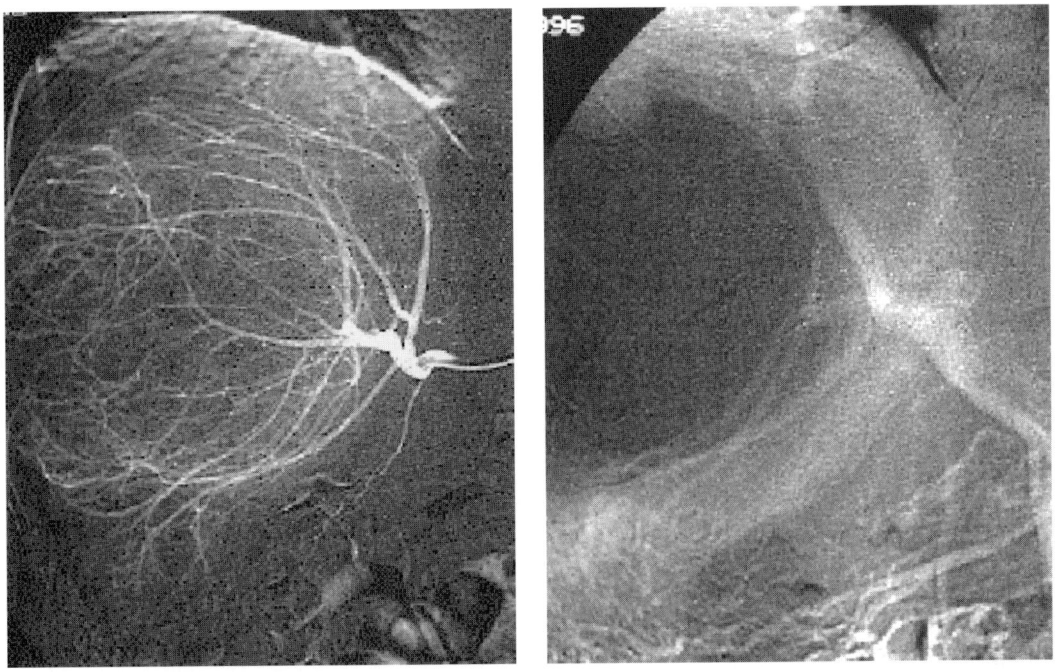

a b

Fig. 25.25a,b. Hepatic subselective DSA. Liver metastases from colorectal cancer. **a** Arterial phase. Central hypervascular lesion in the right lobe, fully supplied by hepatic arteries. Newly formed vessels in the lesion. **b** Portal venous phase. The lesion appears as a "black hole", without any supply by the portal venous system

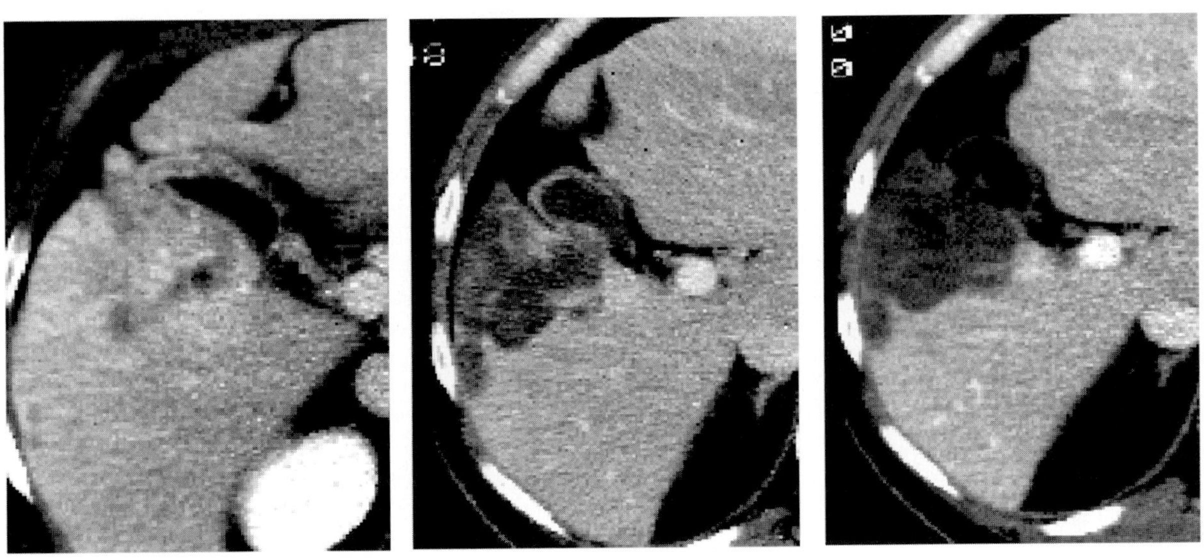

a,b c

Fig. 25.26a–c. Liver metastases from gallbladder cancer treated with HHP. **a** CT before the treatment: lesions near the external wall of the gallbladder. **b** CT control 35 days after first HHP: extensive necrosis of the lesions with remnants of viable tissue. **c** CT 35 days after second HHP: progression of the necrosis with disappearance of remnants

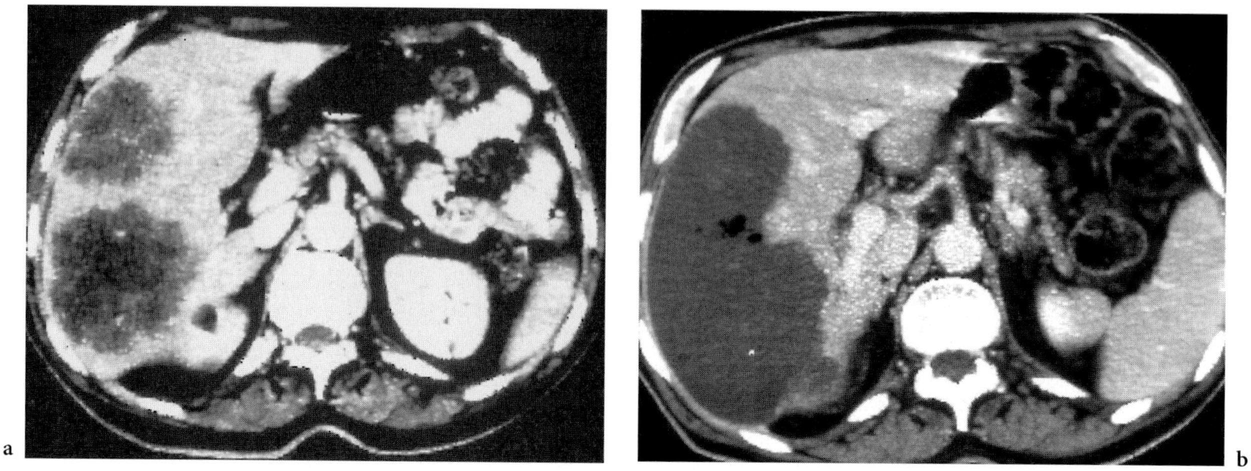

Fig. 25.27a,b. Liver metastases from colorectal cancer treated with HHP. **a** CT before the treatment: large lesions occupying most of the central right lobe. **b** CT control 35 days after HHP: extensive necrosis of the lesions without evidence of remnants of viable tissue

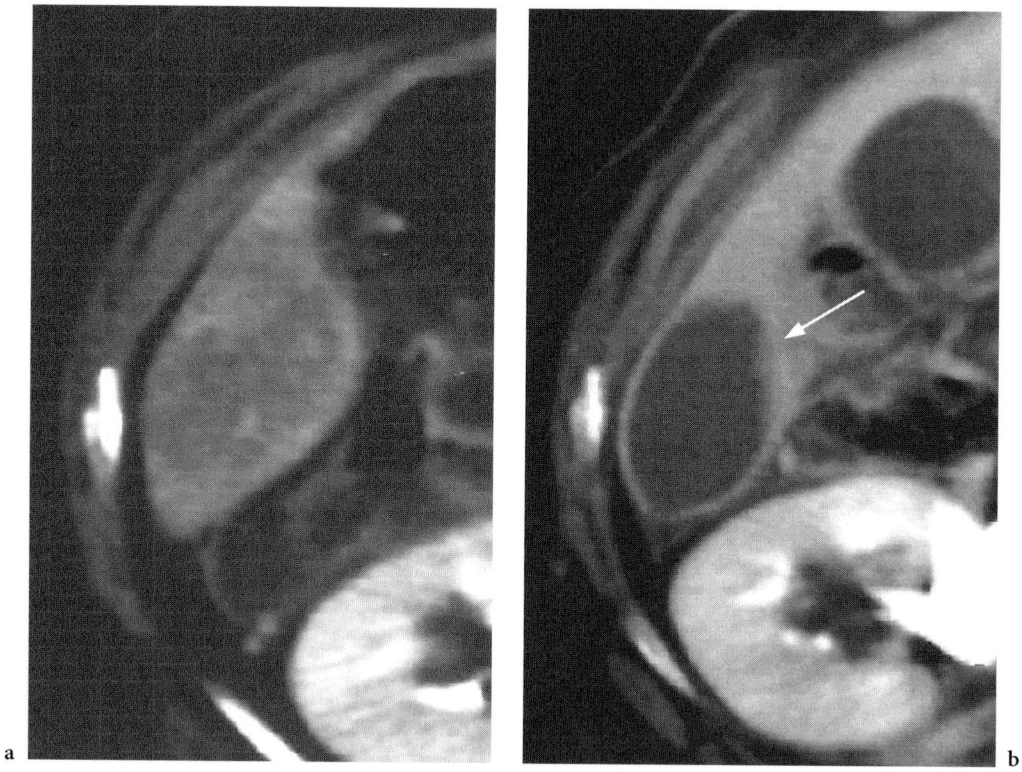

Fig. 25.28a,b. Liver metastases from colorectal cancer treated with HHP. **a** CT before the treatment: a lesion in the fifth segment of the right lobe. **b** CT control after HHP: extensive necrosis of the lesions, with remnants of viable tissue on the outer wall *(arrow)*

Fig. 25.30a–d. Liver metastases from colorectal cancer treated with HHP. **a,b** CT before the treatment: lesions in the left lobe. **c,d** CT controls after HHP: extensive necrosis of the lesions, with remnants of viable tissue ▷

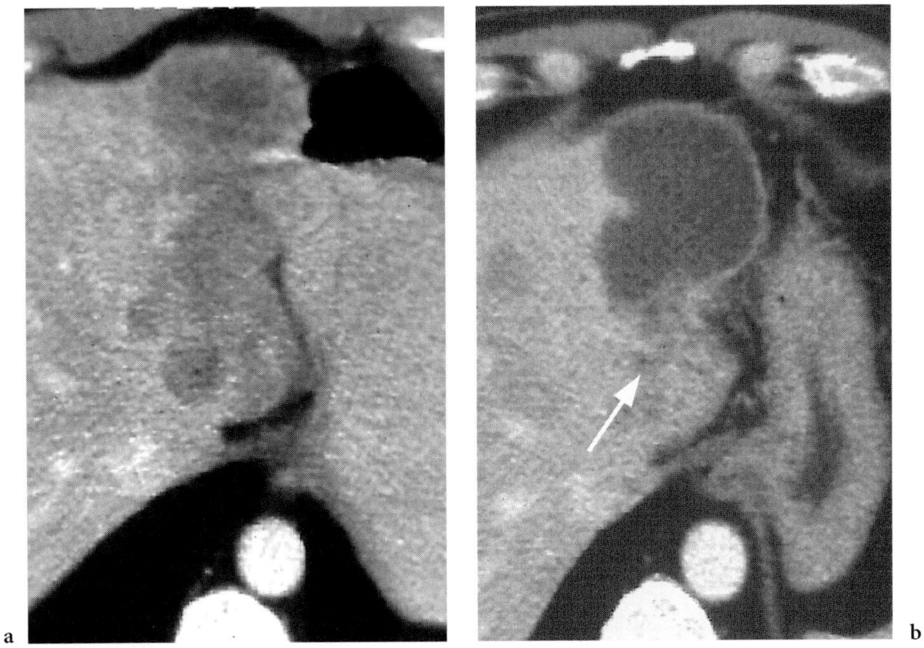

Fig. 25.29a,b. Liver metastases from colorectal cancer treated with HHP. **a** CT before the treatment: lesions in the left lobe. **b** CT control after HHP: extensive necrosis of the lesions, with remnants of viable tissue on the lower zone *(arrow)*

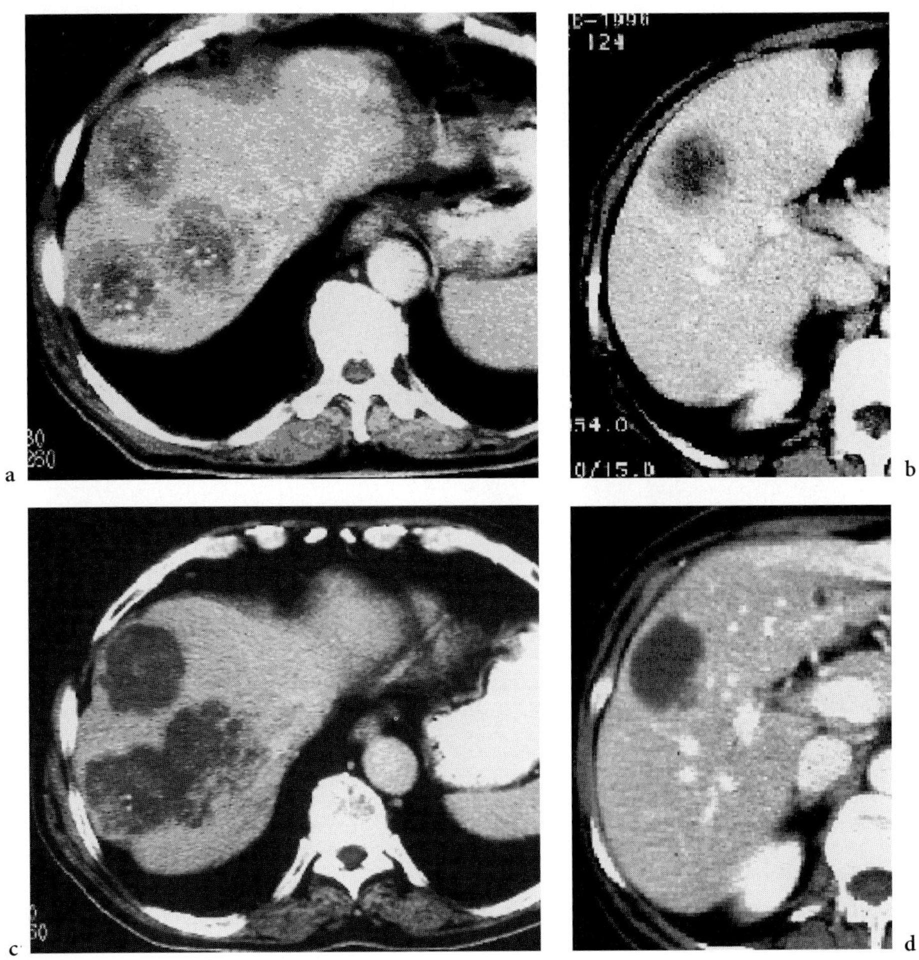

a,b

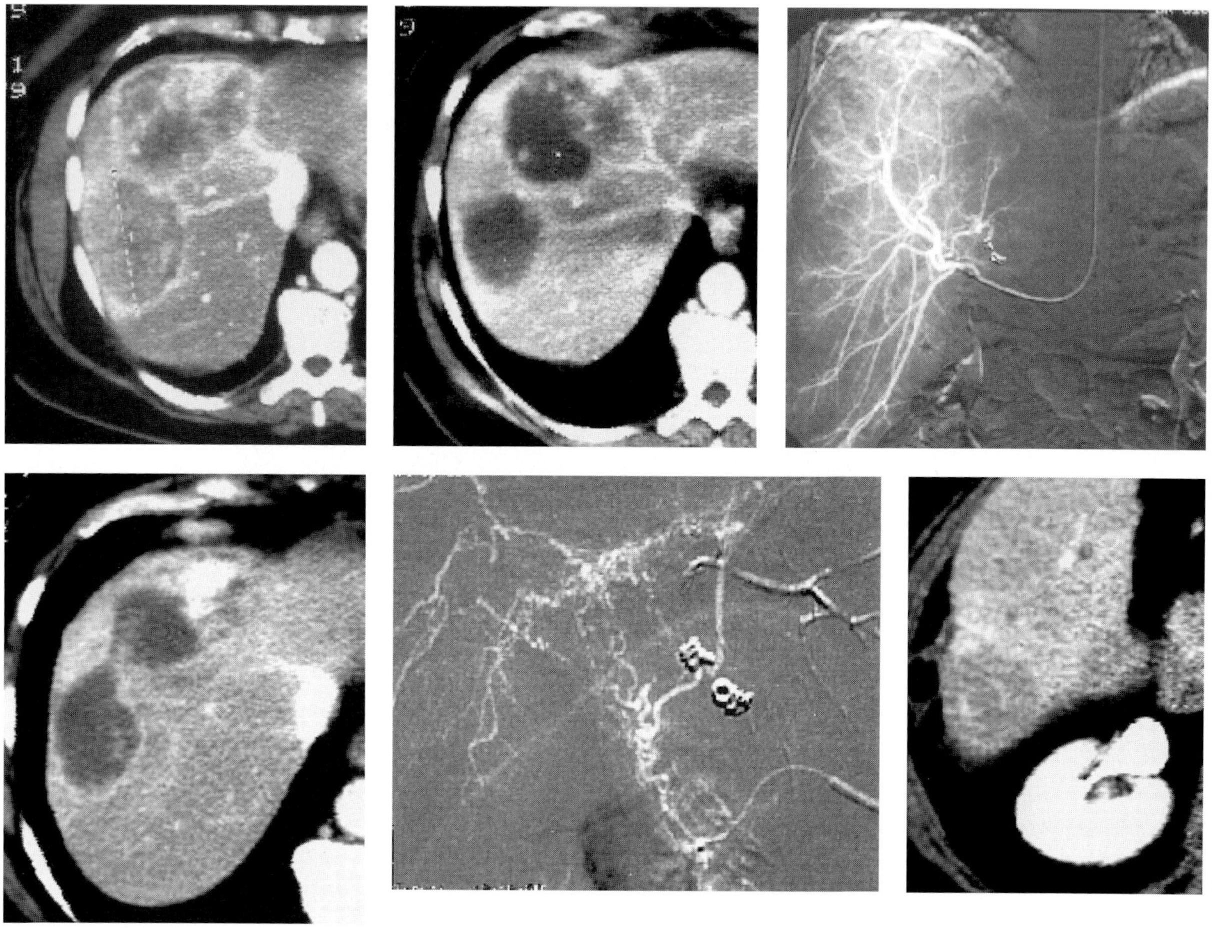

c

d,e

f

Fig. 25.31a–f. Liver metastases from colorectal cancer treated with two sessions of HHP. **a** CT before the treatment: lesions in the upper right lobe. **b** CT control 35 days after the first HHP: partial response with extensive necrosis. **c** DSA: further HHP procedure three months later. **d** CT control 35 days after: positive response confirmed by shrinking of the lesions and signs of calcification. **e** Thrombosis of the hepatic artery after a third HHP session. Coaxial catheter introduced in collateral vessels to perform Lp-TACE. **f** CT control four months later: recurrence in the fifth segment of the liver, programmed for thermoablation

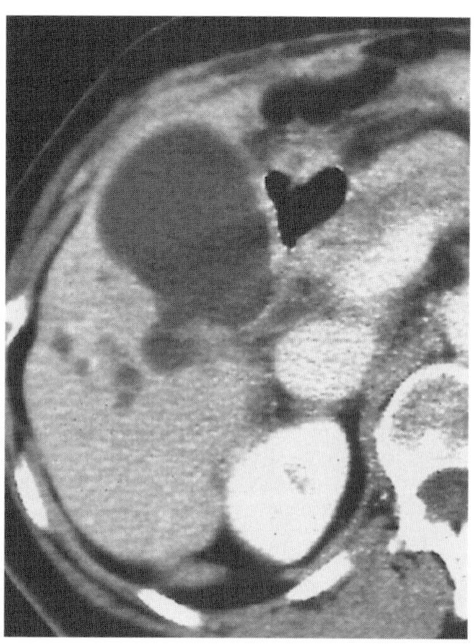

Fig. 25.32. Ischemic cholecystopathy following HHP. Enlargement of the gall-bladder

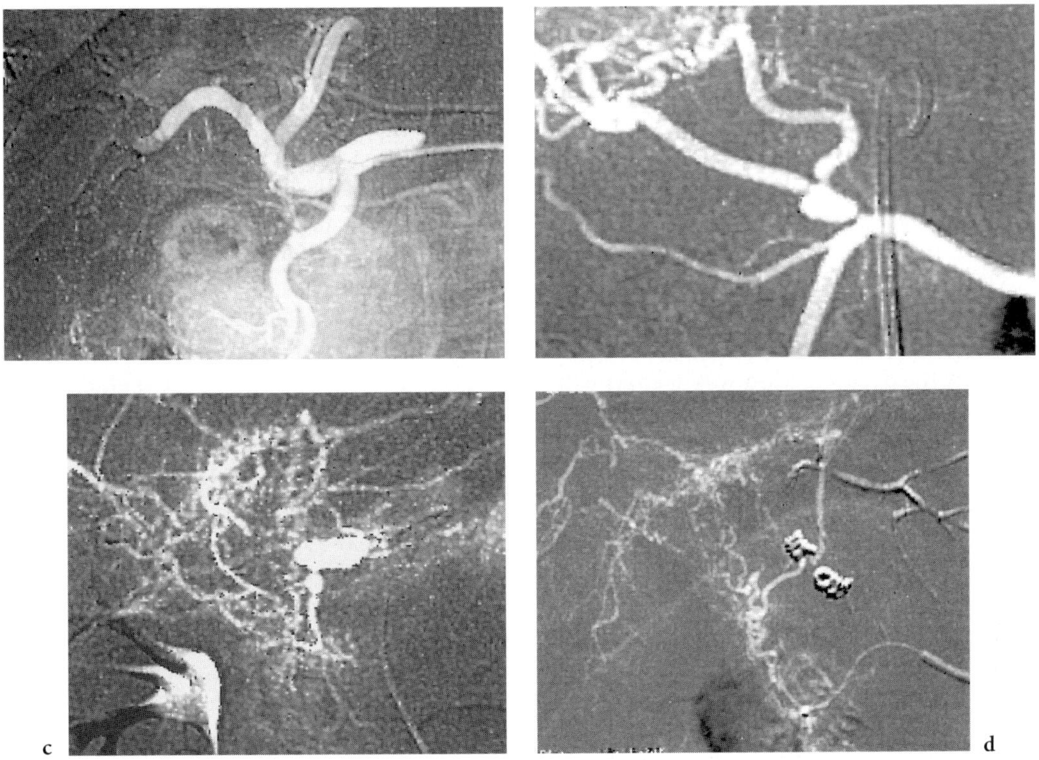

Fig. 25.33a–d. Iatrogenic arteriopathies after HHP. **a** Dissection of the hepatic artery. **b** Stenosis with pseudoaneurysm observed three months after the first treatment. **c** Thrombosis of the hepatic artery. **d** Whole thrombosis of the arterial hepatic system appeared after the third treatment

25.6 Drug Targeting

The most important limit of AIC in treating hypovascular liver metastases is the low targeting of the drug. Only a fraction of the drug itself flows into the tumoral tissue if metastases are vascularized as or less than normal tissue, and most of the therapeutic action is lost. Two negative effects result: first, that adverse reactions are induced on normal liver tissue; second, that a higher dose is needed to obtain a positive response, enhancing the damage on the normal liver. To improve the targeting of drug so sparing normal tissue DSM have been used initially as previously reported.

Angiotensin II (Inoue et al. 1997) and noradrenaline (Sato 1994) were seen to enhance drug delivery in AIC for hepatic tumors if injected, either by the intravenous or the intraarterial method. The theoretical purpose of the so called induced hypertensive chemotherapy is to increase the blood flow in the tumor so improving delivery of anticancer drug and targeting to tumor tissue.

During hypertension induced by drugs the blood flow in both primary and secondary liver tumors did not change, while blood flow in liver parenchyma decreases (Taniguchi et al. 1996): as a result, a relative increase in tumor blood flow appears.

Delivery of cytotoxic microspheres to liver tumors using DSM-TACE may be improved by manipulating the tumor to the normal liver blood flow ratio using angiotensin II (AT-II) (Leen et al. 1993).

Measuring hepatic arterial blood flow (HABF) in patients with colorectal liver metastases during and after an intraarterial infusion of AT-II (15 μg in 3 ml of saline over 90 s), HABF was reduced by 70–76% within 30 s of the start of AT-II infusion, recovered rapidly from the end of the infusion, and increased by up to 20% above the baseline for approximately 2 min (Leen et al. 1993). The median increase in tumor normal tissue ratio following angiotensin II infusion was by a factor of 2.8 (Goldberg et al. 1989, 1991c). Angiotensin II may also be given, as noradrenaline, through a peripheral vein by a microinfusion pump. When systolic pressure rose to about 140 to 150 mmHg, drug can be delivered through an implanted port or by bolus injection (Iwasaki et al. 1996). Increased blood flow following AT-II infusion may then increase the exposure of tumor to therapeutic agents (Hemingway et al. 1992). Two-route chemotherapy under AT-II induced hypertension using a totally implanted injection port system for liver metastases derived from digestive cancers was used by Hokita et al (1989).

As for DSM, the intraarterial infusion of noradrenaline (AT-II is not available in Western countries) has been employed by us to improve the targeting of Lipiodol in hypovascular liver metastases. A significant increase of the accumulation was seen as compared to the basal injection (Figs. 25.34, 25.35).

25.7 Combined Techniques

To obtain results in the therapy of tumors, all available techniques should be theoretically associated and used at their best. Nevertheless, available studies on combined techniques do not always offer satisfactory results. Combining TAE, radiotherapy, immunotherapy, and infusion chemotherapy with hyperthermia in 45 cases with liver metastases, Nagata et al. (1997) obtained at CT control 3% of complete responses and 38% of partial, with 29% progression of the disease. Combined hepatic irradiation and hepatic artery infusion even if well tolerated (Miller et al. 1989) seem not to improve survival (Wiley et al. 1989; Ajlouni et al. 1990).

As regards the relationship between resective surgery and AIC, a treatment including neo-adjuvant locoregional immuno-chemotherapy, surgical resection and adjuvant locoregional immuno-chemotherapy has been used by Lygidakis et al. (1997) in patients with unresectable liver tumors, with an amazing 5-year survival rate of 65% and overall response rate of 80% (Suzuki et al. 1987).

Adjuvant chemotherapy following complete surgical resection of the primary tumor has been suggested (Saltz 1991). Some authors believe that in

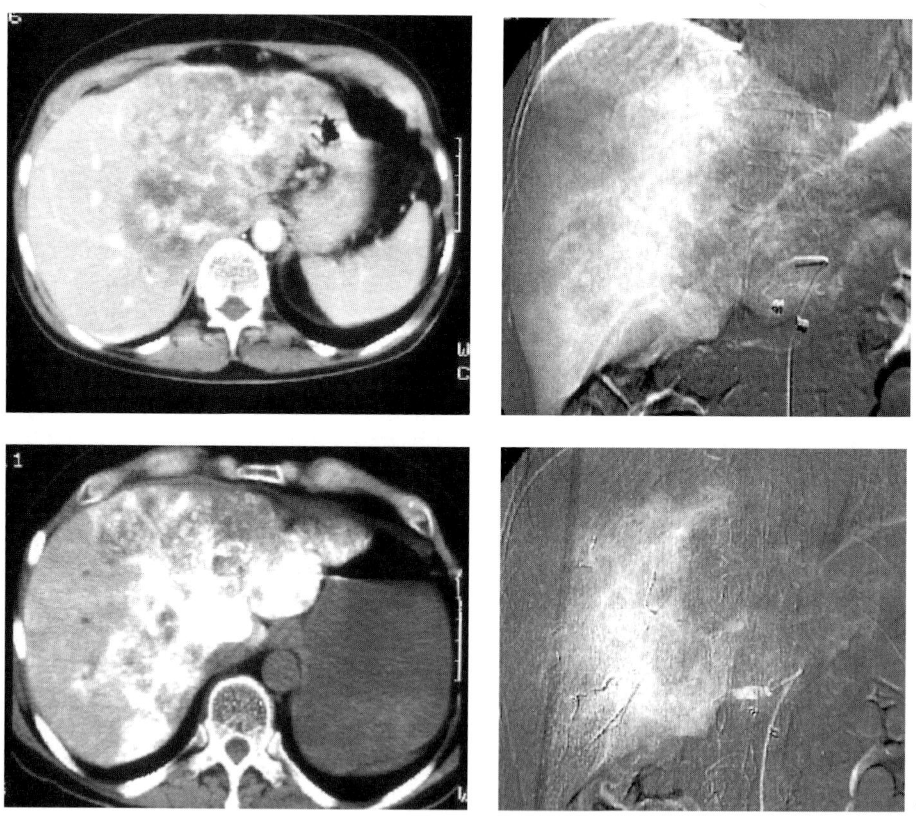

a b c d

Fig. 25.34a–d. Liver metastases from colorectal cancer treated with Lp-TACE. **a** CT before the treatment: extensive metastases in the medial right and left lobe. **b** Hepatic arteriography: large central hypovascular lesion with hyperperfusion of the normal liver tissue. **c** CT control after Lp-TACE: uptake of Lipiodol in the neoplastic tissue. **d** DSA control: reversal of flow from the normal tissue to the outer wall of the tumor lesions after intraarterial injection of noradrenaline

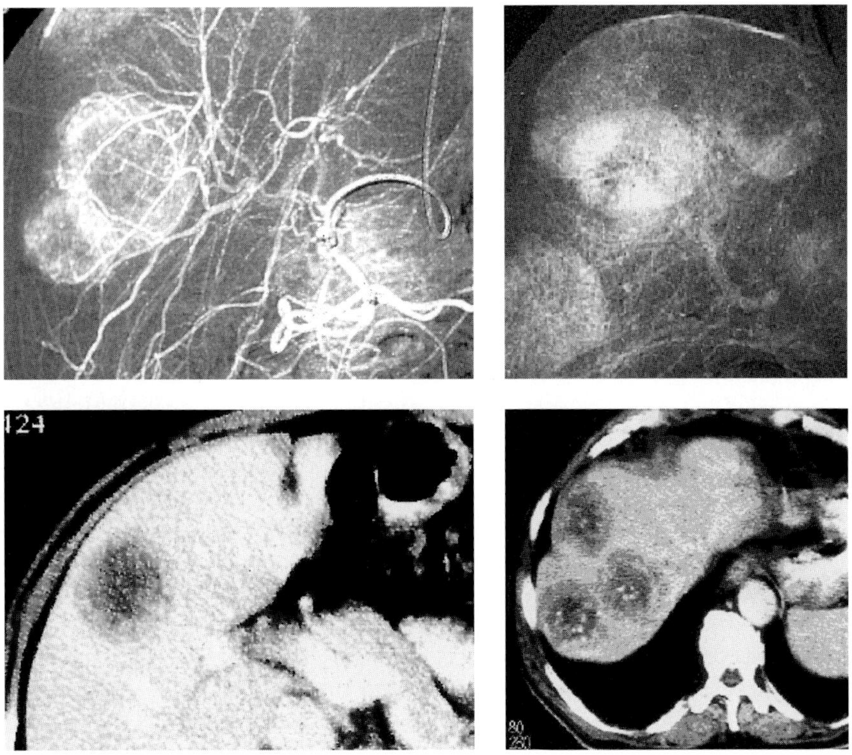

Fig. 25.35a–d. Hypervascular liver metastases from colorectal cancer. **a,b** DSA: hyperperfusion of the lesions in the arterial phase. **c,d** CT: middle zone of the lesions less perfused as compared to normal liver tissue in portal phase. The center is completely necrotic

hepatectomy after neoadjuvant AIC for metastases many problems remain to be resolved and that efficacy is doubtful. A postoperative adjuvant chemotherapy should be considered after hepatic resection for colorectal metastases, following the decreased incidence of recurrent disease (Curley et al. 1993) in patients who received adjuvant AIC compared with historical controls treated with surgery alone.

A strong cytoreductive approach to the treatment of multiple liver metastases isolated to the liver has been introduced by Sugarbaker and Steves (1993), using an induction chemotherapy to achieve a response or stabilize disease in the liver. Patients are then selected for surgery, and a complete response may be achieved through the use of cytoreductive techniques. The reported median survival greatly exceeds in their experience that reported for AIC alone.

No reports are still available with regard to the results of therapies combining US-guided thermoablation or laser therapy and locoregional treatments such as Port-a-Cath AIC, TACE or HHP.

Complex highly invasive procedures have been reported such as isolated liver perfusion (Ravikumar and Dixon 1996) and isolated regional liver perfusion with tumor necrosis factor-alpha followed by hyperthermic melphalan perfusion (Hafstrom et al. 1994). A definitive conclusion on clinical efficacy is still not possible.

25.8 Discussion

Anatomic dye injection studies of the blood supply of colorectal hepatic metastases confirm that tumors are supplied predominantly by the hepatic artery (Sigurdson et al. 1987; Goldberg et al. 1991a). AIC should then increase the local drug concentration and consequently the frequency of morphological response. One milligram of a drug injected in the hepatic artery is equivalent during the first pass to 6–12 mg injected intravenously (Koyanagi 1994). AIC may also relieve adverse reactions, less frequent at lower doses and related to the total dose given. The first pass effect is maximized, and it should be underlined that morphological response depends mainly on the first pass of the drug (TAGUCHI 1994).

Vascularity is a capital prognostic factor for AIC, and the frequency of hypervascular liver metastases showing complete and partial responses to locoregional treatments is much higher than that of hypovascular lesions. If metastases are hyperperfused as compared to normal tissue (NAKAMURA 1992), AIC results in a significantly greater drug delivery to tumor, inducing of course an improved tumor response (LORENZ et al. 1989). Liver metastases, however, especially colorectal, are more often hypovascular.

An exact criterion for the measurement of morphological responses to AIC should also be established. Responses are commonly evaluated quantifying the percentage of hepatic replacement (PHR), but in DWORKIN's opinion (1995) the volume of metastases should instead be used either to assess the extent of disease or the effect of treatment. Only disappearance of the lesion is considered in oncological practice as a complete response, and the reduction of less than 50% if compared to the starting volume, observed by aftertreatment CT, MRI or US controls, as a partial response. This criterion should be accepted in the case of small lesions and if long-term controls are programmed; however, in large lesions a short-term disappearance may not be achieved. A complete necrosis of the lesion during a short-term CT or MRI control (as programmed in HHP) together with the absence of tumor enhanced tissue should be therefore also considered as a complete response, and a loss of the enhanced viable tissue of more than 50% considered as a partial response.

Both disappearance and complete necrosis of the lesions should be confirmed by biopsy, obtained either with US or CT guidance or occasionally in course of resection, but in US/CT guided biopsies multiple approaches are needed and moreover only a positive result could be considered, a negative result being a possible false negative especially in large lesions.

It should be stressed that the apparently "complete" responses following AIC are in most cases a false CT negative: viable cells in the other wall of the lesions often persist assuring a short-term recurrence, microscopically corresponding to the remnants well visualized in partial responses.

In diffuse or multifocal liver metastases not suitable for surgery or with the so called "cosmetic" techniques such as thermoablation or similar, systemic chemotherapy has been the standard treatment. Nevertheless, responses to systemic chemotherapy are reported as poor (ARAI et al. 1997) and AIC was then expected to improve the results. A significant prolongation of the overall survival in intraarterially treated patients compared with controls who received conventional symptom palliation was demonstrated by ALLEN-MERSH et al. (1994), but this report cannot be considered as a comparison with systemic chemotherapy. Prospective randomized trials comparing systemic chemotherapy AIC with the standard bolus dose of 5-fluorouracil (KEMENY et al. 1993), with regional infusion therapy via surgically implanted pumps (PENTECOST 1993) or with hepatic artery chemotherapy with fluorodeoxyuride (SUGARBAKER and STEVES 1993) found increased response rates, although the impact on survival has been minimal. Trials carried out in the late 1980s reported by ARAI (1994) confirmed that AIC had no significant impact on survival of patients with liver metastases if compared with systemic chemotherapy.

On the other hand, AOKI et al. (1991) found that the survival duration was significantly longer in the intraarterial group by the Wilcoxon generalized test and the Cox Mantel test ($P<0.01$).

A conclusion on the hypothetic advantage on survival in patients treated with AIC compared with systemic chemotherapy has therefore not yet been demonstrated even if a good control in the short period may be easily accepted by the high rate of morphological responses (ICHIKAWA et al. 1992).

ARAI (1994) stressed moreover that AIC and similar techniques were not mature in older reports using Port-a-Caths, the incidence of hepatic arterial thrombosis or displacement of the distal tip of the catheter being so high as to prevent a prolonged treatment, which appears the most important factor in obtaining a longer survival. The influence of technical devices was also underestimated. In AIC the technical support has a strong influence, and devices and techniques have actually been highly improved compared to the late 1980s.

No standardized schedules of systemic chemotherapy were accepted for the treatment of colorectal cancer, and drugs have been used in AIC at a dosage similar to or less than a systemic dose without pharmacokinetic bases and knowledge of the optimal dosage and the optimal infusion rate of each drug. Clinical pharmacokinetics should then be better studied and the optimal dosage and schedule of each drug revealed.

Finally, in liver metastases the prognosis depends on several factors other than metastases themselves, first of all the presence or not of extrahepatic lesions (YAMASHITA et al. 1990). It is at first mandatory therefore to associate with every AIC technique systemic chemotherapy. It should be then specified how long liver metastases can be controlled and in how many patients the death caused by liver metastases can be prevented by AIC. If survival may be prolonged from the expected period ended by liver metastases without AIC treatment to the survival period ended by extrahepatic lesions, AIC will be judged to be a valuable treatment.

Every AIC procedure has its advantages and disadvantages.

As previously reported, isolated TAE, except in emergency cases such as hemoperitoneum in ruptured HHC, should not be used to treat malignant hepatic lesions. There is no reason to perform a percutaneous invasive approach for oncological purposes avoiding the exploitation of the highly effective cytoreductive action of hyperconcentrated drugs. Only combined techniques such as chemoembolizations should be therefore employed.

As regards Port-a-Caths, a discussion about the criteria of preference between percutaneous or surgical placement is unnecessary. Percutaneous placement is less expensive, involves a shorter time of hospitalization, may be performed even with day-hospital management and is less invasive (ARAI et al 1997; GROSSO et al 1997). If placement is technically correct, there is no reason to suppose that clinical or morphological results will differ. The risk of displacement of the catheters is higher for percutaneous implants than for surgical, but only percutaneous Port-a-Caths can be easily removed or changed. The axillary approach is, in our personal experience, to be preferred.

Complications such as pocket infections and hepatic artery thrombosis may often occur using both techniques. The global rate of complications seems in any case lower in percutaneous implants (ARAI et al. 1997) than in surgical implants (DAVITTI et al. 1992) and the drop-out rate of the first group is the lowest (9%) (ARAI 1994). In our personal experience of 122 percutaneous implants, a drop-out rate of 27% occurred: we therefore believe, after two years experience of percutaneous Port-a-Caths, a long-term infusion quietly prolonged for more than 16 weeks (four months) to be uncommon.

The clinical efficacy of an indwelling catheter strictly depends on this precise placement. The homogeneous liver perfusion should be confirmed by CT and a badly placed catheter always at once replaced or changed so avoiding complications such as gastric ulcers, pancreatitis or splenic embolization and sparing the patient an unhelpful drug therapy. Changes of arterial blood flow patterns and then of drug distribution by the patients' posture due to the slow flow rate, assessed by SONE et al. (1993), may cause unequal perfusion and therefore unequal response.

Chemoembolizations have also been proved to be effective in the treatment of hepatic metastases from the colon cancer, especially from the standpoint of response rate, and may be considered beneficial even in heavily pretreated patients (LINKS et al. 1993) who have failed systemic chemotherapy. Patients should have a good performance status and metastatic disease confined to the liver (SANZ-ALTAMIRA et al. 1997).

Either Lp-TACE or DSM-TACE have shown evidence of a high-rate tumor response, due both to tissue hyperconcentration of the drug and the long contact time between the agent and the tumor tissue. Lipiodol embolization is not as complete as DSM embolization, and some blood flow is maintained in the tumor tissue. Embolization with gelatin sponge should always therefore complete the injection of the Lipiodolized drug. In chemoembolizations, a high rate of post-procedure syndrome occurs, and portal patency is the first criterion of recruitment.

In hypoxic perfusion (HHP) (as in DSM-TACE or Lp-TACE), the delayed washout of intratumor blood flow with stagnation and the increase of the time of contact between the tumor and the drug are the main factors for the high rate of response (KAMEYAMA et al. 1993). It must be emphasized, however, that HHP is typically a one-step procedure: a progressive decrease of the efficacy appears after further sessions, together with a higher rate of hepatic arterial thrombosis than every other AIC procedure. A single session should only be then performed, but the high rate of positive responses obtained in a short time suggests that HHP probably has, among AIC techniques, the most efficacious cytoreductive effect.

A comparison between clinical efficacy of AIC procedures is difficult especially because of the wide variety of techniques. Almost every combination of drugs and delivery has been tested, and it appears very difficult to arrive at any valuable conclusion. The number of variables such as primary cancer, stage of the disease, previous treatments, duration and number of the sessions, drugs, doses and delivery is so high as to prevent any certainty. This is particularly true for AIC with Port-a-Cath: chemoembolizations are less difficult to standardize.

If we compare the best results of arterial infusion, chemoembolizations and HHP in colorectal metastases, a surprising frequency rate of positive morphological responses (78%) should be emphasized using percutaneous Port-a-Cath and high-dose intermittent weekly infusion (Arai's technique), together with 70% of prevention of hepatic death and the highest overall median survival time of 25.8 months.

DSM-TACE showed a similar frequency of response of 76.2% in colorectal metastases (Fujimoto et al. 1993), but a lower frequency (60%) in breast metastases (De Dycker and Timmermann 1991). The overall survival was only 12 months for breast and 12±5.9 months for colorectal metastases.

Using Lp-TACE, 43% of positive responses occurred in our personal experience, in accordance with Yamashita et al. (1989) (46%) but not with Gorich et al. (1993) (60–80%) and Inoue et al. (1989) (59%). The reported overall survival has been 13.83 months (Tanada et al. 1996) and 11.1 months (Inoue et al. 1989). In a comparison between continuous AIC and Lp-TACE, Tanada et al. (1996) suggested a better response rate for AIC even if without any significant difference in survival, so confirming the slightly lower efficacy of Lp-TACE compared to other therapies.

Hypoxic perfusion (HHP) showed in our personal experience (Roversi et al. 1997) a response rate of 80%, corresponding to the results of AIC with Port-a-Cath using Arai's schedule and of DSM-TACE (Fujimoto et al. 1993), but higher than of Lp-TACE, suggesting a better cytoreductive effect.

Various primitive cancers, previous treatments, number of lesions and of clinical status and no randomization have prevented the buildup of a significant survival curve in patients treated with HHP, but in only 7% of our monitored patients has the cause of death been a progression of the intrahepatic disease. A high rate of responses is not necessarily a valid prerequisite for a longer survival in liver metastases because, as reported by Arai (1994), prognosis depends on several factors other than metastases themselves such as the presence or not of extrahepatic lesions. Moreover, the confirmed strong cytoreductive effect of HHP is also a short-term effect, the majority of patients with apparently complete response showing recurrences of the intrahepatic disease in recent CT studies.

After a two-years experience with isolated HHP we therefore believe it mandatory to always combine a long-term AIC (using a percutaneous Port-a-Cath) with HHP to maximize the long-term hepatic control and to limit intrahepatic recurrences, and systemic chemotherapy for the control of extrahepatic disease.

Except Lp-TACE, showing slightly lower results than those of Port-a-Cath infusion, DSM-TACE and HHP, all AIC reported techniques may achieve a hypothetic highest frequency of positive responses of about 80%, at least in colorectal liver metastases. In any case, if the reported overall median survival time of 25.8 months is confirmed, the intermittent hepatic arterial infusion through Port-a-Caths of high-dose 5-FU on a weekly schedule (Arai et al. 1997) actually appears the most clinically valuable AIC treatment for hepatic metastases, the reported results on survival greatly exceeding those obtained with continuous infusion and chemoembolizations, with a corresponding frequency of positive morphological results. This could then become the standard schedule of AIC for liver metastases.

Percutaneous US-guide thermoablation or laser therapy should be also associated, in order to decrease the amount of the tumoral tissue improving the cytoreductive action of the therapy. A systemic treatment is finally needed for metastatic liver cancer, as well as for regional control of lesions (Tomita 1994).

References

Ajlouni MI, Merrick HW, Skeel RT, Dobelbower RR Jr (1990) Concomitant radiation therapy and constant infusion FUdR for unresectable hepatic metastases. Am J Clin Oncol Cancer Clin Trials 13:532–535

Allen-Mersh TG, Earlam S, Fordy C, Abrams K, Houghton J (1994) Quality of life and survival with continuous hepatic-artery floxuridine infusion for colorectal liver metastases. Lancet 344:1255–1260

Aoki T, Kimura K, Koyanaga Y, et al (1991) Hepatic infusion-chemotherapy for liver metastases from stomach cancer-comparative study for intraarterial group and non-intraaterial group. JpnJCancerChemother 18:2133–2136

Aoki F, Mori T, Takahashi K, Moriyama Y, Tanaka S, Takahashi T (1993) Two cases of intrahepatic biloma during hepatic arterial infusion chemotherapy proved by CT-scan. Jpn J Cancer Chemother 20:1713–1716

Arai Y (1994) Current arterial infusion chemotherapy for liver metastases and required studies. Jpn J Cancer Chemother 20: 1179–1183

Arai Y, Sone Y, Inaba Y, et al (1993) Intermittent hepatic arterial infusion of high-dose 5-FU for liver metastases from colorectal cancer. Jpn J Cancer Chemother 20:1527–1530

Arai Y, Inaba Y, Takeuchi Y, Ariyoshi Y (1997) Intermittent hepatic arterial infusion of high-dose 5FU on a weekly schedule for liver metastases from colorectal cancer. Cancer Chemother Pharmacol 40:526–530

Araki T, Hihara T, Kachi K, et al (1989) Newly developed transarterial chemoembolization material: CDDP-lipiodol suspension. Gastrointest Radiol 14:46–48

Bilbao-Jaureguizar JI, Fernandez-Virgos A, Rodriquez-Cabello J, San-Julian-Artola MP, Fonseca-Cruz R, Longo-Areso JM (1991) Infusion de quimioterapia intraarterial por colaterales extrahepaticas en obstruccion de tronco celiaco. A proposito de un caso. Radiologia 33:489–491

Chuang VP, Wallace S (1981) Hepatic artery embolization in the treatment of hepatic neoplasms. Radiology 140:51–58

Civalleri D, Scopinaro G, Balletto N, et al (1989) Changes in vascularity of liver tumours after hepatic arterial embolization with degradable starch microspheres.Br J Surg 76:699–703

Clark RA, Gallant TE (1987) Bile duct strictures associated with hepatic arterial infusion chemotherapy. Gastrointest Radiol 12:148–151

Coldwell DM, Mortimer JE (1991) Hepatic Artery embolization in the treatment of hepatic malignancies. Reg Cancer Treat 3:298–301

Curley SA, Roh MS, Chase JL, Hohn DC, Johnson FE, Organ CH Jr (1993) Adjuvant hepatic arterial infusion chemotherapy after curative resection of colorectal liver metastases. Am J Surg 166:743–748

Davitti B, Fiorentini G, Guglielminetti D, et al (1992) Complications of port-catheter systems for intra-arterial hepatic chemotherapy: report of 78 patients. Reg Cancer Treat 5:163–166

Dazzi C, Fiorentini G, Davitti B, et al (1994) High-dose intra-arterial plus intraperitoneal chemotherapy combined with hemofiltration in liver metastases from colorectal cancer.Tumori 80:204–208

De Dycker RP, Timmermann J (1991) Combined intraarterial hepatic infusion of degradable starch microspheres and cytostatics in the treatment of breast cancer liver metastases. Reg Cancer Treat 3:302–304

Doyon D (1974) L'embolization arterielle hepatique dans les tumeurs malignes du foie. Journ Radiol Electrol 17:593–603

Duprat G, Charnsangavej C, Wallace S, Carrasco CH (1988) Inferior phrenic artery embolization in the treatment of hepatic neoplasms. Acta Radiol 29:427–429

Dworkin MJ, Burke D, Earlam S, Fordy C, Allen Mersh TG (1995) Measurement of response to treatment in colorectal liver metastases. Br J Cancer British Journal of Cancer 71:873–876

Fujimoto S (1994) Clinical evaluation of albumin microspheres containing anticancer drugs in primary hepatoma and metastatic liver cancer. Jpn J Cancer Chemother 20:998–1003

Fujimoto S, Koike S, Takahashi M, et al (1993) Intra-arterial infusion chemotherapy with degradable starch microspheres and mitomycin C for unresectable hepatic metastasis from gastrointestinal cancer. Reg Cancer Treat 6:7–11

Goldberg JA, Fenner J, Bessent RG, et al (1989) Clinical evaluation of angiotensin II enhanced perfusion scintigraphy in metastatic liver disease. Nucl Med Commun 10:557–566

Goldberg JA, Thomson JAK, McCurrach G, et al (1991a) Arteriovenous shunting in patients with colorectal liver metastases. Br J Cancer 63:466–468

Goldberg JA, Willmott NS, Anderson JH, et al (1991b) The biodegradation of albumin microspheres used for regional chemotherapy in patients with colorectal liver metastases. Nucl Med Commun 12:57–63

Goldberg JA, Murray T, Kerr DJ, et al (1991c) The use of angiotensin II as a potential method of targeting cytotoxic microspheres in patients with intrahepatic tumour. Br J Cancer 63:308–310

Goldstein HM, Wallace S, Anderson JH, Bree RL, Gianturco C (1976) Transcatheter occlusion of abdominal tumors. Radiology 120:539–545

Gorich J, Hasan I, Sittek H, et al (1993) Embolization of primary and secondary liver tumors. Radiol Diagn 34:289–303

Gorich J, Rilinger N, Sokiranski R, et al (1996) Embolization of liver neoplasms in patients with occluded celiac trunk. Reg Cancer Treat 9:79–82

Grosso M, Zanon C, Zanon M (1997) Posizionamento percutaneo di cateteri intrarteriosi con reservoir per infusione sottocutanea. Radiol Med 94:226–232

Hafstrom L, Holmberg SB, Lindner P, et al (1994) Isolated regional liver perfusion with tumour necrosis factor-alpha followed by hyperthermic melphalan perfusion. Reg Cancer Treat 7:172–176

Hanssen LE, Schrumpf E, Jacobsen MB, et al (1991) Extended experience with recombinant alpha -2b interferon with or without hepatic artery embolization in the treatment of midgut carcinoid tumours. A preliminary report. Acta Oncol 30:523–527

Hemingway DM, Angerson WJ, Anderson JH, Goldberg JA, McArdle CS, Cooke TG (1992) Monitoring blood flow to colorectal liver metastases using laser Doppler flowmetry: the effect of angiotensin II. Br J Cancer 66:958–960

Hoefer RA Jr, Falk RL, Howell RS, Seeger J (1990) Computed tomographic arteriography of the liver following chronic intra-arterial FdUrd: a case illustrating multiple perfusion abnormalities. Reg Cancer Treat 3:19–22

Hokita S, Takao S, Tokushige M, Maenohara S, Aikou T, Shimazu H (1989) Two-route chemotherapy under AT-II induced hypertension using totally implanted injection port system for liver metastases derived from digestive cancers. Jpn J Cancer Chemother 16:2901–2904

Hoogewoud H-M (1994) La chimio-embolisation hepatique. Med Hyg 52:1544–1548

Ichikawa W, Nihei Z, Sawai S, et al (1992) Efficacy of intra-arterial infusion chemotherapy for metastatic liver tumors of the colon cancer. Reg Cancer Treat 5:154–158

Inoue H, Kobayashi H, Itoh Y, Shinohara-S (1989) Treatment of liver metastases by arterial injection of adriamycin/mitomycin C lipiodol suspension. Acta Radiol 30: 603–608

Inoue Y, Nakamura H, Takashima S, Yamazaki K, Toyoshima H, Iwasaki M (1991)Biloma following transcatheter oily chemoembolization. Radiat Med 9:57–60

Inoue Y, Machida K, Honda N, et al (1997) Effect of Angiotensin II on arteriovenous shunting assessed by hepatic arterial perfusion scintigraphy. Am J Clin Oncol Cancer Clin Trials 20:237–241

Itano S, Hirai K, Yoshida T, et al (1993) Complication of gastro duodenum with intra-hepatic arterial infusion chemotherapy using implantable reservoir system for hepatic tumors. Jpn J Cancer Chemother 20:1512–1515

Iwasaki Y, Kitamura M, Arai K (1996) Induced hypertensive chemotherapy with angiotensin II for liver metastases from gastric cancer. Jpn J Cancer Chemother 23:1558–1560

Chung JW, Park J, Im JG, Han JK, Han MC (1993) Pulmonary

oil embolism after transcatheter oily chemoembolization of hepatocellular carcinoma. Radiology 187:689–693

Chung JW, Park J, Han JK, et al (1996) Hepatic tumors: predisposing factors for complications of transcatheter oily chemoembolization. Radiology 198:33–40

Kameoka S, Seshimo A, Hamano K (1995) Hepatic atrophy due to intra-arterial chemotherapy for liver metastasis. J Tokyo Women's Med Coll 65:855–859

Kameyama M, Fukuda I, Imaoka S, et al (1988) Transcatheter arterial chemoembolization for liver metastases of colorectal cancer (Lipiodol cisplatin sandwich therapy). Jpn J Cancer Chemother 15:2510–2513

Kameyama M, Fukuda I, Imaoka S, et al (1989) Stagnation of liver blood and effectiveness of intraarterial chemotherapy for metastatic colorectal cancer. Jpn J Cancer Chemother 16:2894–2896

Kameyama M, Imaoka S, Fukuda I, et al (1993) Delayed washout of intratumor blood flow is associated with good response to intraarterial chemoembolization for liver metastasis of colorectal cancer. Surgery 114:97–101

Kemeny N, Lokich JJ, Anderson N, Ahlgren JD (1993) Recent advances in the treatment of advanced colorectal cancer. Cancer 71:9–18

Kimoto T, Nagasue N, Kohno H, et al (1995) Repeated hepatic dearterialization for unresectable liver metastases from gastric cancer: review of five cases. HPB Surg 8:175–180

Kitada M, Shibata T, Takami M, et al (1993) Liver metastases from breast cancer: survival and an attempt at cauterization and thermocoagulation therapy combined with selective intra- arterial infusion chemotherapy. Jpn J Cancer Chemother 20:1601–1604

Kobayashi H, Inoue H, Shimada J, et al (1987) Intra-arterial injection of adriamycin/mitomycin C lipiodol suspension in liver metastases. Acta Radiol 28:275–280

Kohno S, Oda Y, Toya N, et al (1995) Evaluation of 5-FU, leucovorin, etoposide, and cisplatin (FLEP) chemotherapy by hepatic artery injection in the treatment of multiple liver metastases from gastric cancer. Jpn J Cancer Chemother 22:695–698

Koike S, Fujimoto S, Guhji M, et al (1988) Repeated intra-arterial chemotherapy combined with mitomycin c and degradable starch microspheres for inoperable metastatic hepatic cancer. JpnJ Cancer Chemother 15:2601–2605

Koike S, Fujimoto S, Guhji M, et al (1989) Effect of degradable starch microspheres (DSM) on hepatic hemodynamics. Jpn J Cancer Chemother 16:2818–2821

Kondo M (1994) Chemo-embolization with DSM against hepatic malignancies. Jpn J Cancer Chemother 20:1186–1190

Konno T (1994) Basic and clinical use of arterial injection therapy with oily anticancer agents. Jpn J Cancer Chemother 20: 1190–1194

Koyanagi Y (1994) Low-dose intermittent arterial infusion therapy. Jpn J Cancer Chemother 20: 1198–1202

Kuroda C, Sakurai M, Monden M, et al (1989) Transcatheter arterial embolization for metastatic liver tumors: a study in resected cases. Cardiovasc Intervent Radiol 12:72–75

Lang EK, Brown CL Jr (1993) Colorectal metastases to the liver: selective chemoembolization. Radiology 189:417–422

Leen E, Angerson WJ, Warren H, et al (1993) Hepatic arterial haemodynamics changes following intra-arterial angiotensin II infusion: duplex/color Doppler sonography. Clin Radiol 47:321–324

Links M, Ross W, Clingan P, et al (1993) Treatment of liver metastases with intra arterial Lipiodol – Adriamycin. Reg Cancer Treat 6:121–124

Lorenz M, Herrmann G, Kirkowa Reimann M, et al (1989) Temporary chemoembolization of colorectal liver metastases with degradable starch microspheres. Eur J Surg Oncol 15:453–462

Lygidakis NJ, Thodorakopoulou M, Dedemadi G, et al (1997) Resection of unresectable secondary liver tumors – New frontiers in liver surgery. Hepatogastroenterology 44:1632–1640

Maeda K (1994) Transcatheter arterial embolization in liver metastases from colorectal cancer. Jpn J Cancer Chemother 20: 1045–1055

Mavor AID, Parkin A, Riley A, et al (1987) Initial clinical experience with degradable starch microspheres. Nucl Med Commun 8:1011–1018

Miller DL, Carrasquillo JA, Lutz RJ, Chang AE Hepatic perfusion during hepatic artery infusion chemotherapy: evaluation with perfusion CT and perfusion scintigraphy. J Comput Assist Tomogr 13:958–964

Morandi C, Colopi S, Arai Y, et al (1998) Posizionamento percutaneo di catetere di Port nell'arteria epatica per la chemioterapia delle metastasi secondo la tecnica di Arai. Radiol Med 95:357–361

Mori M, Hidaka K, Mashima H, Katano M, Kishikawa T, Hisatsugu T (1993) Clinical study on the effect of continuous transarterial infusion chemotherapy of CDDP for metastatic liver tumors. Jpn J Cancer Chemother 20:1547–1550

Nagata Y, Hiraoka M, Nishimura Y, et al (1997) Clinical results of radiofrequency hyperthermia for malignant liver tumors. Int J Radiat Oncol Biol Phys 38:359–365

Nakagawa H, Kobayashi K, Tono T, et al (1996) Combination with intra-hepatic arterial infusion of low dose cisplatin and oral administration of high dose doxyfluridine for patients with liver metastases of gastric cancer. Jpn J Cancer Chemother 23:783–785

Nakamura K (1992) Hepatic blood flow in patients treated by continuous hepatic artery infusion chemotherapy. Jpn J Nucl Med 29:377–383

Nakamura H (1994) Liver chemoembolization. Jpn J Cancer Chemother 20:1159–1165

Nakamura H, Hashimoto T, Oi H, Sawada S, Furui S (1991) Prevention of gastric complications in hepatic arterial chemoembolization. Balloon catheter occlusion technique. Acta Radiol 32:81–82

Nakayama T, Tamaki Y, Tohno K, et al (1993) Continuous intra-hepatic-arterial infusion of low dose 5-fluorouracil for colorectal cancer patients with unresectable liver metastases. Jpn J Cancer Chemother 20:1504–1506

Nobin A, Mansson B, Lunderquist A (1989) Evaluation of temporary liver dearterialization and embolization in patients with metastatic carcinoid tumor. Acta Oncol 28:419–424

Noda M, Kusunoki M, Yanagi H, Yamamura T, Utsunomiya J (1996) Hepatic artery-biliary fistula during infusion chemotherapy.Hepatogastroenterology 43:1387–1389

Ohori M, Umekita N, Maeshiro T, Miyamoto S, Yamada F, Awane Y (1996) Common bile duct fistula caused by hepatic arterial infusion chemotherapy. Jpn J Cancer Chemother 23:1565–1567

Pentecost MJ (1993) Transcatheter treatment of hepatic metastases. AJR 160:1171–1175

Perring S, Hind R, Fleming J, Birch S, Batty V, Taylor I (1994) Dosimetric assessment of radiolabelled lipiodol as a potential therapeutic agent in colorectal liver metastases using combined CT and SPECT. Nucl Med Commun 15:34–38

Piperkova E, Kurteva G, Grueva A, Braikow N, Kurtev P (1994) Role of (99 m)Tc-albumin microspheres for assessment of vascularisation of liver metastases in patients with colorectal carcinoma. Radiol Diagn 35:323–327

Ravikumar TS, Dixon-K (1996) Isolated liver perfusion for liver metastases: pharmacokinetic advantage? Surg Oncol Clin North Am 5:443–449

Richardet J P, Lons T, Sibony M, et al (1994) Sclerosing cholangitis after oily hepatic arterial chemoembolisation. Gastroenterol Clin Biol 18:168–171

Ross WB, Morris DL, Clingan PR (1996) Major upper gastrointestinal haemorrhage associated with hepatic arterial chemoperfusion. Aust New Zealand J Surg 66:816–819

Roth J, Wallner B, Safi F (1989) Arterial perfusion abnormalities of the liver after hepatic arterial infusion chemotherapy and their correlation with changes in the metastases: evaluation with CT and angiography. AJR 153:751–754

Roversi R (1996) Perfusione antiblastica del fegato in ipossia. Interventional Radiology in Oncology, Milan, Italy, pp 35–49

Roversi R, Cavallo G, Ricci S, Rossi G, Roversi M, Fiorentini GM (1997) Perfusione antiblastica ipossica con blocco di flusso nella terapia delle metastasi epatiche: risultati preliminari. Radiol Med 93:410–417

Sakamoto Y, Fujita M, Ota J, Sugiyama R, Sugimoto T, Taguchi T (1993) Enhancing effects of degradable starch microspheres on experimental intra- arterial chemotherapy with adriamycin in nude rat models with human gastric cancer xenografts. Reg Cancer Treat 6:12–18

Saltz L (1991) Drug treatment of colorectal cancer: current status. Drugs 42:616–627

Sanz Altamira PM, Spence LD, Huberman MS, et al (1997) Selective chemoembolization in the management of hepatic metastases in refractory colorectal carcinoma: a phase II trial. Dis Colon Rectum 40:770–775

Sasaki Y (1994) Sandwich therapy with Lipiodol and cisplatin in hepatocellular carcinoma Jpn J Cancer Chemother 20: 1022–1030

Sato T (1994) Intrarterial cancer chemotherapy. Jpn J Cancer Chemother 20: 1145–1150

Sato S, Nabeyama A, Nakashima A, et al (1992) A case of recurrent liver tumor from gastric cancer responding remarkably to hepatic arterial infusion of doses large mitomycin C and 5-fluorouracil. Jpn J Cancer Chemother 19:537–539

Satoh O, Sakaguchi H, Yoshioka T, et al (1990) Transarterial hepatic embolization for metastatic liver cancers; with reference to 17 cases of survivals for more than 2 years. Jpn J Clin Radiol 35:345–352

Sawada S, Fujiwara Y, Koyama T, et al (1992) Percutaneous transfemoral arterial infusion chemotherapy for metastatic liver tumors – Placement of 3 Fr balloon catheters. Radiat Med 10:6–12

Schneebaum S, Walker MJ, Young D, Farrar WB, Minton JP, Gardner B (1994) The regional treatment of liver metastases from breast cancer. J Surg Oncol 55:26–32

Seki H, Kimura M, Kamura T, Miura T, Yoshimura N, Sakai K (1996) Hepatic perfusion abnormalities during treatment with hepatic arterial infusion chemotherapy: value of CT arteriography using an implantable port system. J Comput Assist Tomogr 20:343–348

Shida H, Ban K, Matsumoto M, et al (1995) Continuous intraarterial infusion of 5-fluorouracil plus leucovorin for liver metastases from colorectal cancer. Jpn J Cancer Chemother 22:221–225

Shuto K, Okazumi S, Takayama W, et al (1997) Evaluation of CTA for arterial infusion chemotherapy for liver metastasis from colorectal cancer. Jpn J Cancer Chemother 24:1749–1752

Sidibe S, Rougier P, Lumbroso J, et al (1989)Controles de perfusion par angioscintigraphie lors des chimiotherapies intra-arterielles hepatiques. Presse Med 18:2045–2049

Sigurdson ER, Ridge JA, Kemeny N, Daly JM (1987) Tumor and liver drug uptake following hepatic artery and portal vein infusion. J Clin Oncol 5:1836–1840

Sone Y, Arai Y, Mukaijo T, Nakatsuka A, Sasaki F, Kido C (1993) Changes of arterial blood flow patterns by patients' posture during hepatic arterial infusion chemotherapy assessed by (99m) Tc-MAA perfusion scintigraphy. Kakuigaku 30:1353–1358

Soulen MC (1997) Chemoembolization of hepatic malignancies. Semin Intervent Radiol 14:305–311

Starkhammar H, Hakansson L (1987) Effect of starch microspheres on the passage of labelled erythrocytes and a low molecular weight marker through the liver. Acta Oncol 26:361–365

Starkhammar H, Hakansson L, Morales O, Svedberg J (1987) Intra-arterial mitomycin c treatment of unresectable liver tumours. Preliminary results on the effect of degradable starch microspheres. Acta Oncol 26:295–300

Stephens FO (1992) Proposal for management of colorectal metastases with hepatic artery 5-FU infusion followed by portal vein FUDR. Reg Cancer Treat 5:146–153

Sugarbaker PH, Steves MA (1993) A cytoreductive approach to treatment of multiple liver metastases. J Surg Oncol 53:161–165

Sugimoto E (1994) Value of transcatheter arterial embolization using lipiodol for hepatic metastases. J Saitama Med Sch 21:185–191

Sugimoto T, Ku Y, Tominaga M, et al (1997) A case of multiple colonic liver metastases treated successfully with percutaneous isolated liver chemoperfusion using cisplatin. Jpn J Cancer Chemother 24:1753–1756

Sullivan RD (1963) Continuous AIC of human liver cancer using 5-fluoro-2-deoxyuridine. Proc Am Assoc Cencer Res 4:66–78

Suzuki Y, Sano A, Hatabu H, et al (1992) Transcatheter arterial infusion of adriamycin-lipiodol suspension to the patients with metastatic liver tumor. Jpn J Cancer Chemother 19:323–326

Suzuki S, Arai K, Arai H, et al (1997) Prognosis of hepatic metastasis from colorectal cancer following hepatic resection and arterial infusion chemotherapy – Assessment from the percentage of tumor involved area. Jpn J Cancer Chemother 24:1699–1702

Taguchi T (1994) Arterial Infusion Chemotherapy. Jpn J Cancer Chemother 20:1031–1039

Takayasu K, Shima Y, Muramatsu Y, et al (1987) Hepatocellular carcinoma: treatment with intraarterial iodized oil with and without chemotherapeutic agents. Radiology 163:345–351

Tanada M, Saeki T, Takashima S, Mogami H, Hyoudou I, Jinno K (1996) Intrahepatic arterial infusion chemotherapy for the colon cancer patients with liver metastases – A comparison of arterial embolization chemotherapy versus continuous arterial infusion chemotherapy. Jpn J Cancer Chemother 23:1440–1442

Tanada M, Yokoyama N, Kurita A, et al (1997) Histological effect of arterial embolization chemotherapy for metastatic liver tumors from colorectal cancer – Report of cases of hepatectomy after arterial embolization chemotherapy. Jpn J Cancer Chemother 24:1745–1748

Tanaka Y, Yamamoto K, Murata T, Nagata K (1992) Effects of multimodal treatment and hyperthermia on hepatic tumors. Cancer Chemother Pharmacol 31:111–114

Taniguchi H, Koyama H, Masuyama M, et al (1996) Angiotensin-II-induced hypertension chemotherapy: Evaluation of hepatic blood flow with oxygen-15 PET. J Nucl Med 37:1522–1523

Teder H, Johansson C J (1993) The effect of different dosages of degradable starch microspheres (Spherex registered) on the distribution of doxorubicin regionally administered to the rat. Anticancer Res 13:2161–2164

Theicher BA, Lazo JS, Sartorelli AC (1981) Classification of antineoplastic agents by their selective toxicities toward oxygenated and hypoxic tumor cells. Cancer 41:73–78

Therasse E, Breittmayer F, Roche A, et al (1993) Transcatheter chemoembolization of progressive carcinoid liver metastasis. Radiology 189:541–547

Tomita M (1994) Arterial infusion chemotherapy and transcatheter arterial embolization (TAE) therapy for primary and metastatic malignant liver tumors. Jpn J Cancer Chemother 20:1011–1018

Tsuji Y, Katsuki Y, Yasuda T, Nishimura A, Shinohara M (1993) Intra-arterial chemotherapy with 5-FU (weekly high dose 5-FU HAI) for the prevention of tumor recurrence in residual liver after hepatic resection of metastasis from colorectal cancer. Jpn J Cancer Chemother 20:1520–1523

Tsujitani S, Watanabe A, Kakeji Y, et al (1991) Hepatic recurrence not prevented with low-dosage long-term intraportal 5-FU infusion after resection of colorectal liver metastasis. Eur J Surg Oncol 15:526–529

Tsuruta S, Mitsuoka S, Tajima H, et al (1990) Hepatic bile cyst, as a side effect of transcatheter oily chemoembolization: report of a case. Acta Hepatol Jap 31:576–580

Une Y, Uchino J, Yasuhara M, et al (1993) Intra-arterial infusion chemotherapy on unresectable hepatocellular carcinoma under occlusion of hepatic arterial flow. Clin Ther 15:347–354

Vogl TJ, Mack MG, Straub R, Roggan A, Felix R (1997) Magnetic resonance imaging – Guided abdominal interventional radiology: laser-induced thermotherapy of liver metastases. Endoscopy 29:577–583

Wacker F, Fobbe F, Boese Landgraf J, Wagner A (1995) Pseudothrombosierung Der Arteria Hepatica Communis Bei Der Regionalen Chemotherapie Von Lebermetastasen. ROFO 162:538–540

Wacker FK, Boese Landgraf J, Wagner A, Albrecht D, Wolf KJ, Fobbe F (1997) Minimally invasive catheter implantation for regional chemotherapy of the liver: a new percutaneous transsubclavian approach. Cardiovasc Intervent Radiol 20:128–132

Wallace S, Carrasco CH, Charnsangavej C, Richli WR, Wright K, Gianturco C (1990) Hepatic artery infusion and chemoembolization in the management of liver metastases. Cardiovasc Intervent Radiol 13:153–160

Wiley AL Jr, Wirtanen GW, Stephenson JA, Ramirez G, Demets D, Lee JW (1989) Combined hepatic artery 5-fluorouracil and irradiation of liver metastases. A randomized study. Cancer 64:1783–1789

Yamamoto M, Miura K, Iizuka H, Yamamoto Y, Fujii H (1993) Application of subcutaneously implanted infusion pump for continuous infusion of IL-2 and intermittent Doxorubicin injections to hepatic artery in advanced hepatocellular carcinoma. Reg Cancer Treat 6:125–130

Yamamura T, Hanai A, Oikawa H, et al (1993) Arterial infusion chemotherapy of 5-FU and leucovorin for patients with liver metastases from cololectal cancer. Jpn J Cancer Chemother 20:1516–1519

Yamashita Y, Takahashi M, Bussaka H, Fukushima S, Kawaguchi T, Nakano M (1989) Intraarterial infusion of 5-fluoro-2-deoxyuridine-C8 dissolved in a lymphographic agent in malignant liver tumors: a preliminary report. Cancer 64:2437–2444

Yamashita Y, Takahashi M, Koga Y, et al (1990) Prognostic factors in liver metastases after transcatheter arterial embolization or arterial infusion. Acta Radiol 31:269–274

Zeiss J, Merrick HW, Savolaine ER, Woldenberg LS, Kim K, Schlembach PJ (1990) Fatty liver change as a result of hepatic artery infusion chemotherapy. Am J Clin Oncol Cancer Clin Trials 13:156–160

26 Cryotherapy of Liver Metastases

A. Giovagnoni, A. Paganini, G. Valeri, P. Busilacchi, and E. Lezoche

CONTENTS

26.1 Introduction

Cryosurgery has been recognized as a promising new modality for treatment of malignant tumors of the liver. This technique was originally employed to treat superficial tumors; however, the development of new cryosurgical instrumentation and imaging modalities to monitor cryotherapy treatment has allowed the application of cryosurgery to freeze tumor tissue deep within the parenchyma (Onik et al. 1993; Polk et al. 1995; Ramming 1995). Currently cryotherapy is widely used in ophthalmology, dermatology, neurosurgery, urology, hepatic surgery and several other clinical applications.

In the liver, the aim of this local curative procedure is to induce tumor cells necrosis using subzero temperatures with a greater preservation of surrounding normal parenchyma than traditional segmentectomy or lobectomy (Busch and Kemeny 1995; Fong et al. 1995; Ramming 1995; Shafir et al. 1996).

Cryosurgery, the "in situ freezing of cancer", is considered a safe and effective treatment used in patients who would not be candidates for traditional hepatic resection because of bilobar disease or a poor overall clinical condition and/or limited hepatic functional reserve. In addition, tumors adjacent to the major vessels can be treated without sacrificing the vasculature. Patients with liver-only hepatic tumors are evaluated for possible cryosurgical treatment (McCall et al. 1995).

The presence of extrahepatic disease is generally considered a contraindication for the operation although patients with colorectal liver metastases and one or two isolated lung metastases may undergo the operation, provided they will subsequently be able to sustain a curative lung metastasectomy. Moreover, curative treatment of all the hepatic tumor tissue that is identified on preoperative and intraoperative imaging should be achieved by cryoablation alone or combined with liver resection. Cryosurgery was originally applied in the treatment of liver tumor using laparotomic preparation of the liver because of the technical characteristics of cryoprobe, which cannot allow a percutaneous approach.

With the refinement of cryosurgical instrumentation, laparoscopic cryoablation has been proposed and the indication extended to the treatment of patients with isolated hepatic tumors (Cuschieri et al. 1995). Very recently a new percutaneously insertable and MR-compatible cryoprobe for interstitial cryotherapy of the liver has been utilized in animal models, giving new opportunities for the non-surgical treatment of liver tumors (Zhou et al. 1993).

Preliminary clinical results in using cryotherapy for the treatment of multiple liver metastases show a 5-year survival rate similar to that achieved with traditional hepatic resection, with a significant reduc-

A. Giovagnoni, MD; MR Center F. Angelini, Department of Radiology, University of Ancona, Torrette, I-60020 Ancona, Italy
A. Paganini, MD; Department of Surgical Sciences, University of Ancona, Umberto I Hospital, Largo Cappelli 1, I-60020 Ancona, Italy
G. Valeri, MD; MR Center F. Angelini, Department of Radiology, University of Ancona, Torrette, I-60020 Ancona, Italy
P. Busilacchi, MD; Department of Radiology, Umberto I Hospital, Largo Cappelli 1, I-60020 Ancona, Italy
E. Lezoche, MD; Department of Surgical Sciences, University of Ancona, Umberto I Hospital, Largo Cappelli 1, I-60020 Ancona, Italy

tion of morbidity compared to traditional surgical treatment (RAVIKUMAR et al. 1991a,b; ZHOU et al. 1993).

26.2 Surgical Techniques

26.2.1 Open Cryoablation

The patient is placed on the operative table in a supine position and a standard subcostal bilateral incision is employed to gain access to the abdominal cavity, which is explored to rule out the presence of macroscopic tumor deposits outside the liver. The demonstration of metastatic hepatoduodenal lymph nodes at intraoperative frozen section is not considered a contraindication to hepatic cryoablation provided an accurate lymphadenectomy is performed, which is extended up to the celiac trunk. The entire liver parenchyma is scanned by intraoperative ultrasound with a 5.5- and a 7.5-MHz probe to confirm the presence of the previously diagnosed lesions, to define their relations with vascular and biliary structures and to identify any lesion smaller than 1 cm that may not have been detected by preoperative imaging techniques. After defining the complete map of the distribution of the hepatic lesions, a surgical treatment plan is decided upon (KANE 1993; RAVIKUMAR et al. 1994).

The indication for cryoablation is to treat multiple isolated lesions with diameters ranging between a few millimeters up to 6–7 cm, located deep in the liver parenchyma, either on one side or on both sides of the liver.

Intraoperative ultrasound is employed to accurately identify the path that the cryoprobe will have to follow, to avoid damaging important structures. Once this is identified, a fine 18G needle with an external sheath is positioned under the ultrasound control inside the lesion using Seldinger's technique.

With the external shaft left in place the needle is removed, a guide-wire is introduced inside the external sheath and is advanced until its J tip is seen exiting in the middle of the tumor nodule. The external sheath of the needle is then removed and a dilating probe with external cannula is advanced over the guide-wire and is positioned inside the lesion. The diameter of the dilating probe and of the cryoprobe that will be employed (3 or 8 mm in diameter) depends on the size of the lesion that has to be treated. The 3 mm probe creates a 5 cm ice-ball in its largest diameter, with a tumor-free zone of up to 4 cm. The 8 mm probe creates a 7 cm ice-ball with a tumor-free zone of up to 6 cm. The reason a tumoricidal temperature is obtained in a smaller ice-ball volume is due to the temperature gradient inside the ice-ball increasing by 10°C/mm of tissue with increasing distance from the probe. Larger or irregularly shaped lesions may be treated by a combination of cryoprobes placed in an asymmetrical position inside the tumor nodule so that the respective ice-balls will fuse with each other to eventually create a single ice-ball of larger diameter. After removing the dilating probe together with the guide wire, the cannula remains positioned with its distal end in the middle of the nodule. Next, a blunt cryoprobe is introduced inside the cannula and is advanced towards the center of the nodule. After the correct position of the cryoprobe has been verified by ultrasound

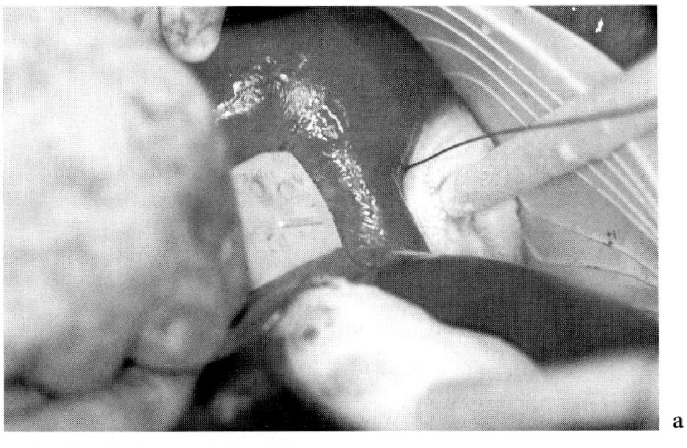

a

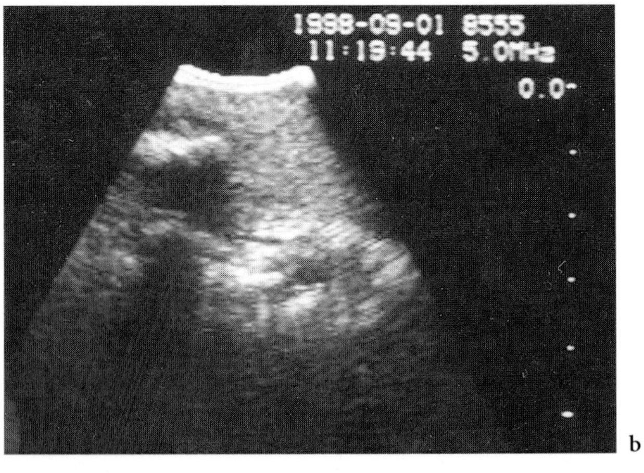

b

Fig. 26.1a,b. Intraoperative ultrasound (IOUS) is employed to verify the correct position of the cryoprobe and to monitor the ice-ball formation. **a** Open cryoablation: surgical view. **b** IOUS image of ice-ball formation. Cyoprobes, thermocouples, sonographic probe and ice-balls are evident

(Fig. 26.1), the external cannula is retracted and the freezing process is begun. The development of an ice-ball around the probe is visualized on the ultrasound screen by the appearance of a hyperechoic rim with posterior acoustic shadowing.

Cryoablation of a lesion located close to a major vessel is free from consequences because the vessel protects itself from freezing by means of its high blood flow ("heat sink effect").

The bile ducts have no protection from freezing and therefore lesions close to a major bile duct should not be treated with a cryoprobe to reduce the risks of the patient developing a postoperative biliary fistula. Lesions in the proximity of major bile ducts are preferably resected.

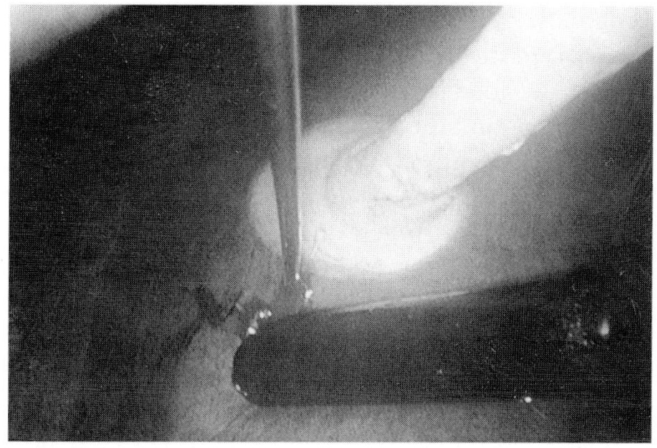

Fig. 26.2, Laparoscopic cryoablation. The refinement of cryosurgical instrumentation has opened up the laparoscopic approach for the cryoablation procedure

26.2.2 Laparoscopic Cryoablation

The selection criteria for laparoscopic cryoablation of a primary or secondary hepatic tumor are the presence of a number of nodules equal to or less than 3 up to 5 cm in diameter. Lesion location in segments VII and VIII is not a contraindication to laparoscopic cryoablation. Pneumoperitoneum is established with standard techniques. The first 10–12 mm trocar is positioned in the right upper quadrant along the mid-clavicular line and the peritoneal cavity is explored with a 45° forward oblique viewing telescope, to exclude any sign of extrahepatic abdominal involvement. Another 10–12 mm trocar is positioned on the right along the anterior axillary line for intraoperative laparoscopic ultrasound. A 6.5 MHz laparoscopic ultrasound probe with an articulating distal extremity is introduced from the lateral trocar and is employed to scan the entire surface of the liver in a systematic manner (Lezoche et al. 1998). The position of the subsequent trocars is decided according to the number of lesions that have to be treated and their location.

The total number of trocars that are employed has to take into account the fact that two trocars, one for the telescope and one for the ultrasound probe, have to be available at all times during the operation to monitor the freezing process (Fig. 26.2). Tumor nodules located in anterior liver segments (III, IVb, V and VIII) are reached with the cryoprobes directly from the anterior surface of the liver with no hepatic preparation. Instead, tumors located in segments II, VI, VII and the apex of segments IVa and VIII require some liver preparation to avoid freezing of perihepatic tissues, such as the diaphragm.

Under laparoscopic vision with ultrasound control, a 5 mm blunt laparoscopic cryoprobe (40 cm in length) is introduced by direct puncture into the liver and directed towards the middle of the nodule to be treated (CMS Accuprobe System, Cryomedical Sciences, Inc., Rockville, MD, USA). As with open cryoablation, laparoscopic cryoprobe introduction is also done free-handed and has to be performed with extreme caution.

The maximum diameter of the ice-ball that develops around the tip of the 5 mm cryoprobe is 6 cm with a tumor-free zone of 5 cm, which is the maximum diameter that we choose to treat by laparoscopic cryoablation. More than one cryoprobe is employed to treat irregularly shaped lesions. In this case, as in open cryoablation, the probes are positioned in an asymmetrical position with respect to the center of the lesion, so that the expanding iceballs eventually join one another to include the entire lesion and an adequate margin of normal liver tissue (1–1.5 cm).

26.3 Cryoablation

The process of cryoablation is identical for the open and for the laparoscopic procedures; therefore it will be described as a single procedure. When the cryoprobe is in the correct position, liquid nitrogen is circulated to rapidly decrease the temperature of the surrounding liver tissue to –100°C, when the cryoprobe sticks into the lesion. The other cryoprobes are then positioned with the same technique inside the lesion. Ideally, the freezing process should be activated simultaneously, unless a different hepatic exposure is required. When all the cryoprobes that can be activated at the same time are in the correct position liquid nitrogen is again circulated through the probes until the temperature of the tissue decreases from −100°C to −196°C. The development of the ice-ball is visualized on the ultrasound screen by the appearance of a hyperechoic rim with posterior acoustic shadowing.

The freezing process continues for 15–20 min during which time the ice-ball expands until its diameter becomes larger than the tumor diameter by 1 cm on each side. A thermocouple may be introduced inside the liver (through a separate 18G percutaneous cannula during laparoscopic cryoablation), and its tip is positioned into macroscopically normal liver tissue close to the nodule. Devitalization of the tissue is demonstrated when the temperature of the thermocouple which is external to the nodule decreases to −40°C. Occasionally more than one thermocouple may be employed. Additional cryoprobes may be positioned in the liver nodule when in doubt about the efficacy of cryodestruction at one particular point of the nodule. After the first freezing process is completed the lesion is allowed to thaw. Thawing may be followed by a second freeze of up to 15 min, which is more effective than a single freeze (Litvinenko 1994; Stewart et al. 1995).

The cryoprobes are actively warmed during the second thawing to remove them when the tissue is still frozen and the solid track can be plugged more easily with regenerated cellulose mesh (Tabotamp, Johnson & Johnson, USA). This is then sealed with cyanoacrylate glue. An original method that we have developed to achieve hemostasis is to irrigate the cellulose mesh with saline and to apply high frequency electrocautery which is transmitted along the cellulose plug to promote its adhesion inside the track. Complete ablation of the tumor nodule may be demonstrated after thawing is completed, when the thawed tumor nodule, the thawed normal liver parenchyma, and the surrounding normal liver tissue demonstrate a different echogenic pattern.

During thawing, parenchymal splits on the liver surface are occasionally observed when the ice-ball reached Glisson's capsule, and these may be a source of hemorrhage. If this is the case, hemostasis must be rapidly obtained because brisk bleeding may ensue and may require conversion to open surgery during the laparoscopic procedure (Polk et al. 1995).

During the operation, patient monitoring includes measurements of intraarterial pressure, central venous pressure and temperature. A pharmacological increase of the glomerular filtration has been observed to facilitate the elimination of the products of cryodestruction that are released in the bloodstream during and immediately after the operation.

Double freezing is more cryodestructive than single freezing but may give rise to severe thrombocytopenia. Thrombocytopenia correlates with hepatocellular injury and reaches its lowest level (more than 50% decrease) by the second postoperative day, after which it gradually returns to normal.

Both during the operation and immediately after, a rapid increase in the serum levels of tumor markers and hepatocellular enzyme (AST, ALT, LDH, bilirubin) are observed but these return to a normal level by the second-third postoperative day.

Cryoablation induces cell necrosis by several mechanisms: intra- and extracellular ice formation; solute-solvent shifts causing cell dehydration and membrane ruptures; and small vessel obliteration with resulting hypoxia. Tumor cells and normal hepatocytes are destroyed with approximately equal efficacy by freezing (Bischof et al. 1993; Tacke et al. 1998; Rubinsky et al. 1966).

Interruption of the hyperenhancing line around the cryolesion was observed when large vessels were directed towards the zone of freezing, near to the boundary of the cryolesion. A small amount of parenchyma was seen surrounding these vessels and interrupting the freeze front line. This phenomenon is possibly due to the relatively high temperature maintained by the blood flow in the surrounding tissues, with subsequent limitation of their damage.

Several factors can influence the ability of the tissue to be damaged by freezing. Most important are the thermal history (e.g., freezing rate, minimum temperature and the period during which the tissue is maintained at the lowest temperature, heating effects from local blood flow and metabolism).

A recent study performed on animals demonstrated a difference in size of frozen and damaged regions, when tissues with different metabolism and vascularization were frozen. Greater cellular dehydration occurs in normal human liver, followed by metastasis from colon carcinoma and finally by primary hepatic tumors. This consideration suggests that relapse should be expected in these regions, peripherally to major vessels.

The necrotic remains of hepatic tumors treated with cryoablation and surrounding normal tissues that are destroyed are left in situ to be reabsorbed with progressive reduction in size of cryolesion within 3 to 6 months (shrinkage).

Histological analysis of cryolesions resected (cryo-assisted surgical resection) showed a preservation of cellular architecture of the normal liver parenchyma and metastatic nodule with peripheral sinusoid enlargement (Fig. 26.3). In a period of 6 days a coagulative necrosis replaced the metastatic nodule and healthy frozen parenchyma. All blood vessels less than 0.5 mm in diameter within the necrotic region were thrombosed; at the same time, at the periphery of the cryolesion, a thin wall of granulation tissue with neovascularity, regenerating bile ducts and progressive shrinkage of sinusoidal enlargement characteristic of the early post-treatment phase were found. The parenchyma cells, intracellular architecture and blood vessels in the surrounding liver were not affected.

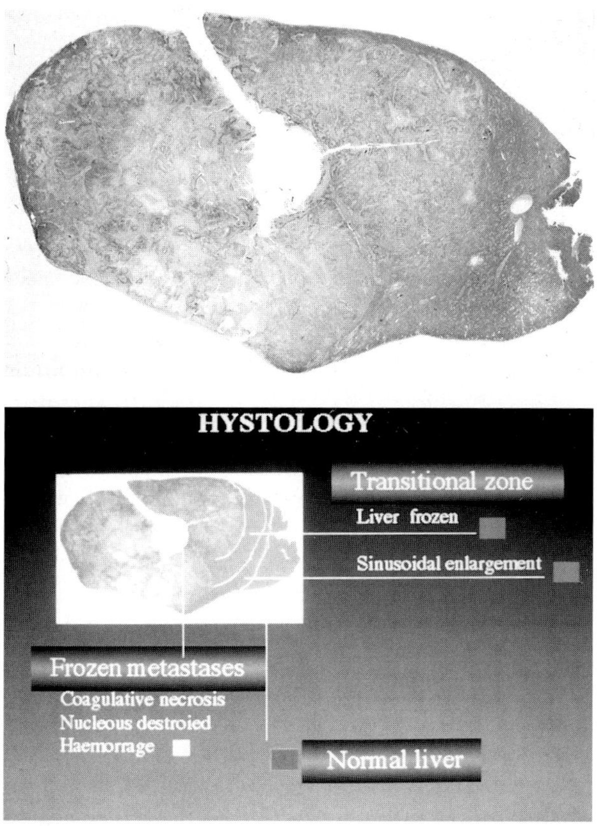

a b

Fig. 26.3a,b. Pathologic findings of cryolesion resected (cryoassisted resection). **a** Macrohistologic inclusion. **b** Scheme of pathologic specimen. Immediately after the freezing process, the architecture of metastases remains unmodified; in a period of 6 days from treatment, the coagulative necrosis replaces the metastatic nodule and healthy frozen liver parenchyma

26.4 Therapeutic Response and Follow-up Protocol

The therapeutic response of cryosurgery can be assessed on the basis of findings from different imaging modalities like ultrasonography (US) and power Doppler-US (PD-US), CT, and MR imaging. Hepatic lesion which undergoes cryosurgery is usually named, conventionally, cryolesion. Complete response is considered in cases in which cryolesion volume is larger than the treated lesion and there is no evidence of residual viable tumor tissue. Partial or minor response is defined as persistence of small (>70% or <70% of necrotic rate respectively of tumor volume) areas of residual tumor.

Follow-up protocol included abdominal US, spiral CT and MRI performed 1 week, 1 and 3 months after the procedure and at a 3-month interval thereafter. The main goal of the first imaging examination 1 week post-treatment is to detect the possible early complications of the procedure and to verify the extension and the localization of the cryolesion.

Right-pleural effusions with possible basal ateliectasis and peri-hepatic fluid collections which do not require drainage and lasted a couple of weeks represents the most frequent (about 45% of cases) complications of the procedure in the early postoperative period. Severe bleeding from the liver surface, intralesion hematoma or abscesses which require drainage, biliary fistula, biliary obstruction and portal thrombosis are uncommon complications of cryotherapy occurring in patients with large nodules.

In the other later examinations included in the protocol follow-up, patients are studied to diagnose recurrences of the treated tumors (i.e., local recurrence), recurrences caused by the evidence of new intrahepatic lesions or extrahepatic metastasis.

Unrelated to tomographic scan modalities (CT, US or MRI), three different shapes of cryolesions were seen at post-treatment exams: round-shaped, wedge-shaped and tear-drop-shaped cryolesions (Figs. 26.4–26.6). These findings are independent of the size, histology or technical approach utilized for cryoablation (open vs laparoscopic) and depend on the course and the orientation of the cryoprobe within the liver parenchyma. Particularly for the tear-drop-shaped cryolesion, a possible vascular thrombosis with subsequent hepatic infarction is evoked (Kuszyk et al. 1996). US is widely used intraoperatively, and is very effective in measuring the diameter of frozen solid hepatic tissue. In the days immediately after the treatment, US could play an important role in identifying early complications of the procedure such as intrahepatic hematoma, perihepatic fluid collection, and portal thrombosis.

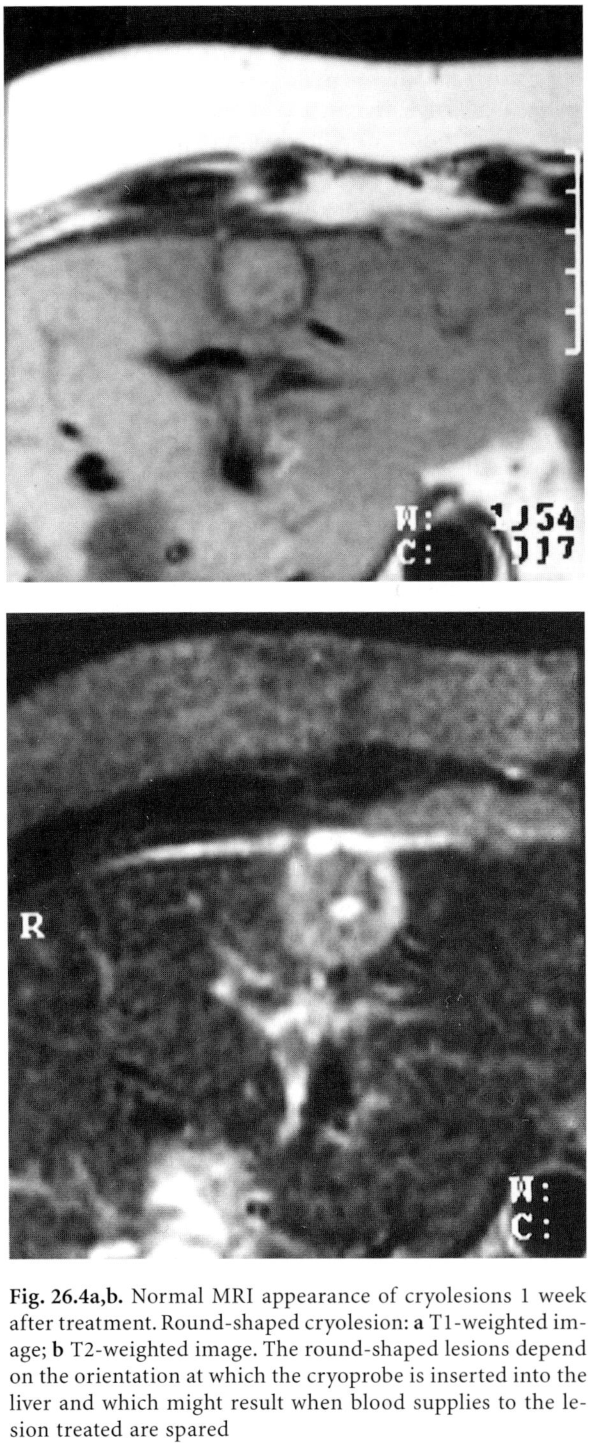

a

b

Fig. 26.4a,b. Normal MRI appearance of cryolesions 1 week after treatment. Round-shaped cryolesion: **a** T1-weighted image; **b** T2-weighted image. The round-shaped lesions depend on the orientation at which the cryoprobe is inserted into the liver and which might result when blood supplies to the lesion treated are spared

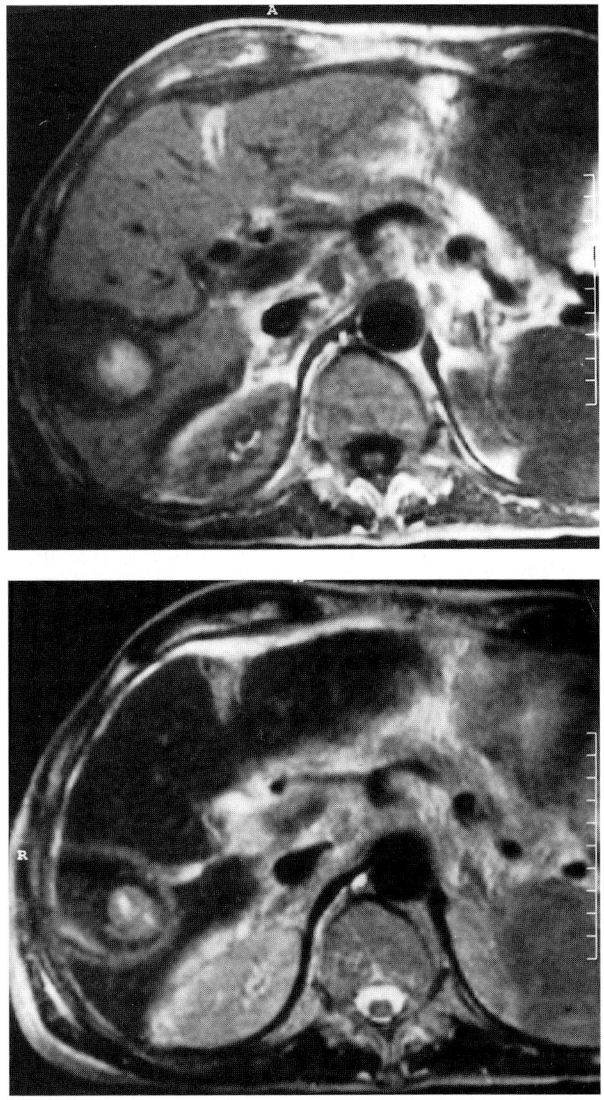

a

b

Fig. 26.5a,b. Normal MRI aspect of cryolesions 1 week after treatment. Tear-drop-shaped cryolesion: **a** T1-weighted image; **b** T2-weighted image. The tear-drop-shaped lesions present a similar origin as described for the round cryolesion; the shape depends on the cryoprobe pathway

The normal US appearance of cryolesions shows mainly dishomogeneous-hyperechoic areas surrounded by a hypoechoic rim which separates them from normal hepatic parenchyma (Fig. 26.7) (Lam et al. 1995). This finding is related to the presence of a coagulative necrosis and new-formation hematoma in the center of cryolesion where the cryoprobe was located, which causes a great quantity of interfaces responsible for the strong hyperechogenicity and the sinusoidal dilatation in the periphery of the lesions as histologically demonstrated.

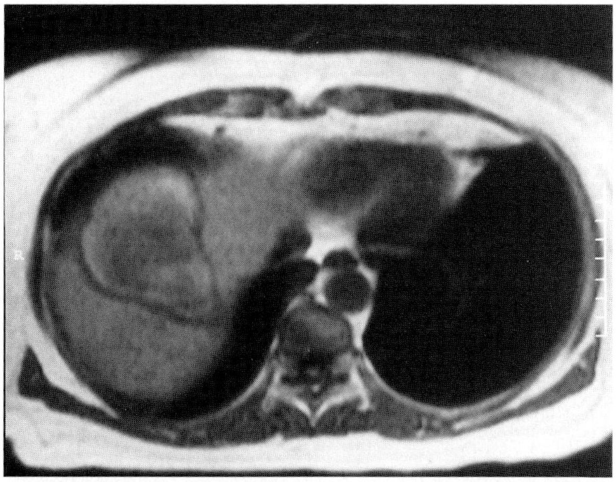

a

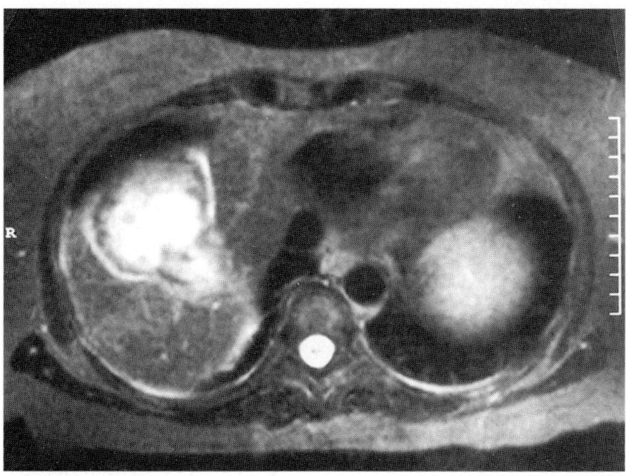

b

Fig. 26.6a,b. Normal MRI aspect of cryolesions 1 week after treatment. Wedge-shaped cryolesion: **a** T1-weighted image; **b** T2-weighted image. The cryoprobe may present some uninsulated tracts; in this condition the resulting cryolesion might extend to the liver surface regardless of either the depth of the tumor that is treated or the cryoprobe orientation. Moreover, an obliteration of both the arterial and portal venous branch could provoke hepatic infarction

As time passes the cryolesion tend to get organized, with a progressive reduction in size, assuming an echographic aspect of complex mass due to phenomena of fibrotic and colliquative degeneration inside the lesion. The progressive "shrinkage" of the cryolesion and the changes in echogenicity of the surrounding liver parenchyma, reducing liver-lesion contrast, make the diagnostic accuracy of the US scans very poor.

In the case of local recurrence which might develop several months after the procedure, US appears unable to identify the neoplastic area inside the cryolesion. For this purpose, a great contribution to the study of the hepatic lesion treated with local ablation procedures has been made by the introduction of the echocontrast agents.

Color-power Doppler (CPD) and more recently contrast-enhanced CPD increase the diagnostic possibility of the US in identifying both the extension of cryolesion and the possible local recurrence.

The cryolesion appears as an avascular area with a increase of CPD signal at the periphery due to sinusoidal dilatation and granulation tissue formation (Fig. 26.8). In the case of local recurrence, a very small vessel within the mass treated could be demonstrated using contrast enhanced CPD (Fig. 26.9). The presence of intralesional or perilesional vascular spots, which are uncertain for disease recurrences, should be considered as the possible target for US guided biopsy for histologic proof.

Computed tomography was extensively used in the follow-up of cryoablation of liver tumors (Kuszyk et al. 1996; McLoughlin et al. 1995) (Fig. 26.10). Contrast enhanced CT shows, in the early period after cryoablation, a well defined non-enhanced region of frozen tissues that is of lower attenuation than normal liver. The tracks from the recently inserted cryoprobes and small gas bubbles, which are irregularly distributed trough the frozen area, may be also visible on CT.

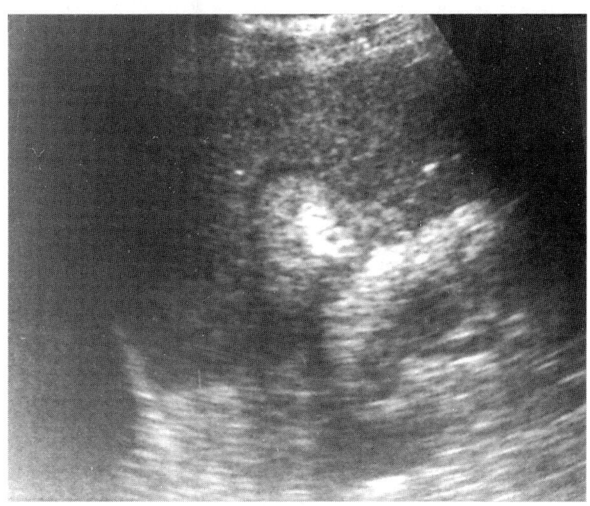

Fig. 26.7. Ultrasonography of cryolesion 3 weeks after treatment. A wedge shaped area corresponding to cryolesion is shown. Three main layers are evident from center to periphery: central hyperechoic zone (hole produced by cryoprobe) corresponding to hemorrhage and necrotic tissues; dishomogeneous hypoechoic area of coagulative necrosis within the metastatic lesions; peripheral hypoechoic rim relating to sinusoidal enlargement and granulation tissues

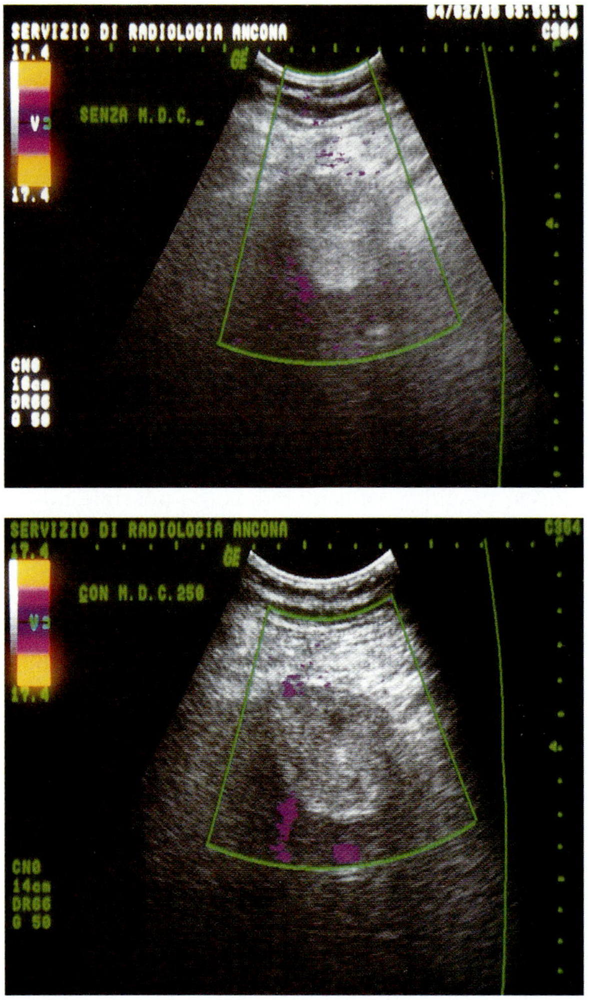

a

b

Fig. 26.8a,b. Color power Doppler ultrasonography. Complete response 2 months after cryoablation. **a** The cryolesion appears as a hyperechoic mass with any power Doppler signals inside. **b** After echocontrast agent e.v. injected no changes in PD signals are demonstrated

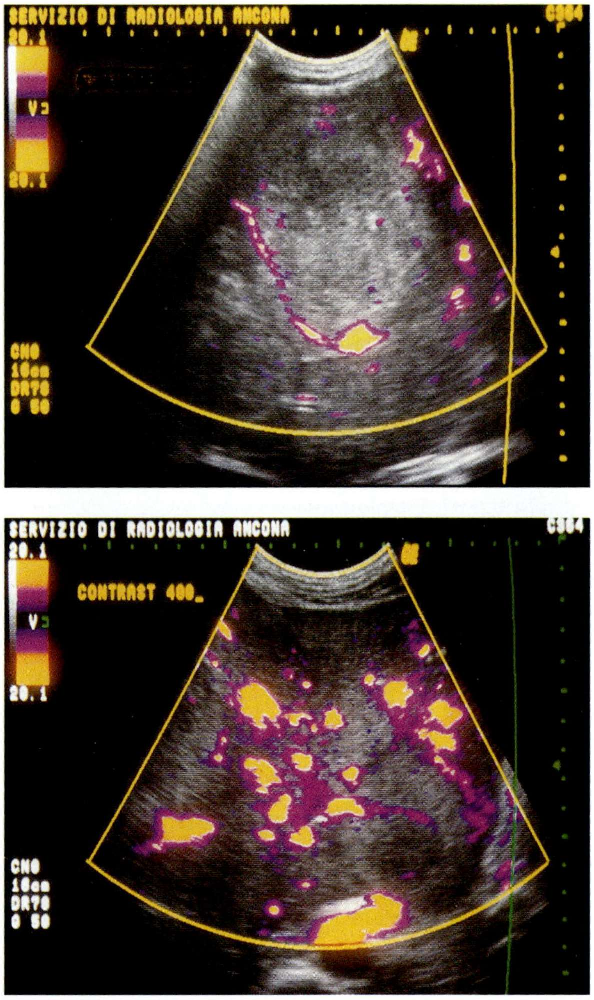

a

b

Fig. 26.9a,b. Color power Doppler ultrasonography. Partial response 6 months after cryoablation. **a** The cryolesion appears as a dishomogeneous area with initial small vascular spots on power Doppler signal. **b** After echocontrast agent i.v. injected, a dramatic increase of the vascular spots in the recurrency area is demonstrated

Air is introduced along the insertion path of the probe or may be present as a result of tissue necrosis; these bubbles usually disappear after several weeks. Higher attenuation areas within the cryolesions are indicative of hemorrhage. When the region of cryotherapy lies near the liver surface, there may be subcapsular extension of the cryonecrotic region. Cryolesion shows peripheral enhancement which is observed in the venous and equilibrium phase after contrast delivery (McLoughlin et al. 1995). In the case of local recurrence, contrast enhanced-CT might show the evidence of a focal area of contrast enhancement within the cryolesion never detected by previous examination.

CT findings, however, are often unspecific, and the distinction between a normal CT appearance of the cryolesion and the possible early complications is critical in many cases. In particular, using CT intralesional hemorrhage or abscess present a similar CT aspect (avascular area with hyperenhancing peripheral rim) with wedge-shaped or round-shaped cryolesion.

For this reason, more recently, MRI has been used for follow-up purposes either in the early period after cryoablation and during cryoablation (Giovagnoni et al. 1997a,b). On MRI, cryolesion, on T1-weighted images, appears as a dishomogeneous area slighty hyperintense or isointense compared to a 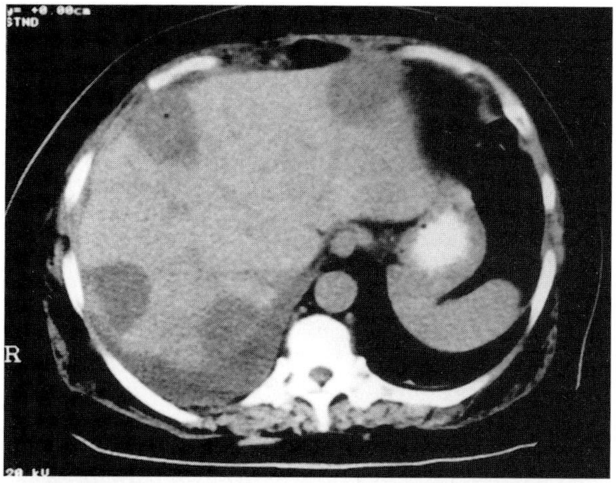

Fig. 26.10a–c. Multiple cryolesions (1 week after treatment). **a** Unenhanced CT. **b** MRI GE T1-weighted image, pre-contrast. **c** MRI GE T1-weighted dynamic images, post i.v. injection of Gd-DTPA (0.1 mmol/kg). Multiple avascular unenhanced areas corresponding to cryolesions are appreciable both at CT and MRI, relating to central coagulative necrosis and indicate successful treatment. A peripheral rim of enhancement is evident in late phase corresponding to sinusoidal enlargement

b 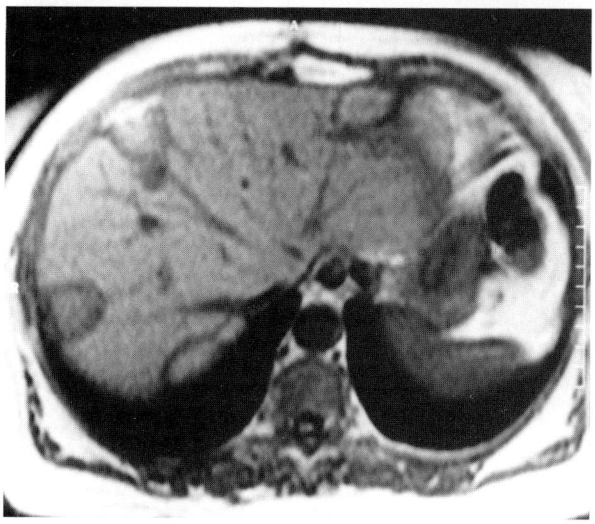

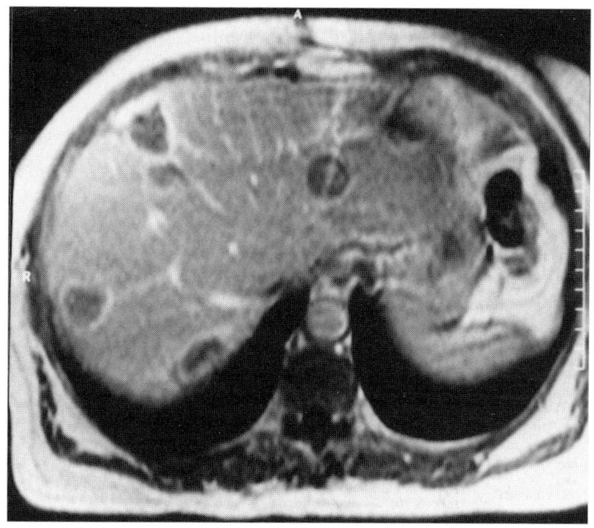 c

health parenchyma; less frequently the cryolesion remains hypointense with a signal intensity similar to metastases at pre-treatment (Matsumoto et al. 1992).

On T2-weighted images, the signal intensity of the cryolesions is low with respect to normal parenchyma, with demonstration of a series of layers within the cryolesion corresponding to the different zones histologically identified. On dynamic contrast enhanced T1-weighted images, the cryolesions appeared as a avascular non-enhanced area with a hyperintense peripheral rim of enhancement (Fig. 26.10). Multiple foci of absent signal intensity in both T1-weighted and T2-weighted images, interpreted as gas bubbles, are often demonstrated.

Interruption of hyperenhancing line around the cryolesion was observed when large vessels were directed towards the zone of freezing, near to the boundary of the cryolesion (Fig. 26.11). A small amount of parenchyma was seen surrounding these vessels and interrupting the freeze front line. This phenomenon is possibly due to the relatively high temperature maintained by the blood flow in the surrounding tissues, with subsequent limitation of their damage. In the case of complete response, a progressive shrinkage of the cryolesion is evident at three to five months (Fig. 26.12); during this period, the cryolesion maintains both avascular unenhanced behavior at dynamic contrast scans and a relative hypointensity on T2-weighted images compared to surrounding parenchyma.

Conversely the local recurrence is evident as a focal area of increase of signal intensity on T2W images which correspond to a hyperenhanced focal nodule in post Gd-chelate T1-weighted images (Fig. 26.13). MRI has demonstrated its usefulness in dif-

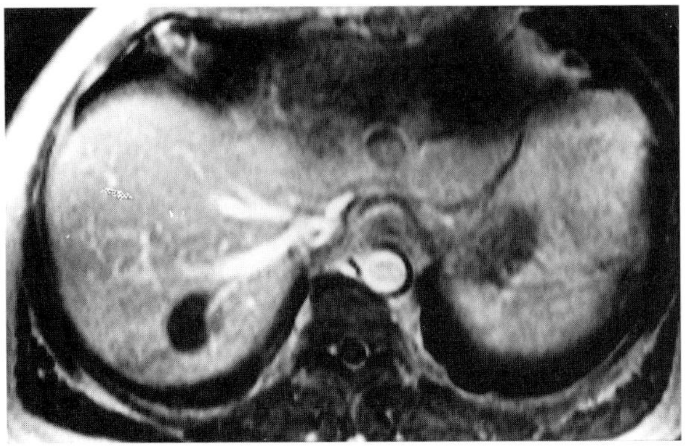

Fig. 26.11. Patient with hepatic cryolesion 1 month after treatment. GE T1-weighted enhanced images (venous phase). The peripheral rim is interrupted, since a portal branch is close to the lesion and a small amount of undamaged tissue is present. These regions should be carefully monitored as areas at risk for possible relapse

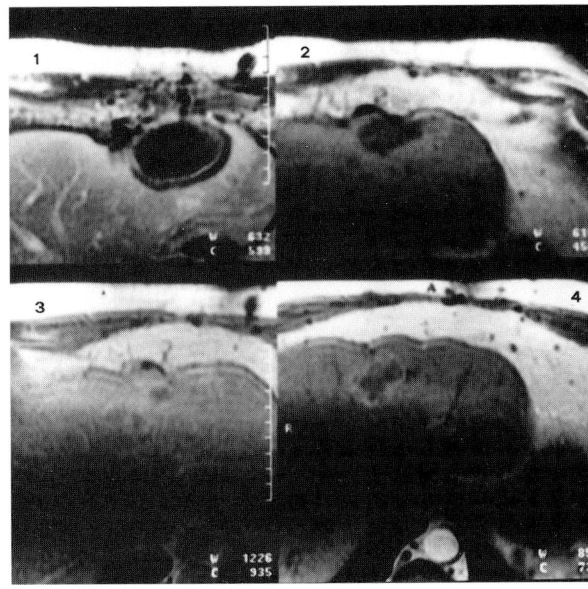

Fig. 26.13. Dynamic contrast enhanced MR images of hepatic cryolesion. Progressive reduction in size of cryolesion (*1, 2, 3*) (shrinkage) at 1, 3, 9 months after treatment. One year follow-up (*4*) shows an increase in size of lesion with dishomogeneous peripheral enhancement relating to recurrence of metastastic disease

ferentiating the normal appearance of cryolesion and more frequently serious complications of the procedure such as intralesional hemorrhages or abscess. In these cases MRI gives more information compared to the other imaging modalities regarding the presence, size and extension of fluid collection, relationship with biliary tract and blood vessels, offering important elements for the choice of the best therapeutic approach.

Very recently the use of superparamagnetic iron oxide hepatobiliary contrast agent (Endorem, Guerbet, France) has been utilized in follow-up of patients with liver metastases treated with cryoablation (Giovagnoni et al. 1997b). The use of contrast agents increase the sensitivity of MRI in the detection of new focal liver lesions; conversely the lack of enhancement of the cryolesion does not allow the differentiation between cryolesion with local recurrence and completely successfully treated metastases.

Cryosurgery should be considered another modality of treatment in patients who are not candidates for traditional hepatic resection, because of

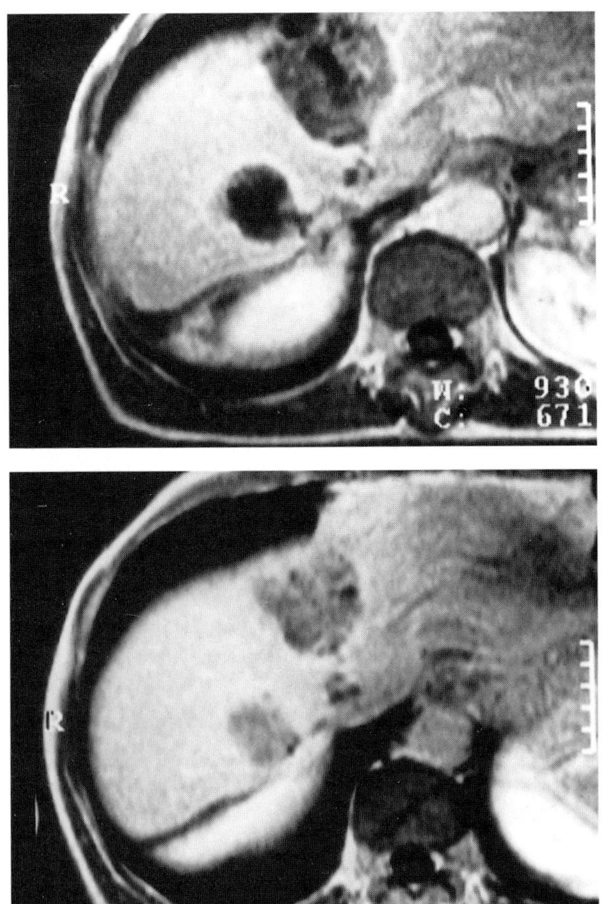

a

b

Fig. 26.12a,b. Patient with hepatic cryolesions. **a** MRI contrast enhanced (i.v. injection of Gd-DTPA 0.1 mmol/kg). T1-weighted image 1 month after treatment. Normal MRI appearance of cryolesion; avascular area with hyperenhancing rim are demonstrated. **b** Contrast enhanced T1-weighted images, 4 months post-treatment. A reduction in size of cryolesion compared to previous examinations is evident. The lesions, however, show a dishomogeneous enhancement in late phase; this finding suggests unsuccessful treatment local with recurrence multiplicity, anatomic location, the patient's condition or limited hepatic reserve. Although the preliminary data are of great interest, the clinical efficacy of this procedure is far from being defined and more survival trials should be done.

References

Bischof J, Christov K, Rubinsky B (1993) A morphological study of cooling rate response in normal and neoplastic human liver tissue: cryosurgical implications. Cryobiology 30:482–92

Busch E, Kemeny MM (1995) Colorectal cancer: hepatic-directed therapy: the role of surgery, regional chemotherapy, and novel modalities. Semin Oncol 22:494–508

Cuschieri A, Crosthwaite G, Shimi S, et al (1995) Hepatic cryotherapy for liver tumors. Development and clinical evaluation of a high-efficiency insulated multineedle probe system for open and laparoscopic use. Surg Endosc 9:483–489

Fong Y, Blumgart LH, Cohen AM (1995) Surgical treatment of colorectal metastases to the liver. CA Cancer J Clin 45:50–62

Giovagnoni A, Paci E, Valeri G, et al (1997a) Follow up MRI of hepatic metastases after cryosurgery. Eur Rad 7:S201–207

Giovagnoni A, Paci E, Valeri G, et al (1997) MRI follow up after cryosurgery of focal liver lesions: use of paramagnetic iron oxide contrast agent. MAGMA 5 126:394–399

Kane RA (1993) Ultrasound-guided hepatic cryosurgery for tumor ablation. Semin Intervent Radiol 10:132–142

Kuszyk BS, Choti MA, Urban BA, et al (1996) Hepatic tumors treated by cryosurgery: normal CT appearance. AJR 165:363–368

Lam CM, Shimi SM, Cuschieri A (1995) Ultrasonographic characterization of hepatic cryolesions. An ex vivo study. Arch Surg 130 10):1068–1072

Lezoche E, Paganini A, Campagnacci P, et al (1998) Ultrasound-guided laparoscopic cryoablation of hepatic tumors: preliminary report. World J Surg 22:829–835

Litvinenko AA (1994) Character and dynamics of structural changes in the liver under the effects of low temperature. Klin Khir 10:51–54

Matsumoto R, Oshio K, Jolesz FA (1992) Monitoring of laser and freezing-induced ablation in the liver with T1-weighted MR imaging. Magn Res Med 2:555–562

McCall Jl, Booth MW, Morris DL (1995) Hepatic cryotherapy for metastatic liver tumours. Br J Hosp Med 54:378–381

McLoughlin RF, Saliken JF, McKinnon G, Wiseman D, Temple W (1995) CT of the liver after cryotherapy of hepatic metastases: imaging findings. AJR Am J Roengtenol 165:329–332

Onik GM, Atkinson D, Zemel R, Weaver ML (1993) Cryosurgery of liver cancer. Semin Surg Oncol 9:309–317

Polk W, Fong Y, Karpeh M, Blumgart LH (1995) A technique for the use of cryosurgery to assist hepatic resection. J Am Coll Surg 180:171–176

Ramming KP (1995) Cryosurgery: the coming of the surgical ice age? J Surg Oncol 58:147–148

Ravikumar TS, Kane R, Cady B, Jenkins R, Clouse M, Sleele G (1991a) A 5-year study of cryosurgery in the treatment ol liver tumors. Arch Surg 126:1520–1524

Ravikumar TS, Steele G, Kane R, King V (1991b) Experimental and clinical observations on hepatic cryosurgery for colorectal metastases. Cancer 51:6323–6327

Ravikumar TS, Buenaventura S, Salem RR, D'Andrea B (1994) Intraoperative ultrasonography of liver: detection of occult liver tumors and treatment by cryosurgery. Cancer Detect Prev 18:131–138

Rubinsky B, Gilbert JC, Roos MS, Pease GR, Brennan KM, Onik GM (1996) Tissue correlation after MRI-guided cryosurgery in dog prostate. In: Proceedings of the International Society for Magnetic Resonance in Medicine. Fourth Scientific Meeting and Exhibition. New York, USA, vol 3, p 59.

Shafir M, Shapiro R, Sung M, Warner R, Sicular A, Klipfel A (1996) Cryoablation of unresectable malignant liver tumors. Am J Surgery 171:27–31

Stewart GJ, Preketes A, Horton M, Ross WB, Morris DL (1995) Hepatic cryotherapy: double-freeze cycles achieve greater hepatocellular injury in man. Crybiology 32:215–219

Tacke J, Adam G, Spetzeen R, Bruskseh K, et al (1998) MR-guided interstizial cryotherapy of the liver with a novel nitrogen-cooled cryoprobe. MRM 39:354–360

Zhou XD, Tang ZY, Yu YQ, et al (1993) The role of cryosurgery in the treatment of hepatic cancer: a report of 113 cases. J Cancer Res Clin Oncol 120:100–102

IV Special Topics

27 Pediatric Tumors of the Liver

P. Tomà, G. Lucigrai, and M. Oddone

CONTENTS

27.1 Introduction

Liver tumors are rare in children, representing 1.5–3% of all tumors (Kramarova et al. 1996; Newman 1997; Stocker et al. 1998; Tschappeler 1993; Vos 1995). They usually present with abdominal distension, occasionally with pain, fever, pallor, anemia or jaundice. The main problem is the differentiation between benign (Luks et al. 1991) and malignant tumors. About 60% of liver tumors are malignant. Alpha-fetoprotein serum level is an essential test in diagnosis and follow-up of a liver tumor. It is elevated in about 90% of hepatoblastoma (HB) and 80% of hepatocellular carcinoma (HCC) (Brunelle et al. 1994; Cohen 1992).

P. Tomà, MD; Chief, Department of Radiology, G. Gaslini Children's Research Hospital, Largo G. Gaslini 5, I-16148 Genoa, Italy
G. Lucigrai, MD; Department of Radiology, G. Gaslini Children's Research Hospital, Largo G. Gaslini 5, I-16148 Genoa, Italy
M. Oddone, MD; Department of Radiology, G. Gaslini Children's Research Hospital, Largo G. Gaslini 5, I-16148 Genoa, Italy

Current imaging techniques play an important role in diagnosis, staging (Cohen et al. 1996), therapeutic decision and follow-up (Bowman and Riely 1996; Donnelly and Bisset 1998; Weimann et al. 1997). The first imaging modality to be done in a child with a large liver is ultrasonography (US), because of its large accessibility and higher sensitivity.

US usually differentiates, with the clinical presentation, tumors from other liver lesions, such as abscesses, hematoma, hydatid cysts, focal fatty infiltration and cirrhotic nodules. Tumors of the right adrenal gland are differentiated from liver tumors on the position of the inferior vena cava, easily assessed by US: the vein is displaced anteriorly by a right adrenal tumor and posteriorly by a liver tumor. US is often sufficient to make the diagnosis of solitary or multiple angioma of the liver. Cystic tumors such as cystic lymphangiomas are so characteristic that they do not need any further imaging. No truly cystic tumors are malignant. When the tumor is solid and secretes high levels of alpha-fetoprotein (Ohama et al.1997), the prognosis is directly related to the resectability (Achilleos et al. 1996; Okada et al. 1998). A precise preoperative workup is necessary by CT; we emphasize the role of spiral CT with 3D reconstruction (Frush et al. 1997; Herzberg et al. 1998; Plumley et al. 1995), magnetic resonance imaging (MRI) (Buetow et al. 1997b; Siegel and Luker 1996), and angiography. When alpha-fetoprotein levels are normal, the exact nature of the tumor may be difficult to assess by imaging techniques only. Diagnosis is frequently made on liver biopsy.

27.2 Benign Tumors

27.2.1 Hemangioma

This is the most frequent liver tumor in infancy. The female to male ratio is about 2:1 (Brunelle et al.

1994). It may present itself as a solitary form or as a diffuse one. The term "cavernous hemangioma" is usually applied only to focal, well defined lesions, whereas "infantile hemangioendothelioma" is generally used to describe more diffuse lesions, particularly in newborns (Davenport et al. 1995). Clinical presentation and evolution are different: multiple hepatic hemangiomas in most cases occur after a free interval after birth (generally 1 week), whereas solitary hemangiomas are usually diagnosed at birth (Kane et al. 1997). Liver hemangiomas can be discovered antenatally (De Bievre et al. 1994; Samuel and Spitz 1995); intrauterine bleeding with bloody amniotic fluid, severe anemia, congestive heart failure and hydrops fetalis were described (Fok et al. 1996; Wu and Teng 1994).

They have a natural tendency to slow fibrolipomatous involution (18 months to 8 years), often after a period of rapid growth (6–8 months) and a variable long-standing florid period. Regression of solitary hemangiomas is more rapid, starting before the third month and calcifications are more frequent than in multiple forms (Brunelle et al. 1994). An exclusive involvement of the extrahepatic biliary tree with hepatomegaly and obstructive jaundice is reported (Maksimak et al. 1990). The pathogenesis is not yet understood; a rare familial occurrence suggesting an autosomal dominant inheritance is reported (Blei et al. 1998; Moser et al. 1998).

Histologically they are characterized by endothelial proliferation, increased turnover of mast cells, and progressive perivascular deposition of fibrofatty tissue. Infantile hemangioendothelioma and cavernous hemangioma differ from the size of the vascular spaces, capillary in the former, larger blood-filled in the latter.

The diagnosis is strongly suspected in an infant with hepatomegaly, cutaneous hemangiomas and cardiac failure: liver US is not necessary as a routine test in children with several immature angiomas, but without the other signs (Lorette et al. 1996). Other severe complications may occur, including consumptive coagulopathy (Kasabach-Merrit syndrome characterized by an atypical histology "infantile kaposiform hemangioendothelioma"), hemoperitoneum, and late recurrence, suggestive of malignant degeneration (Awan et al. 1996). Alpha-fetoprotein may be highly elevated in preterm infants (Lehrnbecher et al. 1996).

Cardiac failure is more frequent in multiple than in solitary hemangiomas, whereas thrombopenia is more frequent in solitary forms. The overall prognosis of multiple hemangiomas is pejorative compared with solitary ones. A rare combination of testicular feminization (Morris S.) with disseminated liver hemangiomatosis is described (Nedkova et al. 1996).

On US (Siegel 1995), liver hemangioma presents itself either as a solid heterogeneous mass or as a huge tumoral hepatomegaly with multiple nodules which are more often hypoechoic. The differential diagnosis mainly includes metastatic neuroblastoma (Pepper's syndrome), when the lesions are multiple, hepatoblastoma in solitary forms and the rare hemangiopericytoma (Flores-Stadler et al. 1997). In both types of hemangioma, color and/or power Doppler show an increased centripetal vascularization, sometimes with fistulas, with enlarged hepatic artery and veins and proximal aorta while pulsed Doppler demonstrates high flow velocity (80–90 cm/s) and a low resistance index (RI: 0.4–0.7) (Fig. 27.1). With the fibrolipomatous involution the RI progressively increases.

If diagnosis remains uncertain, CT has to be performed demonstrating, after bolus injection, marked peripheral enhancement of the hemangioma, identified as a low-attenuation lesion on unenhanced scans. Subsequent images show progressive centripetal opacification, and on delayed scans extending to at least 30 min there is complete isodense fill-in of the lesion compared to normal liver parenchyma (Fig. 27.2). Some variations on this pattern have been described.

MRI is a good imaging modality. Hemangiomas have a high signal intensity on heavily T2 weighted images. Dynamic contrast-enhanced GRE imaging confirms the diagnosis with 100% specificity and 95% accuracy, based on a pathognomonic nodular, globular enhancement pattern, with progressive centripetal filling-in, within 5–30 min.

An early "blush" on Tc-99m RBC hepatic scintigraphy is another diagnostic feature of this type of lesion (Park et al. 1996).

Angiography is nowadays only performed as a prelude to therapeutic embolization in the case of complications of the diffuse form (Fig. 27.3). It shows dilated feeding arteries, large draining hepatic veins, and multiple well-limited nodules with capillary staining, peripheral in the early phase, homogeneous in the late phase (Brunelle et al. 1994). Systemic high dose steroid administration is the first choice of therapy with a response rate of around 30 to 60%. Interferon alpha-2a or 2b also shows encouraging results. The response to therapy may be evaluated by pulsed Doppler of the proximal aorta: reduction in flow (Bruce et al. 1995; Perez Payarols et al. 1995). Also MRI may be useful for monitoring

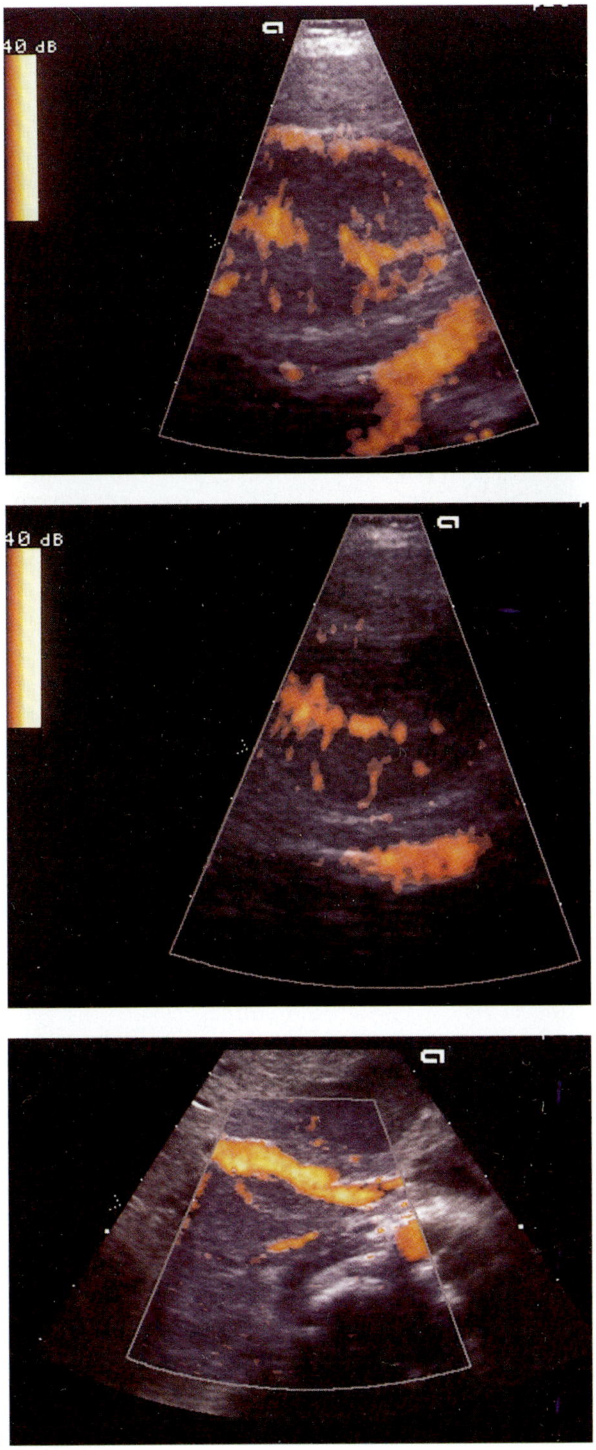

a b c

Fig. 27.1a–c. Hepatic hemangioendothelioma in a newborn. Evaluation of a hypoechogenic nodule with power Doppler (a,b) shows the typical centripetal vascularization. The hepatic artery is bigger than normal (c)

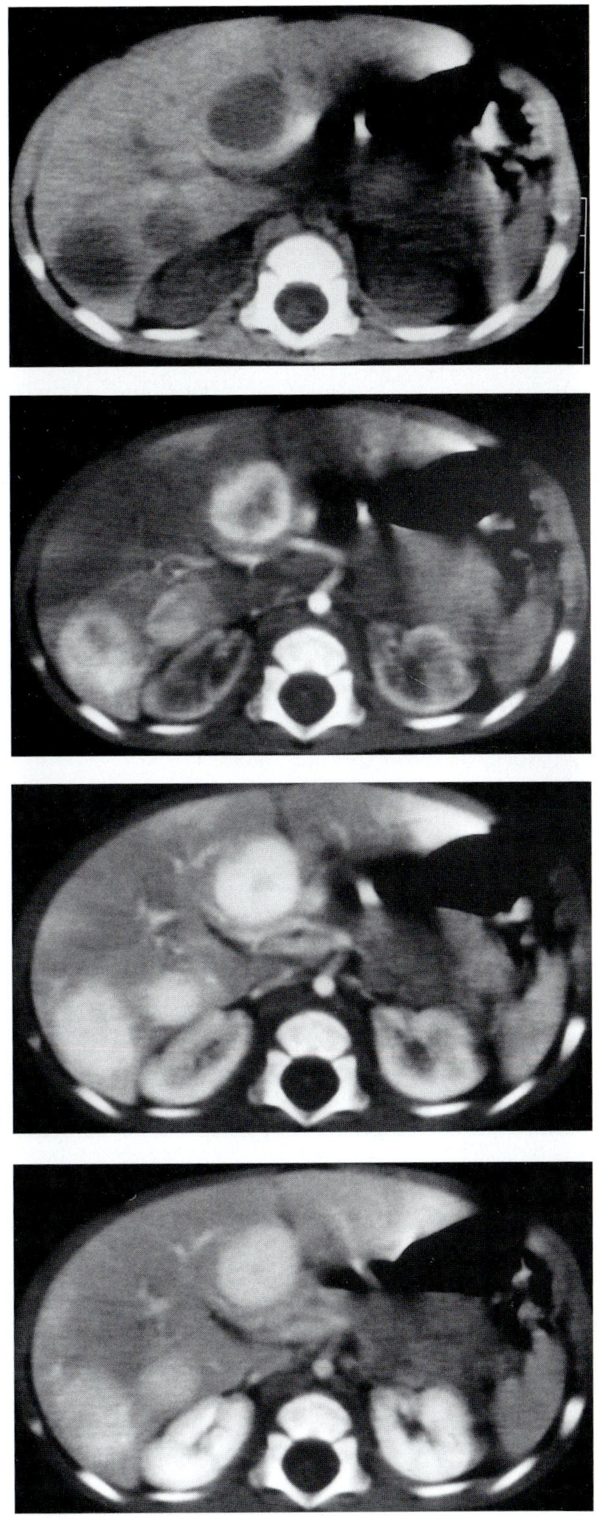

a b c d

Fig. 27.2a–d. Hepatic hemangioendothelioma in a newborn (same case). CT without contrast medium (a) shows multiple hypointense nodules. Dynamic scans after contrast medium show an evident peripheral ring (30 s) (b), a progressive centripetal enhancement (1 min, 30 s) (c), and a homogeneous opacification of the masses (3 min) (d)

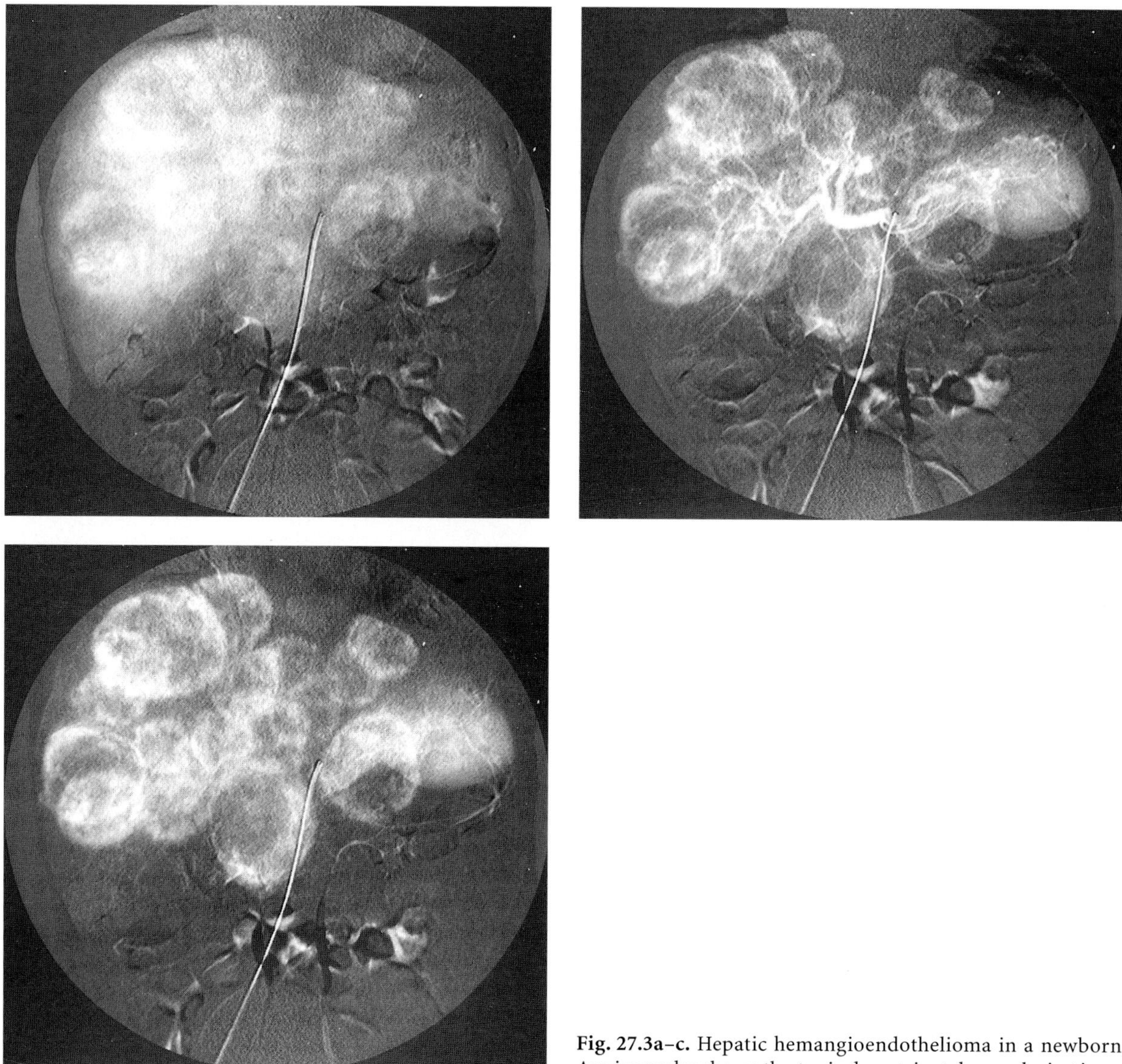

Fig. 27.3a–c. Hepatic hemangioendothelioma in a newborn. Angiography shows the typical centripetal vascularization

therapy: decrease in lesion size and subsequently in number and reduction of the signal intensity on T2-weighted images (Chung et al. 1996; Stover et al. 1995). Embolization and/or surgery (Samuel and Spitz 1995) is performed as the last resort (Iyer et al. 1996).

The so called cavernous hemangiomas that affect older children and adolescents are usually an incidental postmortem finding. Occasionally, they present themselves with hepatomegaly. On US they are homogeneous and hyperechoic if degeneration or fibrosis have not occurred. A definitive diagnosis requires another imaging study, such as contrast enhanced CT or MRI (Nelson and Chezmar 1990).

27.2.2 Mesenchymal Hamartoma

This seems to be a developmental anomaly rather than a true neoplasm, composed of a mixture of hepatocytes, abnormal bile ducts and immature mesenchyme in variable portions (Alwaidh et al. 1997; Lai et al. 1996). Mesenchymal hamartoma may be solid, but most are either partially or totally cystic (Das et al. 1997; George et al. 1994; Motiwale et al. 1996). It has a marked male predominance. Clinical presentation most frequently occurs between 4 months and 2 years of age and is characterized by an asymptomatic, sometimes very large, right upper quadrant mass, sometimes with severe unexplained apnea (Balmer et al. 1996). Symptoms, if they occur, are related to mass effect on adjacent organs. The inferior vena cava may be obstructed. The tumor may be diagnosed prenatally by US (Bejvan et al. 1997; Ruiz et al. 1995; Singh et al. 1996; Tovbin et al. 1997). This tumor has a good prognosis and is usually cured by excision. The natural history of mesenchymal hamartoma of the liver is poorly understood. A link with the hepatic undifferentiated sarcoma is suggested (Lauwers et al. 1997). Cases of spontaneous involution and resolution are reported (Barnhart et al. 1997).

Sonography very often demonstrates a large, predominantly cystic hepatic mass, with thin echogenic septa (Fig. 27.4). A hepatic origin of the lesion is not always evident. The solid subtype usually demonstrates increased echogenicity compared to normal liver parenchyma. The large solid components are relatively vascular. The typical CT or MR appearance of the mesenchymal hamartoma is a large, usually well defined, multilocular cystic mass (Fig. 27.5). Septations of variable thickness and calcifications may be identified on CT. Solid components enhance after administration of intravenous contrast material (Wholey and Wojno 1994).

27.2.3 Adenoma

Hepatocellular adenoma (HCA) is a relatively rare lesion more often associated with glycogen storage

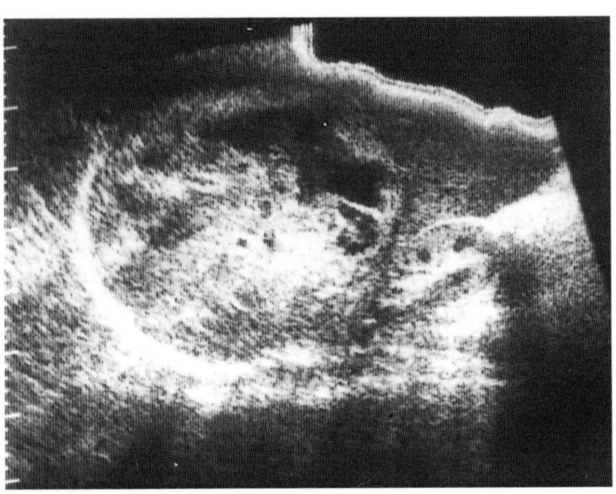

Fig. 27.4. Mesenchymatous hamartoma in a 6-year-old boy. US show a complex mass extensively occupying the right lobe of the liver

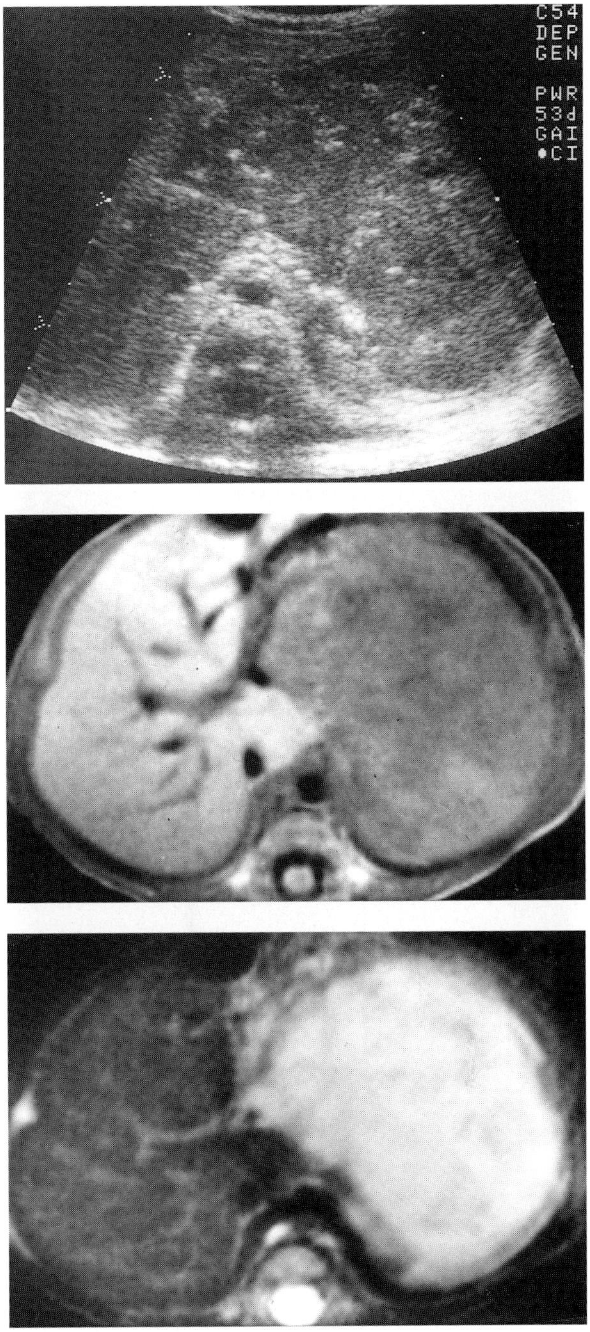

a

b

c

Fig. 27.5a–c. Mesenchymatous hamartoma in a 5-month-old baby. US (**a**) shows a voluminous left hepatic mass with hyperechogenic spots inside (calcifications) and without liquid areas. SE T1-weighted (**b**) and SE T2-weighted (**c**) MR scans show a clear hypersignal of the mass on T2

disease type I, less often type III and rarely type IV (Alshak et al. 1994; Brunelle et al. 1984; Labrune et al. 1997), Fanconi's anemia (due to anabolic steroid treatment) (Garel et al. 1981), Hurler's disease, severe combined immunodeficiency, and some

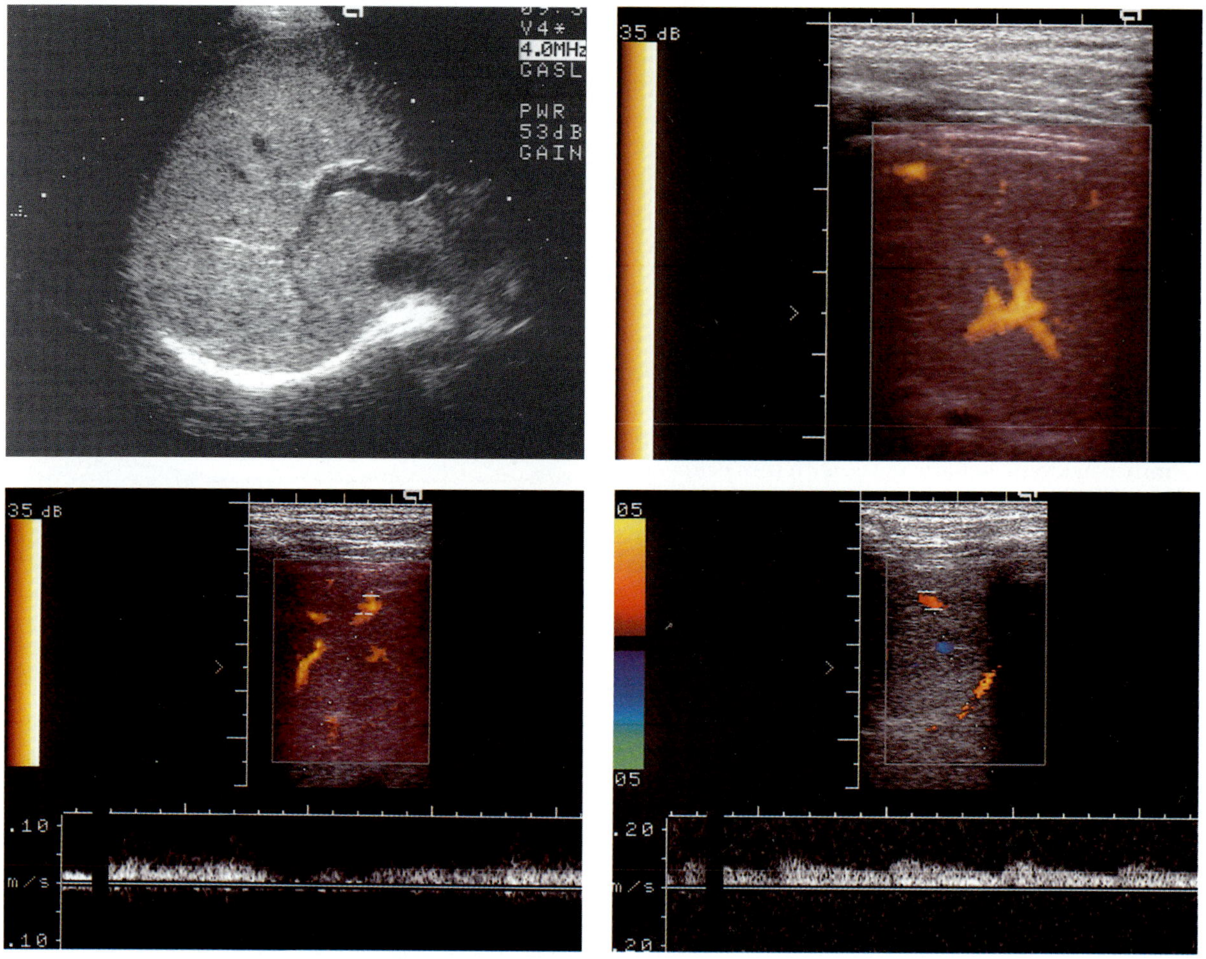

a b c d

Fig. 27.6a–d. Adenoma in a 7-year-old girl. US show a well circumscribed isoechoic mass in the right lobe of the liver **(a)**. Power Doppler shows the vascularization of the tumor **(b)** while pulsed Doppler examination shows the venous spectrum of the intratumoral vessels **(c)** associated with pulsatile peripheral flow **(d)**

progestative drugs (Resnick et al. 1995) or other disease (Bala et al. 1997). A few cases in otherwise healthy children have been reported (Bourliere-Najean et al. 1989; Milillo et al. 1997). Histologically it consists of normal liver cells.

The lesion rarely achieves sufficient size to produce symptoms and, in many cases, it is discovered incidentally on imaging studies performed for other reasons. These tumors, usually solitary, but rarely multiple (Gokhale and Whitington 1996), may be seen because of complications: hemorrhagic infarction, necrosis, and rupture with hemoperitoneum, and infection. Degeneration into HCC is possible.

On US the echogenicity is variable and areas of central hemorrhage and calcifications are suggestive. The lesion is usually well circumscribed and may be iso- or hypoechoic. If bleeding occurs, adenoma can be hyperechoic or can have a mixed echo pattern (Lee et al. 1994). Color/power Doppler shows intratumoral vessels with a venous spectrum (none with an arterial Doppler wave form), associated with either pulsatile and continuous peripheral flow; this pattern allows the differentiation with focal nodular hyperplasia (Fig. 27.6) (Bartolozzi et al. 1997).

The typical CT (Sty et al. 1992) appearance is of low-attenuation masses, best visualized on unenhanced scans. Heterogeneous enhancement is usually identified after intravenous contrast agent administration. Hemorrhage in the lesion may produce a central area of increased attenuation on nonenhanced scans.

Hepatic adenomas are often isointense to normal liver parenchyma on T1-weighted MR, with a hypointense rim (Sty et al. 1992). Since these tumors often contain fat, they may range in signal intensity on T1-weighted images from mildly hypointense to high signal intensity. HCA is mildly hyperintense and somewhat heterogeneous on T2 weighted images (Fig. 27.7). Most frequently hemorrhage appears as a region of mixed high signal intensity on T1- and T2-weighted images (EDELMAN et al. 1996). Embolization is performed on emergency basis because of bleeding.

27.2.4
Focal Nodular Hyperplasia

This is a benign epithelial tumor that likely represents a local hyperplastic response of normal hepatocytes to a congenital vascular anomaly (BUETOW et al. 1996; GUARISO et al. 1998). It is reported in all pediatric age groups with a female predominance. It is generally a unique, large-lobulated, well defined and hypervascular mass, characterized pathologically by a central dense fibrous scar from which septa containing proliferating bile ducts and blood vessels radiate. Among the septa there are normal hepatocytes. It is most frequently detected as an incidental finding during radiologic investigations. Symptomatic patients complain of an abdominal mass or abdominal pain investigations. The association of a portocaval shunt is significant compared to other tumors (SAKATOKU et al. 1996). The prenatal diagnosis by US has been reported (PETRIKOVSKY et al. 1994); in one case the infant was antenatally exposed to steroids (PRASAD et al. 1995). Focal nodular hyperplasia (FNH) resulting in secondary polycythemia and stained positively for erythropoietin by immunohistochemistry has been recently described (SANDLER et al. 1997).

On US (BUETOW et al. 1996), FNH is homogeneous, generally isoechoic, and in some cases has a central fibrotic scar which is hyperechoic and may demonstrate hypervascularity on color Doppler. In some cases, color Doppler will reveal a central hypervascular nidus, corresponding to the scar that was not visualized on gray-scale images. In 25% of cases the vessels follow a typical stellate pattern: several small-sized arteries which originate from a single, central, large vessel. In contrast with the pattern of HCA, central continuous flow is never depicted. Large draining vessels may be identified in the periphery at the tumor margins (pulsatile flow is also evident). Power Doppler imaging is superior to conventional color Doppler sonography in the depiction of the intratumoral flow (BARTOLOZZI et al. 1997). It enables detection of flow also in lesions

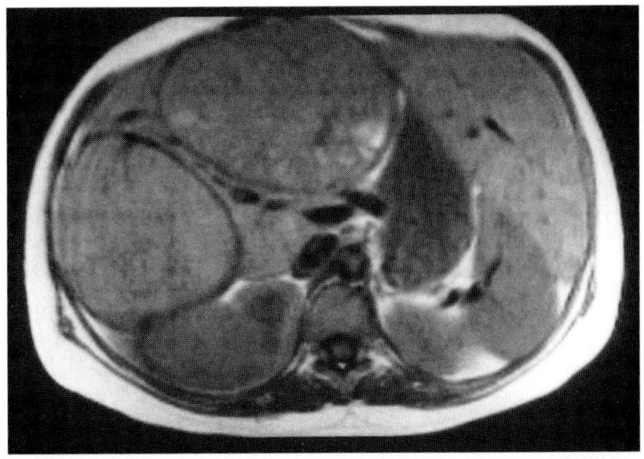
a

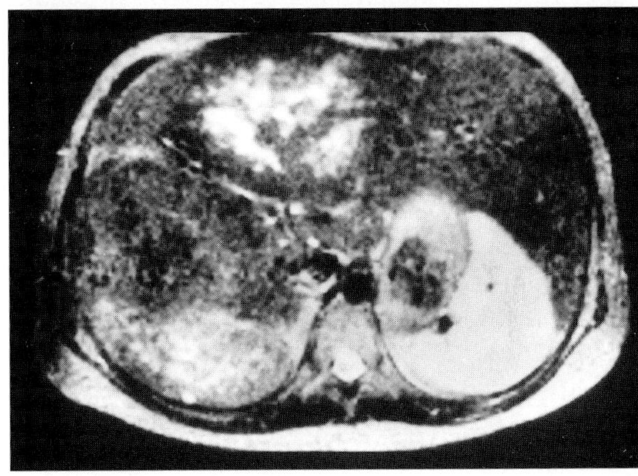
b

Fig. 27.7a,b. Multiple adenomas in glycogenosis. Young adult: MRI, SE T1-weighted (**a**) and SE T2-weighted (**b**) scans. Multiple isointense nodules (T1) with some hyperintense spots inside (fat). Inhomogeneous signal enhancement on T2

smaller than 3 cm. These US characteristics may overlap with those of well-differentiated hepatocellular carcinomas.

On unenhanced CT, FNH appears as a homogeneous, slightly hypoattenuating or isoattenuating mass. A central hypoattenuating scar may be visualized in one-third of cases, small and subtle. On MR images (TOMÀ et al. 1990), the lesion is generally of low-intermediate signal intensity on T1 weighted images and mildly increased signal intensity on T2 weighted images. The central scar is generally hypointense on T1 weighted images, and slightly hyperintense on T2 weighted images. Neither the presence of scar nor its features is diagnostic of FNH.

The tumor is the second benign hepatic lesion which can be identified on the basis of their virtually pathognomonic enhancement profile on CT and MRI. Correct timing of the arterial phase data acquisition is crucial for a confident diagnosis. The mainly arterial supply of the lesion is reflected by very early and homogeneous enhancement (within the first 30 s) followed by rapid wash-out and equilibration with surrounding hepatic parenchyma (90 s after intravenous injection of contrast material). Only the centrally located scar demonstrates late enhancement on the equilibrium phase images (Fig. 27.8) (Buetow et al. 1996). CT has the highest diagnostic accuracy (De Gaetano et al. 1996). Unfortunately, the features of focal nodular hyperplasia may also be seen with a well-differentiated small hepatocellular carcinoma, a fibrolamellar carcinoma, an adenoma and a hyperplastic nodule (Shamsi et al. 1993). Normal or increased uptake on a Tc-99m sulfur colloid scan (about 50%) is extremely helpful in supporting the diagnosis of FNH (Buetow et al. 1996).

A multimodality approach is essential; imaging follow-up, needle biopsy, or even surgical resection may be required in some cases (Buetow et al. 1996). Angiography is performed to reduce, by embolization, the vascularization and volume of the tumor (Reymond et al. 1995). It shows a hypervascular tumor with one or two enlarged arteries giving branches from the periphery to the center of the tumor. Dilated veins are seen at the periphery and there is a massive opacification of hepatic veins on the late films. This type of vascularization gives the impression that the tumor is embedded in a vascular net (Brunelle et al. 1994). All branches of the portal vein are present and patent.

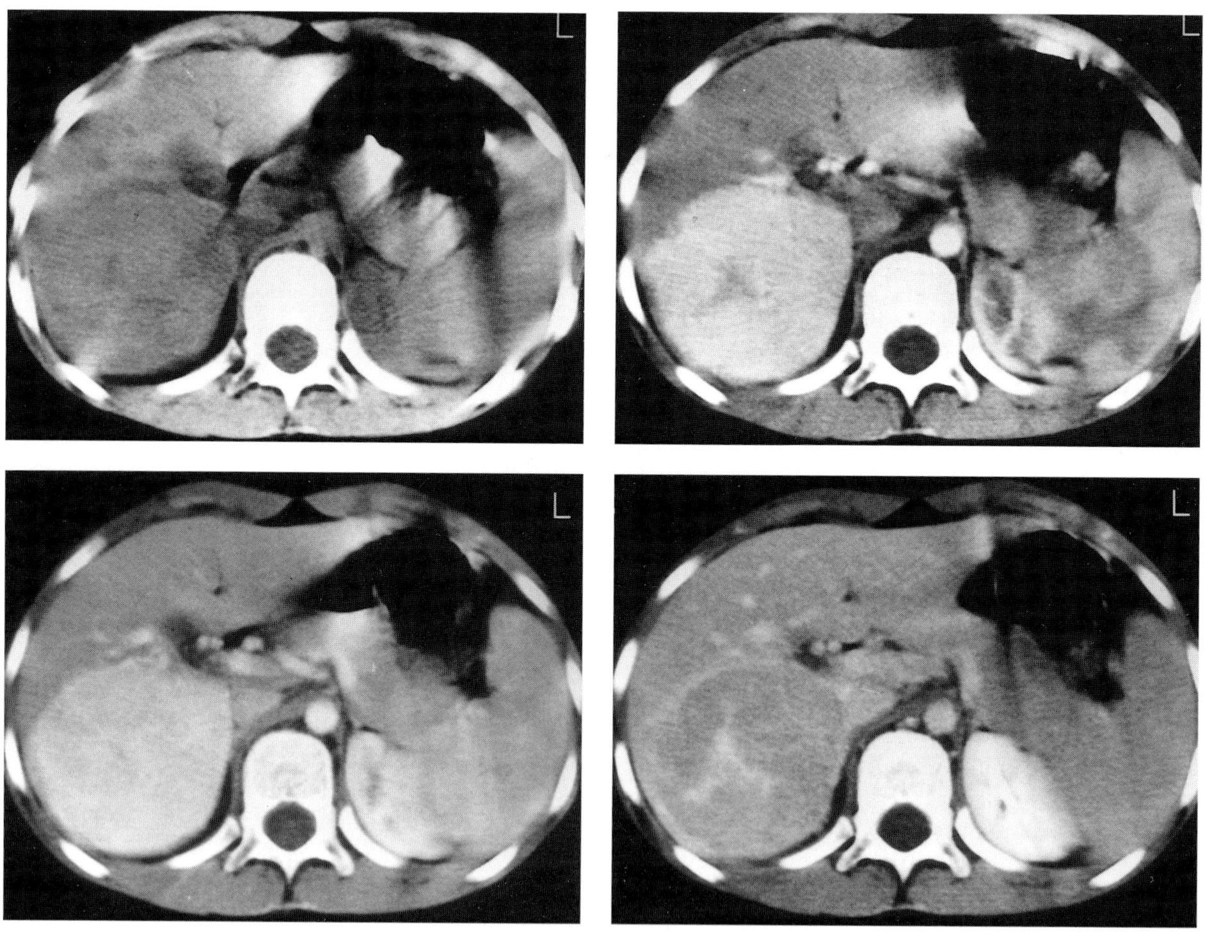

Fig. 27.8a–d. Focal nodular hyperplasia in a 9-year-old boy. CT without contrast medium (**a**) shows a hepatic right mass slightly hypodense with a central zone of lower density (*scar*). Dynamic CT scans after contrast medium (**b–d**) show enhancement of the mass (not of the central scar) at 1 min (**b**); homogeneous enhancement of the mass at 2 min (**c**) and late enhancement of the scar that appears hyperdense compared to the mass at 6 min (**d**)

27.2.5 Other Benign Tumors

Other primary benign hepatic tumors are quite rare. These include teratoma, lymphangioma, epithelioma, epidermoid cyst, and lipoma (angiomyolipoma with/without tuberous sclerosis) (BEN-IZHAK et al. 1995; MONGA et al. 1994). Rare tumors arise from the biliary tract (papilloma, cystadenoma, and fibroma) (BARZILAI and LERNER 1997). Papillomatosis of the gallbladder associated with metachromatic leukodystrophy was described (FOCK et al. 1995); it presents itself as a cystic mass (OAK et al. 1997). Areas of preexisting benign cystadenoma were found in patients with cystadenocarcinoma (DEVANEY et al. 1994). Lymphangioma is a congenital malformation of the lymphatic channels. Sonography shows a multilocular, hypoechoic mass. Solid areas may be noted (Fig. 27.9).

Nodular regenerative hyperplasia (NHR) of the liver is a condition of unknown origin, rarely occurring in children (DALL'IGNA et al. 1996; MORAN et al. 1991), usually accidentally discovered, described in association with a variety of clinical conditions (myelo-lymphoproliferative disorders, Donohue's syndrome, DIC, rheumatic diseases) and drugs (anticonvulsants). It is considered a "tumor-like lesion" and should not be confused with regenerative nodules associated with cirrhosis. NHR may be associated with portal hypertension in one-half of cases (DACHMAN et al. 1987b): obliteration of many small portal veins. It was found in fetuses that exhibited several other malformations (GALDEANO and DRUT 1991). Histologically it consists of single or multiple regenerative foci of hyperplastic hepatocytes without fibrous septa among the nodules (CANO-RUIZ et al. 1985). Probably NHR is a secondary and non-specific tissue adaptation to heterogeneous distribution of blood flow; an intrahepatic microvascular mechanism has been considered most likely pathogenetically (PEREZ RUIZ et al. 1991). Neither surgical removal nor other treatment is needed. Possible pathogenetic relationships with HCC have been described (NZEAKO et al. 1996).

The nodules may take up technetium sulfur colloid and have variable echogenicity on US (more often hyperechoic). They are hypodense on CT with/without significant enhancement (DACHMAN et al. 1987b; FENG et al. 1991). On MRI the lesions are iso/hypointense. Hyperechoic lesions on US or hypodense lesions on TC, barely or not seen on MRI, can be indicative of NHR in an appropriate clinical setting (CASILLAS et al. 1997).

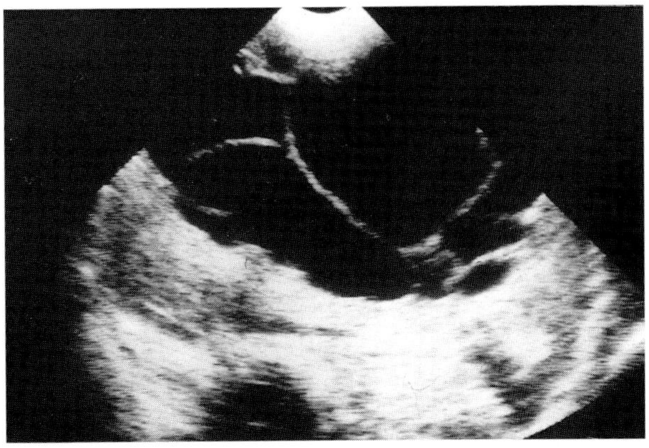

Fig. 27.9. Cystic lymphangioma in a 3-year-old child: US shows a big multilocular cystic mass in the right lobe of the liver

27.3 Primary Malignant Tumors

27.3.1 Hepatoblastoma

This is the most frequent malignant tumor after neuroblastoma and Wilms' tumor, and occurs in children younger than 5 years of age (COHEN 1992). Approximately 50% to 60% of cases are identified before 1 year of age (STY et al. 1992; MARTINEZ IBANEZ et al. 1986). Various conditions are associated with an increased risk of HB: hemihypertrophy (RATTAN et al. 1995), Beckwith-Wiedemann syndrome, polycystic kidneys, diaphragmatic hernia, Meckel's diverticulum, neonatal hepatitis, trisomy 18 (TERAGUCHI et al. 1997), familial adenomatous polyposis and various metabolic disorders (BOVE et al. 1996; GIARDIELLO et al. 1996; STY et al. 1992; TSAI et al. 1996). The risk of HB for low birth weight children may be inherently high, especially for lower birth weights, and the recent rapid increasing trend (5.2%) in incidence over the past two decades (DOUGLASS 1997; ROSS 1997; ROSS and GURNEY 1998) may be the result of an increase in the number of more immature infants with a more sensitive liver and also more frequent exposure to risk factors related to perinatal treatment (RIBONS and SLOVIS 1998; TANIMURA et al. 1998). The HB with unfavorable biologic behavior develops in children who are extremely premature at birth (IKEDA et al.1998).

There is a slightly increased incidence in boys. A possible association between in vitro fertilization and the tumor is suggested (TOREN et al. 1995). The child usually presents an asymptomatic right upper quadrant mass. In some cases, pain, fever, anorexia, vomiting, weight loss, and jaundice may be present. Alpha-fetoprotein serum levels are elevated in more than 90% of cases and therefore diagnosis is easy. Extramedullary hematopoiesis is a characteristic feature of HB; it is induced by intratumoral production of cytokines (von Schweinitz et al. 1995). A variety of paraneoplastic syndromes has been described (male sexual precocity, hypoglycemia, hypercalcemia, etc.) (Cohen 1992).

Prognosis depends on resectability of the lesion (Geiger 1996; von Schweinitz et al. 1994). Marked reduction of volume is obtained with chemotherapy (90% of HB is resectable after chemotherapy) (Ehrlich et al. 1997; Reynolds 1995; Stringer et al. 1995). The increased actual half-life of alpha-fetoprotein indicates residual active tumor after surgical resection (Han et al. 1997).

It is usually, on US, a solid, unique, heterogeneous mass with lobulated margins, calcifications and areas of necrosis. Amputation or thrombosis of portal or hepatic veins is strongly suggestive of the diagnosis (Fig. 27.10) (Brunelle et al. 1994; Dachman et al. 1987a). Multicentric, diffuse and multicystic forms can be seen.

CT and/or MRI are performed at diagnosis and before surgery to assess the precise extension of the lesion (Pariente 1994; Sty et al. 1992). Most HB demonstrate decreased attenuation compared to surrounding liver on unenhanced CT. The margins are well defined, but the internal architecture is inhomogeneous, due to areas of hemorrhage or necrosis. Calcifications are well identified. Contrast en-

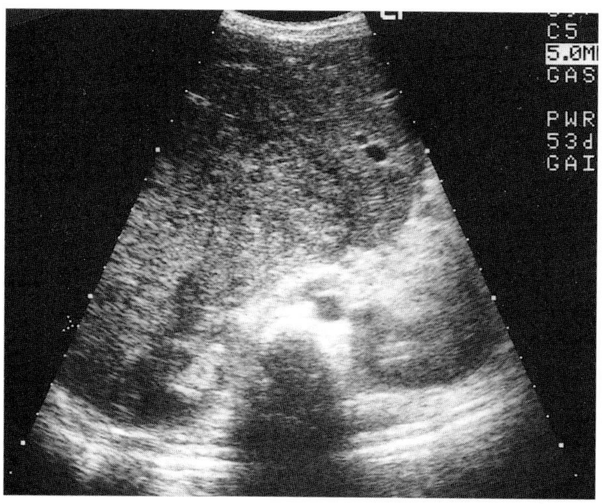

a

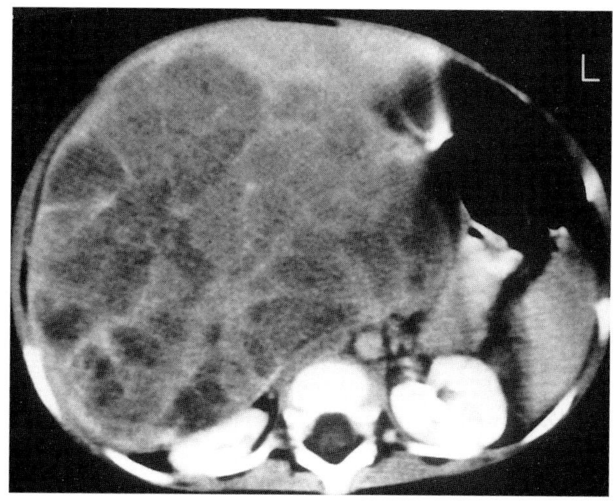

b

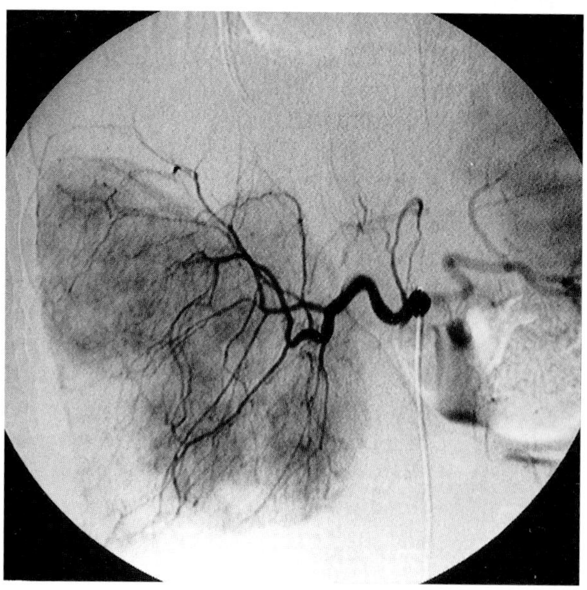

c

Fig. 27.10a–d. Hepatoblastoma in a 2-year-old child. Both US (**a**) and CT after contrast medium (**b**) show a voluminous, inhomogeneous mass in the right lobe of the liver. Hepatic arteriography (**c**) performed 5 months later confirms the presence of the voluminous hypervascular mass in the 5th, 6th and 7th segments of the liver.

hancement is usually less than that of normal liver parenchyma. Pulmonary metastases may be identified by CT.

HB is more often hypointense to normal liver on T1 weighted MR images (Fig. 27.11). Internal areas of hyperintensity correspond to subacute hemorrhage. On T2 weighted images these tumors are hyperintense and inhomogeneous. Hypointense bands correspond to areas of fibrosis and lobulation, and signal voids to calcifications.

Angiography (Brunelle et al. 1994) is still performed before surgery when the tumor is close to the hepatic hilum or when there is suspicion of portal cavernoma. Most of these tumors are hypervascular: neovascularity, irregular vessel margins, and encased vessels are present. The typical large size of these neoplasms may produce significant vascular displacement or occlusion. Thrombosis of the portal vein trunk or of the proximal branches leads to development of a cavernous hepatopetal network which may contraindicate or complicate surgery.

a

b

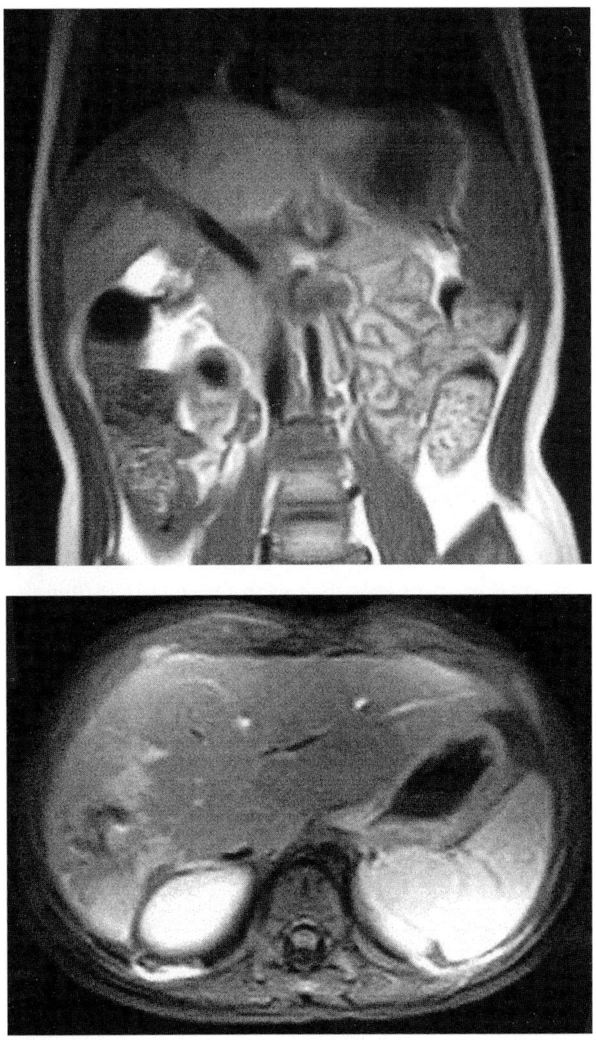

Fig. 27.11a,b. Hepatoblastoma in a 4-year-old child. Coronal T1-weighted (**a**) and axial T1-weighted (fat pre-saturation) after Gd-DOTA (**b**) MR scans. In the right hepatic lobe is evident an inhomogeneous, hypointense area showing low enhancement after infusion of Gd-DOTA. The typical interruption of the right portal branch is evident

27.3.2 Hepatocellular Carcinoma

This is rarer than HB and usually arises in children older than 4 years. There are two peaks of incidence in children, the first one occurring at approximately 4 years of age and the second one in adolescence (Moore et al. 1997; Sty et al. 1992). There is a slight male dominance. The tumor usually arises in children with chronic liver diseases (Siegel 1995). They include cirrhosis (biliary atresia, hepatitis, Byler's disease, Niemann-Pick disease) (Kohno et al. 1995; Jaskiewicz et al. 1995; Pennington et al. 1996), HCA (particularly in glycogen storage disease), tyrosinemia (major risk after 3 years of age), and neonatal hemochromatosis (Esquivel et al. 1994; Oliveira et al. 1998). It may be associated with Gardner's syndrome or familial adenomatous polyposis (Gruner et al. 1998). Association with dermatomyositis was described (Leaute et al. 1995). The clinical presentation is a palpable right upper quadrant mass, sometimes associated with pain or discomfort. Alpha-fetoprotein serum level is increased in less than 80% of cases. The tumor is more often multicentric and invasive than HB.

Most tumors are hyperechoic relative to normal parenchyma and heterogeneous. Cystic areas are uncommon. Vascular invasion or occlusion may be identified sonographically and suggests the diagnosis of malignancy (Fig. 27.12) (Siegel 1995). High-velocity Doppler signals have been reported, probably due to large pressure gradients related to arteriovenous shunting in the lesion. Blood flow within and around the tumor is observed in more than 75% of HCC on color-flow imaging (Lin et al. 1997; Numata et al. 1993; Siegel 1995). HCC in children and adolescents carries a much poorer prognosis compared to HB (Douglass 1997) as chemotherapy causes no response.

Treatment is only surgical: resection or transplantation. A complete work-up is mandatory including CT of the chest, MRI, and, in doubtful cases, CT after intra-arterial injection of Lipiodol (Pariente 1994).

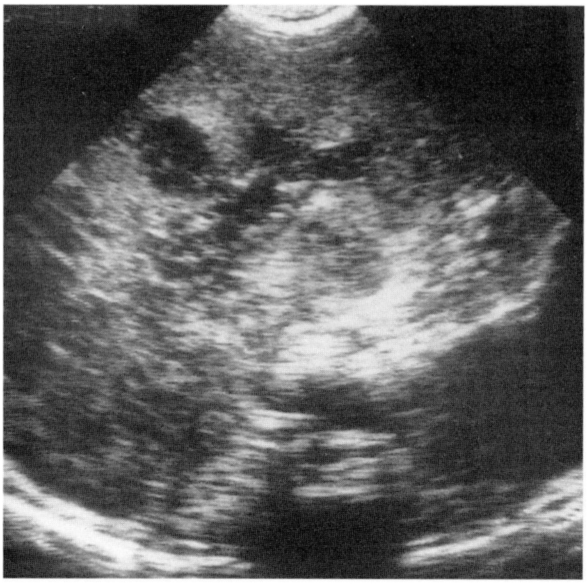

a

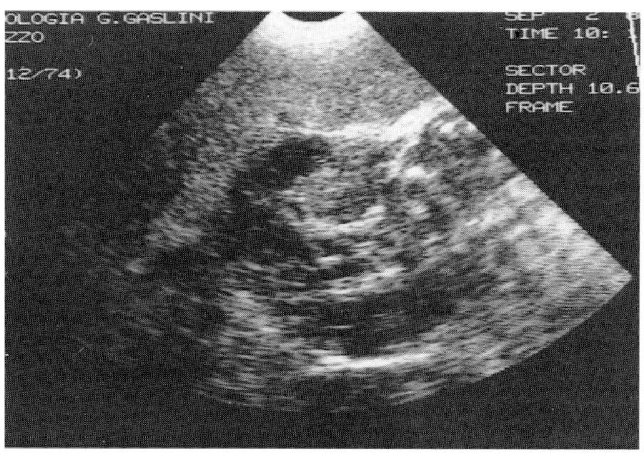

b

Fig. 27.12a,b. Hepatocarcinoma in a 12-year-old boy affected by hepatitis B. Transversal (**a**) and oblique longitudinal along the portal vein (**b**) US sections show the neoplastic thrombosis of the fork and the principal section of the portal vein. Surrounding liver appears inhomogeneous due to the presence of the tumor

MRI appears to be quite sensitive for the detection of HCC, relatively hypointense on T1 weighted images, and invariably hyperintense on T2 weighted images. Other MR findings are pseudocapsule formation, intratumoral septa, daughter nodules, fatty degeneration in the tumor, and vascular invasion (Sty et al. 1992).

A distinct histological variant of HCC with a more favorable outcome occurs in the non-cirrhotic liver of older children and young adults (mean age: 17 years) and has been called fibrolamellar hepatocarcinoma (Brunelle et al. 1994; Cohen 1992; Hayaski et al. 1988; Stevens et al. 1995; Sty et al. 1992). There is no distinctive radiological findings to enable a conclusive diagnosis. Diagnosis can be made preoperatively on percutaneous liver biopsy. The mass may be surrounded by a zone of FNH (arterial supply most probably derived from the tumor) (Saxena et al. 1994).

Gallbladder carcinoma is an extremely rare tumor in childhood. We have found only six cases in the literature. Most of them were associated with an ethnic group: the Navajo Indians. A case associated with achondroplasia was reported (Eire et al. 1995). Also a case of obstructive jaundice resulting from adenocarcinoma of the ampulla of Vater in an 11-year-old boy was described (Andiran et al. 1997).

27.3.3 Sarcoma

Hepatic sarcomas are rare in children, including several types. Rhabdomyosarcoma (RMS) may originate in the major bile ducts (hepatobiliary RMS) with a botryoid appearance, biliary tract dilatation and jaundice. When it arises from the distal intrahepatic duct, it is indistinguishable from other primary neoplasms of the liver (Brunelle et al. 1994; Buetow et al. 1997a; Cohen 1992; Moon et al. 1994; Ros et al. 1986; Sty et al. 1992). The tumor (1% of all pediatric RMS) occurs in infants and children between two and five years old, but some cases are described at 5 months and 11 years. A very slight male predominance was reported.

It grows insidiously and frequently causes weight loss, intermittent jaundice with fever, hepatomegaly, constipation, nausea, and vomiting accompanied by elevation of bilirubin and alkaline phosphatase. Not surprisingly, some of the cases have been initially misdiagnosed as infectious hepatitis.

RMS occurs usually as a large (mean tumor diameter: 13 cm), solitary, spherical mass that is located in the right lobe of the liver. US shows a predominantly echogenic mass with some anechoic spaces of various shapes: the rapid growth is probably responsible for the areas of hemorrhagic necrosis and subsequent cystic degeneration. Sometimes US will show a typical pattern of a tumor mass within the hilum surrounded by fluid areas: this pattern should be suggestive of an intraluminal biliary tumor. Sometimes it may be mistaken for a choledocal cyst (Sanz et al. 1997) (Fig. 27.13).

The increased water content within the abundant myxoid stroma accounts for the attenuation lower than that of soft tissue on CT scans and high signal

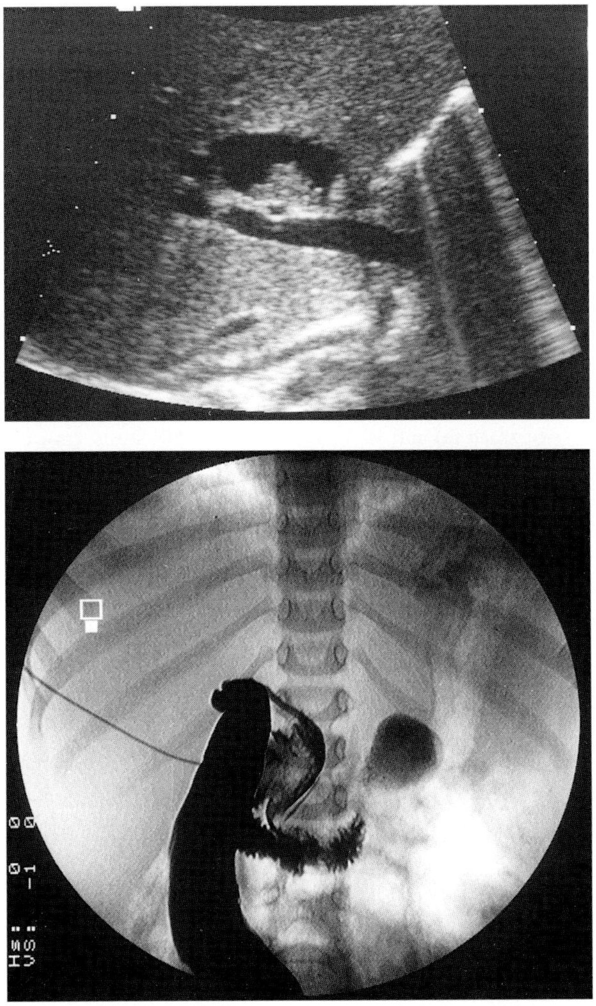
a

a

Fig. 27.13a,b. Rhabdomyosarcoma of the biliary tract in a 4-year-old child. US (a) shows a dilatation of the terminal choledochus with vegetation inside. Percutaneous cholecystography (b) confirms the dilatation with a "minus" in the terminal tract

intensity on T2 weighted MR images (MR cholangiography is a promising tool for evaluation of the major bile ducts in children). Enhancing peripheral rim, representing fibrous pseudocapsule of the tumor, was occasionally found, but there is no consistent pattern of contrast enhancement. CT (chest, abdomen, pelvis) allows the tumor to be staged and shows hepatic metastases and retroperitoneal or hilar adenopathy. Metastases are also found with some frequency in the chest, on peritoneal surfaces, including the omentum, mesentery and diaphragm and in bones. Gallium or thallium scintigraphy (with or without bone scintigraphy) could be performed to assess for metastatic disease. Percutaneous transhepatic cholangiography and (PTC) biliary drainage may be required when there is obstructive jaundice. The typical finding at PTC is the presence of extensive, often bizarre, filling defects corresponding to ductal tumor (Roebuck et al.1998).

Smooth muscle spindle cells neoplasm seem to be particularly frequent in immunocompromised children. The development of leiomyosarcomas, occurring in the allograft itself, is described in pediatric liver recipients (Penn 1996). Hepatobiliary leiomyomas and leiomyosarcomas have been described in HIV infected children (Levin et al. 1994; Tomà et al. 1997).

Hepatic undifferentiated (embryonal) sarcoma (UES) is the fourth or fifth most common liver tumor in the pediatric population. It is composed of spindle- and stellate-shaped sarcomatous cells, closely packed in whirls or sheets or scattered loosely in a myxoid ground substance. At pathologic and US examination UES is predominantly solid (mean, 83% of volume). Conversely, CT shows low attenuation in 88% of the tumor volume and T2 weighted MR images show high signal intensity (equal to that of CSF) in 89% of the masses (Fig. 27.14). The increased water content within the abundant myxoid stroma of UES accounts for the CT and MRI patterns (Buetow et al. 1997a; Yoon et al. 1997). UES may arise in a mesenchymal hamartoma (De Chadarevian et al. 1994; Lauwers et al. 1997).

Pediatric hepatic angiosarcomas have been described (Mistry et al. 1995). In some cases the clinico-pathological features may suggest a link with benign hemangioendothelioma (Awan et al. 1996).

Infantile choriocarcinoma (Kim et al. 1993) is a rare liver tumor that develops in the placenta and spreads to the child. The mass is hypervascularized with a clinical pattern of developing anemia, liver tumor, rapid progression to death and maternal choriocarcinoma (Andreitchouk et al. 1996; Kishkurno et al. 1997; Picton et al. 1995). Estimation of hCG may be diagnostic. The MRI findings are: low signal intensity with internal foci of high signal (repeated hemorrhage) on T1 and high signal with internal foci of low signal on T2 (Sashi et al. 1996).

27.3.4 Epithelioid Hemangioendothelioma

This is a very uncommon malignant type of vascular tumor, mainly reported in adults. It may occur in older girls as a diffuse mass invading hepatic veins and causing Budd-Chiari syndrome (Fig. 27.15)

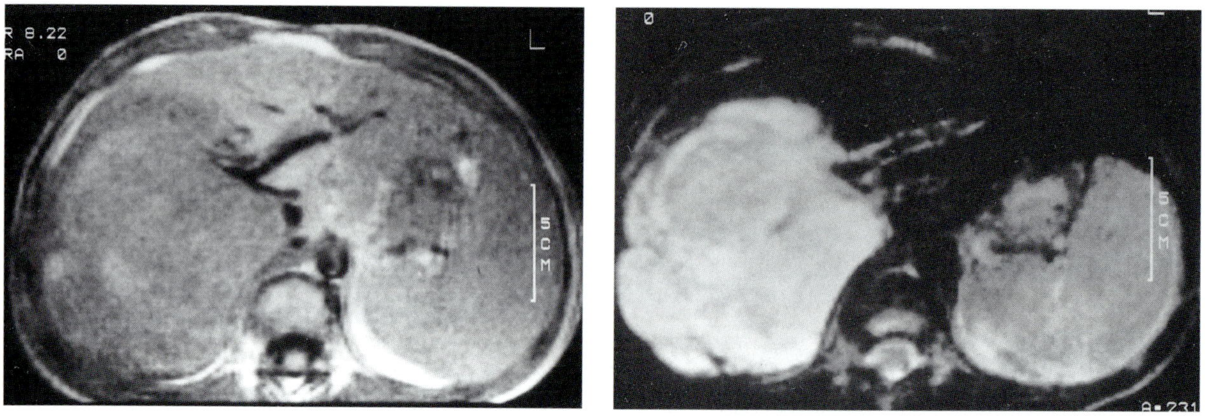

Fig. 27.14a,b. Undifferentiated sarcoma in a 12-year-old boy. SE T1-weighted (**a**) and SE T2-weighted (**b**) MRI scans show the clear hypersignal of the mass on T2 scan. The evident amputation of a portal branch is a typical sign of malignancy

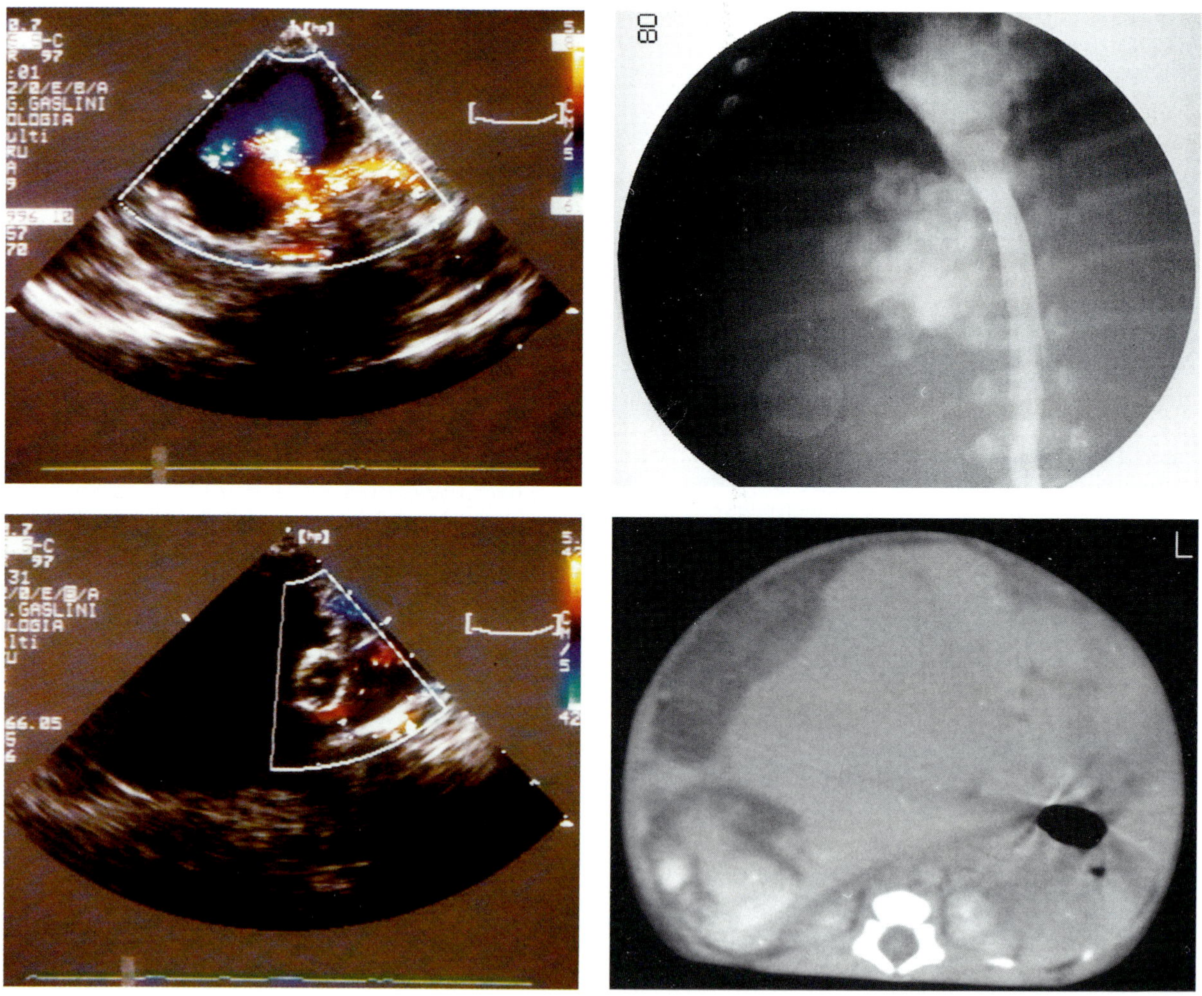

Fig. 27.15a–d. Epithelioid hemangioma in a newborn with prenatal diagnosis of cystic intrahepatic mass. Color Doppler shows that the liquid intrahepatic mass, involving hepatic veins, is communicating with inferior vena cava (**a**). This is confirmed by cavography (**b**). A small balloon located in the communication between inferior vena cava and liver (**c**) stopped the flow and permitted the performance of a surgical intervention (the patient died). CT shows the widespread liver destruction (**d**)

(Brunelle et al. 1994; Han et al. 1998; Hase et al. 1995; Siegel 1995; Wong and Masel 1995; Pethe et al. 1995; Poggiani et al. 1998).

27.4 Metastatic Disease

Virtually all malignant neoplasms of childhood, with the general exception of central nervous system tumors, can metastasize to the liver (Fig. 27.16) (Mahl et al. 1997). The most frequent ones are due to Wilms' tumor, neuroblastoma or rhabdomyosarcoma. They presents themselves on US as nodules more often hypoechoic with hepatomegaly and variable, diffuse distortion of parenchymal echo texture.

Among infants, neuroblastoma is the most common source of hepatic metastases. Stage IV-S, in infants younger than 6 months of age, is associated with extensive hepatic metastasis (Pepper's syndrome) (Fig. 27.17). Hepatomegaly may be massive despite a small, seldom evident primary lesion. This type of neuroblastoma has a better prognosis than neuroblastoma presenting in older children and has a tendency to a spontaneous regression with complete healing in most cases: the survival probability is about 79% (Claviez et al. 1996). Long-standing cases of hepatopathy are described; probably, both the liver infiltration and the chemotherapy (provided for patients initially diagnosed as critically ill) play a role in this process (Claviez et al. 1996). The very young IV-S patients (age <4 weeks at diagnosis) are at high risk of dying of respiratory complications as a result of massive hepatomegaly (Hsu et al. 1996; van Noesel et al 1997).

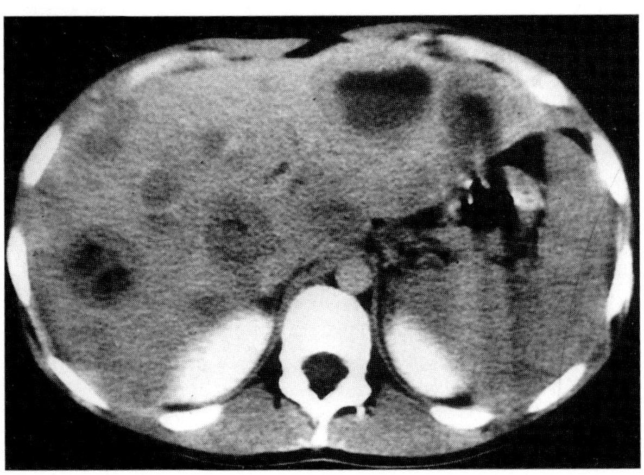

Fig. 27.16. Carcinoid metastasis in a 9-year-old boy. CT without contrast medium shows multiple hypointense nodules with evident colliquative aspects

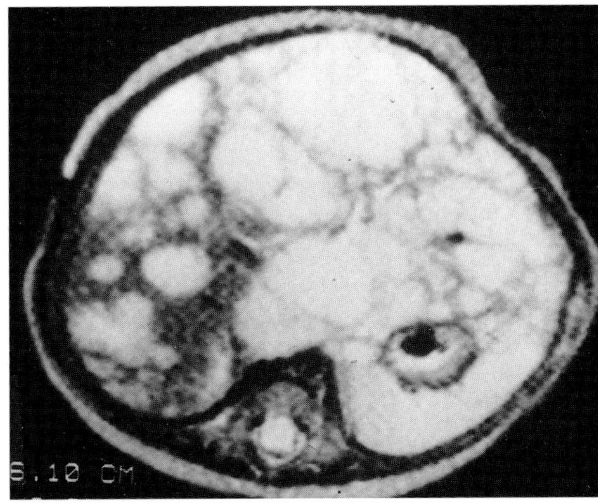

Fig. 27.17. 4S neuroblastoma in a 1-month-old baby. SE T2-weighted MR scan. Diffuse metastasization of the liver. Metastasis appears clearly hyperintense

In children older than 6 months to 1 year of age, neuroblastoma most commonly metastasizes to bone marrow, bones, and lymph nodes. Hepatic metastases can occur in advanced disease. The disease progression to stage 4 is strongly related to the presence of biologic markers in the tumor (Hachitanda and Hata 1996; van Noesel et al 1997).

Leukemia and lymphoma may also present a diffuse liver enlargement or multiple hypoechoic nodules. A high incidence of allograft involvement by lymphoma is reported (Penn 1996).

CT generally is more sensitive than sonography for the detection of hepatic metastasis, most frequently identified as multiple low-attenuation areas on unenhanced scans (Cohen 1992; Sty et al. 1992). Both neuroblastoma and metastatic Wilms' tumor usually produce inhomogeneous enhancement. Calcifications are sometimes evident in metastatic neuroblastoma.

Hepatic involvement with lymphoma may be identified as poorly defined, low-attenuation lesions with irregular margins. All imaging modalities are very poor for identification of lymphoma in the liver and spleen. CT is probably better than ultrasound with an overall sensitivity of probably no more than 40% (Cohen 1992). MRI has been reported to be not better than CT or showing the disease in more spleens than CT. Lymphoma tissue has a T1 and T2 relaxation time similar to normal spleen, and tumor is best identified on T2 weighted images as a mottled appearance in the organ, because of the presence of associated fibrosis, hemorrhage, edema, or necrosis (Figs. 27.18, 27.19) (Cohen 1992).

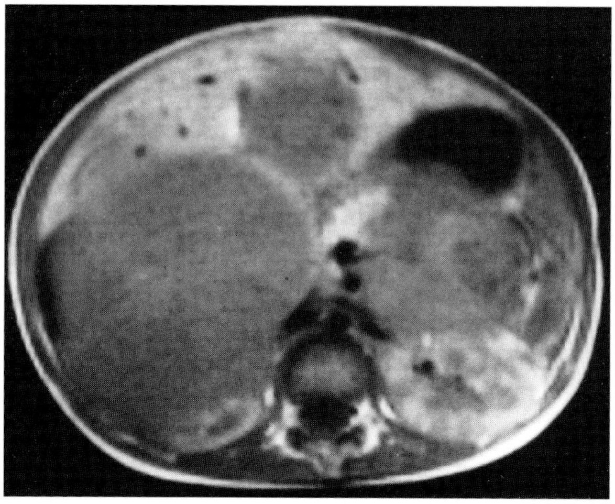

Fig. 27.18. Non-Hodgkin's lymphoma in a 5-year-old boy. SE T1-weighted MR section shows 2 voluminous hypointense hepatic nodules. Note the presence of another extrahepatic prerenal left nodule and the diffuse infiltration of the left kidney

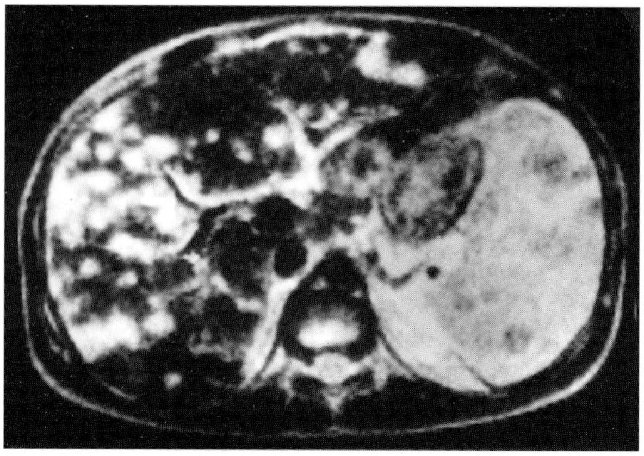

Fig. 27.19. Non-Hodgkin's lymphoma in a 14-year-old girl. SE T2-weighted MR scan shows a diffuse infiltration of the liver and spleen. The lesions appear hyperintense in the liver and hypointense in the spleen

References

Achilleos OA, Buist LJ, Kelly DA, et al (1996) Unresectable hepatic tumors in childhood and the role of liver transplantation. J Pediatr Surg 31:1563–1567

Alshak NS, Cocjin J, Podesta L, et al (1994) Hepatocellular adenoma in glycogen storage disease type IV. Arch Pathol Lab Med 118:88–91

Alwaidh MH, Woodhall CR, Carty HT (1997) Mesenchymal hamartoma of the liver: a case report. Pediatr Radiol 27:247–249

Andiran F, Tanyel FC, Kale G, et al (1997) Obstructive jaundice resulting from adenocarcinoma of the ampulla of Vater in an 11-year-old boy. J Pediatr Surg 32:636–637

Andreitchouk AE, Takahashi O, Kodama H, et al (1996) Choriocarcinoma in infant and mother: a case report. J Obstet Gynaecol Res 22:585–588

Awan S, Davenport M, Portmann B, et al. (1996) Angiosarcoma of the liver in children. J Pediatr Surg 31:1729–1732

Bala S, Wunsch PH, Ballhausen WG (1997) Childhood hepatocellular adenoma in familial adenomatous polyposis: mutations in adenomatous polyposis coli gene and p53. Gastroenterology 112:919–922

Balmer B, Le Coultre C, Feldges A, et al (1996) Mesenchymal liver hamartoma in a newborn; case report. Eur J Pediatr Surg 6:303–305

Barnhart DC, Hirschl RB, Garver KA, et al (1997) Conservative management of mesenchymal hamartoma of the liver. J Pediatr Surg 32:1495–1498

Bartolozzi C, Lencioni R, Paolicchi A, et al (1997) Differentiation of hepatocellular adenoma and focal nodular hyperplasia of the liver: comparison of power Doppler imaging and conventional color Doppler sonography. Eur Radiol 7:1410–1415

Barzilai M, Lerner A (1997) Gallbladder polyps in children: a rare condition. Pediatr Radiol 27:54–56

Bejvan SM, Winter TC, Shields LE, et al (1997) Prenatal evaluation of mesenchymal hamartoma of the liver: gray scale and power Doppler sonographic imaging. J Ultrasound Med 16:227–229

Ben-Izhak O, Groissman G, Lichtig C (1995) Hepatic angiomyolipoma in childhood: association with tuberous sclerosis. Pediatr Pathol Lab Med 15:213–217

Blei F, Walter J, Orlow SJ, et al (1998) Familial segregation of hemangiomas and vascular malformations as an autosomal dominant trait. Arch Dermatol 134:718–722

Bourliere-Najean B, Panuel M, Guy SJM, et al (1989) Spontaneous liver adenoma in a child. Pediatr Radiol 20:95

Bove KE, Soukup S, Ballard ET, et al (1996) Hepatoblastoma in a child with trisomy 18: cytogenetics, liver anomalies, and literature review. Pediatr Pathol Lab Med 16:253–262

Bowman LC, Riely CA (1996) Management of pediatric liver tumors. Surg Oncol Clin N Am 5:451–459

Bruce S, Downe L, Devonald K, et al (1995) Noninvasive investigation of infantile hepatic hemangioma: a case study. Pediatrics 95:595–597

Brunelle F, Tammam S, Odievre M, et al (1984) Liver adenomas in glycogen storage disease in children. Pediatr Radiol 14:94–101

Brunelle F, Pariente D, Chaumont P (1994) Hepatic tumors. In: Brunelle F, Pariente D, Chaumont P (eds) Liver disease in children. An atlas of angiography and cholangiography. Springer-Verlag, London Berlin, pp 53–93

Buetow PC, Pantongrag-Brown L, Buck JL, et al (1996) Focal nodular hyperplasia of the liver: radiologic-pathologic correlation. RadioGraphics 16:369–388

Buetow PC, Buck JL, Pantongrag-Brown L, et al (1997a) Undifferentiated (embryonal) sarcoma of the liver: pathologic basis of imaging findings in 28 cases. Radiology 203:779–783

Buetow PC, Rao P, Marshall WH (1997b) Imaging of pediatric liver tumors. Magn Reson Imaging Clin N Am 5:397–413

Cano-Ruiz A, Martin-Scapa MA, Larraona JL, et al (1985) Laparoscopic findings in seven patients with nodular regenerative hyperplasia of the liver. Am J Gastroenterol 80:796–800

Casillas C, Marti-Bonmati L, Galant J (1997)Pseudotumoral presentation of nodular regenerative hyperplasia of the liver: imaging in five patients including MR imaging. Eur Radiol 7:654–658

Chung T, Hoffer FA, Burrows PE, et al(1996) MR imaging of hepatic hemangiomas of infancy and changes seen with interferon alpha-2a treatment. Pediatr Radiol 26:341–348

Claviez A, Hero B, Schneppenheim R, et al (1996) Hepatopathy in patients with stage 4 S neuroblastoma. Klin Padiatr 208:221–228

Cohen MD (1992) Liver Tumors. In: Cohen MD (ed) Imaging of children with cancer. Mosby Year Book, St.Louis Baltimore, pp 20–42

Cohen MD, Bugaieski EM, Haliloglu M, et al (1996) Visual presentation of the staging of pediatric solid tumors. Radiographics 16:523–545

Dachman AH, Pakter RL, Ros PR, et al (1987a) Hepatoblastoma: radiologic-pathologic correlation in 50 cases. Radiology 164:15–19

Dachman AH, Ros PR, Goodman ZD, et al (1987b) Nodular regenerative hyperplasia of the liver: clinical and radiologic observations. AJR 148:717–722

Dall'Igna P, Cecchetto G, Perilongo G, et al (1996) Nodular regenerative hyperplasia of the liver: description of two cases. Med Pediatr Oncol 26:190–195

Das PC, Rao PL, Radhakrishna K (1997) Cystic hamartoma of the liver in children. J Indian Med Assoc 95:517–518

Davenport M, Hansen L, Heaton ND, et al (1995) Hemangioendothelioma of the liver in infants. J Pediatr Surg 30:44–48

De Bievre P, Dufour P, Lefebvre C, et al (1994) Prenatal diagnosis of hepatic hemangioendothelioma. A propos of a case. J Gynecol Obstet Biol Reprod (Paris) 23:435–439

De Chadarevian JP, Pawel BR, Faerber EN, et al (1994) Undifferentiated (embryonal) sarcoma arising in conjunction with mesenchymal hamartoma of the liver. Mod Pathol 7:490–493

De Gaetano A, De Franco A, Maresca G (1996) The integrated diagnosis of hepatic focal nodular hyperplasia: echography, color Doppler, computed tomography and magnetic resonance compared. Radiol Med 91:258–269

Devaney K, Goodman ZD, Ishak KG (1994) Hepatobiliary cystadenoma and cystadenocarcinoma. A light microscopic and immunohistochemical study of 70 patients. Am J Surg Pathol 18:1078–1091

Donnelly LF, Bisset GS 3rd (1998) Pediatric hepatic imaging. Radiol Clin North Am 36:413–427

Douglass EC (1997) Hepatic malignancies in childhood and adolescence (hepatoblastoma, hepatocellular carcinoma, and embryonal sarcoma). Cancer Treat Res 92:201–212

Edelman RR, Hesselink JR, Zlatkin MB (1996) Clinical magnetic resonance imaging. WB Saunders Company, Philadelphia London Toronto

Ehrlich PF, Greenberg ML, Filler RM (1997) Improved long-term survival with preoperative chemotherapy for hepatoblastoma. J Pediatr Surg 32:999–1002

Eire PF, Pintos E, Jardon JA, et al (1995) Gallbladder carcinoma in an achondroplastic boy. Eur J Pediatr Surg 5:313–314

Esquivel CO, Gutierrez C, Cox KL, et al (1994) Hepatocellular carcinoma and liver cell dysplasia in children with chronic liver disease. J Pediatr Surg 29:1465–1469

Feng WJ, Takayasu K, Konda C, et al (1991) CT of nodular hyperplasia of the liver in non-Hodgkin lymphoma. J Comput Assist Tomogr 15:1031–1034

Flores-Stadler EM, Chou P, Walterhouse D, et al (1997) Hemangiopericytoma of the liver: immunohistochemical observations, expression of angiogenic factors, and review of the literature. J Pediatr Hematol Oncol 19:449–454

Fock JM, Begeer JH, Prins TR (1995) Metachromatic leukodystrophy and coincidental finding of papillomatosis of the gallbladder. A case report. Neuropediatrics 26:55–56

Fok TF, Chan MS, Metreweli C, et al (1996) Hepatic haemangioendothelioma presenting with early heart failure in a newborn: treatment with hepatic artery embolization and interferon. Acta Paediatr 85:1373–1375

Frush DP, Siegel MJ, Bisset GS 3rd (1997) Challenges of pediatric spiral CT. From the RSNA refresher courses. RadioGraphics 17:939–959

Galdeano S, Drut R (1991) Nodular regenerative hyperplasia of fetal liver: a report of two cases. Pediatr Pathol 11:479–485

Garel L, Kalifa G, Buriot D, et al (1981) Multiple adenomas of the liver and Fanconi's anemia. Ann Radiol 24:53–54

Geiger JD (1996) Surgery for hepatoblastoma in children. Curr Opin Pediatr 8:276–282

George JC, Cohen MD, Tarver RD, et al (1994) Ruptured cystic mesenchymal hamartoma: an unusual cause of neonatal ascites. Pediatr Radiol 24:304–305

Giardiello FM, Petersen GM, Brensinger JD, et al (1996) Hepatoblastoma and APC gene mutation in familial adenomatous polyposis. Gut 39:867–869

Gokhale R, Whitington PF (1996) Hepatic adenomatosis in an adolescent. J Pediatr Gastroenterol Nutr 23:482–486

Gruner BA, DeNapoli TS, Andrews W, et al(1998) Hepatocellular carcinoma in children associated with Gardner syndrome or familial adenomatous polyposis. J Pediatr Hematol Oncol 20:274–278

Guariso G, Fiorio S, Altavilla G, et al (1998) Congenital absence of the portal vein associated with focal nodular hyperplasia of the liver and cystic dysplasia of the kidney. Eur J Pediatr 157:287–290

Hachitanda Y, Hata J (1996) Stage IVS neuroblastoma: a clinical, histological, and biological analysis of 45 cases. Hum Pathol 27:1135–1138

Han SJ, Tsai CC, Tsai HM, et al (1998) Infantile hemangioendothelioma with a highly elevated serum alpha-fetoprotein level. Hepatogastroenterology 45:459–461

Han SJ, Yoo S, Choi SH, et al (1997) Actual half-life of alpha-fetoprotein as a prognostic tool in pediatric malignant tumors. Pediatr Surg Int 12:599–602

Hase T, Kodama M, Kishida A, et al (1995) Successful management of infantile hepatic hilar hemangioendothelioma with obstructive jaundice and consumption coagulopathy. J Pediatr Surg 30:1485–1487

Hayaski N, Yamamoto K, Tamaki N, et al (1988) Fibrolamellar hepatocellular carcinoma: pitfalls in non operative diagnosis. Radiology 167:25–30

Herzberg C, Maas R, Bucheler E (1998) Liver tumors in children: spiral CT findings and differential diagnostic classification. Aktuelle Radiol 8:109–113

Hsu LL, Evans AE, D'Angio GJ (1996) Hepatomegaly in neuroblastoma stage 4S: criteria for treatment of the vulnerable neonate. Med Pediatr Oncol 27:521–528

Ikeda H, Hachitanda Y, Tanimura M, et al (1998) Development of unfavorable hepatoblastoma in children of very low birth weight: results of a surgical and pathologic review. Cancer 82:1789–1796

Iyer CP, Stanley P, Mahour GH (1996) Hepatic hemangiomas in infants and children: a review of 30 cases. Am Surg 62:356–360

Jaskiewicz K, Banach L, Izycka E (1995) Hepatocellular carcinoma in young patients: histology, cellular differentiation, HBV infection and oncoprotein p53. Anticancer Res 15:2723–2725

Kane JW, Page-Salyards W, Perry CR (1997) Congenital hepatic hemangioma in the neonate. MCN Am J Matern Child Nurs 22:187–193

Kim SN, Chi JG, Kim YW, et al (1993) Neonatal choriocarcinoma of liver. Pediatr Pathol 13:723–730

Kishkurno S, Ishida A, Takahashi Y, et al (1997) A case of neonatal choriocarcinoma. Am J Perinatol 14:79–82

Kohno M, Kitatani H, Wada H, et al (1995) Hepatocellular carcinoma complicating biliary cirrhosis caused by biliary atresia: report of a case. J Pediatr Surg 30:1713–1716

Kramarova E, Stiller CA (1996) The international classification of childhood cancer. Int J Cancer 68:759–765

Labrune P, Trioche P, Duvaltier I, et al (1997) Hepatocellular adenomas in glycogen storage disease type I and III: a series of 43 patients and review of the literature. J Pediatr Gastroenterol Nutr 24:276–279

Lai FM, Jayakumar CR, Saw L, et al (1996) Hepatic mesenchymal hamartoma: a case report and radiological findings. Singapore Med J 37:226–228

Lauwers GY, Grant LD, Donnelly WH, et al (1997) Hepatic undifferentiated (embryonal) sarcoma arising in a mesenchymal hamartoma. Am J Surg Pathol 21:1248–1254

Leaute-Labreze C, Perel Y, Taieb A (1995) Childhood dermatomyositis associated with hepatocarcinoma. N Engl J Med 133:1083

Lee P, Mather S, Owens C, et al (1994) Hepatic ultrasound findings in the glycogen storage diseases. Br J Radiol 67:1062–1066

Lehrnbecher T, Frauendienst-Egger G, Schrod L (1996) Haemangioendothelioma in a preterm infant associated with highly elevated alpha-fetoprotein. Eur J Pediatr 155:423–424

Levin TL, Adam HM, van Hoeven KH, et al (1994) Hepatic spindle cell tumors in HIV positive children. Pediatr Radiol 24:78–79

Lin ZY, Wang LY, Wang JH, et al (1997) Clinical utility of color Doppler sonography in the differentiation of hepatocellular carcinoma from metastases and hemangioma. J Ultrasound Med 16:51–58

Lorette G, Georgesco G, Sirinelli D, et al (1996) Cutaneous immature hemangioma and hepatic angioma: there is no frequent association. Ann Dermatol Venereol 123:789–790

Luks FI, Yazbeck S, Brandt ML, et al (1991) Benign liver tumors in children: a 25-year experience. J Pediatr Surg 26:1326–1330

Mahl M, Schonfeld J, Lange R, et al (1997) Carcinoid syndrome. Recurrent upper abdominal pain, diarrhea and flush in a 15-year-old girl. Med Klin 92:739–743

Maksimak M, Wilt E, Colley AT, et al (1990) Hemangioendothelioma of the hepatobiliary system: the classic and the unusual. J Pediatr Gastroenterol Nutr 10:131–137

Martinez Ibanez V, Marques Gubern A, De Diego M, et al (1996) Hepatoblastoma today. Our experience. J Cir Pediatr 9:10–12

Milillo F, Romio P, Promenzio CM, et al (1997) Solitary hepatocellular adenoma in infancy. Pediatr Med Chir 19:125–126

Mistry RC, Deshpande RK, Chinoy R, et al (1995) Undifferentiated embryonal sarcoma of the liver in childhood. Indian J Cancer 32:175–178

Monga G, Ramponi A, Falzoni PU et al (1994) Renal and hepatic angiomyolipomas in a child without evidence of tuberous sclerosis. Pathol Res Pract 190:1208–1211

Moon WK, Kim WS, Kim IO, et al (1994) Undifferentiated embryonal sarcoma of the liver: US and CT findings. Pediatr Radiol 24:500–503

Moore SW, Hesseling PB, Wessels G, et al (1997) Hepatocellular carcinoma in children. Pediatr Surg Int 12:266–270

Moran CA, Mullick FG, Ishak KG (1991) Nodular regenerative hyperplasia of the liver in children. Am J Surg Pathol 15:449–454

Moser C, Hany A, Spiegel R (1998) Familial giant hemangiomas of the liver. Study of a family and review of the literature. Schweiz Rundsch Med Prax 87:461–468

Motiwale SS, Karmarkar SJ, Oak SN, et al (1996) Cystic mesenchymal hamartoma of the liver – a rare condition. Indian J Cancer 33:157–160

Nedkova V, Kovacheva K, Tanchev S, et al (1996) The testicular feminization syndrome combined with disseminated hemangiomatosis. Akush Ginekol 35:35–37

Nelson R, Chezmar JL (1990) Diagnostic approach to hepatic hemangiomas. Radiology 176:11–13

Newman KD (1997) Hepatic tumors in children. Semin Pediatr Surg 6:38–41

Numata K, Tanaka K, Mitsui K, et al (1993) Flow characteristics of hepatic tumors at color Doppler sonography: correlation with arteriographic findings. AJR 160:515–521

Nzeako UC, Goodman ZD, Ishak KG (1996) Hepatocellular carcinoma and nodular regenerative hyperplasia: possible pathogenetic relationship. Am J Gastroenterol 91:879–884

Oak S, Rao S, Karmarkar S, et al (1997) Papillomatosis of the gallbladder in metachromatic leukodystrophy. Pediatr Surg Int 12:424–425

Ohama K, Nagase H, Ogino K, et al (1997) Alpha-fetoprotein (AFP) levels in normal children. Eur J Pediatr Surg 7:267–269

Okada A, Fukuzawa M, Oue T, et al (1998) Thirty-eight years experience of malignant hepatic tumors in infants and childhood. Eur J Pediatr Surg 8:17–22

Oliveira MG, Fernandes A, Silva AC, et al (1998) A case of neonatal haemochromatosis. Acta Paediatr 87:102–104

Pariente D (1994) Liver tumours. In: Carty H, Brunelle F, Shaw D, Kendall B (eds) Imaging Children. Churchill Livingstone, Edinburgh, pp 500–514

Park CH, Hwang HS, Hong J, et al (1996) Giant infantile hemangioendothelioma of the liver. Scintigraphic diagnosis. Clin Nucl Med 21:293–295

Penn I (1996) Posttransplantation de novo tumors in liver allograft recipients.Liver Transpl Surg 2:52–59

Pennington DJ, Sivit CJ, Chandra RS (1996) Hepatocellular carcinoma in a child with Niemann-Pick disease: imaging findings. Pediatr Radiol 26:220–221

Perez Payarols J, Pardo Masferrer J, Gomez Bellvert C (1995) Treatment of life-threatening infantile hemangiomas with vincristine. N Engl J Med 333:69–72

Perez Ruiz F, Orte Martinez FJ, Zea Mendoza AC, et al (1991) Nodular regenerative hyperplasia of the liver in rheumatic diseases: report of seven cases and review of the literature. Semin Arthritis Rheum 21:47–54

Pethe VV, Kalgutkar AD, Mondkar J, et al (1995) Hepatic hemangioendothelioma of infancy with congestive cardiac failure – report of a case. Indian J Cancer 32:186–188

Petrikovsky BM, Cohen HL, Scimeca P, et al (1994) Prenatal diagnosis of focal nodular hyperplasia of the liver. Prenat Diagn 14:406–409

Picton SV, Bose-Haider B, Lendon M, et al (1995) Simultaneous choriocarcinoma in mother and newborn infant. Med Pediatr Oncol 25:475–478

Plumley DA, Grosfeld JL, Kopecky KK, et al (1995) The role of spiral (helical) computerized tomography with three-dimensional reconstruction in pediatric solid tumors. J Pediatr Surg 30:317–321

Poggiani C, Auriemma A, Bellan C, et al (1998) A case of congenital hepatic hemangioendothelioma treated with prednisone: the echographic changes and Doppler study. Minerva Pediatr 50:91–96

Prasad VK, Aronson DC, Gerald WL, et al (1995) Hepatic focal nodular hyperplasia in infant antenatally exposed to steroids. Lancet 346:371–373

Rattan KN, Sharma A, Singh Y, et al (1995) Hepatoblastoma associated with congenital hemihypertrophy. Indian Pediatr 32:1308–1309

Resnick MB, Kozakewich HP, Perez-Atayde AR (1995) Hepatic adenoma in the pediatric age group. Clinicopathological observations and assessment of cell proliferative activity. Am J Surg Pathol 19:1181–1190

Reymond D, Plaschkes J, Luthy AR, et al (1995) Focal nodular hyperplasia of the liver in children: review of follow-up and outcome. J Pediatr Surg 30:1590–1593

Reynolds M (1995) Conversion of unresectable to resectable hepatoblastoma and long-term follow-up study. World J Surg 19:814–816

Ribons LA, Slovis TL (1998) Hepatoblastoma and birth weight. J Pediatr 132:750–755

Roebuck DJ, Yang WT, Lam WW, et al (1998) Hepatobiliary rhabdomyosarcoma in children: diagnostic radiology. Pediatr Radiol 28:101–108

Ros PR, Olmsted WW, Dachman AH, et al (1986) Undifferentiated (embryonal) sarcoma of the liver: radiologic and pathologic correlations. Radiology 161:141–145

Ross JA (1997) Hepatoblastoma and birth weight: too little, too big, or just right? J Pediatr 130:516–517

Ross JA, Gurney JG (1998) Hepatoblastoma incidence in the United States from 1973 to 1992. Med Pediatr Oncol 30:141–142

Ruiz MF, Vera P, de La Fuente G, et al (1995) Cystic hamartoma: prenatal diagnosis and follow-up of newborn infants. Rev Chil Obstet Ginecol 60:211–216

Sakatoku H, Hirokawa Y, Inoue M, et al (1996) Focal nodular hyperplasia in an adolescent with glycogen storage disease type I with mesocaval shunt operation in childhood: a case report and review of the literature. Acta Paediatr Jpn 38:172–175

Samuel M, Spitz L (1995) Infantile hepatic hemangioendothelioma: the role of surgery. J Pediatr Surg 30:1425–1429

Sandler A, Rivlin L, Filler R, et al (1997) Polycythemia secondary to focal nodular hyperplasia. J Pediatr Surg 32:1386–1387

Sanz N, De Mingo L, Florez F, et al (1997) Rhabdomyosarcoma of the biliary tree. Pediatr Surg Int 12:200–201

Sashi R, Sato K, Hirano H, et al (1996) Infantile choriocarcinoma: a case report with MRI, angiography and bone scintigraphy. Pediatr Radiol 26:869–870

Saxena R, Humphreys S, Williams R, et al (1994) Nodular hyperplasia surrounding fibrolamellar carcinoma: a zone of arterialized liver parenchyma. Histopathology 25:275–278

Shamsi K, De Schepper A, Degryse H, et al (1993) Focal nodular hyperplasia of the liver: radiologic findings. Abdom Imaging 18:32–38

Siegel MJ (1995) Liver and biliary tract: hepatic mass lesions. In: Siegel MJ (ed) Pediatric sonography, 2nd edn. Raven Press, New York, pp 181–191

Siegel MJ, Luker GD (1996) MR imaging of the liver in children. Magn Reson Imaging Clin N Am 4:637–656

Singh ZN, Ray R, Sarode VR, et al (1996) Congenital mesenchymal hamartoma of liver. Indian Pediatr 33:415–417

Stevens WR, Johnson CD, Stephens DH, et al (1995) Fibrolamellar hepatocellular carcinoma: stage at presentation and results of aggressive surgical management. AJR 164:1153–1158

Stocker JT (1998) An approach to handling pediatric liver tumors. Am J Clin Pathol 109(4 Suppl 1):S67-S72

Stover B, Laubenberger J, Niemeyer C, et al (1995) Haemangiomatosis in children: value of MRI during therapy. Pediatr Radiol 25:123–126

Stringer MD, Hennayake S, Howard ER, et al (1995) Improved outcome for children with hepatoblastoma. Br J Surg 82:386–391

Sty JR, Wells RG, Starshak RJ, et al (1992) The hepatobiliary system: neoplasms. In: Sty JR, Wells RG, Starshak RJ, et al (eds) Diagnostic imaging of infants and children. Aspen Publishers, Inc., Gaithersburg, Maryland, pp 280–293

Tanimura M, Matsui I, Abe J, et al (1998) Increased risk of hepatoblastoma among immature children with a lower birth weight. Cancer Res 58:3032–3035

Teraguchi M, Nogi S, Ikemoto Y, et al (1997) Multiple hepatoblastomas associated with trisomy 18 in a 3-year-old girl. Pediatr Hematol Oncol 14:463–467

Tomà P, Taccone A, Martinoli C (1990) MRI of hepatic focal nodular hyperplasia: a report of two new cases in the pediatric age group. Pediatr Radiol 20:267–269

Tomà P, Loy A, Pastorino C, et al (1997) Leiomyomas of the gallbladder and splenic calcifications in an HIV-infected child. Pediatr Radiol 27:92–94

Toren A, Sharon N, Mandel M, et al (1995) Two embryonal cancers after in vitro fertilization. Cancer 76:2372–2374

Tovbin J, Segal M, Tavori I, et al (1997) Hepatic mesenchymal hamartoma: a pediatric tumor that may be diagnosed prenatally. Ultrasound Obstet Gynecol 10:63–65

Tsai SY, Jeng YM, Hwu WL, et al (1996) Hepatoblastoma in an infant with Beckwith-Wiedemann Syndrome. J Formos Med Assoc 95:180–183

Tschappeler H (1993) Liver tumors in children. Radiologe 33:679–684

van Noesel MM, Hahlen K, Hakvoort-Cammel FG, et al (1997) Neuroblastoma 4 S: a heterogeneous disease with variable risk factors and treatment strategies. Cancer 80:834–843

von Schweinitz D, Wischmeyer P, Leuschner I, et al (1994) Clinico-pathological criteria with prognostic relevance in hepatoblastoma. Eur J Cancer 30 A:1052–1058

von Schweinitz D, Schmidt D, Fuchs J, et al (1995) Extramedullary hematopoiesis and intratumoral production of cytokines in childhood hepatoblastoma. Pediatr Res 38:555–563

Vos A (1995) Primary liver tumours in children. Eur J Surg Oncol 21:101–105

Weimann A, Ringe B, Klempnauer J, et al (1997) Benign liver tumors: differential diagnosis and indications for surgery. World J Surg 21:983–990

Wholey MH, Wojno KJ (1994) Pediatric hepatic mesenchymal hamartoma demonstrated on plain film, ultrasound and MRI, and correlated with pathology. Pediatr Radiol 24:143–144

Wong DC, Masel JP (1995) Infantile hepatic haemangioendothelioma. Australas Radiol 39:140–144

Wu TJ, Teng RJ (1994) Diffuse neonatal haemangiomatosis with intra-uterine haemorrhage and hydrops fetalis: a case report. Eur J Pediatr 153:759–761

Yoon W, Kim JK, Kang HK (1997) Hepatic undifferentiated embryonal sarcoma: MR findings. J Comput Assist Tomogr 21:100–102

28 Diagnostic Imaging in Liver Transplantation

D.A. Leung, T. Pfammatter, and B. Marincek

CONTENTS

28.1 Introduction

The advances in solid organ transplantation achieved in the last 2 decades have seen liver transplantation become a realistic treatment option for patients with hepatic failure. Technical improvements, careful patient selection and particularly the use of cyclosporin have elevated survival rates to 83% at 1 year and 75% at 4 years (Starzl et al. 1989a,b). A wide range of acute and chronic hepatic diseases are presently treated by transplantation. Excellent results have been reported in patients with cryptogenic cirrhosis, chronic active autoimmune or viral (hepatitis C virus) hepatitis, alcoholic cirrhosis, inborn metabolic disorders such as hemochromatosis and Wilson's disease, as well as cholestatic diseases such as primary biliary cirrhosis, sclerosing cholangitis and biliary atresia. Other common indications include postnecrotic cirrhosis, acute liver failure due to viral hepatitis and drugs, as well as Budd-Chiari syndrome.

Liver transplantation in the presence of hepatocellular carcinoma or cholangiocarcinoma is more controversial because of the risk of recurrence (Pichlymayr et al. 1989). A small percentage of patients with occult tumor who undergo liver transplantation is inevitable, and many surgeons treat patients with known hepatocellular carcinoma, dependent on the tumor stage. The use of liver transplantation to treat unresectable cancer is the subject of investigation, often in combination with adjuvant chemotherapy or other treatment protocols. Another controversial indication for liver transplantation is cirrhosis due to hepatitis B infection. Although there is no reliable way of preventing recurrence, some patients have shown a benefit from the procedure.

Absolute contraindications to hepatic transplantation include AIDS, metastatic hepatocellular carcinoma, non-neuroendocrine liver metastases, active alcohol or intravenous drug abuse, as well as severe cardiopulmonary disease. Conditions such as portal or mesenteric venous thrombosis, previous shunt operations to relieve variceal hemorrhage and scarring from multiple abdominal operations are no longer considered contraindications to transplantation.

Abdominal imaging and interventional radiological procedures are an integral part of any liver transplantation program. Preoperative imaging is used to target patients suitable for transplantation and to identify anatomic abnormalities which may alter surgical technique (Zajko et al. 1988). Following transplantation, imaging techniques are necessary to monitor the graft and assess complications. These

D.A. Leung, MD; Department of Radiology, Zürich University Hospital, Rämistrasse 100, CH-8091 Zürich, Switzerland
T. Pfammatter, MD; Department of Radiology, Zürich University Hospital, Rämistrasse 100, CH-8091 Zürich, Switzerland
B. Marincek, MD; Professor and Chairman, Department of Radiology, Zürich University Hospital, Rämistrasse 100, CH-8091 Zürich, Switzerland

include surgical, biliary and vascular complications as well as post-transplant or recurrent malignancy. Interventional procedures play an important role in the management of several complications. Also transjugular intrahepatic portosystemic shunt procedures are sometimes used as a temporizing measure in patients awaiting transplantation (LaBerge et al. 1993).

Orthotopic liver transplantation represents the most commonly employed procedure but other surgical techniques do exist. "Split liver" techniques, where one donor organ is used for two recipients, were developed in an effort to overcome the shortage of donor organs and to transplant portions of adult livers into children. Alternatively, a portion of a liver from a living relative can be used for transplantation. A further development has been ectopic transplantation of an auxiliary liver without removal of the native liver, which may be used in reversible acute liver failure (Heaton et al. 1995). However, this text will focus on the dominant technique of orthotopic hepatic transplantation and discuss both pretransplant imaging as well as post-transplant assessment and treatment of complications.

28.2 Pre-transplant Imaging

Pre-transplant imaging is involved not with diagnosing specific liver diseases, but with recognizing the sequelae of long-standing disease. Careful patient selection is mandated by the general shortage of donor livers as well as the significant morbidity and mortality and high costs associated with liver transplantation. Pretransplant abdominal imaging plays an important role in identifying contraindications to transplantation and anatomic abnormalities and variants that may alter the surgical approach.

Pathologic conditions that require preoperative assessment include primary and secondary malignancy that may preclude transplantation (Ferris et al. 1995) as well as vascular abnormalities (Zajko et al. 1985a; Cardella and Amplatz 1987) such as portal thrombosis which requires operative thrombectomy or venous grafting. Here the extent of portal thrombosis determines surgical planning. Short segment thromboses are treated with thrombectomy or short interposition vein grafts. If the thrombosed segment is long, donor iliac veins must be harvested for portal reconstruction or venous jump grafting between the superior mesenteric vein and the portal vein. Other vascular pathologies which require identification include stenotic celiac artery lesions and caval abnormalities. Since hepatic arterial inflow represents the sole blood supply to the post-transplant bile ducts, obstruction of the celiac axis must be alleviated to avoid biliary complications. This is usually achieved by using a donor iliac arterial graft which is anastomosed with the recipient aorta. The identification of several vascular anatomic variants may also impact surgical planning. Mismatches in donor and recipient vascular size will potentially require altered anastomotic techniques.

Liver transplantation in the presence of a primary hepatic malignancy remains a controversial topic. Experience has been acquired on the risk of recurrence since early liver transplants were performed on patients with unresectable primary and metastatic malignancy because of the lack of portal hypertension and hence reduced surgical mortality. Tumor stage is the major factor determining recurrence of hepatocellular carcinomas following transplantation. It has been shown that lesions under 4 cm may be cured by transplantation. The challenge for radiologists is to correctly stage hepatocellular carcinomas preoperatively and to identify negative prognostic factors (Karani and Williams 1993). Other than tumor size, these include vascular invasion, bilobed distribution of lesions and the presence of regional lymph node metastases. Patients with extrahepatic metastasis of primary hepatobiliary malignancy are not candidates for transplantation. Likewise, with the exception of some neuroendocrine tumors, patients with liver metastases are refused transplantation.

28.2.1 Duplex Sonography

Duplex sonography is probably the most important imaging modality prior to transplantation and is obtained on all transplant candidates (Longley et al. 1988). The examination involves Doppler examination of portal and hepatic veins as well as real-time B-mode imaging of hepatic parenchyma and bile ducts.

Of great importance to the surgeon is the evaluation of portal vein patency and size since these factors can alter surgical technique. The presence of extrahepatic portal and mesenteric venous thrombosis may even prohibit transplantation. The extrahepatic portal vein normally measures 8 to 12 mm in cross-section and should have a minimum diameter of 4 or

5 mm to enable successful portal anastomosis. Thrombus in the portal vein is seen on B-mode imaging as echogenic intraluminal material. Cavernous transformation is recognized as a racemose conglomerate of collaterals in the position of the porta hepatis and must not be mistaken for a patent portal vein. The presence of portal thrombosis should increase suspicion of malignancy as up to half of patients with hepatocellular carcinoma have vascular invasion and thrombosis (Freeny et al. 1992). Normal portal venous flow is hepatopedal and monophasic, which is well demonstrated by duplex Doppler examination. Hepatofugal flow is an indication of portal hypertension. Other changes of portal hypertension which are readily detected by sonography include ascites, splenomegaly and venous collaterals. The patency and size of the hepatic veins as well as the retrohepatic inferior vena cava must also be established preoperatively. This is of particular importance in children with biliary atresia who often have associated abnormalities of the inferior vena cava. Usually duplex examination will also include confirmation of hepatic arterial in-flow. Any vascular abnormality revealed by duplex sonography is further evaluated with magnetic resonance imaging (MRI) and MR angiography (Finn et al. 1991; Nghiem et al. 1995) or conventional angiography.

Gray scale sonographic imaging of the hepatic parenchyma is an excellent method of detecting focal liver lesions. Of utmost importance is the pretransplant visualization of hepatomas which, as explained earlier, has significant implications on the prognosis and hence the decision to operate. Sonographic evaluation may be insufficient in patients with advanced cirrhosis because of diffuse parenchymal hyperechogenicity caused by fatty infiltration and fibrosis. In these cases, MRI or CT is required to rule out malignant hepatic lesions.

28.2.2 Computed Tomography

CT can answer many of the questions asked of imaging studies in the evaluation of patients for liver transplantation. The most important role of CT is the detection of primary malignant hepatobiliary masses as an appendage to duplex sonography (Wernecke et al. 1991). Nevertheless, CT also supplies useful information for size-matching donor and recipient livers and vascular structures as well as providing an abdominal survey for extrahepatic malignancy (Nghiem 1995).

In noncirrhotic livers, malignant lesions usually appear as hypovascular masses and are therefore best detected using contrast-enhanced CT. However, in severely cirrhotic livers this relationship may be reversed. Further, primary and metastatic lesions which are hypervascular may appear isodense to liver parenchyma on venous phase imaging and are more apparent on noncontrast CT. The introduction of helical CT allowed imaging in the arterial and portovenous phase using only one contrast bolus. Arterial phase CT is useful for depicting vascular anatomy as well as evaluating vascular invasion by malignant tumors. Hence, CT evaluation of the pretransplant liver usually takes a triphasic approach including an unenhanced scan followed by arterial and portovenous imaging (Hollett et al. 1995).

It has been shown that liver-lesion conspicuity is maximized by using CT arterial portography (Heiken et al. 1989). With this technique, contrast is injected through a catheter in the splenic or superior mesenteric arteries and CT scanning of the liver is timed to coincide with the first pass of portal venous contrast. Because of its invasive nature, this technique is only employed in selected cases, for example for the differential indication of transplantation versus resection.

28.2.3 MR Imaging

MR imaging is not routinely used in the evaluation of candidates for liver transplantation. Presently, it is used when sonography and CT are indeterminate and in patients with severe allergies to iodinated contrast. MRI is at least as sensitive as CT in the detection of hepatomas (Winter et al. 1994) and more specific in the characterization of benign liver lesions. Apart from lengthy examination times and higher costs, the only disadvantage of MRI is that it does not provide a total abdominal survey including evaluation of extrahepatic disease. However, MRI offers several advantages. The assessment of vascular structures using flow-sensitive techniques and contrast-enhanced 3D MR angiography offers the possibility of evaluating the portal vein in terms of patency and flow direction (Nghiem et al. 1995) as well as obtaining a relatively detailed map of arterial anatomy for preoperative planning purposes. Moreover, using heavily T2-weighted pulse sequences, MR cholangiography can render high resolution images of the biliary tree, potentially obviating the need for invasive cholangiography, which may be required in patients with biliary disease such as sclerosing cholangitis. Hence, MRI offers the possibility of a "one-stop-shop" pretransplant assessment of all imaging aspects pertaining to pretransplant evaluation. At present, however, neither the efficacy nor the cost-effectiveness of such an approach has been investigated. In any event, MRI will increasingly become an important tool in the imaging assessment liver transplant candidates.

28.2.4 Invasive Techniques

Invasive diagnostic techniques that may be used in the preoperative evaluation for liver transplantation include angiography (Zajko et al. 1985a; Cardella and Amplatz 1987), cholangiography as well as percutaneous or transjugular biopsy (LaBerge et al. 1993).

As mentioned earlier, angiography is generally employed if noninvasive imaging studies reveal evidence of a vascular abnormality which may alter surgical technique or even preclude transplantation. Pretransplant angiography may be required to confirm portal vein patency or better demonstrate arterial anatomic variants. If conventional indirect portography does not allow adequate visualization of the portal venous system, dual catheter injection into the splenic and superior mesenteric arteries, wedged hepatic venography or direct portography may be indicated. Rarely, inferior cava venography is used to evaluate caval abnormalities preoperatively. However, with rapid improvements in noninvasive vascular imaging, particularly MR angiography, the need for preoperative catheter angiography is diminishing.

Like angiography, cholangiography is rarely necessary in the preoperative assessment of liver transplantation candidates and is reserved for patients with known or suspected sclerosing cholangitis. However, even in these patients the differentiation between benign duct strictures and cholangiocarcinoma may be difficult. Brush biopsy during endoscopic retrograde cholangiography can also be useful to exclude malignancy.

Hepatic lesions which are not adequately characterized by imaging techniques require biopsy. This is generally performed using ultrasound or CT guidance. Random biopsy of diffuse liver disease may be indicated in patients with an unknown cause of liver failure or in order to establish the extent of underlying cirrhosis in non-neoplastic disease. For this purpose, transjugular biopsy has been shown to yield fewer complications than the percutaneous approach.

In patients with advanced cirrhosis, transjugular intrahepatic porto-systemic shunt can be a useful temporizing procedure to maintain portal patency or lower portal venous pressure and control variceal bleeding while awaiting transplant organ availability (Freedman et al. 1993).

28.3 Surgical Considerations

Orthotopic liver transplantation requires four vascular anastomoses including the suprahepatic and infrahepatic vena cava, the portal vein and the hepatic artery as well as one biliary anastomosis. The suprahepatic and infrahepatic anastomoses are made first. These are usually end-to-end anastomoses but alternative techniques may be used depending on the given anatomic status. For example, absence of the recipient intrahepatic inferior verra cava (IVC) or size discrepancy between donor and recipient IVC is overcome by forming a "piggyback" anastomosis in which the infrahepatic donor inferior vena cava is sutured closed and the suprahepatic donor inferior vena cava is anastomosed to the recipient hepatic venous confluens (Fig. 28.1). After

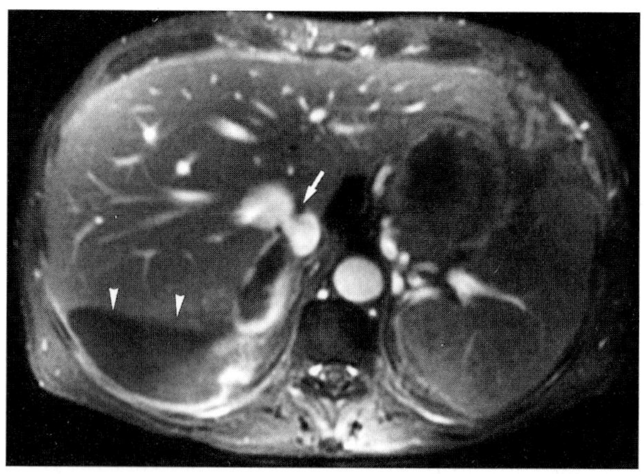

Fig. 28.1. Gadolinium-enhanced T1-weighted axial spin echo image shows "piggyback" anastomosis (*arrow*). Due to size discrepancy between donor and recipient inferior vena cava, the infrahepatic donor inferior vena cava is sutured closed and the suprahepatic donor inferior vena cava is anastomosed to the recipient hepatic venous confluens. A subhepatic hematoma (*arrowheads*) with an enhancing capsule is also visualized

the caval anastomoses have been established, the hepatic artery anastomosis is fashioned. In patients with normal vascular anatomy, the anastomosis is usually made between the donor common hepatic-splenic artery bifurcation or the celiac trunk and the recipient right and left hepatic artery bifurcation or the gastroduodenal-proper hepatic artery bifurcation. If either the donor or the recipient has a dual arterial blood supply from the celiac and superior mesenteric arteries, the larger artery is generally used for the anastomosis. Alternatively, two anastomoses can be made. In the presence of a celiac axis stenosis or discrepancy between donor and recipient artery size, a donor iliac artery homograft may be needed. The portal vein anastomosis is typically an end-to-end connection between donor and recipient extrahepatic portal veins. An iliac venous homograft may be needed in cases of extensive portal and mesenteric thrombosis.

The ideal biliary anastomosis following cholecystectomy is a choledocho-choledochostomy between the donor common bile duct and the recipient common hepatic duct. A T-tube is usually left in place for 3 months providing access for cholangiography and biliary procedures. If the recipient common hepatic duct is diseased as in patients with sclerosing cholangitis or biliary atresia, or if it is too short, a choledochojejunostomy is performed with or without an internal biliary stent.

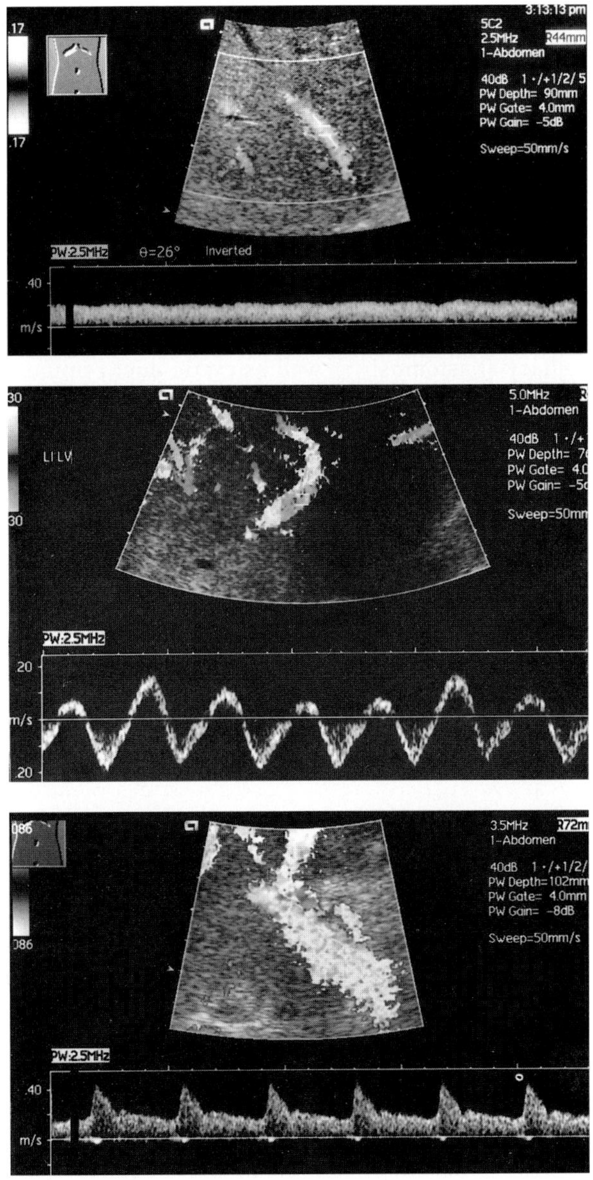

Fig. 28.2a–c. Normal post-transplant Doppler waveforms from the portal vein (**a**), hepatic vein (**b**) and hepatic artery (**c**)

28.4 Post-transplant Imaging

28.4.1 Monitoring the Liver Transplant

28.4.1.1 Duplex Sonography

Duplex sonography is the most important modality for screening the liver transplant and is performed routinely in the immediate postoperative setting as well as in the mid and long-term follow-up (Letourneau et al. 1987). The duplex examination involves evaluation of the patency of the hepatic artery, portal vein, hepatic veins and inferior vena cava (Fig. 28.2) as well as B-mode assessment of the liver parenchyma and bile ducts. Anastomotic sites are evaluated whenever possible. This can sometimes be difficult in the case of the hepatic artery anastomosis, especially in the immediate postoperative period. However, Doppler waveforms from the main right and left hepatic arteries as well as intrahepatic arteries can generally be obtained. The normal hepatic artery waveform is a low-impedance pattern with constant diastolic flow. Hepatic vein waveforms are similar to those in the inferior vena cava and show a period phasic pattern reflecting flow velocity changes during the cardiac cycle. The normal portal vein has a continuous hepatopetal flow with minor variations due to respiration (Fig. 28.2).

Real-time gray-scale imaging of the liver transplant is performed to assess the homogeneity of the liver parenchyma and to rule out bile duct dilatation. Small perihepatic seromas or hematomas are common in the early postoperative period and usually resolve within several days (Fig. 28.3). If fluid collections fail to resolve or even enlarge, the possibility of superinfection or bile leak should be considered.

28.4.1.2
Cholangiography

Cholangiography usually allows identification of the biliary anastomosis as well as cystic duct remnants (Fig. 28.4). The anastomosis and the intrahepatic bile ducts should be evaluated for the presence of strictures or bile leakage. Intrahepatic ducts should taper normally. In general, cholangiography is performed initially only one or two weeks after transplantation. On follow-up, both donor and recipient bile ducts show a slight increase in diameter (Campbell et al. 1992). The duct-duct anastomosis should not be significantly narrowed (Fig. 28.4).

28.4.1.3
Computed Tomography

CT is not routinely performed in the post-transplant setting unless complications are suspected or if sonography provides insufficient visualization. CT allows exquisite assessment of liver parenchyma and bile ducts. In about 60% of patients, low attenuation periportal tracking (Fig. 28.5) is evident on CT after transplantation (Dupuy et al. 1991). Once thought to represent rejection, it has since been shown that these low-attenuation collars dilatated lymphatic vessels as a result of severed lymphatic drainage at the time of transplantation and do not represent imminent rejection or a diminished prognosis (Marincek et al. 1986; Kaplan et al. 1989). As with ultrasound, small perihepatic fluid collections are often visualized several days after transplantation (Fig. 28.5). These may require image-assisted aspiration or drainage if they persist or undergo superinfection.

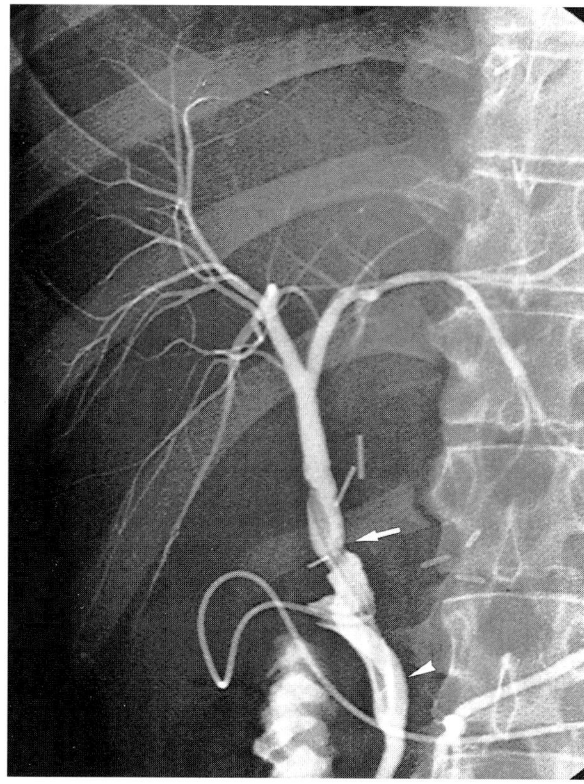

Fig. 28.4. Normal post-transplant T-tube cholangiogram showing the choledocho-choledochostomy (*arrow*) and the cystic duct remnant (*arrowhead*)

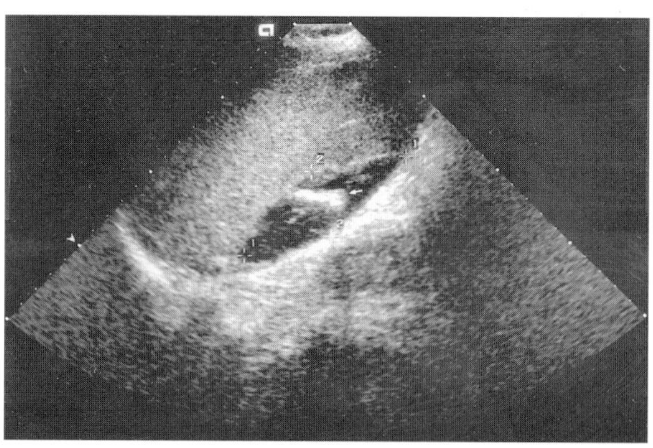

Fig. 28.3. B-mode ultrasound image shows elliptical subcapsular hematoma with echogenic material representing fibrin (*arrow*)

28.4.2
Vascular Complications

Vascular complications are reported in approximately 9% of patients with liver transplants and are considered the most common significant postoperative complications (Dalen et al. 1987; Langnas et al. 1991). Early recognition and treatment are crucial to graft survival. Since clinical presentation can vary from mildly elevated hepatic function tests to fulminant hepatic failure, imaging studies are needed to detect or rule out vascular abnormalities. The mainstay of post-transplant screening is duplex sonography. Catheter angiography is employed to confirm duplex findings or when sonographic evaluation is insufficient. Invasive vascular access may also be used to administer therapy in some instances. Arterial complications include hepatic artery stenosis and thrombosis, hepatic artery pseudoaneurysms as well as arteriovenous fistulas. Venous complications are less common and include stenosis and thrombosis of the portal vein or inferior vena cava.

28.4.2.1 Arterial Complications

28.4.2.1.1 Hepatic Artery Stenosis and Thrombosis

Hepatic artery thrombosis is the most common vascular complication after liver transplantation and is reported in approximately 6% of adults and up to 18% of children. Graft ischemia causes biliary leaks and strictures as well as hepatic infarction. Clinical presentation is very variable including elevated liver function tests in the asymptomatic patient, delayed bile leak, septicemia and fulminant hepatic necrosis. The latter requires early retransplantation for survival. Risk factors for the development of hepatic artery thrombosis include ABO incompatibility, prolonged cold ischemia times and small caliber vessels such as in pediatric patients.

Duplex sonography is the ideal noninvasive screening modality for detecting hepatic artery occlusion and stenosis and as such for identifying patients who require further evaluation with catheter arteriography (Flint et al. 1988). Hepatic artery stenosis (Fig. 28.6) is important to identify because it is treatable by balloon angioplasty (Raby et al. 1991; Orons and Zajko 1995) and if left untreated may progress to thrombosis. Conversely, the early detection of hepatic artery thrombosis (Figs. 28.7, 28.8) allows retransplantation before the development of severe hepatic failure or overwhelming sepsis.

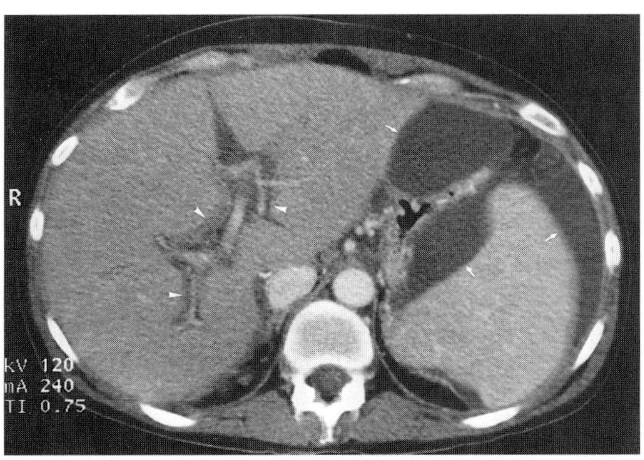

Fig. 28.5. Contrast-enhanced CT demonstrates hypodense periportal collars (*arrowheads*) thought to represent lymph stasis as a result of severed lymphatics during transplantation. Perihepatic and perisplenic fluid collections are also visualized (*arrows*)

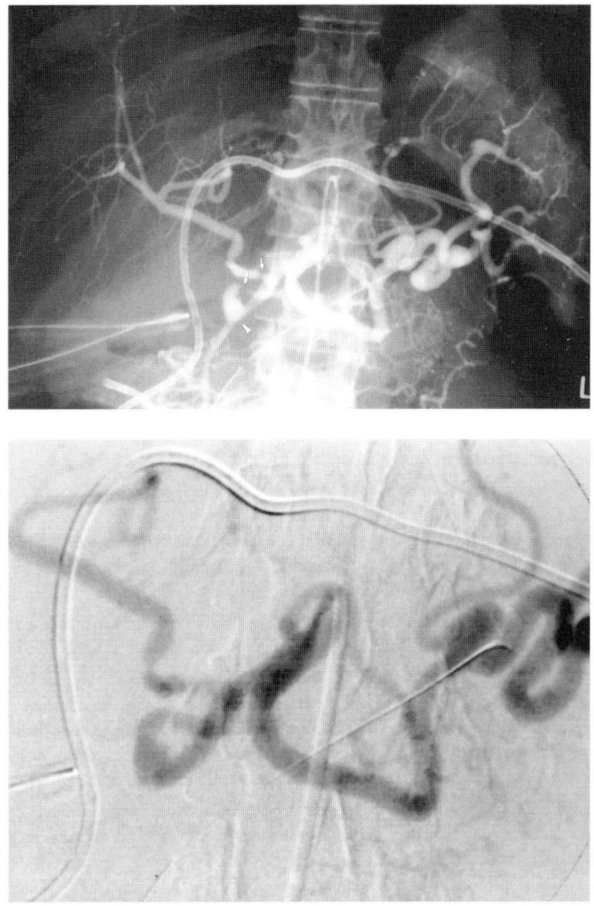

a b

Fig. 28.6a,b. Cut-film celiac angiogram (**a**) shows two donor hepatic artery stenoses (*arrows*) distal to the arterial anastomosis (*arrowhead*). Digital subtraction angiogram (**b**) following balloon dilatation

Diagnosis of hepatic artery thrombosis is made when there is an absence of Doppler-detectable proper hepatic or intrahepatic flow signal. The Doppler findings of hepatic artery stenosis are an increase in peak systolic velocity at the site of stenosis with turbulence-induced spectral broadening distally. However, reliance on direct visualization of the flow alterations at the site of the stenosis may be associated with false-negative interpretations. Therefore, more consistently obtainable intrahepatic Doppler waveforms should also be analyzed for evidence of proximal arterial obstruction (Dodd et al. 1994). Distal to a significant stenosis, a resistive index of less than 0.5 or a systolic acceleration time greater than 0.8 s is highly suggestive of stenosis. The same

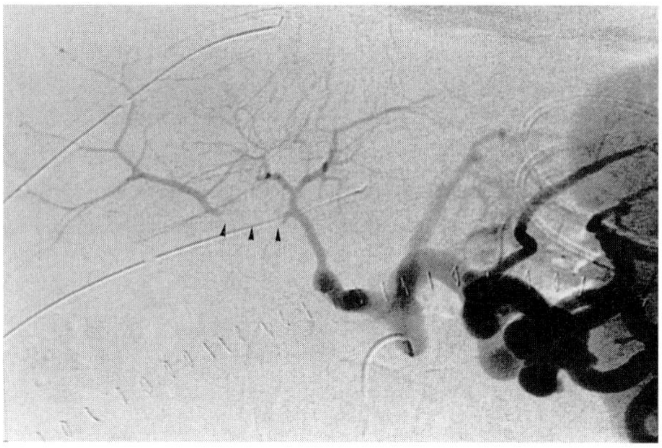

Fig. 28.7. Digital subtraction angiogram shows thrombosis of the donor right hepatic artery (*arrowheads*)

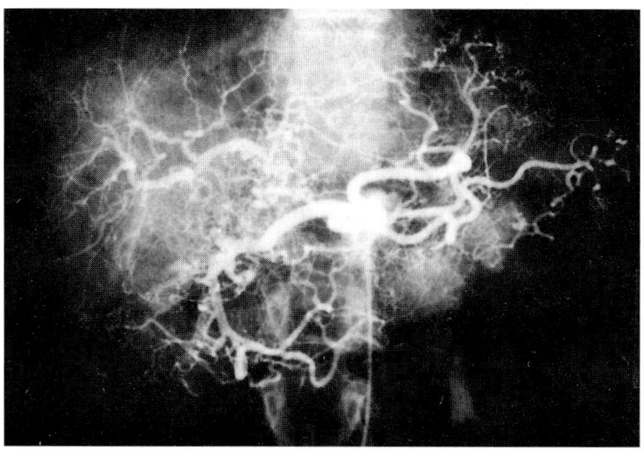

Fig. 28.8. Celiac angiogram demonstrates chronic hepatic artery thrombosis with formation of multiple collateral vessels

intrahepatic tardus/parvus waveform is seen in cases of hepatic artery thrombosis associated with collateral flow to the graft (DODD et al. 1994). Hence, evidence of such a flow signal from an intrahepatic artery should alert the examiner to a proximal arterial obstruction and prompt further angiographic evaluation.

Ultrasound or CT should be used to evaluate the liver parenchyma in patients with hepatic artery thrombosis. If hepatic infarction is seen on either ultrasound or CT (Fig. 28.9), it is almost always a significant event (COOK and CROFTON 1997). Infarctions are usually peripheral and wedge-shaped but may appear as centrally located round lesions. With time, cystic components develop which may become infected and require percutaneous drainage. Contrast-enhanced CT is slightly superior to ultrasound for detecting hepatic infarction. Frequently, portal venous gas is seen on CT in the infarcted segment.

Cholangiographic findings of hepatic artery thrombosis are the result of ischemia and include nonanastomotic bile leak and stricture (ORONS et al. 1995). Ultimately, bile duct necrosis causes dilatation into large irregular cystic spaces.

Hepatic artery thrombosis is often a devastating event which is associated with high mortality rates without retransplantation (LERUT et al. 1988; ZAJKO et al. 1988). In an attempt to postpone surgery, some investigators have proposed urgent revascularization with urokinase and/or stent placement (HIDALGO et al. 1989; MARUJO et al. 1991; VORWERK et al. 1994). Unfortunately, thrombolytic therapy is contraindicated in many patients with hepatic artery thrombosis because of the temporal proximity of the liver transplantation and the occurrence of hepatic artery thrombosis.

Hepatic artery stenosis, on the other hand, can be successfully treated with percutaneous transluminal angioplasty (Fig. 28.6), thus obviating the need for retransplantation in some patients. Stenoses that occur in the immediate postoperative phase are likely associated with surgical technique and thus require surgical revision. Balloon dilatation should not be performed until at least 10 days or 2 weeks postoperatively to avoid rupture of the arterial suture line. Several reports have shown clinical improvement in patients who have undergone balloon dilatation of hepatic artery stenoses (RABY et al. 1991; ORONS and ZAJKO 1995). However, long-term success appears to be related to graft function at the time of presentation rather than the technical success of the procedure.

28.4.2.1.2
HEPATIC ARTERY PSEUDOANEURYSM

Hepatic artery pseudoaneurysm is an uncommon complication of liver transplantation which causes hematobilia, hemoperitoneum and gastrointestinal bleeding that may be life-threatening. The most common site for pseudoaneurysm formation is the arterial anastomosis. The rest are intrahepatic lesions following percutaneous biopsy or biliary drainage procedures. Pseudoaneurysms can be detected using contrast-enhanced CT or ultrasound, with CT being the more sensitive technique (ZAJKO et al. 1989). With ultrasound, all perianastomotic fluid collections should be examined by color Doppler for evidence of turbulent arterial flow (TOBBEN et al. 1988).

Most extrahepatic anastomotic pseudoaneurysms are the result of technical failure and thus require surgical revision. Intrahepatic pseudoaneurysms, on the other hand, are generally acces-

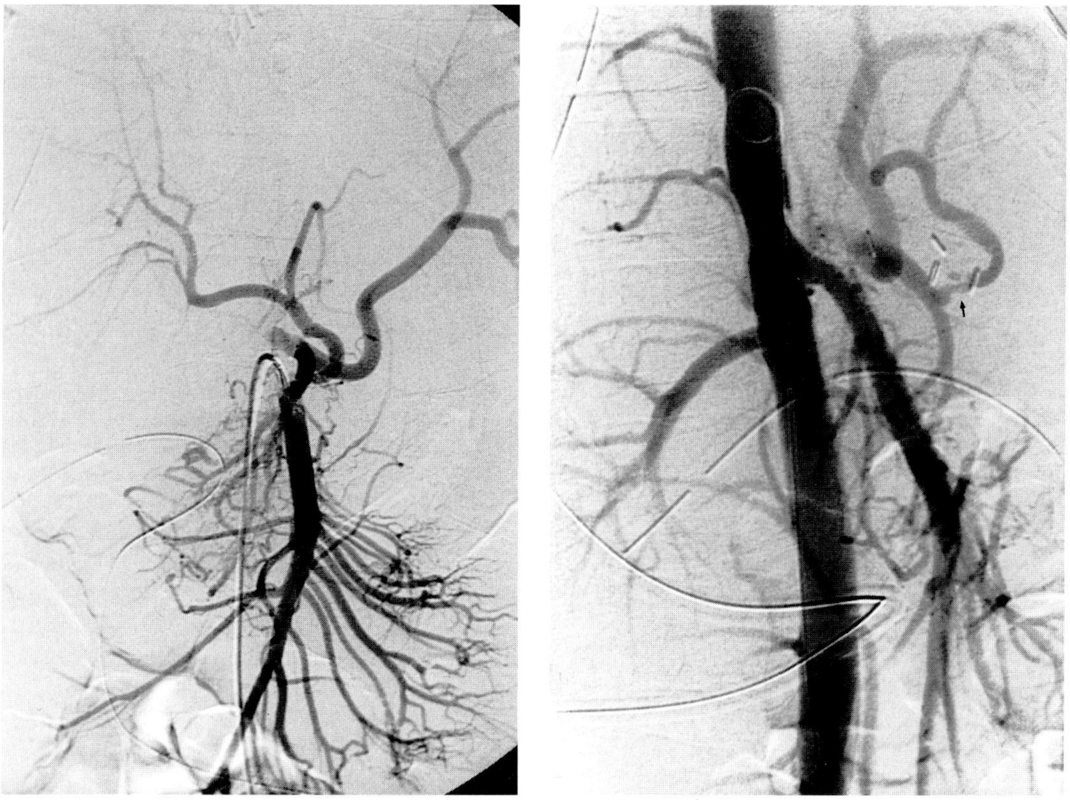

a b

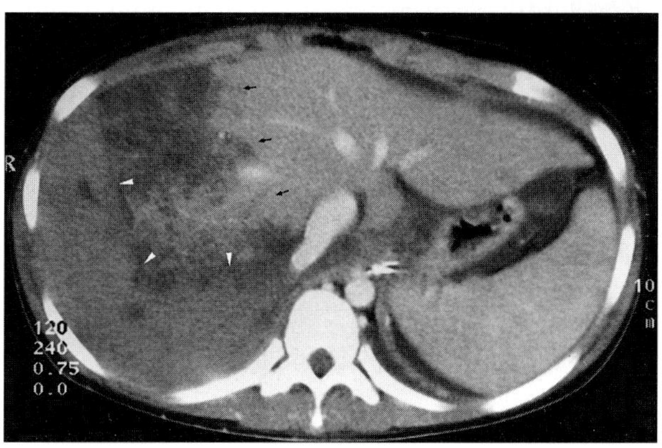

c

Fig. 28.9a–c. Superior mesenteric angiogram (**a**) shows opacification of the celiac artery via the gastroduodenal artery indicative of proximal celiac trunk occlusion. Lateral aortogram (**b**) confirms occlusion of the celiac axis and displays an additional stenosis at the hepatic artery anastomosis (*arrow*). Contrast-enhanced CT (**c**) in the same patient shows hypodense hepatic infarction of the right lobe (*arrows*) as well as a large hyperdense perihepatic hematoma (*arrowheads*)

sible by endovascular techniques for transcatheter embolization (Orons and Zajko 1995).

28.4.2.2 Portal Vein Complications

Portal vein stenosis and thrombosis are relatively rare complications of hepatic transplantation, occurring in under 3% of transplants (Lerut et al.1987a; Marujo et al. 1991). As with hepatic artery stenosis, portal vein stenosis occurs most commonly at the anastomosis. If symptomatic, portal vein stenosis and thrombosis present with elevated liver function tests as well as symptoms and signs of portal hypertension such as variceal hemorrhage, ascites and splenomegaly. Portal vein thrombosis is readily identified on noninvasive imaging studies including sonography, CT and MRI. The presumptive diagnosis of portal vein stenosis can be made by duplex sonography if turbulent flow within the portal vein is demonstrated (Fig. 28.10). However, definitive diagnosis is made angiographically using superior mesenteric and/or splenic catheterization (Fig. 28.10). Pressure gradient measurements should be made to assess the hemodynamic significance of the stenosis.

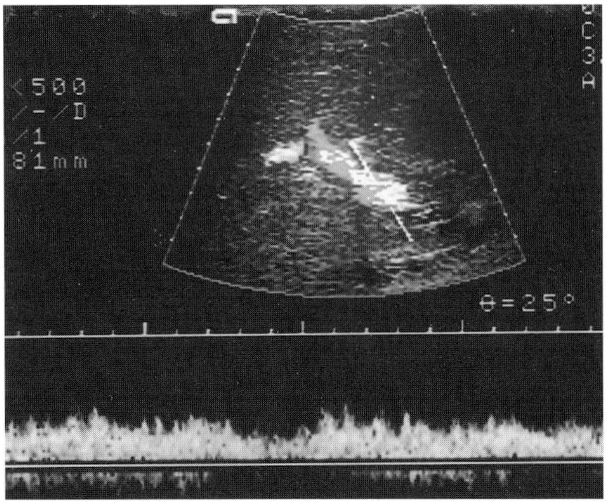
a

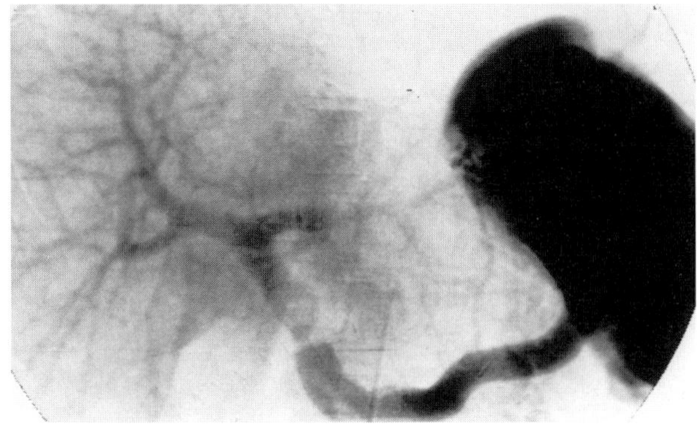
b

Fig. 28.10a,b. Doppler examination of the portal vein (**a**) demonstrates evidence of turbulent flow. Indirect splenoportography confirms portal vein stenosis at the portal anastomosis (**b**)

Portal vein thrombosis (Fig. 28.11) usually requires surgical thrombectomy, venous grafting or retransplantation. Several reports have shown good results with use of transhepatic balloon dilation for the treatment of portal vein stenosis (RABY et al. 1991; ZAJKO et al. 1994).

28.4.2.3 Inferior Vena Cava Complications

Stenosis of the inferior vena cava is a rare complication of hepatic transplantation and has been reported in 0.8% to 2.8% of transplants (LERUT et al. 1988). Suprahepatic caval stenosis causes hepatic venous obstruction and may lead to Budd-Chiari syndrome (Fig. 28.12). Caval stenosis can occur in the early postoperative phase or several years after transplantation. Discrepancy in the size of the donor and recipient inferior vena cava as well as suprahepatic caval kinking have been implicated as causes of caval stenosis. In the long term, fibrosis, chronic thrombus and neointimal hyperplasia are the likely causes of delayed caval stenosis. Retransplantation has been reported to increase the risk of suprahepatic caval stenosis because of the increased fibrosis around the suprahepatic caval anastomosis (Fig. 28.13). Thrombosis of the inferior vena cava is a rare postoperative event in transplant recipients. However, if left unrecognized, caval thrombosis will develop in many patients with obstruction of the inferior vena cava and may extend into the hepatic veins. Early recognition and treatment of caval stenosis is therefore crucial to prevent this serious event.

Ultrasound and CT may show pleural effusion, ascites, hepatosplenomegaly and dilation of the inferior vena cava as sequelae of significant caval stenosis. Doppler examination of hepatic veins may demonstrate flow reversal and absence of periodicity in the hepatic venous waveform. Definitive diagnosis, however, is based on cavography and pressure gradient measurements.

Caval stenosis can be successfully treated by balloon dilatation or stent placement (ZAJKO et al. 1994; PFAMMATTER et al. 1997) (Fig. 28.13). As with venous obstructions at other sites, repeated interventions may be necessary to maintain venous patency.

28.4.3 Biliary Complications

Bile duct complications are a significant cause of post-transplant morbidity and mortality. Children have a higher rate than adults of biliary complications with the overall incidence being 13% to 25% of liver transplant recipients (LERUT et al. 1987b). Factors that significantly impact on the development and extent of biliary complications include cold ischemia times, surgical anastomosis and vascular insufficiency. Most bile duct complications occur within the first three months following transplantation although some strictures and stones may become apparent years later.

Biliary complications can be broadly divided into bile leak and bile obstruction. Bile leak is caused by technical failure at the T-tube site or at the duct-duct anastomosis and by hepatic artery thrombosis at nonanastomotic sites. Bile obstruction can also be divided into anastomotic and nonanastomotic strictures with causes other than technical failure, being ischemia-induced stricture, stones, mucocele of the cystic duct remnant and recurrent malignancy.

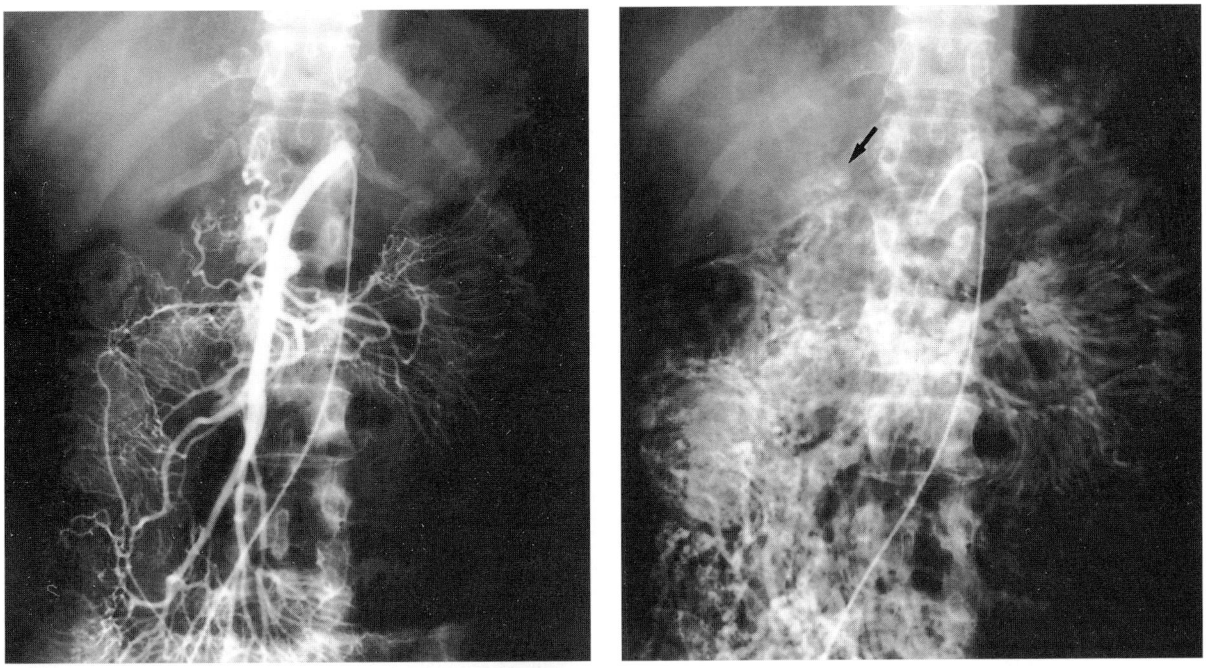

a b

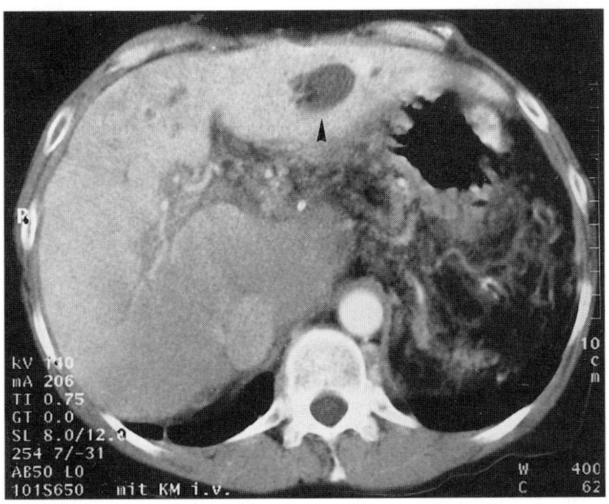

c

Fig. 28.11a–c. Arterial (**a**) and portal venous (**b**) phases of superior mesenteric angiogram show chronic portal vein thrombosis with collateral vessels in the porta hepatis (*arrow*) eight months after hepatic transplantation. Cavernous transformation of the porta hepatis is well demonstrated on contrast-enhanced CT (**c**). An intrahepatic biloma in the left liver lobe is also visualized (*arrowhead*)

Cholangiography is the mainstay for diagnosing biliary complications. Ultrasound and CT are useful for demonstrating secondary findings such as biloma and bile duct dilatation but are not sensitive for detection of early bile duct abnormalities (Zemel et al. 1988). MR cholangiography is a noninvasive alternative to cholangiography and is particularly useful in patients who do not have a T-tube in place.

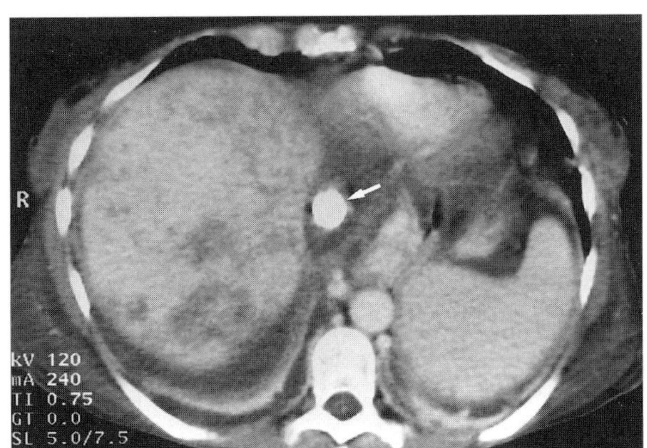

Fig. 28.12. Contrast-enhanced CT shows classic findings of Budd-Chiari syndrome in a liver transplant recipient with heterogeneous parenchymal enhancement. A stent has been placed in the inferior vena cava (*arrow*)

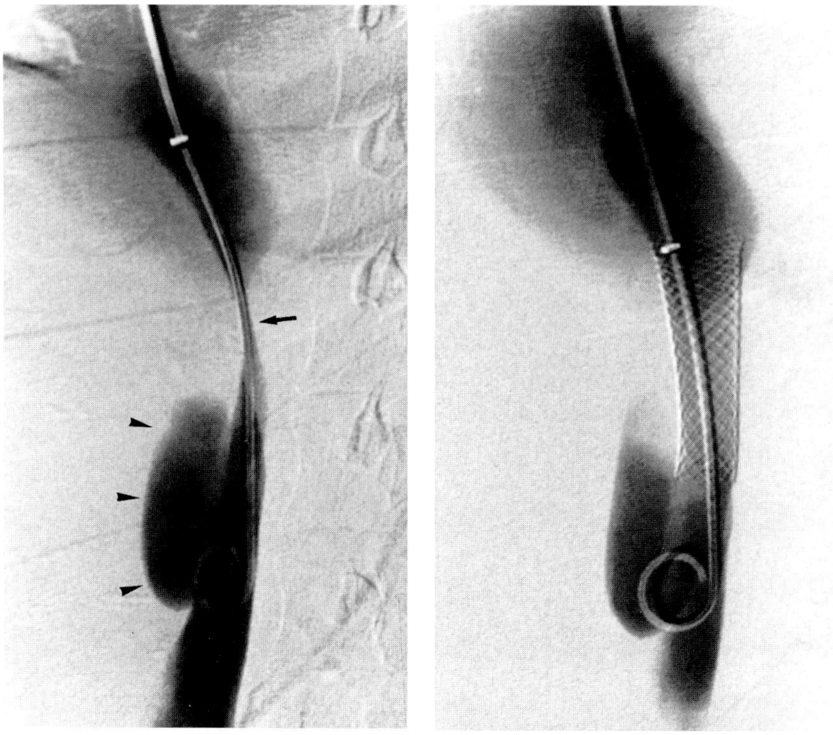

a b

Fig. 28.13a,b. Inferior cavogram (a) shows suprahepatic caval stenosis (*arrow*) proximal to a "piggyback" anastomosis (*arrowheads*) in a patient who underwent hepatic retransplantation. The stenosis was treated by placement of a stent (b)

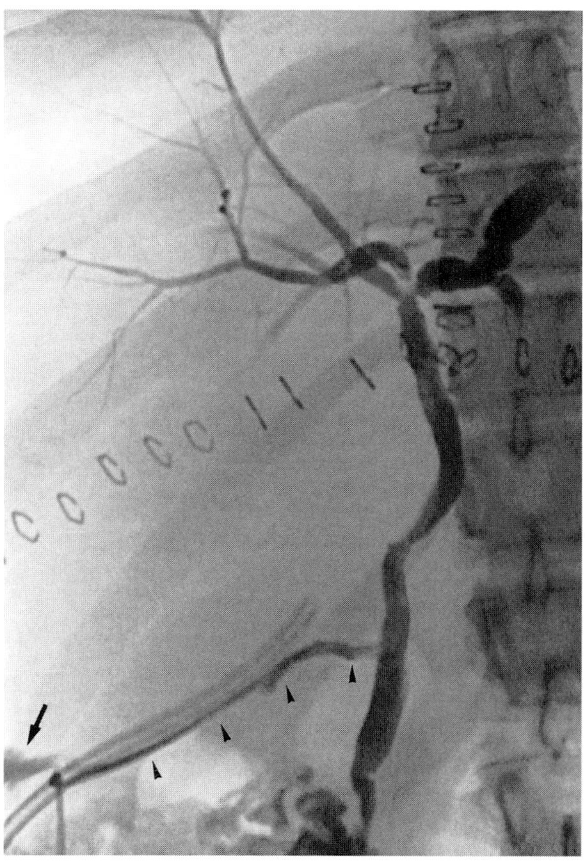

a

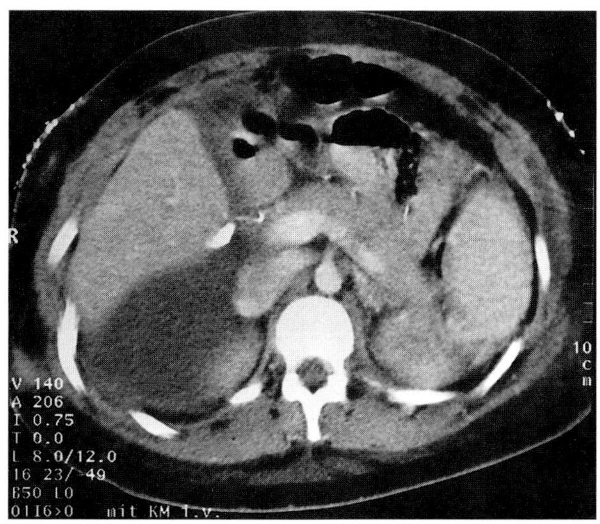

b

Fig. 28.14a,b. Cholangiography (a) three weeks after liver transplantation shows a bile leak at the T-tube site with contrast tracking along the T-tube (*arrowheads*) and forming a lateral subhepatic fluid collection (*arrow*). The associated subhepatic biloma is well demonstrated on contrast-enhanced CT (b)

28.4.3.1
Bile Duct Leaks

28.4.3.1.1
T-Tube Site

The T-tube site is the most common location of bile leakage and is almost always due to a technical problem (Sheng et al. 1994). Usually, the bile leaks are small and occur parallel to the T-tube (Fig. 28.14) but may also arise following accidental or nonaccidental tube removal. At cholangiography the bile leaks are readily recognized as linear areas of contrast extravasation. Larger leaks may form a subhepatic fluid collection which can be demonstrated using ultrasound or CT (Fig. 28.14).

Because of the immunocompromised status of the transplant patient, bile leaks pose a serious threat of infection, potentially causing bile peritonitis, infected biloma or bacteremia (Tzakis et al. 1985; Zajko et al. 1987a). CT or ultrasound guided needle aspiration or drainage procedures may be required in these cases. Small T-tube bile leaks usually resolve spontaneously. If cholangiography demonstrates a persistent leak or if fluid collections enlarge, some sort of intervention may be necessary. Corrective procedures include surgical revision, transhepatic biliary drainage and endoscopic sphincterotomy with percutaneous drainage of biloma (Zajko et al. 1987a; Ward et al. 1991).

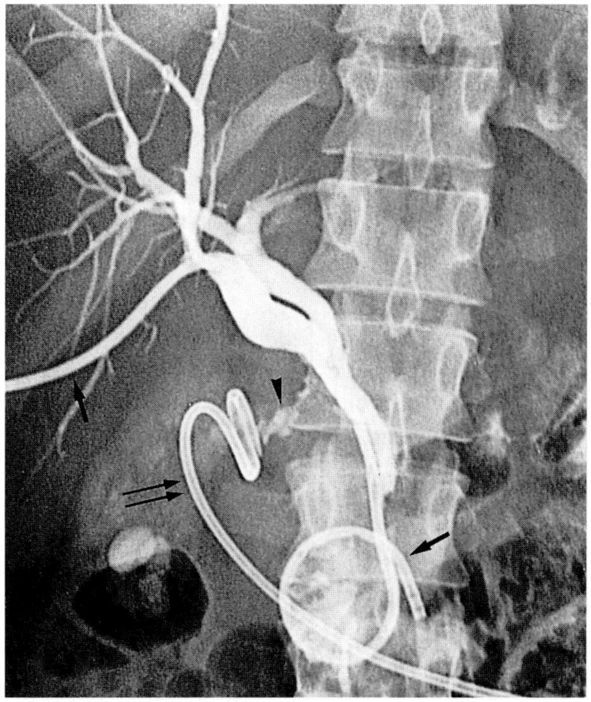

Fig. 28.15. Post-transplant cholangiogram shows contrast extravasation (*arrowhead*) due to anastomotic bile leak which has been treated by percutaneous transhepatic biliary drainage (*arrows*) as well as percutaneous drainage of subhepatic biloma (*double arrow*)

28.4.3.1.2
Anastomotic

Anastomotic bile leak can be the result of technical failure or hepatic artery thrombosis. The latter must always be ruled out angiographically. At cholangiography, contrast extravasation from the anastomosis (Fig. 28.15) can be seen with formation of an extrahepatic fluid collection (Zajko et al. 1985b; Sheng et al. 1994). As with T-tube site leaks, there is a serious threat of infection, especially since anastomotic leaks occur in the early postoperative period. Anastomotic leaks usually require surgical revision although some leaks may respond to the combination of percutaneous biliary drainage or transhepatic biliary stenting (Fig. 28.15).

28.4.3.1.3
Nonanastomotic

Nonanastamotic intrahepatic bile leaks and the formation of bilomas are considered serious findings because they are usually associated with bile duct necrosis as a result of ischemia. The incidence of hepatic artery thrombosis in patients with nonanastomotic bile leak has been reported to be 89% (Zajko et al. 1987b). Angiographic confirmation of hepatic artery patency is therefore a primary concern. Bile leaks caused by hepatic artery thrombosis are usually in the hilar region but may be intrahepatic. Cholangiography may demonstrate bile leaks and strictures with formation of large irregular fluid collections representing distended necrotic bile ducts.

Leaks and bilomas frequently become infected in patients with hepatic artery occlusion and thus necessitate percutaneous drainage as a temporizing measure. Ultimately, however, most patients with this serious complication will require retransplantation although percutaneous drainage has provided long-term yield in some children. This is because collateral blood supply can develop in pediatric recipients following hepatic artery thrombosis (Tzakis et al. 1985; Kaplan et al. 1990).

28.4.3.2 Biliary Obstruction

28.4.3.2.1

Anastomotic Strictures

Anastomotic bile duct strictures are usually caused by fibrosis and scarring and can occur from weeks to years after liver transplantation (Zajko et al. 1988). Unlike nonanastomotic strictures, anastomotic strictures are rarely associated with hepatic artery thrombosis (Fig. 28.16). Mild anastomotic narrowing is often seen at cholangiography but is usually clinically insignificant. If proximal dilatation of bile ducts is observed and there is delayed bile duct emptying, percutaneous biliary drainage should be performed. Biliary stones may form in patients with delayed stricture formation and can become lodged at the stricture site. Good results have been reported with balloon dilatation of anastomotic biliary strictures with a 6-month patency rate of 80% and a 5-year patency rate of 60% (Ward et al. 1990; Zajko et al. 1995).

28.4.3.2.2

Nonanastomotic Strictures

Similar to nonanastomotic bile leak, nonanastomotic stricture is usually caused by ischemia of the donor bile ducts. Causes include hepatic ar-

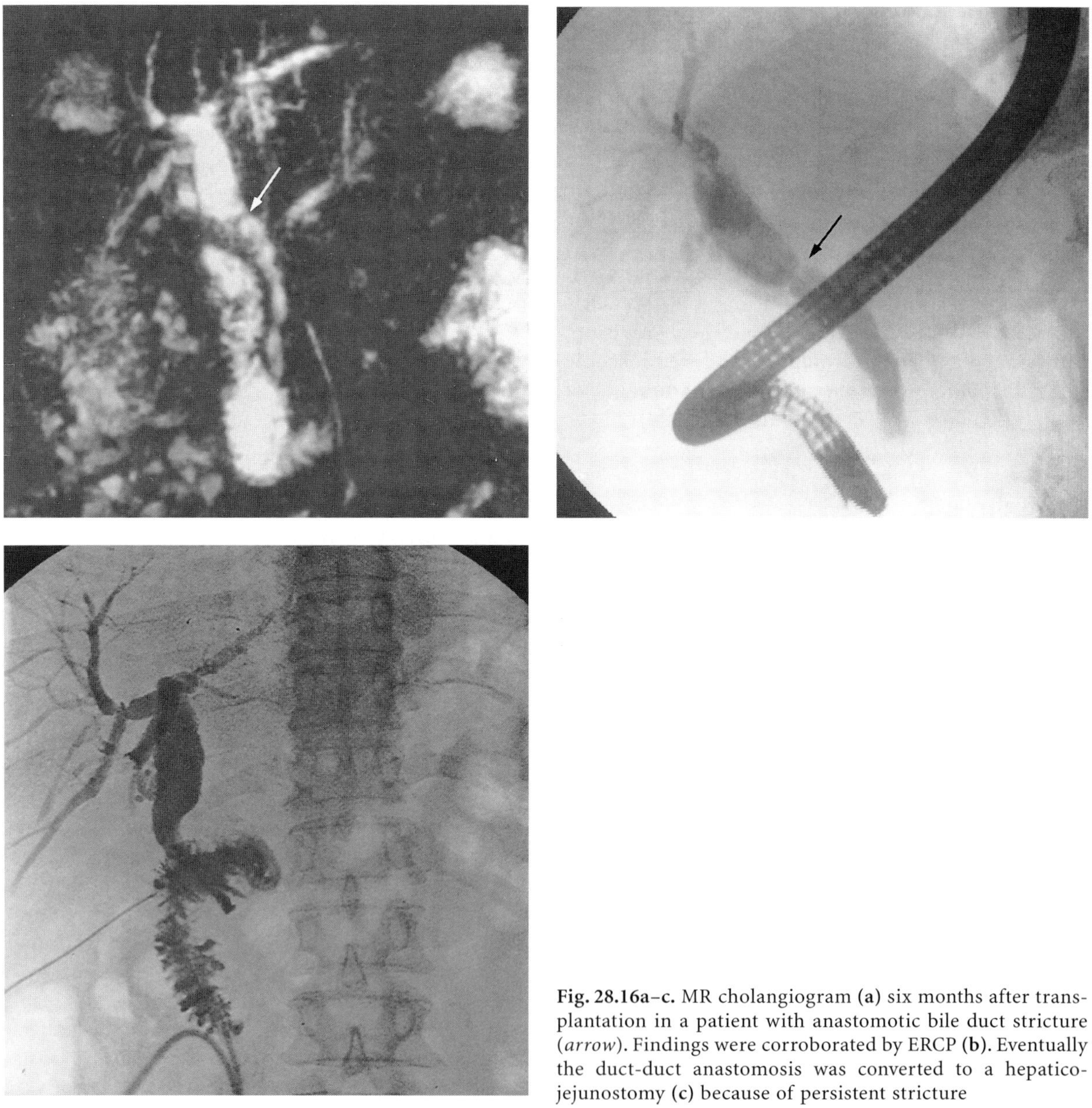

a b c

Fig. 28.16a–c. MR cholangiogram (**a**) six months after transplantation in a patient with anastomotic bile duct stricture (*arrow*). Findings were corroborated by ERCP (**b**). Eventually the duct-duct anastomosis was converted to a hepaticojejunostomy (**c**) because of persistent stricture tery thrombosis, long cold ischemia times, ABO blood type incompatibility of donor and recipient and chronic ductopenic rejection (ZAJKO et al. 1987b; KAPLAN et al. 1990).

The hepatic artery represents the sole arterial blood supply to donor livers since collaterals to the native liver via the gastroduodenal artery are severed during transplantation. Hepatic artery thrombosis is therefore a major ischemic insult to bile ducts, usually resulting in necrosis with associated leaks, strictures and biloma formation in the region of the biliary hilus. This course generally requires percutaneous drainage as a temporizing measure followed eventually by retransplantation. Strictures caused by prolonged cold ischemia times of the donor liver may have a similar appearance to those of hepatic artery thrombosis. In both cases, strictures develop from 3 weeks to 3 months after transplantation.

Strictures caused by ductopenic rejection, on the other hand, are the result of an arteriopathy and do not develop until several months after transplantation. Unlike with hepatic artery thrombosis, strictures resulting from lesser ischemic insults tend to be focal and firm rather than necrotic (WARD et al. 1990, 1994). With improved immunosuppressive therapy, bile duct strictures from ductopenic rejection are being observed less frequently.

Cholangiography is the primary diagnostic modality for diagnosing bile duct stricture (Fig. 28.17). Doppler or angiographic assessment of hepatic artery patency is important in any patient with nonanastomotic bile duct stricture or leak. Several investigators have reported good results with balloon dilatation (Fig. 28.18) and stenting of nonanastomotic strictures (WARD et al. 1990; ZAJKO et al. 1995), especially in patients with causes other than hepatic artery thrombosis and ductopenic rejection.

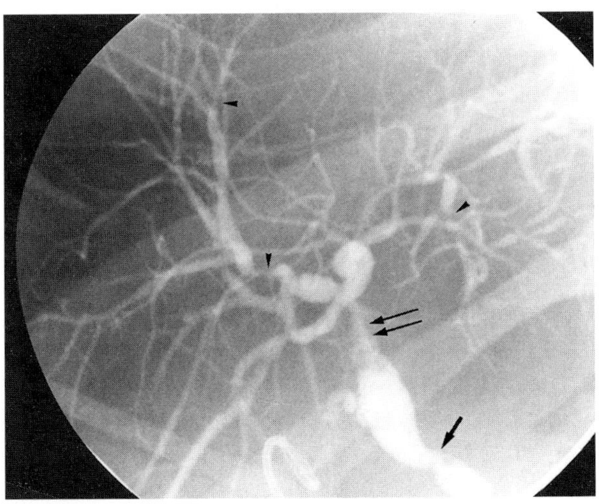

Fig. 28.17. Cholangiogram in a patient with hepatic artery thrombosis shows mild anastomotic stricture (*arrow*) and significant nonanastomotic stricture in the region of the hilus (*double arrow*) as well as other intrahepatic sites (*arrowheads*)

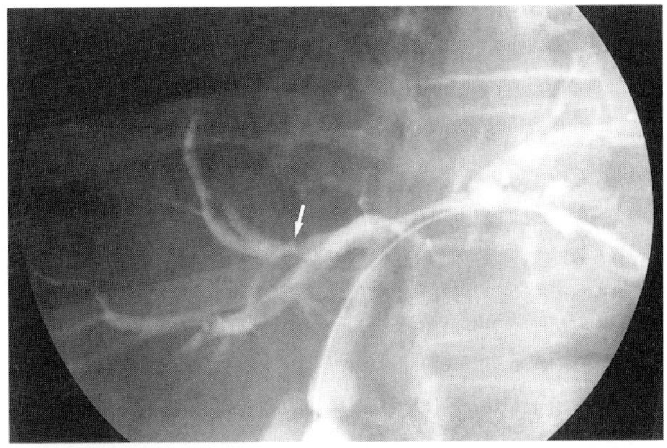

a

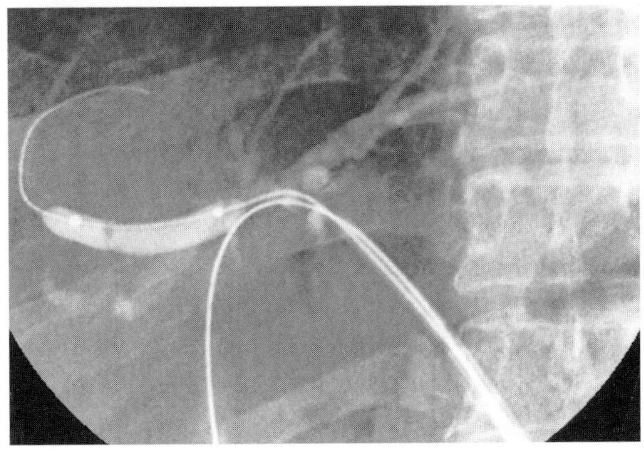

b

Fig. 28.18a,b. Cholangiogram (**a**) shows nonanastomotic intrahepatic bile duct stricture (*arrow*) which was treated by balloon dilatation (**b**)

28.4.3.2.3
OTHER CAUSES

Biliary obstruction may be caused by a malpositioned T-tube or an inspissated surgical stent. Stents may fail to migrate into the small bowl or become lodged in the anastomosis, thus requiring endoscopic or percutaneous removal. Obstructing calculi (Fig. 28.19) can also usually be removed or crushed percutaneously using a Dormia basket.

A rare cause of bile duct obstruction is a mucocele of the remnant donor cystic duct (ZAJKO et al. 1990). This occurs when the remnant cystic duct is obstructed by the duct-duct anastomosis causing mu-

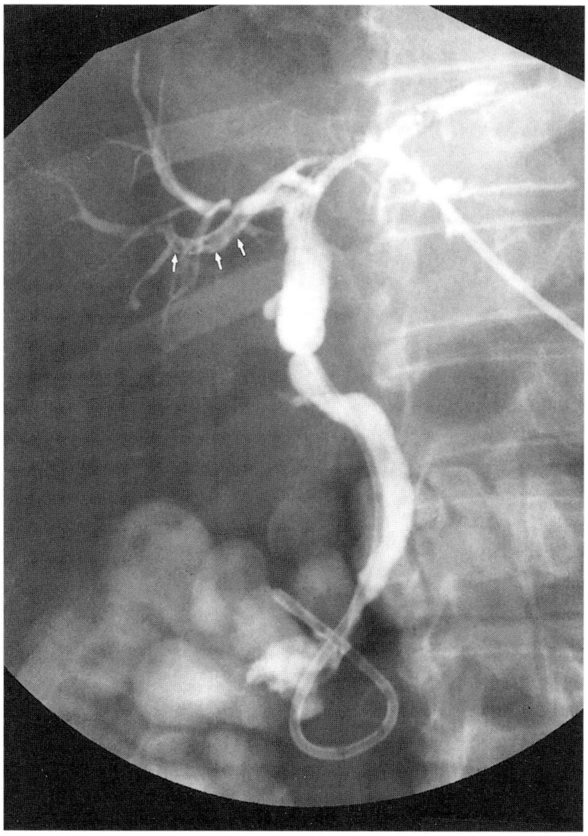

Fig. 28.19. Cholangiogram in a liver transplant recipient with anastomotic and nonanastomotic strictures shows filling defects (*arrows*) in the right hepatic duct representing bile duct calculi

cous accumulation. A rounded mass eventually develops and causes extrinsic compression of the donor common hepatic duct. CT and ultrasound show a well-defined cystic mass adjacent to the anastomosis.

Recurrent malignancy of the donor bile ducts occurs in at least two-thirds of patients with cholangiocarcinoma and may be hilar, intrahepatic or both (Herbener et al. 1988). Transhepatic brush biopsies may be useful to confirm the diagnosis.

Finally, bile duct obstruction may be caused by redundancy and kinking of the donor and recipient extrahepatic bile ducts. This generally requires surgical revision.

28.4.4 Abdominal Complications

The risk of abdominal complications associated with major abdominal surgery exist in liver transplant recipients. Postoperative perihepatic fluid collections occur commonly and include seromas, hematomas and bilomas (Wood et al. 1985). These are readily recognized at ultrasound and CT. Hematomas may be differentiated from other fluid collections if they are hyperdense on CT (Figs. 28.9, 28.20) in the early phase or if they contain echogenic fibrin on ultrasound (Fig. 28.3) in the chronic phase. Bilomas are generally difficult to differentiate from seromas without aspiration. If a persistent fluid collection is found to be a biloma, cholangiography should be performed to identify the site of bile leakage and the patency of the hepatic artery should be assessed ultrasonographically. Owing to the immunocompromised status of liver transplant patients, the risk of superinfection of perihepatic fluid collections (Fig. 28.21) is considerable. These can usually be definitively treated by percutaneous drainage (Kaplan et al. 1990).

Other rare abdominal complications of liver transplantation include adrenal hemorrhage, acute pancreatitis and colonic complications. Colonic perforation may be infectious but is usually the result of direct surgical injury. Pneumatosis cystoides coli has been reported to occur in liver transplant recipients but is of doubtful clinical significance (Andorsky 1990). Acute pancreatitis is an uncommon occurrence following transplantation or after biliary drainage and has a CT and ultrasound appearance similar to that of nontransplant patients. Hemorrhage of the right adrenal gland as a result of surgical ligation of the right adrenal vein while removing a portion of the inferior vena cava is a further possible complication but is rarely of clinical signifi-

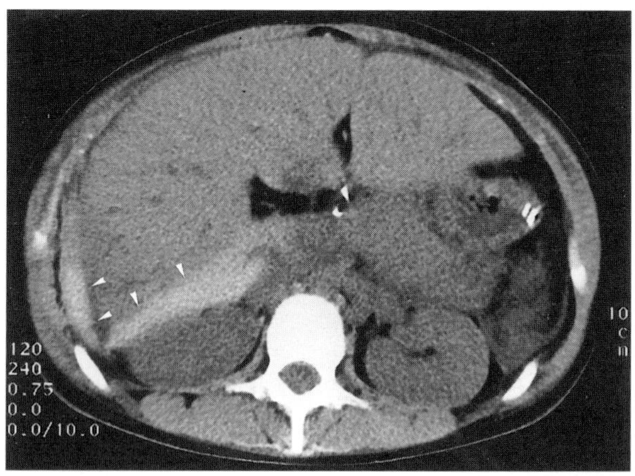

Fig. 28.20. Unenhanced CT performed several days after orthotopic liver transplantation shows hyperdense perihepatic hematoma (*arrowheads*)

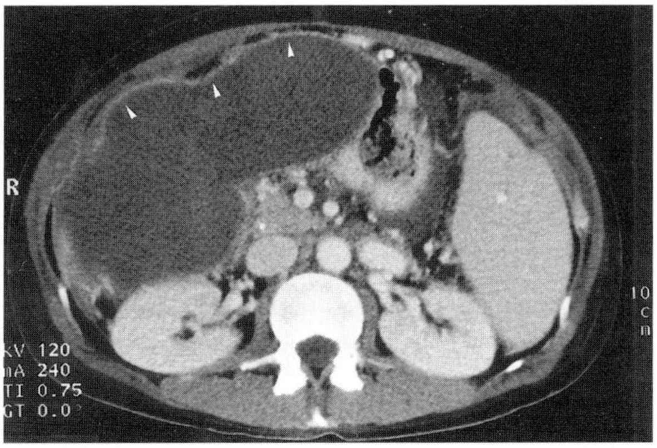

Fig. 28.21. Contrast-enhanced CT demonstrates infected subhepatic biloma with enhancing capsule (*arrowheads*)

cance (BOWEN et al. 1990). Adrenal hemorrhage is easily identified with both CT and ultrasound.

28.4.5 Risk of Malignancy

Organ transplant patients are at an increased risk of developing malignancies. The majority are basal and squamous cell skin malignancies as well as lymphomas (STIEBER et al. 1991; DODD et al. 1992). The development of post-transplant lymphoproliferative disease is associated with cyclosporin therapy which inhibits suppressor T cells and allows proliferation of B cells. There also appears to be an association with Epstein-Barr virus (HARRIS et al. 1987). The imaging of post-transplant lymphoproliferative disease is essentially the same as that of non-Hodgkin's lymphoma and, as such, any body tissue including the transplanted organ may be involved. The most common sites are lymph nodes and the gastrointestinal tract.

Liver transplant patients with a history of inflammatory bowel disease and primary sclerosing cholangitis appear to have an increased risk of developing colorectal carcinoma (BLEDAY et al. 1993). Patients who have undergone hepatic transplantation for hepatocellular malignancy may develop recurrent or metastatic disease, with the risk of recurrence being linked to the preoperative stage. However, patients with incidental preoperatively undetected hepatocellular carcinoma have a low risk of recurrent disease.

References

Andorsky RI (1990) Pneumatosis cytoides intestinalis after organ transplantation. Am J Gastroenterol 85:189–194

Bleday R, Lee E, Jessurun, et al (1993) Increased risk of early colorectal neoplasms after hepatic transplant in patients with inflammatory bowel disease. Dis Colon Rectum 36:908–912

Bowen A, Keslar PJ, Newman B, et al (1990) Adrenal hemorrhage after liver transplantation. Radiology 176:85–88

Campbell WL, Foster RG, Miller WJ, et al (1992) Changes in extrahepatic bile duct caliber in liver transplant recipients without evidence of biliary obstruction. Am J Roentgenol 158:997–1000

Cardella J, Amplatz K (1987) Preoperative angiographic evaluation of prospective liver recipients. Radiol Clin North Am 17:105–122

Cook GJR, Crofton ME (1997) Hepatic artery thrombosis and infarction: evolution of the ultrasound appearances in liver transplant recipients. British J Radiol 70:248–251

Dalen K, Day DL, Ascher NL, et al (1987) Imaging of vascular complications after hepatic transplantation. Am J Roetgenol 150:1285–1290

Dodd GD III, Greenler DP, Confer SR (1992) Thoracic and abdominal manifestations of lymphoma occurring in the immunocompromised patient. Radiol Clin North Am 30:597–610

Dodd GD III, Memel DS, Zajko AB, et al (1994) Hepatic artery stenosis and thrombosis in transplant recipients: Doppler diagnosis with resistive index and systolic acceleration time. Radiology 192:657–661

Dupuy D, Costello P, Lewis D, et al (1991) Abdominal CT findings after liver transplantation in 66 patients. Am J Roentgenol 156:1167–1170

Ferris JV, Marsh W, Little AF (1995) Presurgical evaluation of the liver transplant candidate. Radiol Clin North Am 33:497–520

Finn JP, Edelmann RR, Jenkins RL, et al (1991) Liver transplantation: MR angiography with surgical validation. Radiology 179:265–271

Flint EW, Sumkin JH, Zajko AB, et al (1988) Duplex sonography of hepatic artery thrombosis after liver transplantation. Am J Roentgenol 151:1167–1170

Freedmann AM, Sanyal Aj, Tisnado J (1993) Results with percutaneous transjugular intrahepatic portosystemic stent-shunts for the control of variceal hemorrhage in patients awaiting liver transplantation. Transplant Proc 25:1087–1089

Freeny P, Baron R, Teefey S (1992) Hepatocellular carcinoma: reduced frequency of typical findings with dynamic contrast-enhanced CT in a non-Asian population. Radiology 182:143–148

Harris K, Schwartz, M, Slasky B, et al (1987) Posttransplantation cyclosporine-induces lymphoproliferative disorders: clinical and radiologic manifestations. Radiology 162:697–700

Heaton ND, Corbally M, Rela M, et al (1995) Surgical techniques of segmental reduction, split and auxiliary liver transplantation. In: Williams R, Portmann B, Tan KC (eds) The proactive of liver transplantation. Churchill Livingstone, London, p 143

Heiken J, Weymann P, Lee J, et al (1989) Detection of focal hepatic masses: prospective evaluation with CT, delayed

CT, CT during arterial portography, and MR imaging. Radiology 171:47–51

Herbener T, Zajko AB, Koneru B, et al (1988) Recurrent cholangiocarcinoma in the biliary tree after liver transplantation. Radiology 167:349–354

Hidalgo EG, Abad J, Canterero JM, et al (1989) High dose intraarterial urokinase for the treatment of hepatic artery thrombosis in liver transplantation. Hepatogastroenterology 36:529–533

Hollett MD, Jeffrey RB Jr, Nino-Murcia M, et al (1995) Dual-phase helical CT of the liver: value of arterial phase scans in the detection of small (1.5 cm) malignant hepatic neoplasms. Am J Roentgenol 164:879–884

Kaplan SB, Sumkin JH, Campbell WL (1989) Periportal low-attenuation areas on CT: value as evidence of liver transplant rejection. Am J Roentgenol 152:285–287

Kaplan SB, Zajko AB, Koneru B (1990) Hepatic bilomas due to hepatic artery thrombosis in liver transplant recipients: percutaneous drainage and clinical outcome. Radiology 174:1031–1035

Karani J, Williams R (1993) The staging of hepatocellular carcinoma. Clin Radiol 48:297–301

LaBerge J, Ring E, Gordon R, et al (1993) Creation of transjugular intrahepatic portosystemic shunts with the wallstent endoprosthesis: results in 100 patients. Radiology 187:297–301

Lerut JP, Tzakis AG, Bron KM, et al (1987a) Complications of venous reconstruction in human orthotopic liver transplantation. Ann Surg 205:404–414

Lerut JP, Gordon RD, Iwatsuki S, et al (1987b) Biliary tract complications in human orthotopic liver transplantation. Transplantation 43:47–51

Lerut JP, Gordon RD, Iwatsuki E, et al (1988) Human orthotopic liver transplantation: surgical aspects in 393 consecutive grafts. Transplant Proc 20:603–606

Letourneau JG, Day DL, Ascher NL, et al (1987) Abdominal sonography after hepatic transplantation: results in 36 patients. Am J Roentgenol 149:299–306

Longley D, Skolnick M, Zajko A (1988) Duplex Doppler sonography in the evaluation of adult patients before and after liver transplantation. Am J Roentgenol 151:687–696

Marincek B, Barbier PA, Becker CD, et al (1986) CT appearance of impaired lymphatic drainage in liver transplants. Am J Roetgenol 147:519–523

Marujo WC, Langnas AN, Wood RP, et al (1991) Vascular complications following orthotopic liver transplantation: outcome and role of urgent revascularization. Transplant Proc 23:1484–1486

Nghiem H (1995) Imaging of hepatic transplantation. Radiol Clin North Am 36:429–443

Nghiem H, Winter T III, Mountford M, et al (1995) Evaluation of the portal venous system before liver transplantation: value of phase-contrast MR angiography. Am J Roentgenol 164:871–878

Orons P, Zajko A (1995) Angiography and interventional procedures in liver transplantion. Radiol Clin North Am 33:541–558

Orons P, Sheng R, Zajko AB (1995) Hepatic artery stenosis in liver transplant recipients: prevalence and cholangiographic appearance of associated biliary complications. Am J Roentgenol 165:1145–1149

Pfammatter T, Williams DM, Lane KL, et al (1997) Suprahepatic caval anastomotic stenosis complicating orthotopic liver transplantation: treatment with percutaneous transluminal angioplasty, wallstent placement, or both. Am J Roentgenol 168:477–480

Pichlymayr R, Ringe B, Wittekind C, et al (1989) Hepatic grafting for malignant liver tumors. Transplant Proc 21:2403–2405

Raby N, Karani J, Thomas S, et al (1991) Stenoses of vascular anastomoses after hepatic transplantation: treatment with balloon angioplasty. Am J Roentgenol 175:167–171

Sheng R, Sammon JK, Zajko AB, et al (1994) Bile leak after hepatic transplantation: cholangiographic features, prevalence and clinical outcome. Radiology 192:413–416

Starzl T, Demetris A, van Thiel D (1989a) Liver Transplantation part 1. New Engl J Med 321:1014–1021

Starzl T, Demetris A, van Thiel D (1989b) Liver Transplantation part 2. New Engl J Med 321:1092–1099

Stieber AC, Boillot O, Scotti-Foglieni C, et al (1991) The surgical implications of posttransplant lymphoproliferative disorders. Transplant Proc 23:1477–1479

Tobben PJ, Zajko AB, Sumkin JH, et al (1988) Pseudoaneurysms complicating organ transplantation: roles of CT, duplex sonography, and angiography. Ragiology 169:65–70

Tzakis AG, Gordon RD, Shaw BW, et al (1985) Clinical presentation of hepatic artery thrombosis after liver transplantation in the cyclosporine era. Transplantation 40:667–671

Vorwerk D, Günther RW, Klever P (1994) Angioplasty and stent placement for treatment of hepatic artery thrombosis following liver transplantation. J Vasc Intervent Radiol 5:309–312

Ward EM (1994) Radiology in liver transplantation. In:Margulis and Burhenne (eds) Alimentary tract Radiology. Mosby, St. Louis p1736

Ward EM, Kiely MJ, Maus TP, et al (1990) Hilar biliary strictures after liver transplantation: cholangiography and percutaneous treatment. Radiology 177:259–263

Ward EM, Wiesner RH, Hughes RH, et al (1991) Persistent bile leak after liver transplantation: biloma drainage and endoscopic retrograde cholangiopancreatographic sphincterotomy. Radiology 179:719–724

Wernecke K, Rummeny E, Bongartz G (1991) Detection of hepatic masses in patients with carcinoma: comparative sensitivities of sonography, CT and MR imaging. Am J Roentgenol 157:731–739

Winter T, Takayasu K, Muramatsu Y, et al (1994) Early advanced hepatocellular carcinoma: evaluation of CT and MR appearance with pathologic correlation. Radiology 192:379–387

Wood RP, Shaw, BW, Starzl TE (1985) Extrahepatic complications of liver transplantation. Semin Liver Dis 5:377–384

Zajko AB, Bron K, Starzl T, et al (1985a) Angiography of liver transplantation patients. Radiology 157:305–311

Zajko AB, Campbell WL, Bron KM, et al (1985b) Cholangiography and interventional biliary radiology in adult liver transplantation. Am J Roentgenol 144:127–131

Zajko AB, Bron KM, Orons PD, et al (1987a) Percutaneous transhepatic cholangiography and biliary drainage after liver transplantation: a five-year experience. Gastrointest Radiol 12:137–142

Zajko AB, Campbell WL, Logsdon GA, et al (1987b) Colangiographic findings in hepatic artery occlusion after liver transplantation. Am J Roentgenol 149:485–489

Zajko AB, Campbell WL, Bronk M, et al (1988) Diagnostic and

interventional radiology in liver transplantation. Gastroenterol Clin North Am 17:105–143

Zajko AB, Tobben, P, Equivel C, et al (1989) Pseudoaneurysms following orthotopic liver transplantation: clinical and radiologic manifestations. Transplant Proc 21:2457–2459

Zajko AB, Bennet MJ, Campbell WL, et al (1990) Mucocele of the cystic duct remnant in eight liver transplant recipients: findings at cholangiography, CT and US. Radiology 167:691–693

Zajko AB, Sheng R, Bron KM, et al (1994) Percutaneous transluminal angioplasty of venous anastomotic stenoses complicating liver transplantation: intermediate-term results. J Vasc Intervent Radiol 5:121–123

Zajko AB, Sheng R, Zetti G, et al (1995) Transhepatic balloon dilatation of biliary strictures in liver transplant patients: a 10 year experience. J Vasc Intervent Radiol 6: 79–84

Zemel G, Zajko AB, Skolnick ML, et al (1988) The role of sonography and transhepatic cholangiography in the diagnosis of biliary complications after liver transplantation. Am J Roentgenol 151:943–948

29 Specific MR Contrast Media for Liver Imaging

F. Terrier, J.P. Vallée, S. Pochon, N. Howarth, and C.D. Becker

CONTENTS

29.1 Introduction

The two major goals of magnetic resonance imaging (MRI) of the liver are cancer detection and tissue characterization. However, in this respect, MRI has a strong competitor, namely computed tomography (CT). Indeed, with the advent of the spiral technique and a better understanding of the pharmacokinetics of iodinated contrast media, highly optimized CT imaging protocols, such as double-phase spiral CT, have been established in clinical practice. This has resulted in greatly improved liver imaging. Focal lesions less than 1 cm are now routinely detected with CT (Hollett et al. 1995). However, although sensitivity in detecting focal liver lesions is the first requisite of an imaging procedure, characterization of small lesions is also of great importance, because of the high prevalence (>20%) of benign hepatic tumors, particularly hemangiomas, in the general adult population (Karhunen 1986). Unfortunately, characterization of such small liver lesions with CT is often difficult (Hanafusa et al. 1995). Even common liver cysts, when less than 10 mm in size, can be troublesome. In fact, we now encounter the same problems with liver CT as those we have already been facing with chest CT. Thanks to the exquisite resolution obtained in CT imaging of the lung parenchyma, small peripheral nodules, a few mm in size, are frequently detected. In a given patient, it is often impossible to decide with certainty whether they represent benign lesions, such as granulomas, or malignant lesions, such as metastases. This is of concern, particularly in a patient with a known malignancy, because the presence or absence of lung metastases may be crucial in the choice of an appropriate therapy. One further aspect to consider is that percutaneous biopsy of these small lesions, in the lung as in the liver, can be difficult with a low yield for cytologic or histologic diagnosis.

Problems of characterization of focal liver lesions with CT are not limited only to nodules of small size. The differential diagnosis of hypervascular tumors, such as focal nodular hyperplasia, adenoma or well-differentiated hepatocellular carcinoma, even larger than 1 cm, can sometimes be difficult, despite the use of state-of-the-art double-spiral CT. Some hemangiomas may present as hypervascular lesions (Hanafusa et al. 1995, 1997; Semelka et al. 1994), lacking the well-known pathognomonic feature of nodular enhancement (Gaa et al. 1991; Quinn and Benjamin 1992; Leslie 1995a,b). They are then almost indistinguishable from other hypervascular tumors, such as hypervascular metastases for example.

Therefore, there is still plenty of room for improvement in liver imaging despite the advent of spiral CT!

F. Terrier, MD; Professor and Chairman, Department of Radiology, University Hospital of Geneva, Micheli-du-Crest 24, CH-1211 Geneva 14, Switzerland

J.P. Vallée, MD; Department of Radiology, University Hospital of Geneva, Micheli-du-Crest 24, CH-1211 Geneva 14, Switzerland

S. Pochon, PhD; Bracco Research, CH-1211 Geneva 14, Switzerland

N. Howarth, MD; Department of Radiology, University Hospital of Geneva, Micheli-du-Crest 24, CH-1211 Geneva 14, Switzerland

C.D. Becker, MD; Head, Unit of Abdominal and Gynecological Radiology, University Hospital of Geneva, Micheli-du-Crest 24, CH-1211 Geneva 14, Switzerland

MRI is increasingly used today in liver imaging in the hope of not only increasing sensitivity, but mostly to improve characterization of focal lesions.

For tissue characterization with MRI, various qualitative criteria (e.g., size, outline, homogeneity of signal intensity, etc.) and quantitative parameters (e.g., signal intensity ratios, relaxation times) have been proposed and the importance of T2-weighted images has been emphasized. Unfortunately, tissue characterization with unenhanced MRI is unreliable, particularly at high field strength, because of overlap in the qualitative criteria and the quantitative parameters of focal liver lesions.

For this reason, there is now a consensus that use of contrast media is mandatory in liver MRI, both for the sake of improved detection and characterization of focal lesions. Up to now, the contrast media which have been most frequently used are non-specific gadolinium chelates. However, these contrast media, which diffuse rapidly into the extracellular space, provide similar information to iodinated contrast media used with CT. Therefore, although the diagnostic accuracy of liver MRI, using high-field strength, state-of-the-art equipment allowing fast scanning and dynamic studies after intravenous bolus injection of non-specific gadolinium chelates is already considered superior to that of CT, liver-specific contrast media have been developed and others are still under development. The aim is to further improve the diagnostic value of MRI, in terms both of detection and, even more importantly, of characterization.

29.2 Classification of Contrast Media for Liver Imaging

One can classify contrast media on the basis of their biodistribution. We will consider the mechanisms by which they alter signal intensity later. The contrast media we are interested in are all injected intravenously (although some of them can also be injected intraarterially, for example directly into the hepatic artery or the superior mesenteric artery). Therefore, all of them are transported by the blood circulation to their target, the liver. From the intravascular space, however, they diffuse differently, according to the class they belong to.

The so-called non-specific MRI contrast media, which are gadolinium chelates (of which several are now approved for clinical use: Gd-DTPA, Magnevist; Gd-DOTA, Dotarem; Gd-DTPA-BMA, Omniscan; Gd-HP-DO3 A, ProHance) diffuse rapidly into the interstitial space. They show a behavior which is similar to iodinated contrast media used for CT. They do not penetrate into intact cells, at least not significantly, and are eliminated through the kidneys.

On the other hand, the so-called specific contrast media show several types of behavior, according to their biodistribution (Low 1997; Hahn and Saini 1998).

RES-specific contrast media are particles, such as superparamagnetic iron oxides, which are phagocytosed by the reticulo-endothelial system (RES) (Peterstein et al. 1996). Physico-chemical properties, such as particle size and coating determine into which cells of the RES (liver, spleen, lymph nodes, bone marrow) they are preferentially phagocytosed and the rate of their clearance. Hepatocyte-specific contrast media are internalized into hepatocytes (Giovagnoni and Paci 1996). Such contrast media are taken into hepatocytes by several mechanisms, explaining why there are several types of such contrast media, with different properties. Up to now, at least three of them have already been used in patients: manganese-DPDP, gadolinium-BOPTA and gadolinium-EOB-DTPA. All three are eliminated in part with bile, allowing opacification of the biliary tree. A fourth one, asialoglycoprotein-SPIO, has been studied only in animals up to now, but it is also discussed below, because its mechanism of uptake in hepatocytes and its effect on image contrast are completely different from the other three.

Finally, tumor-specific contrast media can be taken up specifically in tumors, through mechanisms which are not well understood. One example is metalloporphyrins which accumulate in necrotic tissues.

Whereas the mechanism by which iodinated contrast media alter radio-density is unique, namely X-ray attenuation, MRI contrast agents affect signal intensity through several parameters. Thus, some contrast media affect (shorten) mostly the T1 relaxation time. However, at high dose, they also shorten the T2 relaxation time. Other contrast media, mostly the particulate ones, influence predominantly the T2* relaxation time, because they greatly disturb the local magnetic field. The latter usually (but not always!) also have a T1 effect at low dose. It is also important to be aware that unlike iodinated contrast media, the effect of which is a direct one (the molecules of the contrast medium attenuate the X-ray, depending on their concentration), MRI contrast media have an indirect effect. They influence the relaxation times of the water molecules of the tissues in which they are present. This has an important consequence. The effect of a contrast medium visible on the image depends not only on its concentration in the tissue, but also on the basic magnetic properties of the latter.

In the following sections, we will describe in more detail the different types of hepato-specific contrast media.

29.3 RES-Specific Contrast Media

Iron oxide-based RES-specific contrast media have been extensively studied experimentally and are now routinely used in several centers. The first "in-vivo" results were published in 1985 (Wolf et al. 1985). Over the following years, several investigators reported the use of superparamagnetic iron oxides as MRI contrast agents (Saini et al. 1987). Early clinical trials were conducted at the Massachusetts General Hospital in 1987 (Stark et al. 1988; Ferrucci and Stark 1990).

Once injected intravenously, these particulate agents are rapidly removed (plasma half-life of around 15 min) from the circulation by the macrophage monocytic phagocytic system (or RES) of the body. In this regard, the Kupffer cells in the liver play a dominant role. They line the liver sinusoids and are thus in direct contact with blood. Although they represent less than 10% of the liver volume, they normally contribute more than 80% of the blood filtering function of the entire RES of the body (Biozzi and Stiffel 1965). They can phagocytose and degrade proteins and lipids. They neutralize certain drugs and foreign molecules. They clear the portal blood of bacteria, viruses, endotoxins, and immune complexes. As already mentioned, they take up intravenously administered SPIO particles, which are then catabolized through various iron metabolic pathways.

Iron-oxide based MRI contrast media contain a magnetically responsive core (magnetite), which is made up of one or many aggregates of individual iron oxide crystals. To achieve stability of the colloidal solution, surface molecules have to be attached to the magnetic core. In addition, a target specific molecule can be bound to the complex to direct the contrast medium to a certain receptor or antigenic site.

Biodistribution of iron oxide preparations is largely determined by particle size and by molecules attached to the particle surface (Weissleder and Papisov 1992; Peterstein et al. 1996). Medium sized and large particles (>30 nm) tend to accumulate in spleen and lung, while small particles (<30 nm) accumulate significantly in liver, bone marrow, and lymph nodes. Small neutrally charged particles preferably distribute to lymph nodes, whereas positively charged compounds of the same size are rapidly taken up in the liver. SPIO particles with galactose terminals are predominantly captured by hepatocytes via the asialoglycoprotein receptor (see below); dextran-coated particles are phagocytosed by macrophages (including Kupffer cells).

A suspension of homogeneously dispersed SPIO is characterized by high T1 and T2 relaxivity (Chambon et al. 1993). Josephson et al. (1988) have shown that the T1 relaxivity of SPIO particles requires intimate contact between water molecules and the surface of the iron oxides. As the T1 relaxivity is a function of the surface area, it increases when the particles are dispersed in the solvent and not concentrated in a small volume. Conversely, as clustering of SPIO particles occurring at high concentrations decreases the surface of iron oxide in contact with water molecules, the T1 relaxivity decreases. Therefore, a T1 effect (brightening on MR images) predominates at low concentrations.

The T2 effect (darkening on MR images) produced by SPIO particles is caused by dipole-dipole interactions and magnetic susceptibility. The latter is the major relaxation mechanism at high concentration and usually predominates in the normal liver parenchyma. Indeed, SPIO particles are taken up by the cells of the RES and concentrated in lysosomes in the form of clusters. In this configuration, the small particles generate a strong heterogeneity in the local magnetic field. The proton spins of water molecules diffusing across these local magnetic gradients experience a rapid dephasing, and consequently their apparent T2, i.e. T2*, is significantly shortened (Majumdar et al. 1988, 1989; Rozneman et al. 1990; Muller et al. 1991). This effect is so potent, that even concentrated in a small percentage of the liver volume (i.e., the Kupffer cells), SPIO particles produce complete signal loss from the entire liver. Furthermore, any T1 effect is obscured.

Malignant tumor nodules (hepatocellular carcinomas, metastases) may also contain phagocytosing macrophages, but usually the density of the latter is too low to sequester a detectable amount of SPIO particles. As a result, there is no change in the relax-

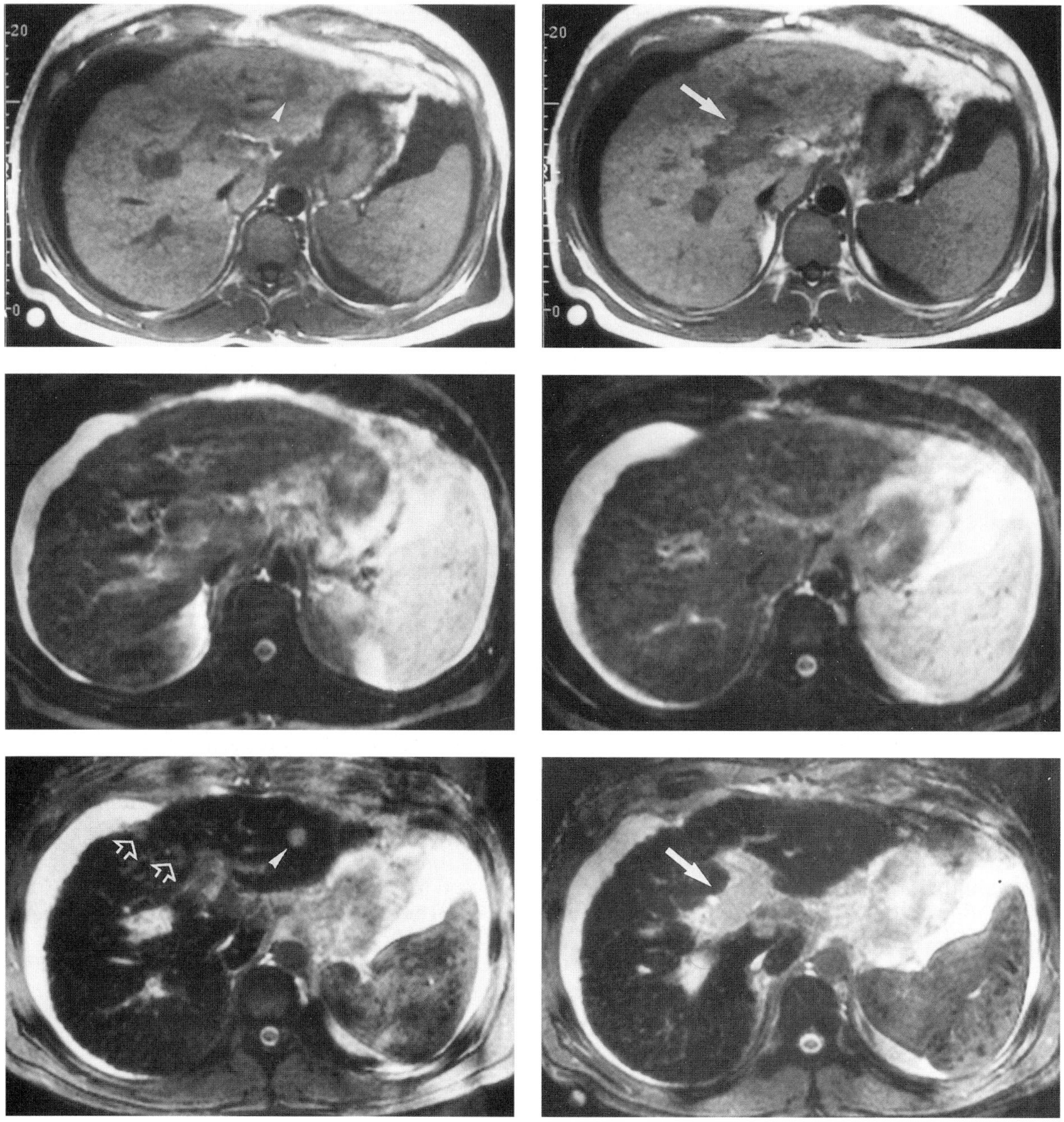

Fig. 29.1a–f. Hepatocellular carcinoma. **a,b** Native T1-weighted spin echo (SE) images. **c,d** Native T2-weighted gradient echo (GE) images. **e,f** Post SPIO T2-weighted GE images. A two-centimeter nodule (*arrowhead*) in the left lobe as well as several smaller nodules (*open arrows*) in segment IV are hardly seen on the native images and are well recognized as bright spots after SPIO administration (**e**). Note liver cirrhosis, ascites, and tumorous portal vein thrombosis (*arrow*)

ation times of tumors, and the signal difference between normal liver tissue and tumor is therefore increased (the nodules appear as bright spots) (Fig. 29.1). In this way, the conspicuity of tumor nodules on MR images, i.e., the sensitivity of MRI in the detection of such nodules, is greatly improved, as shown in several papers (Bellin et al. 1994; Denys et al. 1994; Ros et al.1995; Hagspiel et al. 1995).

The sensitivity of SPIO-enhanced MR is close to that of CT portography and in the same range as double-spiral CT (Senèterre et al. 1996; Strotzer et al. 1997). Besides, SPIO particles are particularly helpful for lesion characterization (Grandin et al. 1995; Vogl et al. 1995, 1996a,b).

The presence of Kupffer cells in lesions like focal nodular hyperplasia and adenoma results in darken-

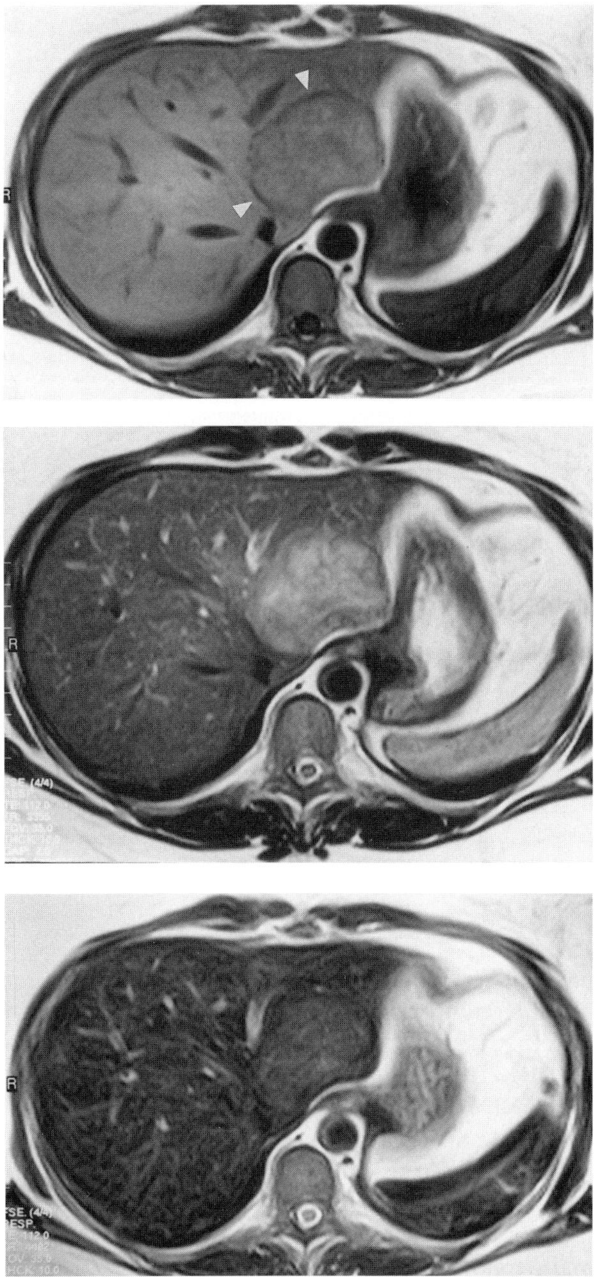

a

b

c

Fig. 29.2a–c. Focal nodular hyperplasia (FNH). **a** Native T1-weighted SE image. **b** Native T2-weighted fast SE image. **c** Post SPIO T2-weighted fast SE image. On **a**, the tumor in segment II is isointense to the normal liver parenchyma, but slightly heterogeneous. At its periphery, one recognizes vessels (*arrowheads*) encircling the tumor like the tyre of a wheel, which is a typical feature of FNH. On **b**, the tumor is moderately hyperintense and has a internal nodular structure. However, a well-defined central stellate structure is not seen. After SPIO administration (**c**), the tumor becomes strongly dark, like surrounding normal liver parenchyma, which indicates the presence of Kupffer cells and its benign nature. However, because a central scar is lacking, we have also considered adenoma in the differential diagnosis, and the patient (a 34 year old woman) was operated upon

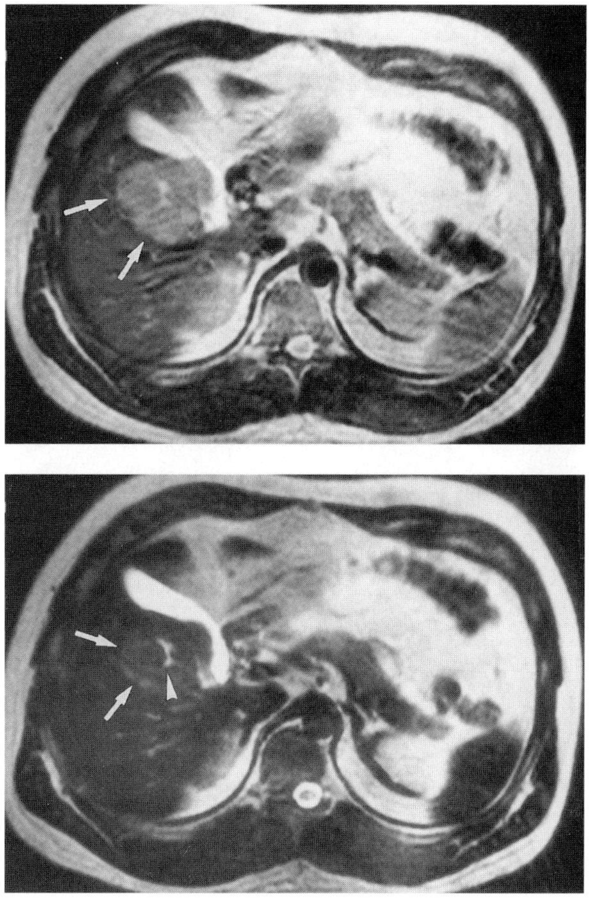

a

b

Fig. 29.3a,b. Focal nodular hyperplasia. **a** Native T2-weighted SE image. **b** Post SPIO T2-weighted. SE image. The central scar (*arrowhead*) appears better on **b**, due to the strong darkening of the nodule (*arrows*) after SPIO administration. In this case, we made a definite diagnosis of FNH. Neither surgery nor biopsy were performed. Even follow-up was not recommended

ing of the tumor on T2 and T2*-weighted images (due to the uptake of SPIO particles), which indicates its benign nature (Vogl 1995, 1996a,b) (Figs. 29.2, 29.3). However, absence of uptake does not exclude a benign liver tumor, nor does scattered uptake exclude the possibility of a highly differentiated hepatocellular carcinoma.

Due to the marked shortening of T2* of liver parenchyma, SPIO particles have been mainly used as a negative contrast agent. Thus, in earlier clinical trials, their effect was evaluated almost exclusively on T2- and T2*-weighted images. More recently, attention has also been given to T1-weighted sequences. Indeed, the latter are very useful for characterization. It has been shown that SPIO particles can greatly influence the T1 relaxation time of hemangiomas and cause strong signal enhancement on T1-

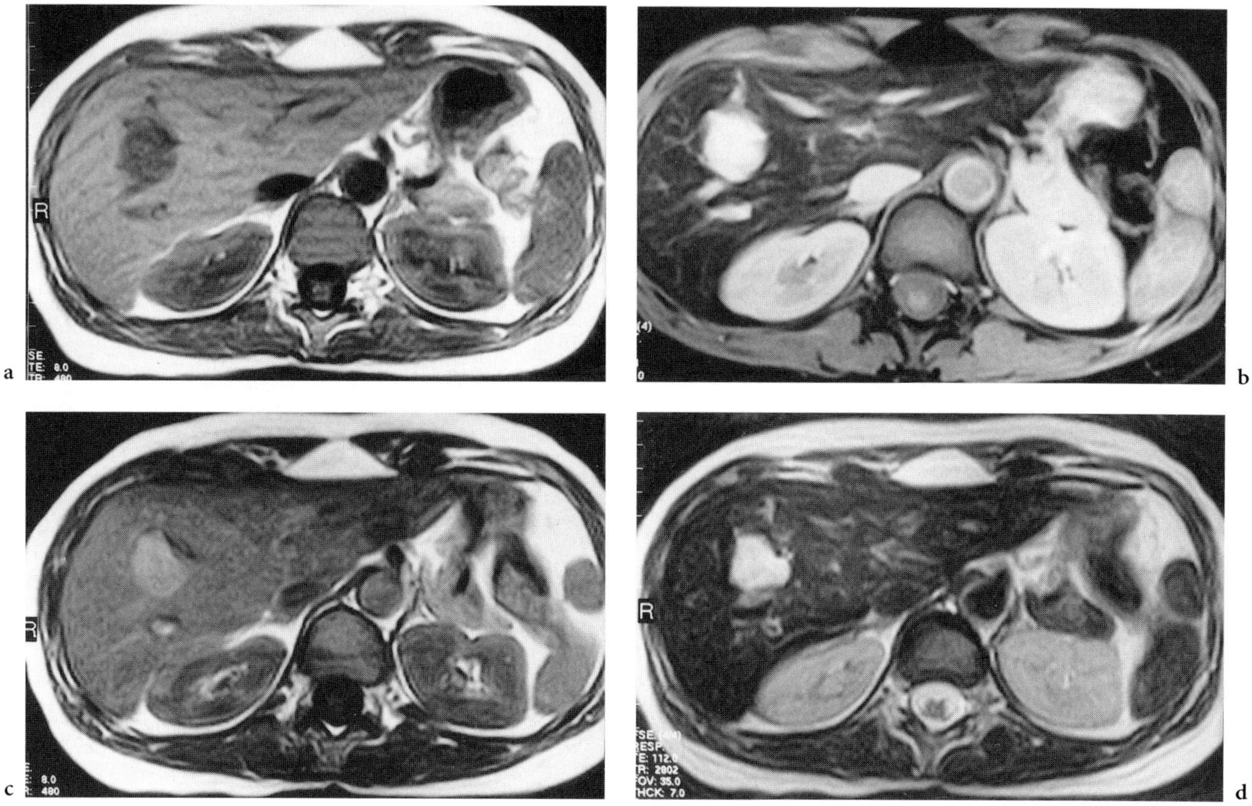

Fig. 29.4a–d. Hemangioma. **a** Native T1-weighted SE image. **b** Native T2 multisegmented echoplanar (EPI) SE image. **c,d** Same sequences as **a** and **b**, after SPIO. Note the strong enhancement of the hemangioma on the T1-weighted image after SPIO administration (**c**)

weighted images (Grangier et al. 1994; Urhahn et al. 1996) (Figs. 29.4–29.6). This behavior is typical for hemangiomas and is due to the fact that SPIO particles are dispersed in low concentration in the vascular lakes of hemangiomas.

The compound which was first introduced into clinical practice is a stable colloidal aqueous suspension of dextran-coated iron oxide particles, designated AMI-25 or Feridex (Advanced Magnetics, Inc., Cambridge, MA, USA). In Europe, it has been commercialized under the name of Endorem (Laboratoire Guerbet, Aulnay-sous-Bois, France). Measured by light scattering, the particle size is distributed between 120 and 180 nm.

The r2 relaxivity in plasma is 0.7×10^5 $(mol/l)^{-1}$ s^{-1} at 37°C at 20 MHz. Under the same conditions, the r1 relaxivity is 0.17×10^5 $(mol/l)^{-1}$ s^{-1}. It is a reddish-brown to black solution, with an iron content of 11.2 mg Fe/ml. Immediately before intravenous use, it is diluted into 100 ml glucose 10%. Then, it is injected slowly as an infusion at a dose of 15 μmol iron/kg body weight, over about 20–30 min. About 70% of the injected dose is taken up by the liver. Imaging is usually performed 40–60 min after the beginning of the injection, but the enhancement lasts as long as 4–7 days.

Side effects are observed in up to 10% of the patients (Laniado and Chachuat 1995). The most frequent complication is lower back pain. However, interruption of the infusion or even administration of medication against pain are necessary in only very few cases. The exact mechanism of lower back pain following injection of SPIO particles is unknown, but the same kind of pain has been noticed previously after intravenous injection of iron preparations as a treatment of anemia. Interestingly, similar back pain is also a typical symptom in acute intravascular hemolysis. More serious side effects, such as arterial hypotension and anaphylactoid reaction, have also rarely occurred after injection of SPIO particles.

As pre-contrast images appear necessary in our experience, we usually remove the patient from the magnet for the contrast medium administration. In the meantime, we can examine another patient. Our current imaging strategy at a field strength of 1.5 T is

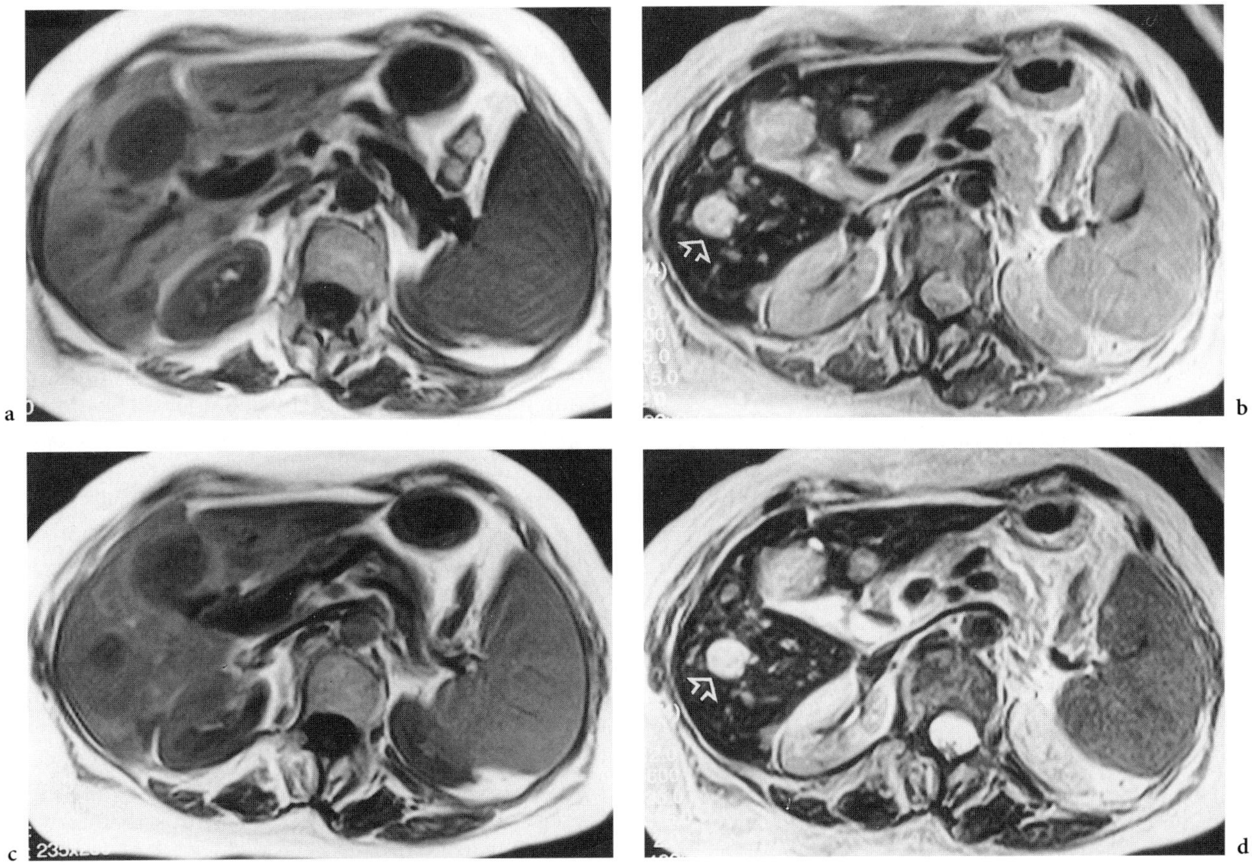

Fig. 29.5a–d. Liver metastases from a neuroendocrine tumor of the pancreas. **a** Native T1-weighted SE image. **b** Native T2-weighted fast SE image. **c,d** Same sequences as **a** and **b**, after SPIO. Multiple nodules, hypointense on **a** and hyperintense on **b**. After SPIO administration no change in the signal intensity of the nodules, neither on T1 (**c**) nor on T2-weighted images (**d**). Note that some of the nodules (*open arrow*) are very hyperintense on T2-weighted images, similar to hemangiomas. The use of SPIO makes the differentiation between metastases and hemangiomas easier

as follows: breathhold T1-weighted gradient echo sequence, respiratory gated moderately T2-weighted fast spin echo sequence, and breathhold T2*-weighted gradient echo sequence (all three before and after administration of SPIO particles).

Other T2* particulate contrast media have been developed. Resovist (SH U 555 A, Schering AG, Berlin, Germany) has the advantage of being injectable as a bolus, so that vascularization of liver tumors can be studied for improved characterization (Vogl 1996a,b, 1997; Kopp et al.1997).

The T1 effect of SPIO particles described above is very helpful for tissue characterization. However, it is often a drawback for lesion detection. In fact, vessels with moderate flow, for example venous structures in the liver, are also positively enhanced with SPIO particles even on T2-weighted sequences. Such vessels lying orthogonal to the imaging plane appear as bright dots, which can be very difficult to differentiate from small solid nodules. Therefore, manufacturers are designing new particles with a very strong T2* effect but without a T1 effect. Using such contrast media, the signal in the vessels disappears, due to the T2* effect, leaving only solid nodules as bright structures (Pochon et al. 1997).

Theoretically, it would appear useful to have a T1 particulate contrast media, in order to have a positive RES-specific contrast. The advantage would be to depend on T1- instead on T2-weighted images, which have a lower signal-to-noise ratio. This would be particularly helpful at low field strengths. Liposomes represent a possible approach to deliver a gadolinium chelate selectively either to the Kupffer cells or to the hepatocytes, depending on the vesicles size and their physical characteristics. The gadolinium chelate can be encapsulated in the aqueous core of the liposomes, or it can also be incorporated into the membranes of the liposomal vesicles

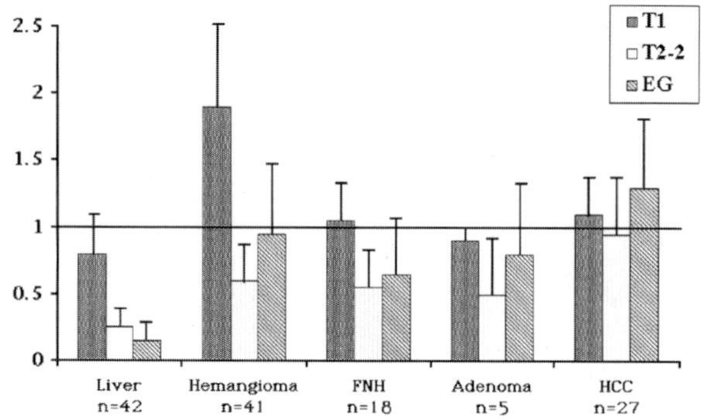

Fig. 29.6. Post-to-precontrast ratio of liver tumors after SPIO (*T1*, T1-weighted SE images, *T2-2*, T2-weighted SE images, second echo; *EG*, T2-weighted gradient echo images). A ratio of 1 indicates no change in the signal intensity after SPIO, a ratio superior of 1, positive enhancement of the tumor (*brightening*), a ratio inferior to 1, negative enhancement (*darkening*). Statistically significant ($P<0.05$) are the changes in liver on T2-2 and EG (*darkening*), in hemangioma on T1 (*brightening*) and T2-2 (*darkening*), in FNH on T2-2 (*darkening*), and in adenoma on T2-2 (*darkening*). According to these results, only hemangiomas show a positive enhancement on T1-weighted SE images after SPIO administration

(Kabalka et al. 1991). Micelles may be a more efficient alternative than liposomes for specifically delivering contrast media.

In addition to the aforementioned SPIO particles, there is a second class of superparamagnetic particles, called ultrasmall superparamagnetic iron oxides (USPIO). They differ from the former by their smaller size (about 20 nm), a longer blood half-life (about 2 h) and a lower r2/r1 relaxivity ratio: 53/24 for USPIO (AMI-227, Sinerem, Laboratoire Guerbet, France) versus 160/40 and 151/25 for SPIO (Ami-25/ Endorem, Laboratoire Guerbet, France, and SH U 555 A /Resovist, Schering AG, Germany, respectively); the units are in $(\text{mmol/l})^{-1}\ s^{-1}$ (Reimer and Tombach 1998). USPIO particles can be used as blood pool agents for MR angiography, due to their persistent T1 effect (Loubeyre et al. 1997). Compared to SPIO particles, they offer additional features for lesion characterization, because they give information on tumor vascularization (Saini et al. 1995; Harisinghani et al. 1997). They also can be made specific to hepatocytes by attaching galactose-terminated polysaccharides on their surface (see below).

29.4 Hepatocyte-Specific Contrast Media

29.4.1 Mn-DPDP

Manganese-DPDP (manganeseII-*N,N'*-dipyridoxyl-ethylene-diamine-*N,N'*-diacetate-5,5'-bisphosphate, manganese dipyridoxal diphosphate, Mangafodipir Trisodium, Nycomed, Wayne, USA) is an analog of vitamin B_6 (pyridoxal 5'-phosphate). It was initially thought to be extracted by the hepatocytes by means of the transport system for this vitamin (Bernardino et al. 1992). However, recent observations did not support this hypothesis (Colet et al. 1998). Because it is a weak chelate of the manganese ion, it dissociates in vivo to give free manganese, which is taken up by the hepatocytes and excreted into the bile. The dipyridoxyl 5'-phosphate ligand is excreted directly through the kidneys. The role of the ligand is to facilitate a slow release of the manganese. The paramagnetic property of manganese, which is a transition metal, derives from its five unpaired electrons (in comparison, gadolinium has seven unpaired electrons). Mn-DPDP is infused intravenously (over 15–20 min) at a dose of 5 µmol/kg bodyweight, and not injected as a bolus, so that patients are usually removed from the magnet between pre- and post-contrast imaging in order to allow contrast medium administration.

Following intravenous injection of Mn-DPDP, liver enhancement occurs as early as after 1 min. The peak of liver enhancement lies between 10 and 30 min after injection (about 100% increase in signal intensity) (Wang 1998). Mn-DPDP is slowly cleared by the liver into the bile with a 50% decrease in the maximal enhancement of the liver approximately 2 h after injection and concomitant increase in signal intensity of the bile (Lim et al. 1992). In patients with cirrhosis, liver enhancement is less intense and may be heterogeneous compared with that of non-cirrhotic livers (Murakami et al.1996).

As a liver-specific contrast medium, Mn-DPDP has been used to improve the conspicuity of focal liver lesions. Because non-hepatocellular tumors lack the ability to selectively take up Mn-DPDP, metastases appear as hypointense lesions within the strongly enhanced liver (Hamm et al. 1992; Aicher et al. 1993; Birnbaum et al. 1994) (Fig. 29.7). A European phase III clinical trial showed that Mn-DPDP-enhanced MRI was superior to unenhanced MRI and to contrast-enhanced CT for the detection of focal

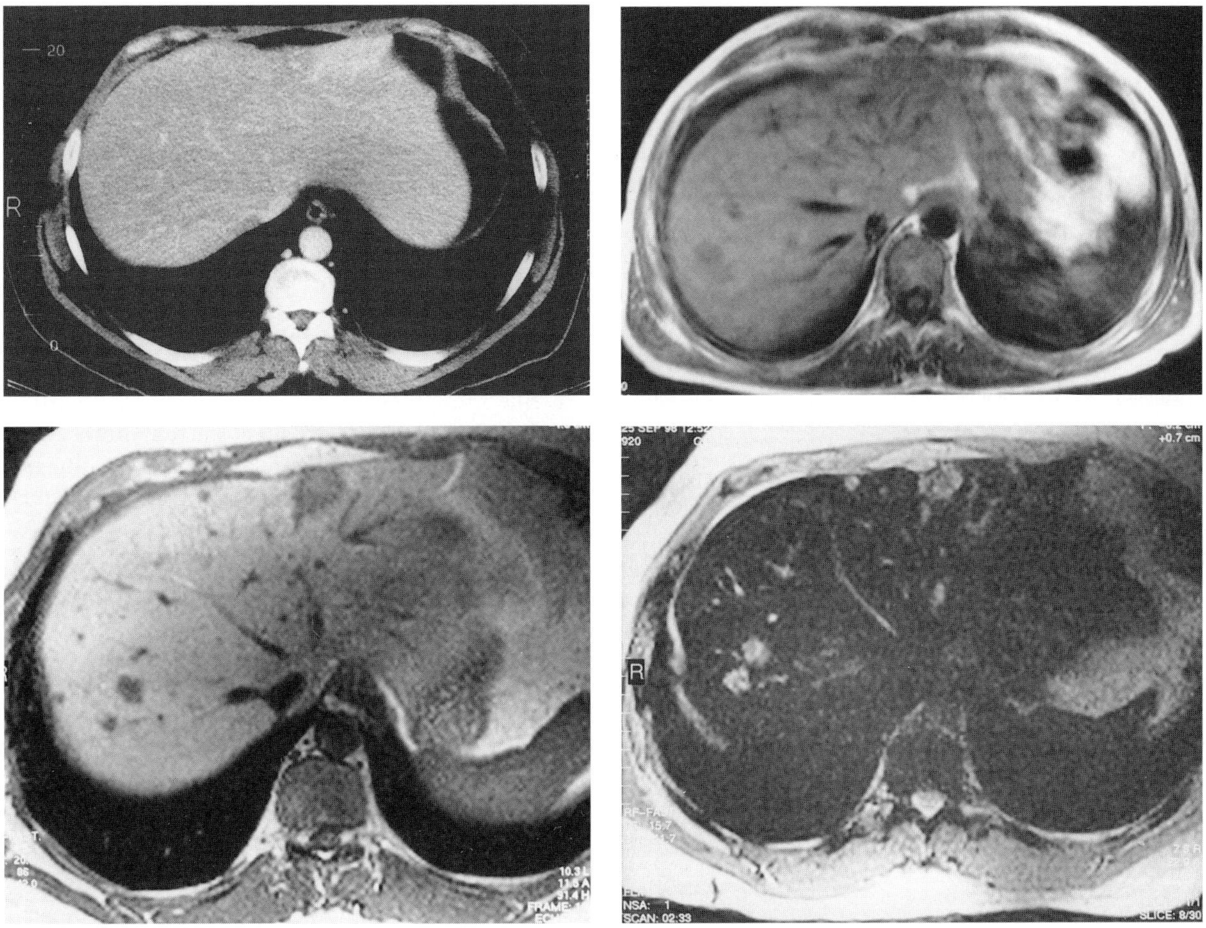

Fig. 29.7a–d. Liver metastases from a colon carcinoma. **a** Post-contrast CT. **b** Native T1-weighted GE image. **c** Post manganese-DPDP T1-weighted GE image. **d** Post SPIO T2-weighted fast SE image (**d** was performed 2 months after **c**). Multiple nodules, not seen on CT (**a**), are detected with MRI. The number of lesions seen on post-contrast images (**c,d**) is much higher than on pre-contrast images (**b**). The advantage of manganese-DPDP over SPIO is that it relies on the use of T1- instead of T2-weighted images and therefore the signal-to-noise ratio is much higher. With both contrast agents, the differentiation between small nodules and vessels lying orthogonal to the image plane is difficult

liver lesions (Rummeny et al. 1997; Wang et al. 1997; Torres et al. 1997)

In addition, in both animal and clinical studies, a rim of peripheral enhancement surrounding some malignant primary and secondary liver tumors has been observed (Rofsky and Earls 1996) (Fig. 29.8). Ni et al. (1993) have attributed this rim, on the basis of histology, to peritumoral malignant infiltration and compression of adjacent liver parenchyma, which impairs biliary drainage and elimination of Mn-DPDP. The presence of this rim, which is best seen on delayed images, is useful in distinguishing metastases from cysts and hemangiomas.

Unlike metastases, hepatocellular tumors maintain some ability to take up Mn-DPDP. Thus, hepatocyte-derived tumors such as well-differentiated hepatocellular carcinomas, regenerating nodules, adenomas and focal nodular hyperplasias show strong enhancement (Vogl et al. 1993; Liou et al. 1994; Rofsky and Earls 1996; Rofsky et al. 1993) (Fig. 29.9). Because these tumors do not contain functioning bile ducts, the Mn-DPDP cannot be excreted. Therefore, the enhancement lasts longer than that of normal liver parenchyma and these tumors become brighter on delayed images.

The positive enhancement of well-differentiated hepatocellular carcinomas persists for more than 48 h, with the highest conspicuity appearing 24 h after the injection. In some tumors, a thin pseudocapsule of low signal intensity can be identified on enhanced images.

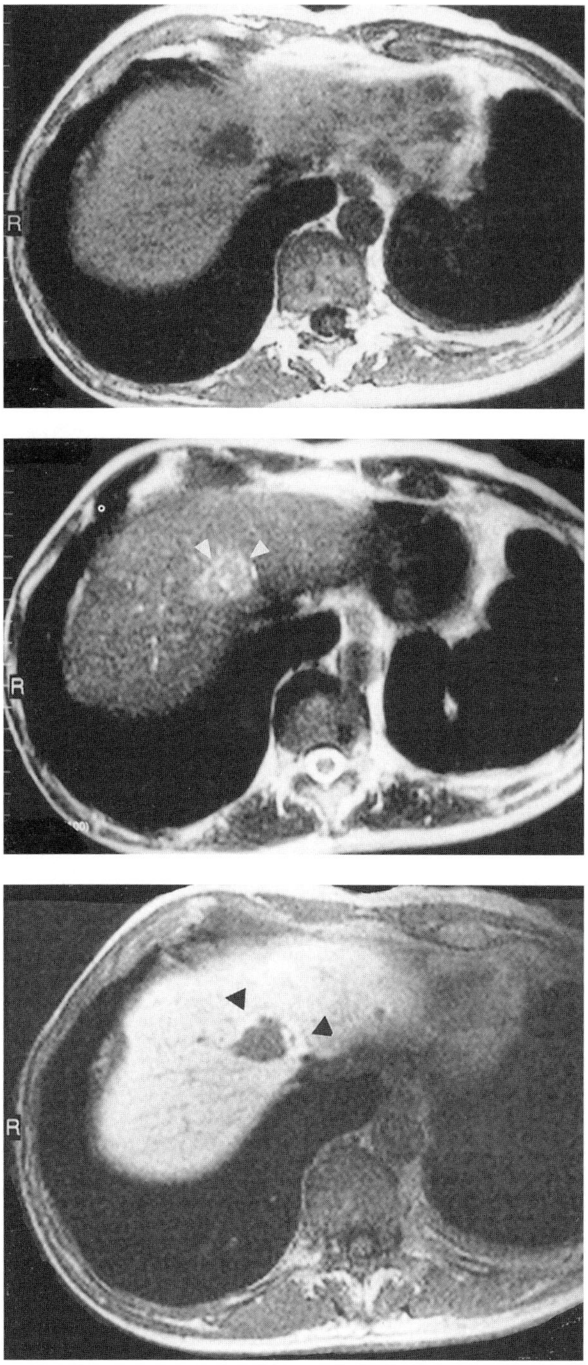

a b c

Fig. 29.8a–c. Liver metastases from a colon carcinoma. **a** Native T1-weighted GE image. **b** Native T2-weighted fast SE image. **c** Post manganese-DPDP T1-weighted GE image. A strongly enhancing rim around the tumor is seen after manganese-DPDP administration (**c**). It corresponds to a faint hyperintense halo on the native T2-weighted image (**b**). Edema and bile retention in compressed peritumoral liver parenchyma explain this aspect

In addition to well-differentiated hepatocellular carcinomas, regenerating nodules, adenomas and focal nodular hyperplasias also show enhancement with Mn-DPDP. In focal nodular hyperplasia, the central scar is well visualized as a hypointense stellate structure on Mn-DPDP enhanced images (Fig. 29.10). Enhancement of benign tumors with Mn-DPDP may simulate the appearance of an hepatocellular carcinoma, therefore complicating image interpretation.

Undifferentiated hepatocellular carcinomas are characterized by a lack of enhancement and therefore, like metastases, a maximal conspicuity within 30 min. This observation suggests that both early (within the first hour) and delayed (at 24 h) images are important to improve detection and characterization of liver tumors.

Although, as discussed above, Mn-DPDP could be of help for the characterization of primary liver tumors, more data are needed before definite conclusions can be drawn. Furthermore, one potential drawback is that hemangiomas and metastases have a similar appearance on enhanced T1-weighted images (hypointense compared to the enhanced liver) (Fig. 29.11). Because Mn-DPDP is injected as an infusion, it cannot be used to study a dynamic effect, such as with the gadolinum chelates. Fortunately, the contrast medium has no influence on T2-weighted images. Thus, tissue characterization is possible using the same criteria as on native T2-weighted images (high, water-like signal intensity of hemangiomas), but, of course, with the same limitations.

A major advantage of Mn-DPDP versus SPIO particles is that lesion detection is based on T1-weighted images rather than on T2-weighted images with poor signal-to-noise ratio. Furthermore, unlike unspecific gadolinium chelates and like the other hepato-specific contrast media, fast imaging is not required, because the imaging window is not just the early phase after contrast medium injection (there is no equilibrium phase as with conventional gadolinium chelates!). Therefore, Mn-DPDP has a potential application with low field MR equipment for liver imaging.

29.4.2 Gd-BOPTA

Gd-BOPTA/dimeg (MultiHance, Bracco Milan, Italy) has the official generic name gadobenate dimeglumine (INN), and its complete chemical name is 1-deoxy-1-(methylamino)-D-glucitol di-

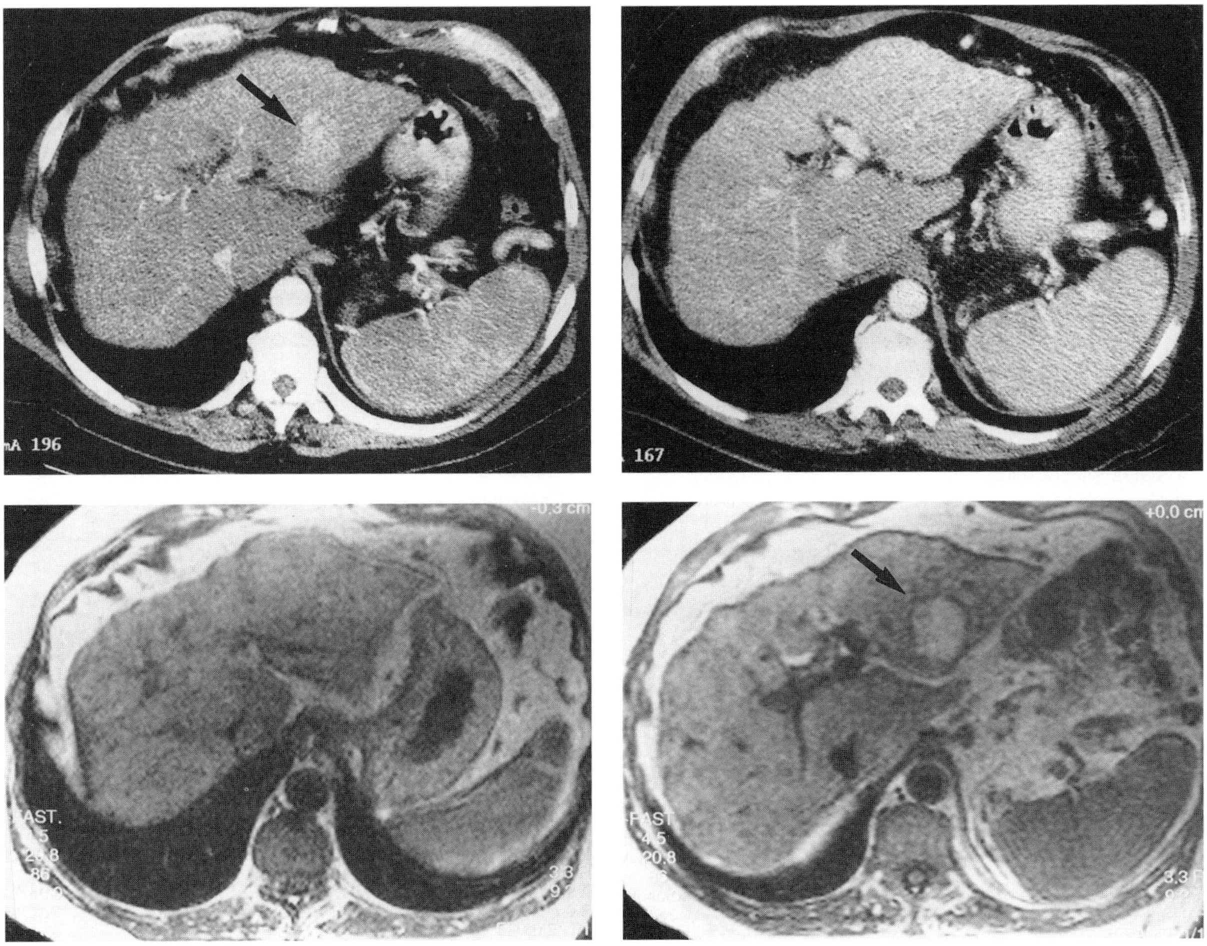

a b c d

Fig. 29.9a–d. Hepatocellular carcinoma. **a** Arterial phase spiral CT. **b** Portal venous phase spiral CT. **c** Native T1-weighted GE image. **d** Post manganese-DPDP T1-weighted GE image. A 3-cm large, enhancing tumor (*arrow*) is seen on the arterial phase spiral CT (**a**) in a patient with liver cirrhosis. Because of rapid wash-out of the contrast agent, it is no longer visible on the portal venous phase (**b**). On MRI, only the post-contrast image (**d**) allows visualization of the tumor (*arrow*). It is characterized by strong uptake of manganese-DPDP as well as the presence of a hypointense capsule

hydrogen [4-carboxy-5,8,11-tris(carboxymethyl)-1-phenyl-2-oxa-5,8,11-triazatridecan-13-oato(5-)] gadolinate (2-) (2:1). Like Gd-EOB-DTPA (see below), it consists essentially of a hydrophilic Gd-DTPA moiety covalently coupled to a lipophilic benzene ring. This complex is amphiphilic and undergoes both hepatobiliary and renal excretion. Its hepatic uptake is thought to occur through the organic anion transport system (the bromosulfophthalein/bilirubin transport system) situated on the membrane of the hepatocytes (De Haen et al. 1995, 1996).

It is injected intravenously as a bolus at a dose of 0.05 or 0.1 mmol/kg body weight. The percentage amount of the administered dose undergoing hepatocyte uptake and subsequent biliary excretion varies among species. Thus, in rats, it is about 50%; in humans, only approximately 2–4% (De Haen and Gozzini 1993). The remainder of the administered dose of Gd-BOPTA undergoes renal filtration and urinary excretion. In spite of the small proportion of Gd-BOPTA that accumulates in hepatocytes, enhancement of liver parenchyma is strong and sustained. As early as 10 min after injection, an increase in liver signal intensity of more than 100% is observed after the injection of 0.1 mmol/kg Gd-BOPTA and persists for more than 2 h (Vogl et al. 1992; Giovagnoni and Paci 1996).

The high relaxivity of Gd-BOPTA within liver tissue is explained by high macromolecular binding of the contrast medium with hepatocyte proteins and membranes (Caudana et al. 1996).

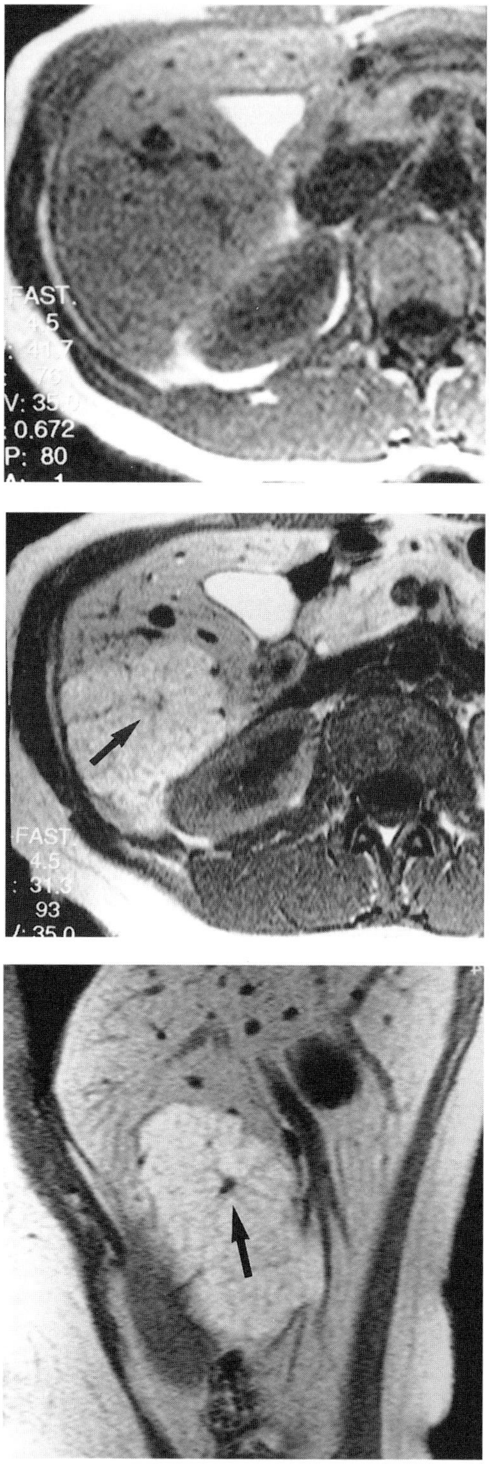

a

b

c

Fig. 29.10a–c. Focal nodular hyperplasia. **a** Native T1-weighted GE image. **b,c** Axial and sagittal post manganese-DPDP T1-weighted GE images. Strongly enhancing tumor after manganese-DPDP administration, showing a characteristic wheel-pattern and a central scar (*arrow*). A definite diagnosis of FNH is possible, based on the internal morphology of the tumor. These features are not seen on the pre-contrast image

Gd-BOPTA serves both as a non-specific extracellular contrast medium on early post-contrast images and as an hepato-specific intracellular contrast medium on delayed images. This dual function facilitates lesion detection and characterization.

In general terms, after administration of a contrast medium, the difference in signal intensity (the image contrast) between a lesion and the surrounding parenchyma is determined by differences in (a) concentration in contrast medium between the lesion and the surrounding liver parenchyma, (b) differences in relaxivity of the contrast medium in the lesion and in the surrounding liver parenchyma, and (c) differences in the intrinsic magnetic properties of the lesion and the surrounding liver parenchyma.

The observed T1 ($T1_{obs}$) of the tissue after administration of a gadolinium chelate can be predicted from the intrinsic T1 of the tissue ($T1_{intr}$) and the concentration dependent T1 of the contrast agent ($T1_c$) as follows:

$$1/T1_{obs} = 1/T1_{intr} + 1/T1_c$$

A similar equation is also valid for the T2 relaxation time.

Among the three aforementioned factors determining the difference in signal intensity between a lesion and the surrounding parenchyma after contrast medium administration, the difference in concentration in the lesion and in the surrounding parenchyma is the most important. Therefore, let us consider it in more detail. As long as the greatest amount of the contrast medium is still in the intravascular space (capillary phase, within 20–30 s from the injection of contrast medium, followed by portal venous phase, approximately 1 min after the injection of contrast medium), lesion and liver enhancement is dominated by the relative size of this space (corresponding to the degree of vascularization). A hypervascular tumor shows a stronger enhancement than a hypovascular one. However, with progressive distribution of the contrast medium into the interstitial space, other parameters become predominant, namely the permeability of the vessels and the relative size of the interstitial space. Thus, viable malignant tumorous tissue usually enhances strongly because of high vascular permeability and large interstitial space. Finally, in the equilibrium phase (i.e., when the contrast medium concentration in the intravascular and the interstitial space of the liver is the same, namely 3 min or more after the injection of contrast medium), the contrast medium concentration in the interstitial space of the tumor is often

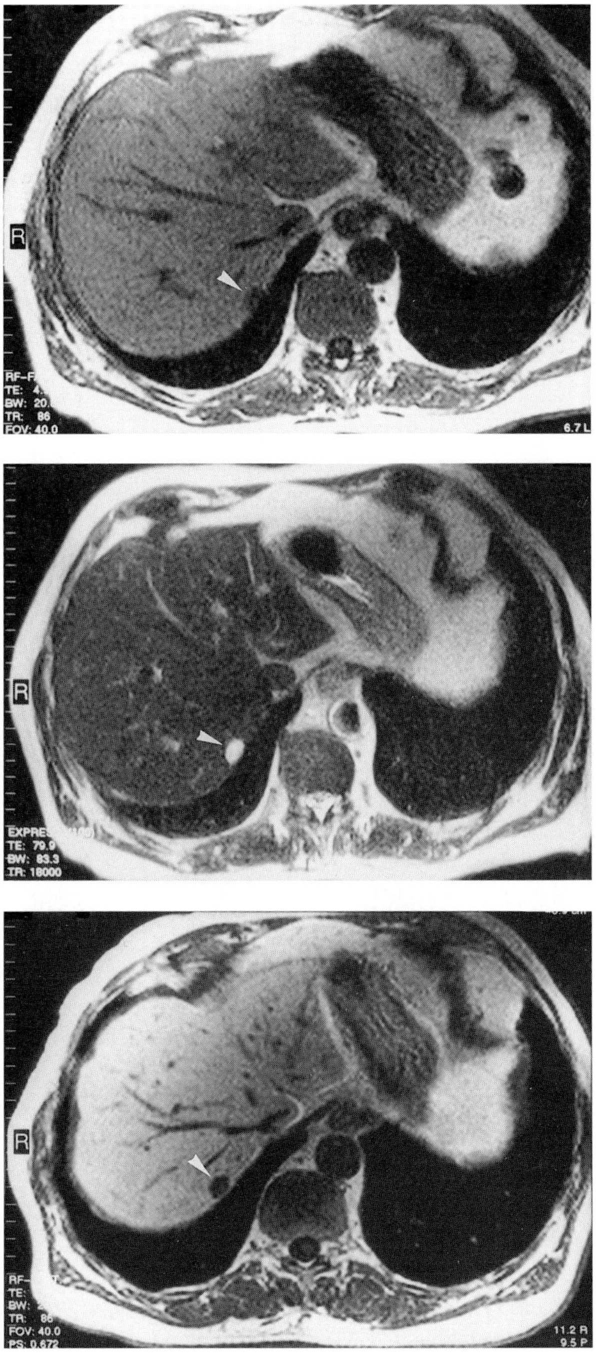

a b c

Fig. 29.11a–c. Hemangioma. **a** Native T1-weighted GE image. **b** Native T2-weighted GE image. **c** Post manganese-DPDP T1-weighted GE image. A 1-cm lesion appears hypointense on **a** and hyperintense on **b**. After administration of manganese-DPDP (**c**), the conspicuity of the lesion is increased because of enhancement of the surrounding liver parenchyma. However, the behavior after manganese-DPDP does not allow characterization of the lesion. Compare to Fig. 29.7

very similar to that of the interstitial space of the liver. Therefore, in this phase, the tumor is easily missed (no difference in image contrast between the tumor and the surrounding liver parenchyma). However, some tumors with a prominent interstitial space, including cholangiocarcinomas, will accumulate more contrast medium than the liver, explaining their increased conspicuity on delayed images. Furthermore, it has been observed that in some malignant tumors, due to increased diffusion of interstitial fluid from the tumor towards the surrounding liver parenchyma, there is a wash-out of the contrast medium at the periphery of the tumor on delayed images. This phenomenon produces a characteristic halo around the tumor, which is highly specific of malignancy (Mahfouz et al. 1994) (Fig. 29.12).

Thanks to the specific uptake of Gd-BOPTA in hepatocytes, there is no equilibrium phase as is the case with non-specific contrast media. With the subsequent wash-out of the contrast medium from the tumor interstitial space, maximal tumor conspicuity is obtained 60–120 min after injection. Thus, on early dynamic images, Gd-BOPTA provides information about patterns of enhancement related to tumor vascularization and thus gives important clues for tumor characterization (Fig. 29.13). Late images allow optimal lesion detection (Fig. 29.14).

In experimental and preliminary clinical studies, the usefulness of Gd-BOPTA for the detection of liver metastases and hepatocellular carcinomas has been demonstrated (Runge et al. 1997; Caudana et al. 1996; Murakami et al. 1996). In phase II and III studies, adverse reactions/events have been observed in 10–15%. In the vast majority, they have been transient, self-limiting and mild in intensity and consisted mostly of hypertension (1.37%), nausea (1.09%) and tachycardia (0.96%) (Hamm 1998).

29.4.3 Gd-EOB-DTPA

Gd-EOB-DTPA [gadolinium(III)-3,6,9-triaza-3,6,9-tris (carboxylmethyl)-4-(4-ethoxybenzyl)-undecandicarboxylic acid, gadolinium-ethoxybenzyl-diethylenetriamine pentacetic acid, Eovist, Schering AG, Berlin, Germany] is characterized by a high affinity for the hepatocytes and an important biliary excretion. It is obtained by covalently linking the ethoxybenzyl moiety to gadolinium-DTPA. The lipophilic EOB moiety facilitates selective hepatocyte uptake and subsequent biliary excretion.

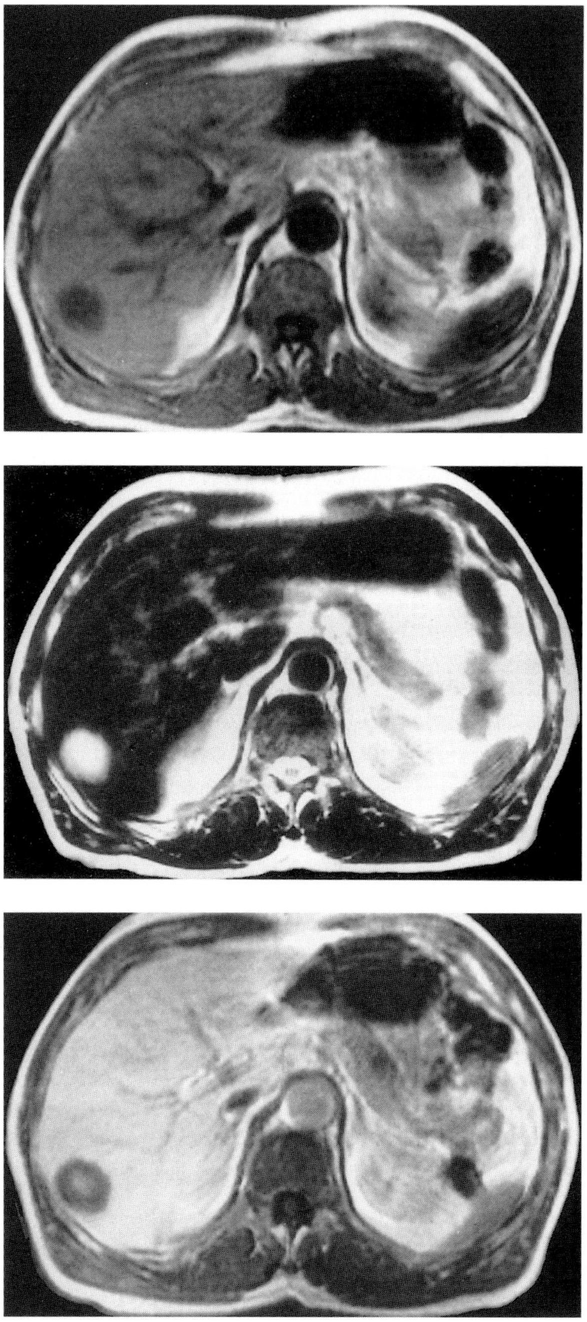

a b c

Fig. 29.12a–c. Liver metastasis from a colon carcinoma. **a** Native T1-weighted SE image. **b** Native T2-weighted SE image. **c** Post gadolinium-BOPTA T1-weighted SE image (delayed image). On **c**, one observes accumulation of the contrast in the center of the nodule, while there is washed-out at the periphery (*halo sign*). This phenomenon is highly specific of a malignant liver tumor, mainly metastasis. The high intensity of the tumor on the native T2-weighted image (**b**) would have made characterization of the tumor difficult if only native images had been acquired (differential diagnosis with a hemangioma!). (Courtesy of Bracco, Milan, Italy)

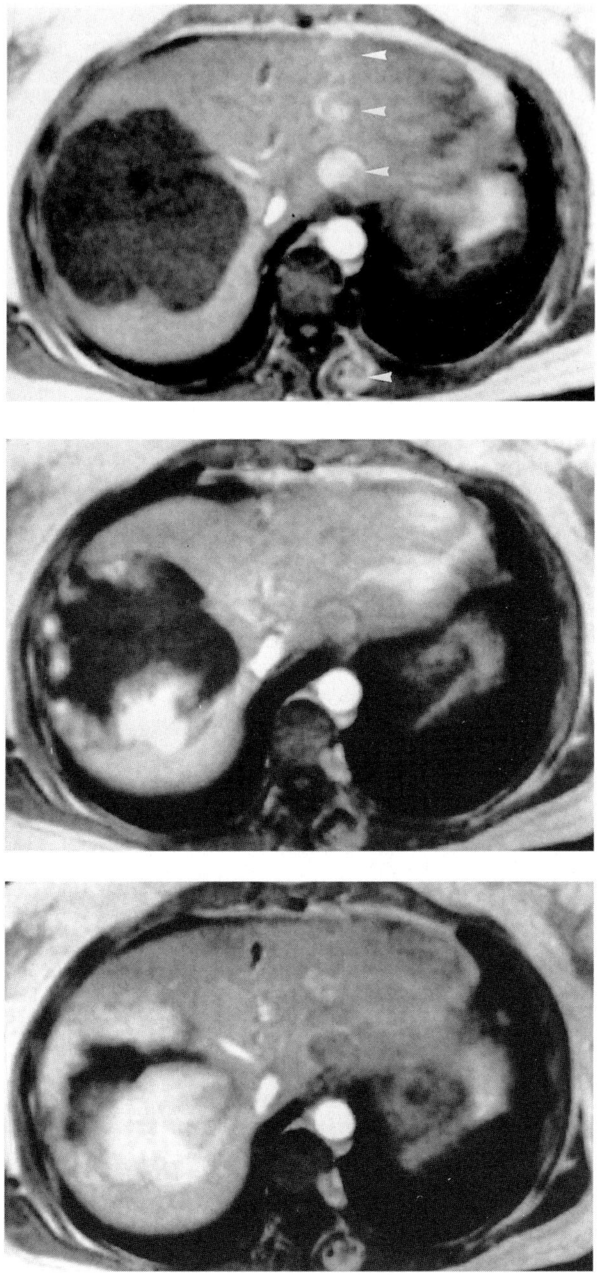

a b c

Fig. 29.13a–c. Hemangioma. **a** Native T1-weighted GE image. **b,c** Post gadolinium-BOPTA T1-weighted GE image at 4 and 9 min, respectively. Typical nodular enhancement of the hemangioma with progressive filling, allowing a definite diagnosis. (Courtesy of Bracco, Milan, Italy)

Hepatocyte uptake of Gd-EOB-DTPA occurs via the same active organic anion transport mechanism as bilirubin, whereas biliary excretion is via a different active transport mechanism (Hamm et al. 1995; Reimer et al. 1996; Schuhman-Gampieri et al. 1992). Compared with unmodified Gd-DTPA, Gd-

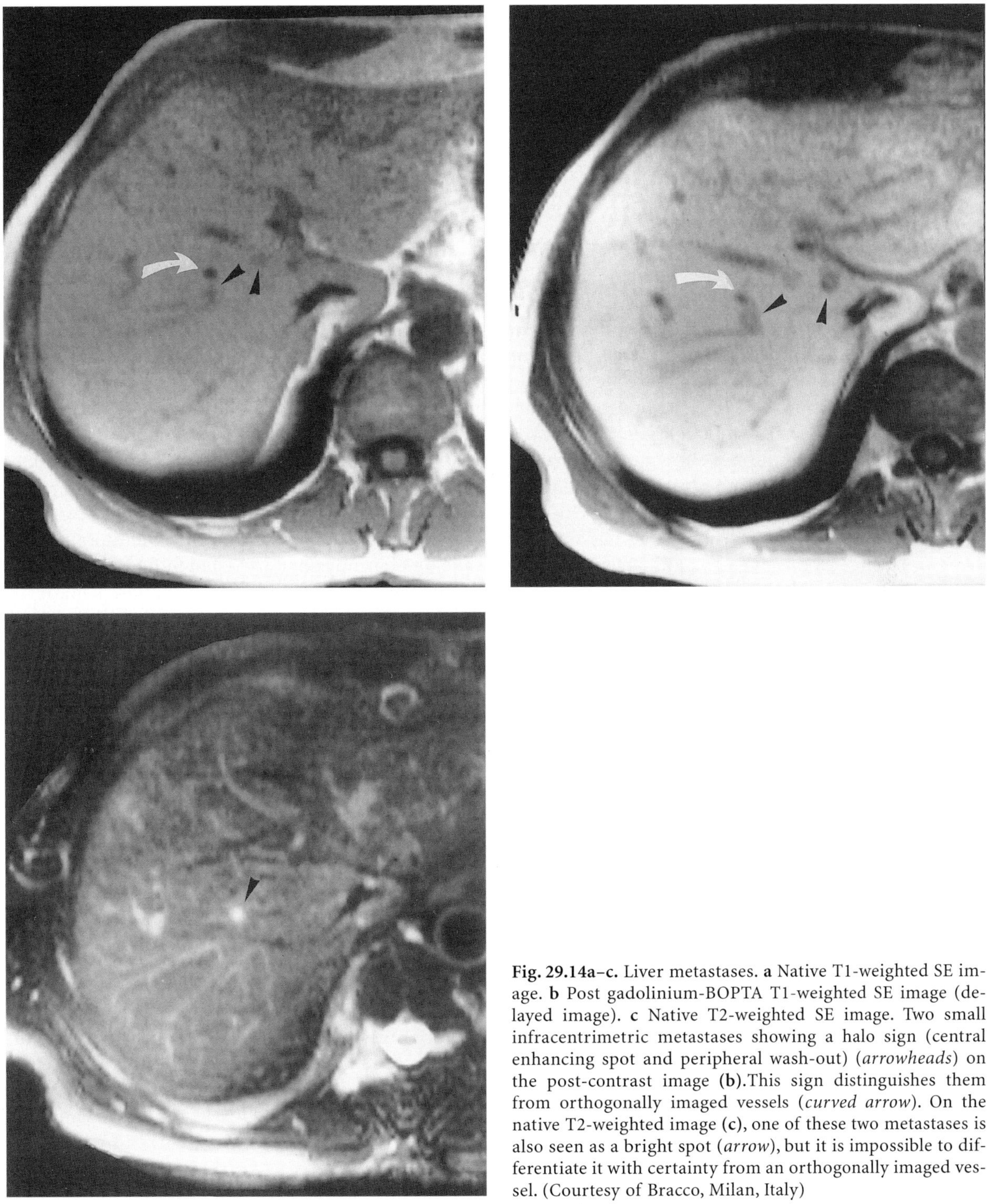

a b c

Fig. 29.14a–c. Liver metastases. **a** Native T1-weighted SE image. **b** Post gadolinium-BOPTA T1-weighted SE image (delayed image). **c** Native T2-weighted SE image. Two small infracentrimetric metastases showing a halo sign (central enhancing spot and peripheral wash-out) (*arrowheads*) on the post-contrast image (**b**).This sign distinguishes them from orthogonally imaged vessels (*curved arrow*). On the native T2-weighted image (**c**), one of these two metastases is also seen as a bright spot (*arrow*), but it is impossible to differentiate it with certainty from an orthogonally imaged vessel. (Courtesy of Bracco, Milan, Italy)

EOB-DTPA produces a fivefold increase in liver tissue relaxivity.

Approximately 50% of the administered dose is excreted in the bile, which is much higher than the biliary excretion of Gd-BOPTA (HAMM et al. 1995). The remainder undergoes renal glomerular filtration and excretion. Biphasic enhancement of normal liver parenchyma occurs after Gd-EOB-DTPA administration. During the initial phase, there is immediate and marked liver enhancement over the first minute, as the contrast medium distributes into the extracellular interstitial space, similar to that observed after Gd-DTPA. During the following hepatobiliary phase, the Gd-EOB-DTPA is taken up by hepatocytes and excreted into the bile. This produces a slower increase in liver enhancement during the next 20 min to reach a plateau of liver signal intensity, which lasts for about 2 h (Hamm et al. 1995; Giovagnoni and Paci 1996).

The appearance of liver lesions depends upon the timing of the image acquisition. Early dynamic imaging during the perfusion phase shows enhancement of lesions in accordance with their degree of vascularity, later with the permeability of their vessels and the size of their interstitial space (Vogl et al. 1996c). Images obtained following the perfusion phase during the hepatobiliary phase depict most liver lesions as hypointense foci within the enhancing liver parenchyma (Reimer et al. 1997).

Hepatocellular carcinomas show initial enhancement with Gd-EOB-DTPA on arterial phase images, independent of histologic tumor grade. On later hepatobiliary phase images, almost all hepatocellular carcinomas show negative enhancement with Gd-EOB-DTPA, unlike with Mn-DPDP (Vogl et al. 1996c). The only exception are highly differentiated hepatocellular carcinomas, which show prolonged positive enhancement. This finding implies that uptake of Gd-EOB-DTPA relies on a higher level of hepatocyte function than Mn-DPDP.

Gd-EOB-DTPA accumulates in focal nodular hyperplasias and adenomas due to the presence of functioning hepatocytes. Prolonged retention of contrast medium is observed on very delayed images, because of dysplasia of the bile duct within these tumors, retarding elimination of the contrast medium (Vogl et al. 1996c).

29.4.4 Asialoglycoprotein-SPIO

Some iron oxide preparations can be delivered to asialoglycoprotein (ASG) receptors on hepatocytes. ASG receptors are physiologically abundant on hepatocytes (400,000–500,000 receptors per cell) and are normally responsible for the clearance of desialylated glycoproteins by the liver (Reimer et al. 1991). ASG receptor specificity of pharmaceuticals can be achieved by attaching them to galactose-terminated polysaccharides, such as arabinogalactan, a branching galactose containing polysaccharide obtained from larch wood. Thus, these compounds bind to hepatocyte cell surface membranes and are then internalized into hepatocytes within lysosomes.

For hepatocyte specific imaging, ultrasmall superparamagnetic iron oxide particles are used as the magnetically active core. Thanks to their small size (around 10 nm in diameter), nonspecific uptake of the particles by the Kupffer cells do not compete with specific accumulation into hepatocytes. Phagocytosis by Kupffer cells is namely size-related, small particles being removed from the blood only very slowly.

Although arabinogalactan-coated ultrasmall superparamagnetic particles are specific for hepatocytes, their underlying mechanism is thus completely different from that of Gd-BOPTA and Gd-EOB-DTPA. They act as T2*-contrast medium, which means that they reduce the signal intensity of normal liver parenchyma, unlike the gadolinium-based hepatospecific contrast media, which increase it (Small et al. 1994). Besides, they are not eliminated into the bile. Malignant primary hepatic tumors lose the expression of the ASG cell surface receptor during malignant degeneration and, therefore, do not take up arabinogalactan-coated SPIO particles.

On the other hand, benign primary hepatic tumors, such as focal nodular hyperplasia and adenoma, express the ASG receptor, which potentially would allow differentiation between benign and malignant tumors.

29.5 Tumor-Specific Contrast Media

Tumor-specific contrast media have been tested in animal studies. Metalloporphyrins have shown moderate accumulation in tumors on delayed images (24–48 h after injection). Today, it seems that this behavior does not rely on a tumor-specific mechanism, but rather on the presence of necrosis (Ni et al. 1997). From CT, it is known that Lipiodol shows a rather specific accumulation in hepatocytic tumors. Up to now, an equivalent of Lipiodol for MRI has not been used, but this would be theoretically feasible.

29.6 Which Contrast Media and Which Imaging Strategy?

The field of tissue-specific contrast media for MRI is currently evolving extremely rapidly. Therefore, it is not surprising that there is as yet no consensus on the best strategy in liver MRI. Several approaches have been put forward, where many factors play a role in the choice a particular imaging center makes, one of them being the privileged contacts it can have with a given contrast medium company! For several years, there has been no doubt that contrast media are mandatory for liver MRI. However, the following questions remain unanswered: what type of contrast media should be used: non-specific or hepato-specific? If hepato-specific contrast media are confirmed as superior to non-specific ones, should RES specific or hepatocyte-specific contrast media be selected? Should the choice of a contrast medium be limited to a single one whatever the indication, or is a tailored approach preferable, depending on the particular indication?

The imaging protocol for a given contrast medium is also a matter of debate. Which is the best timing of imaging after contrast medium administration? These are only some of many unresolved questions.

We can summarize our personal experience, mostly with SPIO particles and Mn DPDP, as follows: we are strongly in favor of using hepato-specific contrast media for liver MRI. Indeed, non-specific contrast media yield the same kind of information as iodinated contrast media. Taking into consideration the advantages and drawbacks of MRI versus state-of-the-art CT, the latter is, at the present time, the preferred modality. Furthermore, because the timing of the imaging sequence after contrast medium administration is so crucial, it is quite demanding to obtain an examination of adequate quality using non-specific contrast media. Doubtless, fast imaging allowing images to be obtained in the arterial phase after administration of non-specific contrast media is very sensitive for hypervascular lesions (such as double-spiral CT with arterial phase). However, hypervascularity is not pathognomonic for a specific entity. This is also true in liver cirrhosis, in which daily practice shows that regenerating nodules can also be hypervascular and thus very similar, in this respect, to small foci of hepatocellular carcinoma. This observation contradicts the commonly expressed view that hypervascularity is a specific sign of malignancy in the setting of liver cirrhosis (Matsui et al. 1991).

Compared to RES-specific contrast media (SPIO particles), hepatocyte-specific (Mn-DPDP) contrast media offer several advantages for lesion detection. The most important is the fact that the imaging sequence relies on T1-weighted images, which have a better signal-to-noise ratio than T2-weighted images. This point favors the use of Mn-DPDP (or other hepatocyte-specific contrast media) for imaging at low field. Besides, Mn-DPDP is very well tolerated, and we have not observed, up to now, any severe adverse reactions. This is confirmed in the literature. To some extent, tumor characterization is also feasible with Mn-DPDP, since uptake by the tumor indicates that the latter originates from hepatocytes. However, differentiation between a well-differentiated hepatocellular carcinoma and a benign tumor is not possible, on the basis of contrast medium uptake only.

On the contrary, in our experience, SPIO particles have been very attractive for tissue characterization. It is our preferred contrast medium to confirm or exclude the diagnosis of hemangioma, when other imaging modalities have not been conclusive (Figs. 29.15, 29.16). For the differential diagnosis between focal nodular hyperplasia, adenoma and hepatocellular carcinoma, SPIO particles give relevant information in the majority of cases, allowing a definite diagnosis (Fig. 29.17). They also allow the better distinction between tumor nodule and surrounding edema, thus yielding more precise information on tumor size and extent than native images (Fig. 29.18).

29.7 Specific Liver Contrast Media for Studying Liver Function

The predominant functions of the liver are the clearance of endo- and xenobiotics, their metabolism and excretion, and the synthesis of biologically important compounds such as clotting factors and albumin. In many diffuse liver diseases, several aspects of liver function are decreased. Measurements of liver function are therefore useful for diagnosis and especially for grading the severity of diffuse liver diseases.

Diffuse liver diseases, including the end-stage of many of them, i.e., liver cirrhosis, are a major health problem. For example, in many European countries, the prevalence of alcoholic liver cirrhosis has been estimated at approximately 3000 per 10^6 population. The mortality rate due to cirrhosis in European countries is between 100 and 400 per 10^6 per year in men and between 40 and 150 per 10^6 per year in women (Rueff 1989).

Hepatic failure is ultimately the major cause of death in patients with severe diffuse liver disease.

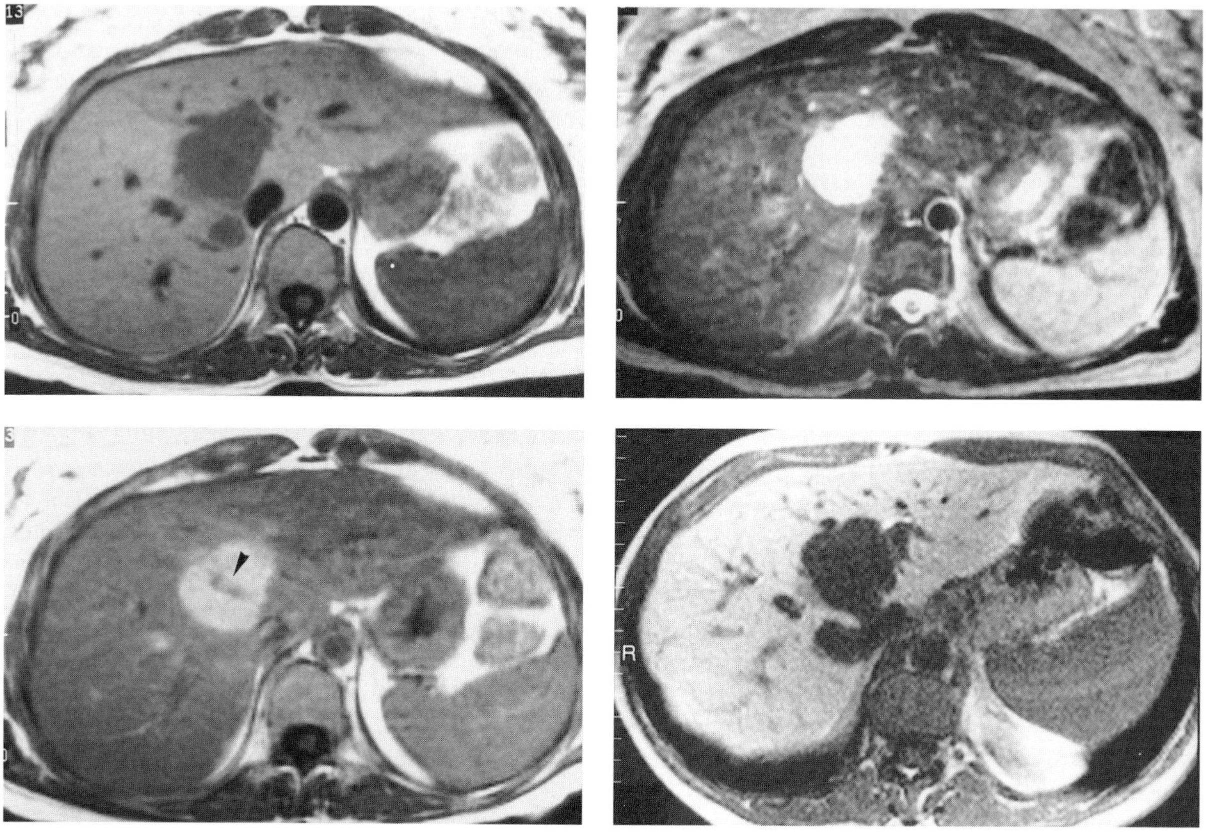

a b c d

Fig. 29.15a–d. Hemangioma. **a** Native T1-weighted SE image. **b** Native T2-weighted SE image. **c** Post SPIO T1-weighted SE image. **d** Post manganese-DPDP T1-weighted GE image. Typical strong positive enhancement of the hemangioma on the T1-weighted image after administration of SPIO (**c**). Note the central hypointense structure, corresponding probably to an area of thrombosis or fibrosis. Manganese-DPDP (**d**) increases the contrast between the hemangioma and the liver parenchyma, but does not give conclusive information for lesion characterization

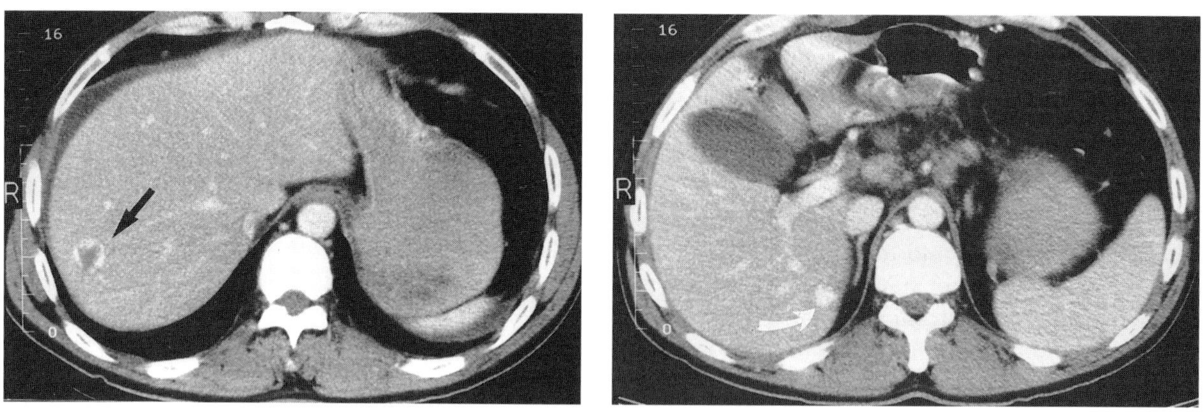

a b

Fig. 29.16a,b

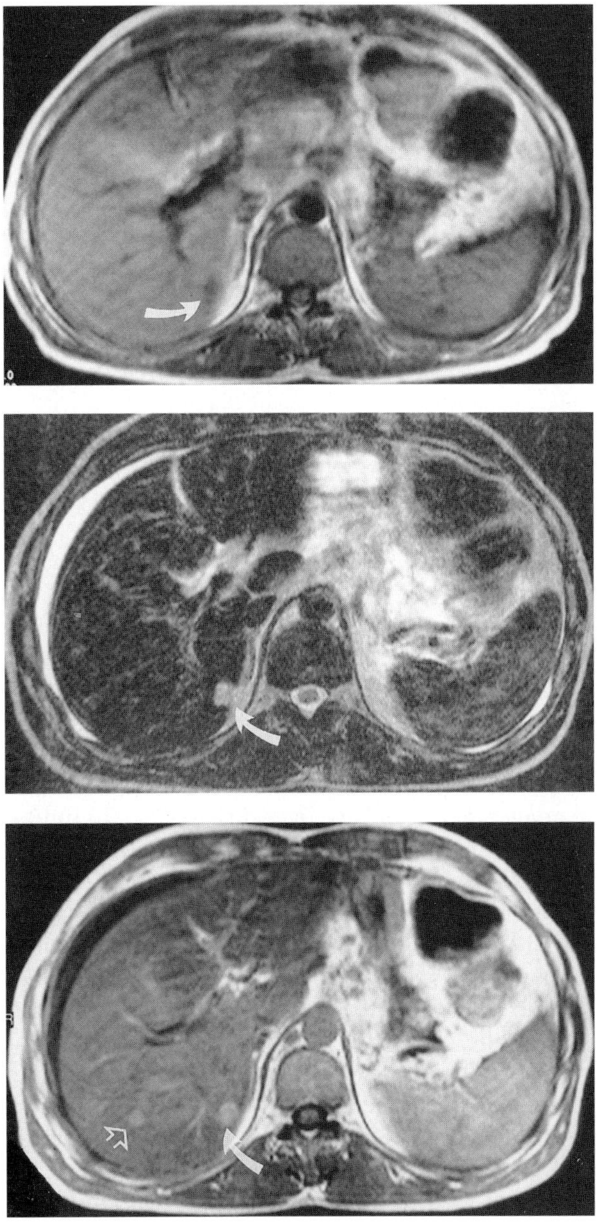

Fig. 29.16a–e. Hemangioma versus metastasis. **a,b** Post contrast spiral CT. **c** Native T1-weighted SE image. **d** Native T2-weighted fast SE image. **e** Post SPIO T1-weighted SE image. In this 46 year old patient with known pancreas carcinoma, spiral CT reveals a characteristic hemangioma in segment VII with nodular enhancement (*arrow in* **a**). A second lesion (*curved arrow in* **b**) shows homogeneous enhancement, so that conclusive diagnosis is not possible (hemangioma or hypervascular metastasis?). On the native T2-weighted image (**d**), the nodule is hyperintense, but less than the cerebrospinal liquid in the vertebral canal, so that a conclusive diagnosis of hemangioma is not possible. After administration of SPIO (**e**), the nodule shows a positive enhancement, allowing the definite diagnosis of hemangioma. Another hemangioma (*open arrow*), not seen on the native image, is seen on the post-SPIO image

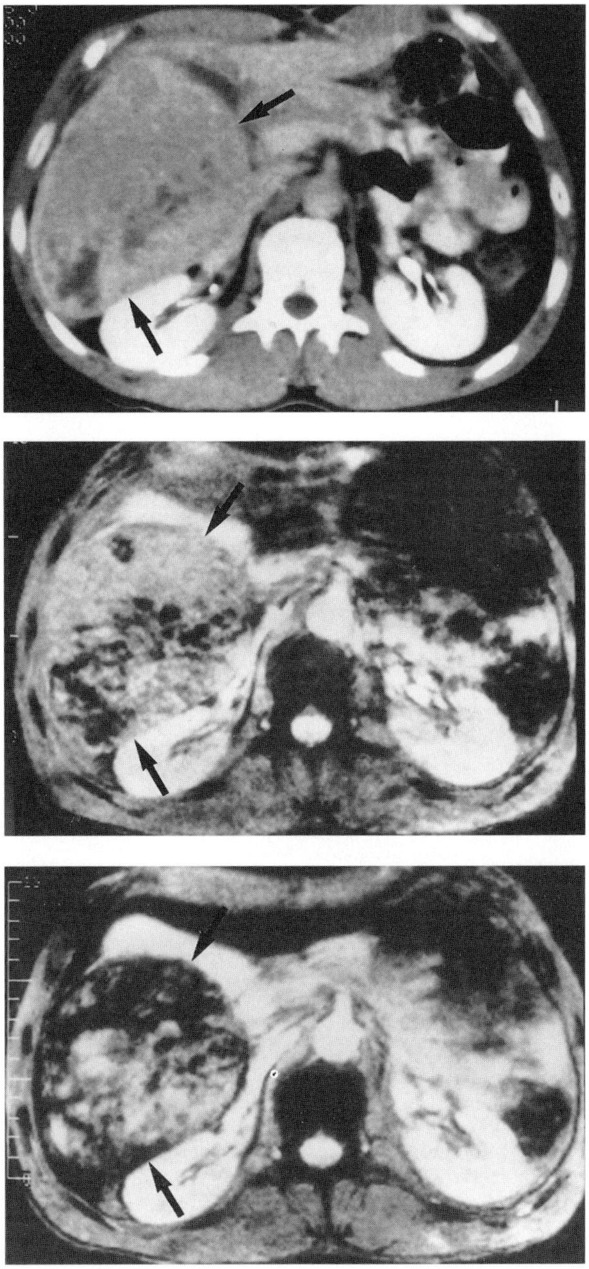

Fig. 29.17a–c. Hyperplastic adenoma with foci of hepatocellular carcinoma. **a** Postcontrast CT. **b** Native T2-weighted fast SE image. **c** Post SPIO T2-weighted fast SE image. In this patient 60 year old with liver cirrhosis, CT (**a**) demonstrates a large heterogeneous tumor hanging from the inferior surface of segment VI. Percutaneous biopsy could not reveal malignant cells and a diagnosis of adenoma was made. On the T2-weighted image (**b**), there are multiple hypointense foci in the tumor, due to old hemorrhages (hemosiderin). After SPIO administration (**c**), the tumor shows heterogeneous uptake, with darkening mostly in its periphery. However, several areas do not present change in signal intensity. The diagnosis of hepatocellular carcinoma was made and the tumor surgically removed. At histology, foci of HCC in a hyperplastic adenoma were demonstrated

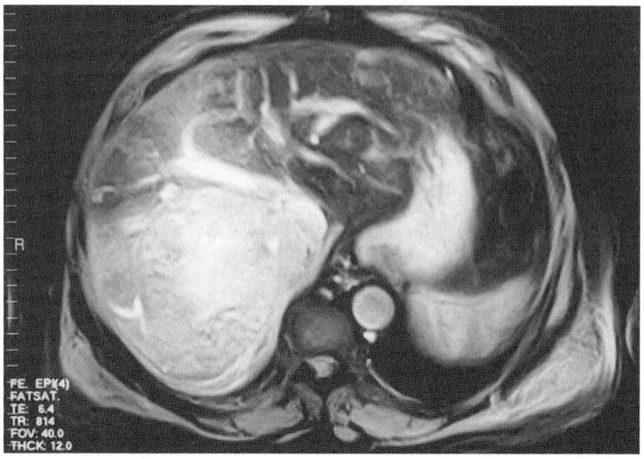

a

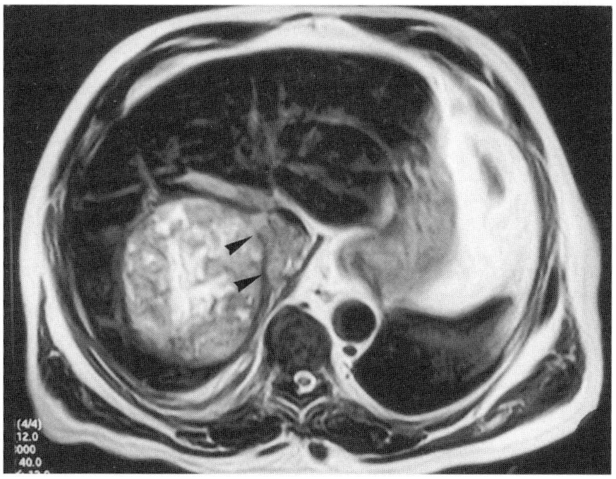

b

Fig. 29.18a,b. Hepatocellular carcinoma. **a** Native T2-weighted multisegmented SE EPI. **b** Post SPIO T2-weighted multisegmented EPI SE images. On the native image (**a**), a large hyperintense tumor is seen in segments VII and VIII. After SPIO administration (**b**), the exact size of the tumor is much better appreciated as well as its internal nodular structure and its infiltration into the inferior vena cava (*arrowheads*). The hyperintensity around the tumor on the native image is due to severe peritumoral edema, reflecting the aggressive nature of the tumor

Therefore, quantification of liver function should improve our understanding of the natural history of diffuse liver diseases and give more precise indices of prognosis and well as the effect of therapeutic interventions (Lauterbur and Preisig 1991).

In addition to laboratory tests (e.g., galactose elimination capacity and lidocaine test), imaging appears as another tool for assessing liver function. Hepatobiliary scintigraphy has been considered for many years as appropriate for studying liver function (Brown et al. 1988; Krishnamurthy and Turner 1990; Doo et al. 1991). However, it is used mainly to assess patency of the biliary tract and, to a lesser extent, for the diagnosis and grading of hepatocellular dysfunction in diffuse liver diseases. Its limitation is related to suboptimal spatial resolution and the lack of data regarding accuracy and reproducibility of functional parameters. Therefore, hepatobiliary scintigraphy is currently used only marginally for evaluating hepatocellular dysfunction. However, the advent of hepato-specific contrast media gives MRI the potential to play a major role in this regard.

MRI offers several advantages over hepatobiliary scintigraphy, the most important being much better spatial resolution. Besides, it is already used in many patients with liver disease because of its ability to give very accurate anatomical information and to detect and characterize focal liver lesions. Therefore, it is reasonable to assume that MRI will gain priority in the investigation of diffuse liver diseases.

The strategy behind the application of nuclear medicine and MRI for functional imaging of the liver is the same, using either the macrophage activity of the liver or cellular mechanisms of bile formation as targets for radiolabeled or magnetically active pharmaceuticals.

In comparison with laboratory tests, the clinical impact of imaging techniques in the diagnosis and management of diffuse liver diseases is still limited (nuclear medicine) or at a research stage (MRI). However, these techniques offer several theoretical advantages for the evaluation of liver function:

- The hepatic uptake of a radiopharmaceutical or a contrast medium and its biliary excretion are measured directly in the liver parenchyma and the bile. Thus, the evaluation of liver function does not rely on the clearance of a compound, i.e., the disappearance from the blood, which may be influenced by extrahepatic factors (for example, extrahepatic catabolism or renal excretion)
- Liver function can be assessed in relation to specific liver areas, whereas laboratory techniques give only global information on the liver as a whole organ. This capability of the imaging techniques may be useful to guide liver biopsy in heterogeneously distributed liver diseases and to determine hepatic reserve before liver resection. By clarifying diagnostic questions, such as the presence of focal fatty liver, unnecessary biopsy attempts can be avoided
- Liver size can be accurately determined, allowing correlation of liver function with liver volume.

The hepatospecific MRI contrast agents described above have been primarily designed for improved detection and characterization of primary and secondary liver tumors. However, because hepatic uptake of these contrast agents relies on the functional integrity of hepatocytes or Kupffer cells, it was assumed from the beginning that they could also provide information on some aspects of organ function and be useful in the diagnosis and management of diffuse liver diseases (YOUNG et al. 1989; TANIMOTO and STARK 1991; SIDHU et al. 1993).

Manganese-DPDP, in particular, has been used experimentally for demonstrating hepatic dysfunction. In rabbits, by monitoring gallbladder enhancement, COLEY et al. (1995) have shown delayed but otherwise normal peak enhancement in segmental biliary occlusion, delayed and diminished enhancement with hepatitis, and absence of enhancement in total biliary occlusion. Using a rat model of acute and chronic ethanol intoxication, SIDHU et al. (1993) could detect hepatic toxicity by measuring the changes of liver signal intensity after administration of Mn-DPDP. Their results suggest that acute, and possibly also chronic ethanol, liver damage at an early stage are reflected in alterations of contrast enhancement with Mn-DPDP.

From preliminary studies, the hepatic uptake of Mn-DPDP does not appear to be reduced by the presence of biliary obstruction in contrast to that of Gd-EOB-DTPA and Gd-BOPTA (CLEMENT et al. 1992; NI et al. 1994, 1995).

In the case of acute hepatitis, the hepatic uptake of Gd-EOB-DTPA and Gd-BOPTA was diminished, suggesting that these agents could be used to evaluate liver function (KIM et al. 1997; MARZOLA et al. 1997).

Because the phagocytic activity of Kupffer cells is related to the functional state of the hepatocytes, diffuse liver diseases, such as hepatitis or liver cirrhosis, cause impairment of the hepatocyte function. This correlation between the functional state of the hepatocytes and the Kupffer cells has been the background for the hypothesis of using SPIO particles as a method of evaluating liver function by imaging (KREFT et al. 1997). Using SPIO particles, TERRIER et al. (1995) have shown a decreased phagocytic activity in the liver following ischemia. CLEMENT et al. (1991) have demonstrated reduced uptake of SPIO particles in carbon tetrachloride induced liver cirrhosis in rats. The same observation was made in patients suffering from cirrhosis or hepatitis (ELIZONDO et al. 1990). MÜHLER et al. (1993) have studied SPIO particles in acute rejection of liver transplants in rats. It has been shown in experimental and clinical work that the decreased phagocytic activity of the Kupffer cells does not compromise the efficacy of SPIO particles for tumor detection in liver cirrhosis (CLEMENT et al. 1991; YAMASHITA et al. 1996; REIMER and TOMBACH 1998).

Arabinogalactan coated ultrasmall superparamagnetic iron oxide (USPIO) particles have also been used to study some aspects of liver functions. Asialoglycoprotein receptors can be used as markers of hepatocyte function (SMALL et al. 1994). Using arabinogalactan-USPIO, REIMER et al. (1991) have demonstrated in rat models a decreased uptake in acute hepatitis, chronic hepatitis, cirrhosis, but not in fatty liver.

29.8 Conclusions

The field of specific contrast media for liver MRI is rapidly evolving and holds great promise. Today, it seems obvious that such contrast media will have a definite role in clinical practice. However, which type of contrast media will finally prevail, and for which indications, is still a matter of intense study and discussion. Such contrast media will improve detection and characterization of focal liver lesions.

One aspect, which appears most exciting, is the use of hepato-specific contrast media for studying and quantifying liver function. Such an application would be of great interest for the diagnosis and prognosis of diffuse liver diseases. Besides, planning a liver resection in a patient with hepatocellular carcinoma and liver cirrhosis is a clinically important and frequent situation, in which evaluation of the functional "hepatic reserve", could have an important impact on patient management. Functional liver imaging using MRI is, however, still in the domain of experimental research and has not yet made a breakthrough into clinical practice.

References

Aicher KP, Laniado M, Kopp AF, Gronewaller E, Duda SH, Claussen CD (1993) Mn-DPDP-enhanced MR imaging of malignant liver lesions: efficacy and safety in 20 patients. JMRI 3:731–737

Bellin MF, Zaim S, Auberton E, et al (1994) Liver metastases: safety and efficacy of detection with superparamagnetic iron oxide in MR imaging. Radiology 193:657–673

Bernardino MR, Young SW, Lee JK, Weinreb JC (1992) Hepatic

MR imaging with Mn-DPDP: safety, image quality, and sensitivity. Radiology 183:53–58

Biozzi G, Stiffel C (1965) The physiopathology of the reticuloendothelial cells of the liver and spleen. In: Popper H, Schaffner E (eds) Progress in liver diseases, vol. 2. Grune & Stratton, New York, pp 166–191

Birnbaum BA, Weinreb JC, Fernandez MP, Brown JJ, Rofsky NM, Young SW (1994) Comparison of contrast enhanced CT and Mn-DPDP enhanced MRI for detection of focal hepatic lesions. Initial findings. Clin Imaging 18:21–27

Brown PH, Juni JE, Liberman DA, Krishnarmurthy GT (1988) Hepatocyte versus biliary disease: a distinction by deconvolutional analysis of technetium-99 m IDA time-activity curves. J Nucl Med 29:623–630

Caudana R, Morana G, Pirovino GP, et al (1996) Focal malignant hepatic lesions: MR imaging enhanced with gadolinium enzyloxypropionictetra-acetate (BOPTA)-preliminary results of a phase II clinical application. Radiology 199:513–520

Chambon C, Clement O, Le Blanche A, Schouman-Claeys E, Frija G (1993) Superparamagnetic iron oxides as positive MR contrast agents: in vitro and in vivo evidence. Magn Res Imag 11:509–519

Clement O, Frija G, Chambon S, et al (1991) Liver tumors in cirrhosis: experimental study with SPIO-enhanced MR imaging. Radiology 180:31–36

Clement O, Muhler A, Vexler V, Berthezène Y, Brasch RC (1992) gadolinium-ethoxybenzyl-DTPA, a new liver-specific magnetic resonance contrast agent: kinetic and enhancement patterns in normal and cholestatic rats. Invest Radiol 184:612–619

Colet JM, Vander Elst L, Muller RN (1998) Dynamic evaluation of the hepatic uptake and clearance of manganese-based MRI contrast agents: a 31P NMR study on the isolated and perfused rat liver. JMRI 8:663–669.

Coley BD, Mattrey RF, Baker KG, Peterson T, Burgan AR (1995) MR imaging assessment of experimental hepatic dysfunction with Mn-DPDP. JMRI 5:11–16

De Haen C, Gozzini L (1993) Soluble-type hepatobiliary contrast agents for MR imaging. JMRI 3: 79–186

De Haen C, Lorusso V, Luzzani F, Tirone P (1995) Hepatic transport of the magnetic resonance imaging contrast agent gadobenate dimeglumine in the rat. Acad Radiol 2:232–238

De Haen C, Lorusso V, Tirone P (1996) Hepatic transport of gadobenate dimeglumine in TR-rats. Acad Radiol 3:S452–S454

Denys A, Arrivé L, Servois V, et al (1994) Hepatic tumors: detection and characterization at 1-T MR imaging enhanced with AMI-25. Radiology 193:665–669

Doo E, Krishnamurthy GT, Eklem MJ, Gilbert S, Brown PH (1991) Quantification of hepatobiliary function as an integral part of imaging with technetium-99m-mebrofenin in health and disease. J Nucl Med 32:48–57

Elizondo G, Weissleder R, Stark DD, et al (1990) Hepatic cirrhosis and hepatitis: MR imaging enhanced with superparamagnetic iron oxide. Radiology 174:797–801

Ferrucci J, Stark DD (1990) Iron oxide-enhanced MR imaging of the liver and spleen: review of the first 5 years. AJR 155:943–950

Gaa J, Saini S, Ferruci JT (1991) Perfusion characteristics of hepatic cavernous hemangioma using intravenous CT angiography (IVCTA). Eur J Radiol 12:228–233

Giovagnoni A, Paci E (1996) Liver III: gadolinium-based hepatobiliary contrast agents (Gd-EOB-DTPA and Gd-BOPTA/Dimeg). Contrast agents for body MR imaging. MRI Clinics N Am 4:61–72

Grandin C, Van Beers BE, Robert A, Gigot JF, Geubel A, Pringot J (1995) Benign hepatocellular tumors: MRI after superparamagnetic iron oxide administration. J Comput Assist Tomogr 19:412–418

Grangier C, Tourniaire J, Mentha G, et al (1994) Enhancement of liver hemangiomas on T1-weighted MR SE images by superparamagnetic iron oxide particles. J Comput Assist Tomogr 18:888–896

Hagspiel KD, Neidl KF, Eichenberger AC, Weder W, Marincek B (1995) Detection of liver metastases: comparison of superparamagnetic iron oxide-enhanced and unenhanced MR imaging at 1.5 T with dynamic CT, intraoperative US, and percutaneous US. Radiology 196:471–478

Hahn PF, Saini S (1998) Liver-specific MR imaging contrast agents. Radiol Clin North Am 36: 287–297

Hamm B (1998) Clinical utility and safety of MultiHance in MRI of liver cancer: results of multicentre studies in Europe and the USA. Multiple Perspectives in MRI Contrast, Milan, pp 23–25

Hamm B, Vogl T, Branding G, Schnell B, Taupitz M, Wolf KJ (1992) Focal liver lesions: MR imaging with Mn-DPDP – initial clinical results in 40 patients. Radiology 182:167–174

Hamm B, Staks T, Muhler A (1995) Phase I clinical evaluation of Gd-EOB-DTPA as a hepatobiliary MR contrast agent: safety, pharmacokinetics, and MR imaging. Radiology 195:785–792

Hanafusa K, Ohashi I, Himeno Y, Suzuki S, Shibuya H (1995) Hepatic hemangioma: findings with two-phase CT. Radiology 196:465–469

Hanafusa K, Ohashi I, Gomi N, Himeno Y, Wakita T, Shibuya H (1997) Differential diagnosis of early homogeneously enhancing hepatocellular carcinoma and hemangioma by two-phase CT. J Comput Assist Tomogr 21:361–368

Harisinghani MG, Saini S, Weissleder R, et al (1997) Differentiation of liver hemangiomas from metastases and hepatocellular carcinoma at MR imaging enhanced with blood-pool contrast agent code-72227. Radiology 202:687–691

Hollett MD, Jeffrey RB Jr, Nino-Murcia M, Jorgensen MJ, Harris DP (1995) Dual-phase helical CT of the liver: value of arterial phase scans in the detection of small (= or <1.5 cm) malignant hepatic neoplasms. AJR 164:879–884

Josephson L, Lewis J, Jacobs P, Hahn PF, Stark DD (1988) The effects of iron oxides on proton relaxivity. MRI 6:647–653

Kabalka GW, Davis MA, Moss TH, et al (1991) Gadolinium-labeled liposomes containing various amphiphilic GD-DTPA derivatives: targeted MRI contrast enhancement agents for the liver. Magn Reson Med 19:406–415

Karhunen PJ (1986) Benign hepatic tumors and tumor like conditions in men. J Clin Pathol 39:183–188

Kim T, Murakami T, Hasuike Y, et al (1997) Experimental hepatic dysfunction: evaluation by MRI with Gd-EOB-DTPA. JMRI 7:683–688

Kopp AF, Laniado M, Dammamm F, et al (1997) MR imaging of the liver with Resovist: safety, efficacy, and pharmacodynamic properties. Radiology 204:749–756

Kreft B, Block B, Dombrowski F, et al (1998) Diagnostic value of a superparamagnetic iron oxide in MR imaging of chronic liver disease in an animal model. AJR 170:661–668

Krishnamurthy GT , Turner FE (1990) Pharmacokinetics and clinical application of technetium 99m-labeled hepatobiliary agents. Seminars Nucl Med 20:130–149

Laniado M, Chachuat A (1995) Verträglichkeitsprofil von Endorem. Radiologe 35 (11 Suppl 2): S266-S270

Lauterbur BH, Preisig R (1992) Quantitation of liver function,. In: McIntyre N, Benhamou JP, Bircher J, Rizzetto M, Rodes J(eds) Oxford Textbook of Clinical Hepatology, vol 1. Oxford University Press, Oxford, pp 309–314

Leslie DF, Johnson CD, Johnson CM, Ilstrup DM, Harmsen WS (1995a) Distinction between cavernous hemangiomas of the liver and hepatic metastases on CT: value of contrast enhancement patterns. AJR 164:625–629

Leslie DF, Johnson CD, MacCarty RL, Ward EM, Ilstrup DM, Harmsen WS (1995b) Single-pass CT of hepatic tumors: value of globular enhancement in distinguishing hemangiomas from hypervascular metastases. AJR 165:1403–1406

Lim KO, Stark DD, Leese PT, Pfefferbaum A, Rocklage SM, Quay SC (1992) Hepatobiliary MR imaging: first human experience with Mn DPDP. Radiology 178:79–82

Liou J, Lee JK, Borrello JA, Brown JJ (1994) Differentiation of hepatomas from nonhepatomatous masses: use of MnDPDP-enhanced MR images. Magn Reson Imaging 12:71–79

Loubeyre P, Zhao S, Canet E, Abidi H, Benderbous S, Revel D (1997) Ultrasmall superparamagnetic iron oxide particles (AMI 227) as a blood pool contrast agent for MR angiography: experimental study in rabbits. JMRI 7:958–962

Low RN (1997) Contrast agents for MR imaging of the liver. JMRI 7:56–67

Mahfouz AE, Hamm B, Wolf KJ (1994) Peripheral washout: a sign of malignancy on dynamic gadolinium-enhanced MR images of focal liver lesions. Radiology 190:49–52

Majumdar S, Zoghbi SS, Pope CF, Gore JC (1988) Quantification of MR relaxation effects of iron oxide particles in liver and spleen. Radiology 169:653–655

Majumdar S, Zoghbi SS, Gore JC (1989) The influence of pulse sequence on the relaxation effects of superparamagnetic iron oxide contrast agents. Magn Res Med 10:289–301

Marzola P, Maggioni F, Vicinanza E, Dapra M, Cavagna FM (1997) Evaluation of the hepatocyte-specific contrast agent gadobenate dimeglumine for MR imaging of acute hepatitis in a rat model. JMRI 7:147–152

Matsui O, Kadoya M, Kameyama T, et al (1991) Benign and malignant nodules in cirrhotic livers: distinction based on blood supply. Radiology 178:493–497

Mühler A, Frerise CE, Kuwatsuru R, et al (1993) Acute liver rejection: evaluation witrh cell-directed MR-contrast agent in a rat transplantation model. Radiology 186:139–146

Muller RN, Gillis P, Moiny F, Roch A (1991) Transverse relaxivity of particulate MRI contrast media: from theories to experiments. Magn Reson Med 22:178–182

Murakami T, Baron RL, Federle MP, et al (1996) Cirrhosis of the liver: MR imaging with mangafodipir trisodium (Mn-DPDP) Radiology 19:567–572

Ni Y, Marchal G, Zhang X, Van Hecke, et al (1993) The uptake of manganese dipyridoxal-diphosphate by chemically induced hepatocellular carcinoma in rats: a correlation between contrast-media-enhanced magnetic resonance imaging, tumor differentiation, and vascularization. Invest Radiol 28:520–528

Ni Y, Marchal G, Lukito G, Yu J, Muhler A, Baert AL (1994) MR imaging evaluation of liver enhancement by Gd-EOB-DTPA in selective and total bile duct obstruction in rats: correlation with serologic, microcholangiographic, and histologic findings. Radiology 190:753–758

Ni Y, Petre C, Lukito G, Marchal G, et al (1995) effect of manganese dipyridoxal diphosphate on liver magnetic resonance imanging and serum bilirubin in rats with removable biliary obstruction. Acad Radiol 2:300–305

Ni Y, Petre C, Miao Y, et al (1997) Magnetic resonance imaging – histomorphologic correlation studies on paramagnetic metalloporphyrins in rat models of necrosis. Invest Radiol 32:770–779

Peterstein J, Saini S, Weissleder R (1996) Liver II: iron oxide-basedreticuloendothelial contrast agents for MR imaging. Contrast agents for body MR imaging. MRI Clin N Am 4:61–72

Pochon S, Hyacinthe R, Terrettaz J, Robert F, Schneider M, Tournier H (1997) Long circulating superparamagnetic particles with high T2 relaxivity. Acta Radiol 412:69–72

Quinn SF, Benjamin GG (1992) Hepatic cavernous hemangiomas: simple diagnostic sign with dynamic bolus CT. Radiology 182:545–548

Reimer P, Tombach B (1998) Hepatic MRI with SPIO: detection and characterization of focal liver lesions. Eur Radiol 8:1198–1204

Reimer P, Weissleder R, Lee AS, Buettner S, Wittenberg J, Brady TJ (1991) Asialoglycoprotein receptor function in benign liver disease: evaluation with MR imaging. Radiology 178:769–774

Reimer P, Rummeny EJ, Shamsi K, et al (1996) Phase II clinical evaluation of Gd-EOB-DTPA: dose, safety aspects, and pulse sequence. Radiology 199:177–183

Reimer P, Rummeny EJ, Daldrup HE, et al (1997) Enhancement characteristics of liver metastases, hepatocellular carcinomas, and hemangiomas with Gd-EOB-DTPA: preliminary results with dynamic MR imaging. Eur Radiol 7:257–280

Rofsky NM, Earls JP (1996) Mangafodipir trisodium injection (Mn-DPDP). A contrast agent for abdominal MR imaging. Magn Reson Imaging Clin N Am 4:73–85

Rofsky NM, Weinreb JC, Bernardino ME, Young SW, Lee JK, Noz ME (1993) Hepatocellular tumors: characterization with Mn-DPDP-enhanced MR imaging. Radiology 188:21–22

Ros PR, Freeny PC, Harms SE, et al (1995) Hepatic MR imaging with ferumoxides: a multicenter clinical trial of safety and efficacy in the detection of focal hepatic lesions. Radiology 196:481–488

Rozneman Y, Zou XM, Kantor HL (1990) Signal loss induced by superparamagnetic iron oxide particles in NMR spin-echo images: the role of diffusion. Magn Res Med 14:31–39

Rueff B (1989) Alcoologie clinique. Paris: Flammarion Médecine-Sciences, pp 83–84

Rummeny EJ, Torres CG, Kurdziel JC, Nilsen G, Op de Beeck B, Lundby B (1997) MnDPDP for MR imaging. Results of an independant image evaluation of the European phase III studies. Acta Radiol 38:638–642

Runge VM, Lee C, Williams NM (1997) Detectability of small

liver metastases with gadolinium BOPTA. Invest Radiol 32:557–565

Saini S, Stark DD, Hahn P, Wittenberg J, Brady TJ, Ferrucci JT Jr (1987) Ferrite particles: a superparamagnetic MR contrast agent for the reticuloendothelial system. Radiology 162:211–216

Saini S, Edelman RR, Sharma P, et al (1995) Blood-pool MR contrast material for detection and characterization of focal hepatic lesions: initial clinial experience with ultrasmall superparamagnetic iron oxide (AMI-227). AJR 164:114 -1152

Schuhman-Gampieri G, Schmitt-Willich H, Press WR, Negishi C, Weinmann HJ, Speck U (1992) Preclinical evaluation of Gd-EOB-DTPA as a contrast agent in MR imaging of the hepatobiliary system. Radiology 183:59–64

Semelka RC, Brown ED, Ascher SM, et al (1994) Hepatic hemangiomas: a multi-institutional study of appearance on T2-weighted and serial gadolinium-enhanced gradient-echo MR images. Radiology 192: 401–406

Senèterre E, Taourel P, Bouvier Y, et al(1996) Detection of hepatic metastases: ferumoxides-enhanced MR imaging versus unenhanced MR imaging and CT during arterial portography. Radiology 200:785–792

Sidhu MK, Muller HH, Aggeler J, Jones AL, Yound SW (1993) Manganese dipyridoxal diphosphate-enhanced magnetic resonance imaging in the evaluation of hepatocye function. Invest Radiol 28:903–910

Small WE, Nelson RS, Sherbourne GM, Bernardino ME (1994) Enhancement effects of a hepatocyte receptor-specific MR contrast agent in an animal model. JMRI 4:325–330

Stark DD, Weissleder R, Elizondo G, et al (1988) Superparamagnetic iron oxide: clinical application as a contrast agent for MR imaging of the liver. Radiology 168:297–301

Strotzer M. Gmeinwieser J, Schmidt J, et al (1997) Diagnosis of liver metastases from colorectal adnocarinoma. Comparison of spiral-CTAP combined with intravenous contrast-enhanced spiral CT and SPIO-enhanced MR combined with plain MR imaging. Acta Radiol 38:986–992

Tanimoto A, Stark DD (1991) Magnetic resonance for liver imaging. Cell-specific contrast agents fail to detect hepatitis. Invest Radiol 26:S139-S141

Terrier F, Tourniaire J, Belenger J, et al (1995) Magnetic resonance imaging with superparamagnetic iron oxide particles to evaluate hepatic macrophage-monocytic phagocytosis after arterial devascularization in minipigs. Acad Radiol 2:565–575

Torres CG, Lundby B, Sterud AT, McGill S, Gordon PB, Bjerknes HS (1997) MnDPDP for MR imaging of the liver. Results from the European phase III studies. Acta Radiol 38:631–637

Urhahn R, Adam G, Busch N, Chen JH, Euringer W, Gunther RW (1996) Superparmagnetische Eisenoxidpartikel: welchen Stellenwert hat der T1-Effekt für die MR-Diagnostik fokaler Leberläsionen? Röfo Fortschr Geb Röntgenstr Neuen Bildgeb Verfahr 165:364–370

Vogl TJ, Pegios W, McMahon C, et al (1992) Gadobenate dimeglumine – a new contrast agent for MR imaging: preliminary evaluation in healthy volunteers. AJR 158:887–892

Vogl TJ, Hamm B, Schnell B, et al (1993) Mn-DPDP enhancement patterns of hepatocellular lesions on MR images. JMRI 3:51–58

Vogl TJ, Hammerstingl R, Keck H, Felix R (1995) Differentialdiagnose von fokalen Leberläsionen mittels MRT unter Verwendung des superparamagnetischen Kontrastmittels Endorem. Radiologe 35:S258-S266

Vogl TJ, Hammerstingl R, Schwarz W, et al (1996a) Magnetic resonance imaging of focal liver lesions. Comparison of the superparamagnetic iron oxide resovist versus gadolinium-DTPA in the same patient. Invest Radiol 31:696–708

Vogl TJ, Hammerstingl R, Schwarz W, et al (1996b) Superparamagnetic iron oxide-enhanced verus gadolinium-enhanced MR imaging for differential diagnosis of focal liver lesions. Radiology 198:881–887

Vogl TJ, Kummel S, Hammerstingl R, et al (1996c) Liver tumors: comparison of MR imaging with Gd-EOB-DTPA and Gd-DTPA. Radiology 200:59–67

Vogl TJ, Schwarz W, Hammerstingl R, et al(1997) Dynamische und statische MRT mitr dem superparamagnetischen MRT-Konstratmittel Resovist zur Darstellung von primären und sekundären Lebertumoren. Röfo Fortschr Geb Röntgenst Neuen Bildgeb Verfahr 167:264–273

Wang C (1998) Mangafodipir trisodium (MnDPDP)-enhanced magnetic resonance imaging of the liver and pancreas. Acta Radiol Suppl 415:1–31

Wang C, Ahlstrom H, Ekholm S, et al (1997) Diagnostic efficacy of MnDPDP in MR imaging of the liver. A phase III multicentre study. Acta Radiol 38:643–649

Weissleder R, Papisov M (1992) Pharmaceutical iron oxides for MR imaging. Reviews of Magnetic Resonance in Medicine 4:1–20

Wolf G, Burnett K, Goldstein E ,et al (1985) Contrast agents for magnetic resonance imaging. In: Kressel H (ed) Magnetic Resonance Annual. Raven Press, New York, pp 231–265

Yamashita Y, Yamamoto H, Hirai A, Yoshimatsu S, Baba Y, Takahashi M (1996) MR imaging enhancement with superparmagnetic iron oxide in chronic liver disease: influence of liver dysfunction and parenchymal pathology. Abdom Imaging 21:318–323

Young SW, Simpson BB, Ratner AV, Matkin C, Carter EA (1989) MRI measurement of hepatocyte toxicity using the new MRI contrast agent manganese dipyridoxal diphosphonate, a manganese/pyridoxal 5-phosphate chelate. Magn Reson Med 10:1–3

30 Imaging Evaluation of Tumor Response

C. Bartolozzi, D. Cioni, F. Donati, G. Granai, and R. Lencioni

CONTENTS

30.1 Introduction

With advances in imaging and surgical techniques, the number of patients undergoing partial hepatectomies for primary or secondary liver tumors have significantly increased during the past decade. Improvements in imaging modalities have contributed to early detection, precise localization and characterization of liver lesions (Menu 1998). Refinements in surgical techniques have reduced both the morbidity and the mortality rates from elective hepatectomy and have allowed surgeons to consider more extensive resections. Nevertheless, in most patients with liver tumors, surgery is not an appropriate option. Patients with primary hepatocellular carcinoma (HCC) are often poor surgical candidates, because of the lack of hepatic reserve resulting from coexisting liver cirrhosis or the presence of multiple lesions at the time of the diagnosis (Lencioni and Bartolozzi 1997; Colombo 1997; Johnson 1997). Also, in most patients with hepatic metastases resection is not feasible because the lesion is adjacent to critical vascular structures or too many segments are involved that resection would not leave enough liver tissue for survival (Steele and Ravikumar 1989).

Therefore, nonsurgical interventional therapies for tumor ablation have gained an increasingly important role in the treatment of liver malignancies (De Sanctis et al. 1998; Lin et al. 1997). These techniques have emerged as powerful therapeutic tools with a constantly growing number of applications (Lin et al. 1997). Two fundamentally different approaches of treatment have been used: (a) the direct percutaneous image-guided approach, in which chemical or thermal ways of tissue destruction are used, as in intratumor injection of alcohol or in radiofrequency or laser thermal ablation; and (b) the intraarterial approach, in which chemotherapeutic agents and embolic materials are injected via a catheter inserted into the branches of the hepatic artery, as in transcatheter arterial embolization or chemoembolization (Lencioni and Bartolozzi 1997; Dalla Palma 1998).

One of the most difficult and troublesome issues of interventional techniques of liver tumor ablation is how to correctly confirm complete necrosis of the treated lesion, which would be equivalent to surgical resection. Although definite proof of the effectiveness would be indicated by the absence of viable tumor cells, it is impossible to know the histologic characteristics of the whole tumor even if repeated biopsies are performed. Thus, biopsy can be considered entirely reliable for evaluating therapeutic efficacy solely when it shows viable malignancy. Serum tumor markers are of limited usefulness for assessing tumor response. Patients with small HCC, in fact, frequently have normal pretreatment levels of alphafetoprotein (AFP). Moreover, tumor markers levels can diminish or return to normal even when the necrosis of the tumor is only partial. Therefore, the evaluation of the therapeutic effect of interventional

C. Bartolozzi, MD; Professor and Chairman, Division of Diagnostic and Interventional Radiology, Department of Oncology, University of Pisa, Via Roma 67, I-56125 Pisa, Italy
D. Cioni, MD; Division of Diagnostic and Interventional Radiology, Department of Oncology, University of Pisa, Via Roma 67, I-56125 Pisa, Italy
F. Donati, MD; Division of Diagnostic and Interventional Radiology, Department of Oncology, University of Pisa, Via Roma 67, I-56125 Pisa, Italy
G. Granai, MD; Division of Diagnostic and Interventional Radiology, Department of Oncology, University of Pisa, Via Roma 67, I-56125 Pisa, Italy
R. Lencioni, MD; Division of Diagnostic and Interventional Radiology, Department of Oncology, University of Pisa, Via Roma 67, I-56125 Pisa, Italy

procedures is based mainly on findings at imaging studies, which should accurately reflect the degree of the treatment and show areas of residual tumor. This is particularly important since in case of incomplete necrosis of the lesion, the treatment can be repeated, and tumor ablation can be further pursued. In this chapter, we discuss the imaging findings and the diagnostic criteria that can be useful to establish the outcome of the most widely used interventional procedures for liver tumor ablation.

30.2 Percutaneous Ethanol Injection

Percutaneous ethanol injection (PEI) is a therapeutic technique that has been established since 1986 (LIVRAGHI et al. 1986). Alcohol enters the cells by diffusion, producing immediate cellular dehydration and protein denaturation, which result in coagulative necrosis of the tumor. In addition, ethanol induces a chemical vasculitis followed by thrombosis of small vessels within and around the tumor. PEI is currently used for treating small, nodular-type HCC lesions less than 3–4 cm in greatest dimension (LENCIONI et al. 1995a, 1997; LIVRAGHI 1998; LIVRAGHI et al. 1995; CASTELLANO et al. 1997; POMPILI et al. 1997; KUMADA et al. 1997), and can be profitably combined with transarterial chemoembolization to treat larger HCC tumors (TANAKA et al. 1992, 1998; BARTOLOZZI et al. 1995; KODA et al. 1994; LENCIONI et al. 1998b; ALLGAIER et al. 1998).

PEI is best administered under US guidance because real-time control allows for a faster procedure, precise centering of the needle in the target, and continuous monitoring of the procedure. This last point is crucial since one must be able to evaluate the distribution of the injected ethanol in order to achieve complete perfusion of the tumor or to detect immediately ethanol leaks outside the lesion, which may cause complications such as injury of the bile ducts or chemical thrombosis of liver vessels adjacent to the tumor (LENCIONI et al. 1995c; LIN et al. 1997). An inherent limitation of gray-scale US, however, is its inability to evaluate the therapeutic effect of treatment. In fact, although PEI usually causes substantial changes in the US pattern of the lesion, it is almost impossible to evaluate with US the necrotic area produced by PEI, owing to the similar appearance of necrosis and viable neoplastic tissue (BARTOLOZZI and LENCIONI 1996). US can be used to demonstrate reduction of tumor size after treatment, which may indicate successful therapy. However, it takes a considerable length of time to evaluate the therapeutic effect of treatment, judging from the reduction of lesion size after treatment.

To achieve information regarding the therapeutic response of the tumor during the course of PEI treatment, the use of color Doppler US is to be recommended. HCC, in fact, is a hypervascular tumor in which color signals with an arterial Doppler spectrum are usually well depicted before treatment, particularly when using the power Doppler mode or injecting microbubble contrast agents to enhance the Doppler signal (LENCIONI et al. 1996; UENO et al. 1998; KIM AY et al. 1998). After successful ablation, color signals become no longer detectable on either unenhanced or contrast-enhanced color Doppler US studies (LENCIONI et al. 1995b; BARTOLOZZI et al. 1998; UENO et al. 1998). In contrast, in lesions containing residual viable tumor, color signals are usually still recognizable. In these cases, the portion of the tumor in which color signals are still detected after therapy closely matches the area of viable cancer as seen on spiral CT scans (Figs. 30.1–30.4). Therefore, contrast-enhanced color Doppler US is also extremely useful in the retreatment of lesions with PEI because it allows for precise targeting of the needle in the viable portion of the tumor (BARTOLOZZI et al. 1998).

Use of color Doppler US, however, is limited because not all native tumors demonstrate a distinct intratumoral blood flow (LENCIONI et al. 1995b; BARTOLOZZI et al. 1998; UENO et al. 1998). Moreover, small portions of viable neoplastic tissue may go undetected even when using the power Doppler mode coupled with contrast agents to maximize color sensitivity. Hence, we do not suggest that color Doppler US should be used as the final diagnostic test for establishing the outcome of therapy. Rather, unenhanced and contrast-enhanced color Doppler US studies could be used to monitor the response of the tumor during the course of PEI treatment. We suggest the performance of an unenhanced color Doppler US study of the lesion immediately before each PEI session: if intratumoral color signals are still depicted, further ethanol should be administered because the presence of residual tumor can be confidently assumed. In this case, unenhanced color Doppler US can also be used to target the viable portions of the tumor during the injection. On the contrary, when no intratumoral blood flow signals are found on the unenhanced color Doppler US, the contrast-enhanced color Doppler US study can be performed to search for residual viable tumor areas undetected

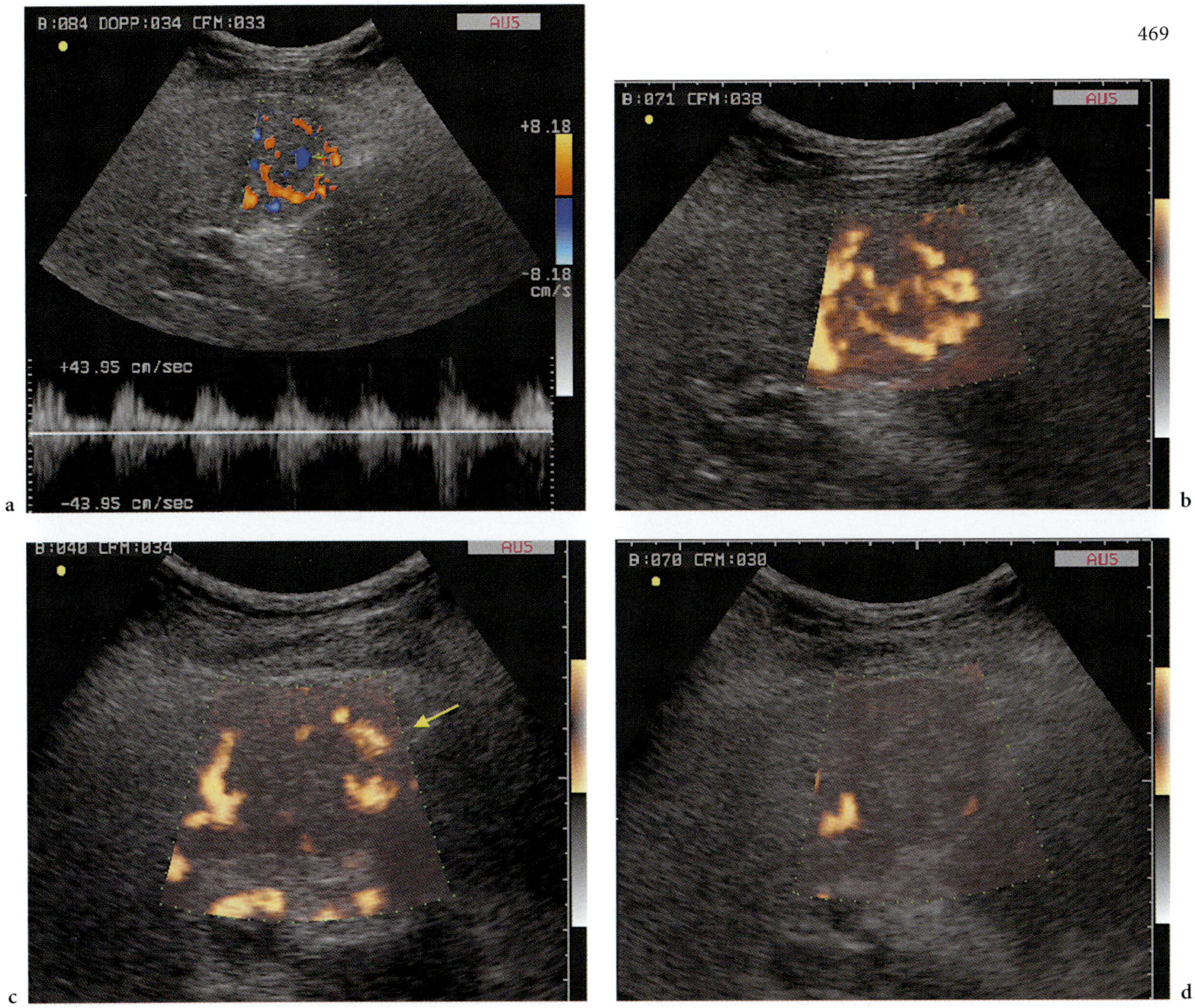

Fig. 30.1a–d. Contrast-enhanced color Doppler US performed before treatment shows hypervascular tumor (**a**). Contrast-enhanced power Doppler imaging better delineates the vascular architecture of the native tumor (**b**). After percutaneous ethanol injection, residual viable tumor is demonstrated by contrast-enhanced power Doppler US in the antero-medial aspect of the tumor (*arrow in* **c**). After additional treatment with percutaneous ethanol injection, targeted in the areas of residual hypervascular tissue, complete absence of flow is demonstrated by contrast-enhanced power Doppler US (**d**)

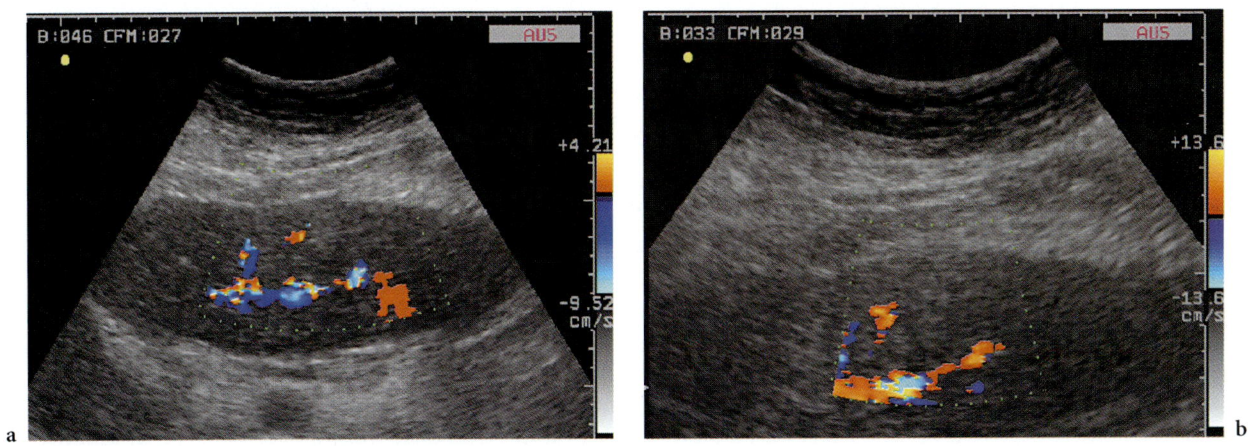

Fig. 30.2a,b. Contrast-enhanced color Doppler US performed after percutaneous ethanol injection shows a small area of residual viable tumor in the anterior aspect of the lesion. After additional ethanol injections, performed with contrast-enhanced color Doppler US guidance, the small viable portion of the tumor is no longer detected on contrast-enhanced color Doppler US (**b**)

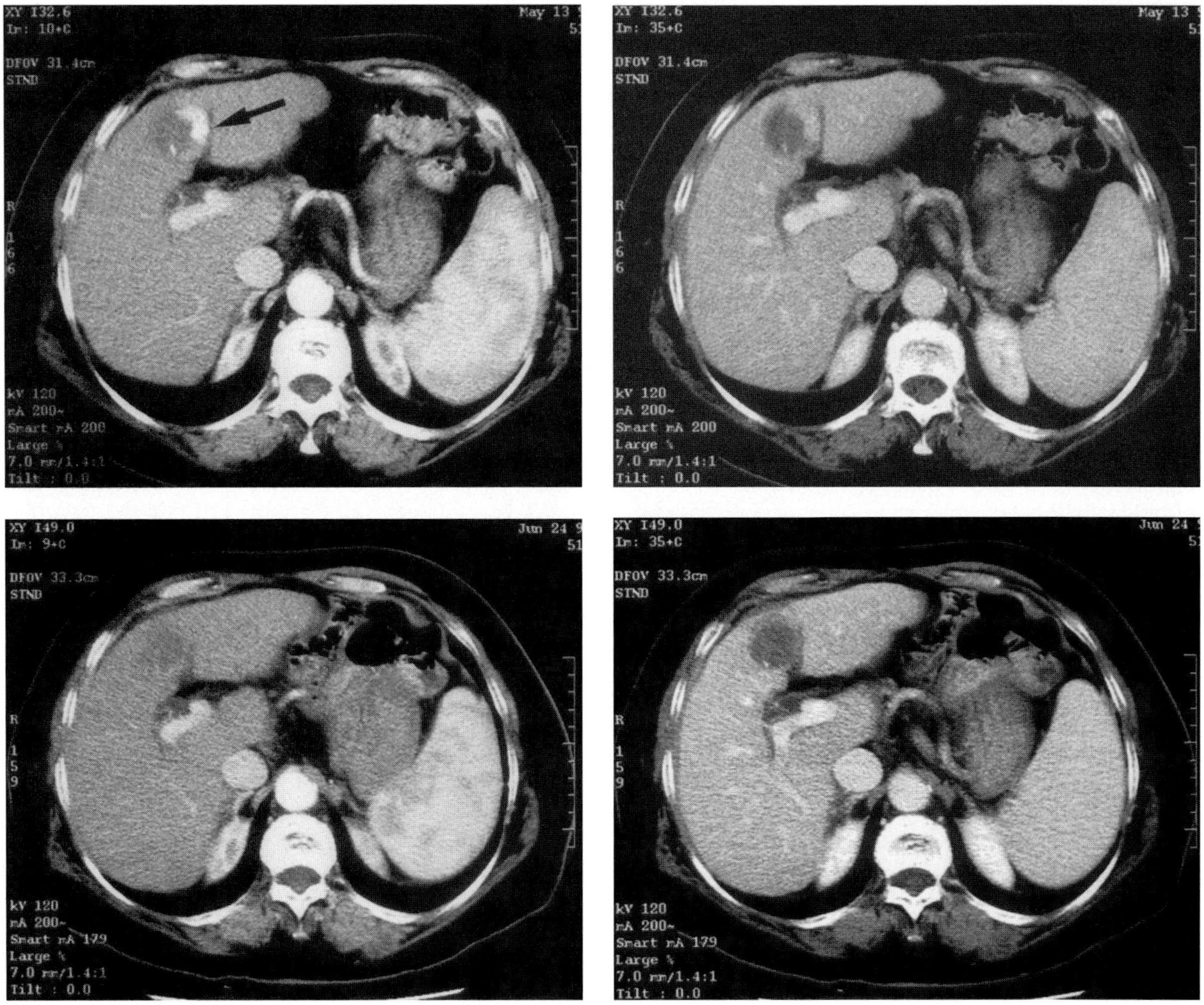

Fig. 30.3a–d. Same case as in Fig. 30.1. Dual-phase spiral CT in the arterial (**a**) and the portal venous phase (**b**) performed after ethanol injection therapy shows residual hypervascular tumor in the antero-medial aspect of the lesion (*arrow in* **a**), corresponding to findings in Fig. 30.1c. Repeated spiral CT in the arterial (**c**) and the portal phase (**d**) after further treatment of the lesion shows complete tumor necrosis, corresponding to findings in Fig. 30.1d

by the unenhanced study and to target these viable portions of the tumor during the injection. When no intratumoral enhancing areas are depicted on contrast-enhanced color Doppler US, further evaluation with spiral CT or dynamic MR imaging can be scheduled to confirm the favorable outcome of treatment and rule out possible false-negative results (Bartolozzi et al. 1998).

Spiral CT and dynamic contrast-enhanced MR imaging, in fact, are recognized as the standard imaging modalities for evaluating the response of HCC to PEI (Bartolozzi et al. 1994a,b; Sironi et al. 1994; Becker et al. 1997). With spiral CT, lesions ablated by PEI appear as hypoattenuating, nonenhancing areas in both the arterial and the portal venous phases (Fig. 30.5) (Bartolozzi and Lencioni 1996; Joseph et al. 1993). On the contrary, in the case of partial necrosis, the areas of residual viable neoplastic tissue can be easily recognized as they stand out in the arterial phase against the faintly enhanced normal liver parenchyma and the unenhanced areas of coagulation necrosis (Fig. 30.6) (Bartolozzi and Lencioni 1996; Joseph et al. 1993).

The enhancement pattern of the tumor-bearing area, however, must be carefully examined to assess the outcome of therapy. In particular, the finding of a wedge-shaped area of increased enhancement during the arterial phase in the vicinity of the treated lesion must be differentiated in terms of whether residual or recurrent infiltrative-type HCC is demonstrated or whether a hyperperfusion abnormality is present. Hyperperfusion abnormalities following

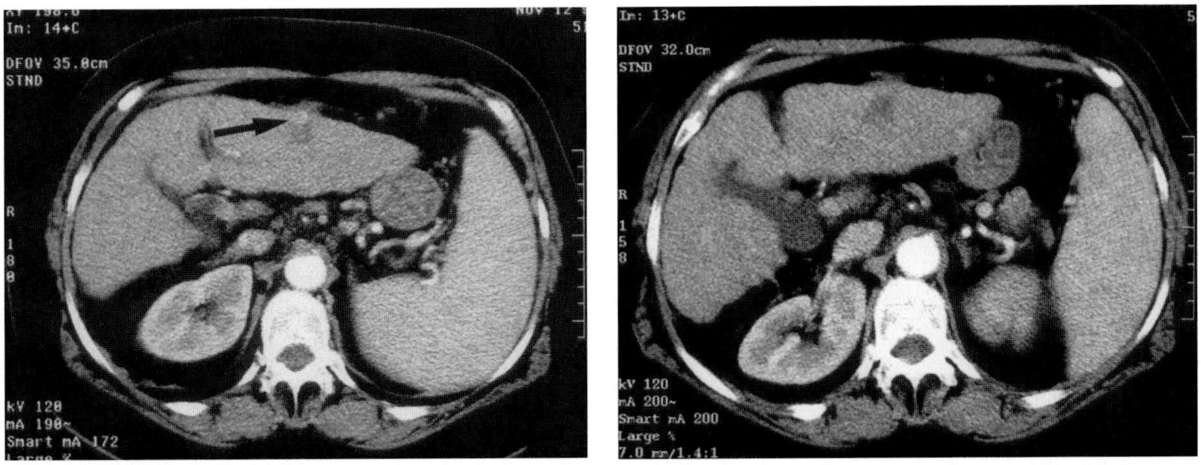

a b

Fig. 30.4a,b. Same case as in Fig. 30.2. **a** Arterial-phase spiral CT performed after ethanol injection therapy shows small area of residual viable tumor (*arrow*), corresponding to findings in Fig. 30.2a. **b** After the second treatment cycle, the enhancing area is no longer depictable on the arterial-phase spiral CT image, corresponding to findings in Fig. 30.2b

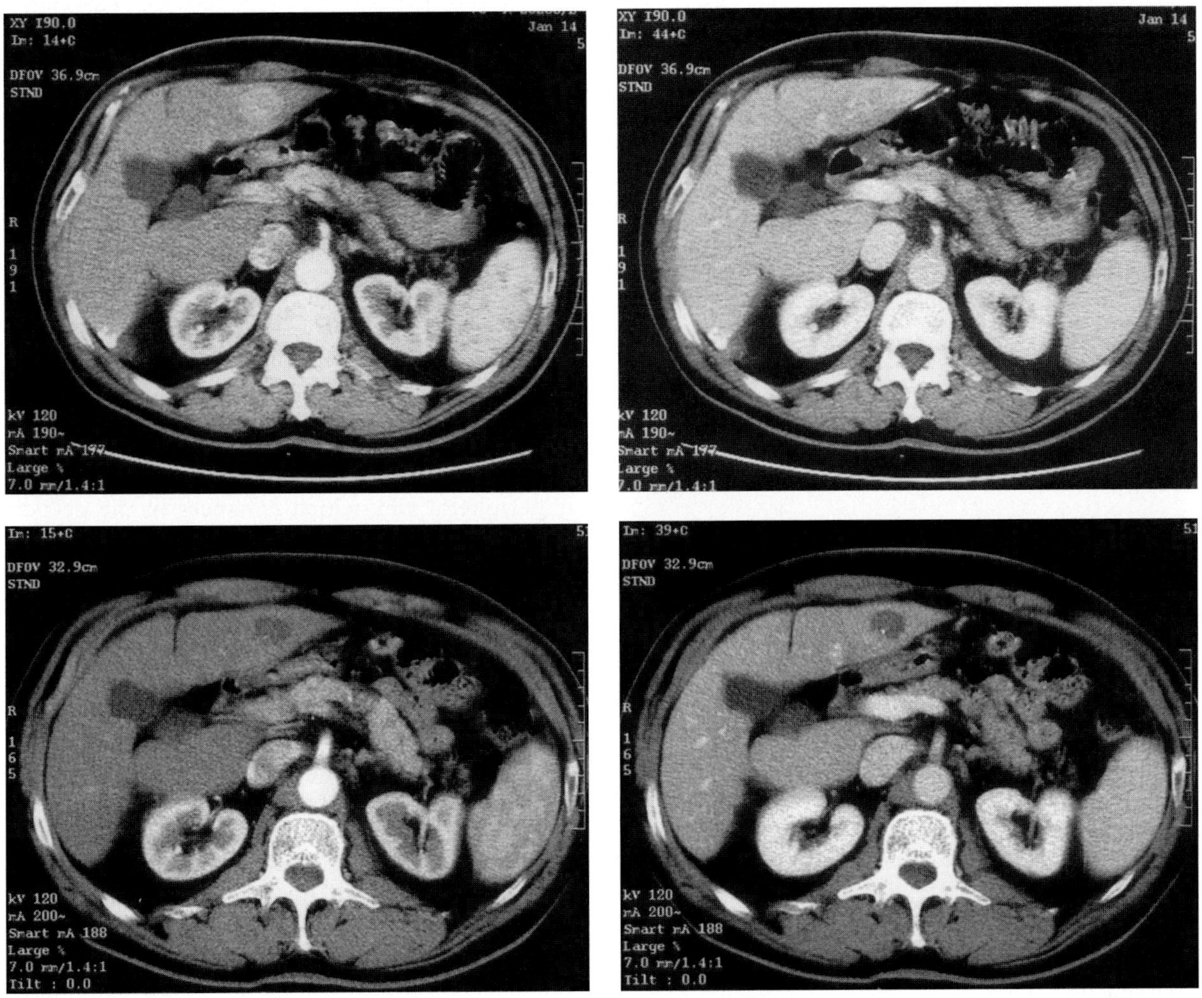

a b c d

Fig. 30.5a–d. Hepatocellular carcinoma with complete necrosis after percutaneous ethanol injection. Before treatment, the lesion is slightly hyperdense in the arterial phase (**a**) and isodense in the portal phase (**b**). After treatment, the tumor is replaced by a hypoattenuating area of coagulation necrosis, which fails to enhance in the arterial (**c**) and the portal venous phase (**d**)

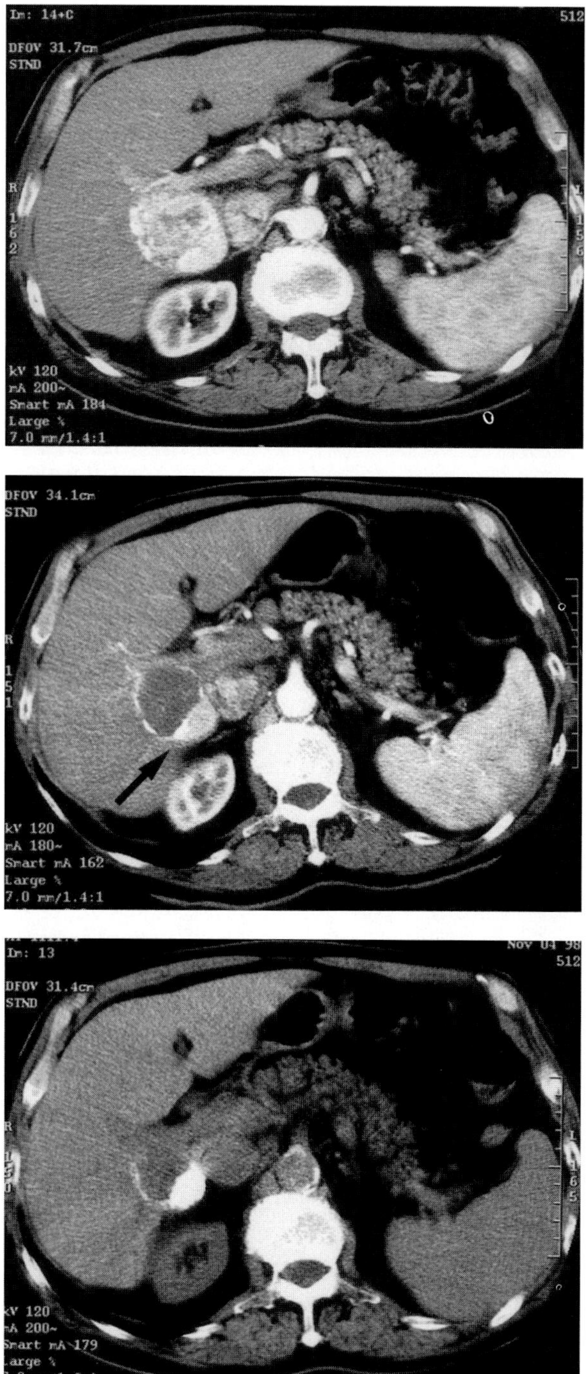

a b c

Fig. 30.6a–c. Hepatocellular carcinoma with partial necrosis after percutaneous ethanol injection. Before treatment, the lesion appears hyperattenuating in the arterial phase (**a**). After ethanol injection therapy, most of the lesion is destroyed and appears hypoattenuating in the arterial phase spiral CT image (**b**). Residual enhancing viable tumor tissue is still present in the postero-medial aspect of the tumor (*arrow in* **b**). After additional treatment with transcatheter arterial chemoembolization, Lipiodol is retained in the viable portion of the tumor (**c**)

PEI may be caused by PEI-induced chemical thrombosis in the peripheral portal vein branches surrounding the lesion or because of microscopic arteriovenous shunts produced by needle injury. Distinction between tumor progression and hyperperfusion abnormalities may be difficult, and requires accurate comparison of pretreatment and posttreatment studies (Yu et al. 1997; Kim TK et al. 1998; Lencioni et al. 1993).

With unenhanced MR imaging, alcohol-induced necrosis is usually shown as a markedly hypointense area on spin-echo T2 weighted images (Bartolozzi et al. 1994a; Sironi et al. 1994). This peculiar feature is due to the strong dehydrating effect of alcohol, which results in a coagulative necrosis of the tumor. Conversely, viable neoplastic tissue that persists after treatment maintains the high signal intensity shown on spin-echo T2 weighted images obtained before treatment and can therefore be recognized as a hyperintense area. To enhance the diagnostic accuracy of MR imaging, the use of dynamic studies after the administration of a paramagnetic contrast agent is to be recommended (Bartolozzi et al. 1994a; Sironi et al. 1994). Dynamic contrast-enhanced MR imaging, like spiral CT, may clearly show the presence of residual viable tumor because of the early arterial uptake of contrast resembling that of native lesions. Necrotic tumor, in contrast, fails to enhance throughout the entire dynamic study (Fig. 30.7) (Fujita et al. 1998).

Also with MR imaging, hepatic parenchymal hyperperfusion abnormalities may be seen adjacent to a treated HCC on dynamic contrast-enhanced MR images (Ito et al. 1995). In addition, a thin and regular peripheral rim, which enhances in the delayed phase, may be detected around the necrotic area produced by PEI. This feature is due to the presence of granulation tissue along the periphery of the treated lesion and should not be misinterpreted as tumor persistence of recurrence (Lencioni et al. 1993, Sironi et al. 1991; Kubota et al. 1989; Sironi et al. 1993; Nagel and Bernardino 1993). In the case of questionable enhancing areas at the periphery of the tumor, MR imaging has an inherent advantage over spiral CT, as additional information can be obtained with the use of tissue-specific MR contrast agents, such as those targeted to the reticulo-endothelial system. Residual or recurrent viable tumor, in fact, does not take up the agent, and can therefore be distinguished from perfusion abnormalities, in which the uptake of reticulo-endothelial system-specific agents is usually normal (Naik et al. 1997; Ros et al. 1995).

The follow-up protocol for HCC patients who underwent PEI includes: US and assays for AFP level at 3-month intervals, and spiral CT or dynamic MR imaging at 6-month intervals. Patients must be studied to diagnose either recurrences of the treated tumors or recurrences caused by the emergence of new nodular lesions (Nishizaki et al. 1997). Complete response is considered to be obtained when no enhancing areas are seen at the level of the treated lesion on contrast-enhanced CT or dynamic MR imaging, reduction in size persisting during the follow-up, and serologic markers remaining stable.

30.3 Transcatheter Arterial Chemoembolization

Transcatheter arterial chemoembolization (TACE) is a therapeutic technique that was developed in the late 1970s by Eastern investigators. Over the last ten years, this procedure has been increasingly used for the treatment of HCC, initially in Asia and then in Europe (Lencioni and Bartolozzi 1997; Groupe d'Etude et de Traitement du Carcinome Hepatocellulaire 1995). The aim of intraarterial chemotherapy is to increase the concentration of anticancer agents within the tumor. Arterial embolization, in contrast, aims at creating tumor necrosis by ischemia and relies on the fact that the main blood supply from HCC comes from arteries while nontumoral hepatic tissue is supplied by the portal vein. In TACE, intraarterial chemotherapy and arterial embolization are combined in an attempt to enhance the anticancer effect of each of the two procedures. TACE allows a drug concentration to be achieved in the tumor 10 to 25 times greater than can be achieved by infusion alone (Lencioni and Bartolozzi 1997). Moreover, up to 85% of the administered drug is trapped in the liver, minimizing systemic toxicity. The use of iodized oil in combination with a chemotherapeutic agent (anticancer-in-oil emulsion) further increases the duration of cancer cell exposure to the drug. The iodized oil droplets deposited in the tumor, in fact, disappear at a slower rate compared with those deposited in the normal liver tissue, and remain for many months within HCC nodules (Tanaka et al. 1992; Bartolozzi et al. 1995; Koda et al. 1994; Lencioni et al. 1998b; Allgaier et al. 1998; Tanaka et al. 1998).

The effect of TACE on liver tumors depends on the morphologic type of the lesion and on its vascular supply. TACE is well indicated for treating hypervascular, encapsulated HCC, which is almost completely fed by hepatic arterial blood and therefore highly responsive to hepatic arterial embolization (Lencioni and Bartolozzi 1997; Choi et al. 1992; Matsui et al. 1993). In contrast, in hypovascular or nonencapsulated tumors or in tumors showing extracapsular invasion of neoplastic cells, TACE often fails to induce complete necrosis of the lesion. In fact tumor cells, either unimpeded by the absence of a capsule or spreading across the capsule itself, invade the adjacent liver parenchyma, thus obtaining additional blood supply from the sinusoidal portal system. TACE represents the treatment of choice for patients with multinodular HCC, provided that the main portal vein branches are not involved in tumor and that tumor replacement of liver parenchyma does not exceed 30–40% (Lencioni and Bartolozzi 1997). Moreover, TACE is used in combination with PEI for the treatment of large, nodular-type HCC (Tanaka et al. 1992; Bartolozzi et al. 1995; Koda et al. 1994; Lencioni et al. 1998b; Lin et al. 1997; Lencioni et al. 1994b).

TACE is usually performed by injecting a mixture of iodized oil and an anticancer drug followed by gelatin sponge particles. The iodized oil (Lipiodol) is the iodinated ethyl ester of the fatty acid of poppy seed oil and contains 37–38% iodine by weight. Since the injection of Lipiodol into the hepatic artery is followed by its selective and prolonged retention within HCC, on unenhanced CT scans performed 3–4 weeks after TACE, treated lesions appear as highly hyperattenuating areas compared with nontumorous liver tissue, from which iodized oil is rapidly washed out. The degree of Lipiodol retention within the lesion as shown by CT helps predict the outcome of therapy: in fact, complete and homogeneous concentration of Lipiodol is usually associated with a favorable response to therapy (Figs. 30.8, 30.9), whereas partial and inhomogeneous retention of iodized oil indicates minor or no response (Figs. 30.10, 30.11) (Choi et al. 1992; Kim TK et al. 1998; Lencioni et al. 1994a).

However, limited persistence of tumor after treatment may sometimes be difficult to assess by CT because the high attenuation of the iodized oil trapped within the lesion does not allow a confident interpretation of contrast-enhanced spiral CT studies (Bartolozzi et al. 1994b; Takayasu et al. 1994; Murayama et al. 1986).

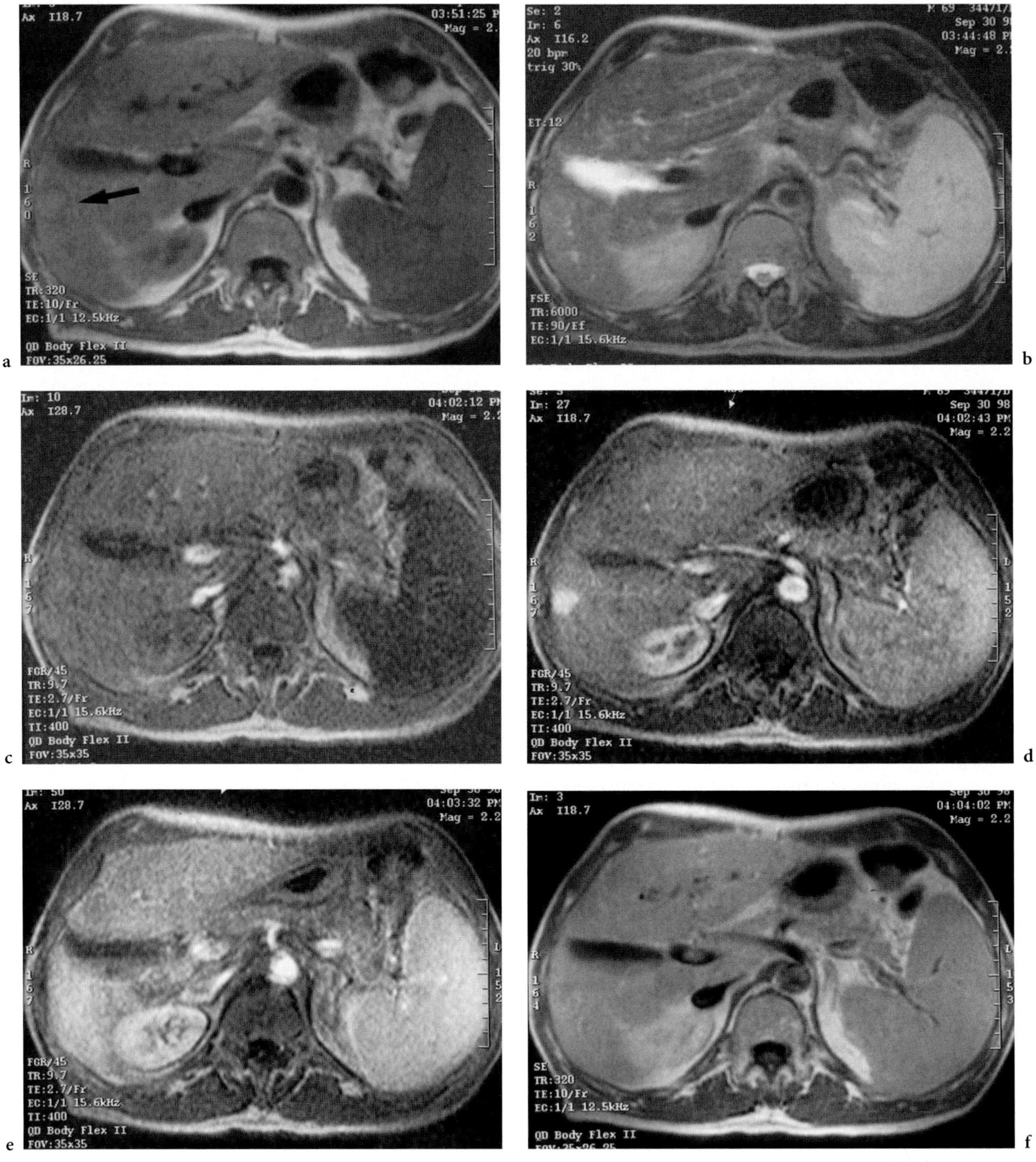

Fig. 30.7a–l. Hepatocellular carcinoma with complete necrosis after percutaneous ethanol injection. Before treatment, the lesion is slightly hyperintense on spin-echo T1-weighted MR image (*arrow in* **a**) and isointense on spin-echo T2-weighted MR image (**b**). The contrast-enhanced dynamic MR study (baseline, **c**; arterial phase, **d**; portal phase, **e**; delayed phase, **f**) confirms uninodular tumor. Note early contrast uptake in the arterial phase image (**d**). After ethanol ablation, the tumor is hyperintense with hypointense halo on spin-echo T1-weighted image (**g**) and definitely hypointense on spin-echo T2-weighted image (**h**). No contrast uptake is seen throughout the dynamic study (baseline, **i**; arterial phase, **j**; portal phase, **k**; delayed phase, **l**). Note peripheral enhancing halo in **l** corresponding to inflammatory reaction along the area of coagulation necrosis

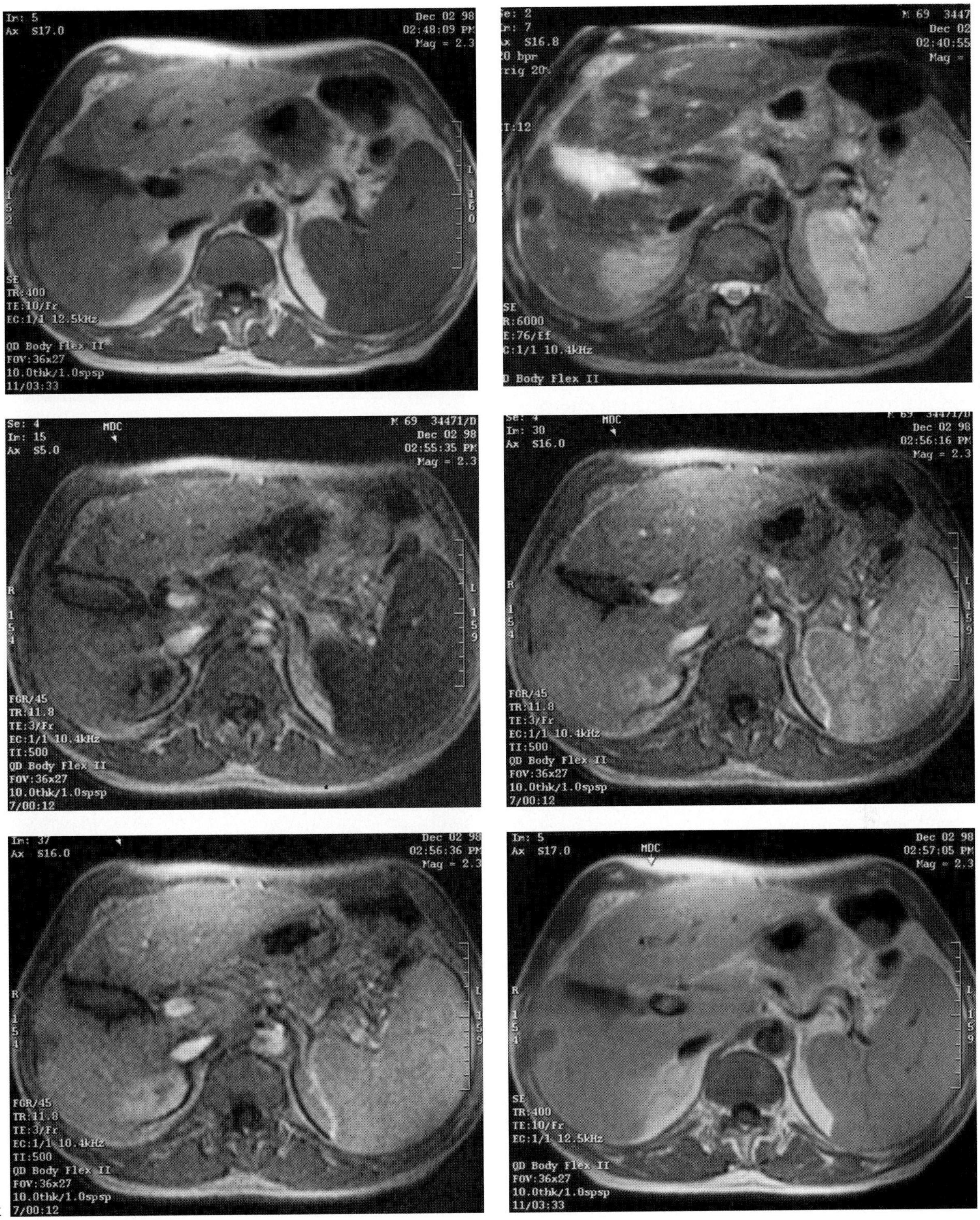

Fig. 30.7g–l (Continued)

MR imaging has a specific advantage over CT in the evaluation of the response to TACE: in fact, the influence of the intratumoral retention of iodized oil on MR signal intensity is minimal. Therefore, the identification of persistent neoplastic tissue within the treated tumors may be easier on contrast-enhanced MR images than on contrast-enhanced spiral CT scans (Fig. 30.12) (Bartolozzi et al. 1994b).

The advantage of MR imaging over spiral CT is even more manifest in lesions treated with a combination of TACE and PEI. In this case, in fact, the coexistence of hyperattenuating areas (due to Lipiodol retention) and hypoattenuating areas (caused by ethanol-induced necrosis) makes the interpretation of the contrast-enhanced CT study very difficult. On the contrary, the different necrotizing effects of TACE and PEI result in the same appearance (absence of enhancement) on dynamic contrast-enhanced MR images, thus making the assessment of the response to therapy easier (Bartolozzi et al. 1994b; Yoshioka et al. 1990).

The standard follow-up protocol for HCC patients who underwent TACE or combined TACE and PEI includes AFP level measurement and contrast-enhanced CT or MR imaging at 3-month intervals. Color Doppler US with administration of echo-enhancers can also be useful in selected cases, but has a limited role in the presence of multinodular disease because of the difficulty of studying multiple lesions and comparing different examinations over time (Kim DE et al. 1998).

30.4 Radiofrequency Thermal Ablation

Radiofrequency (RF) thermal ablation is a percutaneous technique that has been developed during the past few years in an attempt to overcome the limitations of ethanol injection, particularly in the treatment of hepatic metastases (Rossi et al. 1996, 1998; Solbiati et al. 1997a,b; Lencioni et al. 1998a; Solbiati 1998; Goldberg et al. 1998a,b). With this technique, RF waves are used to induce thermal ablation of small hepatic malignancies. An alternating current, in fact, flows from the uninsulated tract of the active electrode to the tissue. Ionic agitation is produced in the tissue around the electrode, as the ions attempt to follow the changes in direction of the alternating current, resulting in frictional heating, which ultimately causes coagulation necrosis of the tumor.

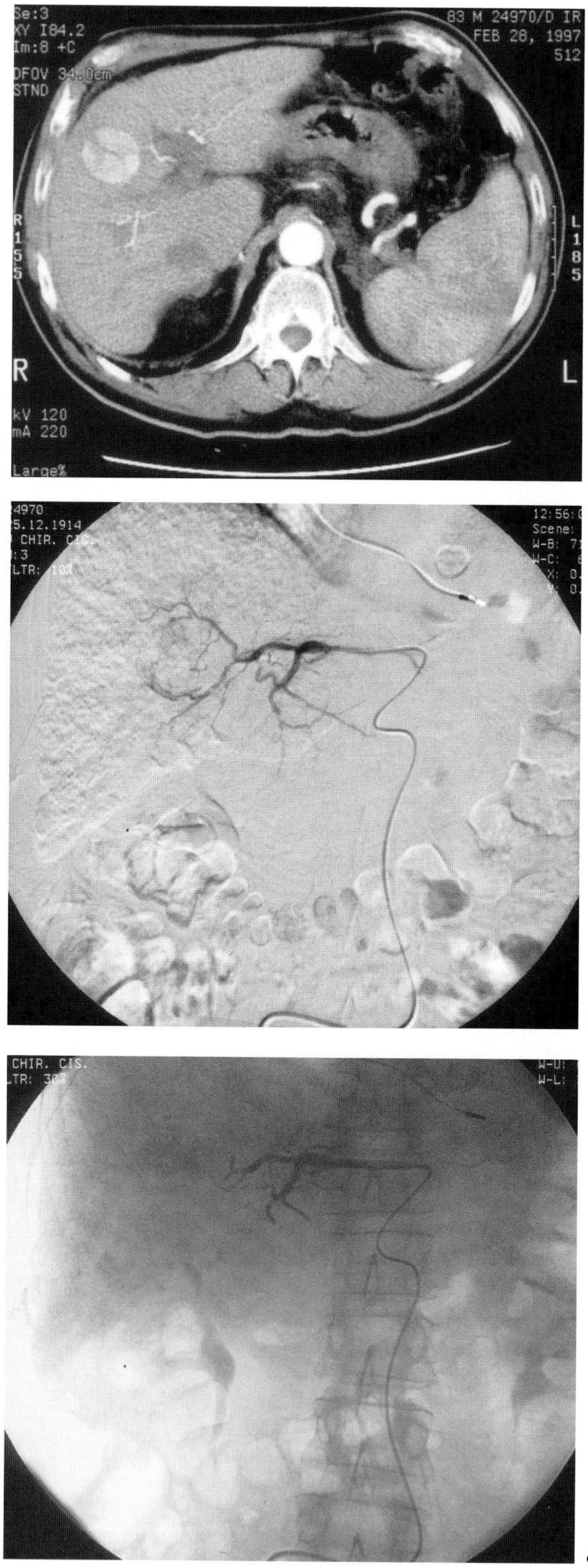

a

b

c

Fig. 30.8 a–c

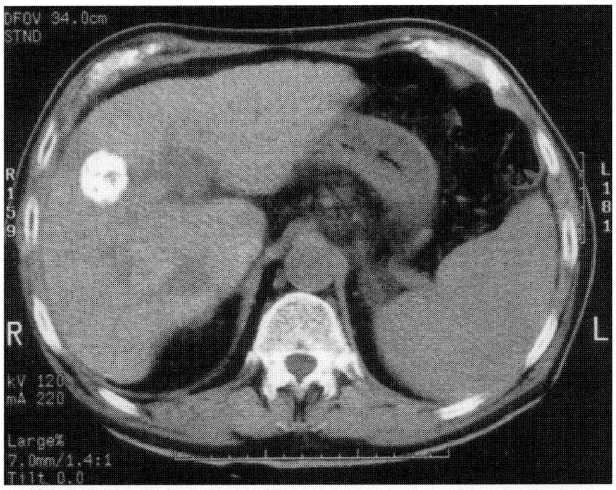

d

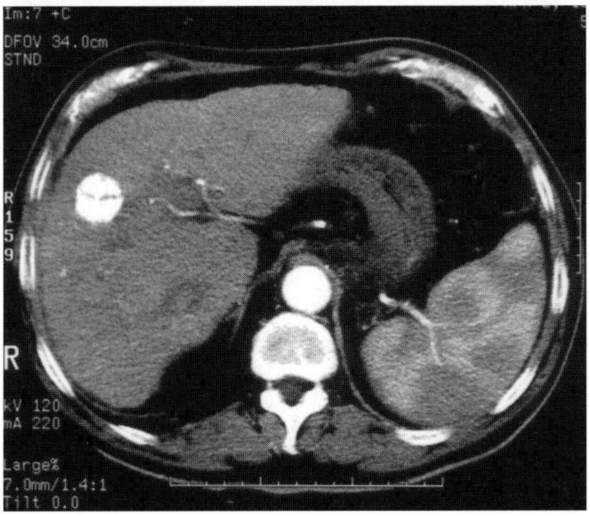

e

Fig. 30.8a–e. Hepatocellular carcinoma treated with transcatheter arterial chemoembolization. **a** Before treatment, spiral CT in the arterial phase shows the lesion as a hyperattenuating nodule. Digital subtraction angiography (**b**) confirms uninodular hypervascular tumor. After chemoembolization, complete devascularization of the tumor is seen angiographically (**c**). CT scan obtained 4 weeks later shows dense and homogeneous retention of iodized oil, suggesting complete tumor response (**d**). No contrast uptake at the periphery of the tumor is demonstrated in the arterial phase image (**e**)

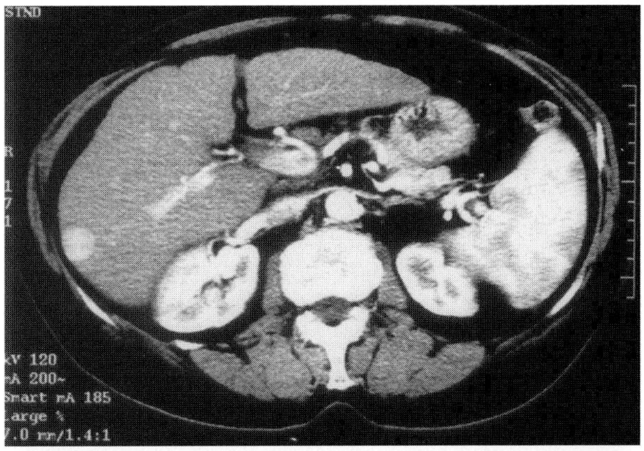

a

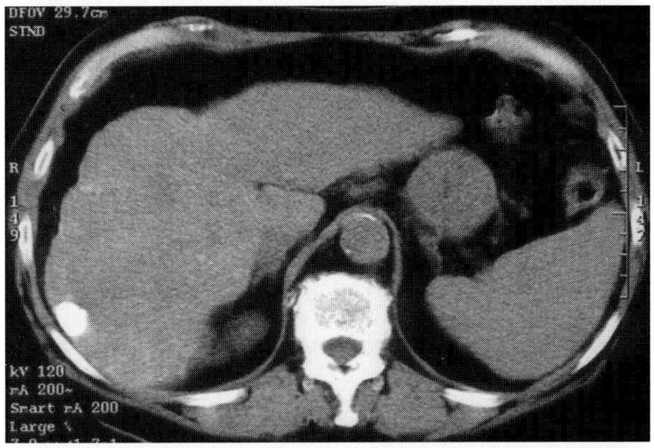

b

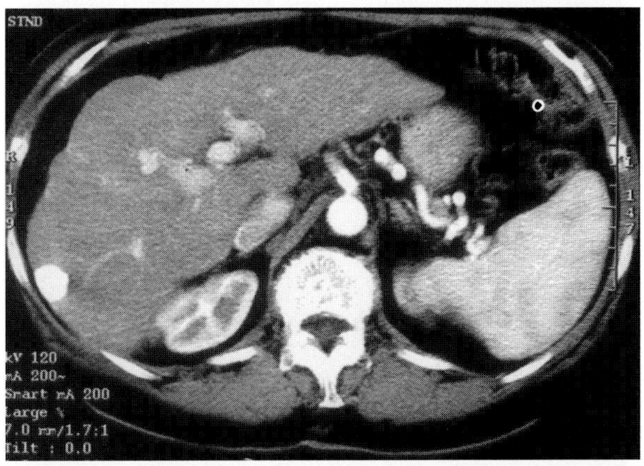

c

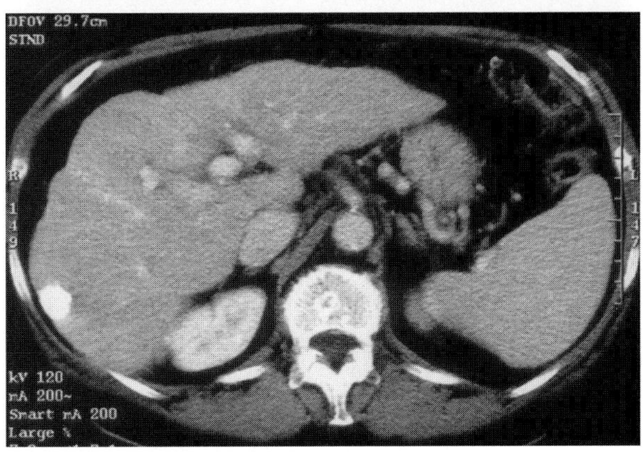

d

Fig. 30.9a–d. Small hepatocellular carcinoma with complete response after chemoembolization. Spiral CT performed before treatment shows the lesion as a hyperattenuating nodule in the arterial phase (**a**). Four weeks after chemoembolization, dense and homogeneous retention of Lipiodol is observed within the tumor on unenhanced CT scan (**b**). No contrast uptake at the periphery of the lesion is detected in the arterial (**c**) and the portal venous phase (**d**)

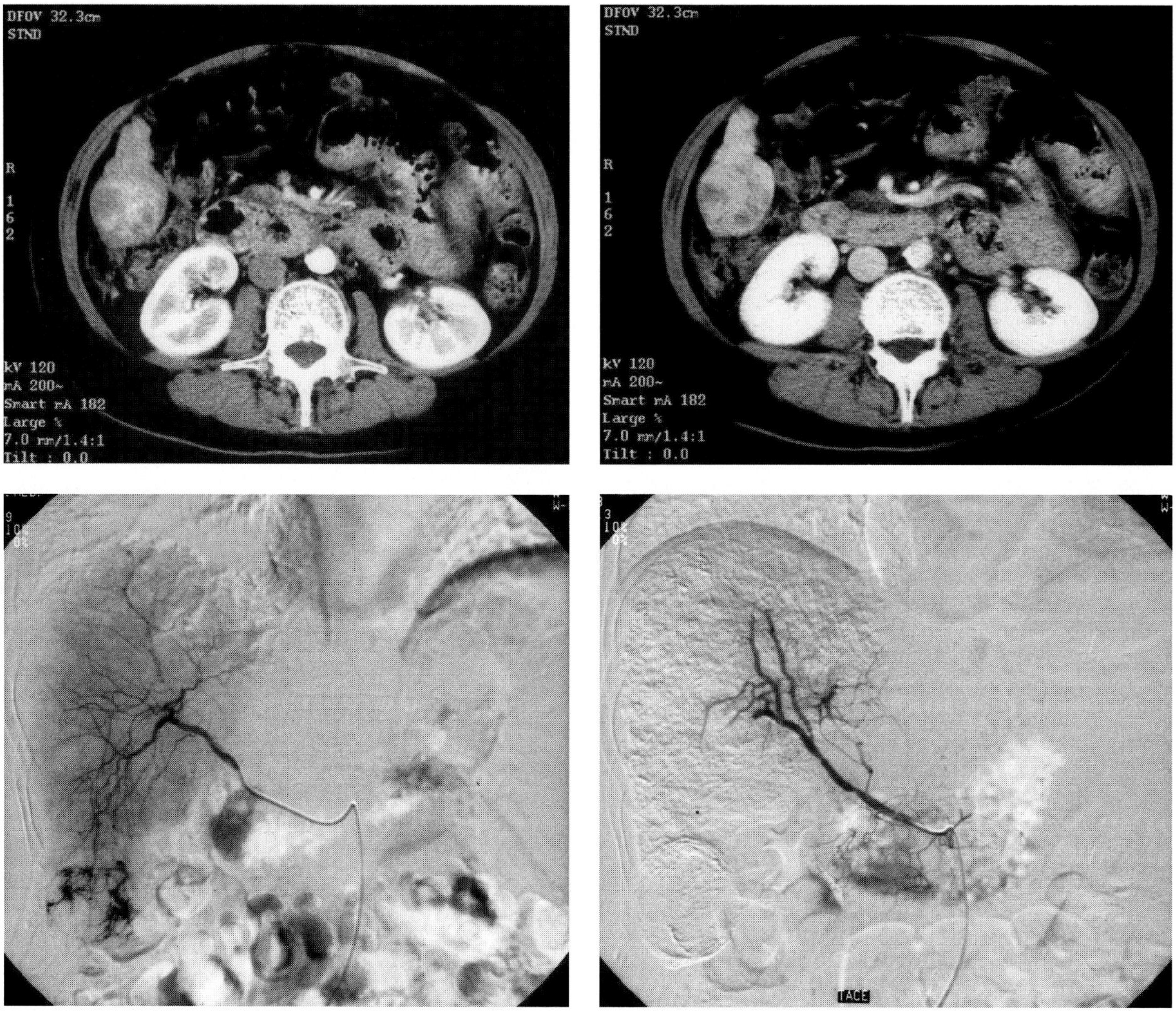

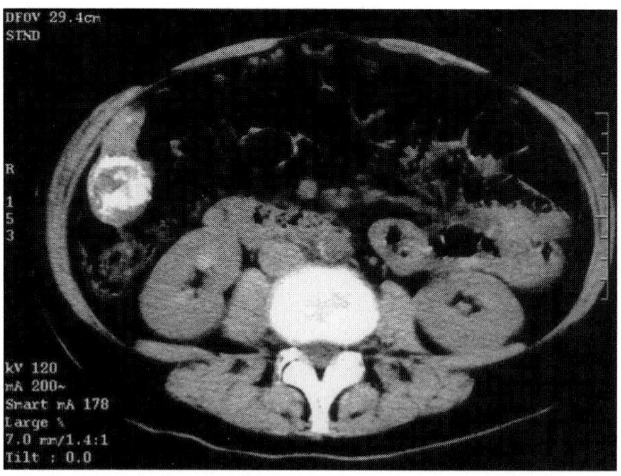

Fig. 30.10a–e. Hepatocellular carcinoma treated with transcatheter arterial chemoembolization. Pretreatment spiral CT in the arterial (**a**) and the portal phase (**b**) demonstrates nodular lesion of the VI hepatic segment. Digital subtraction angiography confirms uninodular tumor with peripheral basket-like neovascularization (**c**). After chemoembolization, tumor devascularization is seen on angiography (**d**). CT scan obtained 4 weeks later shows incomplete and inhomogeneous retention of iodized oil, suggesting partial response (**e**)

RF thermal ablation is a promising and rapidly evolving technique for the treatment of liver malignancies. Until a few years ago, RF treatment performed with a single, unmodified monopolar electrode was capable of producing cylindrical lesions no greater than 1.6 cm in diameter. Recent improvements in the RF technique included the development of expandable electrode needles with multiple retractable lateral exit jackhooks on the tip, and the introduction of high-power generators coupled with

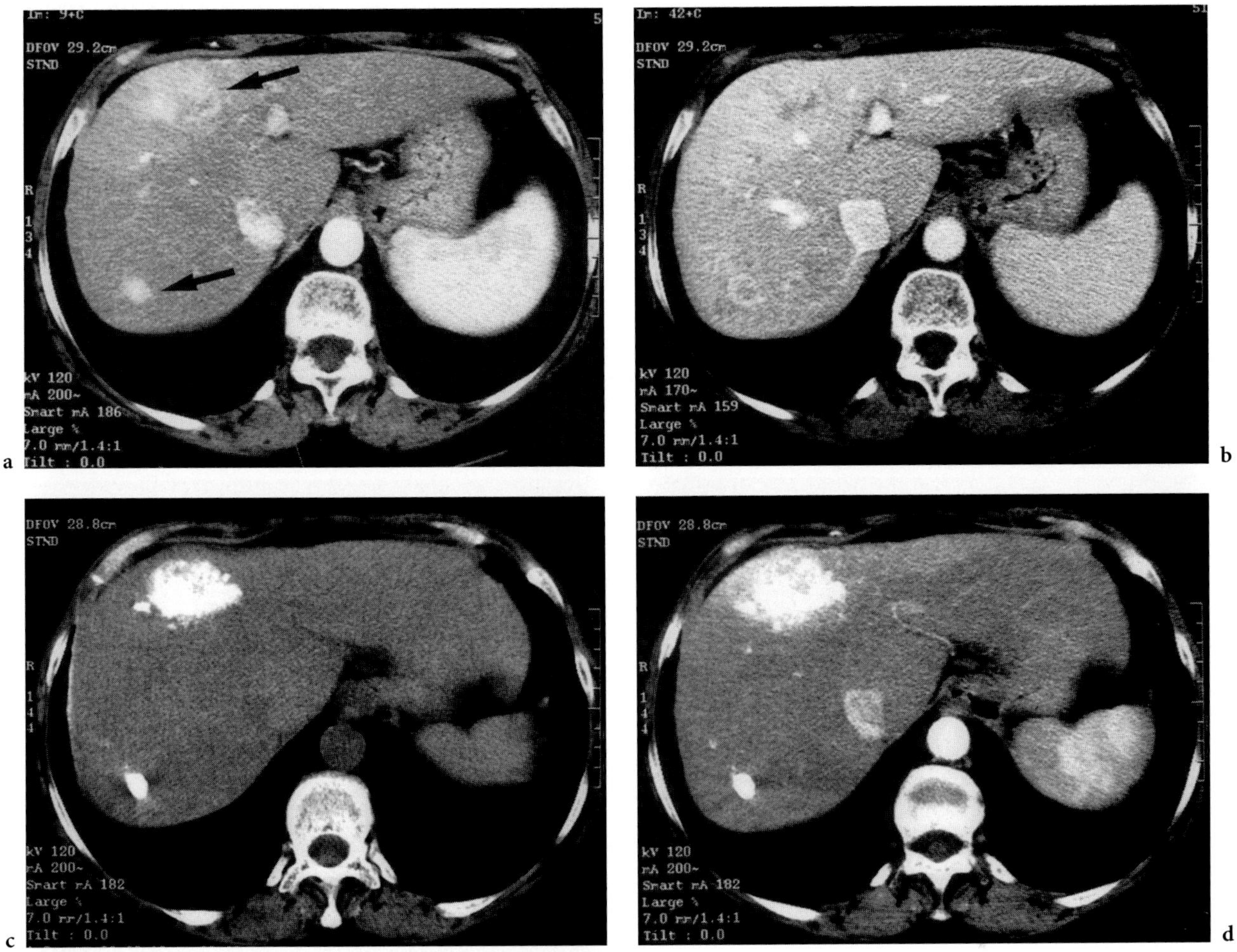

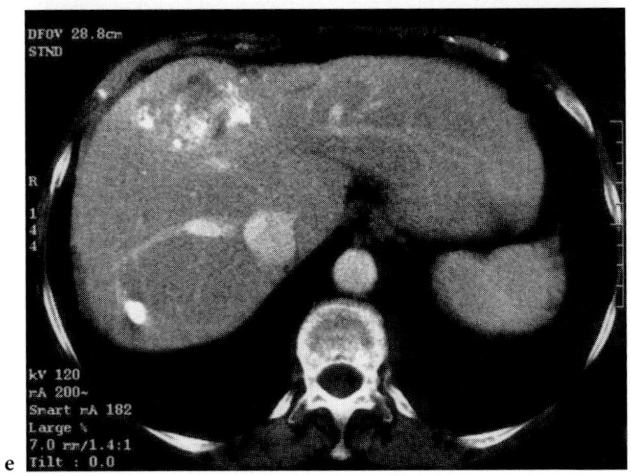

Fig. 30.11a–e. Multinodular hepatocellular carcinoma with complete response after chemoembolization. Spiral CT performed before treatment shows main tumor and satellite lesion (*arrows*) that are hyperdense in the arterial phase (**a**) and iso-hypodense in the portal phase (**b**). On unenhanced CT scan obtained four weeks after chemoembolization, the main tumor shows partial and inhomogeneous retention of iodized oil, while the daughter nodule appears homogeneously hyperattenuating (**c**). Contrast-enhanced images in the arterial (**d**) and the portal (**e**) phases demonstrate residual viable enhancing tumor tissue within the main lesion

dual-lumen, cooled-tip electrode needles (Rossi et al. 1996, 1998; Solbiati et al. 1997a,b; Lencioni et al. 1998a; Goldberg et al. 1998a,b). With these advances, the extent of coagulation necrosis that can be obtained with a single-probe insertion has substantially increased. These generators, in fact, are capable of producing spherical or nearly spherical volumes of thermal necrosis up to 3–4 cm in diameter with a single-probe insertion (Solbiati et al. 1997a,b; Lencioni et al. 1998a; Goldberg et al. 1998a,b).

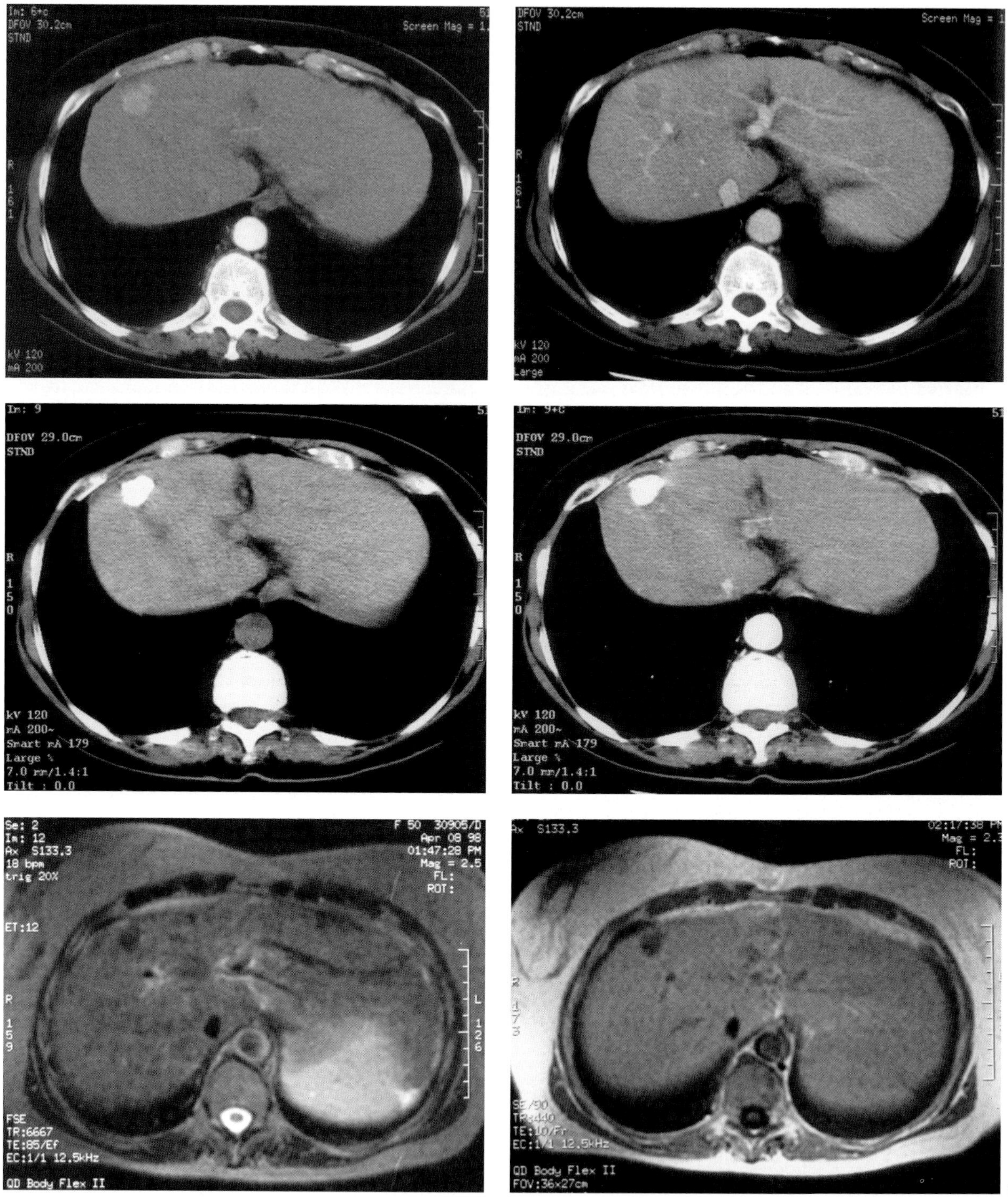

Fig. 30.12a–f. Hepatocellular carcinoma treated with transcatheter arterial chemoembolization. Before treatment, the lesion is hyperattenuating in the arterial phase (**a**) and hypoattenuating in the portal phase (**b**). CT scan obtained 4 weeks after chemoembolization shows dense and homogeneous retention of iodized oil, suggesting complete tumor response (**c**). No contrast uptake at the periphery of the tumor is demonstrated in the arterial phase image (**d**). Fast spin-echo T2-weighted MR image shows the lesion as a hypointense nodule, suggesting coagulative necrosis (**e**). Gd-DTPA-enhanced spin-echo T1-weighted MR image fails to demonstrate contrast uptake by the lesion, confirming complete response (**f**)

Among other interventional methods of local tissue destruction, RF ablation has some inherent advantages. Compared with percutaneous ethanol injection, RF treatment produces a more predictable volume of necrosis at every insertion and is not impaired by the hard consistency of metastatic tissue, which makes ethanol injection ineffective in secondary tumors. With respect to laser photocoagulation, RF treatment is less expensive and seems to create a larger coagulation necrosis volume for each needle insertion, thus simplifying the procedure and shortening the treatment time. Cryosurgery, on the other hand, has disadvantages in that it requires laparotomy to place the probe directly into the lesion and the larger probe size significantly increases the morbidity of the procedure.

The evaluation of the therapeutic effect of the procedure results in different problems according to the histotype of the malignancy. In the case of HCC, in fact, the assessment of tumor response is easier by virtue of the typical hypervascular pattern of this neoplasm. Hence, residual viable tumor tissue after RF therapy can be identified with the different imaging modalities (color Doppler US, spiral CT, or dynamic MR imaging) by using the same diagnostic criteria reported above for lesions treated with PEI. Therefore, contrast-enhanced color and power Doppler US can be useful to monitor the outcome of therapy and, in the case of partial ablation, to target areas of residual viable tumor, whereas spiral CT or dynamic MR imaging should be used as a final diagnostic test to establish the outcome of treatment.

It should be noted that, in the case of HCC, RF treatment tends to produce a volume of thermal necrosis that matches that of the original lesion. This is mainly due to the differences in tissue impedance between tumor interior and surrounding cirrhotic tissue. RF waves do not progress easily outside the lesion because of the reduced conductivity of cirrhotic tissue. As a result, the heat deposition is higher within the tumor, and even lesions exceeding the expected necrosis volume can often be successfully treated. In the case of HCC, the evidence of an unenhancing area replacing the entire lesion at spiral CT or dynamic MR imaging usually indicates successful ablation (Rossi et al. 1996, 1998; Goldberg et al. 1998b).

The same criteria, however, cannot be confidently adopted in the case of metastatic lesions. There are some important differences between metastases and HCC that must be taken into account when assessing treatment outcome. First, metastases (with few exceptions) are hypovascular lesions: hence, residual viable tumor tissue will not stand out in the arterial phase images obtained with spiral CT or dynamic MR imaging, and intratumoral flow will be hardly identified by Doppler US, even by using the power mode in combination with microbubble contrast agents to maximize color sensitivity. Second, metastases do not have a clear lesion-to-liver interface like nodular-type HCC, but tend to strand into the surrounding liver parenchyma: hence, if the necrosis volume produced by RF treatment is nearly equivalent to that of the visible native lesion, tumor recurrence caused by microscopic remains of tumor along the boundary is very likely to occur.

Therefore, to make a confident diagnosis of successful ablation, it is necessary to depict an area of thermal necrosis volume exceeding that of the original lesion, with at least a 0.5-cm "safety margin" of coagulation necrosis in the liver parenchyma all around the lesion (Figs. 30.13–30.15).

This "safety margin" can be obtained in the case of small metastatic lesions because the progression of RF waves outside the lesion is not impaired by the poor conductivity of cirrhotic tissue as in HCC, provided that the lesion is not located close to vascular structures. Flowing blood within the vessels, in fact, acts as a heat sink and substantially limits the necrotizing effect of RF treatment in the adjacent tissue (Solbiati et al. 1997a,b; Lencioni et al. 1998a; Goldberg et al. 1998a,b).

If the imaging assessment of the outcome of therapy is performed shortly after the procedure, spiral CT and dynamic MR imaging may show the presence of a peripheral halo surrounding the treated lesion. This halo, which may be irregular in shape and thickness, enhances predominantly in the arterial phase, and is due to the inflammatory reaction along the periphery of the area of thermal necrosis. It is usually more pronounced in metastases than in HCC, as the injury produced in the liver parenchyma adjacent to the lesion is higher, because the lack of a clear border between tumor and normal liver and the higher conductivity of non-cirrhotic tissue facilitate progression of RF waves into the noncancerous parenchyma (Figs. 30.16, 30.17).

This enhancing halo is depicted for several days after treatment, and usually disappears in later follow-up studies. It is of course of the utmost importance to be aware of this feature to prevent misinterpretation of a peripheral inflammatory reaction associated with a successful ablation as tumor progression. To make a reliable assessment, it is crucial to compare pretreatment and posttreatment studies performed by using the same technical examination

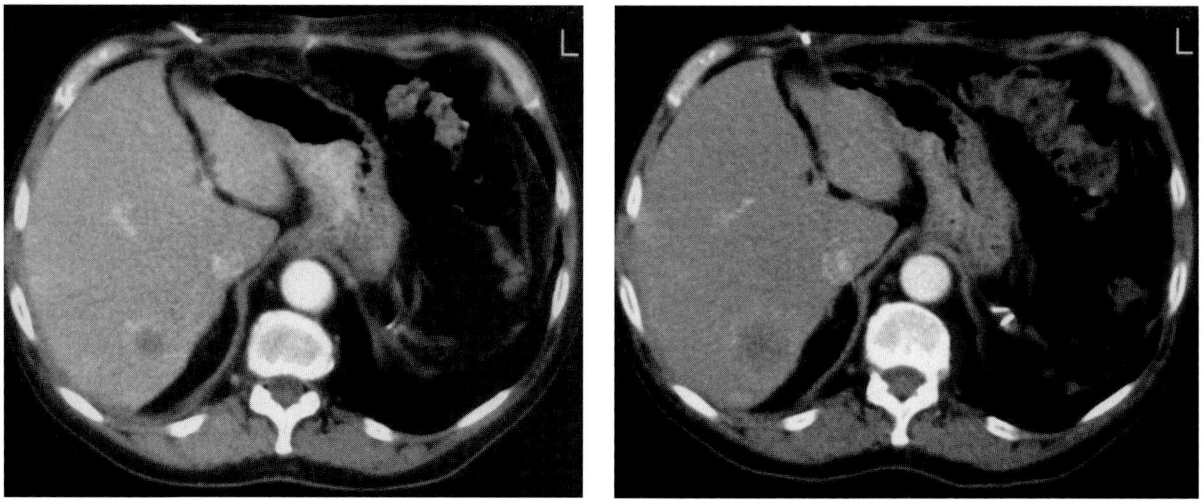

a b

Fig. 30.13a,b. Small hepatic metastasis treated with radiofrequency thermal ablation. Comparison between pretreatment (**a**) and posttreatment CT (**b**) shows an area of coagulation necrosis exceeding the size of the lesion. At least a 0.5-cm safety margin around the lesion is observed

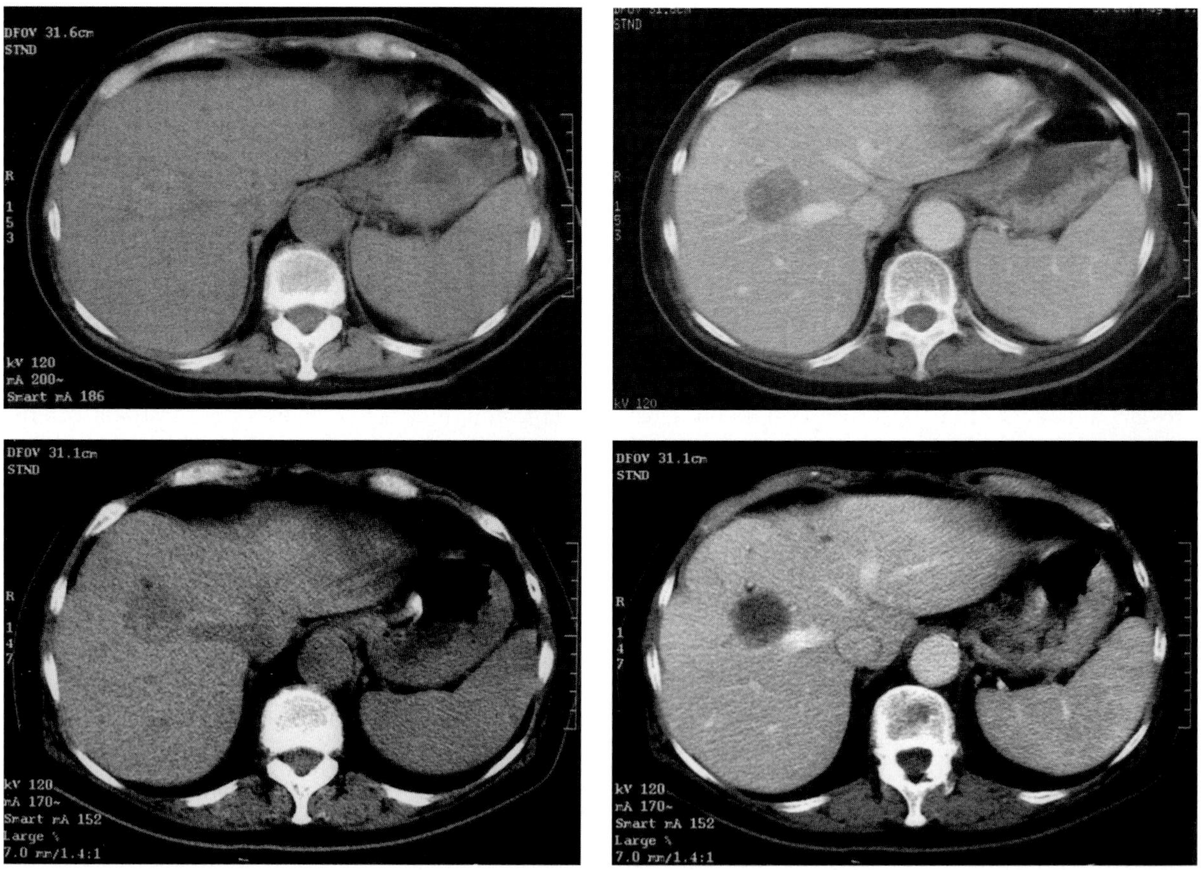

a b c d

Fig. 30.14a–d. Hepatic metastastis treated with radiofrequency thermal ablation. Comparison between CT images obtained before (precontrast, **a**; postcontrast, **b**) and after treatment (precontrast, **c**; postcontrast, **d**) shows an area of coagulation necrosis that matches the native lesion. There is no safety margin around the lesion. Tumor recurrence is predictable on the basis of CT findings

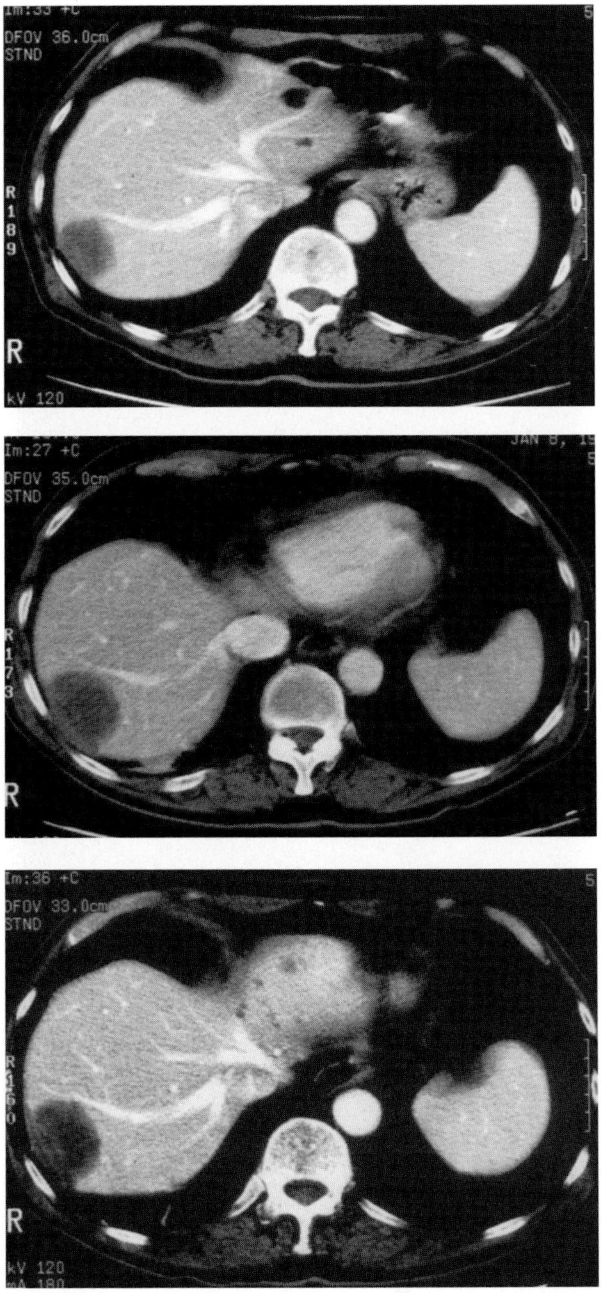

a

b

c

Fig. 30.15a–c. Hepatic metastastis treated with radiofrequency thermal ablation. **a** Pretreatment CT shows solitary metastasis of VII hepatic segment. After radiofrequency thermal ablation, partial necrosis is seen, with residual viable tumor in the antero-lateral aspect of the lesion (**b**). Following repeated radiofrequency ablation, a larger area of necrosis replacing the lesion and part of surrounding parenchyma is depicted (**c**)

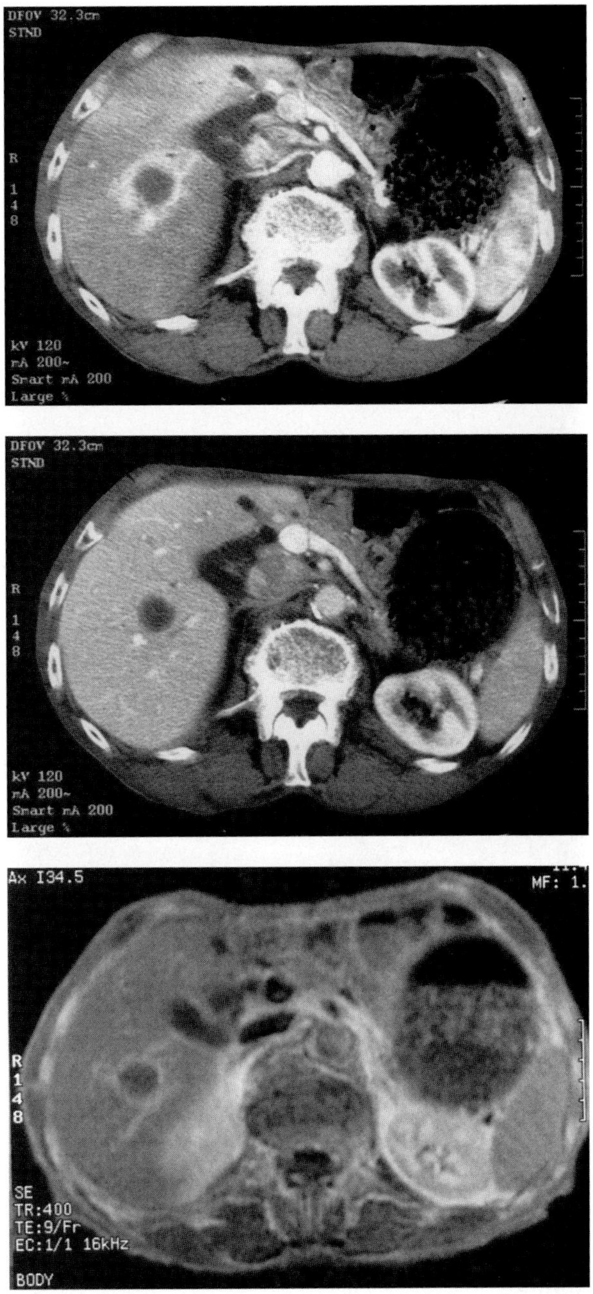

b

b

c

Fig. 30.16a–c Hepatic metastastis treated with radiofrequency thermal ablation. Spiral CT in the arterial (**a**) and the portal phase (**b**), performed two days after the procedure, shows a central area of necrosis with peripheral enhancement due to marked inflammatory reaction. The same feature is less evident in the contrast-enhanced MR image acquired 2 weeks later (**c**)

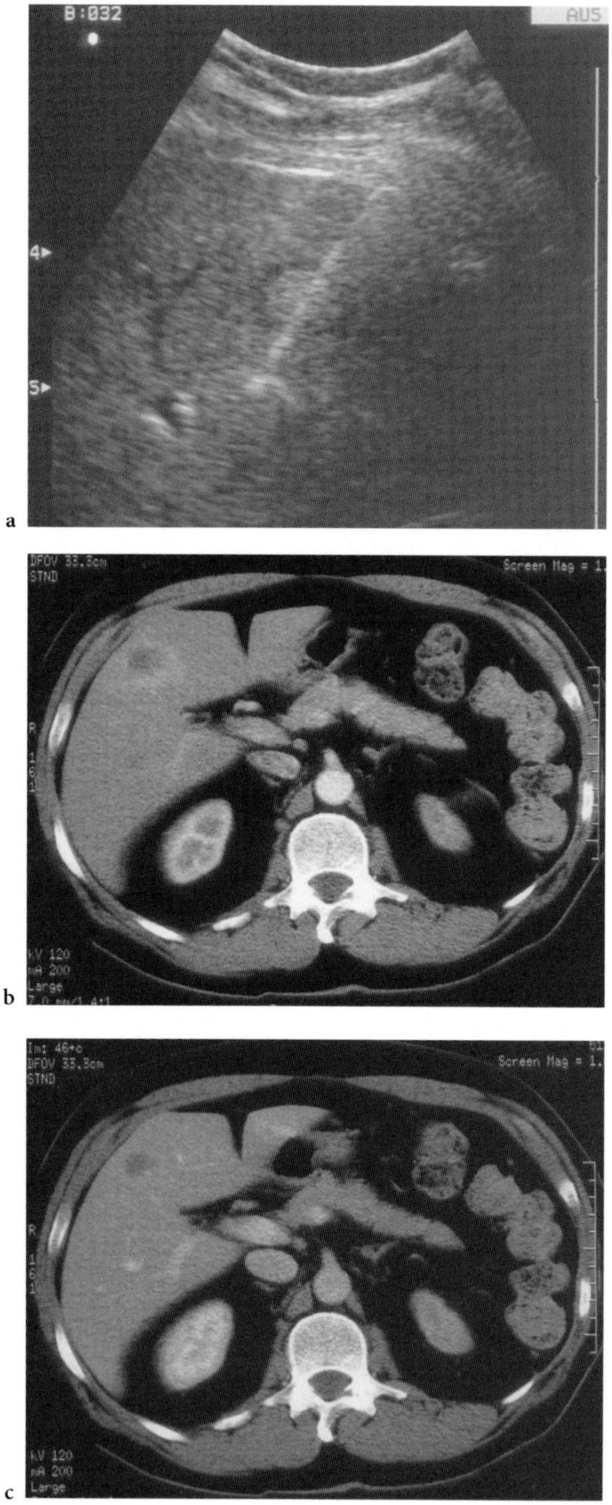

Fig. 30.17a–c. Hepatic metastastis treated with radiofrequency thermal ablation. Ultrasound image acquired at the time of the insertion of the electrode needle (**a**). Dual-phase spiral CT in the arterial (**b**) and the portal phase (**c**) shows hypoattenuating area of necrosis with peripheral enhancement due to inflammatory reaction

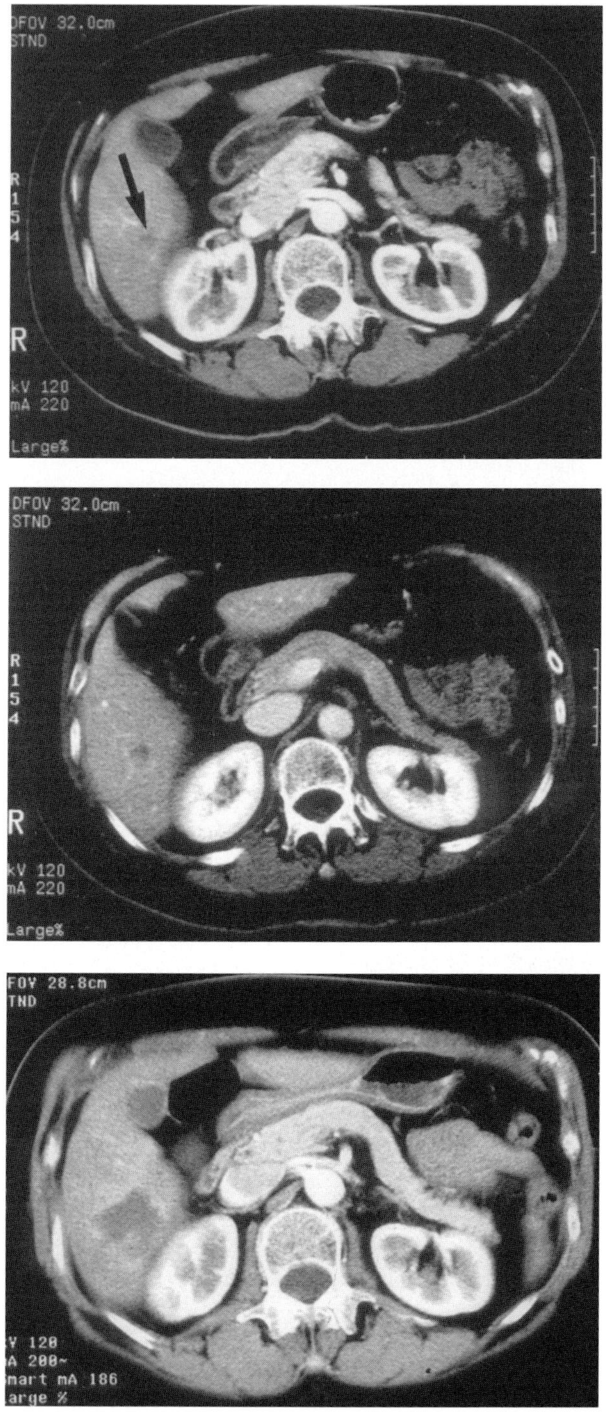

Fig. 30.18a–f. Hepatic metastastis treated with radiofrequency thermal ablation. Before treatment, the small lesion (*arrow*) appears hypoattenuating in both the arterial (**a**) and the portal phase (**b**). After ablation, an area of coagulation replacing the lesion as well as part of surrounding parenchyma is detected (**c**, arterial phase; **d**, portal phase). Follow-up CT study after 6 months confirms complete tumor ablation (**e**, arterial phase; **f**, portal phase)

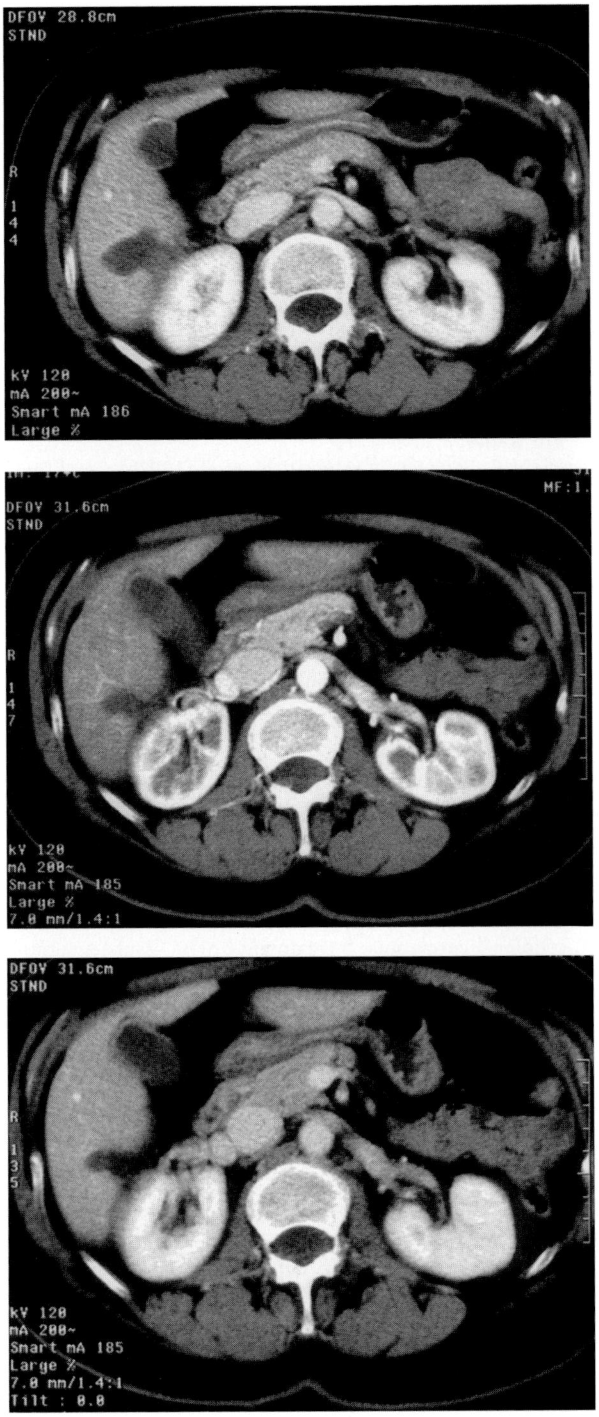

d e f

protocol (Rossi et al. 1996 1998; Solbiati et al. 1997a,b; Lencioni et al. 1998a; Goldberg et al. 1998a,b).

A careful follow-up protocol is to be recommended in the case of metastases treated by RF ablation (Fig. 30.18).

The recurrence of the treated lesion, in fact, is more frequent in metastases than in HCC. In addition, patients with metastases, because of the biology of the disease, are at high risk of developing new intrahepatic lesions or extrahepatic metastases.

References

Allgaier HP, Deibert P, Olschewski M, et al (1998) Survival benefit of patients with inoperable hepatocellular carcinoma treated by a combination of transarterial chemoembolization and percutaneous ethanol injection – a single-center analysis including 132 patients. Int J Cancer 79:601–605

Bartolozzi C, Lencioni R (1996) Ethanol injection for the treatment of hepatic tumours. Eur Radiol 6:682–696

Bartolozzi C, Lencioni R, Caramella D, et al (1994a) Treatment of hepatocellular carcinoma with percutaneous ethanol injection: evaluation with contrast-enhanced MR imaging. AJR 162:827–831

Bartolozzi C, Lencioni R, Caramella D, et al (1994b) Hepatocellular carcinoma: CT and MR features after transcatheter arterial embolization and percutaneous ethanol injection. Radiology 191:123–128

Bartolozzi C, Lencioni R, Caramella D, et al (1995) Treatment of large hepatocellular carcinoma: transcatheter arterial chemoembolization combined with percutaneous ethanol injection versus repeated transcatheter arterial chemoembolization. Radiology 197:812–818

Bartolozzi C, Lencioni R, Ricci P, Paolicchi A, Rossi P, Passariello R (1998) Hepatocellular carcinoma treatment with percutaneous ethanol injection: evaluation with contrast-enhanced color Doppler US. Radiology 209:387–393

Becker CD, Grossholz M, Mentha G, et al (1997) Ablation of hepatocellular carcinoma by percutaneous ethanol injection: imaging findings. Cardiovasc Intervent Radiol 20:204–210

Castellano L, Calandra M, Del Vecchio Blanco C, De Sio I(1997) Predictive factors of survival and intrahepatic recurrence of hepatocellular carcinoma in cirrhosis after percutaneous ethanol injection: analysis of 71 patients. J Hepatol 27:862–870

Choi BI, Kim TK, Han JK, et al (1992) Therapeutic effect of transcatheter oily chemoembolization therapy for encapsulated nodular hepatocellular carcinoma: CT and pathologic findings. Radiology 182:709–713

Colombo M (1997) Treatment of hepatocellular carcinoma. J Viral Hepat 4:S125-S130

Dalla Palma L (1998) Diagnostic imaging and interventional therapy of hepatocellular carcinoma. Br J Radiol 71:808–818

De Sanctis JT, Goldberg SN, Mueller PR (1998) Percutaneous treatment of hepatic neoplasms: a review of current techniques. Cardiovasc Intervent Radiol 21:273–296

Fujita T, Honjo K,Ito K, et al (1998) Dynamic MR follow-up of small hepatocellular carcinoma after percutaneous ethanol injection therapy. J Comput Assist Tomogr 22:379–386

Goldberg SN, Hahn PF, Tanabe KK, et al (1998a)Percutaneous radiofrequency tissue ablation: does perfusion-mediated tissue cooling limit coagulation necrosis? J Vasc Interv Radiol 9:101–111

Goldberg SN, Gazelle GS, Solbiati L, et al (1998b) Ablation of liver tumors using percutaneous RF therapy. AJR 170:1023–1028

Groupe d'Etude et de Traitement du Carcinome Hepatocellulaire (1995) A comparison of lipiodol chemoembolization and conservative treatment for unresectable hepatocellular carcinoma. N Engl J Med 332:1256–1261

Ito K, Honjo K, Fujita T, Awaya H, Mastumoto T, Mastunaga N (1995) Enhanced MR imaging of the liver after ethanol treatment of hepatocellular carcinoma: evaluation of areas of hyperperfusion adjacent to the tumor. AJR 164:1413–1417

Johnson RC (1997) Hepatocellular carcinoma. Hepatogastroenterology 44:307–312

Joseph FB, Baumgartner DA, Bernardino ME (1993) Hepatocellular carcinoma: CT appearance after percutaneous ethanol ablation therapy. Radiology 186:553–556

Kim AY, Choi BI, Kim TK, et al (1998) Hepatocellular carcinoma: power Doppler US with a contrast agent – preliminary results. Radiology 209:135–140

Kim DE, Kim PN, Lee HJ, et al (1998) Vasculature in hepatocellular carcinoma after transcatheter arterial chemoembolization: comparison of power and color Doppler sonography. J Ultrasound Med 17:9–15

Kim TK, Choi BI, Han JK, Chung JW, Park JH, Han MC (1998) Nontumorous arterioportal shunt mimicking hypervascular tumor in cirrhotic liver: two-phase spiral CT findings. Radiology 208:597–603

Koda M, Okamoto K, Miyoshi Y, et al (1994) Combination therapy with transcatheter arterial embolization and percutaneous ethanol injection for advanced hepatocellular carcinoma. Hepatogastroenterology 41:25–29

Kubota Y, Nakano T, Seki T, et al (1989) Validity of MR imaging for monitoring effects of percutaneous ethanol injection for HCC. Hepatogastroenterology 36:262–265

Kumada T, Nakano S, Takeda I, et al (1997) Patterns of recurrence after initial treatment in patients with small hepatocellular carcinoma. Hepatology 25:87–92

Lencioni R, Bartolozzi C (1997) Nonsurgical treatment of hepatocellular carcinoma. Cancer J 10:17–23

Lencioni R, Caramella D, Bartolozzi C (1993) Response of hepatocellular carcinoma to percutaneous ethanol injection: CT and MR evaluation. J Comput Assist Tomogr 17: 723–729

Lencioni R, Caramella D, Vignali C, et al (1994a) Lipiodol-TC in the detection of tumor persistence in hepatocellular carcinoma treated with percutaneous ethanol injection therapy. Acta Radiol 35:323–328

Lencioni R, Vignali C, Caramella D, et al (1994b) Transcatheter arterial embolization followed by percutaneous ethanol injection in the treatment of hepatocellular carcinoma. Cardiovasc Intervent Radiol 17:70–75

Lencioni R, Bartolozzi C, Caramella D, et al (1995a) Treatment of small hepatocellular carcinoma with percutaneous ethanol injection: analysis of prognostic factors in 105 Western patients. Cancer 76:1737–1746

Lencioni R, Caramella D, Bartolozzi C (1995b) Hepatocellular carcinoma: use of color Doppler US to evaluate response to treatment with percutaneous ethanol injection. Radiology 194:113–118

Lencioni R, Caramella D, Sanguinetti F, Battolla L, Falaschi F, Bartolozzi C (1995c) Portal vein thrombosis after percutaneous ethanol injection for hepatocellular carcinoma: value of color Doppler sonography in distinguishing chemical and tumor thrombi. AJR 164:1125–1130

Lencioni R, Pinto F, Armillotta N, Bartolozzi C (1996) Assessment of tumor vascularity in hepatocellular carcinoma: comparison of power Doppler US and color Doppler US. Radiology 201:353–358

Lencioni R, Pinto F, Armillotta N, et al (1997) Long-term results of percutaneous ethanol injection therapy for hepatocellular carcinoma in cirrhosis: a European experience. Eur Radiol 7:514–519

Lencioni R, Goletti O, Armillotta N, et al (1998a) Radio-frequency thermal ablation of liver metastases with a cooled-tip electrode needle: results of a pilot clinical trial. Eur Radiol 8:1205–1211

Lencioni R, Paolicchi A, Moretti M, et al (1998b) Combined transcatheter arterial chemoembolization and percutaneous ethanol injection for the treatment of large hepatocellular carcinoma: local therapeutic effect and long-term survival rate. Eur Radiol 8:439–444

Lin DY, Lin SM, Liaw YF (1997) Non-surgical treatment of hepatocellular carcinoma. J Gastroenterol Hepatol 12:S319-S328

Livraghi T (1998) Percutaneous ethanol injection in the treatment of hepatocellular carcinoma in cirrhosis. Hepatogastroenterology 45(S3):1248–1253

Livraghi T, Festi D, Monti M, et al (1986) US-guided percutaneous alcohol injection of small hepatic and abdominal tumors. Radiology 161:309–312

Livraghi T, Giorgio A, Marin G, et al (1995) Hepatocellular carcinoma and cirrhosis in 746 patients: long-term results of percutaneous ethanol injection. Radiology 197:101–108

Matsui O, Kadoya M, Yoshikawa J, et al (1993) Small hepatocellular carcinoma: treatment with subsegmental transcatheter arterial embolization. Radiology 188:79–83

Menu Y (1998) Hepatocellular carcinoma: radiological findings. Hepatogastroenterology 45(S3):1232–1235

Murayama S, Tsukamoto Y, Watanabe H, Nakata H (1986) Computed tomography of residual hepatomas following transcatheterarterial embolization. J Comput Assist Tomogr 10:969–972

Nagel HS, Bernardino ME (1993) Contrast-enhanced MR imaging of hepatic lesions treated with percutaneous ethanol ablation therapy. Radiology 189:265–270

Naik KS, Ward J, Guthrie JA, et al (1997) Hepatic lesions detection: a comparison of super-paramagnetic ferum oxide (SPIO) enhanced MR imaging and dual-phase helical CT with AFROC analysis. Radiology 205(P):372

Nishizaki T, Takenaka K, Yanaga K, et al (1997) Early detection of recurrent hepatocellular carcinoma. Hepatogastroenterology 44:508–513

Pompili M, Rapaccini GL, De Luca F, et al (1997) Risk factors for intrahepatic recurrence of hepatocellular carcinoma in cirrhotic patients treated by percutaneous ethanol injection. Cancer 79:1501–1508

Ros PR, Freeny PC, Harms SE, et al (1995) Hepatic MR imaging with ferumoxides: a multicenter clinical trial of the safety and efficacy in the detection of focal hepatic lesions. Radiology 196:481–488

Rossi S, Di Stasi M, Buscarini E, et al (1996) Percutaneous RF interstitial thermal ablation in the treatment of hepatic cancer. AJR 167:759–768

Rossi S, Buscarini E, Garbagnati F, et al (1998) Percutaneous treatment of small hepatic tumors by using an expandable RF electrode needle. AJR 170:1015–1022

Sironi S, Livraghi T, Del Maschio A (1991) Small hepatocellular carcinoma treated with percutaneous ethanol injection. MR imaging findings. Radiology 180: 333–336

Sironi S, Livraghi T, Angeli E, et al (1993) Small hepatocellular carcinoma: MR follow-up of treatment with percutaneous ethanol injection. Radiology 187:119–123

Sironi S, De Cobelli F, Livraghi T, et al (1994) Small hepatocellular carcinoma treated with percutaneous ethanol injection: unenhanced and gadolinium-enhanced MR imaging follow-up. Radiology 192:407–412

Solbiati L (1998) New applications of ultrasonography: interventional ultrasound. Eur J Radiol 27:S200-S206

Solbiati L, Goldberg SN, Ierace T, et al (1997a) Hepatic metastases: percutaneous radio-frequency ablation with cooled-tip electrodes. Radiology 205:367–373

Solbiati L, Ierace T, Goldberg SN, et al (1997b) Percutaneous US-guided radio-frequency tissue ablation of liver metastases: treatment and follow up in 16 patients. Radiology 202:195–203

Steele G Jr, Ravikumar TS (1989) Resection of hepatic metastases from colorectal cancer: biological perspectives. Ann Surg 210:127–138

Takayasu K, Moriyama N, Muramatsu Y, et al (1984) Hepatic artery embolization for hepatocellular carcinoma: comparison of CT scans and resected specimens. Radiology 150:661–665

Tanaka K, Nakamura S, Numata K, et al (1992) Hepatocellular carcinoma: treatment with percutaneous ethanol injection and transcatheter arterial embolization. Radiology 185:457–460

Tanaka K, Nakamura S, Numata K, et al (1998) The long term efficacy of combined transcatheter arterial embolization and percutaneous ethanol injection in the treatment of patients with large hepatocellular carcinoma and cirrhosis. Cancer 82:78–85

Ueno N, Tomiyama T, Tano S (1998) Color Doppler sonography-guided ethanol injection therapy for hepatocellular carcinoma. AJR 170:515–519

Yoshioka H, Nakagawa K, Shindou H, et al (1990) MR imaging of the liver before and after transcatheter hepatic chemoembolization for hepatocellular carcinoma. Acta Radiol 31:63–67

Yu JS, Kim KW, Sung KB, Lee JT, Yoo HS (1997) Small arterial-portal venous shunts: a cause of pseudolesions at hepatic imaging. Radiology 203:737–742

31 Ultrasound-Guided Biopsy of Malignant Liver Lesions

L. Buscarini, E. Buscarini, and R. Foroni

CONTENTS

31.1 Introduction

Ultrasonography (US), even associated with other imaging techniques, allows an exhaustive diagnosis of liver lesions only in some cases: however, it is not always possible to distinguish a malignant lesion from a benign one; in a high number of cases diagnosis of histotype is impossible on the basis of imaging examination alone, even when completed by clinical and laboratory criteria. Ultrasound guided biopsy is the method of choice for diagnostic purposes in this field.

L. Buscarini, MD; Chief, Department of Gastroenterology, General Hospital, Cantone del Cristo 40, I-29100 Piacenza Italy
E. Buscarini, MD; Department of Gastroenterology, General Hospital, Cantone del Cristo 40, I-29100 Piacenza Italy
R. Foroni, MD; Department of Pathology, General Hospital, Via Taverna 49, I-29100 Piacenza Italy

31.2 Procedure

31.2.1 Patient

Biopsy is an invasive procedure and should be applied only when a precise even if variable treatment for the patient cannot be achievable with less invasive methods. Preliminary to the biopsy informed consent should be obtained, preferably in written form, where mortality rate and some of the major complications are generally indicated. A detailed list is not useful because if only one of them is forgotten it could represent an element of fault if the forgotten one occurred.

Biopsy can be performed in outpatients if there is no sign of a high risk of bleeding; in this case the patient will remain under observation for two hours at least and will receive a second US observation before the discharge; obviously the patient should have the opportunity to be cared for by a responsible person, to contact the center and to be within easy reach of it (taking no longer than 1 h).

Blood clotting tests: it is mandatory to perform an investigation of the coagulative status, by evaluating at least platelet number, prothrombin time (PT) and partial thromboplastin time (PTT). The values generally accepted for the performance of biopsy are: platelet level not less than 50,000/mm^3; PT not less than 40–50% and PTT within the normal range. However, in patients with severe impairment of blood clotting function who experienced liver biopsy complications, similar results to those in patients without severe coagulopathy were found (Caturelli et al. 1993).

It is very important to point out the necessity of completing this step with an accurate anamnesis of previous bleedings and of eventual intake of drugs altering the coagulation. Assuming antiaggregants or calcium heparin at low dose, it is prudent to postpone the biopsy for the time necessary for drug clearance.

Premedication is not necessary except some very specific cases of anxiety.

31.2.2 Guidance

US guidance allows the performance of quicker and more accurate procedures than does computed tomography (CT). In a recent comparison with CT guidance, US guidance resulted in a significantly shorter room time during performance of a tissue biopsy with cost savings and increase in the number of procedures (SHEAFOR et al. 1998).

Guidance is generally performed by using a dedicated probe or a guidance device (which can be easily sterilized) applied to a normal sector or convex probes (Fig. 31.1); in this way the trajectory is oblique; it is very easy to follow the needle but the distance from the skin to the target is increased; with a perpendicular approach the access to the target is shorter but the visibility of the needle is often less clearer. It is necessary that the lesion coincides with an electronic marker on the US screen.

In the first period of application of US guided biopsy the so called free hand technique was used, and has since been followed by some centers. The probe is covered by a sterile piece of plastic and the needle is inserted close to the probe at an appropriate angle to enter the US beam and to be monitored up to the target (LIVRAGHI 1984). By using a guidance device the diagnostic efficacy of the biopsy is very high also for small lesions (less than 3 cm) (FORNARI et al. 1994).

31.2.3 Choice of Needles

It is possible to use aspiration needles to collect cytological material (the needle caliber is always fine: less than 1 mm) or needles to collect histologic material, which are, in many instances, fine needles even if in selected cases needles with a caliber of more than 1 mm can also be employed.

Cutting needles are Menghini or Tru-cut modified needles; the maneuver is the same as that using the original models. Many automated biopsy needles are commercially available, which can provide a high histologic recovery rate (MOULTON and MOORE 1993). They facilitate the maneuver, particularly for nonexperienced operators.

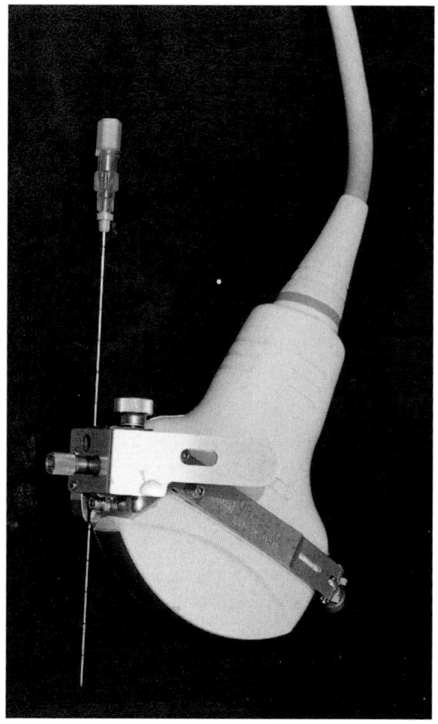

Fig. 31.1. Lateral guidance device applied to a convex probe; the fine needle has been inserted in the guide

We point out that modification of the needle surface (by making the distal part of the outer cannula rough, grooved, hammered, or faceted), made to enhance sonographic detectability (the so called echomarker), entails more potential to drag cells along the outside of the needle during biopsy, as experimentally shown; this observation has suggested caution in the clinical use of needles with an echomarker (BUSCARINI et al. 1997).

31.2.4 Technique

The biopsy is performed without local anesthesia and with normal rules of antisepsis. In a recent report, 357 liver biopsies were performed with the so called free hand technique without using sterile gloves or drapes or covers. Before the procedure the transducer was cleaned with water and 70% alcohol. In a follow-up at six months no patient or operator presented with fever or sepsis and the search for viral immunodeficiency virus antibodies or hepatitis markers remained negative (CATURELLI et al. 1996).

The best approach generally corresponds to the shortest distance to the target; either subcostal or intercostal approaches are possible. Special attention must be given to the needle track. The perforation of colon loops, especially in immunocompromised patients, may cause peritonitis due to dissemination of fecal material; on the other hand, the passage of the needle through the stomach or the small intestine seems to be without consequences. Moreover, it is important to avoid the passage through the main blood vessels and the gallbladder. To avoid hemorrhage complications it is advisable to keep at least 1 cm of normal parenchyma between the liver surface and the lesion (Solbiati et al. 1985). The patient is in the left lateral decubitus or supine postition; after disinfection of the skin with iodized alcohol, the needle is introduced without local anesthesia, inviting the patient to hold the breath or to breathe superficially. Aspiration biopsy is performed by introducing the needle to the target and, after withdrawal of the stylet, by connecting to a syringe generally mounted on a device shaped as a pistol to facilitate the aspiration. The needle performs movements up and down with a variable excursion, according to the diameter of the lesion. It is possible to obtain material also without aspiration but only for capillarity (Fagelman and Chess 1990).

Histology sampling is performed with Menghini modified needles (the needle is placed in the appropriate site for the lesion, according to its dimensions; after placing the syringe in aspiration the needle is advanced for 1–3 cm to obtain a representative tissue sample) or with a Tru-cut needle (the needle is positioned; the inner stylet is advanced and then the sheet, reported on the initial position, will trap the tissue located on the notched stylet). The bioptic apparatus is then retrieved.

31.2.5 Biopsy Material

The optimal cellular material consists of a small amount of soft or semiliquid specimen with as little blood as possible. Cellular material is smeared immediately; a part of the slides is dried with air; a part is placed on ethanol. It is advisable to perform an immediate check of the collected material, by using a rapid staining; in any case it has been shown that two punctures will yield adequate material in most cases (Civardi et al. 1988). The tissue fragments are processed as for any normal biopsy. Cyto-histochemical and/or immunocyto-histochemical reactions are carried out on the obtained material (cells, tissue fragments).

31.2.6 Cost

The economic cost of US guided biopsy with a cutting needle has been calculated to be about US $200 (Livraghi et al. 1993); obviously the cost of aspiration biopsy is less, due to the lower costs of both the needle used and of sample processing. However, the economic impact of US guided biopsy implies a saving of hospitalization days by obtaining a correct diagnosis in a shorter time (Silverman et al 1998; Verbanck et al. 1994).

31.3 Indications and Results

31.3.1 Primary Malignant Liver Tumors

31.3.1.1 Hepatocellular Carcinoma

US guided biopsy is the choice procedure for diagnosis of hepatocellular carcinoma (HCC); only in selected cases can it be substituted by biopsy under laparoscopic control. There is a general agreement that biopsy can be omitted in cases with nodular lesion in cirrhosis accompanied by increase of alpha-fetoprotein (AFP) serum levels to over 200–500 ng/ml. However, according to some authors a nodular lesion in cirrhosis can be considered with a good certainty a HCC and in patients who will undergo liver transplantation fine needle biopsy (FNB) should be omitted even in the absence of AFP modifications, and diagnosis can be performed only on the basis of imaging aspect. It has been pointed out, however, that a second tumor can arise in patients with HCC; B cell lymphoma has been observed in 10/317 patients with HCC (3.1%) (Di Stasi et al. 1994). The contemporary presence of both tumors has also been described (Cavanna et al. 1994).

Biopsy can be carried out either with cytological sampling or with a cutting needle generally with fine caliber. Diagnostic accuracy of cytology is very high with a sensitivity of more than 90% and a specificity of 100% (Bret et al. 1988; Sbolli et al 1990; Buscarini et al. 1990; Pedio et al. 1988; Sangalli et al. 1989).

Cytology identifies different types of HCC: well differentiated, moderately differentiated and poorly differentiated. In well differentiated HCCs the cells are very easily identified as hepatocytes but it could be very difficult to diagnose the malignant transformation (Figs. 31.2–31.4); diagnosis is facilitated by the presence of a large number of naked nuclei which show the same alterations observed in integer cells: dimensional abnormalities, irregular shape, flower aspect, chromatin alterations, and prominent nucleolus (Pedio et al. 1988).

To facilitate differential diagnosis between HCC and dysplastic nodules (according to recent classification) histological sampling, performing if possible a double biopsy into the lesion and outside the lesion, has been suggested (Kondo et al. 1989) or a double sampling with aspiration and with cutting needles to obtain either cytological and histological material (Sangalli et al. 1989) (Fig. 31.5).

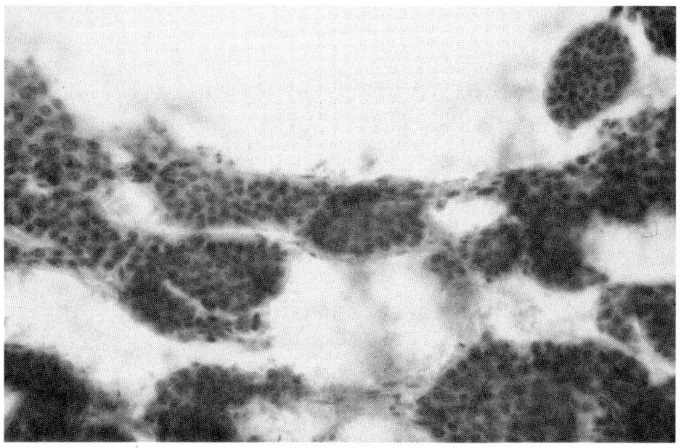

Fig. 31.2. Well differentiated hepatocellular carcinoma. High cellularity with irregular hepatocitic trabeculae, surrounded by spindle endothelial cells. Hepatocytes maintain cellular cohesivity with slight irregularities and infrequent presence of nucleolus. Papanicolau, ×250

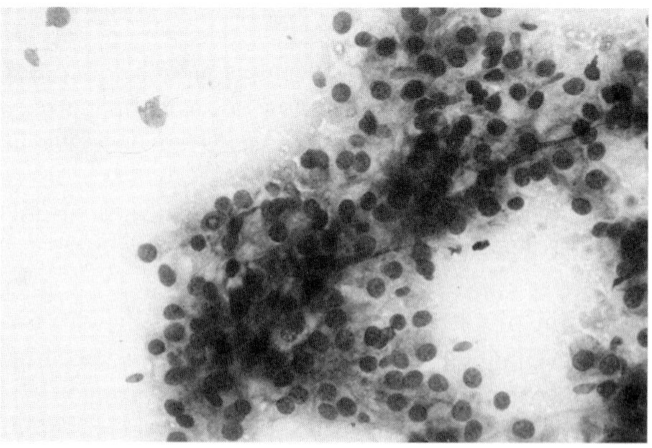

Fig. 31.3. Well differentiated hepatocellular carcinoma. Cluster of hepacytes with slight structural irregularities, sometimes presenting intranuclear vacuoles. Presence of some endothelial cells. May-Grunwald Giemsa, ×400

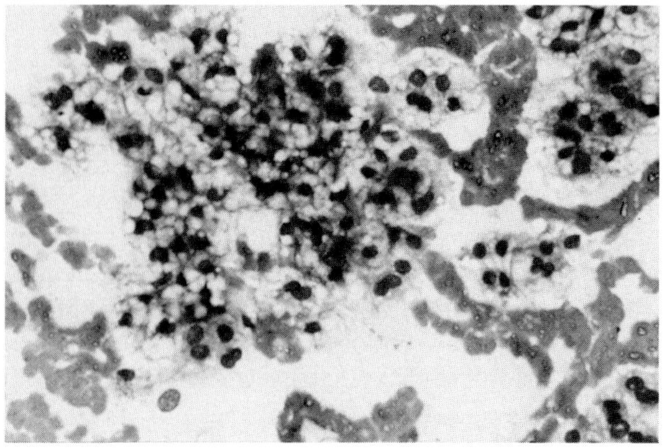

Fig. 31.4. Well differentiated hepatocellular carcinoma, clear cell variety. High cellularity with irregular hepatocyte clusters without important atypias; cytoplasm relatively large, with numerous vacuoles. May-Grunwald Giemsa, ×400

In moderately differentiated HCC the cells can have a relatively large size; nuclear-cytoplasmic ratio is increased with chromatin alterations. Intranuclear cytoplasmic inclusions and intracytoplasmic hyalin globules can be observed (Figs. 31.6, 31.7). Poorly differentiated HCC is characterized by irregular cells, with nuclear pleomorphism, a high nuclear-plasmatic ratio, and prominent nucleoli; naked nuclei can be present (Figs. 31.8, 31.9). Diagnosis of malignancy is easy but the hepatic cellular origin can sometimes represent a difficult diagnostic problem.

A multicenter study was performed collecting a series of 680 patients with HCC double biopsy (aspiration and cutting), showing a higher diagnostic sensitivity than single methods even if smear cytology appears to be a highly effective diagnostic procedure not only in moderately and poorly differentiated but also in well differentiated HCC (Buscarini et al. 1990; Rapaccini et al. 1994).

A recent study has compared the diagnostic value of cytology and microhistology by using a unique sampling with a modified needle which allows a tissue fragment and a cytological sample to be obtained simultaneously. In this situation the cytology showed a higher sensitivity than microhistology but the double examination in turn had a diagnostic sensitivity better than the single examination (Caturelli et al. 1994).

31.3.1.2 Other Primary Malignancies

HCC constituted more than 90% of the cases in a series of primary hepatic tumors from Japan. The

a

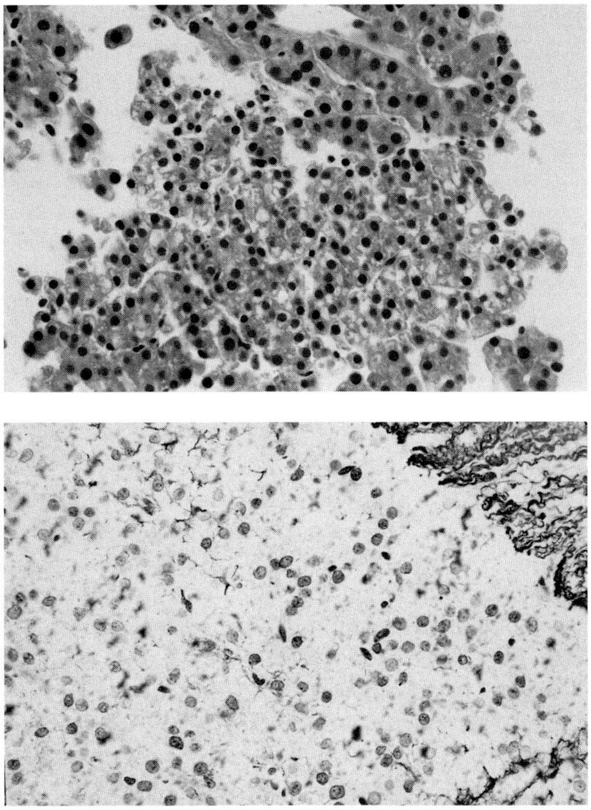

b

Fig. 31.5a,b. Well differentiated hepatocellular carcinoma. **a** Hepatocytic trabeculae have irregular thickness and are not uncommonly surrounded by spindle endothelial cells. Hepatocytes show minimal atypias. Hematoxylin-eosin, ×250. **b** Diagnosis can be proposed by studying the reticulum, which appears practically absent. Gomori, ×400

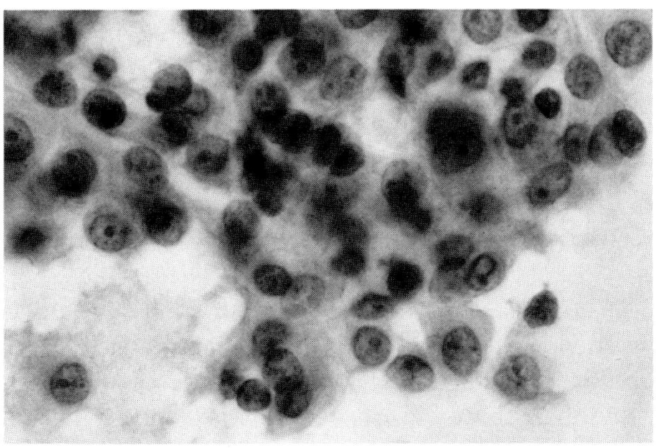

Fig. 31.6. Moderately differentiated hepatocellular carcinoma. Cluster of hepatocytes with evident atypias: thickening and irregularity of nuclear membrane, prominent nucleolus, intranuclear cytoplasmic inclusion, increase of nucleus/cytoplasm rate. The presence of bile globules mixed with tumoral cells concurs to identify the hepatic cellular nature. Papanicolau, ×400

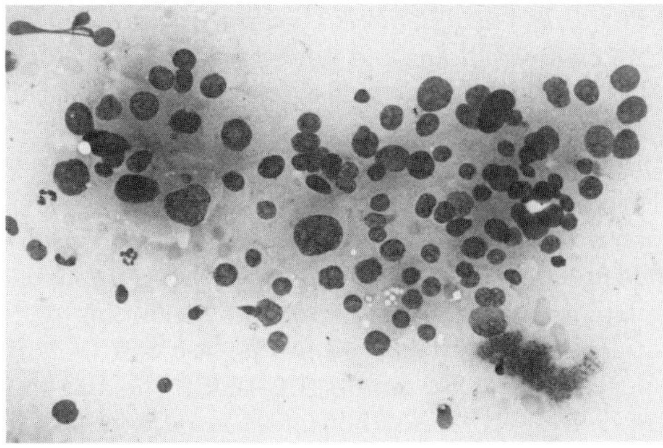

Fig. 31.7. Moderately differentiated hepatocellular carcinoma. Scattered atypical hepatocytes of relatively large size with evident structural disorder and anisocariosis. May-Grunwald Giemsa, ×400

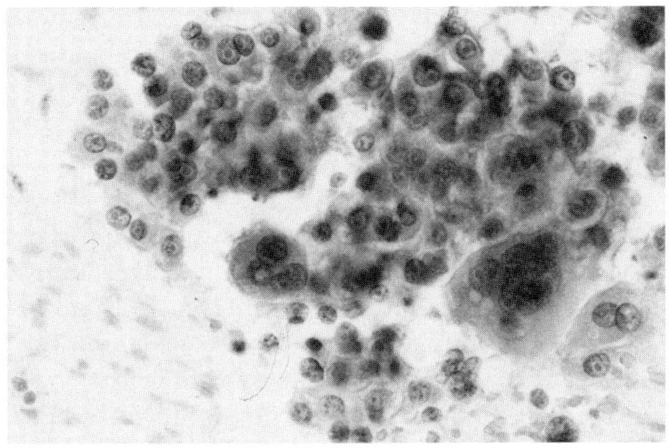

Fig. 31.8. Poorly differentiated hepatocellular carcinoma. Hepatocytes with very atypical features, multinuclearity and prominent nucleoli. The hepatocytic nature is still evident above all due to cytoplasmic characteristics. Papanicolau, ×400

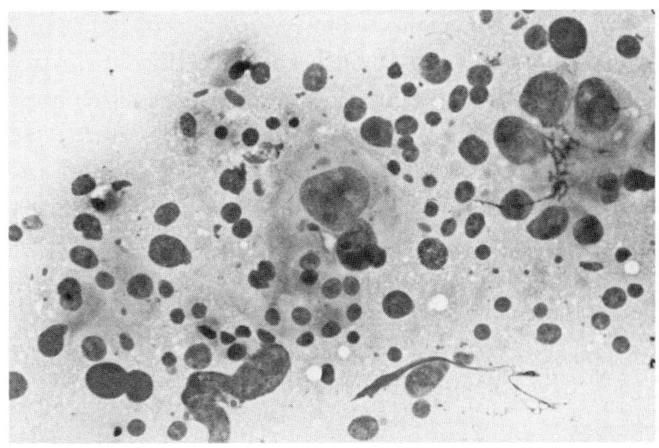

Fig. 31.9. Poorly differentiated hepatocellular carcinoma. Very atypical cells with evident anisocariosis. The observed irregularities, macronucleoli, present also in naked nuclei, multinuclearity and intracytoplasmic jalin globules, permitted the identification of the hepatocytic nature. May-Grunwald Giemsa, ×400

remaining malignancies included intrahepatic cholangiocarcinoma and other rare forms.

31.3.1.2.1
CHOLANGIOCARCINOMA

The prevalence of the tumor in cirrhosis ranges between 14 and 23%; this association probably does not support a pathogenic role of cirrhosis in the development of peripheral cholangiocarcinoma (CC) similar to that established in the case of HCC and suggested in mixed tumors (CC-HCC). The diagnostic value of FNB has so far not been well established (CHERQUI et al. 1995). To distinguish CC from HCC is relatively easy with the help of immuno-histochemistry (KILPATRICK et al. 1993); but it may be difficult to differentiate a metastatic adenocarcinoma from a CC (DEKKER et al. 1989). For these reasons it is advisable in patients suspected of having CC to rule out any primary extrahepatic adenocarcinoma as a possible source of metastasis.

31.3.1.2.2
ANGIOSARCOMA

The tumor is highly vascularized and this characteristic is an important risk factor for liver biopsy (NESHIWAT et al. 1992); in the literature there are cases of death due to biopsy (LIVRAGHI et al. 1997). However, also in recent papers this danger has been erroneously ignored and the possibility of a cytological diagnosis pointed out (CHO et al 1997).

31.3.1.2.3
LEIOMYOSARCOMA

Primary leiomyosarcoma of the liver is a very rare tumor and with imaging findings a correct diagnosis cannot be reached. The smooth muscle nature can be confirmed using various immunohistochemical markers (for actin, desmin, myosin); however, the diagnosis of malignancy in differentiated forms is strictly dependent on the mitotic count and this feature can be identified only by histology examination. In a recent report, in fact, a pathological diagnosis was obtained by using a US-guided biopsy with a coarse needle (CIVARDI et al. 1996).

31.3.2 Liver Metastases

The approach to performing biopsy is different in cases without a previous tumor history or with a previous or simultaneous cancer. Two preliminary observations can help in reaching a correct judgment: in cirrhotic patients a nodular lesion is much more frequently a primary tumor (HCC) than a secondary one (MELATO et al. 1989). A small lesion (less than 1.5 cm in diameter) is probably benign even in an oncologic context (JONES et al. 1992).

From a practical point of view in patients without an oncologic history the detection of a liver nodule is generally followed by a bioptic control; in an oncologic context the biopsy is mandatory only if the diagnosis of metastasis changes in a radical way the therapeutic program. If not, according to recent experience, when the US supports the suspicion of metastasis the judgment is always correct and biopsy could be omitted (KHATTAR et al. 1994).

In a recent retrospective study of a large series of oncologic patients it was observed that a US pattern of malignancy (peritumoral halo, hypoechoic focal lesion, multiple solid nodules) associated with abnormal liver function tests had a positive predictive value of malignancy ranging from 96.2 to 100%. This high specificity supports the possibility of avoiding histologic confirmation when the exact diagnosis has no therapeutic implications (BRUNETON et al. 1997).

According to the literature the diagnostic accuracy of US-guided biopsy is very high for metastasis. In this case the use of cytology is generally sufficient (Fig. 31.10) as shown in a multicenter study: cytology resulted in a greater sensitivity than microhistology and the double biopsy did not improve diagnostic sensitivity. In some instances the routine staining must be completed by immunocytochemical reactions (Figs. 31.11–31.13). The use of coarse needles is reserved only for cases where the sampling of a large amount of material is important for a more detailed diagnosis.

31.4 Complications

The study of complications of liver FNB can be performed by using monoinstitutional series, multicenter surveys and the census of case reports. Obviously these reports do not allow the evaluation of the incidence of the complications but they emphasize some specific aspects that it is important to know. On the other hand, an adverse event that often occurs can be a good index of the frequency of a complication.

In multicenter surveys the complications are related to the whole series of procedures and they are

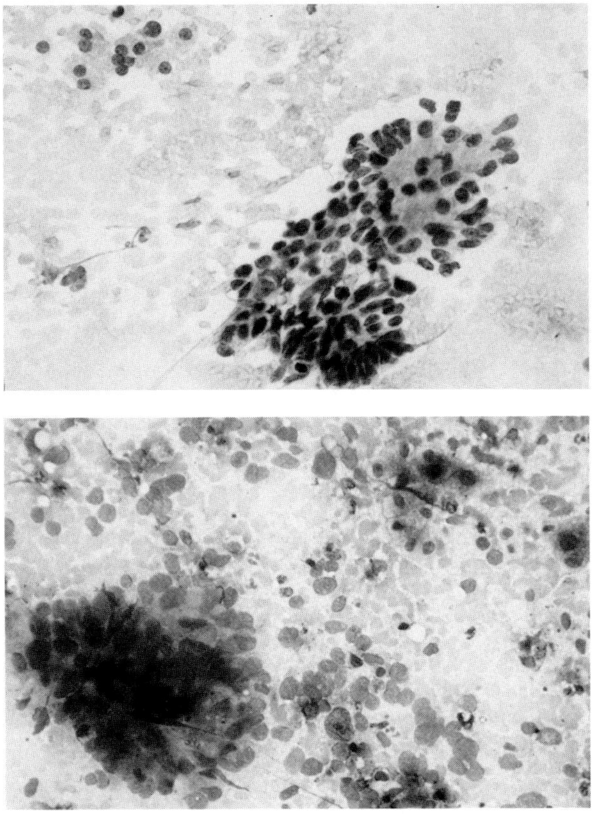

Fig. 31.10a,b. Liver metastasis from colon cancer. The histotype of a liver metastasis can be rarely suggested. However, adenocarcinoma of digestive tract, if well differentiated, shows the typical cell palisade at the periphery of tumoral clusters. Also some normal hepatocytes are present. **a** Papanicolau, ×400; **b** May-Grunwald Giemsa, ×400

not divided into single groups (depending on the target organ or structure). Therefore to find a number of major complications due to liver biopsy does not identify the true risk of the procedure, because the total number of liver biopsies, from which the cases of complications have arisen, is unknown.

Fatal complications: 7 cases of fatal complications after biopsy of HCC have been described all due to hemorrhage, but in only one case did a severe coagulopathy coexist. Three deaths have been described after puncture of angiosarcoma.

Ten fatal complications after biopsy of liver metastasis have been described: 8 cases were due to bleeding. In one of them (metastasis from pancreatic cancer) hemorrhage was due to chronic disseminated intravascular coagulation. In one case death was determined by carcinoid crisis and in the tenth it was of unknown origin (Buscarini and Di Stasi 1996).

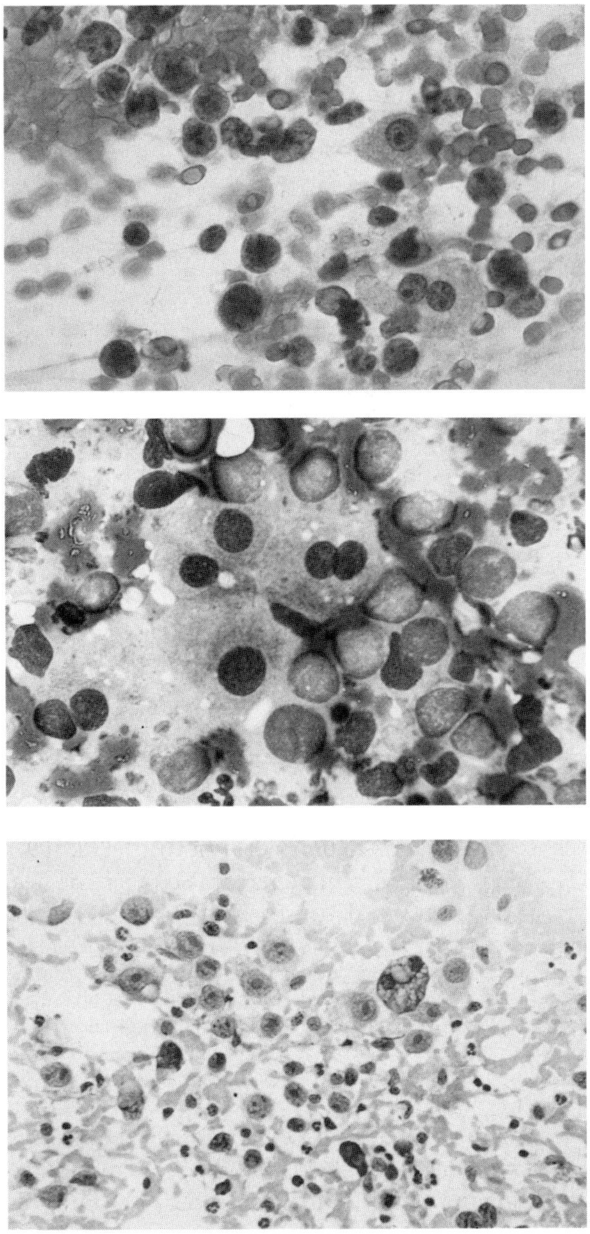

Fig. 31.11a–c. High degree non-Hodgkin's lymphoma. Some reactive hepatocytes are associated with large sized lymphatic cells, frequently with nucleoli. The lymphoid nature can be confirmed by a small panel of immunocytochemical reactions including common leukocytic antigen. L26, UCHL1 and cytokeratin pool: the only two positive cells with this reaction are two normal hepatocytes. **a** Papanicolau, ×1000; **b** May-Grunwald Giemsa, ×1000; **c** cytokeratin pool, ×400

An important major complication following the biopsy of malignant lesions is represented by tumoral seeding along the needle track. Tumor seeding after biopsy is due to spreading of a critical number of cells and their deposition in a favorable microen-

a
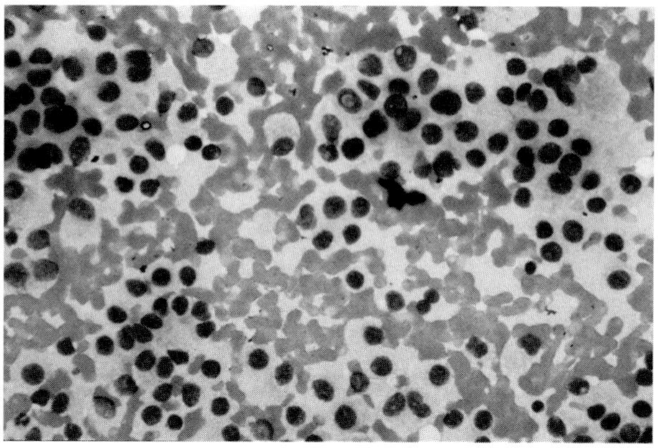

b
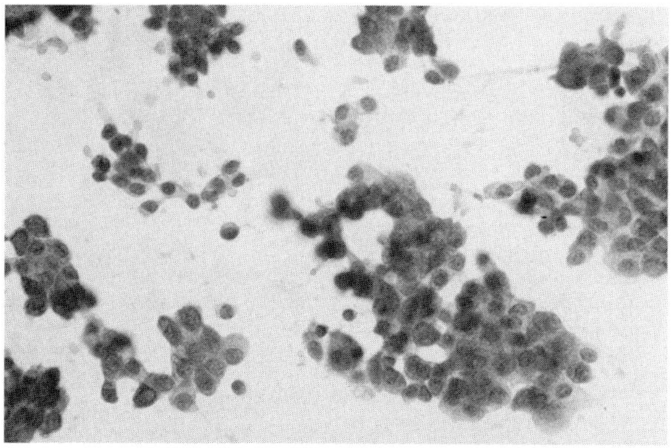

Fig. 31.12a,b. Neuroendocrine tumor localized in the liver. Relatively small sized cells, dissociated or in small clusters, often with a microacinar structure. The absence of relevant atypias, the presence of intracytoplasmic inclusion together with microacinar aggregation allow in many instances the suggestion of the tumor nature only on the basis of routine staining. Immunocytochemical methods allow a sure diagnosis. **a** May-Grunwald Giemsa, ×400; **b** neuronal specific enolase, ×400

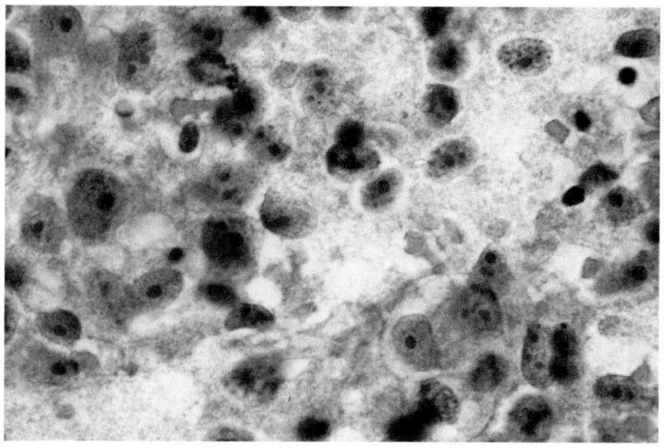

Fig. 31.13. Liver metastasis from prostate cancer. Layer of tumoral cells with strong atypias and with glandular aspects. Knowing the primary tumor, metastasis could be confirmed by routine staining and by two immunocytochemical reactions: for acid prostate phosphates and for prostate specific antigen. Papanicolau, ×400

vironment. The phenomenon depends on several factors: the needle caliber (it has been calculated that doubling the needle caliber increases by 6 times the risk of dissemination); the number of passes performed; the tumor histology that is the cell cohesivity and their ability to produce tumor necrosis factor, which increases the metastasizing capability in the area of damaged tissue; and finally the patient's immune status (Roussel et al. 1989). Tumoral seeding generally involves the subcutis and the omentum. The number of cases of seeding after FN biopsy of HCC collected in the literature are 10.

The seeding appeared a relatively short time after FNB (about 5 months) and as expectation of life in these patients is generally greater the phenomenon could be considered as rare. However, it assumes a relevant clinical impact when the patient is proposed for a radical surgery: resection or graft. In these situations the problem whether to perform a diagnostic biopsy or not is still under discussion.

After biopsy of liver metastases tumoral seeding has been described in 9 cases: in 8/9 cases it was a metastasis due to colon cancer.

Other major nonfatal complications were biliary peritonitis, sepsis, anaphylactic shock, and pneumothorax (Buscarini and Di Stasi 1996).

31.5 Conclusions

FNB of liver malignancies is increasing in popularity. The majority of malignant liver lesions can be correctly diagnosed. Obviously some cases can pose diagnostic problems: in these difficult, even rare, situations the best approach is to use a multidisciplinary team of pathologists, radiologists and clinicians (Pisharodi et al. 1995).

FNB of liver masses offers the advantages of a decreased hospital stay and a lower economic cost. For these reasons FNB has been applied as a first step only on clinical and ultrasound indications. In this way significant economic savings resulted (Verbanck et al. 1994). However, the real problem is to identify according to previous suggestions when FNB is necessary and useful and when it can be omitted. This question in the era of reduction of invasiveness of a medical approach cannot be considered well defined.

References

Bret PM, Labadie M, Bretagnolle M, Paliard P, Fond A, Valette PJ (1988) Hepatocellular carcinoma: diagnosis by percutaneous fine needle biopsy. Gastrointest Radiol 13:253–255

Bruneton JN, Raffaelli CR, Padovani B, Maestro C, Chevallier P, Mourou MY (1997) Etiologic diagnosis of hepatic lesions in cancer patients. Value of ultrasound and liver function tests. Clin Imaging 21:366–371

Buscarini E, Di Stasi M (1996) Complications of abdominal interventional ultrasound. In: Poletto (ed), Milan, pp 34-50

Buscarini L, Fornari F, Bolondi L, et al (1990) Ultrasound-guided fine-needle biopsy of focal liver lesions: technique, diagnostic accuracy and complications. A retrospective study on 2091 biopsies. J Hepatol 11:344–348

Buscarini E, Foroni R, Rossi S, et al (1997) Fine needles with echo markers: increasing cell dragging during biopsy. Acta Cytol 41:1246–1249

Caturelli E, Squillante M, Andriulli A, et al (1993) Fine-needle liver biopsy in patients with severely impaired coagulation. Liver 13:270–273

Caturelli E, Bisceglia M, Fusilli S, Squillante MM, Castelvetere M, Siena DA (1994) Cytological vs microhistological diagnosis of hepatocellular carcinoma. Comparative accuracies in the same fine-needle biopsy specimen. Dig Dis Sci 41:2326–2331

Caturelli E, Giacobbe A, Facciorusso D, et al (1996) Free-hand technique with ordinary antisepsis in abdominal US-guided fine-needle punctures: three-year experience. Radiology 199:721–723

Cavanna L Civardi G, Fornari F, et al (1994) Simultaneous relapse of liver cell carcinoma and non Hodgkin's lymphoma in the liver. Report of a case with diagnosis by ultrasonically guided aspiration biopsy. Acta Cytol 38:451–454

Cherqui D, Tantawi B, Alon R, et al (1995) Intrahepatic cholangiocarcinoma. Results aggressive surgical management. Arch Surg 130:1073–1078

Cho NH, Lee KG, Jeong MG (1997) Cytologic evaluation of primary malignant vascular tumors of the liver. One case of angiosarcoma and hemangioendothelioma. Acta Cytol 41:1468–1476

Civardi G, Fornari F, Cavanna L, Di Stasi M, Sbolli G, Buscarini L (1988) Value of rapid staining and assessment of ultrasound-guided fine needle aspiration biopsy. Acta Cytol 32:552–554

Civardi G, Cavanna L, Iovine E, Buscarini E, Vallisa D, Buscarini L (1996) Diagnostic imaging of primary hepatic leyomiosarcoma: a case report. Ital J Gastroenterol 28:98–101

Dekker A, Kate FJW, Terpstra OT (1989) Cholangiocarcinoma associated with multiple bile-duct hamartomas of the liver. Dig Dis Sci 34:952–958

Di Stasi M, Sbolli G, Fornari F, et al (1994) Extrahepatic primary malignant neoplasms associated with hepatocellular carcinoma: high occurrence of B cell lymphoma. Oncology 51: 459–464.

Fagelman D, Chess Q (1990) Nonaspiration fine-needle cytology of the liver: a new technique for obtaining diagnostic samples. AJR 155:1217–1219

Fornari F, Filice C, Rapaccini GL, et al (1994) Small (< 3 cm) hepatic lesions: results of sonographically guided fine-needle biopsy in 385 patients. Dig Dis Sci 39:2267–2275

Hopper KD, Abendroth CS, Sturtz KW, Matthews YL, Shirk SJ (1992) Fine-needle aspiration biopsy for cytopathologic analysis: utility of syringe handles, automated guns and nonsuction method. Radiology 185:819–824

Jones EC, Chezmar JL, Nelson RC, Bernardino ME (1992) The frequency and significance of small (<15 mm) hepatic lesions detected by CT. AJR 158: 535–539

Khattar SC, Torp-Pedersen ST, Lorentzen T, et al (1994) Liver metastases: is biopsy verification necessary when sonographic assessment is certain? Eur J Ultrasound 1:67–70

Kilpatrick SE, Geisinger KR, Loggie BW, Hopkins III MB (1993) Cytomorphology of combined hepatocellular-cholangiocarcinoma in fine needle aspirates of the liver. A report of two cases. Acta Cytol 37:944–947

Kondo F, Wada K, Nagato Y, et al (1989) Biopsy diagnosis of well-differentiated hepatocellular carcinoma based on a new morphologic criteria. Hepatology 9:751–755

Livraghi T (1984) A simple no-cost technique for real-time biopsy. J Clin Ultrasound 12:60–62

Livraghi T, Belli P, Garavaglia GM, Matricardi L, Torzilli G, Vettori C (1993) Focal nodular hyperplasia of the liver: diagnostic role of smear cytology vs microhistology following ultrasound-guided fine needle biopsy. J Intervent Radiol 8:155–158

Melato M, Laurino L, Mucli E, Valente M, Okuda K (1989) Relationship between cirrhosis, liver cancer, and hepatic metastases. An autopsy study. Cancer 64:455–459

Moulton JS, Moore PT (1993) Coaxial percutaneous biopsy technique with automated biopsy devices: value in improving accuracy and negative predictive value. Radiology 186:515–522

Neshiwat LF, Friedland ML, Shorr-Lesnick B, Feldman S, Glucksman WJ, Russo RD (1992) Hepatic angiosarcoma. Am J Med 93:219–222

Pedio G, Landolt V, Zobeli L, Gut D (1988) Fine needle aspiration of the liver: significance of hepatic naked nuclei in the diagnosis of hepatocellular carcinoma. Acta Cytol 32:437–442

Pisharodi LR, Lavoie R, Bedrossian CWM (1995) Differential diagnosis dilemmas in malignant fine-needle aspirates of liver. A practical approach to final diagnosis. Diagn Cytopathol 12:364–371

Rapaccini GL, Pompili M, Caturelli E, et al (1994) Ultrasound-guided fine-needle biopsy of hepatocellular carcinoma: comparison between smear cytology and microhistology Am J Gastroenterol 89:898–902

Roussel F, Dalion J, Benozio M (1989) The risk of tumoral seeding in needle biopsies. Acta Cytol 33:936–939

Sangalli G, Livraghi T, Giordano F (1989) Fine needle biopsy of hepatocellular carcinoma: improvement in diagnosis by microhistology. Gastroenterology 96:524–526

Sbolli G, Fornari F, Civardi G, et al (1990) Role of ultrasound guided fine needle aspiration biopsy in the diagnosis of hepatocellular carcinoma. Gut 31:1303–1305

Sheafor DH, Paulson EK, Simmons CM, DeLong DM, Nelson RC (1998) Abdominal percutaneous interventional procedures: comparison of CT and US guidance. Radiology 207:705–710

Silverman SG, Deuson TE, Kane N, et al (1998) Percutaneous abdominal biopsy: cost-identification analysis. Radiology 206:429–435

Solbiati L, Livraghi T, De Pra L, Ierace T, Masciadri H, Ravetto C (1985) Fine needle biopsy of hepatic hemangioma with sonographic guidance. AJR 144:471–474

Verbanck JJ, Rutgeerts LJ, Verstraete SF, Vandewiele IA, Deprez JL, De Soete CJ (1994) Cost-benefit analysis of ultrasound-guided punctures in 400 consecutive patients. Europ J Ultrasound 1:223–228

32 Computed Tomography-Guided Percutaneous Biopsy of Malignant Hepatic Lesions

R.D. Redvanly

CONTENTS

32.1 Introduction

Image-guided percutaneous biopsy of a focal hepatic mass is among the most common interventional radiologic procedures performed today. Its increased use is related to advances in cytologic techniques, the safety of smaller biopsy needles, and to imaging methods that allow precise needle placement and monitoring. Most biopsies are performed to confirm suspected malignancy. However, percutaneous biopsy is also used for characterization of benign hepatic lesions and inflammatory masses. An accurate histologic diagnosis can be obtained in more than 90% of cases, even with lesions smaller than 1.5 cm in diameter (Middleton et al. 1997). Because of its accuracy and safety, percutaneous image-guided needle biopsy improves care to the patient and lowers health care cost by eliminating unnecessary surgery, decreasing the need for other diagnostic studies, and shortening the hospital stay and diagnostic workup.

R.D. Redvanly; Assistant Professor, Department of Radiology, Emory University Hospital, 1364 Clifton Road, N.E., Atlanta, GA 30322, USA

Many successful techniques for image-guided percutaneous biopsy have been described. The method for image guidance is primarily dependent upon physician experience and preference, ability to identify the lesion to be biopsied, and availability of imaging technology. This discussion is not meant to be a comprehensive review of all biopsy methods reported in the literature. Rather, I will present the techniques that have been successful in our practice using computed tomography (CT) guidance for biopsy of a focal hepatic lesion.

32.2 Indications and Contraindications

Most image-guided liver biopsies are performed to determine the etiology of a focal hepatic mass. In the patient with an extrahepatic malignancy, biopsy is utilized to determine if a mass represents metastatic disease, determine whether a hepatic mass is a second primary tumor, or to determine whether such a mass represents viable tumor or necrotic tissue after therapy.

The patient with chronic liver disease poses a special problem to the clinician. These patients are at risk for development of hepatocellular carcinoma (HCC). In the setting of end-stage liver disease, foci of HCC are difficult to detect owing to severe alterations in portal hemodynamics and hepatic parenchyma related to areas of regeneration, necrosis, and fatty infiltration. Furthermore, the cirrhotic patient often develops multiple nodular lesions that comprise a spectrum of nodular lesions ranging from regenerative nodules and dysplastic nodules to frankly malignant HCC which are often difficult to distinguish with noninvasive imaging techniques (Choi et al. 1993). Consequently, any solid lesion found within the end-stage cirrhotic liver should be viewed with caution and considered to represent HCC until proved otherwise. Thus, biopsy is often performed in these patients to determine the nature of a solid focal lesion.

Due to increasing use of organ transplantation, intensive chemotherapeutic regimens, and the AIDS epidemic, immunocompromised patients are seen with increased frequency. These patients are at risk for opportunistic infections, but are also at increased risk for development of a variety of neoplasms such as lymphoma and Kaposi's sarcoma. Both opportunistic infections and malignant neoplasms may affect the liver. Because the clinical findings and imaging appearances may be nonspecific, image-guided biopsy is often necessary so that appropriate therapy can be initiated.

The imaging appearance of benign hepatic lesions, such as cavernous hemangiomas, is usually characteristic and can obviate biopsy in most cases. However, some lesions such as hepatic adenomas and focal nodular hyperplasias (FNH) may have features that overlap those of a malignant hepatic lesion. In this situation, determination of a benign or malignant lesion may be difficult based on clinical and radiologic features. In these cases, percutaneous biopsy is useful to determine the etiology of such lesions.

Lastly, some hepatic abscesses can have an atypical presentation. The imaging appearances of a hepatic abscess are quite variable and can mimic that of a necrotic tumor (Halvorsen et al. 1984). Thus, biopsy is necessary to confirm the proper diagnosis and to determine appropriate therapy.

There are two relative contraindications to performing percutaneous liver biopsy. The most common is a bleeding diathesis, although, in most cases, administration of appropriate blood products (vitamin K, platelets, and/or fresh frozen plasma depending on the type of coagulopathy) can improve the patient's hemostasis sufficiently to allow biopsy to be performed. Presently, there are no universal guidelines for assessing a patient's hemostatic function prior to undergoing percutaneous interventional procedures (Silverman, 1991). Since hemorrhage is the most common and potentially life-threatening complication that may occur after percutaneous biopsy, most radiologists screen for coagulation abnormalities in advance (Rapaport 1990; Silverman 1990, 1991). At the very least, one should obtain a hematologic history from the patient. This alone has been shown to be the most accurate predictor of bleeding complications (Erban 1989). Although the indexes of coagulation in the peripheral blood correlate poorly with the risk of bleeding complications following laparoscopic liver biopsy, this is contrary to the experience of others in which thrombocytopenia and prolonged prothrombin time are associated with an increased risk of bleeding following percutaneous liver biopsy (Ewe 1981; Sharma et al. 1982; Gazelle et al. 1992, 1993a). Therefore, a thorough hematologic history and assessment of coagulation parameters should be performed prior to biopsy (Silverman et al. 1990, 1991; Murphy et al. 1993). At our institution, a platelet count and prothrombin time are routinely obtained. As a general rule, a platelet count greater than 50,000/mm^3, a prothrombin time less than 40% above the normal range, and INR less than 1.5 is sufficient.

Since routine coagulation studies will not detect deficiencies in platelet function, it is recommended that aspirin or other non-steroidal antiinflammatory agents be stopped 7–10 days prior to biopsy. Assessment of platelet function with use of a bleeding time is not routinely performed. Instead, we rely on the absence of underlying predisposing conditions such as uremia or myeloproliferative disorders (Silverman et al. 1990).

The second relative contraindication is the uncooperative patient because uncontrolled patient movement hinders accurate needle placement and increases the risk of hepatic laceration and bleeding.

In the past, a moderate to large amount of ascites was considered a contraindication to hepatic biopsy. However, it has been shown that the presence of ascites is not associated with an increased risk of bleeding complications and is not considered a contraindication to biopsy, even in the cirrhotic patient (Fig. 32.1) (Murphy et al. 1988; Little et al. 1996).

32.3 Patient Preparation and Monitoring

Most patients undergoing liver biopsy have a known or suspected malignancy and are concerned about the possible pathologic findings. In addition, patients are apprehensive about physical pain they may experience during the procedure and possible complications. Before the biopsy is performed, the procedure should be explained in simple terms that the patient can understand. The importance of discussing the biopsy procedure with the patient cannot be overemphasized. Establishing good rapport with the patient alleviates many of the patient's anxieties and promotes better patient cooperation during the procedure. The patient should understand why the biopsy is necessary, that these procedures are commonly performed, and that there is a

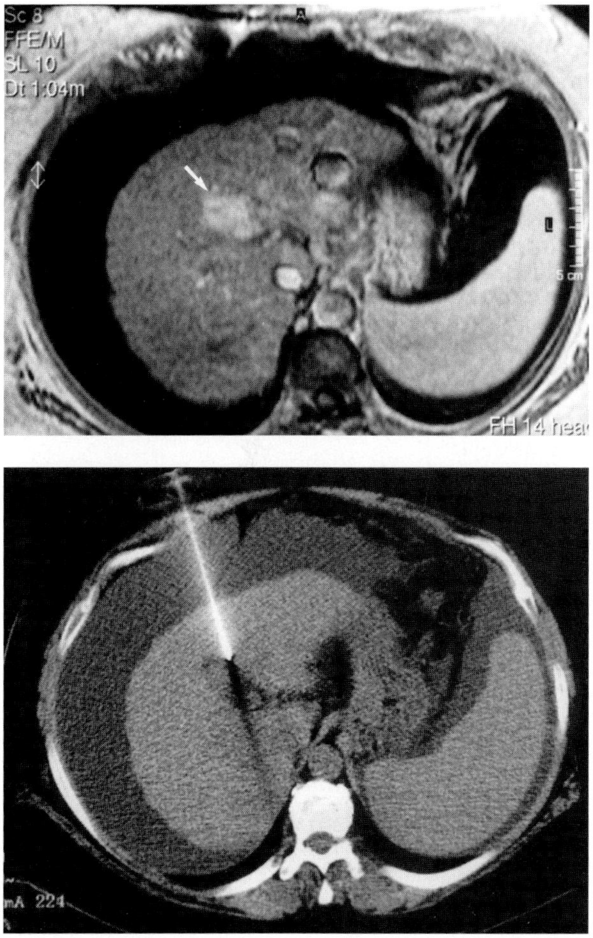

a

b

Fig. 32.1a,b. Percutaneous biopsy of focal mass in a 48-year-old man with cirrhosis and a large amount of ascites. **a** Gadolinium-enhanced T1-weighted gradient-echo image demonstrates an enhancing mass (*arrow*). **b** CT-directed biopsy with needle tip in anterior aspect of lesion. Pathologic evaluation revealed HCC

remote chance of a complication such as bleeding. A brief description of the entire biopsy procedure and reassurance that pain is usually minimal and can be controlled with ample use of local anesthetic help to put the patient at ease. Consequently, most patients are less anxious and understand that their cooperation is important for successful performance of the liver biopsy.

Most liver biopsies can be performed safely with local anesthesia for the control of pain and in an outpatient setting. Premedication with parenteral sedatives or analgesics is not routinely administered unless the patient is extremely anxious or apprehensive. Intravenous access should be established in the event that parenteral analgesics, sedatives, or other medications or fluids are necessary during or after the procedure. Assessment of vital signs should be performed before, during, and after the biopsy so that potential complications are quickly detected and appropriately managed. Use of a nurse to monitor vital signs and administer medications or fluids is very helpful.

32.4 Biopsy Needles

Both needle gauge and tip design are important determinants of the amount and type of specimen obtained (Andriole 1983; Bateson et al. 1980; Gazelle and Haaga, 1991; Haaga et al. 1983; Dahnert et al. 1992). An understanding of the qualities of a biopsy needle allows the radiologist to capitalize on these qualities and obtain increased accuracy while minimizing potential complications.

There are numerous variations in needle tip design, caliber, length, and method of tissue removal that are available for percutaneous biopsy. In general, biopsy needles can be classified as thin-gauge (20–22 gauge) or larger gauge (14–19 gauge) needles. Alternatively, biopsy needles can be classified based on tip design and method of tissue recovery. Thus, for our discussion, needles will be categorized as aspirating needles, cutting needles, and automated spring-loaded biopsy devices.

32.4.1 Aspiration Needles

Biopsy needles with beveled edges, such as a spinal needle or the Chiba needle, and with jagged edges, such as the Franseen needle, are known as aspirating needles. The specimen obtained from these needles is primarily used for cytologic analysis. However, adequate tissue fragments for histologic analysis can usually be obtained with use of an aspiration type needle (Wittenberg et al. 1982).

Thin-gauge needles usually can obtain a sufficient sample for cytologic analysis. Tissue obtained with thinner gauge needles is generally considered to be less reliable for histologic analysis and specific typing of some malignant masses. As a result, use of larger gauge cutting needles is recommended for lesions requiring histologic analysis and subtyping. However, if a proper rotatory motion is used to perform the biopsy, cores of tissue sufficient for histologic analysis can be obtained even from thin-gauge needles. These needles minimize the risk of hemorrhagic complications when sampling vascular lesions. On the other hand, a problem that is occasionally encountered with the use of thinner gauge needles is deflection of the needle tip as it passes through tissue towards a deeply located lesion. Tip deflection causes the needle to "bow". Consequently, if initial needle placement is not within the lesion, subsequent repositioning may be more difficult.

Larger-gauge needles substantially improve the quantity of tissue obtained for both cytologic and histologic analysis (HAAGA et al. 1983; PAGANI 1983; PLECHA et al. 1997). Use of larger needles provides larger specimens and the tissue architecture is more likely to be preserved. As a result, the pathologist can more easily determine the specific type of a benign or malignant hepatic mass. Because more tissue is obtained with a larger gauge needle, fewer passes are usually required (PLECHA et al. 1997). Although the risk of hemorrhage is very low, it is higher than the risk with thinner needles. However, we believe that the use of larger needles is more efficient because more tissue can be recovered with fewer passes, which reduces the chances of complications (PLECHA et al. 1997). In our practice, most liver lesions are biopsied with use of larger gauge needles (18-gauge Chiba or Franseen needles). If the patient has a coagulopathy or if the lesion is hypervascular, a 20-gauge needle is used.

32.4.2 Cutting Needles

Larger gauge needles with cutting surfaces are used mainly to obtain tissue for histologic analysis. These needles obtain a core of tissue that preserves lesion architecture and facilitates histologic analysis (HOPPER et al. 1990). The cutting surface is oriented 90° to the needle shaft. The Tru-Cut needle is a commonly used cutting needle that consists of a slotted stylet needle over which a cutting canula is advanced to secure the tissue.

32.4.3 Automated Spring-Loaded Cutting Needles

A multitude of automated, spring-loaded cutting biopsy devices are available (BERNARDINO 1990; HOPPER et al. 1991). The needle design is similar to other manually operated cutting needles. When the needle is triggered, the inner slotted stylet is thrust forward for 1 to 2 cm, followed immediately by the outer canula which cuts off the tissue sample. These automated devices eliminate the repetitive up-and-down motion necessary for aspiration biopsy. Because the automated device allows a more rapid biopsy, the needle is in the liver for less time. Both of these factors probably account for the fact that most patients find biopsy with an automated device to be less painful than with conventional aspiration biopsy techniques. Most importantly, an intact core of tissue that preserves hepatic architecture is almost always obtained which is easier for the pathologist to interpret (HOPPER et al. 1990, 1991).

32.4.4 Needle Selection

The selection of needle size and type depends on the clinical setting of the biopsy and safety considerations. If a biopsy is performed to confirm metastasis of a known extrahepatic malignancy, then confirmation of the hepatic metastasis can be accomplished with use of thin-gauge aspiration needles. On the other hand, if the type of malignancy is unknown, then use of larger gauge aspiration needles to obtain larger cores of tissue is necessary for reliable diagnosis. The diagnosis of lymphoma, for example, often requires large-gauge cutting needles so that intact cores of tissue are obtained for histologic analysis and flow cytometry. Patient safety is the other major consideration when selecting a needle for biopsy. Thin-gauge needles are used if the patient's coagulation parameters are elevated. Also, smaller gauge needles are preferred for hypervascular lesions and those adjacent to the surface of the liver.

32.5 Site Selection and Sampling Techniques

CT-guided biopsy is quite simple and is generally easier to learn than sonographically guided biopsy. CT is an accurate guidance technique for biopsy of focal liver lesions. It provides excellent depiction of most hepatic masses and provides an accurate image of the needle within the lesion. In fact, the ability to accurately localize the needle tip consistently is an important advantage of the CT-guided method. Additionally, use of contrast-enhanced CT may help identify specific foci of tumor enhancement which should be targeted for biopsy. Until recently, its main limitation was a lack of continuous real-time monitoring of the needle during insertion and biopsy. Presently, several manufacturers provide CT fluoroscopy, which allows for continuous visualization of the needle.

Preliminary CT scans of the liver are obtained to identify the lesion while radiopaque markers are placed on the patient's abdomen to localize an appropriate needle entry site. In general, the scan slice that demonstrates the largest anteroposterior diameter of the lesion is chosen for the biopsy site. The exact path and depth to the proximal aspect of the lesion are then determined from the preliminary images. If the lesion demonstrates central necrosis, the needle is targeted for a peripheral portion of the tumor (Figs. 32.2, 32.3). In most cases, a short and perpendicular needle trajectory to the lesion is preferred. To minimize the chance of bleeding complications, especially in cases of hypervascular lesions or those near the surface of the liver, the needle path should interpose a small cuff of normal liver tissue between the lesion and the liver capsule. Also, one should select a needle path that avoids major vessels.

Once a scan slice is selected, the patient's skin is marked at the appropriate couch index using the laser light guide of the scanner. If the reference catheter is not directly over the lesion, electronic calipers are used to measure the distance between the catheter and the desired skin entry site. The skin is then marked, prepared with povidone-iodine (Betadine), and draped in a sterile manner. The skin and underlying soft tissues are anesthetized with 1% lidocaine. Care should be taken to anesthetize the peritoneum and liver capsule. If the peritoneum and capsule are not adequately anesthetized, the patient may feel some pain during the biopsy and is probably the most common cause of poor patient compliance during the procedure. Proper local anesthesia of the proposed needle path results in a more efficient, comfortable biopsy for the patient, and is more likely to be diagnostic.

To facilitate needle placement, a small skin incision is made with a scalpel, and the skin and underlying soft tissues are separated using a hemostat. With the patient in suspended respiration, the needle is advanced to the predetermined depth, preferably within the proximal aspect of the lesion. Another scan is obtained to confirm proper needle placement. If the needle is not in the lesion, the needle is repositioned until properly placed. Consequently, depending on the experience of the radiologist, multiple needle adjustments may be necessary

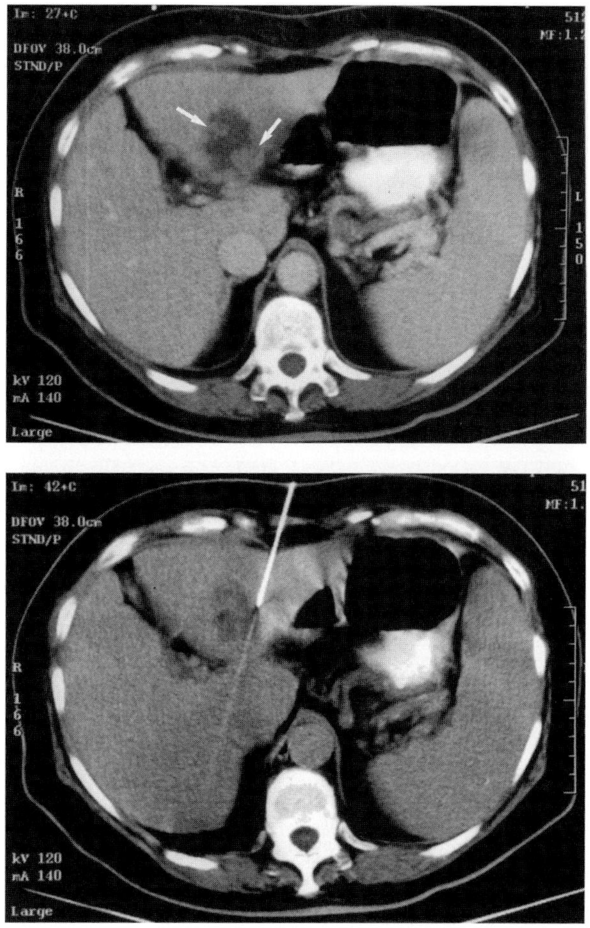

a

b

Fig. 32.2a,b. Percutaneous biopsy of HCC previously treated with ethanol injection. **a** Contrast-enhanced CT reveals enhancing nodularity (*arrows*). **b** Percutaneous biopsy along medial aspect of lesion confirmed persistent viable tumor which was retreated

for precise needle placement. Lastly, to ensure that the needle remains within the lesion during the biopsy, we measure the distance from the needle tip to the distal aspect of the lesion (using electronic calipers) and use this as the maximal depth for needle excursion.

Once within the lesion, the suction aspiration technique or fine-needle aspiration biopsy (FNAB) is utilized for biopsy of the lesion. In brief, the stylet is removed and a 10 cc syringe is attached to the needle. Approximately 5–10 cc of suction is applied and a repetitive in-and-out needle excursion, with a rotatory motion, through the lesion is performed during suspended respiration. Maintaining adequate suction throughout the biopsy is important and has been shown to improve recovery of tissue (Hueftle and Haaga 1986; Hopper et al. 1996; Kinney et al.

a
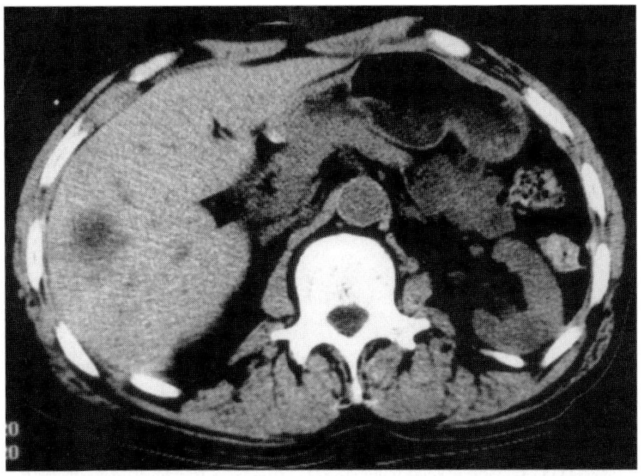

b
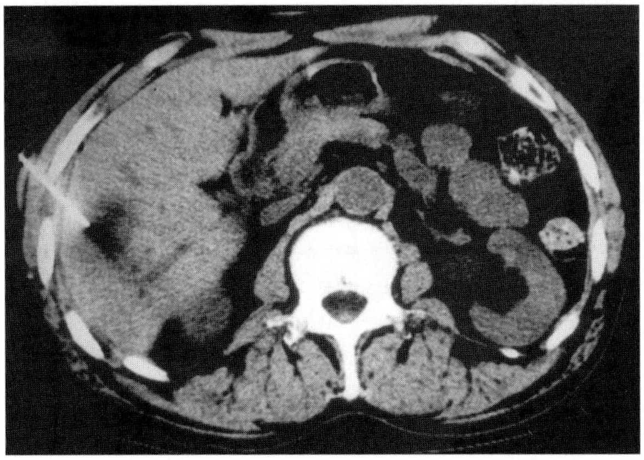

Fig. 32.3a,b. Percutaneous biopsy of necrotic colorectal metastasis. **a** Preliminary unenhanced CT images demonstrate a 3 cm lesion with central necrosis in right lobe of liver. **b** CT-directed biopsy with needle tip placed in periphery of lesion

1993; KREULA 1990). One study demonstrated that at least 5 cc of syringe suction is necessary to obtain 84% of a tissue sample and 10 cc of suction to obtain 94% of the sample (HUEFTLE and HAAGA 1986b). Suction is also maintained during removal of the needle from the biopsy site so that tissue fragments are retained within the needle. In most cases, two to three samples are obtained from various portions of the lesion to ensure adequate sampling of the lesion. For example, the needle may be placed towards the anterior or posterior, left or right, cephalad or caudad aspects of a lesion so that representative sampling is obtained.

It must be emphasized that attention to proper technique is critical for obtaining adequate tissue samples with aspiration biopsy. One study demonstrated that the amount of tissue recovered is related to the number of needle passes and to the depth of the needle excursion during the biopsy (KREULA 1990). In addition, angling the needle between passes in a fan-like manner allows sampling of various portions of the tumor which should diminish the chance for a sampling error (KREULA 1990).

Once the sample has been obtained, the needle is separated from the syringe and the contents of the syringe expelled using a small aliquot of 0.9% sterile saline into a specimen cup containing a 50% ethyl alcohol solution. Tissue fragments are also expelled from the needle into the same specimen cup. In the pathology department, the tissue cores are separated and processed for histologic analysis; the remainder of the aspirate is examined cytologically (LIMBERG et al. 1987). If the biopsy is performed in a patient with suspected hepatic lymphoma, the specimen is placed in a specimen cup containing sterile saline so that the pathologist may perform immunocytologic analysis and flow cytometry.

An alternative sampling technique without syringe aspiration, known as fine needle capillary biopsy (FNCB), has been shown to yield specimens of superior diagnostic quality (FAGELMAN and CHESS 1990). FNCB relies on the physical principle of capillary pressure for advancement of tissue into the needle. Movement of fluid or a mixture of fluid and tissue into a small needle is dependent on capillary tension that is inversely proportional to the diameter of the needle. Thus, the need for aspiration may be eliminated. Some claim that when a diagnostic specimen is obtained, the specimen is superior because FNCB reduces trauma to cells, reduces the number of specimens rendered non-diagnostic because of an abundance of blood, and yields a more concentrated sample of diagnostic cells for the pathologist (FAGELMAN and CHESS 1990b). FNCB is simply performed by removing the stylet from the needle and a pass through the lesion is made with a rapid up-and-down rotatory movement. Although initial reports suggested that FNCB yielded a superior quality of tissue samples, recent studies comparing FNAB and FNCB have demonstrated that less tissue is obtained with the FNCB technique which may result in lower diagnostic accuracy (SAVAGE et al. 1995; HOPPER et al. 1992, 1996; KINNEY et al. 1993).

An additional technique that we have recently incorporated into our practice is the coaxial method (MOULTON and MOORE 1993; HOPPER et al. 1995). With the coaxial technique, a large-gauge needle (e.g., 18-gauge) needle is placed into the lesion. After removal of the stylet, a longer thinner gauge needle is inserted through the larger needle. This technique allows some flexibility for the biopsy. That is, several passes may be made with use of either the suction aspiration method, the nonsuction capillary method, or an automated cutting biopsy device without additional needle repositioning. The final sample can be obtained with the larger gauge needle before its removal from the mass. The coaxial technique has several advantages. First, only a single puncture is made through the liver capsule, which should decrease the risk of hemorrhagic complications. Second, multiple samples of tissue are obtained with a single needle placement. Thirdly, precise needle placement is required only once. For these reasons, the coaxial technique is often utilized in patients who are at increased risk for bleeding complications such as those with severe coagulopathy and ascites (i.e., cirrhotic patients). The only disadvantage to this technique is that all the tissue samples are obtained from the same general area of the lesion. There is also some concern that after the initial pass all subsequent passes tend to follow the same path within the mass which may yield mostly bloody non-diagnostic specimens. This effect can be partially overcome by pushing the hub of the outer, larger needle laterally to redirect the tip. Also, use of a side-exiting coaxial needle allows sampling of different portions of the mass that has not been previously biopsied (Kopecky et al. 1996).

32.6 Post-Biopsy Patient Care

Once the biopsy is completed, the patient is observed in the radiology department for 4–6 h. Most symptoms related to significant post-biopsy hemorrhage are noted within 3 h after the biopsy (Perrault et al. 1978). Therefore, this complication should be detected during routine post procedural observation and these patients could be admitted for further observation or treatment as indicated. Standard post procedure observation includes bedrest for 4–6 h and close monitoring of the biopsy site and vital signs. The patient is asked to lie on the biopsy site, as this local increased pressure helps minimize bleeding from the biopsy site. The radiologist should examine the patient to inspect the biopsy site and review the vital signs. Before discharge, the patient and an accompanying adult are advised of the signs and symptoms of complications. The patient is given the phone number of the radiologist and referring physician so that they may be contacted should a complication develop.

32.7 Specimen Preparation

The pathologist is the single most important factor in obtaining an accurate diagnosis. Methods of tissue sampling, tissue fixation, and tissue processing within the pathology department vary from one institution to another. Thus, it is important to deliver the specimen to the pathologist in the manner that they prefer.

In our experience, cores of tissue are almost always obtained with use of 18- or 20-gauge Chiba needles and with a proper suction aspiration technique. In most cases, our biopsy specimens can be submitted for both histologic and cytologic analysis (Limberg et al. 1987). As a result, our pathologists prefer our specimens placed in a 50% ethyl alcohol solution. This allows the pathologist to process the cores of tissue as cell blocks for histologic analysis. The remaining solution can then be processed for cytology.

In some institutions, the specimens are given directly to the pathologist in the CT suite to make smears as the biopsies are being performed. The advantages of an on-site pathologist are that they can examine the smears to determine if subsequent passes are required for either additional material or ancillary studies. Consequently, the number of passes may be reduced which may reduce the risk for potential bleeding complications. In addition, the pathologist can usually render a preliminary opinion with regard to the nature of the lesion (benign vs. malignant).

32.8 Lesions that Pose Specific Problems

Even in the best of hands, there are some liver lesions that are often problematic for CT-guided biopsy. Specifically, some lesions are difficult to biopsy due to lesion location such as those in the dome of the liver. In addition, certain pathologic features may render some lesions difficult to obtain adequate tissue samples and may be at a higher risk for complications.

Percutaneous biopsy of lesions in the dome of the liver may be particularly difficult with use of CT guidance. In such cases, a steep angle of needle insertion is required to avoid transgressing the pleura and aerated lung (van Sonnenberg et al. 1981). Consequently, multiple needle insertions and needle repositioning are often necessary to determine the correct angle and depth to reach the lesion. Also, multiple scans are necessary to visualize the needle tip. There are a number of alternative methods that may be employed when attempting to biopsy a lesion in the dome of the liver. First, the coaxial technique may be performed in conjunction with a steeply angled needle placement so that additional needle placements can be obviated. Second, the most direct route to the lesion, a transpulmonary path, may be chosen. This technique simplifies the placement of the needle into the lesion and is an effective method for such lesions (Gervaise et al. 1996). That is, by choosing the most direct route to the lesion, lengthy procedures using multiple steeply angled transhepatic needle passes can be avoided. The lesion can be more readily targeted and reached with fewer needle passes and adjustments which may reduce the risk of bleeding. On the other hand is the potential for development of a pneumothorax. In one report using the transpulmonary route, diagnostic accuracy of 93% was achieved and there were no complications (Gervaise et al. 1996). However, the possibility of pneumothorax is real and the risk is probably similar to that with percutaneous lung biopsy. Lastly, use of continuous sonographic guidance instead of CT guidance should be seriously considered. Sonographic guidance is advantageous since it provides real-time monitoring of the needle tip allowing precise placement into these difficult to reach lesions and can avoid transgressing the lung.

Although the detection of small liver lesions may be superior with CT, these lesions may be very difficult to biopsy with CT guidance. That is, the changing position of the liver, which occurs in some patients that are unable to suspend respiration at a reproducible level, can make CT-guided biopsy of small lesions difficult and may result in a lengthy procedure with multiple needle placements and adjustments. However, we have found that this problem can be minimized with adequate coaching of the patient before and during the procedure.

Certain liver lesions because of their vascularity or other pathologic features may make obtaining an adequate tissue sample difficult. For example, lesions such as a cavernous hemangioma with atypical imaging features may occasionally undergo biopsy. In most cases, hemangiomas will be correctly diagnosed based on noninvasive imaging studies and biopsy is unnecessary. Because of the vascular nature of hemangiomas, there is a reluctance to confirm the diagnosis by percutaneous biopsy because of the perceived risk of bleeding complications. However, once the typical hemangioma has been excluded, there is little risk of significant hemorrhage from the atypical variety (Cronan et al. 1988; Heilo and Stennig 1997; Turlington et al. 1991). This is because the features that make their imaging appearance atypical also diminish the potential for significant bleeding complications. Specifically, the atypical hemangiomas tend to be less vascular because of internal fibrosis or thrombosis. In fact, it has been shown that hemangiomas can be safely biopsied with rare complications and a sufficient sample obtained in most cases (Cronan et al. 1988; Heilo and Stennig 1997; Turlington et al. 1991). Consultation with the pathologist is often necessary when the possibility of a hemangioma is a consideration since the diagnosis can be difficult based on cytologic and histologic samples. This is important because tissue samples from cavernous hemangiomas usually contain varying amounts of blood-filled endothelial-lined spaces with a loose connective tissue stroma lacking smooth muscle that may be interpreted as a nondiagnostic biopsy.

Similarly, HCC is a very vascular lesion that typically occurs in the cirrhotic patient whom frequently have coagulopathy and ascites. Though hepatic biopsy can be performed safely in the presence of ascites, caution is warranted when attempting biopsy of a lesion likely to be a HCC. Coagulation parameters should be assessed and corrected if possible with administration of platelets and fresh frozen plasma prior to or during the biopsy. Since normal liver tissue has the ability to tamponade bleeding that occurs after percutaneous biopsy, an oblique needle path through some normal hepatic parenchyma should be attempted for any lesion that is located adjacent to the surface of the liver to minimize potential bleeding complications (Yu et al. 1997). Because nodular lesions occurring within the cirrhotic liver represent a spectrum of abnormalities that include regenerating nodules, dysplastic nodules, and HCC with variable differentiation and grades, the pathologic diagnosis may be difficult (Choi et al. 1993; Wee et al. 1994). In particular, distinction between a nonmalignant lesion such as a regenerative nodule and a well-differentiated HCC can be problematic. Furthermore, distinction between benign hepatocytic tumors, focal nodular hyperplasia and liver cell adenoma, and well-differentiated HCC may also be difficult with cytology and often require histologic analysis of a cell block. Though we routinely use either an 18- or 20-gauge Chiba needle for biopsy of most HCCs, cutting needles are used on occasion so that the architecture of the lesion is preserved for the pathologist. Again, consultation with the pathologist and correlation with imaging studies is important in some cases of suspected HCC.

32.9 Accuracy

CT-guided percutaneous biopsy is highly accurate and is associated with few complications. A recent prospective review of 1000 CT-guided abdominal biopsies at the Mayo Clinic showed that sensitivity was 91.8%, specificity was 98.9%, positive predictive value was 99.7%, and negative predictive value was 73.3% (Welch et al. 1989). Further evaluation of 266 patients undergoing CT-directed biopsy for a focal liver lesion revealed an accuracy of 98.9%. In the liver, only 4 (1.5%) liver biopsies were incorrect and only 2 (0.8%) minor complications were encountered. An analysis of accuracy with regard to lesion size, lesion type, and needle size was not performed in this series. In our experience of approximately 15 years, accuracy in excess of 90% has been achieved for both metastatic lesions as well as for primary malignant neoplasms. This data shows that CT-guided biopsy is a safe, reliable, and accurate technique for diagnosis of a focal hepatic lesion.

Comparison of the effect of needle gauge has shown that the diagnostic accuracy is improved with use of larger needles. In a study comparing use of 18- and 22-gauge aspiration needles, the diagnostic accuracy was superior when 18-gauge needles were used for biopsy (Pagani 1983). In this study, the overall accuracy was 98% for the 18-gauge needle and 84% for the 22-gauge needle.

A review of the literature comparing cutting needles and aspiration needles have generally shown cutting needles to be superior to aspiration type needles. Martino et al. reported a higher accuracy with 14- or 18-gauge cutting needles (91%) versus 22-gauge aspirating needles (69%) in the diagnosis of hepatic malignancy (Martino et al. 1984). Similarly, Ha et al. found that the 14-gauge Tru-Cut needle (90.2%) was superior to a 20-gauge aspiration needle (77.6%) for the diagnosis of hepatic malignancy (Ha et al. 1991). However, both of these studies compared large cutting needles (14- or 18-gauge Tru-Cut needles) to thin-gauge (20- or 22-gauge) aspiration needles and the difference in needle size probably had a significant impact on diagnostic accuracy. On the other hand, a retrospective multicenter analysis of 2091 sonographically guided liver biopsies demonstrated that the overall diagnostic accuracy of 21 to 23 gauge aspirating needles (93%) and 21 to 22-gauge cutting needles (95%) was similar (Buscarini et al. 1990). However, in cases of HCC, use of cutting needle biopsy in addition to FNAB was shown to have a higher sensitivity than FNAB alone (90% vs 98%).

In general, the diagnostic accuracy of CT-guided liver biopsy will vary depending on the inherent characteristics of the lesion, ability to achieve precise needle placement, and the technique of the radiologist performing the biopsy. Negative biopsy results are uncommon. Negative biopsy results may result from a sampling error, an incorrect pathologic diagnosis, or a truly benign lesion. If a biopsy result is contrary to the clinical suspicion, a repeat biopsy is recommended. In these cases, use of sonographic guidance may be advantageous in that precise needle placement and sampling of the lesion could be continuously monitored. In addition, having the pathologist examine the tissue samples during the procedure will ensure that a diagnostic sample is obtained.

32.10 Complications

Major complications after liver biopsy are rare. Hemorrhagic complications, such as hemoperitoneum, intrahepatic hematoma, and subcapsular hematoma, are the most frequently encountered problems. Rarely, intrahepatic arterial pseudoaneurysm may occur following biopsy. Other complications include pneumothorax, bile leakage, and fistula formation between any of the arterial, venous or biliary structures. Death after percutaneous liver biopsy is extremely rare (0.006% to 0.031%) and is usually due to severe hemorrhage (Smith 1991).

The main risk factors for bleeding complications are the size of the needle, the number of passes, the type of lesion biopsied, and the presence of an impairment in hemostasis. Although one would expect larger needles to be associated with a high incidence of complications, it is not clear from the literature whether the complication rate and the incidence of bleeding is actually increased with use of larger needles. One study, in an animal model, comparing different sizes of needles used for biopsy of the liver and kidneys found no significant difference in bleeding among procedures performed with 18 -, 20, and 22-gauge needles, even when anticoagulants were administered (Gazelle et al. 1992). On the other hand, a review of 1000 CT-guided biopsies noted that most complications occurred when large-gauge needles were used, which suggests that use of larger needles may pose a higher risk (Welch et al. 1989). Another study compared CT-guided hepatic biopsy using a 22-gauge cutting needle versus 14- or 18-gauge cutting needles and found a 0.83% complication rate for the thin-gauge cutting needle and a 1.44% complication rate for the larger cutting needles (Martino et al. 1984). Most importantly, these studies demonstrate that the complication rate of CT-guided liver biopsy with a variety of needles is acceptably low.

The risk of complications, though extremely low, is increased for each additional needle pass. That is, each additional pass results in another puncture through the liver capsule and also has the potential to traverse a vessel. Thus, to minimize potential complications, attention to proper biopsy technique and selection of an appropriate biopsy needle is important. Also, the availability of an on-site pathologist to evaluate the adequacy of the tissue sample may decrease the number of passes required.

Hypervascular lesions such as hepatocellular carcinoma and sarcomas potentially have a higher risk of bleeding (Bret et al. 1988). In these cases, inclusion of a small cuff of normal liver between the lesion and the liver capsule minimizes the risk of bleeding (Yu et al. 1997). In addition, alternative biopsy techniques such as use of a protein polymer sheath and embolization of the needle tract have been suggested to decrease the change of bleeding especially in high risk patients with impaired hemostatic function (Gazelle et al. 1993b; Zins et al. 1992; Chisholm et al. 1989; Allison and Adam 1988; Smith et al. 1996).

Minor complications include pain and vasovagal reactions. Some patients may complain of mild transient pain after liver biopsy; reassurance and analgesics are usually effective. Tumor seeding has been reported following biopsy for HCC but is extremely rare with an estimated frequency of 0.003% to 0.009% (Smith 1991).

References

Allison DJ, Adam A (1988) Percutaneous liver biopsy and tract embolization. Radiology 166:261–262

Andriole JG (1983) Biopsy needle characteristics assessed in the laboratory. Radiology 148:659–662

Bateson MC, Hopwood D, Duguid HLD, et al (1980) A comparative trial of liver biopsy needles. J Clin Pathol 133:131–133

Bernardino ME (1990) Automated biopsy devices: significance and safety. Radiology 176:615–666

Bret PM, Labadie M, Bretagnolle M, et al (1988) Hepatocellular carcinoma: diagnosis of percutaneous fine needle biopsy. Gastrointest Radiol 13:253–255

Buscarini, Fornari F, Bolondi L, et al (1990) Ultrasound guided fine needle biopsy of focal liver lesions. Techniques, diagnostic accuracy and complications: a retrospective study of 2091 biopsies. J Hepatol 11:344–348

Chisholm RA, Jones SN, Lees WR (1989) Fibrin sealant as a plug for post liver biopsy needle tract. Clin Radiol 40:627–628

Choi BI, Takayasu K, Han MC (1993) Small hepatocellular carcinomas and associated nodular lesions of the liver: pathology, pathogenesis, and imaging findings. AJR 160:1177–1178

Cronan JJ, Esparza AR, Dorfman GS, et al (1988) Cavernous hemangioma of the liver: role of percutaneous biopsy. Radiology 166:135–138

Dahnert WF, Hoagland MH, Hamper UM, et al (1992) Fine-needle aspiration biopsy of abdominal lesions: diagnostic yield for different needle tip configurations. Radiology 185:263–268

Erban SB, Kinman JL, Schwartz JS (1989) Routine use of the prothrombin and partial thromboplastin times. JAMA 262:2428–2432

Ewe K (1981) Bleeding after liver biopsy does not correlate with indexes of peripheral coagulation. Dig Dis Sci 26:388–393

Fagelman D, Chess Q (1990) Non aspiration fine-needle cytology of the liver; a new technique for obtaining diagnostic samples. AJR 155:1217–1219

Gazelle GS, Haaga JR (1991) Biopsy needle characteristics. Cardiovasc Intervent Radiol 14:13–16

Gazelle GS, Haaga JR, Rowland DY (1992) Effect of needle gauge, level of anticoagulation, and target organ on bleeding associated with aspiration biopsy. Radiology 183:509–513

Gazelle GS, Haaga JR, Rowland DY (1993a) Bleeding due to needle biopsy: effect of venopirin in an animal model and implications for humans. JVIR 4:305–310

Gazelle GS, Haaga JR, Halpern EF (1993b) Hemostatic protein polymer sheath: improvement in hemostasis at percutaneous biopsy in the setting of platelet dysfunction. Radiology 187:269–272

Gervais DA, Gazelle GS, Lu DSK (1996) Technical note. Percutaneous transpulmonary CT-guided liver biopsy: a safe and technically easy approach for lesions located near the diaphragm. AJR 167:482–483

Ha HK, Sachs PB, Haaga JR, et al (1991) CT-guided liver biopsy: an update. Clin Imaging 15:99–104

Haaga JR, LiPuma JP, Bryan PJ (1983) Clinical comparison of small-and large-caliber cutting needles for biopsy. Radiology 146:665–667

Halvorsen RA, Korobkin M, Foster WL, et al (1984) The variable CT appearance of hepatic abscesses. AJR 141:941–946

Heilo A, Stenwig AE (1997) Liver hemangioma: US-guided 18-gauge core-needle biopsy. Radiology 204:719–722

Hopper KD, Baird SE, Reddy VV, et al (1990) Efficacy of automated biopsy guns versus conventional biopsy needles in the pygmy. Radiology 176:671–676

Hopper KD, Abendroth CS, Sturtz KW (1992) Fine-needle aspiration biopsy for cytopathologic analysis: utility of syringe handles, automated guns, and the nonsuction method. Radiology 185:819–824

Hopper KD, Abendroth CS, Sturtz KW, Matthews YL, Stevens LA, Shirk SJ (1991) Automated biopsy devices: a blinded evaluation. Radiology 187:653–660

Hopper KD, Grenko RT, TenHave TR, et al (1995) Percutaneous biopsy of the liver and kidney by using coaxial technique: adequacy of the specimen obtained with three different needles in vitro. AJR 164:221–224

Hopper KD, Grenko RT, Fisher AI, et al (1996) Capillary versus aspiration biopsy: effect of needle size and length on the cytopathological specimen quality. Cardiovasc Intervent Radiol 19:341–344

Hueftle MG, Haaga JR (1986) Technical note. Effect of suction on biopsy sample size. AJR 147:1014–1016

Kinney TB, Lee MJ, Filomena CA (1993) Fine-needle biopsy: prospective comparison of aspiration versus nonaspiration techniques in the abdomen. Radiology 186:549–552

Kopecky KK, Broderick LS, Davidson DS, et al (1996) Side-exiting coaxial needle for aspiration biopsy. AJR 167:661–662

Kreula J (1990) Effect of sampling technique on specimen size in fine needle aspiration. Invest Radiol 25:1294–1299

Limberg B, Hopker WW, Kommerell B (1987) Histologic differential diagnosis of focal liver lesions by ultrasonically guided fine needle biopsy. Gut 28:237–241

Little AF, Ferris JV, Dodd GD III, et al (1996) Image-guided percutaneous hepatic biopsy: effect of ascites on the complication. Radiology 199:79–83

Martino CR, Haaga JR, Bryan PJ, et al (1984) CT-guided liver biopsies: eight years' experience. Radiology 152:755–757

Middleton WD, Hiskes SK, Teefey SA, et al (1997). Small (1.5 cm or less) liver metastases: US-guided biopsy. Radiology 205:729–732

Moulton JS, Moore PT (1993) Coaxial percutaneous biopsy technique with automated biopsy devices: value in improving accuracy and negative predictive value. Radiology 186:515–522

Murphy FB, Barefield KP, Steinberg HV, et al (1988) CT- or sonography-guided biopsy of the liver in the presence of ascites: frequency of complications. AJR 151:485–486

Murphy TP, Dorfman GS, Becker J (1993) Use of preprocedural tests by interventional radiologists. Radiology 186:213–220

Pagani JJ (1983) Biopsy of focal hepatic lesions. Comparison of 18 and 22 gauge needles. Radiology 147:673–675

Plecha DM, Goodwin DW, Rowland DY, et al (1997) Liver biopsy: effects of biopsy needle caliber on bleeding and tissue recovery. Radiology 204:101–104

Perrault J, McGill DB, Ott BJ, et al (1978) Liver biopsy: Complications in 1000 inpatients and outpatients. Gastroenterology 74:103–106

Rapaport SI (1990) Assessing hemostatic function before abdominal interventions. AJR 154:239–240

Savage CA, Hopper KD, Abendroth CS, et al (1995) Fine-needle aspiration biopsy versus fine-needle capillary (nonaspiration) biopsy: in vivo comparison. Radiology 195:815–819

Sharma P, McDonald GB, Banaji M (1982) The risk of bleeding after percutaneous liver biopsy: relation to platelet count. J Clin Gastroenterol 4:451–453

Silverman SG, Mueller PR, Pfister RC (1990) Hemostatic evaluation before abdominal interventions: an overview and proposal. AJR 154:233–238

Silverman SG, Coughlin BF, Seltzer SE, et al (1991) Current use of screening laboratory tests before abdominal interventions: a survey of 603 radiologists. Radiology 181:669–673

Smith EH (1991) Complications of percutaneous abdominal fine-needle biopsy. Radiology 178:253–258

Smith TP, McDermott VG, Ayoub DM, et al (1996) Percutaneous transhepatic liver biopsy with tract embolization. Radiology 198:769–774

Turlington BS, Charboneau JW, Reading CC, et al (1991) Percutaneous needle biopsy of hepatic cavernous hemangiomas. Radiology 181(P):224

van Sonnenberg E, Wittenberg J, Ferrucci JT (1981) Triangulation method for percutaneous needle guidance: the angled approach to upper abdominal masses. AJR 137:757–761

Wee A, Nilsson B, Tan LKA, et al (1994) Fine needle aspiration biopsy of hepatocellular carcinoma. diagnostic dilemma at the ends of the spectrum. Acta Cytol 38:347–354

Welch TJ, Sheedy PF II, Johnson CD, et al (1989) CT-guided biopsy: prospective analysis of 1,000 procedures. Radiology 171:493–496

Wittenberg J, Mueller PR, Ferrucci JT, et al (1982) Percutaneous core biopsy of abdominal tumors using 22 gauge needles: further observations. AJR 139:75–80

Yu SCH, Metrewelli C, Lau WY, et al (1997) Safety of percutaneous biopsy of hepatocellular carcinoma with an 18 gauge automated needle. Clin Radiol 52:907–911

Zins M, Vilgrain V, Gayno S, et al (1992) US-guided percutaneous liver biopsy with plugging of the needle tract: a prospective study in 72 high-risk patients. Radiology 184:841–843

33 Advanced Image Processing

D. Caramella and E. Neri

CONTENTS

33.1 Aims of Image Processing of the Liver

Three-dimensional (3D) visualization of organs or anatomical spaces is considered an important complement to the imaging evaluation of patient candidates for surgery, interventional procedures, or radiotherapy for malignant lesions of the liver.

Surgical interventions can significantly benefit from the preoperative knowledge of the patient's anatomy, for the safety of the intervention and for better therapeutic results. This information can best be provided by imaging techniques that allow the reproduction of the imaged part of the body in a 3D format, such as spiral computed tomography (CT) and magnetic resonance imaging (MRI).

In case of the liver, the 3D study with such diagnostic modalities aims to demonstrate the external surface of the organ and its internal structure. The surface anatomy is given by hepatic lobes (left, right, caudate and quadrate), fissures (umbilical, transverse, right and left sagittal) and fossae (for the inferior vena cava, gallbladder, kidney).

D. Caramella, MD; Division of Diagnostic and Interventional Radiology, Department of Oncology, University of Pisa, Via Roma 67, I-56125 Pisa, Italy

E. Neri, MD; Division of Diagnostic and Interventional Radiology, Department of Oncology, University of Pisa, Via Roma 67, I-56125 Pisa, Italy

The 3D preoperative knowledge of some key surface landmarks helps the surgeon to reach a specific segment for hepatic resections. However, 3D images can provide detailed information about the anatomy of the blood vessels (arterial, portal and venous systems), of the biliary tract, and about the relationships of the liver with the contiguous anatomical structures (colon, pancreas, spleen, etc.) and spaces (peritoneum and retro-peritoneum).

Another important advantage, given by the high sensitivity of spiral CT and MRI for the detection of liver lesions, is represented by the possibility of obtaining volumetric images of hepatic nodules. In this way 3D imaging can be used to represent in a virtual model the lesion position within the liver with respect to the segmental anatomy; furthermore, when the 3D model is created other information regarding the volume and morphology of the nodule can be easily obtained.

The impact of these technical developments on patient management is still under clinical evaluation; however, it is commonly felt that preoperative 3D imaging of the liver has the potential to increase the safety of interventions and ensures an easier communication between radiologists on one hand, and surgeons or clinicians on the other. The presentation of CT or MRI findings with cross-sections is frequently inefficient for communicating the diagnostic observations to surgeons; therefore, 3D reconstruction of the native images makes their interpretation easier and faster with respect to the surgical anatomy.

33.2 Basics of 3D Processing

33.2.1 Introduction

The interest in 3D image processing has been recently renewed by the introduction into clinical practice of fast imaging, provided by spiral CT and

MRI. These diagnostic modalities, by means of dedicated acquisition methods, generate native images that are ideally suited for 3D processing. Although the software technology for image processing is not entirely new, 3D reconstructions and renderings were made feasible in a clinical setting by the spectacular improvements of processing hardware. In fact, the high computational complexity of 3D image processing requires the combination of powerful hardware and software to enable the clinical use of these procedures.

For generating 3D images the computer has to perform three important steps under the guidance of the radiologist. The first step is represented by the generation of the volumetric data set in order to make available the entire volume scanned in a single 3D model. The second step is represented by the segmentation of anatomical structures for their recognition within the volume. The final step is aimed to assign to the resulting 3D image some features that belong to reality, such as depth, shading, light, etc., to simulate a 3D perspective on a bi-dimensional display device such as the computer monitor or a printed image.

33.2.2 Generation of the Volumetric Data-Set

Spiral CT and dedicated MRI sequences provide direct volumetric acquisitions. In the case of spiral CT, the simultaneous X-ray tube rotation and patient transportation ensure a fast and continuous acquisition of raw data; the image reconstruction at selected intervals along the volume is performed in real-time and the data are presented in a cross-sectional format (Kalender et al.1990; Bartolozzi et al. 1998).

In the case of MRI a direct 3D acquisition can be performed by sampling a selected volume of the patient with dedicated sequences. The advantages of this method are represented by an optimal signal-to-noise ratio and the generation of contiguous slices (Meyer et al. 1992; Waggenspack et al. 1993; Bennet et al. 1991). However, the study of the liver with MRI is limited by the movement of the diaphragm with breathing, which is not compatible with the long time required for the acquisition, adversely affecting image quality.

Other types of 3D MRI acquisitions are represented by MR angiography (MRA) and MR cholangiopancreatography (MRCP). Rapid imaging allows contiguous 2D acquisitions or a single 3D acquisition able to enhance the visibility of the blood or the bile (Debatin et al. 1991; Prince 1994; Reinhold and Bret 1996; Miyazaki et al. 1996). Despite this method restricting the MR study to the imaging of fluids, the resulting images are ideal for 3D reconstructions.

The generation of the volumetric data-set is performed by the computer software through the alignment of the native images along the *z*-axis (the longitudinal axis of the patient within the gantry or the magnet). The correct position of the cross-sections along the *z*-axis is essential to maintain the spatial integrity of the scanned volume in the 3D model (Fig. 33.1).

33.2.3 Segmentation

Three-dimensional imaging is a different method for visualizing and analyzing the diagnostic information with respect to axial imaging. In 3D imaging, all the anatomical components of a certain compartment are presented in the same image; therefore a process to differentiate the different organs is extremely important to facilitate the interpretation of their anatomical relationships. This process is called "segmentation".

Different methods for image segmentation are available; some are still under development or under clinical evaluation while others have already been introduced to the market and are installed on commercial diagnostic workstations. The simplest method for performing segmentation is to change the windows and level of 2D or 3D images. This procedure does not require special tools; it is fast and easy to perform in real-time. To enhance the precision of such a method the complement of the image histogram is extremely helpful, since it provides the mathematical classification of the tissues that compose the volume.

More advanced tools for segmentation are available as well. Some methods are strictly dependent on the operator selection, while others are based on the automatic identification of tissues (Bae et al. 1993). A direct method consists of the manual tracing of planes, borders or points on the image in order to select the target anatomical structures (Fig. 33.2). This selection can also be done by setting a certain interval of densities or intensities to which the voxels of the target belong; in this case the operator applies some thresholds to the volume data, and consequently excludes the part of the volume outside the

a b

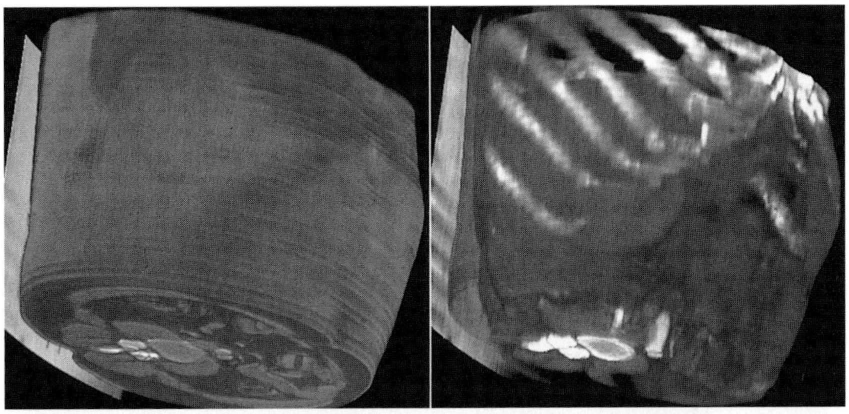

Fig. 33.1a,b. Volume rendering of a spiral CT data-set acquired during a breath-hold for the study of the abdomen. Gray scale coding of the density values distribution can be used for the differentiation of the anatomical structures (**a**) and can be varied by increasing the transparency effect (**b**). Figure 33.4 shows the same data-set coded with the use of colors

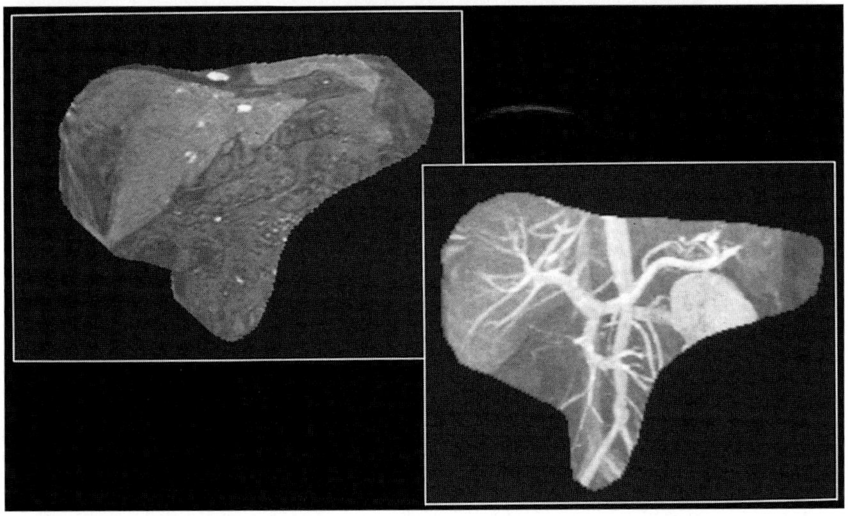

Fig. 33.2 Application of a curvilinear cutting plane to a volumetric MR data-set obtained with a contrast enhanced SPGR sequence for the study of the portal tree. The resulting sub-volume can be processed with MIP. Figure 33.5 shows the same data set after segmentation

selected interval. The setting of the threshold is the critical step of this method, and frequently the incorrect selection of the interval causes the loss of diagnostic information (Neri et al. 1999a). In some situations the threshold segmentation is used to create a surface of the target anatomical structure. The aim of these tools is to reduce the computation time using binary images.

Recently, the increased computation and graphic capability of computers has made feasible volume rendering. The main feature of this processing method is the simultaneous representation of different anatomical structures, with different voxel densities or intensities, within a single volume. Volume rendering is obtained by simulating rays of light, which transverse the volume and are attenuated by its contents. Specific anatomical or pathological structures can therefore be selectively visualized without requiring any time-consuming pre-processing, as opposed to commonly used surface rendering methods (Figs. 33.1, 33.3).

33.2.4 Visualization

When a 3D model is generated and segmented, each anatomical structure must be shown according to its position in the volume, its dimension, its density or intensity, and its morphology. Different attributes are given to different objects that compose the model to better simulate the reality; this can be obtained by assigning gray levels, colors, lighting and shading effects to the objects (Figs. 33.4–33.8).

The last and important parameters of the visualization are the point of view and the perspective through which the final 3D model is presented. The perspective has recently become an important aspect of 3D visualization with the introduction into clinical practice of software tools that simulate endoscopy (Lorensen and Cline 1987). The resulting perspective of the simulation is called "virtual endoscopy". A wide range of clinical applications have been reported for this computer simulated imaging.

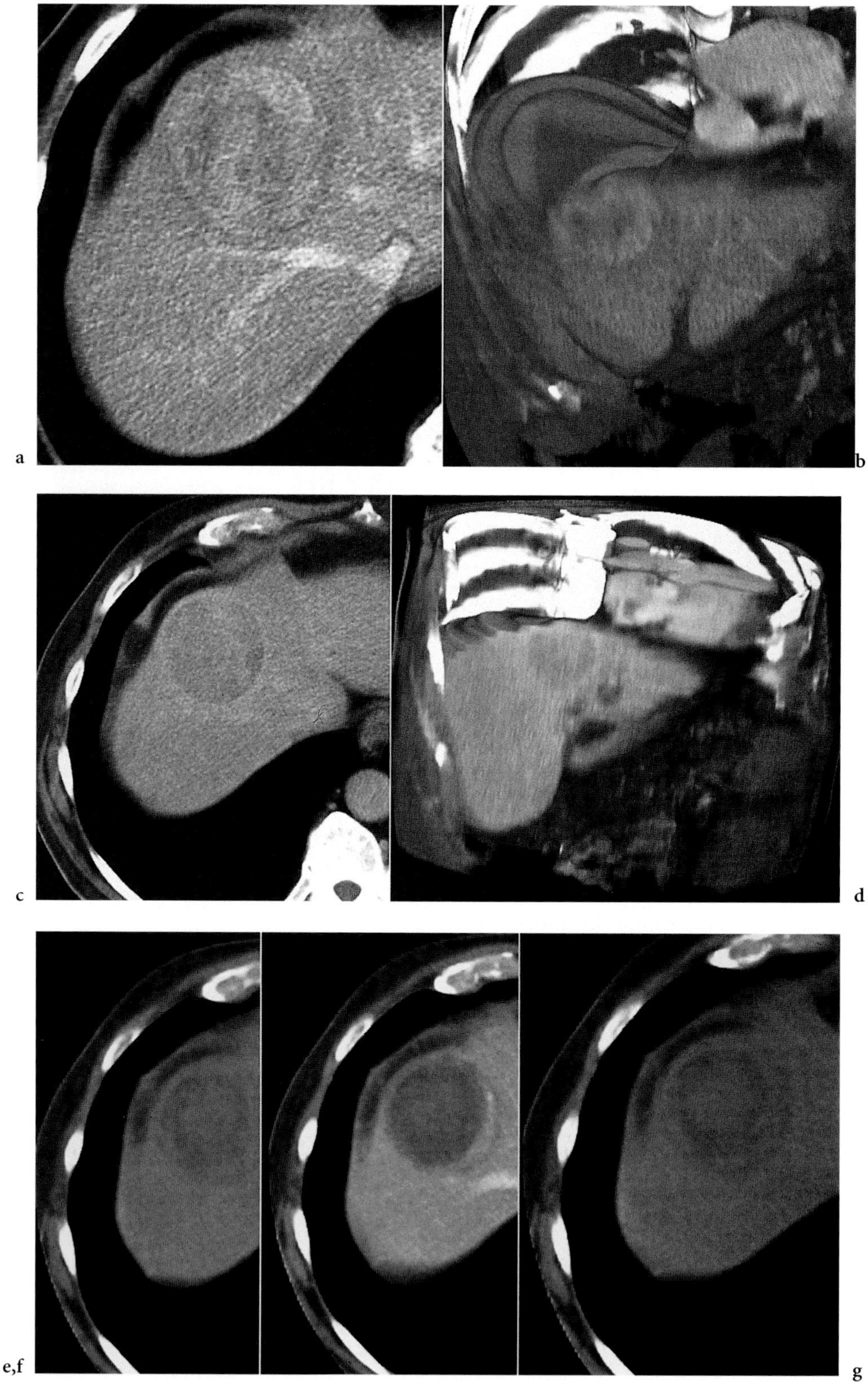

Fig. 33.3a–g. Hepatocellular carcinoma nodule of the eighth hepatic segment. Pre-treatment spiral CT axial scans and volume renderings obtained in the portal phase (**a,b**) and in the delayed venous phase (**c,d**). After radio-frequency thermal ablation, the nodule is imaged by contrast-enhanced spiral CT scans in the arterial (**e**), portal (**f**), and delayed venous phase (**g**). Color coding before and after treatment is shown in Fig. 33.6

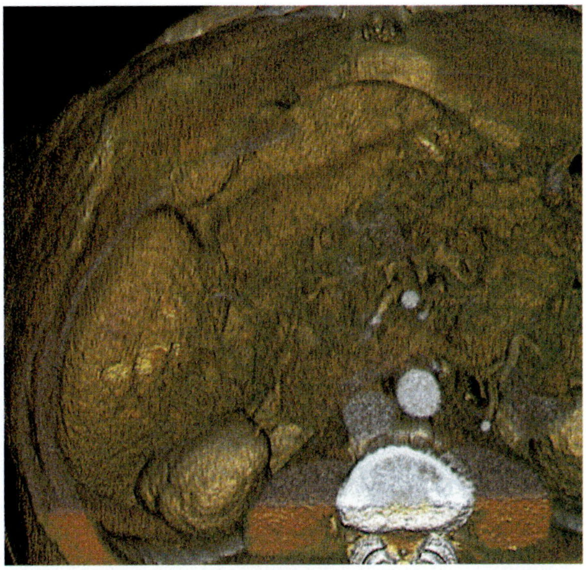

Fig. 33.4. Color coded volume rendering of a spiral CT dataset showing the inferior surface of the liver

a b

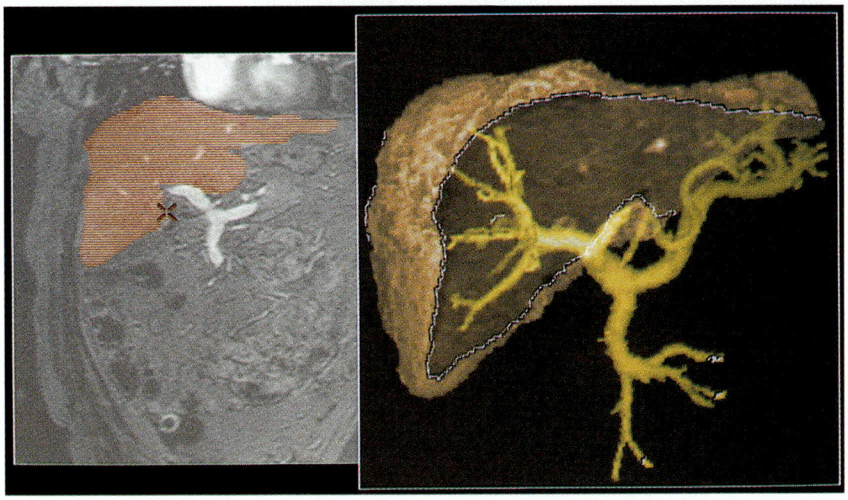

Fig. 33.5a,b. Segmentation of the liver parenchyma achieved by using the region growing method **(a)**. The combination between the resulting 3D model of the liver and the segmented model of the portal tree is shown in **b**

a b

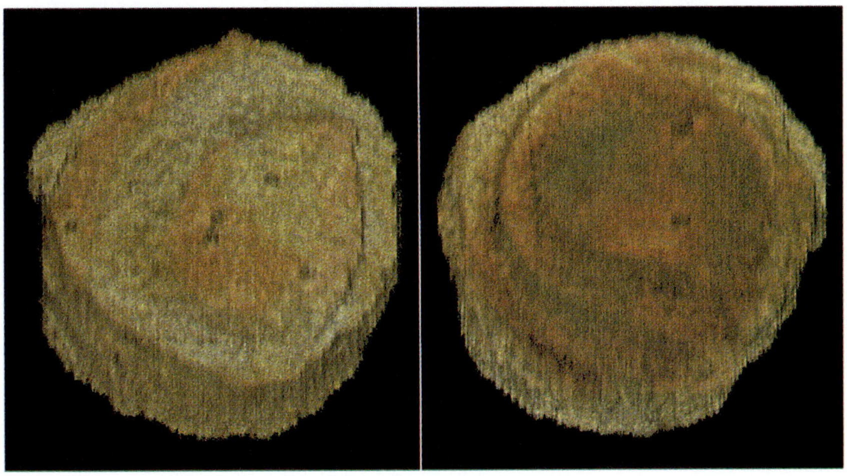

Fig. 33.6a,b. Evaluation of treatment response after radio-frequency thermal ablation. The lesion is segmented and isolated from the liver parenchyma. Before treatment **(a)** there is a clear prevalence of viable tissue (*yellow*), whereas after thermal ablation **(b)**, the necrotic areas (*red and green*) cover the entire lesion

a b c d

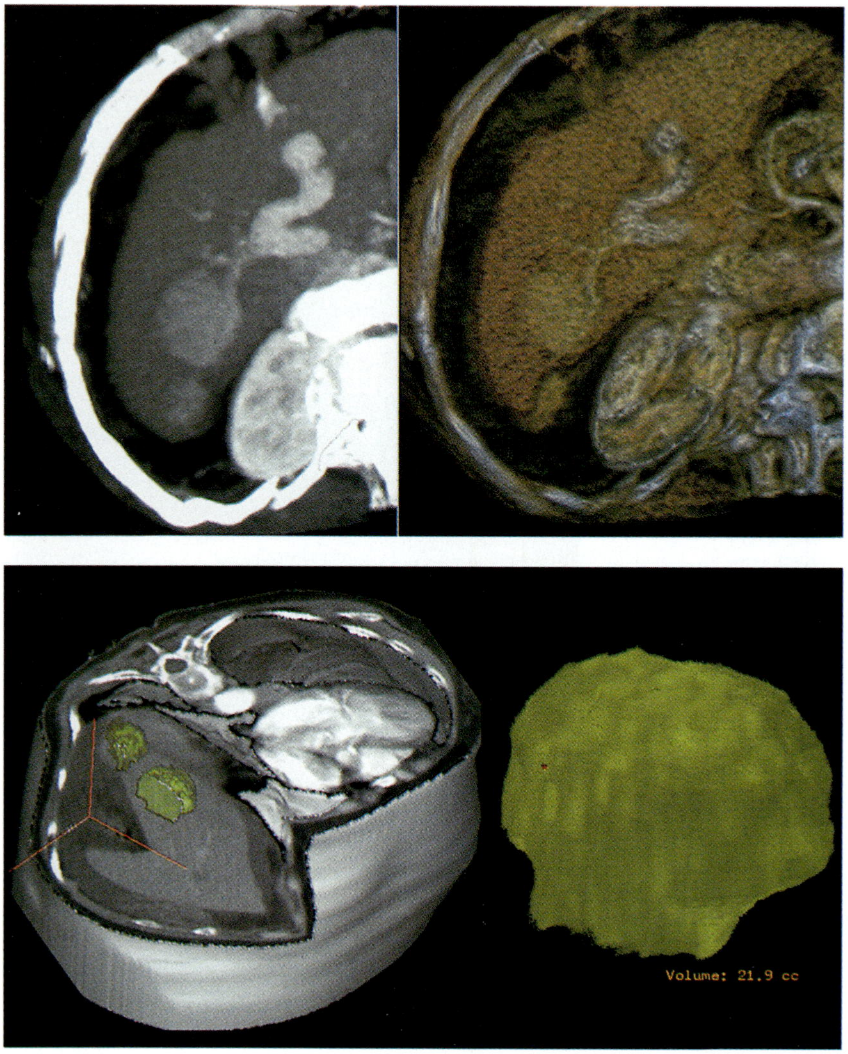

Fig. 33.7a–d. Spiral CT data-set obtained in the portal phase. MIP (**a**) and color coded volume rendering (**b**) demonstrate the position of the hepatocellular carcinoma nodule of the fifth hepatic segment and an adjacent satellite lesion with respect to the portal vessels. After segmentation of the lesions and combination with the volumetric data-set, a surface shaded 3D model is reconstructed (**c**). The volume of the larger nodule can be calculated (**d**)

a b

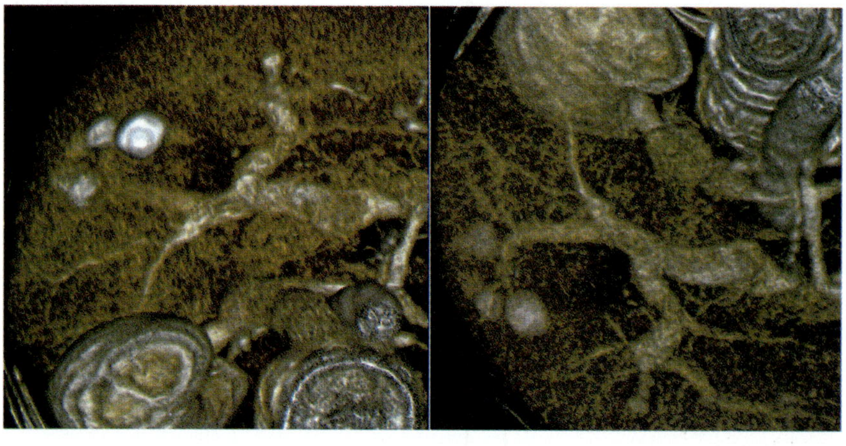

Fig. 33.8a,b. Spiral CT data-set obtained one month after transarterial chemoembolization of hepatocellular carcinoma nodules demonstrating Lipiodol retention in three nodules. Volume rendering of the liver shows the position of the nodules with respect to the portal vessels both in the inferior (**a**) and superior (**b**) views

In the case of the liver, the study of the bile ducts has been reported in particular (Prassopoulos et al. 1998; Dubno et al. 1998; Neri et al. 1999b).

33.3 Imaging Protocols for 3D Liver Studies

Three-dimensional imaging of the liver must be supported by the acquisition of suitable images. Spiral CT and dedicated MRI acquisitions have the technical potential to generate excellent images for volumetric reconstructions. Imaging protocols are designed in order to maximize spatial and temporal resolution for increasing image quality and avoiding motion artifacts. Use of contrast media is helpful to increase contrast resolution and to achieve a precise segmentation.

These requirements are theoretically feasible, but not always easy to comply with in the clinical setting. In fact, patients are sometimes unable to collaborate, time for scanning may not be enough to cover the desired body volume, circulation time varies significantly in different patients (thus causing wrong selection of the scan time). For these reasons 3D rendering sometimes has to be performed with suboptimal images, with increased technical difficulty and with a longer time requirement by the radiologist.

33.3.1 Spiral CT

Spiral CT has two characteristics that are important for 3D imaging: fast scanning and volumetric acquisition. The spiral CT scanning velocity can be exploited for studying the blood vessels, by imaging the patients during the maximum contrast enhancement of the arterial or venous system. In this way spiral CT provides images that resemble those of angiography, and the technique used to obtain such information is called "CT angiography" (CTA).

The principle of arterial and venous enhancement is applied to the study of liver lesions as well, and the typical spiral CT patterns of these tumors are well known. However, although the enhancement variability among the different lesions is important for their characterization, a distinct improvement of spiral CT with respect to conventional CT consists of the volumetric scan in different phases, to best investigate the enhancement of the lesion. Such enhancement can easily be studied on axial images by simultaneously comparing unenhanced, arterial and venous acquisitions. In general two different techniques for liver imaging have been proposed: the biphasic and the three phasic technique. The biphasic technique consists of the first unenhanced scan followed by arterial and portal phase acquisitions of the whole liver. The three phasic technique includes a further scan acquired later, during the venous enhancement (Kemmerer et al. 1998; Nelson et al. 1990; Soyer et al. 1994).

Our spiral CT protocol includes a beam collimation of 5–7 mm, pitch 1–1.4, reconstruction spacing 5–7 mm. We have 1, 3, 5, 7 and 10 mm collimations available. With different equipment the collimation can be further changed (2, 4, 8 mm). The scan delay is 30 s for the arterial phase, 60–70 s for the portal phase and a later scan if required. We do not routinely calculate the circulation time, although this can be necessary in some particular situations (liver transplantation) in which the evaluation of the hepatic artery is important. In these cases, the study of the hepatic artery should be performed using a thin collimation (1–3 mm) and a short reconstruction spacing, in order to increase the longitudinal resolution.

33.3.2 MR Imaging

The main issue of 3D MRI in the study of the liver is how to minimize the effects of motion artifacts due to the patient's breathing. Although many technical solutions have been developed to reduce the influence of motion artifact, the time for 3D imaging with conventional sequences is still longer than the time required for a single breath-hold. Some specific acquisition techniques are being used with increasing frequency in MRI of the liver. Among these techniques, MR angiography (MRA) and MR cholangiopancreatography (MRCP) can have an impact on the 3D study of the liver.

MRA is a well established method for vascular studies. Its most recent development is represented by contrast-enhanced MRA, which is performed by using SPGR sequences with the administration of paramagnetic contrast medium. The acquisition results in the evidence of bright vessels in T1-weighted images, preserving the visibility of liver parenchyma. Such images resemble those of CTA, and are obtained with a similar timing with respect to the bolus injection. In a short time frame (20–30 s) a volumetric acquisition is performed during patient breath-hold, allowing the angiographic study of arterial, portal and/or venous systems.

Another compartment of the liver that can be imaged efficiently with MRI is represented by the biliary tract (Fig. 33.9). In the last few years different authors have reported the use of T2-weighted fast spin echo (FSE) sequences, for the assessment of the biliary tree. These methods are based on breath-hold or non-breath-hold techniques. In both cases the stationary fluid (bile) that fills the biliary ducts shows a high signal intensity on T2-weighted images, but the surrounding structures are not imaged. In these patients the previous intra-muscular administration of scopolamine methyl bromide is useful to avoid peristaltic artifacts, whereas 300–500 ml of water, used as oral contrast agent, improves the visualization of the duodenum.

Imaging protocols include T1-weighted spin-echo axial sequences, FSE T2-weighted, respiratory-triggered, fat-suppressed, axial sequences, and two-dimensional respiratory-triggered, heavily T2-weighted FSE sequences in the coronal plane. In our experience acquisition time ranges between 4 and 6 min for axial and coronal images.

The obtained images can be volume rendered and the internal surface of the biliary tree can be displayed by means of virtual endoscopy (Fig. 33.10).

33.4 3D Reconstruction Tools

The reconstruction methods that can be applied to the study of the liver are essentially represented by multiplanar reconstruction (MPR), multiplanar volume (or subvolume) reconstructions (MPVR), maximum intensity projection (MIP), minimum intensity projection (MinIP), surface shaded display (SSD), virtual endoscopy and volume rendering.

MPR and MPVR consist respectively of the 2D and 3D reformation of data along axial, coronal, sagittal and oblique planes. The vast majority of the commercially available 3D processing software allows the creation of MPR. The advantage of MPR is

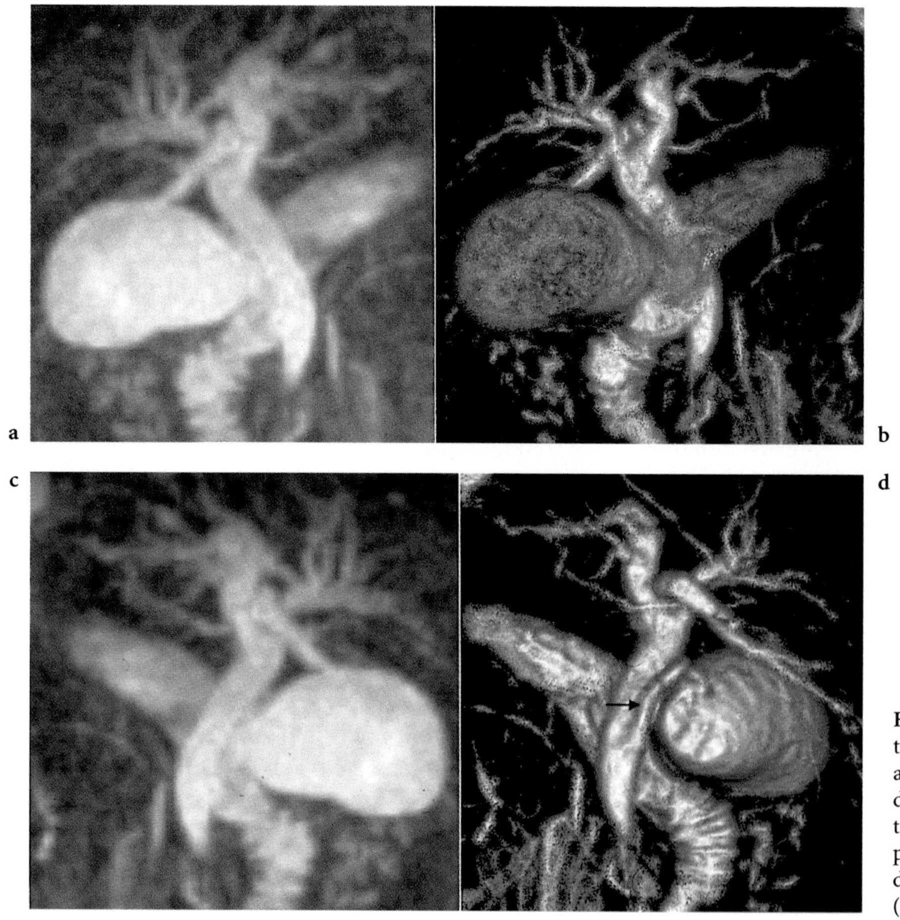

Fig. 33.9a–d. MRCP showing dilatation of common bile duct. MIPs and volume renderings of the data-set are visualized in the anterior **(a,b)** and posterior **(c,d)** perspective. The latter allows the demonstration of the cystic duct (*arrow*)

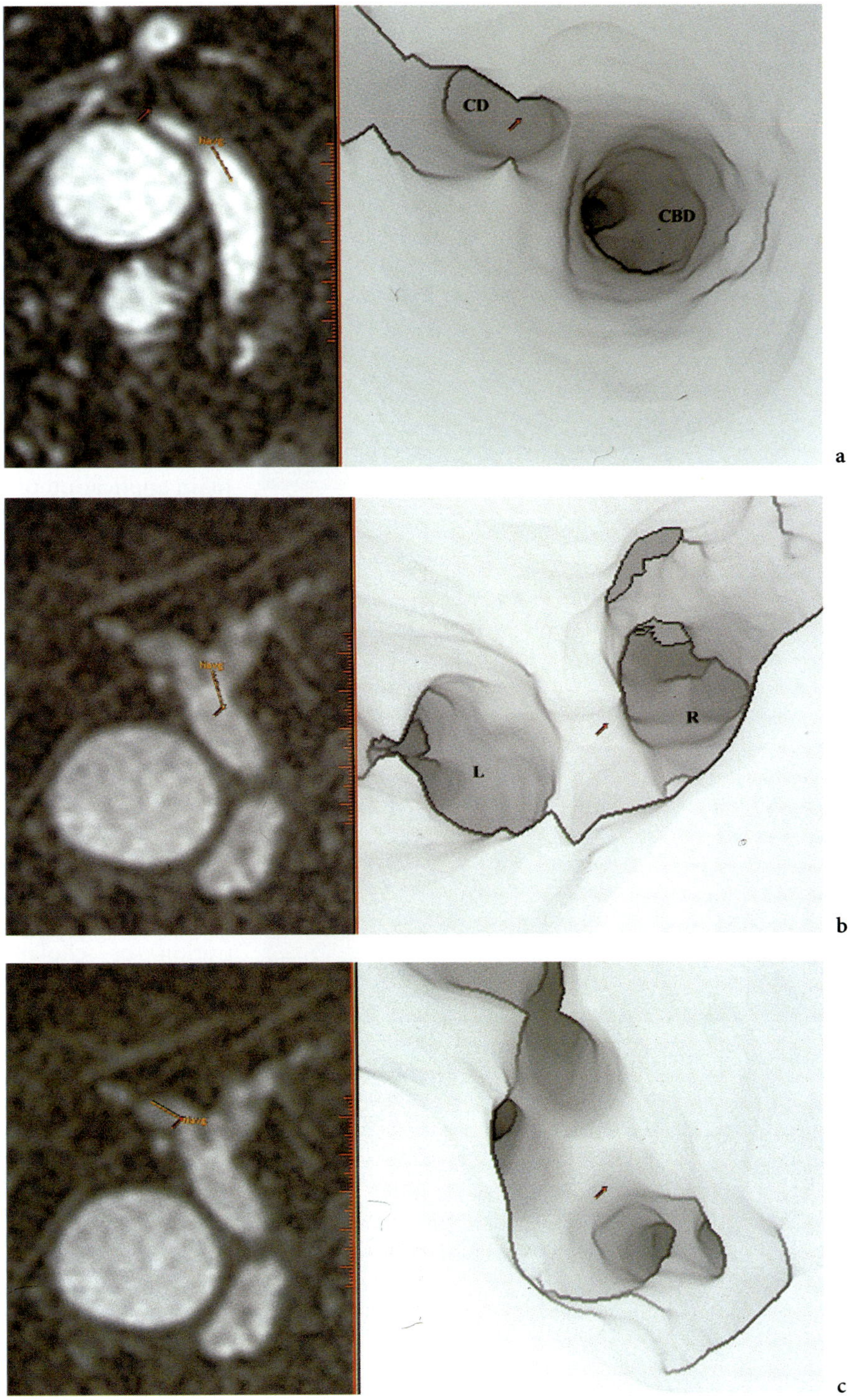

Fig. 33.10a–c. Same case as Fig. 33.9. Virtual endoscopy of the MRCP data-set with a fly-through sequence directed upwards (**a–c**). *CBD*, common bile duct; *CD*, cystic duct; *L*, left hepatic duct; *R*, right hepatic duct

the use of multiple viewing planes crossing through the same point, in order to get spatial information about a single part of the scanned volume. Therefore, the evaluation of liver segmental anatomy, arterial, portal and venous systems, or lesion location, is easier. An extension of MPR is represented by curved planar reconstructions (CPR). This method allows the reformatting of curved planes along the acquired volume and therefore can be used to evaluate curvilinear anatomical structures, such as vessels or stents (Fig. 33.11).

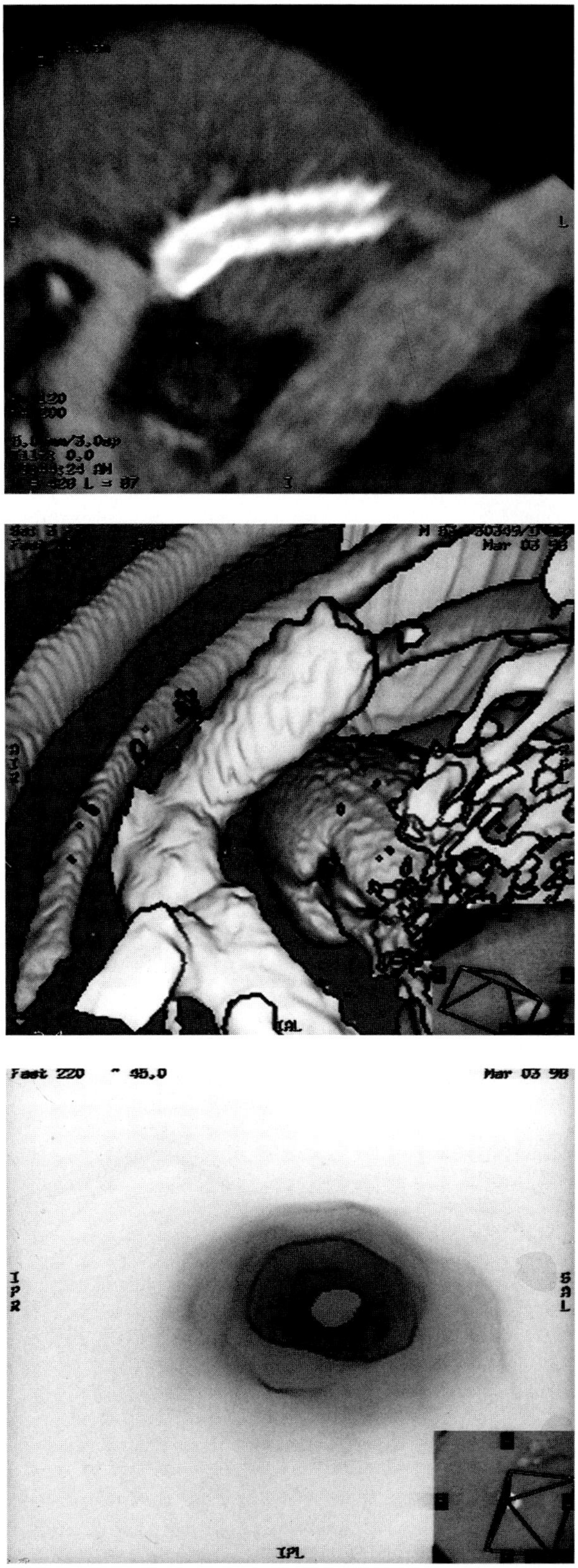

a b c

Fig. 33.11a–c. CTA of the liver after transjugular intrahepatic porto-systemic shunt. CPR of the stent (**a**). Virtual endoscopy fly-around (**b**) and fly-through (**c**) the stent

By using the same planes created with MPR, the thickness of the 2D reformation can be increased to obtain a slab or a subvolume. The subvolume usually includes different anatomical structures of the liver: vessels, parenchyma, and bile ducts. To enhance the appearance of one structure with respect to the others, the MIP, MinIP and VR tools can be applied.

MIP was initially developed for specific application of MR angiography. It produces a 2D representation of the summated signal intensities or CT density of all the pixels along a prescribed line of view. This algorithm is simple and requires few computing resources. However, after the introduction to clinical practice of CTA, MIP has been successfully extended to this technique. The study of the arterial tree is the main application of MIP, and in the case of the liver its use can be extended to the evaluation of the hepatic artery in transplanted patients, to the study of the portal tree in patients with portal thrombosis and to the better location of lesions within the parenchyma (Fig. 33.7). In general MIP allows the highlighting of the brightest structures, so that vessels can be analyzed with particular reference to their course, anatomical distribution and patency.

An important routine application of MIP is the study of the biliary tract with MRCP since it allows the optimal display of the intra- and extrahepatic bile ducts, which have a high signal intensity on T2-weighted FSE sequences. Similarly MIP can be used for CT-cholangiopancreatography after administration of cholangiographic contrast medium (Gillams et al. 1994; Fleischmann et al. 1996; Ludwig et al. 1998; Zeman et al. 1995).

The opposite algorithm is represented by the MinIP. The MinIP enhances the visibility of the structures with lower density or intensity within the volume, as the case of the bile ducts. In fact, MinIP, which was initially proposed for the study of the bronchial tree, has recently found interesting applications in the study of the biliary tract (Raptopoulos et al. 1998). By creating the optimal MPVR along the common bile duct or the intra-hepatic ducts, stenoses or other alterations can be evaluated in a 3D perspective. A drawback of MinIP in the study of the bile ducts is the need to have a major dilatation of these structures in order to enhance their visibility (Fig. 33.12).

SSD images result from a segmentation process that isolates only selected anatomical structures from the background. The process of segmentation can be based on the setting of a threshold (in this case vessels, bone and arterial calcification are best visualized), or on region growing or manual tracing

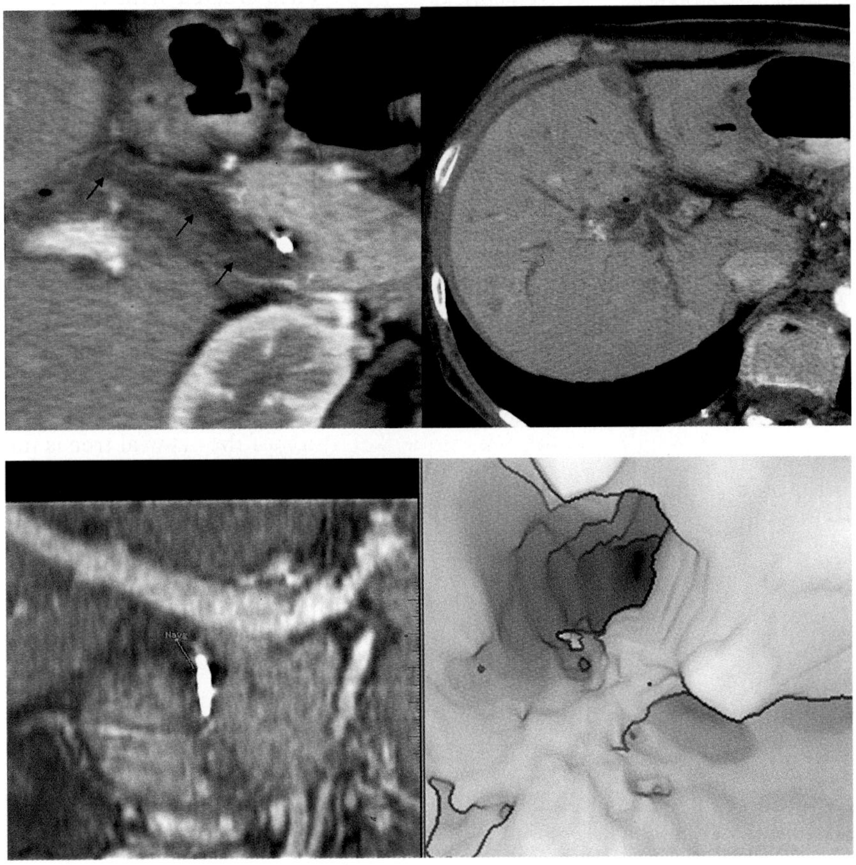

a b c

Fig. 33.12a–c. Spiral CT examination demonstrating obstructive jaundice in a patient with neoplastic stenosis of the common bile duct and biliary drainage. MinIP created with MPVR through the liver parenchyma (**a**) and along the common bile duct (**b**) show dilatation of the intrahepatic and the common bile ducts (*arrows*). Virtual endoscopy of the common bile duct (**c**) displays the dilated lumen and the drainage

methods. Multiple isolated structures can then be combined to better represent the anatomical relationships. Liver lesions can be isolated and then merged with the liver. The use of a different color for each structure allows an easier differentiation (Fig. 33.7) (Stransky et al. 1994; Bjerner et al. 1998).

Virtual endoscopy has been introduced into clinical practice in the past few years, and its first application was reported in the study of the bronchial tree. In this case, the feasibility of virtual endoscopy was due to the easy segmentation of the airways that could be visualized from the inside by surface rendering the walls of the trachea and bronchi. Further applications were found in the study of other organs and tubular structures, such as colon, stomach, paranasal sinuses, larynx, vessels, urinary tract, biliary tract, cerebral ventricles, middle and inner ear, etc. The method can be based on surface or volume rendering techniques.

In the case of the liver, virtual endoscopy permits one to fly-through the bile ducts, the arterial, portal and venous systems, allowing the demonstration of endoluminal masses, stenoses, occlusions, and prostheses (Fig. 33.13).

Volume rendering, which has been already described in this chapter, presents multiple potential applications: study of the anatomy of the liver, demonstration of focal lesions and their characterization with gray scale or color coding, and visualization of the biliary tree and biliary prostheses (Wielopolski et al. 1999). In the latter application, volume rendering allows in particular the evaluation of the morphology, patency and course of biliary stents (Fig. 33.14).

33.5 Clinical Applications

The role of 3D images in the study of liver malignancies is still under clinical evaluation. However, many applications can be envisioned on the basis of the first results reported in the literature. In the field of lesion detection, diagnostic accuracy of CT and MR is primarily dependent on a careful analysis of the axial images acquired during the arterial, portal and delayed phases, by changing window and levels in order to enhance the lesion conspicuity with respect

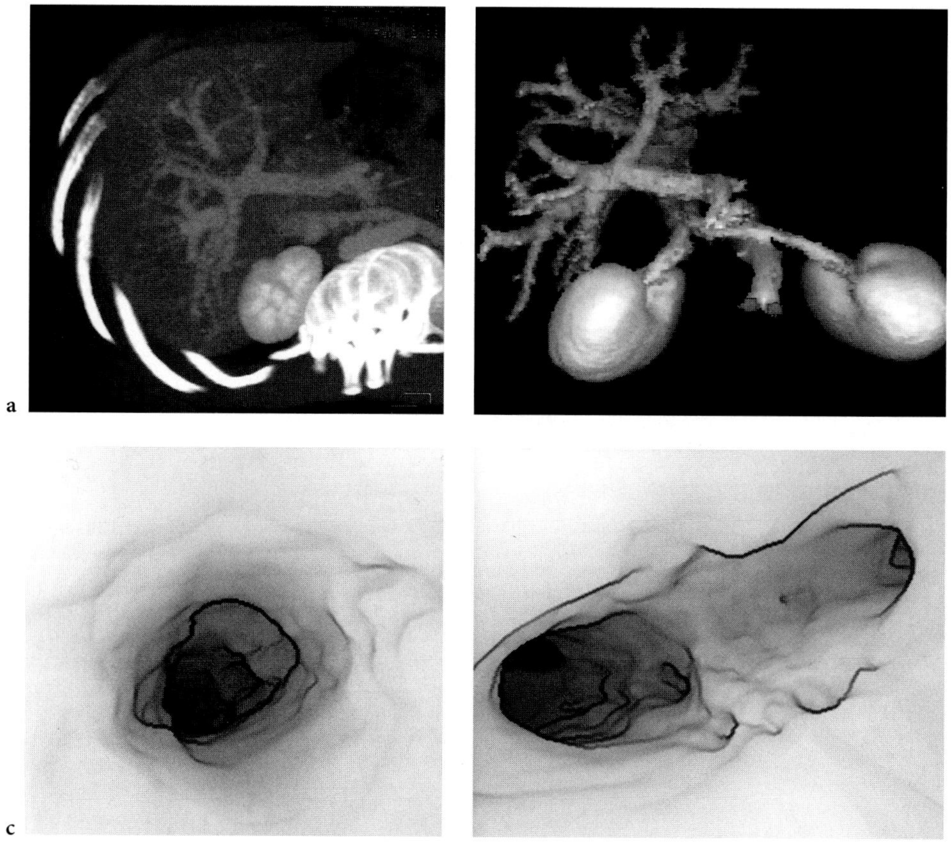

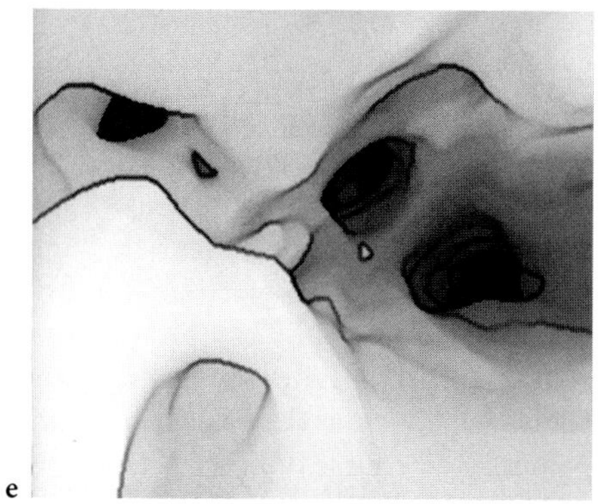

Fig. 33.13a–e. MIP (**a**) and SSD (**b**) of the portal tree. A fly-through sequence is generated along the main trunk of the portal vein (**c**), the portal bifurcation (**d**) and the right intrahepatic branches (**e**)

to the parenchyma. However, 3D images can potentially contribute to increasing the sensitivity of 2D imaging in the presence of enhancing nodules (as in the typical case of hepatocellular carcinoma) (Hawighorst et al. 1999). In these cases the complementary use of MPVR with MIP allows the enhancement of the detectability of the lesions (Fig. 33.7). Moreover, by using volume renderings the lesions can be identified with color coding (Fig. 33.7). A further reason for using these tools is that they enable the complete visualization of vessels, allowing a direct representation of their anatomical position with respect to the lesions. The complementary use of these processing methods is not exceedingly time consuming and can be realistically proposed in a clinical setting (Wilson et al. 1998; Togo et al. 1998; van Leeuwen et al. 1994).

For local tumor staging, visualization of hepatocellular carcinoma nodules in Lipiodol CT data-sets can be facilitated by using 3D reconstruction (Fig. 33.8). In pre-treatment planning (before surgery or locoregional therapies), 3D images can be of assistance by enabling the contemporary visualization of portal and venous vessels, thus allowing the display of the liver segmental anatomy as defined by Couinaud (1986) and Bismuth (1982).

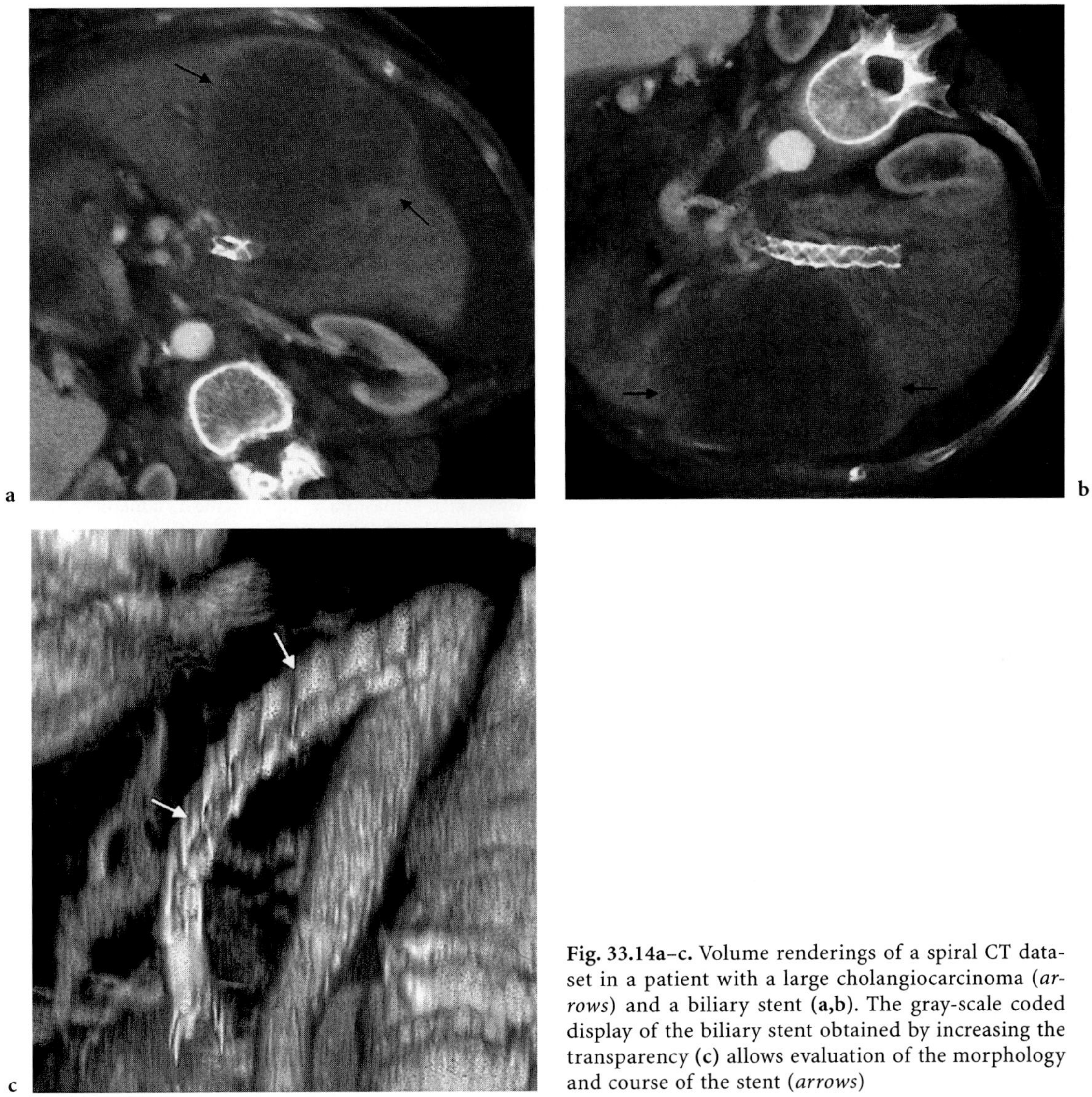

Fig. 33.14a–c. Volume renderings of a spiral CT dataset in a patient with a large cholangiocarcinoma (*arrows*) and a biliary stent (**a,b**). The gray-scale coded display of the biliary stent obtained by increasing the transparency (**c**) allows evaluation of the morphology and course of the stent (*arrows*)

Exploiting these advantages of 3D imaging, more precise segmental hepatectomies can be planned, and the attention of the surgeon can be more easily focused on avoiding damage of the hepatic veins (Waggenspack et al. 1993). If local therapy is planned, 3D visualization permits the identification of the more appropriate path for targeting the lesion within the liver parenchyma (Fig. 33.3).

The knowledge of anatomical details is essential when the patient presents anatomical variants: hepatic veins can have supernumerary branches, early divisions or an uncommon course; portal branches can have an accessory branch that independently arises from the portal vein and contributes to the vascularization of the right posterior segments (VI and VII); bile ducts can have accessory ducts or atresia of intrahepatic branches (van Leeuwen et al. 1994; Kashiwagi et al. 1994).

Three-dimensional reconstructions enable volumetric assessments of anatomical structures. In particular, this can be done for the liver parenchyma by using a careful segmentation (Fig. 33.5). When the patient undergoes hepatectomy, 3D reconstructions allow the quantification of the residual parenchyma and the estimation of the entity and the edge of resection (Togo et al. 1998).

Post-treatment assessment is also useful in cases of follow-up of liver lesion after local therapies (percutaneous ethanol injection, trans-arterial chemoembolization and radiofrequency thermal ablation). A comparison between the pre- and post-treatment imaging of the lesions is able to demonstrate the reduction of the viable tumor tissue in the case of a successful treatment. By applying different segmentation methods (region growing, cutting planes, threshold), the lesion can be isolated from the liver parenchyma; then it can be characterized by color coding and volume renderings. In this way, 3D imaging contributes to the precise estimation of tumor necrosis, and permits the indication of whether or not the treatment has been successful.

References

Bae KT, Giger ML, Chen CT, Kahn CE Jr (1993) Automatic segmentation of liver structure in CT images. Med Phys 20:71–78

Bartolozzi C, Neri E, Caramella D (1998) CT in Vascular Pathologies. Eur Radiol 8:679–684

Bennet WF, Bova JG, Petty L, Martin EW Jr (1991) Preoperative 3D rendering of MR imaging in liver metastases. J Comput Assist Tomogr 15:979–984

Bismuth H (1982) Surgical anatomy and anatomical surgery of the liver. World J Surg 6:3–9

Bjerner T, Johansson L, Haglund U, Ahlstrom H (1998) 3D surface rendering of images from multiple MR pulse sequences in the pre-operative evaluation of hepatic lesions. Acta Radiol 39:698–700

Couinaud C (1986) Anatomie chirurgicale di foie: quelques aspects nouveaux. Chirurgie 112:337–342

Debatin JF, Spritzer CE, Grist TM, et al (1991) Imaging of the Renal Arteries: Value of MR-Angiography. AJR Am J Roentgenol 157:981–990

Dubno B, Debatin JF, Luboldt W, Schmidt M, Hany TF, Bauerfeind P (1998) Virtual MR cholangiography. AJR Am J Roentgenol 171:1547–50

Fleischmann D, Ringl H, Schofl R, et al (1996) Three-dimensional spiral CT cholangiography in patients with suspected obstructive biliary disease: comparison with endoscopic retrograde cholangiography. Radiology 198:861–868

Gillams A, Gardener J, Richards R, Tan AC, Linney A, Lees WR (1994) Three-dimensional computed tomography cholangiography: a new technique for biliary tract imaging. Br J Radiol 67:445–448

Hawighorst H, Schoenberg SO, Knopp MV, Essig M, Miltner P, van Kaick G (1999) Hepatic lesions: morphologic and functional characterization with multiphase breath-hold 3D gadolinium-enhanced MR angiography–initial results. Radiology 210:89–96

Kalender WA, Seissler W, Klots E, Vock P (1990) Spiral volumetric CT with single breath hold technique, continuous transport, and continuous scanner rotation. Radiology 176:181–183

Kashiwagi T, Murakami T, Azuma M, et al (1994) Three-dimensional display of liver, spleen, hepatoma, and blood vessels by MR imaging and computer graphics. Acta Radiol 35:88–89

Kemmerer SR, Mortele KJ, Ros PR (1998) CT scan of the liver. Radiol Clin North Am 36:247–61

Lorensen WE, Cline H (1987) Marching cubes: a high resolution 3D surface construction algorithm. Computer Graphics 21:163–169

Ludwig J, Ritman EL, LaRusso NF, Sheedy PF, Zumpe G (1998) Anatomy of the human biliary system studied by quantitative computer-aided three-dimensional imaging techniques. Hepatology 27:893–9

Meyer CA, Colon E, Provost T, Sherman JL (1992) Delineation of surgical segmental liver anatomy: value of PRISE, an MR fast-scanning technique. AJR Am J Roentgenol 158:299–301

Miyazaki T, Yamashita Y, Tsuchigame T, Yamamoto H, Urata J, Takahashi M (1996) MR cholangiopancreatography using HASTE (half-Fourier acquisition single-shot turbo spin-echo) sequences. AJR Am J Roentgenol 166:1297–1303

Nelson RC, Chezmar JL, Sugarbacker PH, Murray DR, Bernardino ME (1990) Preoperative localisation of focal liver lesions to specific liver segments: utility of CT during arterial portography. Radiology 176:89–94

Neri E, Boraschi P, Braccini G, Caramella D, Perri G, Bartolozzi C (1999a) MR virtual endoscopy of the pancreaticobiliary tract. Magn Reson Imaging 17:59–67

Neri E, Caramella D, Falaschi F, et al (1999b) Virtual CT intravascular endoscopy of the aorta: pierced surface and floating shapes thresholding artifacts. Radiology 212:276–279

Prassopoulos P, Raptopoulus V, Chuttani R, McKee JD, McNicholas MMJ, Sheiman RG (1998) Development of virtual CT cholangiopacreatoscopy. Radiology 209:570–574

Prince MR (1994) Gadolinium-enhanced MR aortography. Radiology 191:155–164

Raptopoulos V, Prassopoulos P, Chuttani R, McNicholas MMJ, Mkee JD, Kressel HY (1998) Multiplanar CT pancreatography and distal cholangiography with minimum intensity projections. Radiology 207:317–324.

Reinhold C, Bret PM (1996) Current status of MR cholangiopancreatography. AJR Am J Roentgenol 166:1285–1295

Soyer P, Bluemke DA, Fishman EK (1994) CT during arterial portography for the preoperative evaluation of hepatic tumors: how, when, and why? AJR Am J Roentgenol 163:1325–31

Stransky G, Weis S, Thaller R, Wenger E, Barousch G (1994) A method for the quantification of the size of liver metastases. Comput Med Imaging Graph 18:175–179

Togo S, Shimada H, Kanemura E, et al (1998) Usefulness of three-dimensional computed tomography for anatomic liver resection: sub-subsegmentectomy. Surgery 123:73–8

van Leeuwen MS, Fernandez MA, van Es HW, Stokking R, Dillon EH, Feldberg MAM (1994) Variations in venous and segmental anatomy of the liver: two- and three-dimensional MR imaging in healthy volunteers. AJR Am J Roentgenol 162:1337–1345

Waggenspack GA, Tabb DR, Tiruchelvam V, Ziegler L, Waltersdorff (1993) Three-dimensional location of hepatic neoplasms with computer generated scissurae recreated from axial CT and MR images. AJR Am J Roentgenol 160:307–309

Wielopolski PA, Gaa J, Wielopolski DR, Oudkerk (1999) Breath-hold MR cholangiopancreatography with three-dimensional, segmented, echo-planar imaging and volume rendering. Radiology 210:247–252

Wilson DL, Carrillo A, Zheng L, Genc A, Duerk JL, Lewin JS (1998) Evaluation of 3D image registration as applied to MR-guided thermal treatment of liver cancer. J Magn Reson Imaging 8:77–84

Zeman RK, Berman PM, Silverman PM, et al (1995) Biliary tract: three-dimensional helical CT without cholangiographic contrast material. Radiology 196:865–867

Subject Index

List of Contributors

Carlo Bartolozzi, MD
Professor and Chairman
Division of Diagnostic and Interventional Radiology
Department of Oncology
University of Pisa
Via Roma 67
I-56125 Pisa
Italy

Christoph D. Becker, MD
Head, Unit of Abdominal and Gynecological Radiology
University Hospital of Geneva
Rue Micheli-du-Crest 24
CH-1211 Geneva 14
Switzerland

Generoso Bevilacqua, MD
Professor and Chairman
Division of Pathology
Department of Oncology
University of Pisa
Via Roma 57
I-56125 Pisa
Italy

Luigi Bolondi, MD
Professor and Chairman
Department of Internal Medicine
S. Orsola Malpighi Hospital
University of Bologna
Via Massarenti 9
I-40138 Bologna
Italy

Concepcio Bru, MD
Department of Radiology
Hospital Clinic, University of Barcelona
Villarroel 170
E-08036 Barcelona
Spain

Jordi Bruix, MD
Chief, Liver Unit
Hospital Clinic, University of Barcelona
Villarroel 170
E-08036 Barcelona
Spain

Francesca Burresi, MD
Department of Radiology
University of Siena, Le Scotte Hospital
Viale Bracci 2
I-53100 Siena
Italy

Elisabetta Buscarini, MD
Department of Gastroenterology
General Hospital
Cantone del Cristo 40
I-29100 Piacenza
Italy

Luigi Buscarini, MD
Professor and Chief
Department of Gastroenterology
General Hospital
Cantone del Cristo 40
I-29100 Piacenza
Italy

Paolo Busilacchi, MD
Department of Radiology
Umberto I Hospital
Largo Cappelli 1
I-60020 Ancona
Italy

Maria Adelaide Caligo, MD
Division of Pathology
Department of Oncology
University of Pisa
Via Roma 57
I-56125 Pisa
Italy

Daniela Campani, MD
Division of Pathology
Department of Oncology
University of Pisa
Via Roma 57
I-56125 Pisa
Italy

Vito Cantisani, MD
Department of Radiology
University of Rome "La Sapienza"
Viale Regina Elena 324
I-00161 Rome
Italy

Davide Caramella, MD
Division of Diagnostic and
Interventional Radiology
Department of Oncology
University of Pisa
Via Roma 67
I-56125 Pisa
Italy

Roberto Caudana, MD
Department of Radiology
University of Verona
Borgo Roma Hospital
Via delle Menetone 10
I-37134 Verona
Italy

Antonio Cicorelli, MD
Division of Diagnostic and Interventional Radiology
Department of Oncology
University of Pisa
Via Roma 67
I-56125 Pisa
Italy

Dania Cioni, MD
Division of Diagnostic and Interventional Radiology
Department of Oncology
University of Pisa
Via Roma 67
I-56125 Pisa
Italy

Corrado Colagrande, MD
Professor, Department of Radiology
A. Gemelli University Hospital
Largo A. Gemelli 8
I-00168 Rome
Italy

Marco Coniglio, MD
Department of Radiology
University of Rome "La Sapienza"
Viale Regina Elena 324
I-00161 Rome
Italy

Pier Franco Conte, MD
Chief, Division of Medical Oncology
Department of Oncology
University of Pisa
Via Roma 57
I-56125 Pisa
Italy

Antonio R. Cotroneo, MD
Professor, Department of Radiology
A. Gemelli University Hospital
Largo A. Gemelli 8
I-00168 Rome
Italy

Luca Cova, MD
Professor, Department of Radiology
General Hospital
Piazzale Solaro 3
Busto Arsizio
I-21052 Varese
Italy

Laura Crocetti, MD
Division of Diagnostic and Interventional Radiology
Department of Oncology
University of Pisa
Via Roma 67
I-56125 Pisa
Italy

Anna M. De Gaetano, MD
Department of Radiology
A. Gemelli University Hospital
Largo A. Gemelli 8
I-00168 Rome
Italy

Marina Dellanoce, MD
Department of Radiology
General Hospital
Piazzale Solaro 3
Busto Arsizio
I-21052 Varese
Italy

Giulio Di Candio, MD
Division of General and Experimental Surgery
Department of Oncology
University of Pisa
Via Paradisa 2
I-56124 Pisa
Italy

Alberto Di Filippo, MD
Department of Radiology
University of Rome "La Sapienza"
Viale Regina Elena 324
I-00161 Rome
Italy

Massimo Di Giulio, MD
Division of Diagnostic and Interventional Radiology
Department of Oncology
University of Pisa
Via Roma 67
I-56125 Pisa
Italy

Francescamaria Donati, MD
Division of Diagnostic and Interventional Radiology
Department of Oncology
University of Pisa
Via Roma 67
I-56125 Pisa
Italy

Irene Esposito, MD
Division of Pathology
Department of Oncology
University of Pisa
Via Roma 57
I-56125 Pisa
Italy

Alfredo Falcone, MD
Division of Medical Oncology
Department of Oncology
University of Pisa
Via Roma 57
I-56125 Pisa
Italy

Cesare Fava, MD
Professor, Department of Radiological Sciences
University of Turin
Via Genova 3
I-10126 Turin
Italy

Francesco Saverio Ferrari, MD
Department of Radiology
University of Siena
Le Scotte Hospital
Viale Bracci 2
I-53100 Siena
Italy

Raoul Foroni, MD
Department of Pathology
General Hospital
Via Taverna 49
I-29100 Piacenza
Italy

Giulia Galletti, MD
Department of Radiology
A. Gemelli University Hospital
Largo A. Gemelli 8
I-00168 Rome
Italy

Francesco Garbagnati, MD
Department of Radiology
National Cancer Institute
Via Venezian 1
I-20100 Milan
Italy

G. Scott Gazelle, MD
Professor, Department of Radiology
Massachusetts General Hospital
Boston, MA 02214
USA

Andrea Giovagnoni, MD
MR Center "F. Angelini"
Department of Radiology
University of Ancona, Torrette
I-60020 Ancona
Italy

S. Nahum Goldberg, MD
Department of Radiology
Beth Israel Deaconess Hospital
Harvard Medical School
330 Brookline Avenue
Boston, MA 02215
USA

Giulia Granai, MD
Division of Diagnostic and
Interventional Radiology
Department of Oncology
University of Pisa
Via Roma 67
I-56125 Pisa
Italy

Walter Franco Grigioni, MD
Professor, Department of Pathology,
Histology and Cytology
F. Addari Institute
S Orsola Malphighi Hospital
Viale Ercolani 4/2
I-40138 Bologna
Italy

Maurizio Grosso, MD
Department of Radiological Sciences
University of Turin
Via Genova 3
I-10126 Turin
Italy

Renate Hammerstingl, MD
Department of Radiology
Johann Wolfgang Goethe University
Theodor-Stern-Kai 7
D-60590 Frankfurt am Main
Germany

Nigel Howarth, MD
Department of Radiology
University Hospital of Geneva
Rue Micheli-du-Crest 24
CH-1211 Geneva 14
Switzerland

Tiziana Ierace, MD
Department of Radiology
General Hospital
Piazzale Solaro 3
Busto Arsizio
I-21052 Varese
Italy

Ramy Kayal, MD
Department of Radiology
University of Rome "La Sapienza"
Viale Regina Elena 324
I-00161 Rome
Italy

Claudia Lattes, MD
Department of Pathology, Histology and Cytology
F. Addari Institute
S. Orsola Malphighi Hospital
Viale Ercolani 4/2
I-40138 Bologna
Italy

Riccardo Lencioni, MD
Division of Diagnostic and Interventional Radiology
Department of Oncology
University of Pisa
Via Roma 67
I-56125 Pisa
Italy

Daniel A. Leung
Department of Radiology
Zürich University Hospital
Rämistrasse 100
CH-8091 Zurich
Switzerland

Emanuele Lezoche, MD
Professor and Chief
Department of Surgical Sciences
University of Ancona
Umberto I Hospital
Largo Cappelli 1
I-60020 Ancona
Italy

Tito Livraghi, MD
Chief, Department of Radiology
General Hospital
Via C. Battisti 23
I-20059 Vimercate (Milan)
Italy

Giorgio Lucigrai, MD
Department of Radiology
G. Gaslini Children's Research Hospital
Largo G. Gaslini 5
I-16148 Genoa
Italy

Riccardo Manfredi, MD
Department of Radiology
A. Gemelli University Hospital
Largo A. Gemelli 8
I-00168 Rome
Italy

Pasquale Marano, MD
Professor and Chairman
Department of Radiology
A. Gemelli University Hospital
Largo A. Gemelli 8
I-00168 Rome
Italy

Giulia Maresca, MD
Professor, Department of Radiology
A. Gemelli University Hospital
Largo A. Gemelli 8
I-00168 Rome
Italy

Borut Marincek, MD
Professor and Chairman
Department of Radiology
Zürich University Hospital
Rämistrasse 100
CH-8091 Zurich
Switzerland

Livia Masi, MD
Department of Internal Medicine
S. Orsola Malpighi Hospital
University of Bologna
Via Massarenti 9
I-40138 Bologna
Italy

Federico Maspes, MD
Department of Radiology
University of Rome "Tor Vergata"
S. Eugenio Hospital
Piazzale dell' Umanesimo 10
I-00143 Rome
Italy

Yves Menu, MD
Professor and Chairman
Department of Radiology
Hôpital Beaujon
100 Boulevard du Général Leclerc
F-92118 Clichy
France

Giovanna Morana, MD
Department of Radiology
University of Verona
Borgo Roma Hospital
Via delle Menetone 10
I-37134 Verona
Italy

Monica Moretti, MD
Division of Diagnostic and Interventional Radiology
Department of Oncology
University of Pisa
Via Roma 67
I-56125 Pisa
Italy

Franco Mosca, MD, FACS
Professor and Chairman
Division of General and Experimental Surgery
Department of Oncology
University of Pisa
Via Paradisa 2
I-56124 Pisa
Italy

Emanuele Neri, MD
Division of Diagnostic and Interventional Radiology
Department of Oncology
University of Pisa
Via Roma 67
I-56125 Pisa
Italy

Mauro Oddone, MD
Department of Radiology
G. Gaslini Children's Research Hospital
Largo G. Gaslini 5
I-16148 Genoa
Italy

Alessandro Paganini, MD
Department of Surgical Sciences
University of Ancona, Umberto I Hospital
Largo Cappelli 1
I-60020 Ancona
Italy

Alessandro Paolicchi, MD
Division of Diagnostic and Interventional Radiology
Department of Oncology
University of Pisa
Via Roma 67
I-56125 Pisa
Italy

Thomas Pfammatter, MD
Department of Radiology
Zürich University Hospital
Rämistrasse 100
CH-8091 Zurich
Switzerland

Elisabetta Pfanner, MD
Division of Medical Oncology
Department of Oncology
University of Pisa
Via Roma 57
I-56125 Pisa
Italy

Andrea Pietrabissa, MD
Division of General and Experimental Surgery
Department of Oncology
University of Pisa
Via Paradisa 2
I-56124 Pisa
Italy

Patrizia Pini, MD
Department of Internal Medicine
S. Orsola Malpighi Hospital
University of Bologna
Via Massarenti 9
I-40138 Bologna
Italy

Gian Franco Pistolesi, MD
Professor and Chairman
Department of Radiology
University of Verona
Borgo Roma Hospital
Via delle Menetone 10
I-37134 Verona
Italy

Giuseppe Pizzi, MD
Department of Radiology
University of Rome "La Sapienza"
Viale Regina Elena 324
I-00161 Rome
Italy

Marco Pocek, MD
Professor, Department of Radiology
University of Rome "Tor Vergata"
S. Eugenio Hospital
Piazzale dell' Umanesimo 10
I-00143 Rome
Italy

Sibylle Pochon, PhD
Bracco Research
CH-1211 Geneva 14
Switzerland

Gianna Poggianti, MD
Department of Radiology
University of Siena
Le Scotte Hospital
Viale Bracci 2
I-53100 Siena
Italy

Gian Ludovico Rapaccini, MD
Professor, Department of Internal Medicine
A. Gemelli University Hospital
Largo A. Gemelli 8
I-00168 Rome
Italy

Richard D. Redvanly, MD
Assistant Professor, Department of Radiology
Emory University School of Medicine
1364 Clifton Road, N.E.
Atlanta, GA 30322
USA

Paolo Ricci, MD
Department of Radiology
University of Rome "La Sapienza"
Viale Regina Elena 324
I-00161 Rome
Italy

Alain Roche, MD
Professor and Chief, Interventional Radiology Section
Department of Medical Imaging
Institut Gustave-Roussy
39 Rue Camille Desmoulins
F-94800 Villejuif
France

Sandro Rossi, MD
Department of Gastroenterology
General Hospital
Cantone del Cristo 40
I-29100 Piacenza
Italy

Rigoantonio Roversi, MD
Professor and Chief, Department of Diagnostic Imaging
and Interventional Radiology
Bellaria-Maggiore Hospital
Via Altura 3
I-40100 Bologna
Italy

Gloria Serafini, MD
Department of Radiology
University of Rome "Tor Vergata"
S. Eugenio Hospital
Piazzale dell' Umanesimo 10
I-00143 Rome
Italy

Giovanni Simonetti, MD
Professor and Chairman, Department of Radiology
University of Rome "Tor Vergata"
S. Eugenio Hospital
Piazzale dell' Umanesimo 10
I-00143 Rome
Italy

Luigi Solbiati, MD
Chief, Department of Radiology
General Hospital
Piazzale Solaro 3
Busto Arsizio
I-21052 Varese
Italy

Paolo Stefani, MD
Professor and Chairman
Department of Radiology
University of Siena, Le Scotte Hospital
Viale Bracci 2
I-53100 Siena
Italy

Ettore Squillaci, MD
Department of Radiology
University of Rome "Tor Vergata"
S. Eugenio Hospital
Piazzale dell' Umanesimo 10
I-00143 Rome
Italy

François Terrier, MD
Professor and Chairman, Department of Radiology
University Hospital of Geneva
Rue Micheli-du-Crest 24
CH-1211 Geneva 14
Switzerland

Paolo Tomà, MD
Chief, Department of Radiology
G. Gaslini Children's Research Hospital
Largo G. Gaslini 5
I-16148 Genoa
Italy

Maurizio Vaccari, MD
Department of Pathology, Histology and Cytology
F. Addari Institute
S Orsola Malphighi Hospital
Viale Ercolani 4/2
I-40138 Bologna
Italy

Gianluca Valeri, MD
MR Center "F. Angelini"
Department of Radiology
University of Ancona, Torrette
I-60020 Ancona
Italy

Jean Paul Vallée, MD
Department of Radiology
University Hospital of Geneva
Rue Micheli-du-Crest 24
CH-1211 Geneva 14
Switzerland

Amorinio Vecchioli, MD
Professor, Department of Radiology
A. Gemelli University Hospital
Largo A. Gemelli 8
I-00168 Rome
Italy

Andrea Veltri, MD
Department of Radiological Sciences
University of Turin
Via Genova 3
I-10126 Turin
Italy

Thomas J. Vogl, MD
Professor, Department of Radiology
Johann Wolfgang Goethe University
Theodor-Stern-Kai 7
D-60590 Frankfurt am Main
Germany

MEDICAL RADIOLOGY
Diagnostic Imaging and Radiation Oncology

Titles in the series already published

DIAGNOSTIC IMAGING

Innovations in Diagnostic Imaging
Edited by J.H. Anderson

Radiology of the Upper Urinary Tract
Edited by E.K. Lang

The Thymus - Diagnostic Imaging, Functions, and Pathologic Anatomy
Edited by E. Walter, E. Willich, and W.R. Webb

Interventional Neuroradiology
Edited by A. Valavanis

Radiology of the Pancreas
Edited by A.L. Baert, co-edited by G. Delorme

Radiology of the Lower Urinary Tract
Edited by E.K. Lang

Magnetic Resonance Angiography
Edited by I.P. Arlart, G.M. Bongartz, and G. Marchal

Contrast-Enhanced MRI of the Breast
S. Heywang-Köbrunner and R. Beck

Spiral CT of the Chest
Edited by M. Rémy-Jardin and J. Rémy

Radiological Diagnosis of Breast Diseases
Edited by M. Friedrich and E.A. Sickles

Radiology of the Trauma
Edited by M. Heller and A. Fink

Biliary Tract Radiology
Edited by P. Rossi

Radiological Imaging of Sports Injuries
Edited by C. Masciocchi

Modern Imaging of the Alimentary Tube
Edited by A. R. Margulis

Diagnosis and Therapy of Spinal Tumors
Edited by P. R. Algra, J. Valk, and J. J. Heimans

Interventional Magnetic Resonance Imaging
Edited by J. F. Debatin and G. Adam

Abdominal and Pelvic MRI
Edited by A. Heuck and M. Reiser

Orthopedic Imaging
Techniques and Applications
Edited by A.M. Davies and H. Pettersson

Radiology of the Female Pelvic Organs
Edited by E.K.Lang

Magnetic Resonance of the Heart and Great Vessels
Clinical Applications
Edited by J. Bogaert, A. J. Duerinckx, and F. E. Rademakers

Modern Head and Neck Imaging
Edited by S. K. Mukherji and J. A. Castelijns

Radiological Imaging of Endocrine Diseases
Edited by J. N. Bruneton in collaboration with B. Padovani and M.-Y. Mourou

Trends in Contrast Media
Edited by H. S. Thomsen, R. N. Muller, and R. F. Mattrey

Functional MRI
Edited by C. T. W. Moonen and P. A. Bandettini

Radiology of the Pancreas
2nd Revised Edition
Edited by A. L. Baert
Co-edited by G. Delorme and L. Van Hoe

Radiology of Peripheral Vascular Diseases
Edited by E. Zeitler

Emergency Pediatric Radiology
Edited by H. Carty

Spiral CT of the Abdomen
Edited by F. Terrier, M. Grossholz, and C. Becker

Liver Malignancies
Diagnostic and Interventional Radiology
Edited by C. Bartolozzi and R. Lencioni

Springer

MEDICAL RADIOLOGY
Diagnostic Imaging and Radiation Oncology

Titles in the series already published

RADIATION ONCOLOGY

Lung Cancer
Edited by C.W. Scarantino

Innovations in Radiation Oncology
Edited by H.R. Withers and L.J. Peters

Radiation Therapy of Head and Neck Cancer
Edited by G.E. Laramore

Gastrointestinal Cancer – Radiation Therapy
Edited by R.R. Dobelbower, Jr.

Radiation Exposure and Occupational Risks
Edited by E. Scherer, C. Streffer, and K.-R. Trott

Radiation Therapy of Benign Diseases - A Clinical Guide
S.E. Order and S.S. Donaldson

Interventional Radiation Therapy Techniques - Brachytherapy
Edited by R. Sauer

Radiopathology of Organs and Tissues
Edited by E. Scherer, C. Streffer, and K.-R. Trott

Concomitant Continuous Infusion Chemotherapy and Radiation
Edited by M. Rotman and C.J. Rosenthal

Intraoperative Radiotherapy – Clinical Experiences and Results
Edited by F.A. Calvo, M. Santos, and L.W. Brady

Radiotherapy of Intraocular and Orbital Tumors
Edited by W.E. Alberti and R.H. Sagerman

Interstitial and Intracavitary Thermoradiotherapy
Edited by M.H. Seegenschmiedt and R. Sauer

Non-Disseminated Breast Cancer
Controversial Issues in Management
Edited by G.H. Fletcher and S.H. Levitt

Current Topics in Clinical Radiobiology of Tumors
Edited by H.-P. Beck-Bornholdt

Practical Approaches to Cancer Invasion and Metastases
A Compendium of Radiation Oncologists' Responses to 40 Histories
Edited by A.R. Kagan with the Assistance of R.J. Steckel

Radiation Therapy in Pediatric Oncology
Edited by J.R. Cassady

Radiation Therapy Physics
Edited by A.R. Smith

Late Sequelae in Oncology
Edited by J. Dunst and R. Sauer

Mediastinal Tumors. Update 1995
Edited by D.E. Wood and C.R. Thomas, Jr.

Thermoradiotherapy and Thermochemotherapy

Volume 1:
Biology, Physiology, and Physics

Volume 2:
Clinical Applications
Edited by M.H. Seegenschmiedt, P. Fessenden, and C.C. Vernon

Carcinoma of the Prostate
Innovations in Management
Edited by Z. Petrovich, L. Baert, and L.W. Brady

Radiation Oncology of Gynecological Cancers
Edited by H.W. Vahrson

Carcinoma of the Bladder
Innovations in Management
Edited by Z. Petrovich, L. Baert, and L.W. Brady

Blood Perfusion and Microenvironment of Human Tumors
Implications for Clinical Radiooncology
Edited by M. Molls and P. Vaupel

Radiation Therapy of Benign Diseases. A Clinical Guide
2nd Revised Edition
S.E. Order and S.S. Donaldson

Carcinoma of the Kidney and Testis, and Rare Urologic Malignancies
Innovations in Management
Edited by Z. Petrovich, L. Baert, and L.W. Brady

Progress and Perspectives in the Treatment of Lung Cancer
Edited by P. Van Houtte, J. Klastersky, and P. Rocmans

Springer

Printing and Binding: Stürtz AG, Würzburg